MW00846303

Scleroderma

Second Edition

John Varga • Christopher P. Denton
Fredrick M. Wigley • Yannick Allanore
Masataka Kuwana
Editors

Scleroderma

From Pathogenesis to Comprehensive Management

Second Edition

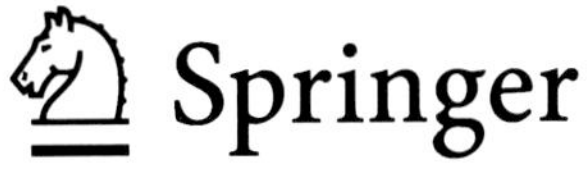

Editors
John Varga
Feinberg School of Medicine
Northwestern University
Chicago, Illinois
USA

Yannick Allanore
Service de Rhumatologie A, INSERMU1016
Universit. Paris Descartes, Hôpital Cochin
Paris
France

Christopher P. Denton
Division of Medicine
Department of Inflammation
Centre for Rheumatology and Connective Tissue Diseases
UCL Division of Medicine, Royal Free Hospital
London
UK

Masataka Kuwana
Department of Allergy and Rheumatology
Nippon Medical School, Graduate School of Medicine
Tokyo
Japan

Fredrick M. Wigley
Johns Hopkins University
Baltimore, Maryland
USA

ISBN 978-3-319-31405-1 ISBN 978-3-319-31407-5 (eBook)
DOI 10.1007/978-3-319-31407-5

Library of Congress Control Number: 2016955861

Printed on acid-free paper

This Springer imprint is published by Springer Nature
The registered company is Springer International Publishing AG Switzerland
The registered company address is Gewerbestrasse 11, 6330 Cham, Switzerland

I gratefully acknowledge Julie, Peter, and Andrew Varga for their unfailing support, patience, and love; my parents who served as my role models; and my patients who teach and inspire me every day.

-John Varga

I am indebted to the ongoing support of my family and the encouragement and guidance from my mentors in rheumatology, especially Dame Carol Black and the late Dr. Barbara Ansell.

-Christopher P. Denton

I am deeply grateful and indebted to Carol, my wife, and my children – Joy and Julie, and family; the entire staff of the Johns Hopkins Scleroderma Center; my colleagues in the Division of Rheumatology and my patients and supporters

-Fredrick M. Wigley

I really appreciate the support and dedication of my family and colleagues at Keio University and Nippon Medical School.

-Masataka Kuwana

I am grateful to all the colleagues and to all the patients who have taught me about systemic sclerosis over the years. I thank all the collaborators with whom we shared basic or clinical research projects, who were always source of inspiration, with special thanks to the EUSTAR network members.

-Yannick Allanore

Foreword

Scleroderma, or systemic sclerosis, is a true multisystem disease that requires integrated multidisciplinary management including rheumatology, cardiology, renal and thoracic medicine and gastroenterology as well as other medical specialties and healthcare professionals. It also has a peculiarly cruel impact on quality of life and the potential to take a dreadful toll on affected patients and their families. No one who has come across the disease in a severe form will ever underestimate its importance or clinical impact. However, it is uncommon and there is a great need for high-quality resources to educate and inform about the disease. I learnt during a medical career dedicated to improving understanding and treatment of scleroderma the tremendous importance of integrated management including all of these disciplines and also that to really advance understanding of scleroderma it was critical to align clinical practice and fundamental clinical and laboratory research.

As a young junior doctor in my first clinical post, I came across scleroderma when a young woman was admitted under my care with scleroderma renal crisis. I was disturbed to learn from the professor of medicine that there was no effective treatment and that she would be dead within 3 months. This was the case, and this incident sowed in my mind the seeds of curiosity about this potentially devastating disease and determination to seek ways to do more. There have been enormous strides in managing scleroderma over the past four decades, and a patient presenting with the same clinical problem to a modern scleroderma unit could expect to survive and have a much better outcome. However, it remains one of the most challenging of the rheumatic diseases and one that still has to reveal much about the underlying cause and mechanism.

I have personally witnessed progress in understanding and managing scleroderma in its diverse forms and would have relished access to this textbook earlier in my career as I established one of the first units in the UK that specializes in scleroderma and later was involved in developing the pulmonary hypertension service in our hospital that has made a major contribution to treatment and improving outcome for patients developing this important complication. In my professional life, I have taken on new challenges over recent years and moved into other areas of academic, medical, and government endeavor. This has focused on the tremendous impact that health issues have on ability to work and participate in society and brings the individual impact of a disease such as scleroderma into sharp focus.

The first edition of this textbook was a masterful integration of basic science and clinical practice, and the second edition builds upon this model but includes new sections, including clinical case summaries, that bridge the gap between the pathology and biological basis of disease and clinical impact. It provides a very clear demonstration of progress in managing major and life-threatening aspects of this disease and highlights the important links between scleroderma and other medical conditions. I am delighted to write this foreword for the second edition of what has emerged as the most comprehensive and up-to-date book on this disease, spanning pathogenesis to clinical management of scleroderma. It more than lives up to expectation and I am sure that it will help prepare and stimulate more healthcare professionals and scientists to work on the disease and further improve treatments and outcome.

Professor Dame Carol Black
Principal of Newnham College, Cambridge, UK
Emeritus Professor of Rheumatology, UCL Division of Medicine, London, UK

Foreword from Bob Saget

I am so honored to have been asked by the Editors to write a foreword for what will shortly become the premier book on scleroderma now in existence …written for doctors, scientists and patients.

Scleroderma is a disease that is very close to my heart, having lost my sister, Gay, to it in 1994 at only 47 years old. She was initially misdiagnosed and treated without full knowledge of the latest clinical trials and forward thinking that can try to help patients stricken with this complex disease.

I have had the pleasure over the years to shoot two short documentaries that were used to raise awareness and to raise much needed funds to support research around the country.

The authors of this book are the forerunners in scleroderma research and clinical trials. The doctors who have written this second new and revised edition are making a significant contribution. One that I trust rheumatologists and doctors who come across scleroderma, no matter their discipline, will take note of and read cover to cover.

I would like to acknowledge all the contributors and thank the editors of this book—the very smartest and passionate Doctors—Dr. John Varga, Dr. Chris Denton, Dr. Yannick Allanore, Dr. Masataka Kuwana, and Dr. Fredrick Wigley.

I became familiar with scleroderma several years before my sister Gay came down with it. Twenty-five years ago I met a woman who was to become one of the dearest friends of my life, Sharon Monsky. She was the founder and then CEO of the Scleroderma Research Foundation. A great woman, mother of three, who'd been stricken with the disease as a young mom.

Sharon cold-called me to perform standup at a benefit in Santa Monica, which she had titled, "Cool Comedy Hot Cuisine." I had never met her before. I knew nothing about scleroderma. She explained the word scleroderma meant "hard skin." She told me that it affects mostly women in the prime of their lives. That it was a difficult disease to pinpoint—some called it "auto-immune," some used the word "vascular," and she also said it occasionally struck people living in the same area and in some rare cases, people in the same family.

The only way to raise money for research was to do what most people do in this situation—have benefits and try to raise the much needed money to fund cutting edge research that goes to helping find a cure, or at the very best, ways to put the disease into some kind of remission in its victims.

Soon as she explained to me what the benefit was, I said "yes" over the phone and since have been involved in her foundation's signature event: a night of comedians and amazing food by chefs and friends—with the idea that the best way to deal with this difficult disease was to try and raise money for research through humor.

The beautiful Robin Williams was the first performer to give of himself to perform for this cause I had yet to have strike my family directly. After I started doing the benefit as a comedian and then its host for twenty-four years, Robin had come to do the event seven times and Top Chefs Susan Feniger and Mary Sue Milliken have been amazing. The first year I performed, Ellen DeGeneres and Rosie O'Donnell were performing as well. It was such a moving night for me personally and I have since hosted it over thirty times to this day. I am also a proud board member of the Scleroderma Research Foundation and these events called "Cool Comedy Hot Cuisine" are the main fundraisers we have to raise money for research.

Just a couple years forward from that first night I did the benefit from that cold-call, my sister Gay had to move back to LA from Bucks County, PA… To move back in with our parents, as a forty-four-year-old woman, so they could help her try and get better medical care than she'd been receiving. She had finally been diagnosed with this disease I had connected with seemingly out of nowhere.

So just three years after I even found out what "scleroderma" was, my sister was sitting in the audience at the benefit, now actually diagnosed as having this orphan disease. One year later, she lost her life to it. I couldn't believe that this happened. It snuck up on her and a year later she was on a decline that ended just two years later. It's how many of us get involved with a cause that cuts us deep to the bone.

I wanted to do something about it. Share our family's story with others and let them know that they aren't alone in this battle that—like any disease, makes you feel completely alone. So, in 1996, I directed a television movie for ABC called, "For Hope," a story "loosely based" on events that "directly" affected my family. The writer was my friend Susan Rice, the producer, the dear Karen Moore. And the cast was extraordinary: Dana Delany, Henry Czerny, Polly Bergen, and Harold Gould basically playing my parents, and Chris Demetral representing my nephew, Adam. And my dear friend, Sharon Monsky, playing "herself." It was a very emotional and fulfilling project, a poignant moment in my life, one that I will always treasure. And through my work with helping to fund research for this disease—coming into contact with so many people who have it –I believe that TV movie helped put scleroderma on the map for some. Still, it's such a long road for the hundreds of thousands of people who have scleroderma in its many incarnations.

Once Sharon passed away thirteen years ago, I knew then I would be working the rest of my life to do whatever I could to help those affected with scleroderma.

Thanks to research, new drugs, and new therapies have since been developed, helping thousands of those struggling with this sometimes fatal disease that there still is no known cure for. Pharmaceutical companies have developed several drugs to deal specifically with the symptoms of scleroderma, mainly the biggest killer of its patients, pulmonary arterial hypertension (PAH), a chronic, progressive, and debilitating rare lung disease that can lead to death or the need for transplantation. So real progress has been made since I started trying to help decades ago.

After the loss of my sister, I have had the good fortune of meeting hundreds, maybe a thousand scleroderma patients—who I feel connected to on a deep level. As though it's some sort of horrific rite of passage to be in "this club." I cannot bear to think of what people go through when their loved ones are hit with this disease that still needs so much attention and funding.

We have all been touched beyond words by all of the comedians who have given their time to perform to get money to support research.

So many dear friends who have been there for me and helped many with scleroderma through the support given to research: Robin Williams, Whoopi Goldberg, Dana Carvey, Jimmy Kimmel, Seth Meyers, John Oliver, Jeff Garlin, Jeff Ross, John Mayer, Jim Gaffigan, Michael Che, Jimmy Fallon, Rodney Dangerfield, Sarah Silverman, Jerry Seinfeld, Conan O'Brien, Craig Ferguson, Jon Stewart, Lily Tomlin, Pat Monahan and Train, The Goo Goo Dolls, Adam Duritz and Counting Crows, and most recently, Andy Cohen, Michael Che and Louie C.K.

No one should have to suffer as my sister Gay did, who lost her life at 47. My heart goes out to the patients and families of those afflicted by this terrible disease—they always say "terrible disease," yet as we all know, there are no "good" ones.

I will spend the rest of my life dedicated to helping support the best medical minds in science as we try to fund what will one day be a day that we all would love to see happen in our lifetime: to find a cure.

I am deeply indebted to all of the doctors, both contributing writers as well as the brilliant editors, all working so diligently in sharing their research and advanced knowledge of a disease that can take so many lives. And thanks to the hard work of these exceptional doctors who have created this book, more lives can be saved, and more progress will be made.

I just want all other doctors around the world to read it, so they are up to date with where we are now, not where we were ten years ago in treating a scleroderma patient. I do believe my sister may have been alive today if the regime of medicine that was cast upon her had the knowledge that is within these pages.

My good fortune is I get to be a small part of this big picture– this book. It is a monumental and defining work and I am so proud to have been asked to write this foreword. And now, enough from me, enjoy reading this, created by the people who are truly making a difference that will change the lives of so many.

Bob Saget

Preface to the First Edition

Scleroderma remains the most enigmatic and challenging of all rheumatic diseases and the one associated with the greatest burden of morbidity and mortality. Despite decades of intense clinical and basic research, and dozens of clinical trials, the causes and pathophysiology of the disease had remained, until recently, largely beyond our grasp, and effective disease modifying therapies are still lacking. The reasons for slow progress in scleroderma are many. They include the remarkable heterogeneity of the disease, its protean and multisystemic manifestations, its low prevalence and orphan disease status, the lack of animal models, low level of public awareness, and so on. Moreover, government investment in scleroderma research has, until recently, lagged behind other comparable diseases; likewise, the pharmaceutical industry has historically viewed scleroderma as a limited market. In the absence of dramatic research advances and faced with disappointing results from clinical trials, a nihilistic attitude toward scleroderma took hold in some circles. Upon receiving a diagnosis of scleroderma, patients were not infrequently informed that "there is no treatment for scleroderma" and denied access to potentially effective interventions or the opportunity to participate in clinical trials.

Fortunately, the scleroderma landscape is now changing rapidly. Indeed, readers of this book will be convinced that the future for scleroderma research and for affected patients has never been brighter. The book highlights the concurrent advances on many fronts that explain this sea-change. Discoveries from the laboratory have led, during the past decade, to the identification and characterization of a plethora of new molecules, pathways, and cell types as critical players in the diverse manifestations of scleroderma. This line of research has been energized by the recent application of "omics" such as genomics and proteomics that allow large-scale, hypothesis-free examination of tens of thousands of molecular components, each representing a potential target for therapy. Increasingly powerful genetic association studies are shedding light on the genetic factors associated with scleroderma, including the identification of specific genes and alleles, and in the near future, of epigenetic changes reflecting the interplay of environment with the genome. Genetic engineering is making it possible to generate complex mouse strains to model particular scleroderma traits such as fibrosis, inflammation, autoimmunity, and vasculopathy. Meticulous evaluation of novel transgenic mice is likely to yield fresh insights into pathogenesis, including the mechanistic bases of distinct disease manifestations. Moreover, innovative animal models provide appealing experimental platforms for preclinical testing of novel anti-inflammatory, vasoprotective, and antifibrotic drugs. The vital bench-to-bedside research continuum is alive, and basic discoveries are translated into clinical trials at an increasingly rapid pace.

Enormously powerful analytic platforms, such as microchip DNA arrays to examine genetic polymorphisms or genome-wide changes at the tissue level, now allow investigators to probe disease heterogeneity at the molecular level. These studies, as elegantly illustrated in this book, reveal a surprising and unsuspected level of complexity and heterogeneity in scleroderma. While new insights often challenge existing paradigms, they open the door for vital progress in disease subclassification and phenotyping that in turn enhances our ability to target specific interventions to predefined patient subsets. They also make it possible to identify and validate novel biomarkers, and to develop novel treatment strategies, including drug repurposing. Integration of laboratory-based reductionist research with hypothesis-free omics surveys on the one hand and patient phenotyping with meticulous clinical, laboratory, serologic, and pathological data collection on the other hand will be vital. Optimal research integration will require real-time coordination among clinical centers and research laboratories and is vitally dependent on shared access to robust registries, databanks, and linked biorepositories. We must be realistic in appreciating the challenges, including the cost, of developing and maintaining requisite infrastructures. These efforts can only succeed with long-term commitment. Steady advances reflect the enthusiasm and dedication of the community of scleroderma researchers, clinicians, advocates, and patients working in tandem with governmental agencies, and, increasingly, the pharmaceutical and biotechnology sectors.

Although truly effective disease-modifying interventions are lacking and a single "magic bullet" for scleroderma is unlikely, disease management is improving, as reflected in better quality of life and survival for patients with scleroderma. The need for comprehensive care to address the totality of the disease is increasingly appreciated. Optimal management should include a holistic approach encompassing nutrition, psychological aspects, exercise, physical and occupational therapy, and sleep optimization to reduce suffering and disability. This book showcases these advances and highlights evidence-based contemporary clinical recommendations, practice guidelines, diagnostic and screening strategies, and innovative approaches to patient care. Each of the chapters is informed by the need to integrate emerging understanding of pathophysiology with the latest advances in clinical practice.

The contributors to this book represent an exceptionally broad spectrum of expertise and come from many countries. Together, the 52 chapters reflect a contemporary global perspective and provide a comprehensive view of scleroderma: where we are and where we are headed. We believe that, having perused this book, the reader will be as impressed as the editors are that we are at the threshold of an era of unprecedented progress in scleroderma.

Finally, a word about the name for the disease that is the subject of this book. Originally called scleroderma, the disease came to be called "progressive systemic sclerosis" and more recently "systemic sclerosis" to illustrate the important role of fibrosis as a hallmark feature and to emphasize the striking systemic nature of the disease. We however use the term "scleroderma" throughout. There are several reasons for this. In conversations with physicians, scientists, and health-care providers around the world, "scleroderma" seems to resonate most of all the alternate terms. Advocacy and patient support groups prefer this term, as do most patients with the diagnosis. Finally, let's face it, "systemic sclerosis" is a mouthful, whereas "scleroderma" is succinct and carries a certain austere elegance. So, while in full recognition that scleroderma is a systemic disease and is not to be confused with localized scleroderma, we have chosen to stick with this name.

Chicago, IL, USA
London, UK
Baltimore, MD, USA

John Varga, MD
Christopher P. Denton, PhD, FRCP
Fredrick M. Wigley, MD

Preface to the Second Edition

We are witnessing significant advances in scleroderma. Perhaps the most challenging to understand and manage of all rheumatic diseases, scleroderma is no longer viewed with bewilderment and a sense of helplessness. Indeed, in the years since the first edition of *Scleroderma: From Pathogenesis to Comprehensive Management* was published, much that we understand about scleroderma has changed. Progress in the science and practice of medicine is occurring rapidly, and new information about scleroderma is accruing at an unprecedented pace. The number of investigators, investigative teams, and research consortia focusing on scleroderma around the globe; the size of the study cohorts; the variety of experimental disease models; and the power and depth of high throughput technologies for data acquisition have all grown exponentially during this time. While this explosion of new information is truly good news for people living with scleroderma as well as students of the disease, it is posing formidable new challenges for anyone seeking to achieve a deeper understanding. The second edition of *Scleroderma: From Pathogenesis to Comprehensive Management* seeks to address these challenges. Our goal is to communicate progress in the field in an up-to-date, authoritative, comprehensive, and accessible manner.

Building on the approach established in the first edition, we present a systematic and critical survey of current knowledge about the epidemiology, genetic basis, pathogenesis, classification, clinical manifestations, evaluation, and management of all aspects of scleroderma. We seek to integrate, to the fullest degree possible, contemporary concepts of pathophysiology and physiology with clinical aspects for each major feature of scleroderma. The book is written with a broad and global readership in mind. We aim to provide a uniquely valuable reference for anyone interested in scleroderma, be they clinicians, investigators, students, or other health professionals. Each chapter is written by distinguished experts in the field, typically representing more than one continent, in order to assure a truly balanced and global perspective. Up-to-date analysis of genetic risk, a very rapidly evolving area, is provided in the context of its impact on understanding pathophysiology, informing disease classification, and identification of innovative therapeutic approaches. Additional chapters discuss the significance and utility of novel and evolving biomarker discovery efforts and how these efforts might yield biomarkers that will have real-life utility in the clinic. The rationale for the use of novel treatments is presented, along with data regarding their efficacy, safety, and appropriate role in patient management. Throughout, each chapter highlights growing awareness of disease heterogeneity and its impact on the practice of individualized "precision" medicine in scleroderma. Finally, for this edition we introduce a series of short clinically oriented chapters that highlight current approaches to common and important disease manifestations. In this way, both clinicians and nonclinician readers can gain a better understanding of the complex challenges of scleroderma and how these challenges are addressed by experts in the field. It is the editors' hope that the second edition of *Scleroderma: From Pathogenesis to Comprehensive Management* will inform and inspire and catalyze new ideas, collaborations, and discoveries that bring us closer to the prevention and cure of scleroderma.

We wish to express our gratitude for the editorial assistance provided by Pam Hill (Baltimore), Elise Paxson (Philadelphia), and Margaret Moore (New York). Without their dedication, hard work, and unfailing patience, this book would not have come to fruition.

Chicago, IL, USA — John Varga
Baltimore, MD, USA — Fred Wigley
London, UK — Christopher Denton
Tokyo, Japan — Masa Kuwana
Paris, France — Yannick Allanore

Abbreviations

6-MP	6-mercaptopurine
6MWT	6-minute walk test
α-SMA	α-smooth muscle actin
ACA	Anticentromere antibodies
ACR	American College of Rheumatology
ACT	Acceptance and commitment therapy
ACTD	Autoimmune connective tissue diseases
ACVR1B	Activin A receptor, type IB
ADAM	Adamalysines
ADHD	Attention deficit hyperactivity disorder
ADM	Antroduodenal manometry
AE	Adverse events
AECA	Antiendothelial cell antibodies
AECG	American-European Conesus Group
AFA	Antifibrillarin antibodies
AGE	Glycation/lipoperoxidation end product
AGTRL2	Angiotensin receptor-like 2
AHA	Antihistone antibodies
AIF1	Allograft inflammatory factor 1
AIH	Autoimmune hepatitis
AKI	Acute kidney injury
ALK	Anti-liver-kidney microsome
AMA	Antimitochondrial antibody
ANA	Antinuclear antibody
ANS	Autonomic nervous system
anti-Scl70	antitopoisomerase 1 antibodies
APC	Antigen-presenting cell or argon plasma coagulation
APRIL	A proliferation-inducing ligand
APS	Antiphospholipid antibody syndrome
ARB	Angiotensin receptor blocker
ARHB	Ras homolog gene family, member B
ASCT	Autologous stem cell transplantation
aSSC	Adult onset systemic sclerosis
AST	Aspartate aminotransferase
ASTIS	Autologous Stem Cell Transplantation International Scleroderma
ATG5	Autophagy-related 5
AUC	Area under the curve
autoAb	Autoantibodies
AV	Atrioventricular
AVNRT	Atrioventricular reentry tachycardia
BAFF	B-cell activating factor
BAL	Bronchoalveolar lavage

BALF	Expanded oligoclonal T cell subsets in affected skin or lungs
BANK1	B cell-specific scaffold protein with ankyrin
BAS	Balloon atrial septostomy
BCR	B cell receptor
BLK	B lymphocyte kinase
BMI	Body mass index
BMPRII	Bone morphogenic protein receptor II
BNP	Brain natriuretic peptide
BP	Blood pressure
BPPV	Benign paroxysmal positional vertigo
BUILD	The Bosentan Use in Interstitial Lung Disease (study)
CACS	Coronary artery calcium score
CAV1	Caveolin 1
CBAA	Calcium-binding amino acid
CBC	Complete blood count
CBT	Cognitive-behavioral therapy
CCP	Cyclic citrullinated peptide
CCP/ACPA	Anticyclic citrullinated peptides
CCR6	Chemokine receptor 6
CDSMP	Chronic Disease Self-Management Program
CES-D	Center for Epidemiologic Studies Depression Scale
cGMP	Cyclic guanosine monophosphate
cGVHD	Chronic graft-versus host disease
CHFS	Cochin hand function scale
CI	Confidence interval or cardiac index
CIDI	Composite International Diagnostic Interview
CIHR	Canadian Institutes of Health Research
CIP	Chronic intestinal pseudo-obstruction
CM	Circumscribed morphea
CMR	Cardiac magnetic resonance
CMV	Cytomegalovirus
CNS	Central nervous system
CO	Carbon monoxide
COL1A2	Alpha 2 chain of collagen I
COL8A1	Alpha 1 chain of collagen VIII
COMP	Cartilage oligomeric protein 1
CPET	Cardiopulmonary exercise test
CPK	Creatine phosphokinase
CREST	Calcinosis, Raynaud's, esophagitis, sclerodactyly, and telangiectasia
CRISS	Combined response index for systemic sclerosis
CRP	C-reactive protein
CSK	c-Src tyrosine kinase
CSR	Cumulative survival rates
CSRG	Canadian scleroderma research group
CT	Computed tomography
CTA	Clinical Trial Application
CTD	Connective tissue disease
CTD-PAH	Connective tissue disease–pulmonary arterial hypertension
CTEPH	Chronic thromboembolic PH
CTGF	Connective tissue growth factor
CTL	Cytotoxic T lymphocyte
CTLA-4	Cytotoxic lymphocyte antigen 4
CVD	Collagen vascular disease

CVD-PAH	Collagen vascular disease–associated pulmonary arterial hypertension
CYC	Cyclophosphamide
DAMP	Damage-associated molecular patterns
DAS	Disease activity score
DASH	Disabilities of the arm, shoulder, and hand
DC	Dendritic cells
DCA	Dichloroacetate
dcSSc	Diffuse cutaneous SSc
DECT	Dual-energy computed tomography
DHFR	Dihydrofolate reductase
DID	Double immunodiffusion
DIP	Distal interphalangeal
DLCO	Diffusion capacity of the lung for carbon monoxide
DM	Dermatomyositis or diabetes mellitus
DMARD	Disease-modifying antirheumatic drug
DNASEIL3	Deoxyribonuclease I-like 3
DNMT	DNA methyltransferase
DNSS	Deutsches Netzwerk für Systemische Sklerodermie
dsDNA	Double stranded DNA
DSG2	Desmoglein-2
DU	Digital ulcer
DZ	Dizygotic
EBV	Epstein Barr virus
EC	Endothelial cell
ECDS	En coup de sabre
ECG	Electrocardiogram
ECM	Extracellular matrix
ECV	Extracellular volume
ED	Erectile dysfunction
EF	Eosinophilic fasciitis
EGD	Esophagogastroduodenoscopy
EGF	Epidermal growth factor
EGG	Electrogastrography
EIA	Enzyme immunoassay
ELAR	European League Against Rheumatism
ELISA	Enzyme-linked immunosorbent assay
ELR	Enzyme-linked receptor
EMG	Electromyogram
EMS	Eosinophilia-myalgia syndrome
ENA	Extractable nuclear antigen
EndoMT	Endothelial-mesenchymal transition
eNOS	Endothelial nitric oxide synthase
eNPV	Estimated net present value
ENT	Ear, nose, and throat
EPC	Endothelial progenitor cell
EPOSS	Outcome measures in pulmonary arterial hypertension related to systemic sclerosis
ERA	Endothelin receptor antagonist
ERK	Extracellular signal-regulated kinase
EScSG	European Scleroderma Study Group
ESR	Erythrocyte sedimentation rate
ESSGAI	European Scleroderma Study Group Activity Index

ESWL	Extracorporeal shock wave lithotripsy
ET-1	Endothelin-1
ET_A	Endothelin receptor type A
ET_B	Endothelin receptor type B
EULAR	European League Against Rheumatism
EUSTAR	EULAR Scleroderma Trials and Research
FBN1	Fibrillin 1
FC	Functional capacity
FDAAA	Food and Drug Administration Amendments Act of 2007
FDG PET	Fluorodeoxyglucose positron emission tomography
FEV1	Forced expiratory volume in 1 s
FGF	Fibroblast growth factor
FHL2	Four and a half LIM domains 2
FIH	First in human
Fli1	Friend leukemia integration 1
FN	Flattening ratio
FN^{EDA}	Fibronectin extracellular domain A
FRQS	Fonds de recherche du Québec
FVC	Forced vital capacity
GAVE	Gastric antral vascular ectasia
GBCS	Gadolinium-based contrast agents
GCGA	Gamma-carboxyglutamic acid
GCP	Good clinical practice
GENISOS	Genetics versus Environment in Scleroderma Outcome study
GERD	Gastroesophageal reflux
GI	Gastrointestinal
GIT	Gastrointestinal tract
GLS	Global longitudinal strain
GLUT	Glucose transporter molecule
GM	Generalized morphea
GMA	Gastric myoelectrical activity
GR	Glucocorticoid receptor
GrB	Granzyme B
GRB10	Growth factor receptor-bound protein 10
GVHD	Graft-versus-host disease
GWAS	Genome-wide association studies
H_2O_2	Hydrogen peroxide
HA	Hyaluronan
HADa	Hospital anxiety depression (anxiety)
HADd	Hospital anxiety depression (depression)
HAMIS	Hand mobility in scleroderma
HAQ-DI	Health assessment questionnaire disability index
HAX-1	HS1-associated protein-1
HDAC	Histone deacetylase
HFI	Hand functional index
HFpEF	Heart failure with preserved ejection fraction
HIF-1α	Hypoxia inducible factor
HLA	Histocompatibility locus antigen or human leukocyte antigen
hPAH	Heritable pulmonary arterial hypertension
HPN	Home parenteral nutrition
HRCT	High-resolution computed tomography
HRM	High-resolution esophageal manometry
HRQOL or HRQL	Health-related quality of life

HSC	Hematopoietic stem cell
hUBF	Human upstream binding factor
ICAM	Intercellular adhesion molecule
ICC	Intraclass correlation coefficient
ICD-9	International Classification of Diseases Version 9
icIL-1RA	IL-1 receptor antagonist
IDDM	Insulin-dependent diabetes mellitus
IDL	Ischemic digital loss
IFN	Interferon
IFN-γ	Interferon-γ
IgG	Immunoglobulin G
IIF	Indirect immunofluorescence
IIP	Idiopathic interstitial pneumonia
IL	Interleukin
ILC	Innate lymphoid cell
ILD	Interstitial lung disease
IMP	Integrated multispecies prediction
IMPRESS	International Multicentric Study on PRegnancy in Systemic Sclerosis
IND	Investigational new drug
iNOS	Inducible nitric oxide synthase
IP	Immunoprecipitation
IPAH	Idiopathic pulmonary arterial hypertension
IPF	Idiopathic pulmonary fibrosis
iPH	Idiopathic-associated pulmonary arterial hypertension
IPSP	Inhibitory postsynaptic potential
IRAK	Interleukin 1 receptor associated kinase-1
IRB	Institutional Review Board
IRF	Interferon regulatory factor or interferon-releasing factor
IRF-7	Interferon regulatory factor 7
iTreg	inducible Treg
IV	Intravenous or intraventricular
IVIG	Intravenous immunoglobulin
jSSc	Juvenile systemic sclerosis
Kco	Diffusion coefficient
KCS	Keratoconjunctivitis sicca
KFT	Keitel functional test
KL6	Krebs von den Lungen-6
KLF5	Krüppel-like factor 5
LBT	Lactulose hydrogen breath test
Lc	Limited cutaneous
lcSSc	Limited cutaneous SSc
LD	Linkage disequilibrium
LES	Lower esophageal sphincter
LKM-1	Liver-kidney-microsomal
LOH	Loss of heterozygosity
LOX	Lysyl oxidase
LPS	Lipopolysaccharide
LV	Left ventricular
LVEDP	Left ventricular end diastolic pressure
LVEF	Left ventricular ejection fraction
M3R	Muscarinic-3 receptor
MAC	Morphea in adults and children (cohort)
MACTAR	McMaster Toronto Arthritis patient preference questionnaire

MCP	Metacarpophalangeal
MCTD	Mixed connective tissue disease
MDC	Macrophage-derived chemokine
mDC	Myeloid DC
MDCT	Multidetector computed tomography
MDD	Major depressive disorder
MDRD	Modification of diet in renal disease
MECP2	Methyl-CpG-binding protein 2
MEF2	Myocyte enhancing factor 2
MHC	Major histocompatibility complex
MHISS	Mouth handicap in systemic sclerosis scale
MINI	Mini-international neuropsychiatric interview
MIP	Macrophage inflammatory protein
mLoSSI	Modified localized scleroderma skin severity index
MMC	Myoelectric complexes
MMF	Mycophenolate mofetil
MMP-1	Matrix metalloproteinase-1
MOA	Mechanism of action
mPAP	Mean pulmonary artery pressure
MPP	Methylprednisolone
MRA	Magnetic resonance angiography
MREc	Magnetic resonance enteroclysis
MREg	Magnetic resonance enterography
MRI	Magnetic resonance imaging
MRSA	Methionine sulfoxide reductase A
MRSB	Methionine sulfoxide reductase B
mRss	Modified Rodnan skin score
MSC	Mesenchymal stem cell
MTX	Methotrexate
MUST	Malnutrition universal screening tool
MVEC	Microvascular endothelial cell
MZ	Monozygotic
NASH	Nonalcoholic steatohepatitis
NBUVB	Narrowband UVB treatment
NCI	National Cancer Institute
NCS	Nerve conduction studies
Nd:YAG	Neodymium-yttrium aluminum garnet
NDA	New drug application
NFD	Nephrogenic fibrosing dermopathy
NFS	Nephrogenic systemic fibrosis
NIH	National Institutes of Health
NIH PROMIS	National Institute of Health Patient-Reported Outcomes Measurement System
NK	Natural killer
NLR	NOD-like receptors
NME	New medical entity
NOS	Nitric oxide synthase
NPWT	Negative pressure wound therapy
NRH	Nodular regenerative hyperplasia
NSAID	Nonsteroidal anti-inflammatory drug
NSF	Nephrogenic systemic fibrosis
NSIP	Nonspecific interstitial pneumonia
NTproBNP	N-terminal brain natriuretic peptide

nTreg	Natural Tregs
NYHA	New York Heart Association
O_2^-	Superoxide anion
OMERACT	Outcome measure in rheumatologic clinical trials
OR	Odds ratio
P1GF	Placenta growth factor
P1NP	Amino-terminal procollagen I
PA	Plasminogen activator
PACK	*P*BC, *A*CA, *C*REST, *K*eratoconjunctivitis sicca
PAH	Pulmonary arterial hypertension
PAMPs	Pathogen-associated molecular pattern molecules
PAP	Pulmonary arterial pressure
PARC	Pulmonary and activation-regulated chemokine
PBC	Primary biliary cirrhosis
PBMC	Peripheral blood mononuclear cells
PCP	Primary care provider
PCWP	Pulmonary capillary wedge pressure
PD	Pharmacodynamics
pDC	Plasmacytoid dendritic cell
PDGFR	Platelet-derived growth factor receptor
PDH	Pyruvate dehydrogenase
PE	Pulmonary embolism
PF	Pulmonary fibrosis
PFT	Pulmonary function test
PH	Pulmonary hypertension
PHA	Progressive hemifacial atrophy
PHAROS	Pulmonary Hypertension Assessment and Recognition of Outcomes in Scleroderma
PHC	Proangiogenic hematopoietic cell
PHQ-9	9-item Patient Health Questionnaire
PICP	Carboxy terminal telopeptide of type I collagen
PIIINP	Amino-terminal III procollagen
PIP	Proximal interphalangeal
PK	Pharmacokinetics
PM	Polymyositis
PN	Parenteral nutrition
PoC	Proof of Concept
POEMS	Polyneuropathy, organomegaly, endocrinopathy, monoclonal gammopathy, and skin changes
PoPH	Portopulmonary hypertension
PPI	Proton pump inhibitors
PreS or PRES	Pediatric Rheumatology European Society
PRS	Parry-Romberg syndrome
PSC	Primary sclerosing cholangitis
PTPN22	Protein tyrosine phosphatase, nonreceptor type 22 (lymphoid)
PTX3	Pentraxin 3
PUVA	Psoralen with UVA
PVOD	Pulmonary veno-occlusive disease
PVR	Pulmonary vascular resistance
QST	Quantitative sensory testing
RA	Rheumatoid arthritis or right atrium
RAGE	Glycation/lipoperoxidation end product receptor
RANTES	Regulated upon activation, normal T-cell expressed and secreted

RAS	Renin-angiotensin system
RCT	Randomized controlled trial
REMS	Risk evaluation and mitigation strategies
RF	Rheumatoid factor
RFA	Radiofrequency ablation
RHC	Right heart catheterization
RLR	RIG-I-like receptors
RNApol3	RNA polymerase III
RNP	Ribonucleoprotein
rNPV	Risk-adjusted net present value
RONS	Reactive oxygen and nitrogen species
ROS	Reactive oxygen species
RP	Raynaud's phenomenon
RT	Rituximab
RV	Right ventricular or residual volume
RVDEV	Right ventricular end-diastolic volume
RVEF	Right ventricular ejection fraction
SAE	Serious adverse events
SaO_2	Arterial oxygen saturation
Schisto-PAH	Schistosomiasis-induced pulmonary arterial hypertension
SCID	Severe combined immunodeficiency
SD	Standard deviation
SDF	Stromal cell-derived factor
SE	Standard error
SERAPHIN	Study with an Endothelin Receptor Antagonist in Pulmonary Arterial Hypertension to Improve Clinical Outcome
SERT	Serotonin transporter
SF-36	Short form-36
SF-6D	Short form-6D
sFlt-1	Soluble fms-like tyrosine kinase-1
SGRQ	Saint George's Respiratory Questionnaire
sHAQ	Scleroderma Health Assessment Questionnaire
SIBO	Small intestine bacterial overgrowth
SIR	Standardized incidence ratio
SLE	Systemic lupus erythematosus
SLS	Scleroderma Lung Study
SLS-II	Second Scleroderma Lung Study
SMA	Smooth muscle antigen
SNHL	Sensorineural hearing loss
SNP	Single nucleotide polymorphism
SOD2	Superoxide dismutase 2
SOX5	SRY (sex determining region Y)-box 5
sPAP	Systemic pulmonary arterial pressure
sPAP	Systolic pulmonary artery pressure
SPARC	Secreted protein acidic and rich in cysteine
SP-B	Surfactant protein B
SPECT	Single-photon emission computed tomography
SPIN	Scleroderma Patient-centered Intervention Network
SRC	Scleroderma renal crisis
SS	Sjögren's syndrome
SSc	Systemic sclerosis
SSc-ILD	Systemic sclerosis–associated interstitial lung disease
SSc-PAH	Systemic sclerosis–associated pulmonary arterial hypertension
SSRI	Selective serotonin reuptake inhibitor

SSS	Stiff skin syndrome
STAT3	Transducer and activator of transcription-3
STAT4	Transcription factor signal transducer and activator of transcription 4
STPR	Skin thickness progression rate
SWAP	Satisfaction with Appearance Scale
^{99m}Tc-DTPA	Technetium-labelled diethylene triamine pentacetate
TAPSE	Tricuspid annular plane systolic excursion
TARC	Thymus and activation regulated chemokine
TCR	T-cell receptor
TdT	Transmission disequilibrium test
TFR	Tendon friction rubs
TGF-beta	Transforming growth factor beta
THY1	Thy-1 cell surface antigen
TIMP	Tissue inhibitor of matrix metalloproteinases
TIN	Tubule-interstitial nephritis
TK	Tyrosine kinase
TLC	Total lung capacity
TLR	Toll-like receptor
TNFAIP3	Tumor necrosis factor, alpha-induced protein 3
TNFSF4	Tumor necrosis factor ligand superfamily, member 4
TNIP1	TNFAIP3 interacting protein 1
TOS	Toxic oil syndrome
TPMT	Thiopurine methyltransferase
TPN	Total parenteral nutrition
TPO	Thyroid peroxidase
TPP	Target product profile
Treg	T regulatory cell
TRIM-21	Tripartite motif family of protein 21
TRJ	Tricuspid regurgitant jet
TSH	Thyroid-stimulating hormone
Tsk-1	Tight skin-1
TSLP	Thymic stromal lymphopoietin
TSP-1	Thrombospondin-1
TSS	Total skin score
UCD	University of California at Davis
UCLA SCTC GIT 2.0	University of California-Scleroderma Clinical Trial Consortium Gastrointestinal Instrument
UDCA	Ursodeoxycholic acid
UIP	Usual interstitial pneumonia
UKFS	UK Functional Score
uPA	Urokinase plasminogen activator
uPAR	Urokinase plasminogen activator receptor
US	Ultrasonography
VA	Volume of ventilated lung
VAS	Visual analogue scale
VCAM	Vascular cell adhesion molecule
VEDOSS	Very early diagnosis of SSc
VEGF	Vascular endothelial cell growth factor
VQ	Ventilation-perfusion
VSM	Vascular smooth muscle
vWF	Von Willebrand factor
WHO	World Health Organization
WML	White matter lesions

Contents

Part IX Case Studies: Approach to Complex Clinical Problems

Contributors

Harsh Agrawal, MD, FACP Department of Internal Medicine, Division of Cardiology, Paul. L. Foster School of Medicine Texas Tech University, El Paso, Texas, USA

Yannick Allanore, MD Service de Rhumatologie A, Université Paris Descartes, Hôpital Cochin, Paris, France

Yoshihide Asano, MD, PhD Department of Dermatology, University of Tokyo Graduate School of Medicine, Tokyo, Japan

Frederic B. Askin, MD Department of Pathology, Johns Hopkins University School of Medicine, Baltimore, MD, USA

Shervin Assassi, MD, MS Division of Rheumatology, University of Texas Health Science Center at Houston, Houston, TX, USA

Jérôme Avouac, MD Rheumatology A Department, Cochin Hospital, Paris Descartes University, Sorbonne Paris Cité, Paris, France

Jammie K. Barnes, MD Department of Internal Medicine – Rheumatology, University of Texas at Houston, Houston, TX, USA

Dame Carol Black Division of Medicine, UCL, London, UK

Francesco Boin, MD Division of Rheumatology, Department of Medicine, University of California San Francisco, San Francisco, CA, USA

Kevin K. Brown, MD Department of Medicine, National Jewish Health, Denver, CO, USA

Maya H. Buch, MBChB, FRCP, PhD Leeds Institute of Rheumatic & Musculoskeletal Medicine, Chapel Allerton Hospital, Leeds, UK

Eliza F. Chakravarty, MD, MS Department of Arthritis and Clinical Immunology, Oklahoma Medical Research Foundation, Oklahoma City, OK, USA

Carlo Chizzolini, MD Immunology and Allergy, Department of Medical Specialties, Geneva University Hospital and School of Medicine, Geneva, Switzerland

Lorinda Chung, MD, MS Department of Medicine and Dermatology (Immunology and Rheumatology Division), Stanford University School of Medicine, Stanford, USA

Palo Alto VA Hospital, Palo Alto, CA, USA

John O. Clarke, MD Division of Gastroenterology & Hepatology, Johns Hopkins University, Baltimore, MD, USA

J. Gerry Coghlan, MD Department of Pulmonary Hypertension, Royal Free Hospital, London, UK

Vincent Cottin, MD, PhD Department of Pulmonology, Reference Center for Rare Pulmonary Diseases, Louis Pradel Hospital, Lyon, France

Vanessa C. Delisle, MSc Lady Davis Institute for Medical Research, McGill University and Jewish General Hospital, Montreal, QC, Canada

Christopher P. Denton, PhD, FRCP Division of Medicine, Department of Inflammation, Centre for Rheumatology and Connective Tissue Diseases, UCL Division of Medicine, Royal Free Hospital, London, UK

Jörg H.W. Distler, MD Department of Internal Medicine, University of Erlangen-Nuremberg, Erlangen-Nuremberg, Germany

Oliver Distler, MD Division of Rheumatology, University Hospital Zurich, Zurich, Switzerland

Rucsandra Dobrota, MD Division of Rheumatology, University Hospital Zurich, Zurich, Switzerland

Department of Internal Medicine and Rheumatology, Carol Davila University of Medicine and Pharmacy, Cantacuzino Hospital, Bucharest, Romania

Robyn T. Domsic, MD, MPH Department of Medicine/Rheumatology and Clinical Immunology, University of Pittsburgh, Pittsburgh, PA, USA

Harrison W. Farber, MD Pulmonary Hypertension Center, Boston University Medical Center, Boston, MA, USA

Carol Feghali-Bostwick, PhD Department of Medicine, Medical University of South Carolina, Charleston, SC, USA

Ivan Foeldvari, MD Hamburg Centre for Pediatric Rheumatology, Head of the Juvenile Scleroderma Working Group (JSScWG), Hamburger Zentrum Für Kinder- und Jugendrheumatologie, Hamburg, Germany

Rina S. Fox, MS, MPH SDSU/UC San Diego Joint Doctoral Program in Clinical Psychology, San Diego, CA, USA

Jaap Fransen, PhD Departments of Rheumatology, Radboud University Nijmegen Medical Center and Sint Maartenskliniek, Nijmegen, The Netherlands

Daniel E. Furst, MD Department of Rheumatology, University of California, Los Angeles, Los Angeles, CA, USA

N. Nazzareno Galié, MD Department of Experimental, Diagnostic and Specialty Medicine-DIMES, University of Bologna, Bologna, Italy

Shadi Gholizadeh, MS, MSc SDSU/UC San Diego Joint Doctoral Program in Clinical Psychology, San Diego, CA, USA

Lauren V. Graham, MD, PhD Department of Dermatology, Northwestern University, McGraw Medical Center, Chicago, IL, USA

Faye N. Hant, DO, MSCR Division of Rheumatology and Immunology, Medical University of South Carolina, Charleston, SC, USA

Elizabeth Harrison, MB, ChB Institute of Inflammation and Repair, University of Manchester, Manchester, UK

Ariane L. Herrick, MD, FRCP Centre for Musculoskeletal Research, Salford Royal NHS Foundation Trust, Manchester Academic Health Science Centre, The University of Manchester, Manchester, UK

Kristin B. Highland, MD, MSCR Department of Pulmonary and Critical Care Medicine, Cleveland Clinic Foundation, Cleveland, OH, USA

Monique Hinchcliff, MD, MS Department of Medicine, Northwestern University, Feinberg School of Medicine, Chicago, IL, USA

Alan Holmes, PhD Drug Discovery Group, Translational Research Office, School of Pharmacy, University College London, London, UK

Marie Hudson, MD, MPH Division of Rheumatology and Lady Davis Institute for Medical Research, Jewish General Hospital, Montréal, QC, Canada

Faculty of Medicine, McGill University, Montréal, QC, Canada

Marc Humbert, MD, PhD Department of Respiratory Medicine, Hôpital Bicêtre, Paris, France

Laura K. Hummers, MD, ScM Department of Medicine and Rheumatology, Johns Hopkins University, Baltimore, MD, USA

Heidi T. Jacobe, MD, MSCS Department of Dermatology, University of Texas Southwestern Medical Center, Dallas, TX, USA

Lisa R. Jewett, MSc Lady Davis Institute for Medical Research, McGill University and Jewish General Hospital, Montreal, QC, Canada

Sergio A. Jimenez, MD Department of Dermatology and Cutaneous Biology, Jefferson Institute of Molecular Medicine, Thomas Jefferson University, Philadelphia, PA, USA

Sindhu R. Johnson, MD, PhD, FRCPC Toronto Scleroderma Program, Mount Sinai Hospital, Toronto Western Hospital, Toronto, ON, Canada

Bashar Kahaleh, MD Division of Rheumatology and Immunology, University of Toledo Medical Center, Toledo, OH, USA

Gregory J. Keir, MBBS, FRACP Department of Respiratory Medicine, Princess Alexandra Hospital, Brisbane, QLD, Australia

Dinesh Khanna, MD, MSc Division of Rheumatology, Department of Internal Medicine, University of Michigan, Ann Arbor, MI, USA

Masataka Kuwana, MD, PhD Department of Allergy and Rheumatology, Nippon Medical School Graduate School of Medicine, Tokyo, Japan

Linda Kwakkenbos, PhD Lady Davis Institute for Medical Research, McGill University and Jewish General Hospital, Montreal, QC, Canada

Robert Lafyatis, MD University of Pittsburgh School of Medicine, Pittsburgh, USA

Simon Lal, PhD, FRCP Intestinal Failure Unit, Salford Royal NHS Foundation Trust, Salford, UK

Edward V. Lally, MD Division of Rheumatology, Rhode Island Hospital, Providence, RI, USA

Brooke Levis, MSc Lady Davis Institute for Medical Research, McGill University and Jewish General Hospital, Montreal, QC, Canada

Ahmad Mahmood, MD Department of Pulmonary Hypertension, Royal Free Hospital, London, UK

J. Mathew Mahoney, PhD Department of Neurological Sciences, University of Vermont, Burlington, VT, USA

Vanessa L. Malcarne, PhD SDSU/UC San Diego Joint Doctoral Program in Clinical Psychology, San Diego, CA, USA

Andrew L. Mammen, MD, PhD National Institutes of Health, National Institutes of Arthritis and Skin and Musculoskeletal Diseases, Bethesda, MD, USA

Mirko Manetti, PhD Section of Anatomy and Histology, Department of Experimental and Clinical Medicine, University of Florence, Florence, Italy

Steven C. Mathai, MD, MHS Division of Pulmonary and Critical Care Medicine, Johns Hopkins University School of Medicine, Baltimore, MD, USA

Marco Matucci-Cerinic, MD, PhD Department of Experimental and Clinical Medicine, Careggi Hospital (AOUC), University of Florence, Florence, Italy

Kimberly Doering Maurer, PhD University of California, San Francisco, CA, USA

Maureen D. Mayes, MD, MPH Division of Rheumatology and Clinical Immunogenetics, University of Texas Health Science Center – Houston, Houston, TX, USA

Thomas A. Medsger, MD Division of Rheumatology, Department of Medicine, University of Pittsburgh, Pittsburgh, PA, USA

Sarah D. Mills SDSU/UC San Diego Joint Doctoral Program in Clinical Psychology, San Diego, CA, USA

Pia Moinzadeh, MD Department of Dermatology and Venerology, University of Cologne, Cologne, Germany

Luc Mouthon, MD, PhD Department of Internal Medicine, Hôpital Cochin, Paris, France

Ulf Müller-Ladner, MD Internal Medicine and Rheumatology, Justus-Liebig University Giessen, Bad Nauheim, Hessia, Germany

Christopher J. Mullin, MD Division of Pulmonary and Critical Care Medicine, Johns Hopkins University School of Medicine, Baltimore, MD, USA

Charles Murray, MA, PhD, FRCP Department of Gastroenterology, Royal Free London NHS TRUST, London, UK

Voon H. Ong, PhD, FRCP Centre for Rheumatology and Connective Tissue Diseases, UCL Medical School Royal Free Hospital, London, UK

Amy S. Paller, MS, MD Department of Dermatology, Northwestern University Feinberg School of Medicine, Chicago, IL, USA

John E. Pandolfino, MD, MS Division of Gastroenterology & Hepatology, Feinberg School of Medicine, Northwestern University, Chicago, IL, USA

Markella Ponticos, PhD Centre for Rheumatology and Connective Tissue Disease, Royal Free Hospital (University College London), London, UK

Janet L. Poole, PhD, OTR/L Occupational Therapy Graduate Program, School of Medicine, University of New Mexico, Albuquerque, NM, USA

Lisa M. Rooper, MD Department of Pathology, Johns Hopkins Hospital, Baltimore, MD, USA

Antony Rosen, MB ChB, BSc Division of Rheumatology, Department of Medicine, The Johns Hopkins Hospital, Baltimore, MD, USA

Ami A. Shah, MD, MHS Clinical and Translational Research, Johns Hopkins Scleroderma Center, Baltimore, MD, USA

Sanjiv J. Shah, MD Northwestern University Feinberg School of Medicine, Chicago, IL, USA

Noëlle S. Sherber, MD Scleroderma Center, Johns Hopkins Hospital, Baltimore, MD, USA

Katherine C. Silver, MD Department of Rheumatology, Medical University of South Carolina, Charleston, SC, USA

Richard M. Silver, MD, MACR Division of Rheumatology and Immunology, Medical University of South Carolina, Charleston, SC, USA

Robert W. Simms, MD Department of Rheumatology, Boston Medical Center and Boston University School of Medicine, Boston, MA, USA

Robert J. Spence, MD, FACS Emeritus, MedStar Good Samaritan Hospital, Baltimore, MD, USA

Virginia Steen, MD Department of Medicine, Rheumatology, Clinical Immunology, and Allergy, Georgetown University Hospital, Washington, DC, USA

Edward P. Stern, MBBS, MRCP Centre for Rheumatology, Royal Free Hospital London, London, UK

Yossra A. Suliman, MD, MSc Department of Rheumatology and Rehabilitation, Assiut University Hospital, Assiut, Egypt

Jaclyn Taroni, PhD Department of Genetics, Geisel School of Medicine at Dartmouth, Hanover, NH, USA

Noelle M. Teske, BA, MSc Department of Dermatology, University of Texas Southwestern Medical Center, Dallax, TX, USA

Brett D. Thombs, PhD Lady Davis Institute for Medical Research, McGill University and Jewish General Hospital, Montreal, QC, Canada

Maria Trojanowska, PhD Department of Medicine, Boston University Medical Center, Boston, MA, USA

Rubin M. Tuder, MD Department of Medicine, Division of Pulmonary Science & Critical Care Medicine, University of Colorado Denver, Aurora, CO, USA

Alan Tyndall, MBBS, FRACP, FRCP (Ed) Department of Rheumatology, University Hospital Basel, Basel, Switzerland

Jacob M. van Laar, MD, PhD Rheumatology and Clinical Immunology, University Medical Center Utrecht, Utrecht, The Netherlands

Frank H.J. van den Hoogen, MD, PhD Department of Rheumatology, Radboud University Nijmegen Medical Center and Sint Maartenskliniek, Nijmegen, The Netherlands

Antonia Valenzuela, MD, MS Department of Medicine, Stanford University, Palo Alto, CA, USA

John Varga, MD John and Nancy Hughes Professor, Feinberg School of Medicine, Northwestern University, Chicago, IL, USA

Athol U. Wells, MD, FRCP Interstitial Lung Disease Unit, National Heart & Lung Institute, London, UK

Michael L. Whitfield, PhD Department of Genetics, Geisel School of Medicine at Dartmouth, Hanover, NH, USA

Fredrick M. Wigley, MD Department of Medicine/Rheumatology, The Johns Hopkins University School of Medicine, Baltimore, MD, USA

Timothy M. Wright, PhD California Institute for Biomedical Research, La Jolla, CA, USA

Part I

Introduction

Historical Perspective of Scleroderma

1

Christopher P. Denton and Marco Matucci-Cerinic

In addition to considering how long a distinct medical entity that we would recognise as scleroderma has been recognised it is useful to place the diagnosis and classification of scleroderma in a historical context. It is clear that there was initially some reluctance to group together all forms of the disease that we would recognise today, and this is perhaps reflective of the advances that have occurred in imaging and laboratory investigation and a greater appreciation of the link between different organ-based manifestations. The milestones in the history of scleroderma bear testimony to the gradual realisation of the heterogeneity of the disorder. For a more detailed discussion of the fascinating history of this disease, the reader is referred to the excellent historical review by Rodnan, the "father" of modern-day clinical scleroderma [1].

Early History

It is often considered that the first description of the systemic disease that we recognise as scleroderma was in 1753 by Cario Curzio (Naples, Italy) (Fig. 1.1). However, a careful review of the reported case suggest the diagnosis may in reality have been *scleroedema* because of the distribution of the skin changes and due to an apparent improvement in the 17-year-old female patient after a combination of therapeutic endeavors that included bloodletting, warm milk, and small doses of elemental mercury. In 1836, Fantonetti (1791–1877), a Milanese physician, became the first to use the term *scleroderma* to designate a disease in an adult. However, it is likely that his patient also had scleroedema. The first convincing case of scleroderma was reported in 1842, and then several other cases were published prior to 1847, a year when interest in the disease greatly increased. By 1860 numerous cases had been reported, and the first articles that attempted to review the disease were published. Maurice Raynaud (1834–1881) described a patient with *sclerodermie* and cold-induced "asphyxie locale" – this was the first description of Raynaud phenomenon in scleroderma. Just as for scleroderma, it has been speculated that the first cases of Raynaud phenomenon may have included individuals with an alternative diagnosis underlying their acrocyanosis and vascular insufficiency. Sir William Osler made the diagnosis of scleroderma while at the Johns Hopkins Hospital between 1891 and 1897. Osler appears to have clearly appreciated the systemic nature of the disease and to recognise the enormous clinical burden that patients with scleroderma endured when he wrote: *In its more aggravated forms diffuse scleroderma is one of the most terrible of all human ills. Like Tithonous, to "whither slowly," and like him to be "beaten down and marred and wasted" until one is literally a mummy, encased in an ever-shrinking, slowly contracting skin of steel, is a fate not pictured in any tragedy, ancient or modern.* Matsui (Japan, 1924) further highlighted the importance of visceral involvement as based on several autopsies that he had performed in individuals that had succumbed to the disease. Goetz (Capetown, 1945) further confirmed the multisystem involvement and suggested the disease be named *progressive systemic sclerosis*. The qualifying term "progressive" was later considered to be inaccurate in some cases that either remained stable or improved or has generally been dropped. It does however serve to highlight the potential severity of the worst forms of the disease. The potential importance of subtypes of scleroderma began in 1964, when Winterbauer reported cases with the CRST (calcinosis, Raynaud's phenomenon, sclerodactyly, and telangiectasias) syndrome. A similar group of patients was reported in 1920, named after the authors, the Thibierge-Weissenbach syndrome. Velayos and colleagues recognised that oesophageal dysmotility was common in these patients; so now it is called the CREST

C.P. Denton, PhD, FRCP (✉)
Division of Medicine, Department of Inflammation, Centre for Rheumatology and Connective Tissue Diseases, UCL Division of Medicine, Royal Free Hospital, London, UK
e-mail: c.denton@ucl.ac.uk

M. Matucci-Cerinic, MD, PhD
Department of Experimental and Clinical Medicine, Careggi Hospital (AOUC), University of Florence, Florence, Italy

J. Varga et al. (eds.), *Scleroderma*, DOI 10.1007/978-3-319-31407-5_1

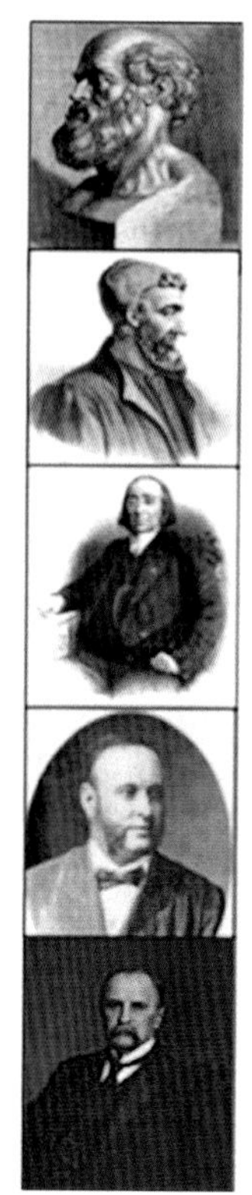

- **Hippocrates and Galen described possible cases of scleroderma**
- **First convincing case published by Curzio (Italy) 1753**

Treatment: "...warm milk, vapor baths, bleeding and small doses of quicksilver. After 11 months the patient's skin had become perfectly soft and flexible." A cure !?

- **Scleroderma first established as a clinical entity, and called 'sclerodermie' by Gintrac 1847**
- **Raynaud's Phenomenon described 1852, and in 1871 associated with scleroderma**
- **Wollers 1892 "According to all observations, scleroderma does not appear to be a disease which threatens life directly." !! But :**
- **Osler 1894 ".. patients are apt to succumb to pulmonary complaints or to nephritis."**

Fig. 1.1 Some of the key historic figures who contributed to the field of scleroderma are listed. Appreciation of the severity of the disease was confounded by clinical variability and absence of unifying diagnostic criteria or investigational modalities

syndrome. In 1969, 58 autopsy cases of scleroderma were compared with matched controls. The organs found to be frequently and significantly involved by this disease were the skin, gastrointestinal tract, lungs, kidneys, skeletal muscle, and pericardium. This report first described the systemic nature of vascular pathology in scleroderma with findings of both kidney and lung arterial changes. Rodnan introduced a clinical method to evaluate the extent of skin disease and correlated this with skin biopsy weight and later with collagen content in the skin. From the same centre in Pittsburgh, Steen and Medsger and others did extensive surveys of large populations of scleroderma patients defining the clinical course and specific subtypes of disease. In the 1980s, a subcommittee of world experts established diagnostic criteria [2], and LeRoy and colleagues [3] suggested the classification of two major subsets of disease defined by skin involvement: *limited* and *diffuse*. Recent work by several investigators has recognised that scleroderma-specific autoantibodies occur that associate with subtypes of disease and can be used to predict disease course. Work in the modern era has revealed details of the pathogenesis of the disease and the recognition that scleroderma is a complex polygenetic autoimmune disease associated with a unique disease process involving tissue fibrosis. Although no drug is yet discovered that can be called a successful disease-modifying agent that controls the underlying disease process, major progress has been made in managing specific organ disease. The discovery of that an angiotensin-converting enzyme inhibitor could reverse the scleroderma renal crisis in the 1970s changed the course of kidney disease and improved the survival of patients. Current therapies for gastrointestinal, cardiac, pulmonary vascular, and interstitial lung disease have improved quality of life and survival. There has been a growing interest in scleroderma around the world and the emergence of specialist centres that now provide effective patient care and scientific interactions with each other and private industry to discover the causes and new treatment for scleroderma. Although uncommon and without effective disease-modifying therapies, the relevance of scleroderma to a broad range of other medical conditions is now fully appreciated, and this has benefited management though translation of treatments into the organ-based complications of scleroderma. In addition, scleroderma (Fig. 1.2) provides a potential platform for the development of anti-fibrotic or vascular therapies that could be beneficial in other commoner diseases that are characterised by vascular insufficiency or extracellular matrix overproduction.

Emergence of Systemic Sclerosis as a Clinical Entity

The appreciation of the spectrum of scleroderma and related disorders over the past 40 years has been a gradual process underpinned by growing expertise in assessment and evaluation of cases and stronger collaboration across medical

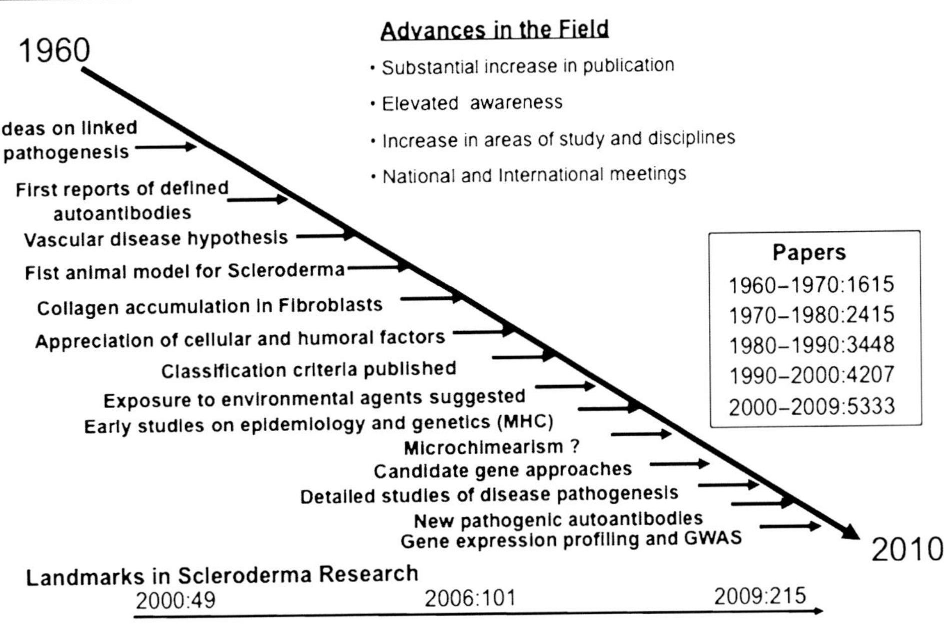

Fig. 1.2 The timeline of translational research into scleroderma illustrates the growing interest in the disease together with better appreciation of its complexity and more candidates for pathogenesis

specialties. This allowed the relationship between systemic sclerosis, localised scleroderma, and other autoimmune rheumatic diseases to become established. Additional recognition of conditions such as eosinophilic fasciitis [4] and environmentally triggered diseases fueled clinical research. Finally, appreciation of the relationship between isolated Raynaud's phenomenon and evolution into connective tissue disease permitted a broadening of the spectrum to encompass what is currently considered the scleroderma spectrum that is covered in this volume.

Recent History

The late twentieth century was a period of tremendous advance in biomedicine, and this is reflected by the growth in understanding of systemic sclerosis. This has occurred in both appreciation of the underlying pathobiology and also the relationship between clinical manifestations of scleroderma and systemic sclerosis (SSc) and other organ-based forms of fibrosis and vascular disease. In this way, SSc provides a paradigm for other commoner medical conditions, and this has fueled clinical and translational research and helped to support further research.

Advances in Scleroderma Biology

Underpinned by the work of LeRoy and others [3], the next generation of researchers has used advances in cell and molecular biology to develop better concepts of pathobiology of SSc that more completely explain the disease. This has most recently included incorporation of genetic and developmental biology, and it is reasonable to assert that models of pathogenesis can now be developed that provide a framework for understanding the disease in its different and diverse forms. Improved outcomes for scleroderma renal crisis emerged in the 1980s, and this provided an important demonstration that SSc was indeed treatable and that outcomes even of the most lethal aspects of the disease could be improved. In a similar time frame, treatments for gastroesophageal disease advanced, with PPIs providing a critical advance in management of upper GI disease. The International Scleroderma Research Workshop was established by Drs. Black and Korn and has provided real stimulus to advance science of SSc and evolve into the area of translational research. This meeting remains preeminent in the field and aims to bring the very best relevant and new science into the arena of scleroderma research.

Progress in Classification Natural History and Clinical Trials Methodology

The past two decades have been a period of clinical progress that has included the development of clinical trials methodology. Important studies have been undertaken; although initially mostly negative these efforts did confirm the feasibility of clinical trials in SSc and led to better understanding of disease natural history. Pooled analysis of these early studies has been essential to better understand trail methods, and this has provided the foundation for current clinical studies. Early templates for trial design were developed and have been updated, and this is exemplified by recent publication of a series of points to consider in scleroderma trials [5]. As in other branches of medicine, the availability of valid trial templates is critical as potential therapeutic approaches emerge. Appreciation of the need for cohort enrichment and clear definition of endpoints has emerged from expert discussion over the past three decades and represents an important achievement in recent scleroderma history.

Classification of SSc was first attempted in 1980 [2] and subset criteria were later developed. The new classification criteria were developed by rigorous methodology and with strong international collaboration and were published in 2013 [6]. These reflected expert practice and a growing understanding of disease heterogeneity, although attempts to define robust criteria for early diagnosis of classification of milder disease proved challenging and no real agreement was reached until much more recently when evidence-based approaches such as the prospective VEDOSS project developed [7].

Important international collaborative groups have emerged including the Scleroderma Clinical Trials Consortium that was established in the 1990s and now have more than 75 member institutions all with a high degree of expertise in clinical research and trails in SSc. This has underpinned recent trials and progress. The first organised group to emerge internationally was the Scleroderma Clinical Trials consortium. This group links expert centres and was set up in the USA but has now become a strong international organisation. More recently the key events internationally have been the establishment of EUSTAR that has developed into an impressive network of scleroderma centres and anchored by a clinical database that is being used for observational clinical research. There are active educational and research programmers, and these are now providing a very powerful research for study and improved understanding of SSc.

Driven by growing interest from clinicians and supported by patients, scientists, and pharmaceutical partners, the World Congress in SSc became established in 2010, and the success of this larger format of international conference for SSc is testament to growing interest in the disease and opportunities for better management and strong engagement with patient organisations. An umbrella organisation for patient groups FESCA has developed in parallel with EUSTAR and the world congress and offers a real hope for the future with opportunities for broader political engagement and support. The World Scleroderma Foundation represents the most recent chapter in the history of international collaboration and enterprise (www.worldsclerodermafoundation.net). It provides potential avenues for larger and more inclusive approaches to education and care for SSc underpinned by highest-quality research and investigation. It is now formally lined to EUSTAR and is underpinned by the successful World SSc Congresses. Thus, the recent history of scleroderma is international, collaborative, and forward looking and represents the start of the next stage in the journey towards understanding the disease and offering better outcomes for patients.

Some of the key events in the history of scleroderma are listed in Table 1.1. This provides an approximate time line that demonstrates the recent progress in understanding the disease, but it is important to observe that the outcome of the

Table 1.1 The landmarks in the history of scleroderma

Date	Person	History of scleroderma
c. 400 BC	Hippocrates	Described an Athenian with indurated unpinchable skin. Insufficient detail to ascertain whether this was scleroderma
1753	Curzio	Description of young woman of Naples with "excessive hardness of the skin" – possibly scleroderma, but probably scleroedema of Buschke
1847	Gintrac	First use of the name "sclérodermie"
1847	Forget	First description of joint involvement in scleroderma
1854	Addison	First description of linear scleroderma
1862	Raynaud	Description of "local asphyxia and symmetrical gangrene of the extremities"
1878	Weber	Coexistence of scleroderma and calcinosis noted
1892	Osler	Tendency for scleroderma patients to die of pulmonary or renal disease noted
1893	Hutchinson	Association of scleroderma and Raynaud's phenomenon noted
1903	Erhmann	Association of scleroderma and dysphagia noted
1910	Thibierge and Weissenbach	"Rediscovery" of the coexistence of scleroderma and calcinosis
1924	Matsui	First clear description of visceral involvement, with sclerosis of lungs, gastrointestinal tract, and kidneys
1943	Weiss	Clear description of myocardial involvement in scleroderma
1945	Goetz	Coined the term "progressive systemic sclerosis"
1964	Winterbauer	Described the CREST subset (calcinosis, Raynaud's, oesophagitis, sclerodactyly, and telangiectasia)
1980	Masi	Preliminary classification criteria for systemic sclerosis published
2001	Medsger and LeRoy	Early scleroderma criteria suggested for minimal skin disease

disease in terms of mortality has substantially improved over the past 20 years and that this has come at a time when there is a much better and more complete appreciation of disease burden from nonlethal manifestations. Thus, many more SSc patients are now living with the disease than are dying from it, and this raises its own important challenges that are considered in detail in the various sections and subsequent chapters of this textbook.

References

1. Rodnan GP, Benedek TG. An historical account of the study of progressive systemic sclerosis (diffuse scleroderma). Ann Intern Med. 1962;57:305–19.
2. Preliminary criteria for the classification of systemic sclerosis (scleroderma). Subcommittee for scleroderma criteria of the American Rheumatism Association Diagnostic and Therapeutic Criteria Committee. Arthritis Rheum. 1980;23:581–90.
3. LeRoy EC, Medsger TA. Criteria for the classification of early systemic sclerosis. J Rheumatol. 2001;28:1573–6.
4. Shulman LE. Diffuse fasciite with hypergammaglobulinemia and eosinophilia: a new syndrome? J Rheumatol. 1974;1 Suppl 1:46–9.
5. Khanna D, Furst DE, Allanore Y, Bae S, Bodukam V, Clements PJ, et al. Twenty-two points to consider for clinical trials in systemic sclerosis, based on EULAR standards. Rheumatology. 2015;54:144–51.
6. van den Hoogen F, Khanna D, Fransen J, Johnson SR, Baron M, Tyndall A, et al. 2013 classification criteria for systemic sclerosis: an American College of Rheumatology/European League against Rheumatism collaborative initiative. Arthritis Rheum. 2013;65(11):2737–47.
7. Matucci-Cerinic M, Allanore Y, Czirják L, Tyndall A, Müller-Ladner U, Denton C, et al. The challenge of early systemic sclerosis for the EULAR Scleroderma Trial and Research group (EUSTAR) community. It is time to cut the Gordian knot and develop a prevention or rescue strategy. Ann Rheum Dis. 2009;68:1377–80.

Part II

Epidemiology, Genetics and Classification

Epidemiology, Environmental, and Infectious Risk Factors

2

Jammie K. Barnes, Luc Mouthon, and Maureen D. Mayes

Systemic sclerosis (SSc) is an autoimmune connective tissue disease characterized by excessive collagen deposition in the skin and internal organs with associated vasculopathy and autoantibody production [1]. Classification of SSc is divided into two main groups: limited and diffuse cutaneous disease [2]. The limited form is characterized by skin thickening that is confined to areas distal to the elbows and knees and generally is associated with less severe internal organ involvement. The diffuse form involves skin thickening proximal to the elbows and the knees as well as distal areas and is associated with more severe organ damage. This chapter will focus on the epidemiology of SSc including both limited and diffuse cutaneous forms.

Incidence and Prevalence of SSc

Reported incidence rates (number of new cases per year) and prevalence estimates (number of total cases) vary widely depending on geographic location and methods of case ascertainment. In 2013, the American College of Rheumatology (ACR) and the European League Against Rheumatism (EULAR) updated classification criteria for SSc [3]. Prior to 2013, the ACR (previously the American Rheumatism Association) published classification criteria in 1980 to distinguish SSc from other connective tissue diseases and to standardize reporting [4]. The absence of a standard classification system for SSc prior to 1980 makes it problematic to interpret occurrence figures for SSc in reports prior to this time.

Reported prevalence figures for definite SSc vary greatly from 30 cases/million (New Zealand, 1979) [5] to 580 cases/million (Alberta, Canada, 1994–2007) [6]. Accordingly, the annual incidence rates also vary widely between 1.96 cases/million from the time period 1950–1973 (New Zealand) [7] to 46 cases/million from the time period 2003–2008 (US managed care population) [8]. Table 2.1, modified and updated from Chifflot et al. [9], summarizes multiple reports of incidence rates and prevalence figures from different geographic locations and time periods reported as unadjusted [5–8, 10–34]. Only studies that included men and women are shown, and only figures for SSc are reported, excluding "scleroderma spectrum disorders."

It is clear from these studies that there are regional variations in reported disease occurrence. This may reflect differences in case definition and/or differences in how complete methods of case ascertainment were. However, the differences may also arise from true variations among regions, and this in turn could be due to differences in exposures to environmental triggers or due to population differences in frequency of susceptibility genes. In addition, regions such as North American and Canada have specific subpopulations, Native Americans and First Nations, respectively, that reportedly have more SSc cases than expected, presumably on the basis of shared genetic risk factors.

Temporal Changes in Incidence Rates

Studies by Medsger et al. [10] and Steen et al. [12] reported changes in the incidence rate (number of new SSc cases per year) over time. Using a hospital record review approach in Tennessee [10], the incidence of SSc was reported to have increased from 0.6 cases/million/year for the years 1947–1952

J.K. Barnes, MD (✉)
Department of Internal Medicine – Rheumatology, University of Texas at Houston, Houston, TX 77030, USA
e-mail: jammie.k.barnes@uth.tmc.edu

L. Mouthon, MD, PhD
Department of Internal Medicine, Hopital Cochin, Paris 75014, France

M.D. Mayes, MD, MPH
Division of Rheumatology and Clinical Immunogenetics, University of Texas Health Science Center – Houston, Houston, TX 77030, USA

J. Varga et al. (eds.), *Scleroderma*, DOI 10.1007/978-3-319-31407-5_2

Table 2.1 Variations of incidence and prevalence of systemic sclerosis by region and time

Reference	Region	Case ascertainment method	Inclusion criteria (n = number of cases)	Study period	Incidence (per million/year)	Prevalence per million	Female/male ratio
North America							
Medsger [10]	Tennessee	Hospital record review	Study specific (n = 60)	1947–1952	0.6	–	1.5:1
					4.5		
				1953–1968	2.7 (entire period)		
				1947–1968			
Michet [11]	Minnesota	Diagnostic retrieval system	ICDA (7th) (n = 13)	1950–1979	10	138	12:1
Steen [12]	Pennsylvania	Hospital record review	ACR + study specific (n = 44)	1963–1972	9.6	–	–
					18.7		
				1973–1982	13.9 (entire period)		
				1963–1982			
Maricq [13]	South Carolina	Multistage population survey	ACR + study specific (n = 2)	1989	–	286	–
Mayes [14]	Michigan	Multiple sources (CR)	ACR and CREST (n = 706)	1989–1991	21	276	4.6:1
Robinson [15]	2 medical/drug claim datasets	ICD diagnostic codes	–	2001–2002	–	300	–
Furst [8]	USA	Medical claims and ICD-9	Diagnosis codes	2003–2008	46	135–184	6.15:1
Bernatsky [16]	Quebec	Hospital and physician billing databases	ICD diagnostic codes	2003	–	443	–
Barnabe [6]	Alberta	Hospital and billing codes	1994–2007	–	508	–	5.8:1
Australia							
Wigley [5]	New Zealand	Hospital record review	Study specific	1950–1973	1.96	–	–
Eason [7]	New Zealand	Hospital record review and specialist practices	ACR (n = 50)	1970–1979	6.3	30	3:1
Englert [17]	Sydney	Hospital record review	ACR + study specific	1974–1988	12	45.2 (1988)	–
Chandran [18]	South Australia	Hospital record review	ACR + study specific + overlap syndrome (n = 215)	1987–1993	–	208	4:1
Roberts-Thomson [19]	South Australia	Multiple sources	ACR + study specific + overlap syndrome (n = 548)	1993	15.1	200	4:1
				1999	22.8	232.4	–
Roberts-Thomson [20]	South Australia	Multiple sources	ACR + study specific (n = 353)	1993–2002	20.4	232.2	–
Japan							
Tamaki [21]	Tokyo	Public health system	ACR (n = 629)	1987	7.2	38	14:1
UK and Europe							
Silman [22]	England (West Midlands)	Multiple sources	Study specific (n = 128)	1986	3.7	31	–
Allcock [23]	England (Newcastle)	Multiple sources	ACR + Leroy/Medsger (n = 80)	2000	–	88	5.2:1
Geirsson [24]	Iceland	Multiple sources	ACR + CREST (n = 18)	1975–1990	3.8	71	8:1
Kaipiainana [25]	Finland	Multiple sources	ACR + CREST (n = 4)	1990	3.7	–	–
Le Guern [26]	France (Seine-St-Denis)	Multiple sources (CR)	ACR + Leroy/Medsger (n = 15)	2001	–	158	11:1

Table 2.1 (continued)

Reference	Region	Case ascertainment method	Inclusion criteria (n = number of cases)	Study period	Incidence (per million/year)	Prevalence per million	Female/male ratio
El Adssi [27]	Lorraine, France	Capture	ACR	2006	–	132.2	6.72:1
		Recapture					
Hoffman-Vold [28]	Norway	Survey	ACR	1999–2009	–	52–144	3.8:1
Alamanos [29]	Greece (northwest)	Multiple sources	ACR + Leroy/Medsger (n = 109)	1981–2002	11	154	8.9:1
Arias-Nunez [30]	Spain (northwest)	Two-stage hospital-based survey	ACR + Leroy/Medsger (n = 78)	1988–2006	23	277	–
	Italy	Retrospective hospital/clinic visit/ICD-9	ACR + Leroy/Medsger	1999–2007	32	254	9.7:1
Monaco [31]	Italy	Survey	ACR				
Sardu [32]	Italy	Survey	ACR	–	–	–	–
Andreasson	Sweden	Register	ACR 1980	–	14	235	3.6:1
South America							
Rosa [34]	Buenos Aires	Med Care Program	ACR + Leroy/Medsger 1999–2004	21.2	296	15:1	

Modified from Chifflot et al. [9]

to 4.5 cases/million/year for the period 1953–1968. Applying a similar approach in Pennsylvania, the incidence of SSc was observed to almost double from 9.6/million/year for the period 1963–1972 to 18.7/million/year for the next decade (1973–1982). However, this latter figure of almost 19/million/year was quite similar to the incidence rate reported in Michigan [14] of 21 new cases/million/year for the study period of 1989–1991 suggesting that the increase in incidence did not continue. A recently published study by Furst et al., utilizing claims data from a large US managed care population, suggested a higher incidence and lower prevalence [8]. This study differed from the earlier Pennsylvania and Michigan-based studies, because it used data from across the USA. However, since this was based on claims rather than record review, there could be coding errors, and it is possible that the incidence rates are inflated because some could have had SSc prior to the study period.

Similarly, incidence figures from New Zealand and Australia suggest an increase over time with an observed incidence that increased from 1.96 for the period 1950 to 1973 to 6.3 in the 1970s, to 12.0 in the period 1974–1988, to 15.1 in 1993, and to 22.8 in 1999 (all incidence figures are per million per year). However, case ascertainment methods also improved during this period making it problematic to interpret these results.

Although taken as a whole these reports are suggestive of increasing incidence, it is difficult to reliably conclude that this is the case, as other changes such as better physician and patient awareness and the establishment of classification criteria for SSc could also account for the apparent increase in identified cases. Finally, incidence figures may change with the application of the 2013 ACR/EULAR criteria since those criteria were established to be more inclusive and to capture cases not previously identified by the 1980 criteria. With respects to that assumption, Andreasson et al. [33] reported incidence and prevalence figures in southern Sweden comparing the 1980 criteria and the 2013 criteria. The incidence rates for 1980 versus 2013 are 14 new cases/million/year for 1980 versus 19/million/year for 2013, and the prevalence estimates are 235 per million in 1980 and 305 per million in 2013. They concluded that application of the 2013 ACR/EULAR criteria results in a 30–40 % higher estimate of SSc incidence and prevalence compared to the previous criteria. It is likely that the new criterion successfully identifies more SSc cases. The above report found that a majority of recognized cases were anticentromere antibody positive and had limited cutaneous disease, some of whom would have been missed in the 1980 criteria. With further epidemiological studies using the new criteria, we should be able to better identify cases of SSc and have a more clear representation of incidence and prevalence. However, this will have to be taken into account in the consideration of temporal changes in disease occurrence.

Geographic Variations in SSc Occurrence

Higher prevalence figures have been consistently reported in North America and Australia as compared to Japan and Europe. Three US studies [13–15] covering the time period 1989–2002 have reported quite similar prevalence figures of 286, 276, and 300 cases/million, respectively, in spite of using dissimilar methods of case ascertainment. The 1989 South Carolina study [13] was population based and used a questionnaire with a physical exam done among the positive responders. This resulted in an estimated prevalence of 286 cases/million for SSc and an estimate of 3,790 cases/million of "scleroderma spectrum disease." This latter prevalence figure is likely related to the inclusion of overlap syndromes and/or primary Raynaud's disease because the questionnaire focused on Raynaud's phenomenon (RP) symptoms. The 2003 Michigan study [14] used five different sources for case finding and used a capture-recapture method of analysis to adjust for incomplete case ascertainment. Based on fairly conservative assumptions for this model, the prevalence estimate was 276 cases/million. A US population-based survey by Robinson et al. [15], which identified cases based on the International Classification of Diseases Version 9 (ICD-9) diagnostic codes as well as two medical and drug claims datasets, reported a prevalence of 300 cases/million in 2002.

In contrast to these three similar estimates, Bernatsky et al. [16] reported a considerably higher prevalence of 443 cases/million in 2003 in the province of Quebec, Canada, using physician billing and hospitalization databases and applying statistical modeling to address issues related to incomplete case ascertainment. Although the use of such administrative databases has value in epidemiology research, it is not yet clear that appropriate statistical models have been developed to provide reliable prevalence estimates.

Similar to the recent US figures noted above, studies from Australia have reported a prevalence of 200 cases/million and 233 cases/million for 1993 and 1999, respectively, using surveys conducted by the same group [19, 20]. However, an earlier study from Sydney [17] had reported a much lower prevalence of 45/million for 1975 and 86/million for 1988. This rather large difference may be explained by different methods of case finding as the earlier figures were based on hospital record review while the latter used multiple sources.

These figures are in marked contrast to incidence and prevalence figures reported in Japan. Tamaki et al. [21] in 1991 reported a survey based on a medical database and reported an incidence rate of 7.2 cases/million/year with a prevalence of 38–53 cases/million.

In the UK, two studies have reported prevalence estimates of 31 cases/million in 1986 [22] and 88 cases/million in 2000 [23].

Two Scandinavian studies have reported remarkably similar incidence rates of 3.8 cases/million/year in Iceland [24] and 3.7 for Finland [25]. Only the Icelandic study provided a prevalence figure of 71 cases/million.

Three studies in Europe have reported occurrence figures, with similar prevalence estimates for France [26] and Greece [29] at 158 and 154 cases/million, respectively. A recent study in northwestern Spain [30] reported a prevalence of 277/million suggesting that there may be a geographic north-south gradient.

In addition, recent incidence and prevalence data from northeastern Italy were found to be higher than reported in various geographical areas (UK, US, Australia) but similar to other Italian studies [31].

The geographic variance may be related to the population in the region. For example Arnett et al. [35] reported a well-defined population of Choctaw Indians in Oklahoma with a high prevalence of SSc estimated at 658.6 cases/million. The prevalence of SSc in the Choctaw group was higher than that reported in other Native Americans in Oklahoma. In addition, SSc disease expression was more uniform among these cases than in the general population, with most Choctaw cases having diffuse cutaneous disease and pulmonary fibrosis. No common exposure was found, but a particular Amerindian histocompatibility locus antigen (HLA) haplotype was identified suggesting a genetic predisposition to disease. In addition, to the Native Americans, the First Nations population in Alberta, Canada, also had a high prevalence reported at 580 cases/million [6]. This high disease occurrence may be related to shared genetic ancestry with associated inherited risk alleles.

Clusters

The phenomenon of clustering in epidemiology refers to a higher than expected number of cases in a defined geographic, occupational, or ethnic population. There have been multiple reports of SSc clustering.

A higher SSc prevalence was reported in boroughs close to major airports near London [36], with an estimated prevalence of 150 cases/million in the three boroughs near the airports, compared to a prevalence of 30.8 cases/million in more distant areas. Although the clusters were seen near the airports, they did not involve airport employees and factors responsible for the clustering were not identified.

Similarly, an increased prevalence of SSc was reported in the town of Woodstock, Ontario, Canada, compared to two nearby communities also in southwestern Ontario [37]. Explanatory factors in terms of occupation and health habits were not identified.

Two other clusters have been reported – one in Western Victoria, Australia [38], and one in rural Italy [39] – but both involved a relatively small number of cases such that population estimates based on these figures may be unreliable.

Survival

Survival rates have recently been reported to have improved significantly compared to earlier published reports. According to Steen and Medsger [40], the 10-year cumulative survival rate improved in their Pittsburg cohort from 54 % in the 1970s to 66 % in the 1990s. Figure 2.1, adapted from Steen and Medsger, illustrates the changes in causes of SSc-related deaths between 1972 and 2001.

Another survival study from a large Italian cohort [41] showed similar improvement in survival rates with survival increasing from 60.6 % in the period 1955–1985 to 78.6 % during 1986–1999.

This improvement in survival is likely related to earlier diagnosis and improvement in treatment, particularly the early detection and effective therapy of scleroderma renal crisis. Steen and Medsger [40] reported changes in organ-specific causes of mortality and found that pulmonary fibrosis and pulmonary hypertension (PH) have now become the leading causes of SSc-related deaths as opposed to SSc renal crisis following the introduction of treatment with angiotensin-converting enzyme inhibitors. Even with higher rates of survival found in these reports, overall survival in SSc remains considerable less than that predicted for age-, sex-, and race-matched controls [14].

Prognostic Factors

In a recent analysis of 234 fatalities from the EUSTAR (EULAR [European League Against Rheumatism] Scleroderma Trials and Research) database, Tyndall et al. [42] reported the following independent risk factors for mortality: proteinuria, pulmonary arterial hypertension (PAH), restrictive pulmonary disease, dyspnea greater than the New York Heart Association Class II, decreased pulmonary diffusion capacity, higher age at onset of Raynaud's phenomenon, and greater modified Rodnan skin score.

In a study from Pennsylvania, early mortality was seen in SSc patients that had significant muscle and cardiac disease, anticentromere antibody negative, and time to first non-Raynaud's phenomenon symptoms [43]. In a Norwegian cohort of SSc patients, factors that trended toward a worse outcome included PH, male sex, diffuse disease, and interstitial lung disease (ILD) [44]. There have been several studies that have found that ILD was a main prognostic factor associated with death [42, 44–49].

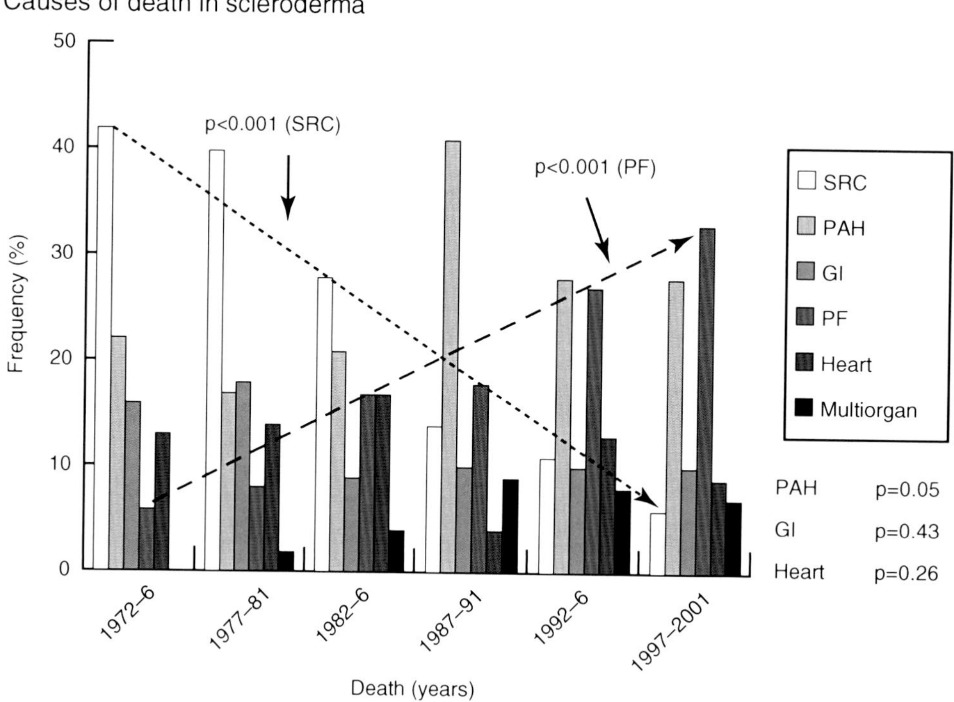

Fig. 2.1 Changes in causes of systemic sclerosis-related deaths between 1972 and 2001. *GI* gastrointestinal, *PAH* pulmonary arterial hypertension, *PF* pulmonary fibrosis, *SRC* scleroderma renal crisis (With permission from Steen and Medsger [40])

Similar results have been reported in studies from South Australia [45], in a meta-analysis from cases from the USA, Europe, and Japan [50], in French Canadians [51], and in cases from the UK [52].

The studies listed above have also found that diffuse skin involvement is associated with a poorer prognosis. A recent report by Domsic et al. [53] suggests that a higher rate of progression of skin thickening (skin thickness progression rate) is a predictor of mortality and early internal organ involvement particularly the development of renal crisis.

With respect to race, African-American patients have higher mortality compared to their white counterparts [14, 54] believed due to more aggressive disease and perhaps due to health care disparities between these groups. In a recent study by Sharif et al. [55], African-American patients had a younger age of onset, higher frequency of digital ulcers and pericarditis and more severe lower gastrointestinal tract involvement. There was also a strong association with anti-fibrillarin antibodies (AFA) and African-American patients. Those patients with AFA compared to African-Americans patients without AFA had less severe lung involvement. However, the presence of AFA did not influence survival in this cohort.

Although SSc has a higher prevalence in females, the risk of death was higher in male patients as seen in several studies [45–47]. In addition to gender, older age was identified as a predictor of mortality [45, 46, 49]. However, in a study from Barcelona, after adjustment was made for population effects of age and sex, the standardized mortality ratio was found to be higher in younger patients [56].

In terms of prognostic factors for mortality, a Japanese study found that gastrointestinal involvement was associated with a worse mortality as was diffuse disease [57]. In addition other studies have found myositis to have an increase hazard ratio for mortality [43, 58].

With respects to PAH and mortality, Chung et al. [59] reported that severely reduced diffusion capacity of the lung for carbon monoxide (DLCO) and functional class IV at the time of PAH diagnosis was associated with a poorer prognosis. In patients with SSc and ILD, the extent of disease found on high-resolution computed tomography was an independent variable that predicted both mortality and ILD progression [60]. Although treatment for PAH is being initiated in SSc patients, to date there are no studies that have clearly demonstrated a survival benefit. What is known currently is that SSc patients being treated for PAH have higher mortality rates than non-SSc patients with PAH [61].

SSc-specific autoantibodies are associated with both risk and survival benefit. For instance, it has been reported that having an anticentromere antibody is associated with a better prognosis [43, 55]. However, having the anti-RNA polymerase III antibody was associated with scleroderma renal crisis and increased mortality [46, 61]. In another study, the presence of anti-topoisomerase or anti-U1 RNP antibodies negatively impacted survival [45]. As noted above, the anti-fibrillarin antibody was associated with African-American patients but did not influence survival [55].

Risk Factors for Susceptibility of SSc

Risk factors for the development of SSc include gender, race, age, family history, birth order, and environmental factors including occupational exposures and possibly infections.

Female Gender

As summarized in Table 2.1, all epidemiology studies that have reported gender have noted that women consistently outnumber men with female to male ratios usually being 4:1–6:1. The reason for this female preponderance is not well understood. There is speculation that the difference may be related to hormones, pregnancy-related events, or gender-specific environmental exposures. There are relatively few published reports that have investigated the relationship of pregnancy with development of SSc. A Swedish population-based study [62] found that nulliparity was associated with an increased risk of SSc (odds ratio [OR] = 1.37, 95 % confidence interval [CI] = 1.22–1.55), whereas increasing parity was associated with a decreased risk. However, the increased risk with lower parity could also be explained, at least in part, by infertility due to subclinical or early disease. A more recent study by Cockrill et al. [63] compared pregnancy histories of SSc patients ($n = 172$) with that of their healthy sisters ($n = 256$) and found a positive association between gravidity and the risk of SSc (OR = 2.8, 95 % CI 1.62–6.61).

Microchimerism, the persistence of fetal cells in maternal tissues, has been proposed as a trigger for SSc or other autoimmune diseases [64], and it has been suggested as an explanation for the increased female to male ratio in these diseases. However, these data remain controversial, and to date the mechanism responsible for this association has not been identified.

Race

In the Michigan study previously noted above, Mayes et al. [14] reported a higher prevalence among African-Americans compared to European-Americans with an adjusted prevalence ratio of 1.15 (95 % CI 1.02–1.30). In addition, the proportion of diffuse disease was higher in black patients versus white patients, and age at diagnosis was earlier (43.8 years for black patients vs. 55.5 years for white patients, $p < 0.001$). In another study, pulmonary fibrosis was more severe at diagnosis among African-Americans than in other ethnic groups [65].

Similar findings were described by Le Guern et al. [26] who reported a prevalence of SSc for non-Europeans (Northern and sub-Saharan African, Asians, and Caribbean ancestries) as 210.8 cases/million versus the prevalence for European Caucasians at 140.2 cases/million. In addition as seen with prior studies, non-Europeans were more likely to have diffuse SSc (34 % vs. 17 %) and ILD (53 % vs. 33 %).

Racial differences in disease susceptibility and expression can be a reflection of genetic differences among groups. Genetic risk factors are discussed in greater detail in another section of this book.

Age at Onset

SSc is rare in childhood. In the Michigan study [14], African-American patients were significantly younger at the time of diagnosis compared with European-American patients ($p < 0.001$). Figure 2.2, adapted from Mayes et al. [14], illustrates peak incidence by race and gender. The peak incidence occurred between the ages of 45 and 54 for African-American women, whereas the peak incidence among white women occurred in the 65–74-year age group. Peak incidence for African-American men was similar to that of African-American women. Among the European-American men, a gradually increasing incidence until the age of 75–84 years was observed.

Familial Risk

In any discussion regarding heritability of disease, it is worthwhile to compare disease frequency between monozygotic (identical) and dizygotic (fraternal) twins in order to distinguish genetic from environmental factors. This is difficult to do in a rare disease and only one such twin study has been reported in SSc. Feghali-Bostwick et al. [66] studied 42 twin pairs (24 monozygotic twin pairs and 18 dizygotic pairs) in which at least one twin had SSc. They reported an overall concordance rate of 4.7 % which did not differ between monozygotic and dizygotic twins. However, the number of twin pairs in this study was relatively small and may have underestimated the recurrence rate.

Although there are several reports of multicase SSc families, there are only four studies that have investigated heritability in a large case cohort. Most recently, Frech et al. [67] studied 1,037 unique SSc cases and, linking the Utah Population Database and billing codes from the

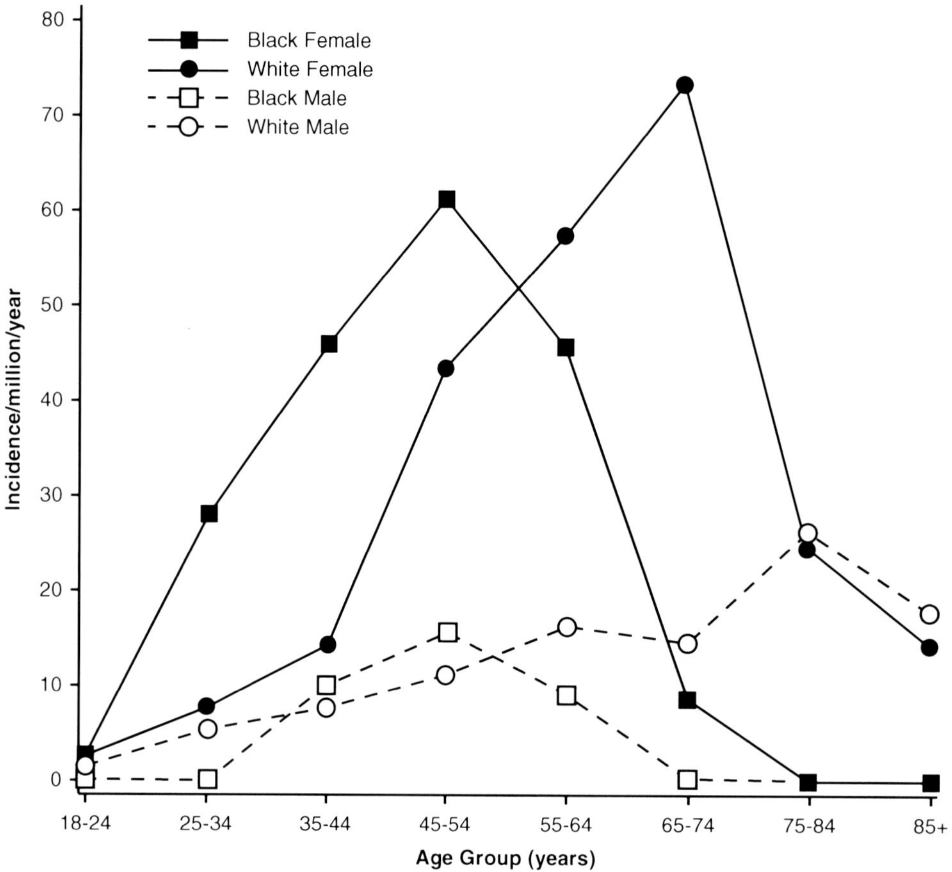

Fig. 2.2 Age-specific incidence of systemic sclerosis by race and sex (Adapted with permission from Mayes et al. [14])

University of Utah Health Science Center Data Warehouse, reported a relative risk of SSc among first-degree relatives as 3.07 (95 % CI 1.25–7.57, $p=0.0148$). In addition, increased relative risks were found for multiple other autoimmune diseases. An Australian study (18) of 353 SSc cases reported a relative risk for SSc among first-degree family members of 14.3 (95 % CI 5.9–34.5) which is remarkably similar to an earlier US study by Arnett et al. [68] of 703 families that found a relative risk of 13 (95 % CI 2.9–48.6, $p<0.001$) for SSc among first-degree family members. In addition, the relative risk among African-American families was greater than among whites in this study, but this difference did not reach statistical significance. A fourth study using cases from Canada and Columbia [69] found increased frequency of multiple autoimmune disease in family members but did not find an increased relative risk for SSc.

To determine if familial scleroderma differed from spontaneously occurring disease, Assassi et al. [70] compared disease type, organ involvement, and autoantibody status among 18 familial SSc cases and 692 sporadic cases. SSc families tended to be concordant for SSc-specific autoantibodies and HLA haplotypes, but otherwise familial SSc did not appear to be a unique disease subset.

Birth Order

Birth order has been found to be a risk factor for allergy and atopy [71] with first-born offspring more likely to have atopic disease than subsequent children in the family. The role of birth order in SSc susceptibility was reported by Cockrill et al. [63] who studied 974 sibships and found that the opposite situation held in scleroderma, that is, the risk of SSc increased with increasing birth order with an odds ratio of 1.25 (95 % CI 1.06–1.50) for birth order 2–5, an odds ratio of 2.22 (95 % CI 1.57–3.15) for birth order 6–9, and odds ratio of 3.53 (95 % CI 1.68–7.45) for birth order 10–15. However, a study by Russo et al. [72] involving 387 SSc cases did not find a statistically significant relationship between SSc and birth order or SSc and parity. The incongruity between these two reports can be resolved only by further studies in multiple cohorts.

Environmental Triggers

Table 2.2 summarizes the well-documented environmental associations with SSc and SSc-like illnesses. Although there have been several case reports of SSc occurring after

Table 2.2 Environmental exposures associated with SSc or SSc-like illnesses

Exposure	Disease	Evidence (reference)
Crystalline silica/silica dust	SSc	Meta-analysis [73, 74]
Solvents	SSc	Meta-analysis [77]
Vinyl chloride monomer	Vinyl chloride disease	Investigation of outbreak [78]
Adulterated cooking oil	Toxic oil syndrome	Investigation of outbreak [79]
Tryptophan	Eosinophilic myalgia syndrome	Investigation of outbreak [80]
Gadolinium	Nephrogenic systemic fibrosis	Multiple case series (review [82, 83])
Drugs		
Bleomycin	Pulmonary fibrosis	Multiple observations (review [85, 86])
Pentazocine	Localized dermal fibrosis at injection site	Multiple observations (review [87])

exposure to various other agents that are not listed here, this table is meant to highlight the few exposures that have been reported in multiple studies and for which an association with SSc can be considered established.

Silica

As noted above, numerous environmental factors have been associated with SSc in case reports and small case series, but few have been verified in case-control studies. One of the most frequently reported exposures to be associated with SSc is silica. Occupational exposure to particulate silica or silica dust occurs in professions such as mining, sandblasting, and pottery. In fact, silica has been associated as a risk factor for several autoimmune diseases including rheumatoid arthritis, systemic lupus erythematosus, and small-vessel vasculitis [73] in addition to SSc. In a meta-analysis published by McCormic et al. [74], the relative risk of developing SSc after exposure to silica was elevated only for men at 3.02 (95 % CI, 1.24–7.35). This association was not seen in women with exposure to silica who had a minimal and insignificant elevation in relative risk of 1.03 % (95 % CI, 0.74–1.44). Although this meta-analysis found considerable heterogeneity among the studies, it does indicate that silica exposure may be a significant risk factor for developing SSc at least in some men.

A prospective study to evaluate the association between SSc and occupational exposure by Marie et al. [75] revealed that silica, white spirit, aromatic solvents, trichloroethylene, ketones, and welding fumes had increased odds ratio for development of SSc. In male patients, a strong association was seen with exposure to the above agents. In female patients, the association was found with white spirit, aromatic solvents, any solvents, and ketones. However, these exposures were reported by a relatively small number of cases, usually men, and thus do not explain the vast majority of SSc cases predominantly women who comprise over 80 % of SSc cases and men who have had no such exposure.

Although case reports suggested an association between silicone breast implants and SSc, multiple studies as described in a meta-analysis by Janowsky et al. [75, 76] concluded that there was in fact no association between SSc and breast implants.

Solvents

Since 1957, there have been over 100 published articles on the possible association between exposure to various chemical solvents and the subsequent development of SSc. A meta-analysis of 11 case-control studies by Kettaneh et al. [77] involving 1,291 cases and 3,335 controls was performed. The conclusion from this meta-analysis is that there is indeed an increased risk of SSc both for men and women and that this risk was greater for male cases than for female cases; for men the odds ratio for solvent exposure was 2.96 (95 % CI 1.893–4.64, $p<0.0001$), and for women the odds ratio was 1.75 (95 % CI 1.48–2.09, $p<0.0001$). The authors were unable to conduct separate analyses for specific solvent subtypes, due to the limited number of studies for each solvent category. The mechanism underlying this association is unclear, but it is thought that solvents could alternative molecules to generate self-antigens that could in turn initiate an autoimmune response.

Exposures and Scleroderma-Like Syndromes

In addition to case reports of SSc occurring after contact with various chemicals, the impetus to study environmental exposures has come from reports of scleroderma-like diseases that have occurred in an epidemic fashion and that have resulted from an identified source.

Vinyl Chloride Disease

In the mid-1960s, a syndrome was described in factory workers employed in the plastics industry involving exposure to vinyl chloride. The workers developed paresthesias, Raynaud's phenomenon, skin thickening, edema of the hands and forearms, pseudo-acropachy, and phalanx acro-osteolysis [78]. The risk of developing these symptoms was related to cumulative exposure over time. Once the association was identified and changes made in the manufacturing process to protect workers, this syndrome has virtually disappeared.

Toxic Oil Syndrome

A review by Posada de la Paz et al. [79] described an epidemic illness that occurred in 1981 in Spain that was a progressive multisystem disease affecting over 20,000 people and resulting in hundreds of deaths. The causative agent was traced to rapeseed oil that had been contaminated with aniline and illicitly sold as cooking oil. People who consumed this toxic oil developed pulmonary edema, myalgias, rash, cardiomyopathy, vasculopathy, and pulmonary hypertension. Once the causative agent was identified and removed from the market, the epidemic resolved.

L-Tryptophan and Eosinophilia-Myalgia Syndrome

Another scleroderma-like illness, the eosinophilia-myalgia syndrome (EMS) [80, 81], occurred in the USA in 1984–1989 and was traced to a nutritional supplement containing L-tryptophan that had a contaminant introduced in the manufacturing process. Characteristics of the illness included sclerodermatous skin thickening, sensorimotor polyneuropathy, proximal myopathy, severe myalgias, and peripheral eosinophilia. The recent study by Marie et al. [75] mentioned above did not find an association between L-tryptophan and defined SSc.

Again, once the causal agent for EMS was identified and removed from the market in 1989, the syndrome essentially disappeared, although sporadic cases are still reported in the absence of apparent ingestion of this supplement.

Gadolinium and Nephrogenic Systemic Fibrosis (See Chap. 9)

Nephrogenic systemic fibrosis (NSF, previously called nephrogenic fibrosing dermopathy) was first reported by Cowper in 2000 ([82], for review see [83]) and characterized by rapidly progressive skin thickening with the early development of flexion contractures affecting the lower extremities more than the upper extremities and typically sparing the face. There can also be internal organ fibrosis involving skeletal muscle, myocardium, and lung. NSF typically occurs following administration of gadolinium contrast material for magnetic resonance imaging in the setting of renal compromise.

Prevention is the best approach, with the avoidance of gadolinium containing agents in at-risk patients, since treatment of established disease is unsatisfactory. Although the underlying pathogenic mechanism remains unclear, it is thought that fibrosis results from activation of the transforming growth factor beta (TGF-beta) pathway [84].

Bleomycin and Pulmonary Fibrosis

Bleomycin is an antineoplastic antibiotic drug used for several types of cancer. A known side effect of this drug is a pneumonitis which can be fatal [85]. The central event is endothelial damage to the pulmonary vasculature, and those who survive this complication usually recover completely with normalization of pulmonary function.

There have been 12 case reports of SSc (fulfilling 1980 classification criteria) occurring in the setting of bleomycin therapy for malignancy [86]. This has led to the development of the bleomycin mouse model as an in vivo system to study pulmonary and lung fibrosis and to test potential agents for the treatment of human disease.

Pentazocine

Repeated injection of pentazocine, a synthetic narcotic analgesic, can cause a local fibrotic reaction affecting dermal, subcutaneous, and muscle layers in the area of administration [87]. This was first reported in 1975 [88] and since has been described in the setting of repetitive and prolonged use typically associated with narcotic abuse. The mechanism is not clear and the changes are usually irreversible.

Infection Risk

The hypothesis that infectious agents play a role in the pathogenesis of autoimmune disease has been extensively studied with mixed results. It has been suggested that the production of SSc-specific autoantibodies results from an antigen-driven response called molecular mimicry [89]. The following will review the suggested role of some infections in the development of SSc, including parvovirus B19, cytomegalovirus (CMV), and *Helicobacter pylori* (*H. pylori*).

Parvovirus B 19 DNA has been detected in the bone marrow of SSc patients ($n = 17$ cases positive for viral DNA out of 29 total cases studied or 17/29) and but not in the bone marrow of healthy individuals ($n = 0/10$) [90]. The SSc patients with bone marrow persistence of parvovirus B 19 DNA had a shorter mean duration of disease and showed more severe perivascular and active endothelial injury than SSc cases without demonstrable viral DNA [91]. Although intriguing, it is difficult to establish a causal link between this common infection and the subsequent development of a rare autoimmune disease.

CMV infection has also been postulated to contribute to SSc pathogenesis because of the virus' ability to infect both endothelial cells and monocytes and persist in a latent form. Interestingly, Lunardi et al. [92] reported that antibodies directed against the CMV-derived protein UL94 cross-reacted with a cell surface membrane protein of endothelial cells inducing apoptosis and activating fibroblasts suggesting a possible role of CMV in the triggering and maintenance of SSc. In fact, human CMV infection has been implicated in the initiation and/or persistence of multiple autoimmune diseases including SSc, systemic lupus erythematosus, rheumatoid arthritis, and others (for review see [93]). Again, there is difficulty in establishing a causal relationship between CMV infection and SSc, since CMV infection is common (found in 60–90 % of healthy adults) whereas SSc is a rare disease.

There has been an increasing amount of interest and research regarding a link between *H. pylori* and SSc. In a 1998 study [94] of patients with primary Raynaud's phenomenon (RP) and coincidental *H. pylori* infection, those patients who were treated and cured of *H. pylori*, reported either complete disappearance of RP or reduction of symptoms. In patients that were not cured of their *H. pylori* infection, RP did not improve. A recent study about the effect of *H. pylori* and disease severity revealed that SSc patients with *H. pylori* infection had a higher severity score compared to those without the disease [95]. However, there is conflicting data about *H. pylori* because other studies have not found a difference in SSc patients with and without the infection or an impact of treatment on Raynaud's phenomenon [96]. Therefore, this remains controversial.

In a similar fashion to CMV, Epstein-Barr virus (EBV) has been associated with SSc [97, 98]. It has been reported that EBV is able to persistently infect human SSc fibroblast in vitro and produce an aberrant innate immune response [98]. However, EBV is also found in a large proportion of the population suggesting that it may play a role but certainly is not the sole contributing factor to the development of SSc.

With respect to chlamydia infection, it has been postulated that such an infection may play a role in SSc as well as other immune-related diseases. However, in one study [99], skin biopsies from patients with SSc and controls were negative for chlamlydia species.

Considering all the evidence to date, although several studies have linked various infectious diseases to SSc, there are conflicting data and a clear, direct association is missing. It is possible, although not yet proven, that infectious agents serve as "cofactors" in disease causation or persistence contributing to both tissue damage (via direct or indirect cellular toxicity) and immune dysregulation (via molecular mimicry or superantigen stimulation). Such considerations remain speculative at present.

Conclusion

Although incidence rates and prevalence estimates vary by region, these figures are fairly similar from recent reports for Europe, the USA, and Australia and suggest that prevalence is in the range of 150–300 cases/million with lower prevalence in Scandinavia, Japan, and the UK.

Incidence rates (number of new cases per year) have apparently increased from the 1940s to the present, but it is not clear if this represents a real increase in disease occurrence or if this is due to improved awareness and earlier diagnosis. The implementation of the 2013 ACR/EULAR classification criteria will lead to identification of more cases than the previous criteria allowed, thus causing an apparent (but not real) increase in incidence and prevalence. This will have to be taken into account in future studies.

Survival in SSc has clearly improved over time, and this improvement is largely related to the introduction of angiotensin-converting enzyme inhibitors for the treatment of scleroderma renal crisis in the early 1980s. ILD and pulmonary vascular disease have replaced renal failure as the most common cause of death. New treatments for both these complications may improve survival, but evidence for this is not yet available.

In terms of fender differences, SSc is more common in women than in men with most reports of female to male ratios of 4:1–6:1.

African-American race and the Choctaw Native American/First Nations ancestry are risk factors for the development of SSc, and African-Americans have more severe disease with an earlier age at onset and worst prognosis.

Familial clustering clearly suggests a genetic contribution, and multiple recent studies, described elsewhere in this book, have begun to identify these factors. The finding that increasing birth order predisposes to SSc is intriguing and suggests that early exposure to infectious and/or other agents may contribute to the development of SSc.

Although the evidence for an association between SSc and environmental exposure to particulate silica and chemical solvents is relatively well-established, these exposures account for only a tiny percentage of all cases. Hence, an environmental trigger(s) for the majority of cases remains unknown. Several agents have been associated with scleroderma-like illnesses, but the relevance to spontaneously occurring SSc is unclear.

Finally, several infectious diseases have been implicated in the development of autoimmune disease; however, to date this remains controversial and no clear association has been demonstrated.

References

1. Bolster MB, Silver RS. Clinical features of systemic sclerosis. In: Hochberg MC, Silman AJ, Smolen JS, Weinblatt ME, Weisman MH, editors. Rheumatology. 5th ed. Philadelphia: Mosby, Elsevier; 2011. p. 1373–86.
2. LeRoy EC, Black C, Fleischmajer R, Jablonska S, Krieg T, Medsger Jr TA, Rowell N, Wollheim F. Scleroderma (systemic sclerosis): classification, subsets and pathogenesis. J Rheumatol. 1988;15(2):202–5.
3. van den Hoogen F, Khanna D, Fransen J, Johnson SR, Baron M, Tyndall A, Matucci-Cerinic M, Naden RP, Medsger TA, Carreira PE, Riemekasten G, Clements PJ, Denton CP, Distler O, Allanore Y, Furst DE, Gabrielli A, Mayes MD, van Laar JM, Seibold JR, Czirjak L, Steen VD, Inanc M, Kowal-Bielecka O, Muller-Ladner U, Valentini G, Veale DJ, Vonk MC, Walker UA, Chung L, Collier DH, Csuka ME, Fessler BJ, Guiducci S, Herrick A, Hsu VM, Jimenez S, Kahaleh B, Merkel PA, Sierakowski A, Silver RM, Simms RW, Varga J, Pope JE. Classification criteria for systemic sclerosis: an American college of rheumatology/European league against rheumatism collaborative initiative. Arthritis Rheum. 2013;72:1747–55.
4. Preliminary criteria for the classification of systemic sclerosis (scleroderma). Subcommittee for scleroderma criteria of the American Rheumatism Association Diagnostic and Therapeutic Criteria Committee. Arthritis Rheum. 1980;23(5):581–90.
5. Wigley R, Borman B. Medical geography and the aetiology of the rare connective tissue diseases in New Zealand. Soc Sci Med Med Geogr. 1980;14(2):175–83.
6. Barnabe C, Joseph L, Belisle P, Labrecque J, Edworthy S, Barr SG, Fritzler M, Svenson LW, Hemmelgarn B, Bernatsky S. Prevalence of systemic lupus erythematous and systemic sclerosis in the First Nations population of Alberta, Canada. Arthritis Care Res. 2012;64(1):138–43.
7. Eason RJ, Tan PL, Gow PJ. Progressive systemic sclerosis in Auckland: a ten year review with emphasis on prognostic features. Aust N Z J Med. 1981;11(6):657–62.
8. Furst DE, Fernandes AW, Iorga SR, Greth W, Bancroft T. Epidemiology of systemic sclerosis in a large US managed care population. J Rheumatol. 2012;39(4):784–6.
9. Chifflot H, Fautrel B, Sordet C, Chatelus E, Sibilia J. Incidence and prevalence of systemic sclerosis: a systematic literature review. Semin Arthritis Rheum. 2008;37:223–35.
10. Medsger Jr TA, Masi AT. Epidemiology of systemic sclerosis (scleroderma). Ann Intern Med. 1971;74:714–21.
11. Michet Jr CJ, McKenna CH, Elveback LR, Kaslow RA, Kurland LT. Epidemiology of systemic lupus erythematosus and other connective tissue diseases in Rochester, Minnesota, 1950 through 1979. Mayo Clin Proc. 1985;60(2):105–13.
12. Steen VD, Oddis CV, Conte CG, Janoski J, Casterline GZ, Medsger Jr TA. Incidence of systemic sclerosis in Allegheny county, Pennsylvania. A twenty-year study of hospital-diagnosed cases, 1963–1982. Arthritis Rheum. 1997;40(3):441–5.
13. Maricq HR, Weinrich MC, Keil JE, Smith EA, Harperl FE, Nussbaum AI, et al. Prevalence of scleroderma spectrum disorders in the general population of South Carolina. Arthritis Rheum. 1989;32:998–1006.
14. Mayes MD, Lacey Jr JV, Beebe-Dimmer J, et al. Prevalence, incidence, survival, and disease characteristics of systemic sclerosis in a large US population. Arthritis Rheum. 2003;48:2246–55.
15. Robinson Jr D, Eisenberg D, Nietert PJ, Doyle M, Bala M, Paramore C, et al. Systemic sclerosis prevalence and comorbidities in the US, 2001–2002. Curr Med Res Opin. 2008;24:1157–66.
16. Bernatsky S, Joseph L, Pineau CA, Belisle P, Hudson M, Clarke AE. Scleroderma prevalence: demographic variations in a population-based sample. Arthritis Rheum. 2009;61(3):400–4.
17. Englert H, Small-McMahon J, Davis K, O'Connor H, Chambers P, Brooks P. Systemic sclerosis prevalence and mortality in Sydney 1974–88. Aust NZ J Med. 1999;29:42–50.
18. Chandran G, Smith M, Ahern MJ, Roberts-Thomson PJ. A study of scleroderma in South Australia: prevalence, subset characteristics and nailfold capillaroscopy. Aust N Z J Med. 1995;25(6):688–94.
19. Roberts-Thomson PJ, Jones M, Hakendorf P, Kencana Dharmapatni AA, Walker JG, MacFarlane JG, Smith MD, Ahern MJ. Scleroderma in South Australia: epidemiological observations of possible pathogenic significance. Intern Med J. 2001;31(4):220–9.
20. Roberts-Thomson PJ, Walker JG, Lu TY, Esterman A, Hakendorf P, Smith MD, et al. Scleroderma in South Australia: further epidemiological observations supporting a stochastic explanation. Intern Med J. 2006;36:489–97.
21. Tamaki T, Mori S, Takehara K. Epidemiological study of patients with systemic sclerosis in Tokyo. Arch Dermatol Res. 1991;283:366–71.
22. Silman A, Jannini S, Symmons D, Bacon P. An epidemiological study of scleroderma in the West Midlands. Br J Rheumatol. 1988;27(4):286–90.
23. Allcock RJ, Forrest I, Corris PA, et al. A study of the prevalence of systemic sclerosis in northeast England. Rheumatology (Oxford). 2004;43:596–602.
24. Geirsson AJ, Steinsson K, Guthmundsson S, Sigurthsson V. Systemic sclerosis in Iceland. A nationwide epidemiological study. Ann Rheum Dis. 1994;53(8):502–5.
25. Kaipiainen-Seppanen O, Aho K. Rare systemic rheumatic and connective tissue diseases in Finland. J Int Med. 1996;240:81–4.
26. Le Guern V, Mahr A, Mouthon L, et al. Prevalence of systemic sclerosis in a French multi-ethnic county. Rheumatology (Oxford). 2004;43:1129–37.
27. Adssi HE, Cirstea D, Virion JM, Guillemin F, de Korwin JD. Estimating the prevalence of systemic sclerosis in the Lorraine Region, France, by the capture-recapture method. J Semin Arthritis Rheum. 2013;42:530–8.
28. Hoffmann-Vold AM, Midtvedt O, Molberg O, Garen T, Gran JT. Prevalence of systemic sclerosis in south-east Norway. Rheumatology. 2012;51:1600–5.
29. Alamanos Y, Voulgari PV, Tsifetaki N, et al. Epidemiology of systemic sclerosis in northwest Greece 1981–2002. Semin Arthritis Rheum. 2005;34:714–20.
30. Arias-Nuñez MC, Llorca J, Vazquez-Rodriguez TR, Gomez-Acebo I, Miranda-Filloy JA, Martin J, Gonzalez-Juanatey C, Gonzalez-Gay MA. Systemic sclerosis in northwestern Spain: a 19-year epidemiologic study. Medicine (Baltimore). 2008;87(5):272–80.
31. Monaco AL, Bruschi M, La Corte R, Volpinari S, Trotta F. Epidemiology of systemic sclerosis in a district of northern Italy. Clin Exp Rheumatol. 2011;29 Suppl 65:S10–4.
32. Sardu C, Cooco E, Mereu A, Massa R, Cuccu A, Marrosu MG, Cantu P. Population based study of 12 autoimmune diseases in Sardina, Italy: prevalence and comorbidity. PLoS ONE. 2012;7(3):e32487.
33. Andreasson K, Saxane T, Bergknut C, Hesselstrand R, Englund M. Prevalence and incidence of systemic sclerosis in southern Sweden: population-based data with case ascertainment using the, 1980 ARA criteria and the proposed ACR-EULAR classification criteria. Ann Rheum Dis. 2014;73:1788–92.
34. Rosa JE, Soriano ER, Narvaez-Ponce L, Castel del Cid C, Imamura PM, Catoggio LJ. Incidence and prevalence of systemic sclerosis in a health care plan in Buenos Aires. J Clin Rheumatol. 2011;17:59–63.
35. Arnett FC, Howard RF, Tan F, et al. Increased prevalence of systemic sclerosis in a Native American tribe in Oklahoma: association with an Amerindian HLA haplotype. Arthritis Rheum. 1996;39:1362–70.

36. Silman AJ, Howard Y, Hicklin AJ, Black C. Geographical clustering of scleroderma in south and west London. Br J Rheumatol. 1990;29:93–6.
37. Thompson AE, Pope JE. Increased prevalence of scleroderma in southwestern Ontario: a cluster analysis. J Rheumatol. 2002;29(9):1867–73.
38. Englert H, Joyner E, Bade R, Thompson M, Morris D, Chambers P, Carroll G, Manolios N. Systemic scleroderma: a spatiotemporal clustering. Intern Med J. 2005;35(4):228–33.
39. Valesini G, Litta A, Bonavita MS, Luan FL, Purpura M, Mariani M, Balsano F. Geographical clustering of scleroderma in a rural area in the province of Rome. Clin Exp Rheumatol. 1993;1(1):41–7.
40. Steen VD, Medsger TA. Changes in the causes of death in systemic sclerosis, 1972–2002. Ann Rheum Dis. 2007;66:940–4.
41. Ferri C, Valentini G, Cozzi F, Sebastiani M, Michelassi C, La Montagna G, Bullo A, Cazzato M, Tirri E, Storino F, Giuggioli D, Cuomo G, Rosada M, Bombardieri S, Todesco S, Tirri G, Systemic Sclerosis Study Group of the Italian Society of Rheumatology (SIR-GSSSc). Systemic sclerosis: demographic, clinical, and serologic features and survival in 1,012 Italian patients. Medicine (Baltimore). 2002;81(2):139–53. PMID: 11889413.
42. Tyndall AJ, Bannert B, Vonk M, et al. Causes and risk factors for death in systemic sclerosis: a study from the EULAR Scleroderma Trials and Research (EUSTAR) database. Ann Rheum Dis. 2010;69:1809–15.
43. Derk CT, Huaman G, Littlejohn J, Otieno F, Jimenez S. Predictors of early mortality in systemic sclerosis: a case-control study comparing early versus late mortality in systemic sclerosis. Rheumatol Int. 2012;32:3841–4.
44. Hoffman-Vold AM, Molberg O, Midtvedt O, Garen T, Gran JT. Survival and causes of death in an unselected and complete cohort of Norwegian patients with systemic sclerosis. J Rheumatol. 2013;40:1127–33.
45. Hissaria P, Lester S, Hakendorf P, Woodman R, Patterson K, Hill C, Ahern MJ, Smith MD, Walker JG, Roberts-Thomson PJ. Survival in scleroderma: results from the population based South Australian Register. Intern Med J. 2010;41(5):381–90 [Epub ahead of print].
46. Strickland G, Pauling J, Cavill C, Shaddick G, McHugh N. Mortality in systemic sclerosis – a single centre study from the UK. Clin Rheumatol. 2013;32:1533–9.
47. Sampaio-Barros PD, Bortoluzzo AB, Marangoni RG, Rocha LF, T. Del Rio AP, Samara AM, Yoshinari NH, Marques-Neto JF. Survival, causes of death, and prognostic factors in systemic sclerosis: analysis of 947 Brazilian patients. J Rheumatol. 2012;39:1971–8.
48. Foocharoen C, Mahakkanukrauh A, Suwannaroj S, Nanagara R. Clinical characteristics and mortality in systemic sclerosis: a comparison between early- and late-referred cases. J Med Assoc Thai. 2014;97(1):28–35.
49. Winstone TA, Assayag D, Wilcox PG, Dunne JV, Hague CJ, Leipsic J, Collard HR, Ryerson CJ. Predictors of mortality and progression in scleroderma – associated interstitial lung disease. Chest. 2014;146(2):422–36.
50. Ioannidis JP, Vlachoyiannopoulos PG, Haidich AB, Medsger Jr TA, Lucas M, Michet CJ, Kuwana M, Yasuoka H, van den Hoogen F, Te Boome L, van Laar JM, Verbeet NL, Matucci-Cerinic M, Georgountzos A, Moutsopoulos HM. Mortality in systemic sclerosis: an international meta-analysis of individual patient data. Am J Med. 2005;118(1):2–10.
51. Scussel-Lonzetti L, Joyal F, Raynauld JP, Roussin A, Rich E, Goulet JR, et al. Predicting mortality in systemic sclerosis: analysis of a cohort of 309 French Canadian patients with emphasis on features at diagnosis as predictive factors for survival. Medicine (Baltimore). 2002;81:154–67.
52. Bryan C, Knight C, Black CM, Silman AJ. Prediction of five-year survival following presentation with scleroderma: development of a simple model using three disease factors at first visit. Arthritis Rheum. 1999;42:2660–5.
53. Domsic RT, Rodriguez-Reyna T, Lucas M, Fertig N, Medsger Jr TA. Skin thickness progression rate: a predictor of mortality and early internal organ involvement in diffuse scleroderma. Ann Rheum Dis. 2011;70(1):104–9. PMIT 20679474.
54. Mendoza F, Derk CT. Systemic sclerosis mortality in the United States: 1999–2002 implications for patient care. J Clin Rheumatol. 2007;13(4):187–92.
55. Sharif R, Fritzler MJ, Mayes MD, Gonzalez EB, McNearney TA, Draeger H, Baron M, the Canadian Scleroderma Research Group, Furst DE, Khanna DK, Del Junco DJ, Molitor JA, Schiopu E, Phillips K, Seibold JR, Silver RM, Simms RW, Genisos Study Group, Perry M, Rojo C, Charles J, Zhou X, Agarwal SK, Reveille JD, Assassi S, Arnett FC. Anti-fibrillarin antibody in African American patients with systemic sclerosis: immunogenetics, clinical features, and survival analysis. J Rheumatol. 2011;38:1622–30.
56. Alba MA, Velasco C, Simeon CP, Fonollosa V, Trapiella L, Egurbide MV, Saez L, Castillo MJ, Callejas JL, Camps MT, Tolosa C, Rios JJ, Freire M, Vargas JA, Espinosa G, RESCLE Registry. Early – versus late-onset systemic sclerosis differences in clinical and outcome in 1037 patients. Medicine. 2014;93(2):73–81.
57. Hasmimoto A, Tejima S, Tono T, Suzuki M, Tanaka S, Matsui T, Tohma S, Endo H, Hirohata S. Predictors of survival and causes of death in Japanese patients with systemic sclerosis. J Rheumatol. 2011;38:1931–9.
58. Foocharoen C, Nanagara R, Kiatchoosakun S, Suwannaroj S, Mahakkanukrauh A. Prognostic factors of mortality and 2-year survival analysis of systemic sclerosis with pulmonary arterial hypertension in Thailand. Int J Rheum Dis. 2011;14:282–9.
59. Chung L, Domsic RT, Lingala B, Alkassab F, Bolster M, Csuka ME, Derk C, Fischer A, Frech T, Furst DE, Gomberg-Maitland M, Hinchcliff M, Hsu V, Hummers LK, Khanna D, Medsger Jr TA, Molitor JA, Preston IR, Schiopu E, Shapiro L, Silver R, Simms R, Varga J, Gordon JK, Steen VK. Survival and predictors of mortality in systemic sclerosis – associated pulmonary arterial hypertension: outcomes from the pulmonary hypertension assessment and recognition of outcomes in scleroderma registry. Arthritis Care Res. 2014;66(3).
60. Chung L, Farber HW, Benza R, Miller DP, Parsons L, Hassoun PM, McGoon M, Nicolls MR, and Zamanian RT. Unique predictors of mortality in patients with pulmonary arterial hypertension associated with systemic sclerosis in the reveal registry. Chest. 2014; Online version http://journal.publications.chestnet.org. epub ahead of print.
61. Hesselstrand R, Scheja A, Wuttge DM. Scleroderma renal crisis in a Swedish systemic sclerosis cohort: survival, renal outcome, and RNA polymerase III antibodies as a risk factor. Scand J Rheumatol. 2012;41(1):39–43.
62. Lambe M, Bjornadal L, Neregard P, Nyren O, Cooper GS. Childbearing and the risk of scleroderma: a population-based study in Sweden. Am J Epidemiol. 2004;159:162–6.
63. Cockrill T, del Junco D, Arnett FC, et al. Separate influences of birth order and gravity/parity on the development of systemic sclerosis. Arthritis Care Res. 2010;62:418–24.
64. Adams Waldorf KM, Nelson JL. Autoimmune disease during pregnancy and the microchimerism legacy of pregnancy. Immunol Invest. 2008;37(5):631–44.
65. McNearney TA, Reveille JD, Fischbach M, Friedman AW, Lisse JR, Goel N, Tan FK, Zhou X, Ahn C, Feghali-Bostwick CA, Fritzler M, Arnett FC, Mayes MD. Pulmonary involvement in systemic sclerosis: associations with genetic, serologic, sociodemographic, and behavioral factors. Arthritis Rheum. 2007;57(2):318–26.
66. Feghali-Bostwick C, Medsger Jr TA, Wright TM. Analysis of systemic sclerosis in twins reveals low concordance for disease and

high concordance for the presence of antinuclear antibodies. Arthritis Rheum. 2003;48:1956–63.
67. Frech T, Khanna D, Markewitz B, Mineau G, Pimentel R, Sawitzke A. Heritability of vasculopathy, autoimmune disease, and fibrosis in systemic sclerosis: a population-based study. Arthritis Rheum. 2010;62(7):2109–16.
68. Arnett FC, Cho M, Chatterjee S, Aquilar MB, Reveille JD, Mayes MD. Familial occurrence frequencies and relative risk for systemic sclerosis (scleroderma) in three United States cohorts. Arthritis Rheum. 2001;44:1359–62.
69. Hudson M, Rojas-Villarraga A, Coral-Alvarado P, López-Guzmán S, Mantilla RD, Chalem P, Baron M, Anaya JM, Canadian Scleroderma Research Group, Colombian Scleroderma Research Group. Polyautoimmunity and familial autoimmunity in systemic sclerosis. J Autoimmun. 2008;31(2):156–9.
70. Assassi S, Arnett FC, Reveille JD, Gourh P, Mayes MD. Clinical, immunologic, and genetic features of familial systemic sclerosis. Arthritis Rheum. 2007;56(6):2031–7.
71. McKeever TM, Lewis SA, Smith C, Collins J, Heatlie H, Frischer M, Hubbard R. Siblings, multiple births, and the incidence of allergic disease: a birth cohort study using the West Midlands general practice research database. Thorax. 2001;56(10):758–62.
72. Russo PA, Lester S, Roberts-Thomson PJ. Systemic sclerosis and birth order and parity. Int J Rheum Dis. 2014;17:557–61.
73. Makol A, Reilly MJ, Rosenman KD. Prevalence of connective tissue disease in silicosis (1985–2006)-a report from the state of Michigan surveillance system for silicosis. Am J Ind Med. 2010;54(4):255–62 [Epub ahead of print].
74. McCormic ZD, Khuder SS, Aryal BK, Ames AL, Khuder SA. Occupational silica exposure as a risk factor for scleroderma: a meta-analysis. Int Arch Occup Environ Health. 2010;83(7):763–9.
75. Marie I, Gehanno JF, Bubenheim M, Duval-Modeste AB, Joly P, Dominique S, Bravard P, Noel D, Cailleux AF, Weber J, Lagoutte P, Benichou J, Levesque H. Prospective study to evaluate the association between systemic sclerosis and occupational exposure and review of the literature. Autoimmun Rev. 2014;13:151–6.
76. Janowsky EC, Kupper LL, Hulka BS. Meta-analyses of the relation between silicone breast implants and the risk of connective-tissue diseases. N Engl J Med. 2000;342:781–90.
77. Kettaneh A, Al Moufti O, Tiev KP, Chayet C, Toledano C, Fabre B, et al. Occupational exposure to solvents and gender-related risk of systemic sclerosis: a metaanalysis of case-control studies. J Rheumatol. 2007;34:97–103.
78. Nicholson WJ, Henneberger PK, Seidman H. Occupational hazards in the VC-PVC industry. Prog Clin Biol Res. 1984;141:155–75.
79. de la Posada PM, Philen RM, Borda AI. Toxic oil syndrome: the perspective after 20 years. Epidemiol Rev. 2001;23(2):231–47.
80. Kilbourne EM, Philen RM, Kamb ML, Falk H. Tryptophan produced by Showa Denko and epidemic eosinophilia-myalgia syndrome. J Rheumatol Suppl. 1996;46:81–8. discussion 89–91. Review.
81. Kaufman LD, Seidman RJ. L-tryptophan-associated eosinophilia-myalgia syndrome: perspective of a new illness. Rheum Dis Clin N Am. 1991;17(2):427–41. Review.
82. Cowper SE, Su LD, Bhawan J, Robin HS, LeBoit PE. Nephrogenic fibrosing dermopathy. Am J Dermatopathol. 2001;23(5):383–93.
83. Chen AY, Zirwas MJ, Heffernan MP. Nephrogenic systemic fibrosis: a review. J Drugs Dermatol. 2010;9(7):829–34. Review.
84. Schieren G, Gambichler T, Skrygan M, Burkert B, Altmeyer P, Rump LC, Kreuter A. Balance of profibrotic and antifibrotic [corrected] signaling in nephrogenic systemic fibrosis skin lesions. Am J Kidney Dis. 2010;55(6):1040–9.
85. Sleijfer S. Bleomycin-induced pneumonitis. Chest. 2001;120(2):617–24. Review.
86. Inaoki M, Kawabata C, Nishijima C, Yoshio N, Kita T. Case of bleomycin-induced scleroderma. J Dermatol. 2012;39(5):482–4. doi:10.1111/j.1346-8138.2011.01301.x. Epub 2011 Sep 28. Review. No abstract available.PMID:21955042].
87. Palestine RF, Millns JL, Spigel GT, Schroeter AL. Skin manifestations of pentazocine abuse. J Am Acad Dermatol. 1980;2(1):47–55.
88. Levin BE, Engel WK. Iatrogenic muscle fibrosis. Arm levitation as an initial sign. JAMA. 1975;234(6):621–4.
89. Radic M, Martinovic Kaliterna D, Radic J. Infectious disease as aetiological factor in the pathogenesis of systemic sclerosis. Neth J Med. 2010;68(11):348–53.
90. Zakrzewska K, Corcioli F, Carlsen KM, Giuggioli D, Fanci R, Rinieri A, Ferri C, Azzi A. Human Parvovirus B 19 (B19V) infection in systemic sclerosis patients. Intervirology. 2009;52:279–82.
91. Magro CM, Nuovo G, Ferri C, Crowson AN, Giuggioli D, Sebastiani M. Parvoviral infection of endothelial cells and stromal fibroblast: a possible pathogenic role in scleroderma. J Cutan Pathol. 2004;31:43–50.
92. Lunardi C, Bason C, Navone R, Millo E, Damonte G, Corrocher R, Puccetti A. Systemic sclerosis immunoglobulin G autoantibodies bind the human cytomegalovirus late protein UL94 and induce apoptosis in human endothelial cells. Nat Med. 2000;6(10):1183–6.
93. Halenius A, Hengel H. Human cytomegalovirus and autoimmune disease. Biomed Res Int. 2014;2014:472978.
94. Gasbarrini A, Massari I, Serricchio M, Tondai P, De Luca A, Franceschi F, Ojetti V, Dal Lago A, Flore R, Santoliquido A, Basbarrini G, Pola P. Helicobacter pylori eradication ameliorates primary Raynaud's phenomenon. Dig Dis Sci. 1998;43(8):1641–5.
95. Radic M, Kaliterna DM, Bonacin D, Vergles JM, Radic J, Fabijanic D, Kovacic V. Is *Helicobacter pylori* infection a risk factor for disease severity in systemic sclerosis? Rheumatol Int. 2013;33:2943–8.
96. Prelipcean CC, Mihai C, Gogălniceanu P, Mitrică D, Drug VL, Stanciu C. Extragastric manifestations of Helicobacter pylori infection. Rev Med Chir Soc Med Nat Iasi. 2007;111(3):575–83. PMID: 18293684, Review.
97. Farina A, Cirone M, York M, Lenna S, Padila C, Mclaughlin S, Faggioni A, Lafyatis R, Trojanowska M, Farina GA. Epstein-Barr virus infection induces aberrant TLR activation pathway and fibroblast-myofibroblast conversion in scleroderma. J Investig Dermatol. 2014;134:954–64.
98. Grossman C, Dovrish Z, Shoenfeld Y, Amital H. Do infections facilitate the emergence of systemic sclerosis? Autoimmun Rev. 2011;10:244–7.
99. Mayes MD, Whittum-Hudson JA, Oszust C, Gerard HC, Hudson AP. Lack of evidence for bacterial infections in skin in patients with systemic sclerosis. Am J Med Sci. 2009;337(4):233–5.

Genetic Factors

3

Shervin Assassi and Yannick Allanore

Introduction

Systemic sclerosis (SSc) is characterized by early vascular damage and immune dysregulation followed by tissue fibrosis affecting many organs, in particular, the skin, lungs, heart, kidneys, and digestive tract. The epidemiological data are consistent to define SSc as an orphan disease. The combination of environmental and stochastic factors converging upon individuals of a particular genetic background seems to contribute to the development of this disease. Subtle combinations and interactions may also contribute to the heterogeneity of the disease that is a hallmark of this condition. We will begin by considering various genetic approaches that can be applied to the study of polygenic diseases and will then move on to the principal factors implicated in this disease, which will be considered in greater detail.

Genetic Approaches to the Study of Polygenic Diseases

There are several possible approaches to demonstrating the existence of a genetic component in the pathogenesis of a complex or polygenic disease. Genetic susceptibility to polygenic diseases is based on a combination of polymorphisms in several genes. These polymorphisms are variations of the coding (exons) and noncoding (introns) regions occurring at various frequencies in the general population. Genomic variations fall into three categories [1]: (1) single-nucleotide polymorphism (SNP) which are single-base-pair changes in nucleotide sequences, (2) insertion and deletions of nucleotides from the DNA, and (3) structural rearrangements that reshuffle the DNA sequence (e.g., chromosome 9 and 22 translocation in Philadelphia gene predisposing to chronic myelogenous leukemia).

S. Assassi, MD, MS (✉)
Division of Rheumatology, University of Texas Health Science Center at Houston, Houston, TX, USA
e-mail: Shervin.Assassi@uth.tmc.edu

Y. Allanore, MD
Service de Rhumatologie A, INSERMU1016,
Universit. Paris Descartes, Hôpital Cochin, Paris, France

Single-Nucleotide Polymorphism (SNP)

SNPs are biallelic, with a given individual carrying one allele inherited from each parent (Fig. 3.1). The nucleotide variations involved are classified as nonsynonymous if it leads to modification of the amino-acid sequence of the encoded protein. A SNP is considered "functional" if the function of the resulting protein is altered in some way. Such alterations, which may involve a gain or a loss of function, are much less frequent in polygenic diseases than in monogenic diseases and are generally not solely responsible for the phenotype in this context. However, such genetic variations may cause subtle differences in protein function or in expression of the corresponding gene with biological implications. They may also contribute to the variability used to define the thresholds separating the normal and pathological ranges. These types of genetic variations are also known as quantitative trait loci. An example, relevant to rheumatic diseases, is the SNPs in urate transporter genes that affect serum uric acid concentrations [2].

There are about ten million SNPs in humans and the rarest SNP alleles have a frequency of at least 1 %. SNPs located in close proximity to each other on the chromosome tend to remain linked or inherited together en block during hereditary transmission. Such a group of associated SNP alleles inherited together as group in a chromosomal region is known as a haplotype. In other words, these associated SNPs have a low frequency of recombination during meiosis. Most chromosomal regions have only a few common haplotypes (each with a frequency of at least 5 %) accounting for most of the genetic diversity between the individuals of a population. A given chromosomal region may contain many SNPs, but

J. Varga et al. (eds.), *Scleroderma*, DOI 10.1007/978-3-319-31407-5_3

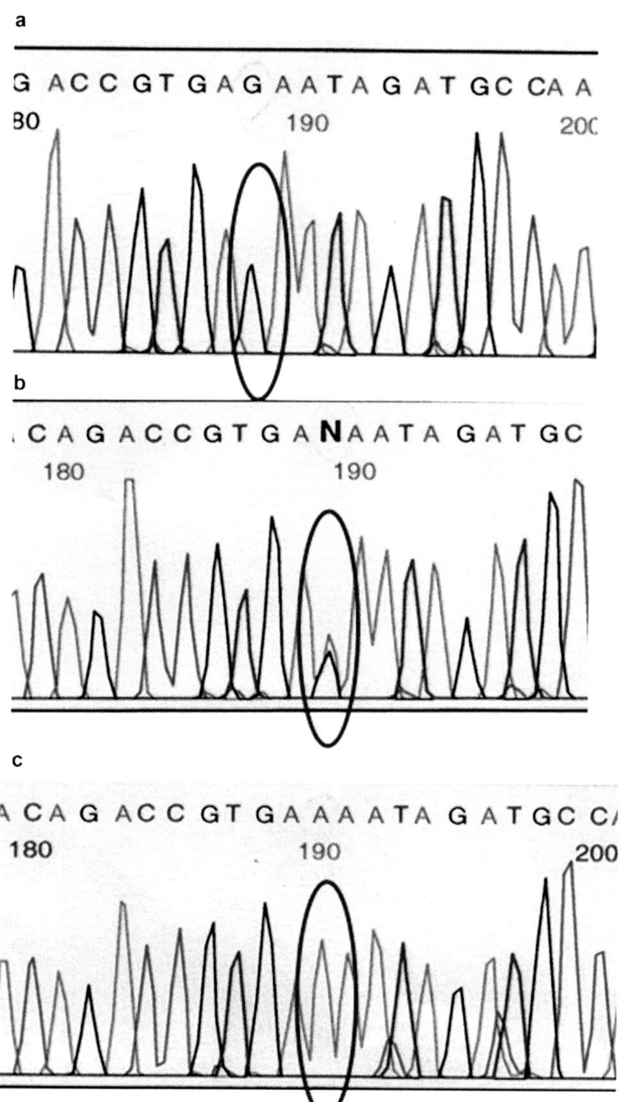

Fig. 3.1 Example of an SNP with the homozygous major allele profile (**a**), and heterozygous (**b**) and homozygous (**c**) minor allele profiles

the identification of only a few of these SNPs may be sufficient to capture the majority of the genetic variation in that region. These regions are called haploblocks.

General Approaches to Genetic Studies

The first type of analysis to be used when investigating the possible existence of a genetic component of a polygenic disease is the family association study. This involves checking for a larger number of cases among the first-degree relatives of patients than in the general population. It is then possible to establish the relative risk of a first-degree relative having the disease above the predicted risk for the general population. A higher frequency among monozygotic than among dizygotic twins may also be sought. Monozygotic twins are genetically identical, whereas dizygotic twins are only as genetically similar as their siblings. Their environment exposure during childhood may be considered identical, making it possible to attribute the resemblances or differences between mono- and dizygotic twins largely due to their genetic background.

Association studies are the most frequently used type of analysis in SSc. The association is sought either in so-called "case-control" studies or through a transmission disequilibrium test (TdT). In case-control studies, the frequency of the allele studied or of the genotype including the suspect allele is compared between patients and controls. Statistical tests are applied to compare the frequencies, after checking that the populations are in Hardy-Weinberg equilibrium (according to which the frequency of alleles and genotypes remains at equilibrium over successive generations). TdT tests require genetic material from both parents and from the affected child (trios). It is rare for all these samples to be available in cases of SSc due to the late onset of disease. This method compares the alleles transmitted to the affected child with the non-transmitted alleles, used as controls. Table 3.1 summarizes the assumptions, advantages, and disadvantages of the abovementioned study designs.

It is also recognized that differences in racial admixture (also known as population stratification) is a confounder that can lead to spurious associations. This is due to different degrees of recombination between genetic markers among the different racial groups. This concept is known as linkage disequilibrium (LD). For example, the extent of LD between groups of genetic markers in ancient populations such as African Yoruban is much lower than that of Northern European Caucasians. Therefore, many of the studies discussed examine subjects only from one racial group (e.g., Northern European Caucasians), analyze each racial group separately, or utilize logistic regression models or other methods to account for differences in race. Moreover, since different races may experience different migration patterns and selection pressures, some associations may not cross ethnic barriers. Therefore, it is paramount that patients and controls are selected from the same population for genetic studies.

Genome-Wide Versus Candidate-Gene Studies

Genome-wide association studies (GWAS) use high-throughput genotyping platforms to examine hundreds of thousands common single-nucleotide polymorphisms (SNPs) at the same time. The advantage of GWAS is that it allows examination of common SNPs in the entire human genome. The genome-wide, non-hypothesis-driven nature of GWAS is an unprecedented opportunity to discover novel, disease-related pathways in an unbiased manner. GWAS

Table 3.1 Study designs for genetic studies in systemic sclerosis

	Case control	Trio (family studies)
Assumptions	Case and controls are recruited from the same population Differences in allele frequencies relate to the disease rather than differences in background population	Disease-related alleles are transmitted in excess of 50 % to affected offspring from heterozygous parents
Advantages	Large numbers of case and control participants can be recruited in a relative short period of time Optimal for studying late-onset, rare diseases	Immune to population stratification Does not require phenotyping of parents
Disadvantages	Prone to biases arising from population stratification (systematic background differences) between case and control populations	Difficult to recruit both parents and offspring in disorders with older age of onset such as systemic sclerosis

relies on the "common disease, common variant" hypothesis, which suggests that genetic influences in many common diseases will be at least in part explained by limited number of allelic variants present in more than 1–5 % of general population. Common variants are either present directly on GWAS arrays or are covered by representative SNPs (tag SNPs) that are in linkage disequilibrium with them. Typically, variation in ten million common SNPs are captured in sufficient density by one million tag SNPs. However, the GWAS approach leads to massive number of comparisons, raising the likelihood for false-positive results. Therefore, more stringent levels of significance are applied, and replication in an independent cohort is mandatory. Furthermore, it is possible that rare allelic variants (frequency <1 %) or other types of genetic variants contribute to the genetic susceptibility of disease. In addition to GWAS, advent of next-generation sequencing technology has enabled more cost-effective and timely sequencing of human genome. The sequencing experiments can examine a specific area of genome, human exome, or the entire genome.

Finally, association studies can be used as part of a "candidate-gene" approach. The candidate genes are identified on the basis of an understanding of, or hypotheses about, the physiopathology of the disease developed during or resulting from studies in vitro, in vivo, or based on animal models of SSc. The aim is to look for differences in frequency between certain polymorphisms of these genes encoding proteins of interest. While this approach is hypothesis driven, it suffers from the major limitation that we have an incomplete or limited knowledge of disease processes. Nevertheless, based on similarities with other autoimmune connective tissue diseases such as systemic lupus erythematosus (SLE) and rheumatoid arthritis (RA), this approach has been crucial in identifying multiple SSc-associated genes.

A critical requirement for these genetic association studies is adequate sample size. In most non-HLA susceptibility genes that have been identified thus far in SSc, SLE, RA, and other autoimmune connective tissue diseases, the odds ratio conferred is usually modest (O.R.<1.5), requiring sample sizes of several thousand subjects in order to detect significant associations.

Another fundamental notion in the genetic approach to complex diseases is the definition of a precise diagnostic profile (phenotype). This is of great importance when trying to optimize research on disease genes. The phenotype is the physical expression of the genotype (the genes responsible). Thus, the definition of genotypic variation depends on correct definition of the phenotype. An imprecise definition increases the background noise in genetic analyses, limiting the likelihood of identifying genes involved in the disease. Furthermore, it is also important to point out that disease manifestations and characteristics (phonome) are only in part determined by genetic factors. Other factors such as environment and stochastic events have also an impact on physiology and morphology of diseases.

Another potential approach would be to deconstruct a complex disease phenotype into a simpler variable as a proxy for the disease which can be more precisely measured. This are readily applied for common disorders. For example, type II diabetes → hemoglobin A1C, or gout → serum uric acid level. This approach is known as quantitative trait loci analysis [4]. In this type of analysis, the phenotype is assumed to be a continuous variable, ideally normally distributed in the population. The SNPs being studied are considered covariates in a polygenic linear regression model.

Application of Genetic Approaches to Systemic Sclerosis

Family Association Studies

Analyses of three American cohorts including 703 families, 11 of which were multiplex for SSc, reported a risk for first-degree relatives of about 13 (10–16, depending on the cohort), with a recurrence rate of 1.6 %, versus 0.026 % for the general population [3]. For brothers and sisters, the risk was estimated at 15 (10–27, depending on the cohort). This risk is the strongest risk factor for the disease established to date but, as concerns individuals, the risk of first-degree descendants having the disease is nonetheless below 1 % [4]. A follow-up study showed that affected first-degree relatives with SSc had significantly more concordance for the SSc-related antibodies and class II HLA haplotypes than expected by chance [5].

Twin Studies

Only one twin study has been carried out to date [6]. This study was based on 42 pairs of twins (24 monozygotic twins) and showed poor concordance with clinical expression of the disease (4.7 %). However, stronger concordance was observed for the presence of antinuclear antibodies: 40 % for dizygotic twins and 90 % for monozygotic twins. These results suggest that genetic predisposition alone is not sufficient for the development of this disease but that susceptibility could lead to a profile of autoantibody production. However, in a complementary study based on the same cohort, molecular concordance was found between the gene expression profiles of cultured dermal fibroblasts and a profibrotic phenotype involving, in particular, the overexpression of genes regulated by TGF-beta, including *ACVR1B* (activin A receptor, type IB), *COL1A2* (alpha 2 chain of collagen I), *COL8A1* (alpha 1 chain of collagen VIII), *SPARC* (secreted protein acidic and rich in cysteine), *CTGF* (connective tissue growth factor) and *THY1* (Thy-1 cell surface antigen), *AGTRL2* (angiotensin receptor-like 2), FHL2 (four and a half LIM domains 2), and *ARHB* (Ras homolog gene family, member B). The overexpression of *COL1A2*, *SPARC*, and *CTGF* was subsequently independently confirmed by RT-qPCR [7].

Genome-Wide Association Studies (GWAS)

There are three GWA studies published so far based on Korean and US populations [8], on European and US Caucasian populations [9] (see Fig. 3.2), and on European population [10] (see Fig. 3.3).

Candidate-Gene Approach and Main Biological Pathways

Candidate-gene studies have been conducted based on their relevance to SSc pathogenesis (i.e., inflammatory, fibrotic, or vascular pathways) or their relevance in other autoimmune diseases. Recently, two Immunochip studies in SSc have been also completed: one investigates a large population of US/European Caucasian decent [11] and another one in an Australian Caucasian population [12]. Immunochip is a SNP microarray containing 195,806 SNPs and 718 insertion-deletions which provides dense coverage for gene regions that were relevant in 11 distinct autoimmune and inflammatory diseases.

Gene Regions Associated with SSc

In this section, we will discuss a selection of gene regions that have been robustly associated with susceptibility to SSc in GWAS or candidate-gene studies. The vast majority of robustly replicated SSc susceptibility loci are involved in innate or adaptive immune system. However, few genes in apoptotic and fibrotic pathways are also emerging. For the

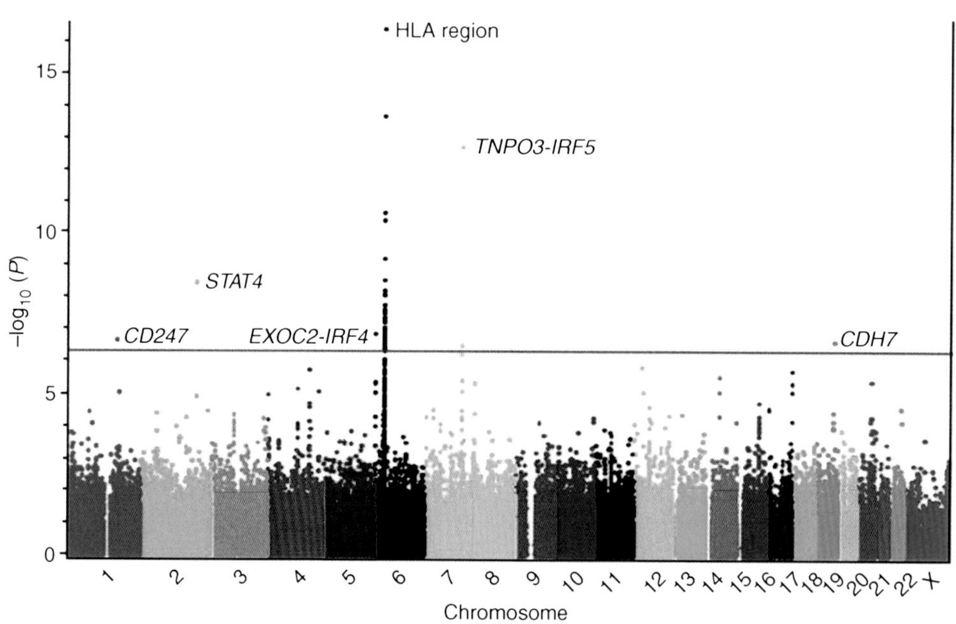

Fig. 3.2 Manhattan plot of the GWAS of 2,346 Caucasian SSc cases and 5,193 healthy controls. The $-\log_{10}$ of the Mantel-Haenszel test *P* value of 279,621 SNPs after genomic control correction is plotted against its physical chromosomal position. Chromosomes are shown in alternate colors. SNPs above the red line represent those with a genome-wide level of significance *P* value of $<5\times10^{-7}$. Note the considerable number of peaks that fall just below genome-wide significance (Figure from Radstake et al. [9], reproduced with permission from the author)

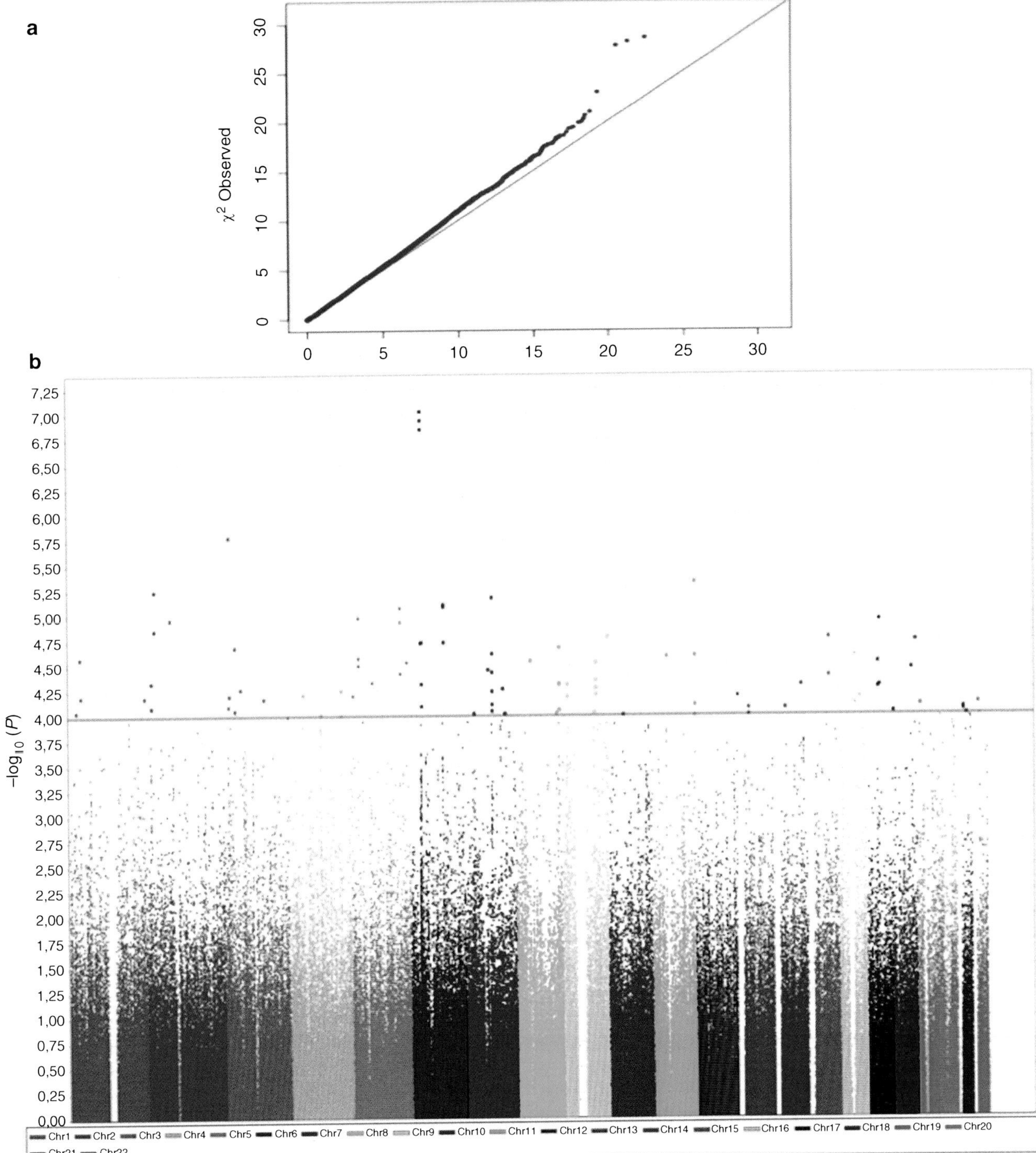

Fig. 3.3 Manhattan plot of the GWAS of 564 Caucasian SSc cases and 1,776 healthy controls (Figure from Allanore et al. [10] © 2011 Allanore et al.)

non-HLA genes, we focused on a selected list of genetic loci that were associated with SSc, its clinical (limited versus diffuse) subtypes, or serological subtypes that fulfilled the following criteria:

(1) The loci were verified in at least two independent cohorts (replication and confirmation cohorts) in one or more studies. (2) The association was not contradicted by a larger subsequent study.

Immune System Regulatory Genes

The Major Histocompatibility Complex and Antigen Presentation

The association between HLA molecules and SSc was established in the 1970s. SSc is associated with class II HLA molecules for which strong genotypic variation has been found between ethnic groups and, in some cases with gender

(*DQA1*05:01* is more strongly associated with the disease in men than in women) [13]. The genotype also varies particularly strongly as a function of the presence of different types of autoantibodies associated with SSc: anti-topoisomerase I (topo) with DRB1*11-*15:02 [14], DQB1*03-*04 [15], DPB1*13:01, and DPB1**09:01 [16] and anti-centromere antibodies (ACA) with DRB1*01:01, DRB1*01:04, DRB1*01:08, DQB1*05:01, and DPB1*04:02 [14, 16].

A large study of HLA class II genes (*DRB1*, *DQB1*, *DQA1*, *DPB1*) was recently carried out in 1,300 SSc cases (961 Caucasians) and 1,000 controls [17]. The strongest associations identified were those with the *DRB1*11:04*, *DQA1*05:01*, and *DQB1*03:01* haplotypes and the *DQB1* allele. However, many other alleles or haplotypes have also been associated with certain subtypes of the disease, particularly those defined on the basis of the presence of autoantibodies. For example, HLA-*DPB1*13:01* had an OR of 14 in comparison of topo + SSc patients to controls. In a similar study, 944 Caucasian SSc patients and 1,320 unaffected controls from Italy and Spain were examined. The association of *DRB1*11:04*, *DQA1*05:01*, and *DQB1*03:01* haplotype with SSc was confirmed in this study [18]. In the first GWAS [8], the strongest association ($P = 8.16 \times 10^{-13}$) identified was that with five SNPs in the *HLA-DPB1* and *-DPB2* regions. A more detailed study of this region subsequently identified rs3128930, rs7763822, and rs7764491 as responsible for this association, particularly in cases of anti-topoisomerase I antibody detection. In the American replication cohort, rs7763822 and rs7764491 were the most strongly associated with SSc. These findings confirm the relevance of HLA-*DPB1* for SSc and especially topo-positivity. In the two additional, large-scale GWAS [9, 10], the strongest association was also that with the class II HLA region on chromosome 6 (Figs. 3.2 and 3.3).

These findings also reflect the considerable differences in HLA genetic background between ethnic groups and the tremendous heterogeneity of the disease itself. Finally, the complex genetic structure of the HLA system in terms of LD complicates fine analyses and the identification of causal variants. The advent of next-generation sequencing technology demonstrates a unique opportunity to investigate this highly polymorphic genomic region.

Innate Immunity

Interferon Pathway (IRF5, IRF7, IRF8) Type I interferon (IFN) is a key mediator of innate immunity and of the normal immune response triggered by microbial infection. IFN stimulates the maturation of monocytes to generate dendritic cells and plasmocytes, immunoglobulin class switching, the cytotoxic activity of natural killer cells and lymphocytes, and the synthesis of chemokines. Various studies, including some based on transcriptomics, have shown a prominent IFN-regulated gene signature in circulating immune cells and skin in SSc [19–21]. Recent studies have generated consistent results, but with several fine points of difference for SSc in terms of the magnitude and prevalence of the IFN signature in SSc compared to lupus patients [22]. In general, the IFN signature is present in only ~50 % of SSc patients, pointing to the molecular heterogeneity of the disease. The hypothesis underlying the presence of the IFN signature is inappropriate activation of the innate immune system during the pathogenesis of SSc. This could occur via activation of pathogen-associated molecular pattern receptors such as toll-like receptors (TLR) [23, 24].

The *IRF5* gene encodes interferon regulatory factor 5, a transcription factor involved in signaling by TLRs and in the activation of type I IFN transcripts. A number of *IFR5* variants have been shown to be associated with SSc, including rs2004640, which creates an alternative splice site leading to the generation of an alternative transcript (exon 1B). This variant was identified by a candidate-gene approach [25], and the homozygous genotype was found to be associated with SSc-related pulmonary fibrosis. Multivariate analyses also showed this association to be significant for the allele and the homozygous genotype, suggesting a role in the severe pulmonary fibrosis phenotype. This finding was also replicated in an independent population from Japan [26]. In a GWAS of 2,296 cases and 5,014 controls [9], three SNPs in the *TNPO3-IRF5* region showed associations with SSc at genome-wide significance level. In a follow-up study, the minor allele of one of those SNPs (rs4728142) was associated with longer survival and higher forced vital capacity. This gene variant was also associated with lower IRF5 transcript levels in monocytes of patients and controls [27]. These data definitively identifies *IRF5* as one of the major susceptibility factors for SSc, playing a key role in type I IFN production and innate immunity.

IRF8 is another interferon regulatory factor that represents a risk locus in SSc. In a GWAS follow-up study examining the susceptibility loci of SSc serological and clinical subtypes, *IRF8* (rs11642873) was associated with limited cutaneous SSc (lcSSc) in the discovery and replication cohorts (OR = 0.75, $p = 2.32E-12$) [28]. This finding has not yet been investigated in an independent study.

These results were corroborated by another study, using an independent sample and that showed association between *IRF8* rs11117432 SNP and SSc susceptibility together with confirming in a meta-analysis the association signal for rs11642873 [29]. Haplotype analyses suggested a stronger association for rs11117432 for a subset of our patients, but a denser genotyping would be required to better narrow a potential causal variant. Furthermore, the latter report indicates that the variant *IRF8* rs11117432 increases IFN-γ whereas decreases IFIT1 gene expression. IRF8 is a nuclear protein, which upon stimulation by pathogen-associated molecular pattern molecules (PAMPs) moves into the cytoplasm and activates NF-kB and TLR signaling pathways, leading to cytokine production thereby regulating inflammatory responses. The consequences of unregulated inflammation are associated with the development of pathologic fibrosis such as that seen in SSc [30].

Interferon regulatory factor 7 (*IRF7*) represents also a susceptibility locus for SSc, specifically for ACA-positive subgroup. A nonsynonymous SNP (rs1131665) located in the exonic region of *IRF7* was associated with ACA-positive SSc in US and European cohorts (overall OR = 0.78, $P_{FDR} = 6.14 \times 10^{-4}$ – the minor allele is protective) [31]. This *IRF7* SNP is also associated with SLE in a concordant direction, and the disease associated variant was associated with higher *IRF7* activity [33]. The association of *IRF7* with SSc has not been confirmed in an independent study.

Toll-Like Receptor 2 (TLR2)

Toll-like receptors as pattern recognition molecules are pivotal elements of innate immunity. A relatively rare, nonsynonymous SNP in *TRL2* (rs5743704) was associated with anti-topo + SSc in two European patient cohorts (overall OR = 2.55, $P < 0.001$). The dendritic cells of SSc patients carrying the risk allele also showed increased IL6 and TNF-α production upon TLR-2 agonist stimulation [34]. The association of *TLR2* with SSc has not been confirmed in an independent study.

Interleukin 1 Receptor-Associated Kinase-1 (IRAK1) and Methyl-CpG-binding Protein 2 (MECP2)

SNPs in the *IRAK1* and *MECP2* have been linked to SSc. Both genes are located on X-chromosome (Xq28 genomic region) which raises the possibility that these risk loci might contribute to female predilection in SSc. IRAK1 has important immune modulatory function by modulating the IL1-induced activation of NF-kB in TLR pathway, whereas MECP2 encodes a nuclear protein that binds specifically to methylated DNA, playing a central role in the transcriptional regulation of methylation-sensitive gene. A nonsynonymous SNP in the *IRAK1* (rs1059702) was associated with diffuse cutaneous SSc (dcSSc) and topo positive in female patients and controls recruited from French and follow-up German/Italian cohorts. Furthermore, this SNP was associated with SSc-related fibrosing alveolitis in addition to dcSSc and topo-positive SSc. These associations remained significant even in case-case comparisons (i.e., dcSSc versus lcSSc, topo- versus ACA-positive SSc, SSc with versus without fibrosing alveolitis) [36]. A follow-up study investigated the above *IRAK1* SNP and four additional SNPs on *MECP2* gene. The IRAK1 SNP rs1059702 and MECP2 rs17435 were both associated specifically with dcSSc in female patients and controls recruited from Spain and follow-up European/US cohorts. However, conditional logistic regression analysis indicated that the association of *IRAK1* rs1059702 with dcSSc was explained by the effect of MECP2 rs17435. These two SNPs were in moderate LD (r^2 0.6). However, only *IRAK1* SNP rs1059702 was associated with presence of fibrosing alveolitis in case-control and case-case comparisons (OR = 1.3, $P_{FDR} = 0.039$; OR = 1.26, $p = 0.025$, respectively) [32].

Adaptive Immunity

CD247 A SNP in the *CD247* gene (the rs2056626) was associated with SSc in the first Caucasian GWAS SSc study (combined analysis: $P = 3.39E^{-9}$; OR 0.86; 95 % CI 0.81–0.90) [9]. This gene encodes the zeta subunit of the T-cell receptor (TCR), which is involved in the formation of the TCR/CD3 complex. This finding was subsequently confirmed in a French independent cohort [35].

Transcription Factor Signal Transducer and Activator of Transcription 4 (STAT4) The gene product of *STAT4* is a member of the STAT family that regulates the expression of many genes. Studies on STAT4 have focused particularly on T lymphocytes and have demonstrated that this molecule is activated by interleukins 12 and 23 and by type I interferon. STAT4 plays an important role in the orientation of T-helper cells towards the Th1 and Th17 pro-inflammatory phenotypes. Several genetic studies have identified associations between variants of the *STAT4* gene and autoimmune diseases. Such an association has been identified, in particular, for an SNP within the third intron, rs7574865, which may induce alternative splicing or other changes to transcription, although its precise role remains to be established.

Two large studies of European populations have independently demonstrated an association between this marker, rs7574865, and the disease [37, 38]. However, one of these studies found that the association was restricted to the limited cutaneous subtype [38], whereas the other found no restriction to a particular cutaneous subtype and instead showed an association with pulmonary fibrosis [37]. Complementary studies in North America [39] and Japan [40] provide support for an association between the *STAT4* gene and SSc, but the variants studied were principally susceptibility factors for the limited cutaneous form and for the presence of ACAs. As for *IRF5*, the association between *STAT4* and the disease has recently been confirmed by whole-genome approach [9, 10], definitively placing *STAT4* on the list of susceptibility factors for SSc.

STAT4 may be as a genetic susceptibility factor not only in SSc but also to other autoimmune diseases. One very challenging question is the real impact of *STAT4* variants on SScc phenotype. A first translational approach has been reported investigating the contribution of *STAT4* in the development of a fibrotic phenotype in two different mouse model of experimental dermal fibrosis [41]. Mice deficient for *stat4* (stat4(−/−)) and wild-type littermates (stat4(+/+)) were injected with bleomycin or NaCl, and the outcome of mice lacking *stat4* was also investigated in the tight-skin (tsk-1) mouse model. *Stat4*(−/−) mice appeared to be protected from bleomycin-induced dermal fibrosis with reduction of dermal thickening (65 ± 3 % reduction, $p = 0.03$), hydroxyproline content (68 ± 5 % decrease, $p = 0.02$), and myofibroblast counts (71 ± 6 % reduction, $p = 0.05$). Moreover, the number of infiltrating leukocytes, and especially T cells, were significantly decreased in lesional skin of *stat4*(−/−) mice (63 ± 5 % reduction of T-cell counts, $p = 0.02$). *Stat4*(−/−) mice also displayed decreased levels of inflammatory cytokines such as TNFα, IL-6, IL-2, and IFNγ in the lesional skin. Consistent with a primary role of STAT4 in inflammation, STAT4 deficiency did not ameliorate fibrosis in *tsk-1* mice. These data demonstrate that the transcription factor STAT4 exerts potent profibrotic effects by controlling T-cell activation, proliferation, and cytokine release. These findings help validate the results of the genetic studies on the role of *STAT4* in the development of SSc and open new avenues for potential innovative therapies.

Tumor Necrosis Factor Ligand Superfamily, Member 4 (TNFSF4)

TNFSF4 encodes OX40 antigen ligand, which is involved in interactions between T cells/antigen presentation and the activation of T and B cells. Variants of this gene are associated with lupus, and a case-control study of 1,059 US Caucasian SSc cases and 698 controls revealed associations for several SNPs of this gene, with specific associations dependent on autoantibody status [43]. This finding was replicated in a study based on a total of 8 European populations of Caucasian ancestry comprising 3,014 patients with SSc and 3,125 healthy controls [44]. A third study examined the association of TNFSF4 SNPs in 1,031 SSc patients and 1,014 controls of French Caucasian ancestry and performed a meta-analysis of all three studies. The meta-analysis confirmed the overall association with SSc but also showed preferential association with the ACA+ subset. The strongest effect was seen with the TNFSF4 SNP rs2205960 (OR 1.33, $p = 0.00013$) [45].

Protein Tyrosine Phosphatase Non-receptor Type 22 (Lymphoid) (PTPN22) *PTPN22* encodes the LYP protein, a tyrosine phosphatase expressed by lymphoid cell lines. This enzyme regulates T-lymphocyte activation by interacting with the effector kinases. It can downregulate the negative selection of T cells in the thymus. The T allele of nonsynonymous SNP rs2476601 (PTPN22*620 W) induces a gain of function, which may prevent the deletion of autoreactive T cells in the thymus or may lead to insufficient activity of Treg cells. The PTPN22*620 W allele is thus involved in various autoimmune diseases and has been shown to be associated, in particular, with type 1 diabetes, lupus, and rheumatoid factor-positive rheumatoid arthritis. An allelic association was found in North American multiethnic patients (905 patients and 656 controls) with topo and ACA antibodies [46]. Subsequently, seven SNPs were studied in a French sample of 659 patients and 504 healthy controls. In 8 % of the patients, an autoimmune disease known to be associated with PTPN22 (e.g., thyroiditis) was discovered. These patients were excluded from the analysis. No allelic or genotype association was reported, but a haplotypic association was found: disease was associated with the haplotype that carried PTPN22*620 W allele ($P = 1.52 \times 10^{-7}$) [47]. Finally, a meta-analysis study with inclusion of above studies and additional European Caucasians patients showed that PTPN22*620 W was associated with SSc (OR = 1.15, $P_{FDR} = 0.03$) and ACA + SSc (OR = 1.22, $P_{FDR} = 0.02$) [48].

B-Cell-Specific Scaffold Protein with Ankyrin (BANK1) Despite the specificity of certain autoantibodies in SSc, the role of B lymphocytes had not been clearly established. Genetic data confirm the probable role of these antibodies in the disease. The *BANK1* gene encodes the B-cell-specific scaffold protein with ankyrin repeats, which acts as a substrate of the LYN tyrosine, phosphorylating the inositol 1,4,5-triphosphate receptors. Two nonsynonymous and functional SNPs of *BANK1* (rs10516487 and rs3733197) were associated with the diffuse cutaneous form of the disease in 1,295 patients and 11,137 controls of French and German Caucasian ancestry [37] and in another European study of 2,380 patients and 3,270 controls [49].

Chemokine Receptor 6 (CCR6) CCR6 protein, the receptor of CCL20, is a surface marker for IL-17-producing TH17 cells. CCR6 is a key factor for recruiting TH17 into target tissue. *CCR6* rs10946216 was associated with topo+ SSc (OR= 1.32 Padj=9E-5) in 3 European populations (France, Italy, and Germany) [50]. This genetic association has not been yet investigated in independent studies. This finding provides support for potential role of Th17 pathways in SSc pathogenesis.

B-lymphocyte Kinase (BLK) The protein encoded by *BLK* transduces the downstream B-cell receptor (BCR) signal. Two variants of the *C8orf13-BLK* region (rs13277113 and rs2736340) were studied in 1,050 Caucasian cases and 694 controls from the USA, and a replication study was carried out in 589 cases and 722 controls from Spain. In the pooled analyses, BLK SNP rs2736340 was associated with SSc and especially with the lcSSc and ACA+ subsets [42]. Furthermore, the SNP rs13277113 was found to be associated with SSc in a Japanese study [51]. In a meta-analysis that included the above studies and additional 1,031 patients and 1,014 controls from France, this SNP was associated with SSc and especially with dcSSc [52].

Tumor Necrosis Factor, Alpha-Induced Protein 3 (TNFAIP3) *TNFAIP3* (6q23) encodes the A20 protein, a zinc-finger protein required for feedback control of the NF-kB (nuclear factor-kB) signaling pathway. Furthermore, A 20 can negatively regulate NLRP3 inflammasome activity [53] as well as Wnt/β-catenin signaling [54]. Three variants of this gene were genotyped in a European sample of 1656 patients and 1311 controls, and the rs5029939 (allele G) marker was identified as associated with the disease (OR 2.08; $P=1.16\text{E-}7$) [55]. Strong associations have also been found with certain phenotypes, including, in particular, the diffuse cutaneous form of the disease (OR 2.71, $P=5.2\text{E-}9$), pulmonary fibrosis (OR 2.26, $P=2.5\text{E-}6$), and pulmonary arterial hypertension (OR 3.11, $P=1.3\text{E-}5$), suggesting a possible role of TNFAIP3 in disease severity. The observed genetic association has not been yet investigated in independent studies, although another *TNFAIP3* SNP was associated with ACA+ SSc in the US/European Immunochip study [11].

TNFAIP3-Interacting Protein 1 (TNIP1) TNIP1 protein downregulates NF-kB signaling in part by interacting with TNAIP3. *TNIP1* SNP rs2233287 was associated with SSc in the discovery and replication cohorts of the European GWAS (pooled OR: 1.31, $p=4.7\text{E-}09$). Furthermore, TNIP1 levels were lower at protein and mRNA levels in the skin tissue of SSc patients compared to unaffected controls. Recombinant TNIP1 abrogated collagen synthesis in SSc and control fibroblasts, showing relevance of this inflammatory molecule for fibrotic response [10]. The association of TNIP1 with SSc was confirmed in an independent US/European study [56].

Autophagy-Related 5 (ATG5) ATG5 protein forms a complex with ATG12 and assists in autophagosomal elongation. Autophagy mediates pathogen degradation and allows cells to clear unwanted cytoplasmic material and to recycle nutrients. It plays a pivotal role in adaptive and innate immunity. *ATG5* SNP rs9373839 was associated with SSc in the recently completed US/European Caucasian Immunochip study, linking SSc pathogenesis to autophagy (pooled OR = 1.19, $p=3.75$ E-8) [11]. The observed genetic association has not been yet investigated in independent studies.

IL12 Signaling Pathways

IL-12 levels are increased in the serum of SSc patients, as well as in the alveolar lavage fluid from patients with SSc-associated interstitial lung disease. IL12 can trigger a pro-inflammatory cell-mediated immunity and Th1 response. Three genes in IL12 signaling pathway were reported to be associated with SSc, implying an important role for this cytokine in SSc pathogenesis.

IL12RB2 intronic SNP rs3790567 was associated with SSc in a GWAS follow-up study of US/European Caucasian patients (OR = 1.17, $p=2.82$ E-9) [57]. Similarly, a SNP in the intergenic region of *SHIP1-IL12A* (rs7758790) was associated with SSc with relatively high OR of 2.57 ($p=1.22$ E-11) in the US/European Caucasian Immunochip study, providing further evidence for importance of IL12 signaling in SSc [11]. Furthermore, an Immunochip follow-up study revealed that *IL12* SNP rs436857 was associated with SSc (pooled OR=0.81 $p=3.9$ E-9) in combined US/European cohorts [58]. The above associations in IL12 signaling pathways have not been yet replicated in independent studies.

Interleukin 21 (IL-21)

IL-21 protein is a potent regulatory cytokine that is expressed in Th2, Th17, and NK cells. The *IL-21* SNP rs6822844, which is located in the flanking 3′-untranslated region of *IL-21*, was associated with SSc in patients of European/US Caucasian decent (pooled OR=0.86, $p=6.6\text{E-}04$) [59]. This genetic association has not been yet replicated in independent studies.

Apoptosis and Cell Fate

Two genes involved in apoptosis and determination of cell fate have been associated with SSc and its clinical subtypes. The prominent role of dysregulated apoptosis in vascular and immune components of SSc pathogenesis raises the importance of below genetic loci for follow-up mechanistic studies.

Deoxyribonuclease I-Like 3 (DNASEIL3)

DNASEIL3 protein plays an important role in DNA fragmentation during apoptosis and in the generation of resected double-strand breaks in immunoglobulin-encoding genes. The nonsynonymous *DNASEIL3* SNP rs35677470 was associated with SSc in the first SSc Immunochip study in patients of European/US Caucasian decent (pooled OR=1.47, $p=3.36\text{E-}16$). The association was strongest in the ACA^{+} SSc (pooled OR = 2.03, $p=4.25$ E-31) [11]. This gene variant results in an Arg-to-Cys amino-acid substitution and loss of a hydrogen bond leading to diminished Dnase activity (Fig. 3.4). This genetic association was confirmed in subsequent Australian Immunochip study [12].

SRY (Sex-Determining Region Y)-Box 5 (SOX5) SOX5 protein is a transcription factor involved in determination of cell fate. A *SOX5* SNP was associated with ACA+ SSc in GWAS follow-up study in US/European Caucasian populations (pooled OR = 1.36, $P=1.39$ E-7) [28]. This finding has not been investigated in independent studies.

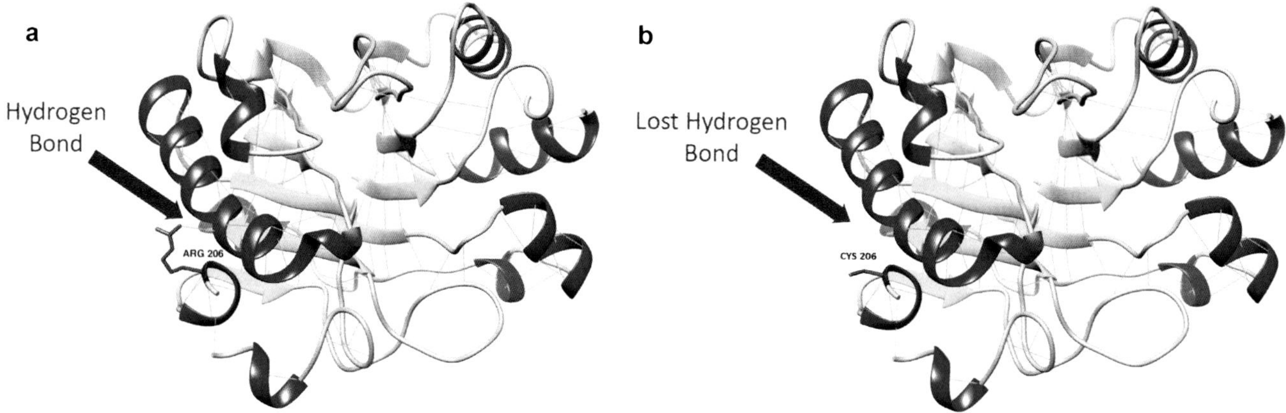

Fig. 3.4 Ribbon representation of the loss of the hydrogen bond as a consequence of the substitution of arginine (**a**, major allele) for cysteine (**b**, minor allele) in the protein coded by *DNASE1L3* due to genetic variation in SNP rs35677470 (Figure reproduced from Mayes et al. [11])

Fibrosis Pathways

Fibrosis is the ultimate end-product of SSc in several prominently affected organs such as skin and lung. Although the majority of SSc susceptibility loci belong to immune regulation pathways, genetic associations with few genes, prominently involved in fibrotic pathways, have been also reported.

c-Src tyrosine kinase (CSK). CSK protein is involved in the regulation of myofibroblast differentiation in vitro and in mouse models by modulating the function of Src kinase [60]. Src kinases are involved in fibrosis by regulating transmission of integrin signaling upon adhesion of fibroblasts to the extracellular matrix and their subsequent differentiation into myofibroblast. *CSK* SNP rs1378942 was associated with SSc in a GWAS follow-up study in US/European Caucasian populations (pooled OR = 1.2, *P* = 5.04E-12) [61]. This finding has not been investigated in independent studies.

Caveolin 1 (CAV1) CAV1 protein is an inhibitor of tissue fibrosis, and decreased CAV1 expression has been thought to contribute to the fibrotic process in SSc. Based on its relevance to SSc pathogenesis, the SNPs with the highest association in *CAV1* in the GWAS of French SSc patients were investigated in an Italian Caucasian cohort. *CAV1* SNP rs959173 was associated with SSc (pooled OR 0.81, 95 %, *p* = 0.0018). Indeed, *CAV1* protein expression levels were significantly higher in skin samples of both patients with SSc and controls carrying the allele that was protective for SSc (rs959173 C) in follow-up Western blot and immunohistochemistry experiments [62]. The observed genetic association has not been yet investigated in independent studies.

Growth Factor Receptor-Bound Protein 10 (GRB10) GRB10 protein interacts with a number of receptor tyrosine kinases and insulin-like growth factor receptors and regulates cell growth. Both tyrosine kinases and insulin-like growth factors have been implicated in SSc pathogenesis. *GRB10* SNP rs12540874 was associated with lc SSc in GWAS follow-up study (OR = 1.15, *P* = 1.27 E-6) [28]. This finding has not been investigated in independent studies.

Conclusion

It is clear from these studies that there is a genetic component to the physiopathology of SSc and major progress has been recently achieved in understanding the genetics of the SSc susceptibility. Multicenter and transnational efforts have allowed the building of large cohorts, which are mandatory to investigate the genetic component in complex disorders. The majority of the risk loci that have been identified and replicated thus far are involved in autoimmune regulation. This finding provides further support for the hypothesis that the inciting immune dysregulations trigger and maintain the fibrotic manifestations of SSc. As in many polygenic diseases, the presence of several polymorphisms in a given individual probably contributes to the risk of the disease, with each polymorphism having only a minimal effect on its own. It is also possible that these genetic loci have a multiplicative effect on disease susceptibility by gene-gene or gene-environment interactions.

The most consistent results to date have been obtained for the autoimmune component, with replication in large studies identifying *HLA*, *IRF5*, *CD247*, and *STAT4*, etc. as the principal genes involved (Table 3.2). Several of these genes are already well-established risk factors for other autoimmune diseases, raising the possibility of shared autoimmunity. Several genetic factors of relatively small effect may cumulatively create a state of susceptibility to autoimmune diseases according to the quantitative threshold concept (reviewed in Cho et al. [63]). Self-reactive B and T cells are a normal component of the immune system. However, they are usually kept in check

Table 3.2 Selected genetic susceptibility loci in systemic sclerosis

Gene	Chr	SNP	Type of study	Comments
TNFSF4 (OX40L)	1q25	rs1234314; rs2205960 rs844648	Candidate gene (American population)	Association particularly with autoantibody status; mainly limited cutaneous Scc
PTPN22	1p13.2	rs2476601	Candidate gene (with replication in an independent population)	Limited to ACA+ or topo+ patients
CD247	1q24.2	rs2056626	Whole genome	
STAT4	2q32	rs7574865	Candidate gene and whole genome	Associated subtype poorly defined
BANK1	4q24	rs10516487 rs3733197 rs17266594	Candidate gene	Only the diffuse cutaneous subtype
HLA class II	6	NA	Candidate gene and whole genome	Causal variant not identified
TNFAIP3	6q23	rs5029939	Candidate gene (European Caucasian population)	Severe phenotype, causal variant not identified
IRF5	7q32	rs2004640	Candidate gene and whole genome	Diffuse cutaneous form and pulmonary fibrosis SSc Survival and risk of ILD
C8orf13/BLK	*8p23-p22*	rs2736340 rs13277113	Candidate gene (with replication in an independent population)	Higher risk if ACA+
IRF8	16q24.1	rs11117432; 11642873	Candidate gene	LcSSc
IRF7	11p15.5	rs1131665	Candidate gene	ACA+
TLR2	4q32	rs5743704	Candidate gene	Topo+
CCR6	6q27	rs10946216	Candidate gene	Topo+
BANK1	4q24	rs10516487; 3733197	Candidate gene	DcSSc
BLK	*8p23-p22*	rs13277113; rs2736340	Candidate gene	
GRB10	7p12.2	rs12540874	Secondary analyses of GWAS	LcSSc
CAV1	*7q31.1*	rs959173	Candidate gene	
SOX5	12p12.1		Secondary analyses of GWAS	ACA+
CSK	15q24.1	rs1378942	Secondary analyses of GWAS	
DNASE1L3	3p14.3	rs35677470	Immunochip	ACA+
ATG5	6q21	rs9373839	Immunochip	
IL12RB2	1p31.3	rs3790567	Secondary analyses of GWAS	
1 L12	12q13.3	rs436857	Immunochip	
IL21	*4q26*	rs6822844	Candidate gene	
IRAK1/MECP2	*Xq28*	IRAK1 rs1059702 MECP2 rs17435	Candidate gene	DcSSc, topo+ ILD

by regulatory mechanisms in the thymus/bone marrow or peripheral blood. In the concept of quantitative threshold, the implicated shared genetic variations in autoimmune diseases lead cumulatively to an impairment of the necessary biological processes for destruction of self-reactive immune cells, leading to autoimmunity. Although the disease manifestations of specific autoimmune diseases vary, the genetic basis for occurrence of autoimmunity seems to overlap among them. It is possible that other triggers such as environmental and stochastic factors further contribute to phenotypic manifestation of a specific autoimmune disease in a susceptible host.

Many of the reported susceptibility SNPs are located in noncoding regions (introns). It is possible that these loci are in LD with SNPs in coding regions. However, there is also increasing evidence that these loci might influence the transcription of regulatory RNAs such as microRNAs or long-noncoding RNAs [64]. These regulatory RNAs might have important biological functions in SSc pathogenesis [65]

Adding complexity to the regulation of gene expression is the fact that gene function is also subject to regulation by epigenetic factors. An epigenetic change is defined as a heritable change in gene expression that does not involve a change in the DNA sequence. Epigenetic mechanisms play an essential role in eukaryotic gene regulation by modifying chromatin structure, which in turn modulates gene expression. These epigenetic changes are reversible, respond to environmental triggers, and vary by cell type [66].

However, this highly complex puzzle is not yet complete, and the so-called missing heritability is still challenging.

This question is a source of ongoing debate and many sources could contribute to it. Possible explanations are the following: (i) Additional common variants with low genetic effects exist, but current GWAS remain underpowered to identify such risk loci (Figs. 3.2 and 3.3). (ii) Rare variants might be involved that cannot be detected with GWAS approach, but direct association mapping through sequencing candidate genes, exomes, or entire genomes can be applied. (iii) Genetic heterogeneity is also likely; genetic studies of clinically more homogeneous subforms of the disease may be targeted. (iv) Interactions between genes or between genes and environment are likely to contribute to the disease risk.

Key Points

- There is a familial risk of systemic sclerosis, with SSc occurring more frequently in families in which cases have already been identified than in the general population.
- Clinical concordance between monozygotic twins is poor, but concordance rates are higher mainly for autoantibodies and fibrotic transcript profile.
- International collaborations have enabled sufficiently powered, genome-wide association studies, leading to discovery of robust and reproducible genetic susceptibility loci.
- The majority of SSc susceptibility loci are involved in innate and adaptive immunity, underscoring the role of immune dysregulation for the SSc pathogenesis.
- The majority of SSc susceptibility loci are located in the intronic areas which might influence directly the transcription of noncoding regulatory RNAs or be in linkage disequilibrium with genetic variants in coding areas.

References

1. Feero WG, Guttmacher AE, Collins FS. Genomic medicine–an updated primary N Engl J Med. 2010;362:2001–11.
2. Vitart V, Rudan I, Hayward C, et al. SLC2A9 is a newly identified urate transporter influencing serum urate concentration, urate excretion and gout. Nat Genet. 2008;40:437–42.
3. Arnett FC, Cho M, Chatterjee S, et al. Familial occurrence frequencies and relative risks for systemic sclerosis (scleroderma) in three United States cohorts. Arthritis Rheum. 2001;44:1359–62.
4. Plomin R, Haworth CMA, Davis OSP. Common disorders are quantitative traits. Nat Rev Genet. 2009;10:872–8.
5. Assassi S, Arnett FC, Reveille JD, Gourh P, Mayes MD. Clinical, immunologic, and genetic features of familial systemic sclerosis. Arthritis Rheum. 2007;56:2031–7.
6. Feghali-Bostwick C, Medsger Jr TA, Wright TM. Analysis of systemic sclerosis in twins reveals low concordance for disease and high concordance for the presence of antinuclear antibodies. Arthritis Rheum. 2003;48:1956–63.
7. Zhou X, Tan FK, Xiong M, et al. Monozygotic twins clinically discordant for scleroderma show concordance for fibroblast gene expression profiles. Arthritis Rheum. 2005;52:3305–14.
8. Zhou X, Lee JE, Arnett FC, Xiong M, Park MY, Yoo YK, et al. HLA-DPB1 and DPB2 are genetic loci for systemic sclerosis: a genome-wide association study in Koreans with replication in North Americans. Arthritis Rheum. 2009;60:3807–14.
9. Radstake TR, Gorlova O, Rueda B, Martin JE, Alizadeh BZ, Palomino-Morales R, et al. Genome-wide association study of systemic sclerosis identifies CD247 as a new susceptibility locus. Nat Genet. 2010;42:426–9.
10. Allanore Y, Saad M, Dieudé P, Avouac J, Distler JH, Amouyel P, et al. Genome-wide scan identifies TNIP1, PSORS1C1, and RHOB as novel risk loci for systemic sclerosis. PLoS Genet. 2011;7(7):e1002091.
11. Mayes MD, Bossini-Castillo L, Gorlova O, Martin JE, Zhou X, Chen WV, et al. Immunochip analysis identifies multiple susceptibility loci for systemic sclerosis. Am J Hum Genet. 2014;94:47–61.
12. Zochling J, Newell F, Charlesworth JC, Leo P, Stankovich J, Cortes A, et al. An Immunochip-based interrogation of scleroderma susceptibility variants identifies a novel association at DNASE1L3. Arthritis Res Ther. 2014;16(5):438.
13. Lambert NC, Distler O, Muller-Ladner U, Tylee TS, Furst DE, Nelson JL. HLA-DQA1 *0501 is associated with diffuse systemic sclerosis in Caucasian men. Arthritis Rheum. 2000;43:2005–10.
14. Kuwana M, Inoko H, Kameda H, Nojima T, Sato S, Nakamura K, et al. Association of human leucocyte antigen class II genes with autoantibody profiles, but not with disease susceptibility in Japanese patients with systemic sclerosis. Intern Med. 1999;38:336–44.
15. Ueki A, Isozaki Y, Tomokuni A, et al. Different distribution of HLA class II alleles in anti-topoisomerase I autoantibody responders between silicosis and systemic sclerosis patients, with a common distinct sequence in the HLA-DQB1 domain. Immunobiology. 2001;204:458–65.
16. Gilchrist FC, Bunn C, Foley PJ, et al. Class II HLA associations with autoantibodies in scleroderma: a highly significant role for HLA-DP. Genes Immun. 2001;2:76–81.
17. Arnett FC, Gourh P, Shete S, Ahn CW, Honey RE, Agarwal SK, et al. Major histocompatibility complex (MHC) class II alleles, haplotypes and epitopes which confer susceptibility or protection in systemic sclerosis: analyses in 1300 Caucasian, African-American and Hispanic cases and 1000 controls. Ann Rheum Dis. 2010;69:822–7.
18. Beretta L, Rueda B, Marchini M, Santaniello A, Simeón CP, Fonollosa V, et al. Analysis of Class II human leucocyte antigens in Italian and Spanish systemic sclerosis. Rheumatology (Oxford). 2012;51:52–9.
19. Tan FK, Zhou X, Mayes MD, Gourh P, Guo X, Marcum C, et al. Signatures of differentially regulated interferon gene expression and vasculotropism in the peripheral blood cells of systemic sclerosis patients. Rheumatology. 2006;45:694–702.
20. York MR, Nagai T, Mangini AJ, Lemaire R, van Seventer JM, Lafyatis R. A macrophage marker, Siglec-1, is increased on circulating monocytes in patients with systemic sclerosis and induced by type I interferons and toll-like receptor agonists. Arthritis Rheum. 2007;56:1010–20.
21. Higgs BW, Liu Z, White B, Zhu W, White WI, Morehouse C, et al. Patients with systemic lupus erythematosus, myositis, rheumatoid arthritis and scleroderma share activation of a common type I interferon pathway. Ann Rheum Dis. 2011;70:2029–36.
22. Assassi S, Mayes MD, Arnett FC, Gourh P, Agarwal SK, McNearney TA, et al. Systemic sclerosis and lupus: points in an

interferon-mediated continuum. Arthritis Rheum. 2010;62:589–98.
23. Farina GA, York MR, Di Marzio M, Collins CA, Meller S, Homey B, et al. Poly(I:C) drives type I IFN- and TGFβ-mediated inflammation and dermal fibrosis simulating altered gene expression in systemic sclerosis. J Invest Derm. 2010;130:2583–93.
24. Agarwal SK, Wu M, Livingston CK, Parks DH, Mayes MD, Arnett FC, Tan FK. Toll-like receptor 3 upregulation by type I interferon in healthy and scleroderma dermal fibroblasts. Arthritis Res Ther. 2011;13(1):R3.
25. Dieudé P, Guedj M, Wipff J, Avouac J, Fajardy I, Diot E, et al. Association between the IRF5 rs2004640 functional polymorphism and systemic sclerosis: a new perspective for pulmonary fibrosis. Arthritis Rheum. 2009;60:225–33.
26. Ito I, Kawaguchi Y, Kawasaki A, Hasegawa M, Ohashi J, Hikami K, et al. Association of a functional polymorphism in the IRF5 region with systemic sclerosis in a Japanese population. Arthritis Rheum. 2009;60:1845–50.
27. Sharif R, Mayes MD, Tan FK, Gorlova OY, Hummers LK, Shah AA, et al. IRF5 polymorphism predicts prognosis in patients with systemic sclerosis. Ann Rheum Dis. 2012;71:1197–202.
28. Gorlova O, Martin JE, Rueda B, Koeleman BP, Ying J, Teruel M, et al. Identification of novel genetic markers associated with clinical phenotypes of systemic sclerosis through a genome-wide association strategy. PLoS Genet. 2011;7(7):e1002178.
29. Arismendi M, Giraud M, Ruzehaji N, Dieudé P, Koumakis E, Ruiz B, et al. Identification of NF-kB and PLCL2 as new susceptibility genes and highlights on a potential role of IRF8 through interferon signature modulation in systemic sclerosis. Arthritis Res Ther. 2015;17:71.
30. Lafyatis R, York M. Innate immunity and inflammation in systemic sclerosis. Curr Opin Rheumatol. 2009;21:617–22.
31. Carmona FD, Gutala R, Simeón CP, Carreira P, Ortego-Centeno N, Vicente-Rabaneda E, et al. Novel identification of the IRF7 region as an anticentromere autoantibody propensity locus in systemic sclerosis. Ann Rheum Dis. 2012;71:114–9.
32. Carmona FD, Cénit MC, Diaz-Gallo LM, Broen JC, Simeón CP, Carreira PE, et al. New insight on the Xq28 association with systemic sclerosis. Ann Rheum Dis. 2013;72:2032–8.
33. Fu Q, Zhao J, Qian X, Wong JL, Kaufman KM, Yu CY, et al. Association of a functional IRF7 variant with systemic lupus erythematosus. Arthritis Rheum. 2011;63:749–54.
34. Broen JC, Bossini-Castillo L, van Bon L, Vonk MC, Knaapen H, Beretta L, et al. A rare polymorphism in the gene for Toll-like receptor 2 is associated with systemic sclerosis phenotype and increases the production of inflammatory mediators. Arthritis Rheum. 2012;64:264–71.
35. Dieudé P, Boileau C, Guedj M, Avouac J, Ruiz B, Hachulla E, et al. Independent replication establishes the CD247 gene as a genetic systemic sclerosis susceptibility factor. Ann Rheum Dis. 2011;70:1695–6.
36. Dieudé P, Bouaziz M, Guedj M, Riemekasten G, Airò P, Müller M, et al. Evidence of the contribution of the X chromosome to systemic sclerosis susceptibility: association with the functional IRAK1 196Phe/532Ser haplotype. Arthritis Rheum. 2011;63:3979–87.
37. Dieude P, Wipff J, Guedj M, Ruiz B, Melchers I, Hachulla E, et al. BANK1 is a genetic risk factor for diffuse cutaneous systemic sclerosis and has additive effects with IRF5 and STAT4. Arthritis Rheum. 2009;60:3447–54.
38. Rueda B, Broen J, Simeon C, Hesselstrand R, Diaz B, Suárez H, et al. The STAT4 gene influences the genetic predisposition to systemic sclerosis phenotype. Hum Mol Genet. 2009;18:2071–7.
39. Gourh P, Agarwal SK, Divecha D, Assassi S, Paz G, Arora-Singh RK, et al. Polymorphisms in TBX21 and STAT4 increase the risk of systemic sclerosis: evidence of possible gene-gene interaction and alterations in Th1/Th2 cytokines. Arthritis Rheum. 2009;60:3794–806.
40. Tsuchiya N, Kawasaki A, Hasegawa M, Fujimoto M, Takehara K, Kawaguchi Y, et al. Association of STAT4 polymorphism with systemic sclerosis in a Japanese population. Ann Rheum Dis. 2009;68:1375–6.
41. Avouac J, Fürnrohr BG, Tomcik M, Palumbo K, Zerr P, Horn A, et al. Inactivation of the transcription factor STAT4 prevents inflammation-driven fibrosis in systemic sclerosis animal models. Arthritis Rheum. 2011;63:800–9.
42. Gourh P, Agarwal SK, Martin E, Divecha D, Rueda B, Bunting H, et al. Association of the C8orf13-BLK region with systemic sclerosis in North-American and European populations. J Autoimmun. 2010;34:155–62.
43. Gourh P, Arnett FC, Tan FK, Assassi S, Divecha D, Paz G, et al. Association of TNFSF4 (OX40L) polymorphisms with susceptibility to systemic sclerosis. Ann Rheum Dis. 2010;69:550–5.
44. Bossini-Castillo L, Broen JC, Simeon CP, Beretta L, Vonk MC, Ortego-Centeno N, et al. A replication study confirms the association of TNFSF4 (OX40L) polymorphisms with systemic sclerosis in a large European cohort. Ann Rheum Dis. 2011;70:638–41.
45. Coustet B, Bouaziz M, Dieudé P, Guedj M, Bossini-Castillo L, Agarwal S, et al. Independent replication and meta analysis of association studies establish TNFSF4 as a susceptibility gene preferentially associated with the subset of anticentromere-positive patients with systemic sclerosis. J Rheumatol. 2012;39:997–1003.
46. Gourh P, Tan FK, Assassi S, Ahn CW, McNearney TA, Fischbach M, et al. Association of the PTPN22 R620W polymorphism with anti-topoisomerase I- and anticentromere antibody-positive systemic sclerosis. Arthritis Rheum. 2006;54:3945–53.
47. Dieude P, Guedj M, Wipff J, Avouac J, Hachulla E, Diot E, et al. The PTPN22 620W allele confers susceptibility to systemic sclerosis: findings of a large case-control study of European Caucasians and a meta-analysis. Arthritis Rheum. 2008;58:2183–8.
48. Diaz-Gallo LM, Gourh P, Broen J, Simeon C, Fonollosa V, Ortego-Centeno N, et al. Analysis of the influence of PTPN22 gene polymorphisms in systemic sclerosis. Ann Rheum Dis. 2011;70:454–62.
49. Rueda B, Gourh P, Broen J, Agarwal SK, Simeon CP, Ortego-Centeno N, et al. BANK1 functional variants are associated with susceptibility to diffuse systemic sclerosis in Caucasians. Ann Rheum Dis. 2010;69:700–5.
50. Koumakis E, Bouaziz M, Dieudé P, Ruiz B, Riemekasten G, Airo P, et al. A regulatory variant in CCR6 is associated with susceptibility to antitopoisomerase-positive systemic sclerosis. Arthritis Rheum. 2013;65:3202–8.
51. Ito I, Kawaguchi Y, Kawasaki A, Hasegawa M, Ohashi J, Kawamoto M, et al. Association of the FAM167A-BLK region with systemic sclerosis. Arthritis Rheum. 2010;62:890–5.
52. Coustet B, Dieudé P, Guedj M, Bouaziz M, Avouac J, Ruiz B, et al. C8orf13-BLK is a genetic risk locus for systemic sclerosis and has additive effects with BANK1: results from a large french cohort and meta-analysis. Arthritis Rheum. 2011;63:2091–6.
53. Vande Walle L, Van Opdenbosch N, Jacques P, Fossoul A, Verheugen E, Vogel P, et al. Negative regulation of the NLRP3 inflammasome by A20 protects against arthritis. Nature. 2014;512:69–7349.
54. Shao L, Oshima S, Duong B, Advincula R, Barrera J, Malynn BA, et al. A20 restricts wnt signaling in intestinal epithelial cells and suppresses colon carcinogenesis. PLoS ONE. 2013;8:e62223.
55. Dieudé P, Guedj M, Wipff J, Ruiz B, Riemekasten G, Matucci-Cerinic M, et al. Association of the TNFAIP3 rs5029939 variant with systemic sclerosis in the European Caucasian population. Ann Rheum Dis. 2010;69:1958–64.
56. Bossini-Castillo L, Martin JE, Broen J, Simeon CP, Beretta L, Gorlova OY, et al. Confirmation of TNIP1 but not RHOB and

PSORS1C1 as systemic sclerosis risk factors in a large independent replication study. Ann Rheum Dis. 2013;72:602–7.
57. Bossini-Castillo L, Martin JE, Broen J, Gorlova O, Simeón CP, Beretta L, et al. A GWAS follow-up study reveals the association of the IL12RB2 gene with systemic sclerosis in Caucasian populations. Hum Mol Genet. 2012;21:926–33.
58. López-Isac E, Bossini-Castillo L, Guerra SG, Denton C, Fonseca C, Assassi S, et al. Identification of IL12RB1 as a novel systemic sclerosis susceptibility locus. Arthritis Rheumatol. 2014;66: 3521–3.
59. Diaz-Gallo LM, Simeon CP, Broen JC, Ortego-Centeno N, Beretta L, Vonk MC, et al. Implication of IL-2/IL-21 region in systemic sclerosis genetic susceptibility. Ann Rheum Dis. 2013;72:1233–8.
60. Skhirtladze C, Distler O, Dees C, Akhmetshina A, Busch N, Venalis P, et al. Src kinases in systemic sclerosis: central roles in fibroblast activation and in skin fibrosis. Arthritis Rheum. 2008;58: 1475–84.
61. Martin JE, Broen JC, Carmona FD, Teruel M, Simeon CP, Vonk MC, et al. Identification of CSK as a systemic sclerosis genetic risk factor through Genome Wide Association Study follow-up. Hum Mol Genet. 2012;21:2825–35.
62. Manetti M, Allanore Y, Saad M, Fatini C, Cohignac V, Guiducci S, et al. Evidence for caveolin-1 as a new susceptibility gene regulating tissue fibrosis in systemic sclerosis. Ann Rheum Dis. 2012;71:1034–41.
63. Cho JH, Gregersen PK. Genomics and the multifactorial nature of human autoimmune disease. N Engl J Med. 2011;365:1612–23.
64. Gardini A, Shiekhattar R. The many faces of long noncoding RNAs. FEBS J. 2015;282(9):1647–57. [Epub ahead of print].
65. Altorok N, Almeshal N, Wang Y, Kahaleh B. Epigenetics, the holy grail in the pathogenesis of systemic sclerosis. Rheumatology (Oxford). 2015;54:1759–70.
66. Ballestar E. Epigenetic alterations in autoimmune rheumatic diseases. Nat Rev Rheumatol. 2011;7:263–71.

Disease Subsets in Clinical Practice

4

Robyn T. Domsic and Thomas A. Medsger Jr.

Why Classify Patients?

Disease classification has two primary purposes [1]. The first is to assure the reader that the author(s) are describing a group of patients with a single condition that can be distinguished from patients without this condition. The second is a phenotypic classification to help categorize patients with a disease into subsets which may have different risks for disease complications or mortality or behave differently from a clinical perspective. For the former, the object in systemic sclerosis (SSc) is to develop criteria which accurately classify groups of patients because they include clinical features which are frequent in SSc patients but are infrequent in patients with other closely related diseases. This is a particularly challenging task, as SSc includes patients with a wide spectrum of clinical and laboratory manifestations.

Generally, classification refers to systematic placement into categories. Classification criteria are not the same as diagnostic criteria, although they can reflect areas along a continuum. Classification criteria were initially proposed to enhance research by developing a systematic approach to creating groups of similar patients. A goal of classification criteria development is to reach high levels of both sensitivity and specificity. However, in this circumstance, 100% sensitivity is rarely achieved. Neither is specificity 100%, as patients with other conditions may, on occasion, satisfy criteria. Diagnostic criteria refer to classification of the individual patient. If the criteria are not satisfied, then a patient cannot be said to have the disease in question. If a patient falls short of satisfying a set of diagnostic criteria for "definite" disease, yet the disease remains the most likely diagnosis, the patient may be said to have "probable" disease.

The rationale for disease subsetting (or phenotyping) is that in disorders with a broad spectrum of clinical manifestations and severity, the natural history and risk of morbidity and mortality may be highly variable. Disease subsetting offers the opportunity to identify patients early in their disease who have a greater likelihood of developing one or another manifestation or complication of the disease and may have a higher risk of morbidity or mortality. Understanding these risks is important for the patient and the managing physician, as organ system surveillance and prompt identification of disease-associated problems can result in appropriate intervention. SSc lends itself to subset classification.

SSc Classification Criteria

The American Rheumatism Association (now American College of Rheumatology) Scleroderma Criteria Cooperative Study authors developed preliminary classification criteria for SSc which were published in 1980 [2]. The final criteria for definite SSc required one major criterion (skin thickening proximal to the metacarpophalangeal joints) or any two of three minor criteria (digital pitting scars, sclerodactyly [skin thickening restricted to the fingers only], or bibasilar pulmonary fibrosis on chest radiograph). These criteria clearly showed that skin thickening is a distinctive feature of SSc. However, the 1980 criteria have been criticized because they fail to identify a group of SSc patients with either limited cutaneous (lc) involvement or no skin thickening (SSc sine scleroderma or ssSSc) [3, 4], resulting in a lower sensitivity than initially reported. In 2013 a joint ACR and European League Against Rheumatism (EULAR) committee published revised classification criteria for SSc [5, 6]. These new criteria (Table 4.1) improved upon the shortcomings of the earlier ACR criteria as they recognized post-1980 advances in the detection of SSc-associated autoantibodies and distinctive

R.T. Domsic, MD, MPH
Department of Medicine/Rheumatology and Clinical Immunology, University of Pittsburgh, Pittsburgh, PA, USA

T.A. Medsger Jr., MD (✉)
Division of Rheumatology, Department of Medicine, University of Pittsburgh, Pittsburgh, PA 15261, USA
e-mail: tam8@pitt.edu

J. Varga et al. (eds.), *Scleroderma*, DOI 10.1007/978-3-319-31407-5_4

Table 4.1 Revised classification criteria for SSc

Item	Sub-item(s)	Weight/score[a]
Skin thickening of the fingers of both hands extending proximal to the metacarpophalangeal joints (sufficient criterion)		9
Skin thickening of the fingers (only count the higher score)	Putty fingers	2
	Sclerodactyly of the fingers (distal to the metacarpophalangeal joints but proximal to the proximal interphalangeal joints)	4
Fingertip lesions (only count the higher score)	Digital tip ulcers	2
	Fingertip pitting scars	3
Telangiectasia		2
Abnormal nailfold capillaries		2
Pulmonary arterial hypertension and/or interstitial lung disease (maximum score is 2)	Pulmonary arterial hypertension	2
	Interstitial lung disease	2
Raynaud phenomenon		3
SSc-related autoantibodies (anticentromere, anti-topoisomerase I [anti-Scl-70], anti-RNA polymerase III) (maximum score is 3)	Anticentromere	3
	Anti-topoisomerase I	
	Anti-RNA polymerase III	

[a]The total score is determined by adding the maximum weight (score) in each category. Patients with a total score of ≥9 are classified as having definite SSc

SSc-abnormalities on nailfold capillaroscopy. All three hallmark features of SSc (fibrosis of the skin and/or internal organs, production of specific autoantibodies, and evidence of vasculopathy) are included. The new criteria have a sensitivity of 91 % and specificity of 92 %. The use of antibodies in the criteria underscores the growing importance of serologic classification, as we discuss later in this chapter [7].

In SSc, it is unclear how often patients with other established connective tissue diseases (CTDs) satisfy SSc classification criteria. This question has not been formally addressed in the medical literature. Using the University of Pittsburgh CTD database, we found that 87 of 1,499 (6 %) definite SSc patients, excluding those diagnosed by one of our physicians with an "overlap syndrome," satisfied the 1982 revised classification criteria for SLE [8]. This high proportion is due to the relatively high percentage of SSc patients who had joint findings, serositis, and/or a positive ANA. Twenty-three (1.3 %) of the 1,499 SSc patients satisfied the 1975 Bohan and Peter diagnostic criteria for definite PM/DM [9].

SSc Subset Classification

Cutaneous Classification

Although several different subset classification systems have been proposed, the most widely accepted clinical method of dividing SSc patients is to separate them based on the distribution of skin thickening into diffuse and limited cutaneous subsets [10]. A patient who during the course of his/her disease has *ever* had skin thickening proximal to the elbows or knees (upper arms, thighs, chest, abdomen, back) is considered to have diffuse SSc. Thus, even patients who have had regression of the skin involvement to fit the limited SSc definition are still classified as having diffuse SSc. Patients with limited SSc have either no skin thickening (sine scleroderma) [11] or skin thickening present only distal to the elbows or knees. Facial and neck skin thickening can occur in either variant and do not influence classification. Several authors have proposed that three [12] or even four [13] cutaneous subsets are more appropriate, but these more complicated subsets do not include distinctive clinical, laboratory, or serologic features that convincingly function better than the simple diffuse versus limited SSc classification.

How Is the Diffuse and Limited SSc Classification Helpful?

The cutaneous distribution method is helpful because the natural history of these subsets is different for both skin and internal organ involvement. From a cutaneous standpoint, progression and extent of skin thickening over time is different (Fig. 4.1) in these two subgroups. Mirroring this, the at-risk time of new internal organ involvement is also different between the limited and diffuse SSc patients [14]. Patients with diffuse SSc tend to develop 90 % of their internal organ involvement during the first 2 years of disease (Fig. 4.2).

Assessment of Cutaneous Disease

The classic bedside method for semiquantitative measurement of skin thickness is the modified Rodnan skin score (mRss) [15], in which the examiner grades skin thickness in each of 17 surface anatomic areas as 0 (no skin thickening) to 3 (severe skin thickening). The maximal value is thus 51. Skin thickness is relatively easy to measure and has good interobserver correlation [16]. The mRss correlates closely with the weight of a core dermal punch biopsy from the same site [17]. It should be noted, however, that skin in SSc patients which is not obviously thickened can be abnormal in other clinical respects (hyperpigmentation, telangiectasias). Furthermore, fibroblasts grown from biopsies of apparently normal skin in SSc patients have been shown to have a biochemical "profile" which more closely resembles scleroderma-affected skin than normal skin [18].

Natural History and Disease Staging in Diffuse SSc

Patients with diffuse SSc have a rapid increase in mRss early in their disease. The skin score typically peaks 12–18 months after the first SSc symptom and improves slowly thereafter, although does not necessarily return to 0 (no skin thickening). The skin thickness progression rate, or STPR, is defined as the total skin score at the time of initial evaluation divided by the time since the first symptom attributable to SSc in years. The STPR is an independent predictor of early mortality and risk of renal crisis in early diffuse SSc [19]. In the Pittsburgh experience, the majority of internal organ involvement in diffuse SSc patients is early, and 90 % of the complications experienced within 5 years of disease onset occur in the first 2 years [20] (Fig. 4.2). The exception to this is pulmonary hypertension, which can occur later in disease. During the phase of rapidly increasing skin thickness in dcSSc, there is also a greater frequency of constitutional findings (fatigue, weight loss), arthralgias/arthritis, palpable tendon/bursal friction rubs, carpal tunnel symptoms, and development of finger joint contractures [21].

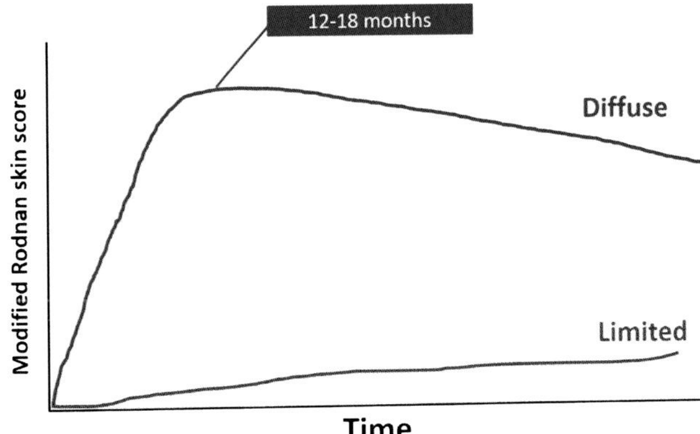

Fig. 4.1 Schematic representation of skin changes over time in diffuse and limited cutaneous SSc. In the majority of patients, maximal skin thickness occurs within 12–18 months from the first symptom attributable to scleroderma

Defining the time of diffuse SSc onset for staging of disease in individual patients is important in reporting groups of patients in the medical literature and in identifying "cutoffs" for enrollment of patients into clinical trials. A number of authors have used the time of first non-Raynaud symptom to define diffuse SSc onset [22–24]. Our opinion is that this is not a good method because Raynaud phenomenon is the first symptom in 40 % of dcSSc patients. In our databank, the first non-Raynaud symptom occurs at a mean of 3 months after the first symptom attributable to SSc in diffuse SSc patients. Thus, if a clinical trial permits entry of patients up to 24 months after disease "onset," a considerable portion of patients will be past the peak of skin thickening, which occurs 7–13 months after the first non-Raynaud symptom (see Fig. 4.1).

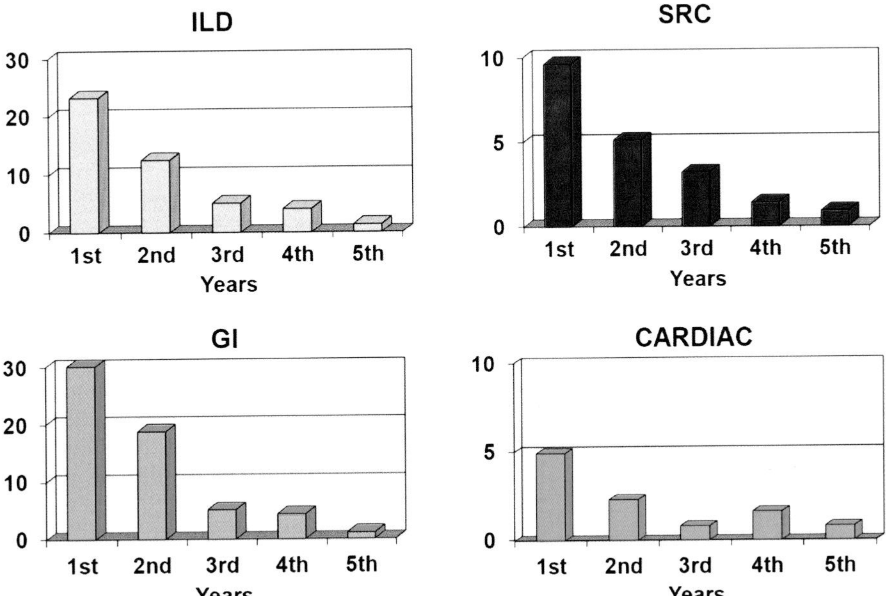

Fig. 4.2 Rate of new internal organ involvement in the first 5 years of diffuse disease. Patients presented with early diffuse SSc (<2 years of symptoms) to the UPMC and University of Pittsburgh Scleroderma Center, 1980–2007

As internal organ involvement typically appears during the first 2 years of disease, one reasonable definition of early diffuse SSc is up to 2 years after the first symptom attributable to SSc (onset) and late diffuse SSc as 5+ years after onset. However, as the majority of skin thickening occurs within the first 18 months of SSc symptoms, an alternative cutaneous-based definition of early diffuse SSc is the first 18 months.

It is incumbent on the managing physician to "stage" his/her patient as "early diffuse," "late diffuse," or, if uncertain, "intermediate diffuse SSc (2–5 years duration)" in order to facilitate appropriate management and counseling of the patient [25]. For example, patients with early diffuse SSc should have careful and routine surveillance for organ involvement, such as blood pressure monitoring for renal crisis. This would be unnecessary in an individual with late dcSSc. A minority of patients who have passed the peak of skin thickening have a "relapse" with redevelopment of increased skin thickening [26]. Such relapses carry all of the internal organ risks associated with the initial increase of skin thickening. The likelihood of later cutaneous exacerbations declines with time even in untreated patients, so that after 10 years, the risk is approximately 5%. Pulmonary hypertension should be screened for in all diffuse SSc patients, regardless of stage.

Natural History and Disease Staging in Limited SSc

In contrast to diffuse SSc, patients with limited SSc have restricted skin thickening distribution (fingers, dorsum of hands, sometimes distal forearms) which does not spread, regardless of how long they are followed, even over decades. In general, limited SSc patients have fewer internal organ complications and better long-term survival in published studies [13]. Distinct from diffuse SSc, patients with limited SSc accumulate their internal organ involvement slowly, sometimes over decades (Fig. 4.3). This means that patients with limited SSc need to be screened for internal organ involvement regardless of how long they have their disease.

Early limited SSc is arbitrarily defined as the first 5 years after the onset of disease. Many such patients will not have seen a physician or had a diagnosis of SSc made during these first 5 years. Raynaud phenomenon with or without digital tip ulceration is most frequently the first symptom, followed by swollen fingers after 1–3 years or even longer. Articular complaints and heartburn often begin during this time period but are typically of minor importance to the patient and not evaluated by the attending physician. Severe finger joint contractures are rare in limited SSc. Serious internal organ involvement in early limited SSc is uncommon. For example, pulmonary fibrosis occurs in fewer than 10% of early limited SSc patients, perhaps in part because many of these individuals have anticentromere antibody, which is seldom associated with interstitial lung disease.

After 10 years of disease, it is more appropriate to use the term late limited SSc. The most obvious difference between late and early limited SSc is that over time, there is an increased frequency of matte-like telangiectasias (face, lips, fingers) and subcutaneous or intracutaneous calcinosis. Skin thickness scores continue to be low or sometimes skin thickness disappears completely. Hand disability in late limited SSc is primarily due to severe Raynaud phe-

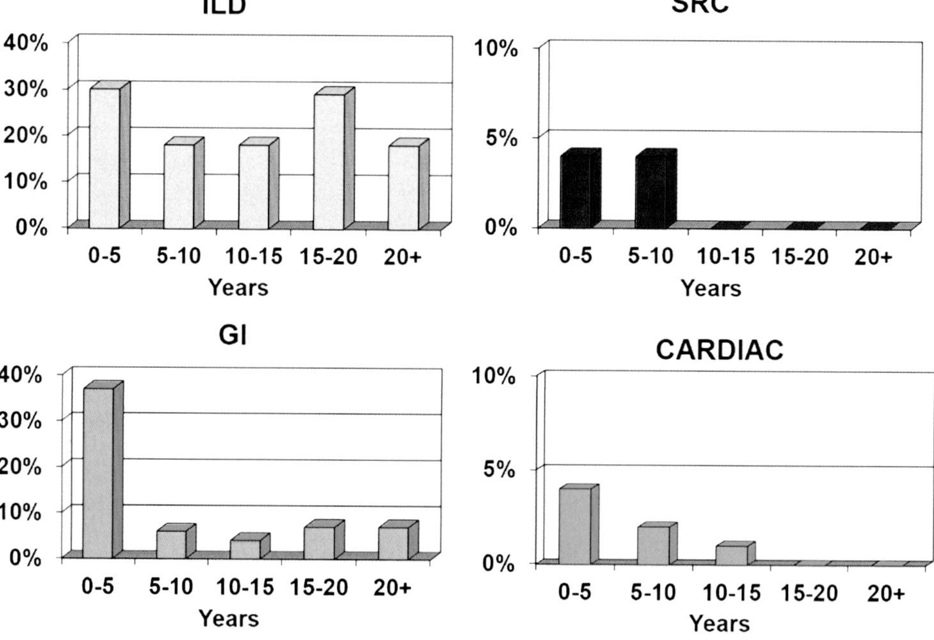

Fig. 4.3 Rate of new internal organ involvement in patients over 20+ years in limited SSc. Patients presented with early limited SSc (<5 years of SSc symptoms) to the UPMC and University of Pittsburgh Scleroderma Center, 1980–2007

nomenon and digital ischemia with digital tip tissue loss and ulcerations. Esophageal symptoms (heartburn, distal dysphagia for solid foods) often persist or worsen as esophageal smooth muscle becomes atrophic and dysfunctional. However, the advent of more effective acid-blocking medical regimens in recent decades has minimized these symptoms and has sharply reduced the frequency of late distal esophageal strictures. Small bowel involvement with diarrhea, weight loss, and episodes of pseudo-obstruction and malabsorption are uncommon but can occur in up to 5 % of late lcSSc patients [27].

The most serious problem in late limited SSc is the development of pulmonary hypertension (PH) in a small minority of patients (approximately 10 %). This complication can occur in SSc patients with long-standing disease (two or more decades) who have had few other disease-related problems.

In late limited SSc patients with coexisting autoimmune diseases, symptoms may be due to the latter conditions rather than due to SSc. Sjogren syndrome can be complicated by polyarthritis, vasculitis affecting the skin (palpable purpura), and peripheral sensory neuropathy or mononeuritis multiplex; such patients most frequently have anti-SSA and/or anti-SSB antibodies and hypocomplementemia [28]. Autoimmune hypothyroidism and primary biliary cirrhosis also occur disproportionately frequently in late limited SSc patients [29, 30].

SSc Sine Scleroderma

SSc sine scleroderma is an uncommon presentation of SSc with classic internal organ manifestations, but no skin thickening. This occurs in <5 % of individuals with SSc [11, 31]. These individuals almost all have Raynaud phenomenon and an SSc-associated serum antibody. The frequency of internal organ involvement and mortality are similar to those in patients with limited SSc [11], and it is felt by most authors that SSc sine scleroderma represents a portion of the spectrum of limited cutaneous SSc. Long-term follow-up of these patients suggests that approximately half will develop some limited skin thickening over time [31].

Overlap Syndromes

It is commonly accepted that there is a subset of SSc patients who demonstrate distinctive features of SSc along with manifestations of other connective tissue diseases, for example, inflammatory myopathies, systemic lupus erythematosus (SLE), or inflammatory arthritides. These patients have frequently been classified as having "overlap syndromes." The concept of overlap syndrome is a difficult one, as there are no accepted guidelines to help managing physicians or clinical investigators define overlaps. When does an SSc patient have SSc-associated polyarthritis and when an overlap with rheumatoid arthritis (RA)? When is polymyositis (PM) an integral part of SSc or a separate CTD? It has been our policy to say that an overlap exists when a patient with definite SSc also satisfies the published classification criteria for SLE [8] or RA [32] or the diagnostic criteria for PM/DM [9]. Although the existence of such patients provides indirect evidence that there are common pathophysiologic processes underlying these rheumatic conditions, further study of these clinically and serologically heterogeneous patients will be necessary for more appropriate classification.

Mixed Connective Tissue Disease

Mixed connective tissue disease (MCTD) was originally described in 1972 and defined by the presence of U1-RNP autoantibody. This was based on the principle that virtually all patients with a U1-RNP antibody had features of SSc, SLE, and PM. Several diagnostic criteria have been published for MCTD [33–37]. The criteria of Alarcon-Segovia and Kahn are felt to be the best. In both the presence of U1-RNP is required. In the Kahn criteria Raynaud plus two of the following is required: swollen fingers, synovitis, or myositis. In the Alarcon-Segovia criteria three of the following features are required (of which synovitis or myositis had to be present): swollen hands, synovitis, myositis, Raynaud, or acrosclerosis.

Although initially a point of debate, MCTD is now generally felt to represent a distinct clinical entity. One difficulty in establishing a diagnosis of MCTD is that the overlapping features can occur sequentially over time, rather than presenting together initially. This often delays a diagnosis of MCTD. The earliest feature is often Raynaud with constitutional symptoms of fatigue, arthralgias, and myalgias. This can lead to an initial differential of undifferentiated connective tissue disease, SLE, or RA. It is frequently later that the more distinctive features emerge (puffy fingers, synovitis, and/or myositis). It should be noted that patients with MCTD may develop prominent features of SLE such as lupus nephritis, although this is uncommon. From a scleroderma spectrum of disease viewpoint, these patients will have typical SSc nailfold capillaroscopy patterns and can develop interstitial lung disease (ILD), PH, and esophageal or small bowel dysmotility. In the case of MCTD, the U1-RNP positivity and SSc-like internal organ risks associated with it can be helpful in patient management.

Classification Based on a Combination of Cutaneous Features and Serum Autoantibodies

The above described SSc cutaneous classification method is very useful, but it is an imperfect system, as clinical organ involvement and outcomes are still heterogenous within the limited and diffuse subsets. Greater specificity regarding the future risk of internal organ involvement may be gained by using a combined cutaneous and serologic classification system. Serum autoantibodies in SSc are described in detail in Chapter 18. For purposes of this discussion, the primary focus is that each of these antibodies is associated with a unique cutaneous subtype and risk profile for internal organ involvement. It is also important to consider that (1) 85–95 % of SSc patients have one of ten SSc-associated serum autoantibodies, (2) seldom (2 %) does a SSc patient have more than one of these antibodies, and (3) different antibodies do not appear over time. One must be cautious, however, with current commercially based ELISA and multiplex antibody assays as it has been our experience that there is a high false-positive anti-Scl-70 rate.

We recommend using the diagram in Fig. 4.4 as a method of placing patients into cutaneous-serologic categories. For each antibody, we have listed those clinical features which are particularly frequent compared with their frequency in other autoantibody subsets. For example, anti-RNA polymerase III antibody is associated with diffuse SSc (90 %) with severe skin thickening (mean maximum mRss in dcSSc patients >30) and a high risk of renal crisis (25 %) [38]. In contrast, anticentromere antibody patients almost all have limited SSc (95 %) and 15 % ultimately develop pulmonary hypertension [39]. For some autoantibodies, the situation is somewhat more complex as they may not as clearly be associated with a cutaneous subtype. For example, anti-topoisomerase (Scl-70) positive patients with diffuse skin thickening have a higher risk of renal and cardiac involvement than do anti-Scl-70 positive limited SSc patients, but the risk of ILD is similar in anti-Scl-70 positive diffuse and limited patients [40].

Clinical-cutaneous disease subsets are clearly associated with different short- and long-term cumulative survival. Table 4.2 depicts the previously unpublished 5- and 10-year cumulative survival rates (CSRs) for 2,500+ SSc patients first evaluated at the University of Pittsburgh Scleroderma Clinic during 1980–2010 from first physician diagnosis of SSc according to cutaneous-serologic subset. Some patient groups are small, making generalizations premature.

Further refinements of the lifetime risk of organ system involvement and the time of onset of these involvements according to autoantibody should be examined in the future. These data will provide managing physicians important information concerning surveillance for complications, regardless of disease stage. Of greatest importance will be the early detection of internal organ involvements which have a high likelihood of progression to disability or death, such as "renal crisis," ILD, and PH, and which can potentially be managed effectively with aggressive ACE inhibitor, anti-inflammatory, immunosuppressive drug, or vasodilator therapies, respectively.

Patient Profiles for SSc Disease Subsetting and Staging

Below are brief patient summaries typical of the combined clinical-serologic profiles described above.

Early Diffuse SSc A 45-year-old woman develops swollen fingers and inflammatory arthralgias affecting the small joints of her hands. Three months later she notes Raynaud

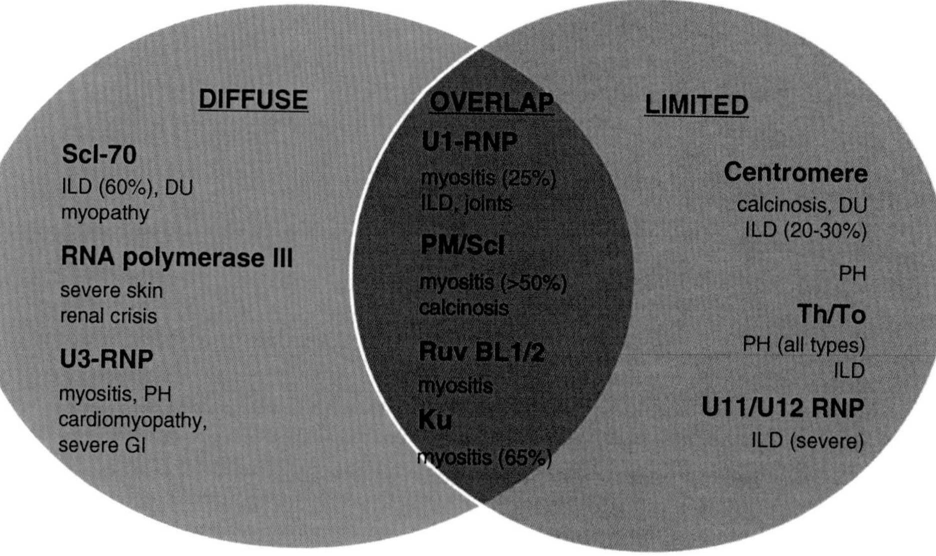

Fig. 4.4 Clinical-serologic classification and internal organ associations

Table 4.2 Cumulative unadjusted survival rates from the UPMC and University of Pittsburgh SSc Center. Survival calculated from SSc diagnosis and presented by cutaneous-serologic subset (first evaluation 1980–2010)

	Diffuse			Limited		
Autoantibody	*N*	5 years (%)	10 years (%)	*N*	5 years (%)	10 years (%)
Scl-70	368	76	57	200	93	78
RNA pol III	549	82	71	74	80	72
ACA	53	90	76	582	86	74
U1-RNP	30	90	78	124	90	82
Ku	10	60	30	12	75	58
U3-RNP	46	74	61	48	81	62
Th/To	4	75	50	180	77	67
PM-Scl	27	95	90	69	95	90
U11/U12	19	62	49	18	83	62

phenomenon. After an additional 2 months, the skin over the dorsum of her hands and forearms becomes thickened, and she has proximal interphalangeal (PIP) joint contractures. Heartburn and fatigue occur next. Eight months after the onset of swollen fingers, she sees her primary care physician, who does an ANA test which is positive at 1:640 with speckled and nucleolar staining.

She is referred to a rheumatologist who makes the diagnosis of SSc 10 months after her first symptom. Physical examination findings include a blood pressure of 120/75, and an mRss of 33 with thickening involving the distal extremities as well as the upper arms, chest, and abdomen. The STPR is rapid at 46 per year [19]. She has palpable wrist extensor and anterior tibial tendon friction rubs and PIP joint contractures. The anti-RNA polymerase III antibody test is positive. HRCT of the chest, echocardiogram, serum creatinine, and urinalysis are all within normal limits. Cine esophagram reveals mild distal esophageal hypomotility.

Late Diffuse SSc A 62-year-old man relocates to another city and sees a new rheumatologist for the first time. Review of his medical records reveals that he developed Raynaud phenomenon at age 47, swollen fingers at age 48, and skin thickening described as "extensive, including the chest and abdomen" later that year. He had flexion contractures of the PIP joints and occasional ulcerations over the dorsal surfaces of the PIP joints. The ANA was positive at 1:160 with speckled and nucleolar staining, and the anti-Scl-70 antibody was positive.

Records after this initial visit were not available. The patient recalls receiving "many medications, none of which seemed to help." He took partial disability for 6 months. He had been told of "a touch of scarring" in the lungs and had mild but nonprogressive dyspnea on exertion. He said that "my esophagus was affected, but acid-blocking drugs controlled heartburn." After several years, skin thickening regressed. In general the patient feels well. He has had no fatigue and is able to work full time as an accountant.

On physical examination he is normotensive. There are faint bibasilar end-inspiratory rales audible. He had an mRss of 6 with 2+ sclerodactyly and 1+ skin thickening of the dorsum of the hands. There are numerous facial telangiectasias. There are several small non-tender digital pitting scars. The PIP joints lacked 20° of extension, and there are healed ulcerations over the PIP joints.

Laboratory studies confirmed the presence of anti-Scl-70 antibody. The erythrocyte sedimentation rate (ESR) and C-reactive protein (CRP) are normal. A high-resolution computed tomography (HRCT) scan of the lungs reveals mild basilar fibrosis with slight honeycombing but without "ground-glass" changes. The forced vital capacity (FVC) is 68 % predicted and DLCO 59 % predicted. Echocardiogram does not show either left or right ventricular dysfunction, and peak systolic pulmonary arterial pressure is estimated as 31 mmHg.

Early Limited Cutaneous SSc A 42-year-old woman noticed painful blanching followed by bluish discoloration of her fingertips on cold exposure beginning in the early fall. At a New Year's Eve party, she had heartburn, which was intermittent thereafter but became more frequent over the next 2 months. In mid-February she developed a small ulceration at the tip of the right index finger. This was quite painful, and she went to her primary care physician. She denied any joint pain or muscle weakness, but attested to morning stiffness of the small joints of her hands for 30–60 min. Her exam was remarkable for a blood pressure of 124/82, periungual erythema, and a small 0.7 cm ulceration on the tip of her right index finger. The primary care provider (PCP) noted blanching of several of the fingertips during the interview. Bloodwork shows a positive ANA, and she was referred to a rheumatologist who found several mat-like telangiectasias on the dorsum of her hands and mild skin thickening of the fingers only. Nailfold capillaroscopy revealed 3+ dilated capillaries with some areas of dropout. There was a digital pitting scar on the left fourth fingertip. Serum testing showed a positive anticentromere antibody. Mild esophageal distal hypomotility was found on cine esophagram. Subsequently, pulmonary function tests, echocardiogram, and electrocardiogram were performed and all were normal.

Late Limited SSc A 54-year-old woman presents to a gastroenterologist for bloating after eating and intermittent bouts of diarrhea which have greatly impacted her quality of life. She has lost 21 lb over the past 6 months. On one occasion she went to an emergency room because of severe abdominal distention. She was told that an abdominal film showed that she was "full of gas and stool." A laxative was prescribed and the symptoms resolved after 1 week. She also complains of daily heartburn for the last 10 years, improved by proton pump inhibitor use. Her past medical history is significant for mild hypertension, hypothyroidism, and Raynaud phenomenon starting around age 40 (14 years previously).

On exam the gastroenterologist notes matte-like telangiectasias on her hands and face. Workup reveals esophagitis/gastritis on esophagogastroduodenoscopy (EGD), as well as delayed gastric emptying and reduced transit time on small bowel follow-through. The gastroenterologist refers her to a rheumatologist because of his concern for possible scleroderma as the cause of her intestinal dysmotility. Further history confirms the presence of SLE in a maternal aunt, and a first cousin has hypothyroidism. The patient notes some mild dyspnea on exertion, but attributes it to lack of exercise due to a demanding job. Physical examination reveals periungual erythema with visibly abnormal nailfold capillaries and sclerodactyly (2+ skin thickening of the fingers bilaterally). She is found to be ANA positive. There is a mild restrictive pattern on pulmonary function tests. High-resolution chest CT shows interstitial fibrosis. Echocardiogram reveals no evidence of pulmonary arterial hypertension.

SSc Sine SSc A 43-year-old woman presents to her PCP for evaluation of progressive dyspnea over the last year. She has a reduced diffusion capacity for carbon monoxide (DLCO) on pulmonary function tests, and an echocardiogram reveals an estimated peak pulmonary arterial systolic pressure of 56 mmHg (normal <40 mmHg). She has normal systolic and diastolic heart function. Electrocardiogram is within normal limits. She is referred to a cardiologist who obtains the additional history of blanching of the fingertips with cold exposure starting after her second pregnancy at age 35. Serum testing reveals the presence of a positive ANA and she is referred to a rheumatologist.

Her review of systems is positive for 10+ years of heartburn and intermittent distal dysphagia for solid foods. She has had to increase her ring size over the last 5 years but denies any skin thickening. Physical examination reveals periungual erythema with visibly abnormal nailfold capillaries and puffy fingers without sclerodactyly. P2 sound is accentuated on auscultation. Additional ANA testing done by immunofluorescence reveals a nucleolar pattern, and the rheumatologist strongly suspects anti-Th/To antibody. Esophageal hypomotility with spontaneous reflux is found on cine esophagram.

Mixed Connective Tissue Disease A 21-year-old college student reported the onset of Raynaud phenomenon and inflammatory polyarthralgias 3 months prior to seeing her PCP. She also had been experiencing low-grade fever and myalgias. The PCP finds no abnormalities on physical examination and a CBC is normal. The ESR and CRP are moderately elevated. He attributes her symptoms to a viral syndrome. When her symptoms have not resolved 6 months later, she returns to her PCP. At this time her aspartate aminotransferase (AST) is abnormal at 52 units/dL (normal <40 units/dL), ALT 69 units/dL (normal <50 units/dL), and alkaline phosphatase normal. Hepatitis panels were negative, and she was referred to a gastroenterologist who ordered an ANA test that returned positive at 1:2560 with speckled nuclear staining. A liver biopsy was performed to evaluate for autoimmune hepatitis and this was normal.

Six months following the biopsy, she developed swelling of the *proximal interphalangeal* (PIP) *join* and *metacarpophalangeal* (MCP) joints. She was referred to a rheumatologist for evaluation of possible RA. She did not complain about muscle weakness, dyspnea, or heartburn. At that time she had MCP and PIP joint polyarthritis, puffy fingers, and skin thickening of the fingers. The neck flexor and shoulder girdle muscles were weak at 4/5. The creatine phosphokinase (CPK) was elevated at 577 units/dL (normal <200 unit/dL). An electromyogram (EMG) suggested inflammatory myopathy and a deltoid muscle biopsy showed changes typical of polymyositis. The cine esophagram was abnormal with mild distal esophageal hypomotility. Pharyngeal swallowing function was normal. A chest x-ray was normal, but a high-resolution CT scan of the lungs revealed bibasilar fibrosis. The FVC was 82% predicted and the DLCO 74% predicted. An echocardiogram was normal. Anti-U1-RNP was positive.

Future Directions

A current limitation of the combined clinical-serologic subset classification is that not all ten SSc-associated serum autoantibodies are easily and accurately available commercially for testing. It is our hope that this may be resolved in the future. Molecular methods such as microarray analysis and gene expression may provide additional information to further refine clinical subsetting and risk stratification in SSc.

References

1. Fries JF, Hochberg MC, Medsger Jr TA, Hunder GG, Bombardier C. Criteria for rheumatic disease. Different types and different functions. The American College of Rheumatology Diagnostic and Therapeutic Criteria Committee. Arthritis Rheum. 1994;37:454–62.
2. Preliminary criteria for the classification of systemic sclerosis (scleroderma). Subcommittee for scleroderma criteria of the American Rheumatism Association Diagnostic and Therapeutic Criteria Committee. Arthritis Rheum. 1980;23:581–90.
3. Lonzetti LS, Joyal F, Raynauld JP, Roussin A, Goulet JR, Rich E, et al. Updating the American College of Rheumatology preliminary classification criteria for systemic sclerosis: addition of severe nailfold capillaroscopy abnormalities markedly increases the sensitivity for limited scleroderma. Arthritis Rheum. 2001;44:735–6.
4. Vayssairat M, Baudot N, Abuaf N, Johanet C. Long-term follow-up study of 164 patients with definite systemic sclerosis: classification considerations. Clin Rheumatol. 1992;11:356–63.
5. van den Hoogen F, Khanna D, Fransen J, Johnson SR, Baron M, Tyndall A, et al. 2013 classification criteria for systemic sclerosis: an American College of Rheumatology/European League against Rheumatism collaborative initiative. Arthritis Rheum. 2013;65:2737–47.
6. van den Hoogen F, Khanna D, Fransen J, Johnson SR, Baron M, Tyndall A, et al. 2013 classification criteria for systemic sclerosis: an American college of rheumatology/European league against rheumatism collaborative initiative. Ann Rheum Dis. 2013;72:1747–55.
7. Matucci-Cerinic M, Allanore Y, Czirjak L, Tyndall A, Muller-Ladner U, Denton C, et al. The challenge of early systemic sclerosis for the EULAR Scleroderma Trial and Research group (EUSTAR) community. It is time to cut the Gordian knot and develop a prevention or rescue strategy. Ann Rheum Dis. 2009;68:1377–80.
8. Tan EM, Cohen AS, Fries JF, Masi AT, McShane DJ, Rothfield NF, et al. The 1982 revised criteria for the classification of systemic lupus erythematosus. Arthritis Rheum. 1982;25:1271–7.
9. Bohan A, Peter JB, Bowman RL, Pearson CM. Computer-assisted analysis of 153 patients with polymyositis and dermatomyositis. Medicine. 1977;56:255–86.
10. LeRoy EC, Black C, Fleischmajer R, Jablonska S, Krieg T, Medsger Jr TA, et al. Scleroderma (systemic sclerosis): classification, subsets and pathogenesis. J Rheumatol. 1988;15:202–5.
11. Poormoghim H, Lucas M, Fertig N, Medsger Jr TA. Systemic sclerosis sine scleroderma: demographic, clinical, and serologic features and survival in forty-eight patients. Arthritis Rheum. 2000;43:444–51.
12. Masi AT. Classification of systemic sclerosis (scleroderma): relationship of cutaneous subgroups in early disease to outcome and serologic reactivity. J Rheumatol. 1988;15:894–8.
13. Giordano M, Valentini G, Migliaresi S, Picillo U, Vatti M. Different antibody patterns and different prognoses in patients with scleroderma with various extent of skin sclerosis. J Rheumatol. 1986;13:911–6.
14. Steen VD, Medsger Jr TA. Epidemiology and natural history of systemic sclerosis. Rheum Dis Clin N Am. 1990;16:1–10.
15. Brennan P, Silman A, Black C, Bernstein R, Coppock J, Maddison P, et al. Reliability of skin involvement measures in scleroderma. The UK Scleroderma Study Group. Br J Rheumatol. 1992;31:457–60.
16. Clements P, Lachenbruch P, Siebold J, White B, Weiner S, Martin R, et al. Inter and intraobserver variability of total skin thickness score (modified Rodnan TSS) in systemic sclerosis. J Rheumatol. 1995;22:1281–5.
17. Rodnan GP, Lipinski E, Luksick J. Skin thickness and collagen content in progressive systemic sclerosis and localized scleroderma. Arthritis Rheum. 1979;22:130–40.
18. Hsu E, Shi H, Jordan RM, Lyons-Weiler J, Pilewski JM, Feghali-Bostwick CA. Lung tissues in patients with systemic sclerosis have gene expression patterns unique to pulmonary fibrosis and pulmonary hypertension. Arthritis Rheum. 2011;63:783–94.
19. Domsic RT, Rodriguez-Reyna T, Lucas M, Fertig N, Medsger Jr TA. Skin thickness progression rate: a predictor of mortality and early internal organ involvement in diffuse scleroderma. Ann Rheum Dis. 2011;70:104–9.
20. Domsic RT, Lucas M, Medsger Jr T. Internal organs are affected very early in diffuse scleroderma: implications for clinical trials (abstract). Clin Exp Rheumatol Scleroderma Care Res. 2010;62(28 Suppl):S-63.
21. Silver R, Medsger Jr T, Bolster M. Systemic sclerosis and scleroderma variants: clinical aspects. In: Koopman W, Moreland LW, editors. Arthritis and allied conditions. 15th ed. Philadelphia: Lippincott Williams & Wilkins; 2005. p. 1633–80.
22. Clements PJ, Furst DE, Wong WK, Mayes M, White B, Wigley F, et al. High-dose versus low-dose D-penicillamine in early diffuse systemic sclerosis: analysis of a two-year, double-blind, randomized, controlled clinical trial. Arthritis Rheum. 1999;42:1194–203.
23. Khanna D, Clements PJ, Furst DE, Korn JH, Ellman M, Rothfield N, et al. Recombinant human relaxin in the treatment of systemic sclerosis with diffuse cutaneous involvement: a randomized, double-blind, placebo-controlled trial. Arthritis Rheum. 2009;60:1102–11.
24. Tashkin DP, Elashoff R, Clements PJ, Goldin J, Roth MD, Furst DE, et al. Cyclophosphamide versus placebo in scleroderma lung disease. N Engl J Med. 2006;354:2655–66.
25. Medsger Jr T. Classification, prognosis. In: Clements P, Furst DE, editors. Systemic sclerosis. 2nd ed. Philadelphia: Lippincott Williams & Wilkins; 2004. p. 17–8.
26. Steen V, Medsger Jr T. Skin flares in systematic sclerosis with diffuse scleroderma (dcSSC). Arthritis Rheum. 2000;43:S319.
27. Rose S, Young MA, Reynolds JC. Gastrointestinal manifestations of scleroderma. Gastroenterol Clin N Am. 1998;27:563–94.
28. Oddis CV, Eisenbeis Jr CH, Reidbord HE, Steen VD, Medsger Jr TA. Vasculitis in systemic sclerosis: association with Sjogren's syndrome and the CREST syndrome variant. J Rheumatol. 1987;14:942–8.
29. Fregeau DR, Leung PS, Coppel RL, McNeilage LJ, Medsger Jr TA, Gershwin ME. Autoantibodies to mitochondria in systemic sclerosis. Frequency and characterization using recombinant cloned autoantigen. Arthritis Rheum. 1988;31:386–92.
30. Gordon MB, Klein I, Dekker A, Rodnan GP, Medsger Jr TA. Thyroid disease in progressive systemic sclerosis: increased frequency of glandular fibrosis and hypothyroidism. Ann Intern Med. 1981;95:431–5.
31. Diab S, Dostrovsky N, Hudson M, Tatibouet S, Fritzler MJ, Baron M, et al. Systemic sclerosis sine scleroderma: a multicenter study of 1417 subjects. J Rheumatol. 2014;41(11):2179–85.
32. Aletaha D, Neogi T, Silman AJ, Funovits J, Felson DT, Bingham 3rd CO, et al. 2010 rheumatoid arthritis classification criteria: an American College of Rheumatology/European League Against Rheumatism collaborative initiative. Ann Rheum Dis. 2010;69:1580–8.
33. Alarcon Segovia D, Villareal M. Classification and diagnostic criteria for mixed connective tissue disease. In: Kasukawa R, Sharp G, editors. Mixed connective tissue disease and anti-nuclear antibodies. Amsterdam: Elsevier; 1987. p. 33.
34. Doria A, Ghirardello A, de Zambiasi P, Ruffatti A, Gambari PF. Japanese diagnostic criteria for mixed connective tissue disease in Caucasian patients. J Rheumatol. 1992;19(2):259–64.
35. Jonsson J, Norberg R. Symptomatology and diagnosis in connective tissue disease. II. Evaluations and follow-up examinations in consequence of a speckled antinuclear immunofluorescence pattern. Scand J Rheumatol. 1978;7:229–36.

36. Kahn M, Appelboom T. Syndrom de Sharp. In: Kahn M, Peltier A, Meyer O, Peiette J, editors. Les maladies systemiques. 3rd ed. Paris: Flammarion; 1991. p. 545.
37. Kasukawa R, Tojo T, Miyawaki S. Preliminary diagnostic criteria for classification of mixed connective tissue disease. In: Kasukawa R, Sharp G, editors. Mixed connective tissue disease and antinuclear antibodies. Amsterdam: Elsevier; 1987. p. 41.
38. Kuwana M, Okano Y, Pandey JP, Silver RM, Fertig N, Medsger Jr TA. Enzyme-linked immunosorbent assay for detection of anti-RNA polymerase III antibody: analytical accuracy and clinical associations in systemic sclerosis. Arthritis Rheum. 2005;52:2425–32.
39. Mitri GM, Lucas M, Fertig N, Steen VD, Medsger Jr TA. A comparison between anti-Th/To- and anticentromere antibody-positive systemic sclerosis patients with limited cutaneous involvement. Arthritis Rheum. 2003;48:203–9.
40. Perera A, Fertig N, Lucas M, Rodriguez-Reyna TS, Hu P, Steen VD, et al. Clinical subsets, skin thickness progression rate, and serum antibody levels in systemic sclerosis patients with anti-topoisomerase I antibody. Arthritis Rheum. 2007;56:2740–6.

Evolving Concepts of Diagnosis and Classification

5

Sindhu R. Johnson, Lorinda Chung, Jaap Fransen, and Frank H.J. Van den Hoogen

Systemic sclerosis (SSc) is a rare connective tissue disease characterized by fibrosis of the skin and internal organs and a vasculopathy affecting the micro- and macrovasculature. The pathogenesis of SSc involves the interplay between vascular injury and dysregulation of the immune response with resultant fibrosis of various target organs. More than 90 % of patients with SSc suffer from Raynaud's phenomenon, a reversible vasospastic disorder induced by cold or stress, which results in typical white, blue, and red color changes of the distal extremities from decreased perfusion [1]. Other clinical features that are common in patients with SSc in addition to cutaneous sclerosis include pulmonary disease (interstitial lung disease and pulmonary hypertension), gastrointestinal dysmotility and malabsorption, digital ulcerations, inflammatory myositis and arthritis, and cardiac and renal disease. There are two main subsets of SSc that are commonly recognized: limited cutaneous SSc and diffuse cutaneous SSc. The two subsets differ in manifestations and in prognosis and presumably to some extent also in their pathogenesis. Although disease-modifying therapies have demonstrated minimal efficacy in SSc [2–6], several organ-specific therapies have emerged over the past couple of decades resulting in improved survival and quality of life. These include angiotensin-converting enzyme (ACE) inhibitors for the treatment of scleroderma renal crisis (SRC) [7] and various agents for the treatment of pulmonary arterial hypertension (PAH), including prostacyclins, endothelin receptor antagonists, and phosphodiesterase-5 inhibitors [8]. The development of successful disease-modifying therapies for SSc is hindered by the heterogeneous clinical manifestations of this disease, also making early diagnosis challenging. Patients with early disease are more likely to respond to targeted therapies, and irreversible organ damage may be prevented. For studying the effects of potential disease-modifying drugs, and for more successful treatment in clinical practice, it is of paramount importance to recognize the presence of SSc early in the disease process. This is equally important for the diagnosis in clinical practice as well as for classification criteria used to include patients in clinical studies. If patients who are classified with SSc are similar to patients who are diagnosed with the disease, then it is straightforward to generalize evidence from clinical studies to those patients who have been diagnosed in practice. Therefore, classification and diagnosis in SSc should be developed toward recognition of SSc early in the disease process. This chapter will review the clinical subsets of SSc, the classification criteria for SSc, and ongoing and future projects for revising and improving classification criteria.

S.R. Johnson, MD, PhD, FRCPC (✉)
Toronto Scleroderma Program, Mount Sinai Hospital, Toronto Western Hospital, Toronto, ON, Canada
e-mail: Sindhu.Johnson@uhn.ca

L. Chung, MD, MS
Department of Medicine and Dermatology (Immunology and Rheumatology Division), Stanford University School of Medicine and the Palo Alto VA Hospital, Palo Alto, CA 94305, USA

J. Fransen, PhD • F.H.J. Van den Hoogen, MD, PhD
Department of Rheumatology, Radboud University Nijmegen Medical Center and Sint Maartenskliniek, Nijmegen, The Netherlands

Classification and Diagnosis

Classification criteria are not synonymous with diagnostic criteria but will almost always mirror the list of criteria that one uses for diagnosis. A clinical diagnosis results from a clinical evaluation for features that suggest the presence (absence) of disease, which ultimately results in the physician making his/her mind up over the probability of the disease (SSc) being present. Therefore, classification according to diagnosis and the diagnostic process in practice are regarded as different. Classification typically has a yes/no

J. Varga et al. (eds.), *Scleroderma*, DOI 10.1007/978-3-319-31407-5_5

form, while diagnosis involves the concept of probability. Since the function of classification criteria is to identify more homogeneous groups of patients (a narrower range of the disease spectrum), classification criteria may exclude some patients with the disease in question (SSc) [9]. Classification of individuals should be determined at the time classification criteria are evaluated and met [10].

Clinical Subsets of Systemic Sclerosis

Original LeRoy Classification

In 1988, an international panel of scleroderma experts convened to define subsets of SSc that are clinically distinguishable [11]. The two subsets were termed diffuse cutaneous (dSSc) and limited cutaneous SSc (lSSc), with the extent of cutaneous sclerosis as the primary differentiating feature. Patients with lSSc have skin involvement that is limited to the hands, forearms, feet, legs below the knees, and face, whereas those with dSSc have also skin involvement proximal to the elbows and knees and/or truncal involvement. The debate as to whether these subsets represent different diseases or a spectrum of the same disease has not entirely been settled. These two subsets follow different disease courses with particular organ manifestations [12, 13] and typically experience different outcomes, with poorer survival rates in patients with dSSc [14]. Patients with dSSc usually develop Raynaud's phenomenon within a year of onset of skin changes, whereas patients with lSSc often experience symptoms of Raynaud's phenomenon for years before cutaneous or internal organ manifestations develop [12]. Together with the often rapid progression of cutaneous sclerosis in patients with dSSc, tendon friction rubs and joint contractures commonly develop [11, 12]. Patients with dSSc are also more likely to develop severe interstitial lung disease (ILD), SRC, or myocardial involvement during the first few years of disease than those with lSSc, who typically have a late onset of pulmonary disease, particularly PAH [12]. These two subsets are also distinguished serologically, with the anticentromere antibody (ACA) associated with lSSc with a specificity of 93 % and the anti-Scl-70 antibody associated with dSSc with a specificity of 82 % [15]. The CREST syndrome, an acronym for calcinosis, Raynaud's phenomenon, esophageal dysmotility, sclerodactyly, and telangiectasias, has been considered a subset of lSSc because of the strong association with ACA [15, 16]. However, because patients with dSSc can present with any of the five features of CREST, the use of this term as a subset of lcSSc can be confusing [17]. The classical two subset (dSSc vs. lSSc) classification scheme has been the most frequently cited, and widely used in registries, clinical studies and therapeutic trials [18].

Three-Subset Cutaneous Model of SSc

Three-subset models of SSc based on extent of skin involvement have been proposed by at least four groups [19–22]. The 3-subset model described by Masi in 1988 included the following subsets: (1) lcSSc with sclerosis of fingers with or without sclerosis of the neck and/or face; (2) intermediate cutaneous SSc (ISSc) with sclerosis of upper and lower limbs, neck, and face, without truncal involvement; and (3) dSSc with truncal and acral involvement as described by LeRoy et al. [11, 22]. Survival analysis in a cohort of Italian patients demonstrated that ISSc patients had survival rates that are midway between those of lcSSc and dSSc [10]. However, a different study in a French Canadian population showed no significant difference in survival between lcSSc and ISSc, but did demonstrate a significant survival difference between patients with lcSSc and dSSc [23]. In addition, anticentromere antibodies have been found to perform best in predicting limited cutaneous involvement in SSc distal to the elbows and knees as opposed to fingers alone [15]. The ISSc subset becomes unnecessary when defining lcSSc more broadly, and therefore, the three-subset model has not been used in the majority of clinical studies. However, the three-subset model highlights the prognostic value of skin involvement, even within lcSSc or dSSc.

Systemic Sclerosis Sine Scleroderma

In 1986, Giordano et al. proposed a four-subset cutaneous classification with the inclusion of a group of patients who lacked any evidence of cutaneous sclerosis but had other systemic features of SSc [21]. This group of patients has been termed SSc sine scleroderma (ssSSc) and has since been further characterized [24]. The largest study of patients with ssSSc performed at University of Pittsburgh defined these patients as follows: a clinical diagnosis of SSc with no skin thickening on physical examination and one or more of the following visceral involvements typical of SSc: distal esophageal or small bowel hypomotility, pulmonary fibrosis, PAH, cardiac involvement, or SRC [24]. In addition, Raynaud's phenomenon or a peripheral vascular equivalent (digital pitting scars, digital tip ulcers or gangrene, abnormal nailfold capillaries), a positive antinuclear antibody (ANA), and the absence of another defined connective tissue disease were considered necessary for the diagnosis of ssSSc. This study compared 48 patients with ssSSc to 507 patients with lSSc as defined by LeRoy et al. No differences were found in the frequencies of individual internal organ involvements, laboratory features, SSc-specific autoantibodies, or survival between the groups. In this study, ssSSc patients were more likely to be ANA positive with other non-SSc-specific autoantibodies than lSSc patients. The authors concluded that ssSSc patients should be considered a form of lSSc rather than a distinct subset [24].

Early SSc Versus Undifferentiated Connective Tissue Disease

Early in the disease course, patients with SSc may present with some symptoms or signs suggestive of the disease, as well as serologic abnormalities, without fulfilling the classification criteria for SSc. These patients may be described as undifferentiated or unclassified connective tissue disease (UCTD). The definition of UCTD includes patients with clinical manifestations suggestive of any CTD and the presence of at least one non-organ-specific autoantibody, such as antinuclear antibodies (ANA) or anti-extractable nuclear antigen antibodies (ENA) [25, 26]. Although the majority of patients with UCTD remain undifferentiated or remit, up to one-third of patients may develop an established CTD within 5 years of follow-up [27]. Evolution into SSc occurs in 8–39 % of those UCTD patients who develop a definite CTD [27, 28]. The most frequent symptom at the onset of UCTD is Raynaud's phenomenon, and 10 % of patients with isolated Raynaud's phenomenon have been shown to progress to SSc [25, 27]. Sclerodactyly and esophageal dysfunction at the onset of UCTD have been identified as significant predictors for evolution into SSc [28]. Therefore, a subset of patients with UCTD may represent those with early SSc, particularly those with sclerodactyly and/or esophageal dysfunction.

Evolution of Mixed Connective Tissue Disease into SSc

Mixed connective tissue disease was initially described by Sharp et al. in 1972 as a disorder displaying clinical features of SLE, SSc, and PM/DM in association with the presence of a high titer of anti-U1-ribonucleoprotein (RNP) antibodies [29]. Debate exists as to whether MCTD represents a distinct disease entity or a variant of individual CTDs [30]. Anti-U1-RNP antibodies occur in approximately 7–21 % of SSc patients and can be present in other CTDs as well [31, 32]. In addition, 55 % of patients initially classified as MCTD can be diagnosed as having one or a combination of two CTDs within 5 years of follow-up [33]. In one study, approximately one-third of MCTD patients evolved into SSc or an SSc overlap syndrome [33]. Therefore, a subset of patients with MCTD may in reality represent early SSc. The identification of predictive factors for the evolution of MCTD into SSc may be useful in recognizing patients who have early SSc.

American Rheumatism Association/ American College of Rheumatology Classification Criteria

Study Design and Description

The intent of the 1980 American College of Rheumatology (ACR) classification criteria for SSc was "to establish a standard for definite or certain disease in order to permit comparison of groups of patients from different centers and to assist in the proper evaluation of the results of clinical investigation and therapeutic trials" [34]. These criteria were not designed to aid in the diagnosis of early disease, but were based on patients who had a diagnosis of definite SSc that was made no longer than 2 years before entry into the study. The study included 264 cases of definite SSc and 413 comparison patients with systemic lupus erythematosus (SLE), polymyositis/dermatomyositis (PM/DM), and Raynaud's phenomenon. Twenty-nine rheumatology centers in the USA, Canada, and Mexico were involved in this multicenter effort. Table 5.1 shows the clinical and laboratory variables originally selected for criteria analysis [34]. Using univariate and multivariate analyses, the goal was to find the fewest items that yielded the highest sensitivity and specificity for SSc.

The final classification criteria are listed in Table 5.2 [34]. Proximal scleroderma, defined as "sclerodermatous involvement proximal to the digits, affecting proximal portions of the extremities, the face, neck, or trunk," was found to be the most useful major criterion with a specificity of 99.8 % differentiating SSc cases from comparison patients. Using multivariate analytic techniques, three minor criteria were identified: (1) sclerodactyly, (2) digital pitting scars of fingertips or loss of substance of the distal finger pad, and (3) bilateral basilar pulmonary fibrosis on chest X-ray. Either the one major criterion or two minor criteria provided a sensitivity of 97 % and specificity of 98 % [34]. The proposed criteria were then externally validated using more than 1,300 case and comparison patients stored in the American Rheumatism Association Medical Information System (ARAMIS) database, yielding a sensitivity of 92 % and a specificity of 96 % [34].

Limitations

As mentioned above, the intent of the criteria was not specifically to identify patients with early SSc, and in fact, 35 patients with probable or early-stage SSc were excluded from the analyses. Therefore, the population of patients who are most likely to benefit from therapeutic interventions, and who should be targeted for enrollment into clinical trials, is not represented by these classification criteria. Several studies have verified the low sensitivity of the ACR classification criteria for early SSc. A study comparing 240 SSc patients

Table 5.1 Clinical and laboratory variables originally selected for criteria for classification of SSc

Clinical variables	Laboratory variables
Sclerodermatous skin changes	LE cell preparation
Any location	FANA, any titer
Sclerodactyly	Latex agglutination, any titer
Proximal scleroderma	X-ray findings
Face or neck	Digital tuft resorption
Bilateral hand edema	Calcinosis, subcutaneous
Digital pitting scars	Bibasilar pulmonary fibrosis
Hand deformity or contractures	Abnormal electromyogram
Abnormal skin pigmentation	Esophageal manometry
Raynaud's phenomenon	Abnormal proximal only
Telangiectasia, fingers	Abnormal distal only
	Abnormal proximal and distal
	Gastrointestinal X-ray
	Esophageal hypomotility proximal only
	Esophageal hypomotility distal only
	Esophageal hypomotility proximal and distal
	Duodenal loop dilatation
	Colonic sacculations
	Skin biopsy with dermal collagen thickening
	Anti-RNP
	Anti-Sm
	ESR
	Serum complement (C3)
	Urine creatine excretion
	SGOT

Modified from Williams et al. [27]
LE lupus erythematosus, *FANA* fluorescent antinuclear antibody, *RNP* ribonucleoprotein, *Sm* Smith, *ESR* erythrocyte sedimentation rate, *SGOT* serum glutamic oxaloacetic transaminase

from the USA and 87 SSc patients from France showed sensitivities of 83 % and 87 % in the two populations, respectively [32]. Nadashkevich et al. reported an even lower sensitivity of 70 % due to the exclusion of patients with early disease who had SSc-specific serologic markers and rapidly progressive disease [35].

In addition to excluding patients with early SSc, the current ACR classification criteria exclude a substantial portion of patients with established mild or limited cutaneous disease. An initial evaluation of the ACR classification criteria in the Pittsburgh SSc cohort found that 41 % of lcSSc did not fulfill the major criterion, and 20 % did not fulfill either the major or two of the three minor criteria [36]. Maricq and Valter reported that only 53 % of their cohort, which included patients with diffuse and intermediate cutaneous involvement, sclerodactyly only, sine sclerosis,

Table 5.2 1980 American rheumatism association criteria for the classification of systemic sclerosis [27]

Major criterion: proximal cutaneous sclerosis
Induration of the skin proximal to the metacarpophalangeal or metatarsophalangeal joints, affecting other parts of the extremities, face, neck, or trunk, usually bilateral, symmetrical, and almost always including sclerodactyly
Minor criteria
1. Sclerodactyly
2. Digital pitting scars of fingertips or loss of substance of the distal finger pad
3. Bibasilar pulmonary fibrosis

One major criterion or two or more minor criteria provide a sensitivity of 97 % and specificity of 98 % for definite systemic sclerosis

UCTD, and CREST, fulfilled the ACR criteria [37]. Ninety-six percent (77/80) of patients in the latter three categories with more mild disease were excluded [37]. Hudson et al. studied a group of SSc patients from the Canadian Scleroderma Research Group who had skin involvement distal to the metacarpophalangeal joints only. Of 101 patients, only 68 (67 %) met the ACR classification criteria [38]. Lonzetti et al. reported an even poorer sensitivity with only one-third of French Canadian patients with lcSSc as diagnosed by expert clinicians fulfilling the 1980 ACR classification criteria [39].

Importance of Revising ACR Classification Criteria

There were several reasons why revision of the ACR classification criteria was necessary and timely. As described above, the poor sensitivity of the ACR Classification Criteria for patients with early SSc limits the identification of patients who may potentially have a greater response to treatment before irreversible damage ensues. Therefore, exclusion of these patients affects early diagnosis in clinical practice, as well as enrollment of appropriate patients in clinical studies and therapeutic trials. The low sensitivity for patients with lcSSc has also resulted in exclusion of a large portion of eligible patients in clinical trials. LcSSc patients may indeed benefit from treatments targeting cutaneous sclerosis, ILD, PAH, Raynaud's phenomenon, and digital ulcerations and should not be excluded from these studies. Technological advances in the past few decades provide an opportunity to improve the sensitivity of the current classification criteria. In particular, the development and widespread availability of tests for SSc-specific autoantibodies and nailfold capillary abnormalities have improved the detection of early SSc and should be incorporated into the revised classification criteria. Data supporting the utility of these tests in the diagnosis of SSc will be discussed below.

Autoantibodies in the Diagnosis of SSc

Autoantibodies are detected in more than 95 % of patients with SSc [40]. Seven SSc-specific autoantibodies have been described, but not all are widely clinically available (Table 5.3). These autoantibodies are rarely detected in patients with other CTDs and very infrequently observed in the general population [15]. These antibodies generally remain stable over time and are mutually exclusive in the majority of patients [15]. Autoantibody status (ACA vs. anti-Scl-70 antibody positivity) has been shown to supersede cutaneous subset (lcSSc vs. dSSc) in predicting the development of particular SSc organ manifestations [13]. Autoantibodies have also been shown to precede the onset of symptoms in SSc and other CTDs, such as SLE, and therefore, they are useful in the early diagnosis of disease [41, 42].

Anticentromere Antibodies

ACA have a high specificity for the limited cutaneous subset of SSc, but 5–7 % of patients with dSSc can have ACA [13, 40]. ACA have been associated with long disease duration at diagnosis with a mean of 8.7 years since first SSc symptom onset at the time of diagnosis [40]. Patients with ACA have a significantly higher prevalence of digital tip ulcers, gangrene, digital tuft resorption, and calcinosis than patients with other SSc-specific autoantibodies, but significantly lower prevalence of arthritis or muscle inflammation [40]. In addition, ACA are associated with the development of isolated pulmonary hypertension [13, 40].

As a diagnostic test for SSc, ACA detected by indirect immunofluorescence show a high degree of specificity, but fairly low sensitivity. Compared with healthy controls, the ACA has a specificity of almost 100 %, but a sensitivity of 33 % [15]. The sensitivity improves to 65 % when comparing the frequency of ACA in patients meeting at least two of five CREST criteria to healthy controls. The sensitivity is 31 % when diagnosing SSc compared with other CTDs, but the specificity remains high at 97.4 %. When compared with patients with primary Raynaud's phenomenon, the sensitivity is 24.1 % and specificity 90 % [15]. Given the overall high specificity for diagnosing SSc and the strong predictive value in determining internal organ involvement, ACA appears to be a good candidate for inclusion in diagnosis or classification of SSc.

Table 5.3 Scleroderma-specific autoantibodies

Anticentromere[a]
Anti-Scl-70 (anti-topoisomerase I)[a]
Anti-PM-Scl[b]
Anti-Th/To[b]
Anti-U3-ribonucleoprotein (antifibrillarin)[b]
Anti-RNA polymerase I/III
Anti-U1-ribonucleoprotein

[a]Clinically available at the majority of centers

[b]Associated with nucleolar staining pattern of antinuclear antibody

Anti-Scl-70 Antibodies

Anti-Scl-70 (also known as anti-topoisomerase I) antibodies are classically associated with diffuse cutaneous disease; however, 31–36 % of SSc patients with anti-Scl-70 antibodies have lcSSc [13]. Anti-Scl-70 positivity is associated with a higher prevalence of arthritis, tendon friction rubs, severe pulmonary fibrosis, severe heart disease, and SRC than other SSc-specific autoantibodies, presumably due to the association of these organ manifestations with diffuse cutaneous disease [40]. Similar to ACA, anti-Scl-70 antibodies also confer a higher risk for compromise of the microvasculature with a high prevalence of digital tip ulcers, gangrene, and digital tuft resorption in patients with anti-Scl-70 antibodies [40]. Unlike diffuse cutaneous involvement, anti-Scl-70 positivity is associated with a higher prevalence of myocardial conduction block and diastolic dysfunction, but a lower prevalence of hypertension, than ACA positivity [13].

Similar to ACA, anti-Scl-70 antibodies detected by immunodiffusion have a very high specificity of 100 % compared with normal controls; however, the sensitivity is only 20.2 % [15]. Compared with patients with other CTDs or primary Raynaud's phenomenon, the specificity remains high at 99.5 % and 98 %, with sensitivity of 26 % and 28 %, respectively [15]. The sensitivity improves to approximately 40 % when compared with normal controls and other CTDs if immunoblotting techniques are used to detect anti-Scl-70 antibodies [15]. Further data on the diagnostic value of anti-Scl-70 antibodies detected by enzyme-linked immunosorbent assays (ELISA) is necessary. The high specificity of anti-Scl-70 antibodies, and the ability to predict organ involvement even better than the diffuse cutaneous subset, makes these antibodies important to consider in revised classification criteria for SSc.

Anti-nucleolar Antibodies

A nucleolar staining pattern of ANA on indirect immunofluorescence can be observed when any of the following SSc-specific autoantibodies is present: anti-PM-Scl, anti-Th/To, anti-U3-RNP (antifibrillarin), and anti-RNA polymerase

(RNAP) I, II, and III. The anti-RNAP antibodies, and in particular anti-RNAP III, demonstrate nucleolar staining only 30–44 % of the time [43, 44]; therefore, nucleolar staining on the ANA is not useful as a screening test for these autoantibodies, and they will be discussed separately. Immunodiffusion to detect anti-PM-Scl antibodies is commercially available, while the other nucleolar autoantibodies are typically detected by immunoprecipitation performed only at certain centers. However, a new ELISA for the detection of antibodies to fibrillarin and PM-Scl was recently described [45]. When evaluated in 50 SSc patients who were negative for ACA and anti-Scl-70 compared with 122 controls (42 SSc positive for ACA or anti-Scl-70, 40 SLE, and 40 rheumatoid arthritis), the antifibrillarin ELISA had a sensitivity of 22 % and specificity of 92.5 %, and the anti-PM-Scl antibody had a sensitivity of 8 % and specificity of 98.8 % [45]. This study, however, did not compare the sensitivity and specificity of the ELISAs to immunoprecipitation.

Anti-PM-Scl antibodies are detected in 3–12.5 % of patients with SSc and are associated with a high prevalence of muscle inflammation [32, 46]. Patients with anti-PM-Scl antibodies also have a high prevalence of severe pulmonary fibrosis and digital ulcers with a lower frequency of PAH [40, 46].

Anti-Th/To antibodies are associated with the limited cutaneous subset and have been reported in up to 24 % of lcSSc patients compared with 2 % of dSSc patients [40]. Patients with these autoantibodies have a high prevalence of pulmonary fibrosis and pulmonary hypertension, as well as severe gastrointestinal involvement [40]. Compared with ACA, lcSSc patients with anti-Th/To antibodies have more subtle skin disease, less severe digital vasculopathy, and a higher prevalence of ILD [47]. The presence of anti-Th/To antibodies in patients with lcSSc portends a poorer prognosis than other SSc-specific autoantibodies [40, 47].

Anti-U3-RNP antibodies are present in 8 % of patients with SSc and are associated with African American race [48]. These autoantibodies are associated with male gender and the diffuse cutaneous subset. SSc patients with these autoantibodies have a high prevalence of pulmonary fibrosis, cardiac, renal, and gastrointestinal involvement [40, 48]. Initial reports did not find an association between anti-U3-RNP antibodies and pulmonary hypertension, but a more recent study found an increased frequency of the combination of ILD and isolated pulmonary hypertension in patients with anti-U3-RNP antibodies [40].

Although anti-nucleolar antibodies have been reported in 15–40 % of patients with SSc, few studies have reported the frequency of these autoantibodies in healthy controls or other CTDs [15]. A recent study indicated that anti-PM-Scl antibodies have a specificity of 96.9 % for SSc when compared with healthy controls and other CTDs, but no patients with PM/DM were included in the comparison group [46]. Anti-Th/To antibodies have been shown to be 98.8 % specific for SSc when compared with other CTDs [49]. However, one report evaluating for antifibrillarin antibodies by radioimmunoassay found that these antibodies were present in a large percentage of patients with MCTD, SLE, rheumatoid arthritis, and Sjogren's syndrome in addition to patients with SSc [50]. The lack of specificity of the radioimmunoassay for antifibrillarin antibodies may not apply to immunoprecipitation methods. Although anti-nucleolar antibodies may be specific for SSc, the variable sensitivity and the lack of widespread commercially available assays for these autoantibodies make them less useful for classification criteria.

Anti-RNA Polymerase Antibodies

Anti-RNAP antibodies detected by immunoprecipitation have been reported in 4–25 % of patients with SSc depending on the population studied [32, 44]. On indirect immunofluorescence, these antibodies typically display a fine-speckled nucleoplasmic stain with additional occasional bright dots, with or without concurrent punctate nucleolar staining [44]. Although anti-RNAP II antibodies are not specific for SSc and have been reported in 9–14 % of patients with SLE and MCTD, antibodies to RNAP I and III detected by immunoprecipitation have a specificity of >99 % for SSc when compared with other CTDs [51]. Anti-RNAP III antibodies are associated with diffuse cutaneous disease and a high prevalence of SRC, but a low frequency of severe pulmonary fibrosis [40]. In recent years, anti-RNAP III antibodies have been detected by ELISA and have become more widely available. Compared with immunoprecipitation, the ELISA has a sensitivity of 91–96 % and specificity of 98–99 % [44, 52]. As a diagnostic test for SSc, the sensitivity and specificity of the ELISA for anti-RNAP III have been reported as 11–17 % and 98–99 %, respectively [52, 53]. The relatively high sensitivity and specificity of anti-RNAP III antibodies for SSc, the strong predictive value of these antibodies for diffuse skin disease and SRC, and the increasing availability of the ELISA assay to test for these antibodies are all reasons that anti-RNAP III antibodies may be considered for inclusion in the revised ACR classification criteria.

Anti-U1-RNP Antibodies

As described above, anti-U1-RNP antibodies are present in high titers in patients with MCTD, but they can also be detected in 7–21 % of patients with SSc [31, 32]. Clinical features associated with the presence of anti-U1-RNP antibodies in patients with SSc include a younger age at disease onset, vasospasm, arthritis, muscle inflammation, and ILD [31, 40]. In patients with lcSSc, the presence of anti-U1-RNP antibodies predicts a better survival when compared with other SSc-specific antibodies [40]. Given the high prevalence of anti-U1-RNP antibodies in patients with MCTD, overlap syndromes, and other CTDs, these antibodies may not be useful in classification criteria for SSc.

Nailfold Capillaroscopy in the Diagnosis of SSc

Nailfold Capillaroscopic Patterns in SSc

Since the 1970s, patients with SSc have been known to demonstrate a distinct pattern of nailfold capillary abnormalities when examined microscopically compared with patients with primary Raynaud's phenomenon and other connective tissue diseases [54, 55]. Maricq et al. initially described the scleroderma pattern of capillary abnormalities using in vivo widefield capillaroscopic techniques. Enlarged and deformed capillary loops surrounded by relatively avascular areas were found in 82 % of patients with SSc and 54 % of patients with MCTD but only 2 % of patients with SLE [55]. One of 11 patients with primary Raynaud's phenomenon showed these changes, but this patient developed SSc 5 months after the initial capillaroscopic examination. Another study found that the presence of the scleroderma pattern of capillary abnormalities predicted the development of SSc in five of ten patients with Raynaud's phenomenon within 9 months to 5 years of follow-up [56]. A more recent study found that approximately 14 % of patients with UCTD had the scleroderma pattern on nailfold capillaroscopy and thus may be at higher risk of progressing to SSc or a related CTD [57].

During the past decade, nailfold videocapillaroscopic techniques have been used to describe three patterns of microangiopathy in SSc that correlate with disease duration: early, active, and late (Fig. 5.1) [58, 59]. The early pattern is characterized by few (fewer than four altered capillaries per millimeter) enlarged or giant capillaries, few capillary hemorrhages, relatively well-preserved capillary distribution, and no evident loss of capillaries. The active pattern demonstrates frequent (more than six altered capillaries per millimeter) giant capillaries, frequent capillary hemorrhages, 20–30 % loss of capillaries, mild (between 4 and 6 altered capillaries per millimeter) disorganization of the capillary architecture, and absent or mild ramified capillaries. The late pattern shows irregular enlargement of the capillaries, few or absent giant capillaries and hemorrhages, and 50–70 % loss of capillaries with large avascular areas, disorganization of the normal capillary array, and ramified or bushy capillaries [58, 59]. The late pattern was shown to be associated with older age and longer duration of Raynaud's phenomenon and SSc when compared with the early and active patterns [59]. Therefore, the early capillaroscopic changes of enlarged and giant capillaries, along with hemorrhages, likely represent the earliest microvascular changes observed in patients with SSc or related diseases, and may be useful in the early diagnosis of SSc.

Office Capillaroscopy

Although widefield microscopy and nailfold videocapillaroscopy provide detailed images of the nailfolds and have excellent inter- and intra-rater reliability in the detection of giant capillaries, microhemorrhages, and capillary loss [60], these modalities are not widely available and require specific training to use the instruments. The ophthalmoscope is a widely accessible instrument that has been used to assess for nailfold capillary abnormalities in the office setting with the application of a drop of oil or immersion gel to the nailfold surface. One study showed that the ophthalmoscope detected giant capillaries, severe avascular areas (loss of more than six capillaries), and bushy capillaries with 100 % correlation with the stereomicroscope [61]. However, another study showed only moderate agreement between use of the ophthalmoscope and the microscope in detecting dilated and giant capillaries (kappa 0.63 and 0.52, respectively), with poor agreement in the detection of avascular areas (defined as any confluent area free of capillary loops) (kappa <0.1) [62]. The latter study also showed moderate inter- and intra-rater reliability for the ophthalmoscopic detection of dilated (kappa 0.43 and 0.61) and giant (kappa 0.54 and 0.56) capillaries with poor reliability for detection of avascular areas (kappa 0.19 and 0.31) [62].

The dermatoscope is a handheld, battery-powered instrument used by dermatologists to assess pigmented and other skin lesions. The most current models use a polarized light source that eliminates reflection from the skin surface and therefore do not require the application of oil or immersion gel. When compared with the standard microscope, the dermatoscope has shown excellent agreement for the detection of dilated capillaries (kappa 0.93), megacapillaries (kappa 0.97), avascular areas (kappa 0.93), and microhemorrhages (kappa 0.94) [63]. The inter- and intra-rater reliability using the dermatoscope was better than that of the ophthalmoscope for detecting dilated (kappa 0.63 and 0.71) and giant (kappa 0.4 and 0.55) capillaries but was also poor for the detection of avascular areas (kappa 0.2 and 0.4) [62]. The dermatoscope is relatively inexpensive and is easy to use with a mean capillaroscopic examination time of 4 min [63]. When used to differentiate patients with SSc from healthy controls, the presence of two or more enlarged capillaries in one or more fingers as detected by the dermatoscope showed a sensitivity of 83 % and specificity of 100 % for the diagnosis of SSc [64]. Hudson et al. assessed the effect of the addition of capillaroscopic changes detected by the dermatoscope to the sensitivity of the ACR criteria in a population of SSc patients with skin involvement distal to the metacarpophalangeal

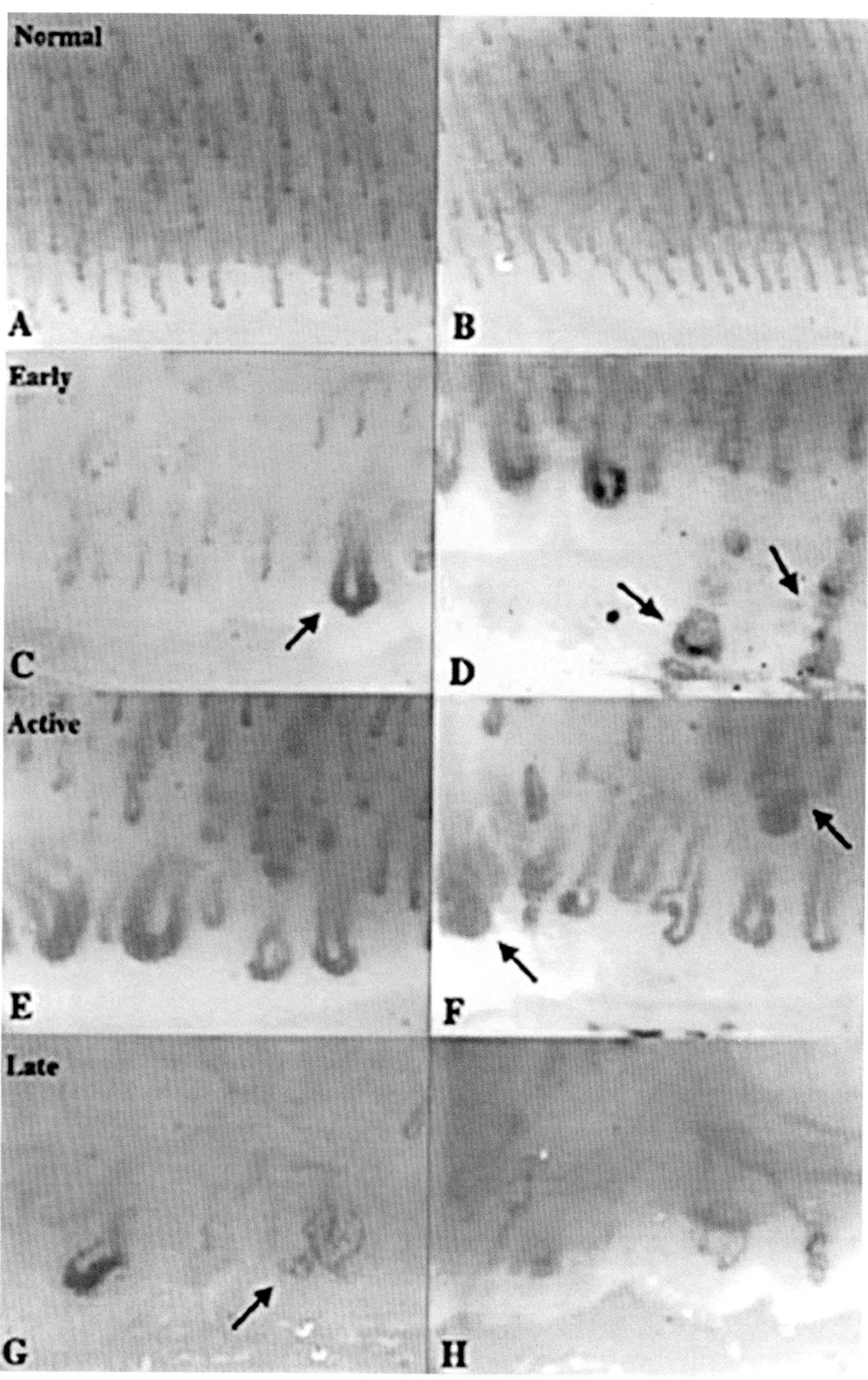

Fig. 5.1 Early, active, and late nailfold capillaroscopic patterns observed in systemic sclerosis

joints (with or without face involvement) [38]. They found that the sensitivity improved from 67 to 91 %, with further improvement to 99 % if visible mat-like telangiectasias were added [38]. Capillaroscopic evaluation using the dermatoscope may provide a feasible technique for clinicians and researchers to assess patients with early microvascular changes consistent with the scleroderma pattern.

Autoantibodies and Capillaroscopic Abnormalities May Predict the Onset of SSc

Several studies have shown that the combination of autoantibodies and nailfold capillaroscopic abnormalities may be helpful in the early detection of SSc and related diseases in patients presenting with Raynaud's phenomenon. The annual incidence of transition from primary Raynaud's phenomenon to secondary Raynaud's phenomenon has been shown to be 1 %, with ANA > 1:160 at presentation increasing the risk of developing secondary Raynaud's phenomenon by more than 68-fold [65]. In this study, after a mean follow-up period of 11.2 ± 3.9 years, the prevalence of transition from primary to secondary Raynaud's phenomenon was in 14.9 % of cases [65]. Another study found that the addition of serial nailfold videocapillaroscopic examinations identified a similar percentage of patients transitioning from primary to secondary Raynaud's phenomenon over a shorter follow-up time of 29.4 ± 10 months [66]. Therefore, the addition of nailfold capillaroscopic examination to standard evaluations, including autoantibody assessments, likely permits the earlier detection of secondary Raynaud's phenomenon. Another study of 152 patients with sclerodactyly and Raynaud's phenomenon found that the addition of dilated capillaries visualized by stereomicroscope improved the sensitivity of ACR criteria for the diagnosis of SSc from 33.6 to 74.3 % [39]. This was further improved to 82.9 % with the addition of avascular areas detected by stereomicroscope, 88.8 % with the addition of visible nailfold telangiectasias, and 91.5 % with the addition of ACA [39]. A recent study evaluated a cohort of 586 patients with Raynaud's phenomenon and found that 12.6 % (*n* = 74) of these patients progressed to definite SSc over a median follow-up time of 4.6 years [67]. Only 24 (32 %) of these patients fulfilled the ACR criteria for SSc. The strongest independent predictors for the development of definite SSc were positive ANA, SSc-specific autoantibodies (anti-Scl-70, anti-Th/To, ACA or anti-RNAP III), and a scleroderma pattern on nailfold capillaroscopy using stereomicroscope [67]. The combination of the presence of abnormal findings on nailfold capillaroscopy and SSc-specific autoantibody at baseline was associated with a 60-fold increased risk for the development of definite SSc, with a sensitivity of 47 %. The presence of abnormal capillaroscopy and/or SSc-specific autoantibody at baseline improved the sensitivity to 89 % with a negative predictive value of 98 % [67]. In other words, patients with Raynaud's and normal findings on nailfold capillaroscopy and negative SSc-specific autoantibodies had a probability of only 1.6 % to have SSc 10 years later; quite in contrast, patients with Raynaud's and SSc pattern on nailfold capillaroscopy and positive SSc-specific autoantibodies had a 73 % probability to have developed SSc in the course of 10 years. This illustrates how the patient profile informs clinicians about the probability of SSc being present (becoming manifest). These studies support the usefulness of SSc-specific autoantibodies and nailfold capillaroscopic abnormalities in the early diagnosis of SSc and in the revised classification criteria.

Recently Proposed Classification Criteria for SSc

Multiple different classification criteria have been proposed for SSc over the past several decades [18, 68]. Here we will discuss the most widely accepted criteria proposed since 2000.

LeRoy and Medsger Criteria

In 2001, LeRoy and Medsger proposed a classification system extending the criteria originally published by LeRoy in 1988 [69]. Taking advantage of the SSc-specific autoantibodies and nailfold capillaroscopy to detect vascular changes suggestive for connective tissue diseases, Leroy and Medsger suggested to extend the classification criteria to include "early" cases of SSc still without skin manifestations. Criteria for limited SSc (lSSc or "pre-SSc" or "unclassifiable SSc") can be fulfilled by patients with Raynaud's phenomenon plus an SSc-type nailfold capillary pattern and/or SSc-specific autoantibodies (Table 5.4a) [69]. Patients with lSSc must have either (1) objective documentation of Raynaud's phenomenon (direct observation or direct measurement of response to cold) plus either abnormal widefield nailfold capillaroscopy or SSc-specific autoantibodies (ACA, anti-Scl-70, antifibrillarin, anti-PM-Scl, anti-fibrillin, or anti-RNAP I or III in a titer of 1:100 or higher) or (2) subjective symptoms of Raynaud's phenomenon plus abnormal widefield nailfold capillaroscopy and SSc-specific autoantibodies [69]. Patients with lSSc can have overlap features, thus capturing patients with UCTD and MCTD who have prominent sclerodermatous features. Patients with lSSc who also have cutaneous manifestations of SSc are again subdivided into the limited cutaneous (lcSSc) and diffuse cutaneous (dSSc) forms (Table 5.4b) [69]. These subsets are differentiated from patients with diffuse fasciitis and eosinophilia who have proximal cutaneous changes but do not have Raynaud's phenomenon, abnormal nailfold capillaries, autoantibodies, or distal cutaneous changes. A small retrospective Swiss study found that 33/49 (67 %) of SSc patients fulfilled the ACR classification criteria for SSc [70]. When using the amended LeRoy and Medsger criteria, this improved to 80 % [70]. The study by Lonzetti et al. also included a group of 152 lSSc patients with Raynaud's phenomenon, but these patients also had sclerodactyly [39]. When adding nailfold capillary abnormalities and positive ACA to the ACR classification criteria, the sensitivity for diagnosis of SSc improved from 33.6 to 91.5 % [39]. The amended LeRoy and Medsger criteria certainly improve the sensitivity of the ACR classification criteria but exclude a small percentage of patients with SSc who lack Raynaud's phenomenon. Studies

Table 5.4 LeRoy and Medsger criteria for the classification of early systemic sclerosis (SSc)

A. Proposed criteria for limited forms of SSc (lSSc)
Raynaud's phenomenon (RP), objectively documented by:
1. Direct observation of any two of:
(a). Pallor (well-demarcated whitening of acral skin)
(b). Cyanosis (dusky blueness, which disappears on rewarming)
(c). Suffusion (well-demarcated redness)
Or 2. Direct measurement of response to cold by:
(a). Objective evidence of delayed recovery after cold challenge
(b). Nielsen test or equivalent
Plus 1. Abnormal widefield nailfold capillaroscopy (dilation and/or avascular areas)
Or 2. SSc selective autoantibodies (anticentromere, anti-Scl-70, antifibrillarin, anti-PM-Scl, anti-fibrillin, or anti-RNA polymerase I or III in a titer of 1:100 or higher)
If RP is subjective only, both SSc capillary pattern and SSc selective autoantibodies (in titer > 1:100) are required to define lSSc. LSSc can overlap with any other disease
B. Constellations of criteria for diagnosis of SSc
1. LSSc: defined in A above
2. LcSSc: criteria for lSSc + distal cutaneous changes
3. DSSc: criteria for lSSc + proximal cutaneous changes
4. Diffuse fasciitis with eosinophilia (DFE): proximal cutaneous changes without criteria for lSSc or lcSSc

Modified from Bauersachs and Lssner [63]

Table 5.5 Maricq and Valter proposed classification of scleroderma spectrum disorders

Group	Classification criteria definitions
I Diffuse scleroderma disorder[a]	Skin involvement proximal to elbows/knees; includes trunk
II Intermediate scleroderma disorder[a]	Skin involvement proximal to MCP/MTP, distal to elbows/knees; trunk not involved
III Digital scleroderma disorder	Sclerodactyly only; meets ACR minor criteria, but excludes those without skin involvement
IV Scleroderma sine sclerosis	Scleroderma capillary pattern or pitting scars and visceral involvement; no ACA; no telangiectasias
V UCTD-scleroderma disorder	UCTD with scleroderma features; no ACA; no telangiectasias
VI "CREST"	No skin involvement or sclerodactyly only; telangiectasias required with one or more other acronyms; or ACA is required with any two or more acronyms

Modified from Venables [30]

MCP metacarpophalangeal, *MTP* metatarsophalangeal, *ACR* American College of Rheumatology, *ACA* anticentromere antibodies, *UCTD* undifferentiated connective tissue disease, *CREST* calcinosis, Raynaud's phenomenon, esophageal dysmotility, sclerodactyly, telangiectasias

[a]Groups I and II were subdivided into two categories: (a) without and (b) with CREST features

indicate that approximately 10% of patients with SSc do not suffer from Raynaud's phenomenon [1, 37]. Patients most likely to be excluded by these criteria are those who do not have sclerodactyly or cutaneous sclerosis, but have internal organ disease consistent with SSc and SSc-specific autoantibodies or nailfold capillary abnormalities.

Maricq and Valter Criteria

In 2004, Maricq and Valter proposed another set of classification criteria for SSc with six different categories (Table 5.5) [37]. The first three groups are divided based on the extent of cutaneous sclerosis. The fourth category includes patients with scleroderma sine sclerosis who have internal organ involvement and scleroderma pattern nailfold capillary changes or pitting scars but no ACA or telangiectasias. The fifth group includes patients with UCTD with sclerodermatous features but no ACA or telangiectasias. The last category includes patients who fulfill the CREST criteria with telangiectasias plus one or more of the other acronyms or ACA plus two or more of the acronyms [37]. Using these classification criteria, Maricq and Valter were able to capture 77/165 (47%) patients with mild or early forms of SSc who were excluded from the ACR classification criteria [37]. Unlike the LeRoy and Medsger criteria, these criteria do not require the presence of Raynaud's phenomenon, thus increasing the sensitivity for SSc. However, the Maricq and Valter criteria only include the assessment of one SSc-specific autoantibody (ACA), which may compromise sensitivity. In addition, these criteria have not been externally validated and have been criticized for being too complicated.

Nadashkevich, Davis, and Fritzler Criteria

Nadashkevich et al. proposed another set of classification criteria in 2004 through a three-phase study [71]. The first phase involved 752 Ukrainian patients assessed between 1987 and 1994 who were diagnosed with SSc (n=170, 38% dSSc, 56% lcSSc, 6% overlap), SLE (n=170), RA (n=170), PM/DM (n=20), Sjogren's syndrome (n=23), isolated Raynaud's phenomenon (n=88), diabetes mellitus (n=100), eosinophilic fasciitis (n=5), and generalized morphea (n=6). In this cohort, the sensitivity of the ACR classification criteria for SSc was only 71.2% [71]. In the proposed criteria, classification as SSc was based on the presence of Raynaud's phenomenon and/or sclerodactyly or nonpitting digital edema plus one of 13 other SSc-related clinical manifestations. This phase identified 8 of the 15 clinical criteria as sufficient to identify all patients with SSc if at least 3 of the 8 criteria were fulfilled. None of the controls had more than two of the clinical criteria. Phase IIA of the study validated the initial set of eight clinical criteria in an indepen-

Table 5.6 Nadashkevich, Davis, and Fritzler proposed criteria for systemic sclerosis (SSc)

Criterion	Comments
Autoantibodies	Anticentromere, anti-Scl-70, or antifibrillarin
Bibasilar pulmonary fibrosis	Detected by chest radiograph
Contracture	Permanent limitation of joint motion
Dermal thickening proximal to wrists	Defined by the modified Rodnan skin score [66]
Calcinosis cutis	Detected by X-ray, crystallographic/chemical analysis
Raynaud's phenomenon	By patient's history or physician's observation
Esophageal distal hypomotility	Detected by cine/video barium esophagram or endoscopy
Sclerodactyly	Symmetric tightening of skin or nonpitting edema of digits
Telangiectasias	Common locations: digits, face, lips, tongue

Modified from Hirschl et al. [65]. Three or more of these criteria are necessary for a diagnosis of SSc

dent cohort of 99 Canadian SSc patients and 138 controls with SLE, RA, PM/DM, and Sjogren's syndrome evaluated between 1995 and 1997 [71]. In the external validation study, the criteria had a sensitivity of 99 % (compared with a sensitivity of 69.7 % using ACR criteria) and specificity of 100 % for the diagnosis of SSc. In phase IIB, various autoantibodies were assessed to add to the proposed criteria with the hopes of increasing sensitivity further. Ultimately, the presence of ACA (detected by indirect immunofluorescence), anti-Scl-70 antibodies (detected by double immunodiffusion), or antifibrillarin antibodies (detected by immunoprecipitation) was added as a final criterion [71]. Phase III of the study reviewed the SSc and isolated Raynaud's phenomenon patients in phase I to develop the final set of classification criteria, requiring three or more criteria for a diagnosis of definite of SSc (Table 5.6) [71]. Although the authors demonstrate superb sensitivity and specificity of their proposed classification criteria, other independent validation studies have not been performed [35]. Although this set of classification criteria does account for patients without Raynaud's phenomenon, abnormal nailfold capillaroscopic examination and other SSc-specific autoantibodies (i.e., Anti-RNAP III) were not included in the criteria.

Criteria from the Canadian Scleroderma Research Group

In 2007, Hudson et al. proposed a revision to the ACR classification criteria using data from the Canadian Scleroderma Research Group (CSRG) [38]. The authors proposed the addition of nailfold capillary abnormalities as assessed by the handheld dermatoscope (dilated or giant capillary loops or avascular areas) plus visible mat-like telangiectasias to the ACR classification criteria. Using the proposed criteria, the sensitivity to identify SSc patients with skin involvement distal to the metacarpophalangeal joints improved from 67 % to 99 % [38]. However, this study did not include controls, and therefore, the specificity of the proposed criteria was not assessed. Since SSc-specific autoantibodies and Raynaud's phenomenon were not included, the specificity of this classification system may be lower than other proposed criteria.

In 2010, Hudson, Fritzler and Baron published diagnostic criteria for SSc to aid the clinician in recognizing salient features of SSc rather than to classify patients for observational studies or clinical trials [72]. Of 1,048 SSc patients from the CSRG, 127 (12 %) did not fulfill the ACR classification criteria. Using regression tree analysis, the authors identified the presence of Raynaud's phenomenon, skin thickening proximal to the fingers, mat-like telangiectasias, and SSc-specific autoantibodies (ACA and anti-Scl-70) as providing 97 % sensitivity for the diagnosis of SSc [72]. Again this study did not include controls to assess specificity. A combination of the two sets of criteria proposed by Hudson et al. might be useful in the revision of the ACR classification criteria.

Modern Era of SSc Classification Criteria

Very Early Diagnosis of Systemic Sclerosis (VEDOSS)

The very early diagnosis of systemic sclerosis (VEDOSS) project of the European League Against Rheumatism Scleroderma Trials and Research group (EUSTAR) aims at early diagnosis of SSc. Early SSc may be suspected on the basis of Raynaud's phenomenon, autoantibodies, and SSc capillaroscopic pattern [69]. Presumably, also puffy fingers or early signs of sclerodactyly or one of the other early symptoms of SSc are to be considered in early diagnosis. For clinical purposes, the aim is to have criteria for the diagnosis of very early SSc. The criteria that are proposed are provisional (Fig. 5.2) and need to be validated: (a) initially through a Delphi technique, (b) thereafter perhaps using already available datasets, but (c) of critical importance, through prospective studies [18]. Prospective studies are needed for validation of proposed diagnostic criteria. Moreover, prospective studies do inform the clinician what the exact probabilities are that a patient may or may not have (or develop) SSc. In the VEDOSS cohort, patients are included with an increased probability of SSc; patients with Raynaud's phenomenon and/or puffy fingers who are positive for ANA are considered to be at risk (Fig. 5.3). The other items that were judged as most relevant for the diagnosis of SSc were sclerodactyly, abnormal capillaroscopy, positive ACA, and positive anti-Scl-70 antibodies (Table 5.7). If a sufficient number of

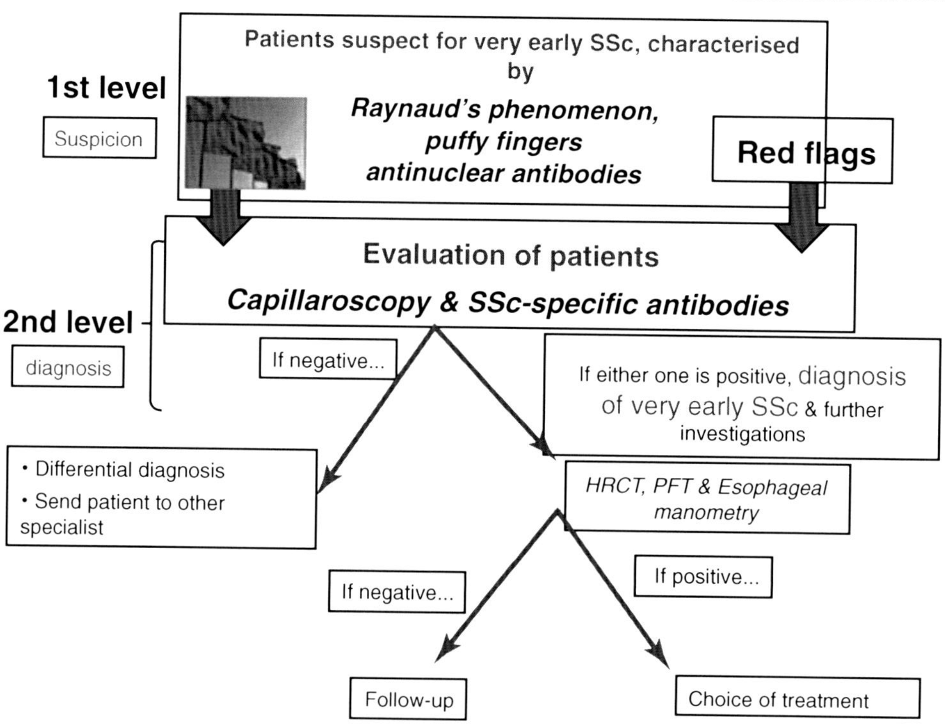

Fig. 5.2 Algorithm to diagnose patients with very early systemic sclerosis

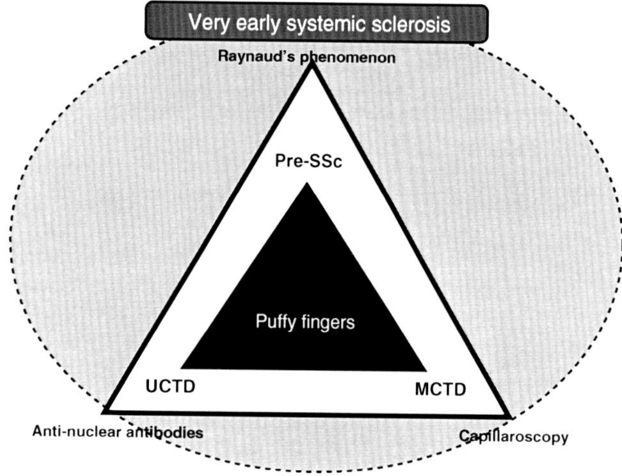

Fig. 5.3 Pyramid depiction of very early diagnosis of systemic sclerosis (SSc)

Table 5.7 Criteria for very early diagnosis of systemic sclerosis (SSc) determined by Delphi Consensus from EUSTAR

	Criteria selected by experts
Criteria considered as having a high clinical relevance for the very early diagnosis of SSc	Raynaud's phenomenon
Criteria considered as leading to an early referral	Puffy swollen digits turning into sclerodactyly
	Abnormal capillaroscopy with scleroderma pattern
	Positive anticentromere antibodies
	Positive anti-topoisomerase I antibodies
	Raynaud's phenomenon
	Puffy fingers
	Positive antinuclear antibodies

Modified from Walker et al. [68]
EUSTAR European League Against Rheumatism Scleroderma Trials and Research group

patients are included with a sufficiently long follow-up time (i.e., at least 5 years), then the best predictors and the probabilities of having/developing SSc can be determined.

ACR-EULAR Classification Criteria

The aim of the ACR-EULAR classification criteria for SSc working group was to develop classification criteria for inclusion of patients in clinical studies that met the demands of early recognition of SSc, include new knowledge gained over the preceding decades (e.g., importance of vascular manifestations, SSc-specific autoantibodies), and use a rigorous methodologic approach. Signs and symptoms (items) that should be considered to be included in the criteria were proposed through 2 independent Delphi exercises in Europe and North America; 168 items were scored for their importance. Low scoring criteria were discarded leaving 102 criteria [73, 74]. Through use of nominal group technique with 16 international experts, the proposed criteria were reduced to 23. Using cases and controls from databases from Madrid, Berlin, Toronto, Pittsburgh, Canadian Scleroderma Research Group, and 1,000 Faces of Lupus cohorts, these

Table 5.8 Performance characteristics of the ACR-EULAR criteria compared to the 1980 criteria

Cohort	ACR-EULAR criteria sensitivity (95 % CI)	ACR-EULAR criteria specificity (95 % CI)	1980 criteria sensitivity (95 % CI)	1980 criteria specificity (95 % CI)
Internal validation				
Derivation cohort	95 % (90 %, 98 %)	93 % (86 %, 97 %)	80 % (72 %, 87 %)	77 % (68 %, 84 %)
Validation cohort	91 % (87 %, 94 %)	92 % (86 %, 96 %)	75 % (70 %, 80 %)	72 % (64 %, 79 %)
≤3 years disease duration	91 % (86 %, 96 %)	90 % (70 %, 99 %)	75 % (70 %, 80 %)	72 % (63 %, 79 %)
External validation				
Alhajeri et al. 2015	98 %	NA	88 %	NA
Limited cutaneous SSc	99 %	NA	86 %	NA
≤ 3 years disease duration	99 %	NA	85 %	NA
Hoffmann-Vold et al. 2015	96 % (93 %, 97 %)	90 % (85 %, 94 %)	75 %	NA

Modified from Johnson [80]

criteria were found to have face, discriminant, and construct validity [75]. The 23 candidate criteria were further reduced and weighted and a threshold for classification identified using multicriteria decision analysis [75].

- Presence of "skin thickening sparing the fingers" was made an exclusionary criterion. If this is present, the classification criteria should not be applied, because if there is scleroderma that is not affecting the fingers, presence of a similar disease not being SSc is far more likely.
- "Skin thickening of the fingers extending proximally to the metacarpophalangeal joints" was a sufficient criterion. If present, the individual can be classified as systemic sclerosis.
- Acro-osteolysis, pitting scars, and digital ulcers were grouped under the heading "fingertip lesions."
- Systemic sclerosis-specific antibodies were also grouped under one criterion.

Antinuclear antibody, esophageal reflux, digital pulp loss, forced vital capacity, dysphagia, and diffusing capacity were removed due to poor ability to distinguish cases from controls, minimal added value in classification (low weight), or insufficient reliability in the clinical setting. This methodologic approach facilitated a system of classification that produced a measure of probability that an individual with certain features can be classified as systemic sclerosis. The draft classification system and weights were then tested against a range of cases that reflected low to high probability of having systemic sclerosis rated by experts. A total score of 9 or more was identified as the threshold with the least misclassification [76, 77].

The criteria set performance was tested in cases and controls from 10 European and 13 North American centers. The controls reflected conditions that could be confused with SSc and included scleromyxedema, graft-versus-host disease, undifferentiated connective tissue disease, dermatomyositis, nephrogenic sclerosing fibrosis, polymyositis, eosinophilic fasciitis, mixed connective tissue disease, and generalized morphea. As they did not provide added value in sensitivity or specificity, esophageal dilation, calcinosis cutis, acro-osteolysis, finger flexion contractures, tendon or bursal friction rubs, and renal crisis were removed. The new criteria have improved sensitivity and specificity compared to the 1980 and LeRoy/Medsger criteria and classify more individuals with early and limited disease. This has been independently replicated in other cohorts [78, 79] (Table 5.8).

The ACR-EULAR criteria have largely been lauded for their improved performance characteristics and large collaborative international effort. However, it is worth noting that it has also received some criticism [80]. Pragmatic criticisms are the use of a numeric additive point system requiring the use of "mental mathematics" and concerns that there remain too many criteria. Attempts to further reduce the number of criteria and simplify the weighting resulted in reduced sensitivity and specificity [81]. The new SSc classification criteria reflect a trade-off between a comprehensive system versus a feasible one that is easy to use [82]. An online tool is available to aid in calculation of the score (http://rheuminfo.com/physician-tools/ssc-calculator).

A second criticism relates to use of the criteria in individuals with mixed connective tissue disease [78]. The 1980 criteria investigators excluded MCTD patients from the derivation processes as they felt that it was "virtually impossible" to distinguish from SSc [82]. For the new criteria, the criteria testing, derivation, and validation cohorts included MCTD patients. Since many MCTD patients are SSc predominant in their clinical features, it was decided that these criteria could be applied to MCTD when considering enrollment into an SSc study [81]. A Norwegian cohort of 178 MCTD patients reported 10 % fulfilled the new criteria [78]. However, this cohort study did not collect data on abnormal nailfold capillaries or telangiectasias; therefore, 10 % may be an underestimate [82].

Conclusions

It is clear that these hallmarks of the SSc pathogenic process play an important role in the recognition (diagnosis, classification) of SSc. The 1980 ARA criteria were not intended for diagnostic purposes, did not include CREST-type patients, and made no attempt to deal with disease heterogeneity [83]. In 1988, it was proposed by LeRoy to subdivide SSc into limited and diffuse subsets, which is widely accepted [11, 84]. Although the difference between lcSSc and dSSc is largely based on the extent of skin involvement, these subtypes differ in clinical course and in prognosis and may differ to a certain degree in their pathogenesis. The latter is supported by the fact that different autoantibodies are strongly associated with each subtype of SSc.

Developed using a rigorous methodologic approach, the new ACR-EULAR classification criteria for SSc emphasize the vasculopathic manifestations and include the early manifestation of puffy fingers. The new criteria have improved sensitivity and specificity, particularly among cases with early, mild, and/or limited disease. We may now include more individuals with SSc into clinical trials and are hopefully closer to achieving new goals of preventing disease progression and inducing remission. The new classification criteria set has shifted the way we think of SSc, ushering in a new era.

References

1. Block JA, Sequeira W. Raynaud's phenomenon. Lancet. 2001;357(9273):2042–8.
2. Clements PJ, Furst DE, Wong WK, et al. High-dose versus low-dose D-penicillamine in early diffuse systemic sclerosis: analysis of a two-year, double-blind, randomized, controlled clinical trial. Arthritis Rheum. 1999;42(6):1194–203.
3. Pope JE, Bellamy N, Seibold JR, et al. A randomized, controlled trial of methotrexate versus placebo in early diffuse scleroderma. Arthritis Rheum. 2001;44(6):1351–8.
4. Denton C, Merkel P, Furst D, et al. Recombinant human anti-transforming growth factor beta1 antibody therapy in systemic sclerosis: a multicenter, randomized, placebo-controlled phase I/II trial of CAT-192. Arthritis Rheum. 2007;56(1):323–33.
5. Postlethwaite A, Wong W, Clements P, et al. A multicenter, randomized, double-blind, placebo-controlled trial of oral type I collagen treatment in patients with diffuse cutaneous systemic sclerosis: I. oral type I collagen does not improve skin in all patients, but may improve skin in late-phase disease. Arthritis Rheum. 2008;58(6):1810–22.
6. Khanna D, Clements P, Furst D, et al. Recombinant human relaxin in the treatment of systemic sclerosis with diffuse cutaneous involvement: a randomized, double-blind, placebo-controlled trial. Arthritis Rheum. 2009;60(4):1102–11.
7. Rhew E, Barr W. Scleroderma renal crisis: new insights and developments. Curr Rheumatol Rep. 2004;6(2):129–36.
8. Mathai S, Hassoun P. Therapy for pulmonary arterial hypertension associated with systemic sclerosis. Curr Opin Rheumatol. 2009;21(6):642–8.
9. Aggarwal R, Ringold S, Khanna D, Neogi T, Johnson SR, Miller A, et al. Distinctions between diagnostic and classification criteria. Arthritis Care Res (Hoboken). 2015;67(7):891–7.
10. Johnson SR, Laxer RM. Classification in systemic sclerosis. J Rheumatol. 2006;33(5):840–1.
11. LeRoy EC, Black C, Fleischmajer R, et al. Scleroderma (systemic sclerosis): classification, subsets and pathogenesis. J Rheumatol. 1988;15(2):202–5.
12. Medsger T. Natural history of systemic sclerosis and the assessment of disease activity, severity, functional status, and psychologic well-being. Rheum Dis Clin N Am. 2003;29(2):255–73. vi.
13. Walker UA, Tyndall A, Czirjk L, et al. Clinical risk assessment of organ manifestations in systemic sclerosis: a report from the EULAR Scleroderma Trials and Research group database. Ann Rheum Dis. 2007;66(6):754–63.
14. Ferri C, Valentini G, Cozzi F, et al. Systemic sclerosis: demographic, clinical, and serologic features and survival in 1,012 Italian patients. Medicine. 2002;81(2):139–53.
15. Reveille J, Solomon D. Evidence-based guidelines for the use of immunologic tests: anticentromere, Scl-70, and nucleolar antibodies. Arthritis Rheum. 2003;49(3):399–412.
16. Tan EM, Rodnan GP, Garcia I, Moroi Y, Fritzler MJ, Peebles C. Diversity of antinuclear antibodies in progressive systemic sclerosis. Anti-centromere antibody and its relationship to CREST syndrome. Arthritis Rheum. 1980;23(6):617–25.
17. Wigley FM. When is scleroderma really scleroderma? J Rheumatol. 2001;28(7):1471–3.
18. Johnson SR, Feldman BM, Hawker GA. Classification criteria for systemic sclerosis subsets. J Rheumatol. 2007;34(9):1855–63.
19. Barnett AJ, Coventry DA. Scleroderma. 1. Clinical features, course of illness and response to treatment in 61 cases. Med J Aust. 1969;1(19):992–1001.
20. Rodnan GP, Jablonska S, Medsger TA. Classification and nomenclature of progressive systemic sclerosis. Clin Rheum Dis. 1979;5(1):5–13.
21. Giordano M, Valentini G, Migliaresi S, Picillo U, Vatti M. Different antibody patterns and different prognoses in patients with scleroderma with various extent of skin sclerosis. J Rheumatol. 1986;13(5):911–6.
22. Masi AT. Classification of systemic sclerosis (scleroderma): relationship of cutaneous subgroups in early disease to outcome and serologic reactivity. J Rheumatol. 1988;15(6):894–8.
23. Scussel-Lonzetti L, Joyal F, Raynauld J-P, et al. Predicting mortality in systemic sclerosis: analysis of a cohort of 309 French Canadian patients with emphasis on features at diagnosis as predictive factors for survival. Medicine. 2002;81(2):154–67.
24. Poormoghim H, Lucas M, Fertig N, Medsger TA. Systemic sclerosis sine scleroderma: demographic, clinical, and serologic features and survival in forty-eight patients. Arthritis Rheum. 2000;43(2):444–51.
25. Williams HJ, Alarcon GS, Joks R, et al. Early undifferentiated connective tissue disease (CTD). VI. An inception cohort after 10 years: disease remissions and changes in diagnoses in well established and undifferentiated CTD. J Rheumatol. 1999;26(4):816–25.
26. Mosca M, Tavoni A, Neri R, Bencivelli W, Bombardieri S. Undifferentiated connective tissue diseases: the clinical and serological profiles of 91 patients followed for at least 1 year. Lupus. 1998;7(2):95–100.
27. Bodolay E, Csiki Z, Szekanecz Z, et al. Five-year follow-up of 665 Hungarian patients with undifferentiated connective tissue disease (UCTD). Clin Exp Rheumatol. 2003;21(3):313–20.
28. Danieli MG, Fraticelli P, Salvi A, Gabrielli A, Danieli G. Undifferentiated connective tissue disease: natural history and evolution into definite CTD assessed in 84 patients initially diagnosed as early UCTD. Clin Rheumatol. 1998;17(3):195–201.
29. Sharp GC, Irvin WS, Tan EM, Gould RG, Holman HR. Mixed connective tissue disease–an apparently distinct rheumatic disease syndrome associated with a specific antibody to an extractable nuclear antigen (ENA). Am J Med. 1972;52(2):148–59.
30. Venables PJW. Mixed connective tissue disease. Lupus. 2006;15(3):132–7.
31. Hesselstrand R, Scheja A, Shen GQ, Wiik A, Akesson A. The association of antinuclear antibodies with organ involvement and survival in systemic sclerosis. Rheumatology. 2003;42(4):534–40.

32. Meyer O, Fertig N, Lucas M, Somogyi N, Medsger T. Disease subsets, antinuclear antibody profile, and clinical features in 127 French and 247 US adult patients with systemic sclerosis. J Rheumatol. 2007;34(1):104–9.
33. van den Hoogen FH, Spronk PE, Boerbooms AM, et al. Long-term follow-up of 46 patients with anti-(U1)snRNP antibodies. Br J Rheumatol. 1994;33(12):1117–20.
34. Masi, et al. Preliminary criteria for the classification of systemic sclerosis (scleroderma). Subcommittee for scleroderma criteria of the American Rheumatism Association Diagnostic and Therapeutic Criteria Committee. Arthritis Rheum. 1980;23(5):581–90.
35. Nadashkevich O, Davis P, Fritzler MJ. Revising the classification criteria for systemic sclerosis. Arthritis Rheum. 2006;55(6):992–3.
36. Hachulla E, Launay D. Diagnosis and classification of systemic sclerosis. Clin Rev Allergy Immunol. 2011;40(2):78–83.
37. Maricq HR, Valter I. A working classification of scleroderma spectrum disorders: a proposal and the results of testing on a sample of patients. Clin Exp Rheumatol. 2004;22(3 Suppl 33):S5–13.
38. Hudson M, Taillefer S, Steele R, et al. Improving the sensitivity of the American College of Rheumatology classification criteria for systemic sclerosis. Clin Exp Rheumatol. 2007;25(5):754–7.
39. Lonzetti LS, Joyal F, Raynauld JP, et al. Updating the American College of Rheumatology preliminary classification criteria for systemic sclerosis: addition of severe nailfold capillaroscopy abnormalities markedly increases the sensitivity for limited scleroderma. Arthritis Rheum. 2001;44(3):735–6.
40. Steen V. Autoantibodies in systemic sclerosis. Semin Arthritis Rheum. 2005;35(1):35–42.
41. Steen VD, Powell DL, Medsger TA. Clinical correlations and prognosis based on serum autoantibodies in patients with systemic sclerosis. Arthritis Rheum. 1988;31(2):196–203.
42. Arbuckle M, McClain M, Rubertone M, et al. Development of autoantibodies before the clinical onset of systemic lupus erythematosus. N Engl J Med. 2003;349(16):1526–33.
43. Yamasaki Y, Honkanen-Scott M, Hernandez L, et al. Nucleolar staining cannot be used as a screening test for the scleroderma marker anti-RNA polymerase I/III antibodies. Arthritis Rheum. 2006;54(9):3051–6.
44. Parker JC, Burlingame RW, Webb TT, Bunn CC. Anti-RNA polymerase III antibodies in patients with systemic sclerosis detected by indirect immunofluorescence and ELISA. Rheumatology. 2008;47(7):976–9.
45. Villalta D, Morozzi G, Tampoia M, et al. Antibodies to fibrillarin, PM-Scl and RNA polymerase III detected by ELISA assays in patients with systemic sclerosis. Clin Chim Acta. 2010;411(9–10):710–3.
46. Hanke K, Brckner C, Dhnrich C, et al. Antibodies against PM/Scl-75 and PM/Scl-100 are independent markers for different subsets of systemic sclerosis patients. Arthritis Res Ther. 2009;11(1):R22.
47. Mitri G, Lucas M, Fertig N, Steen V, Medsger T. A comparison between anti-Th/To- and anticentromere antibody-positive systemic sclerosis patients with limited cutaneous involvement. Arthritis Rheum. 2003;48(1):203–9.
48. Arnett FC, Reveille JD, Goldstein R, et al. Autoantibodies to fibrillarin in systemic sclerosis (scleroderma). An immunogenetic, serologic, and clinical analysis. Arthritis Rheum. 1996;39(7):1151–60.
49. Okano Y, Medsger TA. Autoantibody to Th ribonucleoprotein (nucleolar 7–2 RNA protein particle) in patients with systemic sclerosis. Arthritis Rheum. 1990;33(12):1822–8.
50. Kasturi KN, Hatakeyama A, Spiera H, Bona CA. Antifibrillarin autoantibodies present in systemic sclerosis and other connective tissue diseases interact with similar epitopes. J Exp Med. 1995;181(3):1027–36.
51. Satoh M, Ajmani AK, Ogasawara T, et al. Autoantibodies to RNA polymerase II are common in systemic lupus erythematosus and overlap syndrome. Specific recognition of the phosphorylated (IIO) form by a subset of human sera. J Clin Invest. 1994;94(5):1981–9.
52. Kuwana M, Okano Y, Pandey J, Silver R, Fertig N, Medsger T. Enzyme-linked immunosorbent assay for detection of anti-RNA polymerase III antibody: analytical accuracy and clinical associations in systemic sclerosis. Arthritis Rheum. 2005;52(8):2425–32.
53. Satoh T, Ishikawa O, Ihn H, et al. Clinical usefulness of anti-RNA polymerase III antibody measurement by enzyme-linked immunosorbent assay. Rheumatology. 2009;48(12):1570–4.
54. Maricq HR, LeRoy EC. Patterns of finger capillary abnormalities in connective tissue disease by "wide-field" microscopy. Arthritis Rheum. 1973;16(5):619–28.
55. Maricq HR, LeRoy EC, D'Angelo WA, et al. Diagnostic potential of in vivo capillary microscopy in scleroderma and related disorders. Arthritis Rheum. 1980;23(2):183–9.
56. Maricq HR, Weinberger AB, LeRoy EC. Early detection of scleroderma-spectrum disorders by in vivo capillary microscopy: a prospective study of patients with Raynaud's phenomenon. J Rheumatol. 1982;9(2):289–91.
57. Nagy Z, Czirjk L. Nailfold digital capillaroscopy in 447 patients with connective tissue disease and Raynaud's disease. J Eur Acad Dermatol Venereol. 2004;18(1):62–8.
58. Cutolo M, Sulli A, Pizzorni C, Accardo S. Nailfold videocapillaroscopy assessment of microvascular damage in systemic sclerosis. J Rheumatol. 2000;27(1):155–60.
59. Cutolo M, Pizzorni C, Tuccio M, et al. Nailfold videocapillaroscopic patterns and serum autoantibodies in systemic sclerosis. Rheumatology. 2004;43(6):719–26.
60. Smith V, Pizzorni C, De Keyser F, et al. Reliability of the qualitative and semiquantitative nailfold videocapillaroscopy assessment in a systemic sclerosis cohort: a two-centre study. Ann Rheum Dis. 2010;69(6):1092–6.
61. Anders HJ, Sigl T, Schattenkirchner M. Differentiation between primary and secondary Raynaud's phenomenon: a prospective study comparing nailfold capillaroscopy using an ophthalmoscope or stereomicroscope. Ann Rheum Dis. 2001;60(4):407–9.
62. Baron M, Bell M, Bookman A, et al. Office capillaroscopy in systemic sclerosis. Clin Rheumatol. 2007;26(8):1268–74.
63. Bauersachs RM, Lssner F. The poor man's capillary microscope. A novel technique for the assessment of capillary morphology. Ann Rheum Dis. 1997;56(7):435–7.
64. Muroi E, Hara T, Yanaba K, et al. A portable dermatoscope for easy, rapid examination of periungual nailfold capillary changes in patients with systemic sclerosis. Rheumatol Int. 2010;31:1601–6.
65. Hirschl M, Hirschl K, Lenz M, Katzenschlager R, Hutter H-P, Kundi M. Transition from primary Raynaud's phenomenon to secondary Raynaud's phenomenon identified by diagnosis of an associated disease: results of ten years of prospective surveillance. Arthritis Rheum. 2006;54(6):1974–81.
66. Cutolo M, Pizzorni C, Sulli A. Identification of transition from primary Raynaud's phenomenon to secondary Raynaud's phenomenon by nailfold videocapillaroscopy: comment on the article by Hirschl et al. Arthritis Rheum. 2007;56(6):2102–3.
67. Koenig M, Joyal F, Fritzler M, et al. Autoantibodies and microvascular damage are independent predictive factors for the progression of Raynaud's phenomenon to systemic sclerosis: a twenty-year prospective study of 586 patients, with validation of proposed criteria for early systemic sclerosis. Arthritis Rheum. 2008;58(12):3902–12.
68. Walker J, Pope J, Baron M, et al. The development of systemic sclerosis classification criteria. Clin Rheumatol. 2007;26(9):1401–9.
69. LeRoy EC, Medsger TA. Criteria for the classification of early systemic sclerosis. J Rheumatol. 2001;28(7):1573–6.
70. Ziswiler H-R, Urech R, Balmer J, Ostensen M, Mierau R, Villiger P. Clinical diagnosis compared to classification criteria in a cohort of 54 patients with systemic sclerosis and associated disorders. Swiss Med Wkly. 2007;137(41–42):586–90.
71. Nadashkevich O, Davis P, Fritzler M. A proposal of criteria for the classification of systemic sclerosis. Med Sci Monit. 2004;10(11):CR615–21.

72. Hudson M, Fritzler M, Baron M. Systemic sclerosis: establishing diagnostic criteria. Medicine. 2010;89(3):159–65.
73. Fransen J, Johnson SR, van den Hoogen F, Baron M, Allanore Y, Carreira PE, et al. Items for developing revised classification criteria in systemic sclerosis: results of a consensus exercise. Arthritis Care Res (Hoboken). 2012;64(3):351–7.
74. Coulter C, Baron M, Pope JE. A Delphi exercise and cluster analysis to aid in the development of potential classification criteria for systemic sclerosis using SSc experts and databases. Clin Exp Rheumatol. 2013;31(2 Suppl 76):24–30.
75. Johnson SR, Fransen J, Khanna D, Baron M, van den Hoogen F, Medsger Jr TA, et al. Validation of potential classification criteria for systemic sclerosis. Arthritis Care Res (Hoboken). 2012;64(3):358–67.
76. van den Hoogen F, Khanna D, Fransen J, Johnson SR, Baron M, Tyndall A, et al. 2013 classification criteria for systemic sclerosis: an American College of Rheumatology/European League against Rheumatism collaborative initiative. Arthritis Rheum. 2013;65(11):2737–47.
77. van den Hoogen F, Khanna D, Fransen J, Johnson SR, Baron M, Tyndall A, et al. 2013 classification criteria for systemic sclerosis: an American college of rheumatology/European league against rheumatism collaborative initiative. Ann Rheum Dis. 2013;72(11):1747–55.
78. Hoffmann-Vold AM, Gunnarsson R, Garen T, Midtvedt O, Molberg O. Performance of the 2013 American College of Rheumatology/European League against rheumatism classification criteria for systemic sclerosis (SSc) in large, well-defined cohorts of SSc and mixed connective tissue disease. J Rheumatol. 2015;42(1):60–3.
79. Alhajeri H, Hudson M, Fritzler M, Pope J, Tatibouet S, Markland J, et al. The 2013 ACR/EULAR classification criteria for systemic sclerosis out-perform the 1980 criteria. Data from the Canadian Scleroderma Research Group. Arthritis Care Res (Hoboken). 2015;67(4):582–7.
80. Johnson SR. New ACR EULAR guidelines for systemic sclerosis classification. Curr Rheum Rev. 2015;17(5):32.
81. van den Hoogen F, Khanna D, Fransen J, Johnson SR, Baron M, Tyndall A, et al. 2013 classification criteria for systemic sclerosis: an American college of rheumatology/European league against rheumatism collaborative initiative. Ann Rheum Dis. 2013;72(11):1747–55.
82. Pope JE. Systemic sclerosis classification: a rose by any other name would smell as sweet? J Rheumatol. 2015;42(1):11–3.
83. Wollheim F. Classification of systemic sclerosis: visions and reality. Rheumatology. 2005;44(10):1212–6.
84. Johnson SR, Goek ON, Singh-Grewal D, et al. Classification criteria in rheumatic diseases: a review of mathodologic properties. Arthritis Rheum. 2007;57(7):1119–33.

Overlap Syndromes

6

Pia Moinzadeh and Christopher P. Denton

Definition/Classification

Systemic sclerosis (SSc) overlap syndrome is a term used to describe a very heterogeneous group of patients with features of different connective tissue diseases, combined with clinical signs of SSc [1–3].

Up to now, no firm classification criteria for SSc overlap syndromes are established, but it is generally considered when musculoskeletal involvement or features of other rheumatic diseases are significantly greater than usually found in general SSc patients [4].

SSc and each of the other connective tissue disorder itself are already heterogeneous. SSc patients have been diagnosed in the past with established disease, using the American College of Rheumatology (ACR) preliminary criteria, published in 1980 [5] and now based on the improved/amended EULAR/ACR criteria [6]. LeRoy et al. has published in 1988 the most widely used classification system for defining the major SSc forms, namely, those patients suffering from limited (lcSSc) and diffuse SSc (dcSSc), depending on the extent of skin thickening [7]. This classification system has been used in clinical practice and clinical trials and has been the basis for many patient registries worldwide [8].

Other autoimmune rheumatic disorders are classified depending on internationally accepted classification systems, including autoantibodies, such as anti-double-stranded DNA (dsDNA) and anti-Smith antigen (Sm) for patients suffering from systemic lupus erythematosus (SLE) [2, 9], detection of rheumatoid factor (RF) for rheumatoid arthritis [10, 11] and anti-smooth muscle antigen (SMA) and anti-liver/kidney microsome (LKM) bodies for autoimmune hepatitis [2, 12].

P. Moinzadeh, MD
Department of Dermatology and Venerology, University of Cologne, Cologne, RNW 50937, Germany

C.P. Denton, PhD, FRCP (✉)
Division of Medicine, Department of Inflammation, Centre for Rheumatology and Connective Tissue Diseases, UCL Division of Medicine, Royal Free Hospital, London, UK
e-mail: c.denton@ucl.ac.uk

Epidemiology

SSc overlap syndromes represent the third major subgroup of SSc, and epidemiological studies report divergent frequencies (incidence and prevalence rates are not reported yet) of overlap subgroups, ranging between 10 and 38 % (see Table 6.1) [1, 3, 4, 18].

The most common SSc overlap syndromes are SSc/myositis (polymyositis (PM) or dermatomyositis (DM)), SSc/rheumatoid arthritis (RA), SSc/Sjogren's (SS) and SSc/systemic lupus erythematosus (SLE) overlap syndromes. SSc may also occur together with other organ-specific autoimmune diseases, such as autoimmune hepatitis/primary biliary cirrhosis (PBC), autoimmune thyroiditis, sarcoidosis and antiphospholipid syndrome and (see Table 6.2).

Pakozdi et al. reported recently that 20 % of the patients attending the Centre for Rheumatology at the Royal Free Hospital had overlapping features with other rheumatologic diseases. Of these, 43 % overlapped with polymyositis/dermatomyositis, 8 % with systemic lupus erythematosus (SLE), 17 % with Sjogren's syndrome and 32 % with rheumatoid arthritis [4]. The German Deutsches Netzwerk für Systemische Sklerodermie (DNSS) has reported that 10 % of the registered patients suffered from SSc overlap syndromes [18].

A recent meta-analysis has revealed that the mean age at diagnosis of patients with SSc overlap syndromes was 47.6 (+2.6) years and that it was found more often in European patients than in patients from North America [19].

Balbir-Gurman reported that the overall mortality in their SSc overlap cohort did not differ from other SSc patients [3]. Depending on different geographical regions/centres, a wide range of frequencies of SSc overlap syndromes have been reported (see Table 6.3).

J. Varga et al. (eds.), *Scleroderma*, DOI 10.1007/978-3-319-31407-5_6

Table 6.1 SSc overlap syndromes and associated autoantibodies

SSc overlap syndrome	Autoantibodies directed against
Mixed connective tissue disease	Anti-U1snRNP (specific), found in 75–90 % of MCTD patients [13, 14]
SSc/myositis overlap syndrome	Anti-PmScl (specific) [15]
	Anti-Ku, anti-U1RNP, anti-Scl70, anti-Jo1, anti-Ro/SSA, anti-U3RNP and anti-RNA-polymerase have also been reported [1]
	Anti-RuvBL1/2 antibody is a new SSc-related autoantibody, associated with muscle involvement and diffuse skin thickening [16]
SSc/rheumatoid arthritis overlap syndrome	High titres of RF (60–72 %), ACPA (prevalence of 64 %) [1]
	ACPA more frequent in patients with RA features in SSc patients [4]
	Anti-Scl-70 and anti-ACA antibodies have been reported [4]
	COMP level may become a nonspecific marker for joint involvement [17]
SSc/Sjogren's overlap syndrome	Anti-Ro/SSA and anti-La/SSB have been reported [1, 4]
	Clearly more often associated with anti-ACA [1, 4]
SSc/SLE overlap syndrome	Anti-dsDNA together with anti-Scl70 antibodies has been reported [1]
	Also single cases with anti-ACA and anti-PmScl have been reported [1]

Table 6.2 Rare cases of SSc overlap syndromes [3]

SSc overlap syndrome with	Definition
Antiphospholipid syndrome	Incidence varies between 7 % and 13 % [3]
	The presence of lupus anticoagulant, anti-cardiolipid or anti-ß2-glycoprotein-1 antibodies has been reported in SSc patients [3] and has been associated with severe ischemia, PAH, digital loss, and thromboembolism
Sarcoidosis	Very rare variant of SSc overlap syndrome
	Elevated temperature, weight loss and bihilar adenopathy have been shown in SSc sarcoidosis overlap syndromes
	Lung and lymph node biopsy is necessary to define the disease [3]
PBC	Prevalence ranges between 7 and 15 %
	Mostly associated with lcSSc
	Positive ACA in PBC patients reveals a higher risk for lcSSc
	Often clinically silent, but anti-mitochondrial antibodies, elevation of cholestatic enzymes and hyperglobulinemia are possible [3]

Table 6.3 Frequencies of different SSc overlap syndromes [1]

SSc overlap syndrome		Total
Patients with SSc	118 [20], 719 [21], 1,483 [22], 165 [3], 1,700 [4], 2,425 [15]	6,610 [1]
SSc overlap syndromes	32.2 % [20], 38 % [21], 10.9 % [22], 24.2 % [3], 20 % [4], 9.2 % [15]	16.2 % [1]
SSc/PM or SSc/DM overlap syndrome	5.3 % [20], 47.5 % [3], 42.8 % [4], 60.1 % [15]	44.6 % [1]
SSc/Sjogren's overlap syndrome	26.3 % [20], 18 % [21], 42.5 % [3], 16.8 % [4]	18.5 % [1]
SSc/rheumatoid arthritis overlap syndrome	8 % [20], 21.1 % [21], 15.4 % [3], 32 % [4], 6.2 % [15]	19.3 % [1]

Pathogenesis

Up to date, knowledge about the pathogenesis of SSc overlap syndromes is still not fully elucidated. The question, why some patients develop only one connective tissue disease and other patients a combination of clinical features of different rheumatic diseases, has not been answered yet. Possibly, a common or overlapping genetic susceptibility plays an important role. Genetic studies have shown the existence of some susceptibility genes, which predispose to multiple other autoimmune diseases [19]. Koumakis E has reported recently that a regulatory gene located in TNFAIP3 region is associated with a higher risk to develop SSc polyautoimmunity [19, 23].

SSc Overlap Subgroups and Clinical Features

Clinical features of SSc overlap syndrome patients are very heterogeneous; patients classified as SSc overlap syndrome usually present with skin sclerosis typically for limited SSc, although organ manifestations clearly separate these patients as distinct subset [18]. A German study showed that patients suffering from SSc overlap syndromes developed significantly earlier and more often an involvement of the musculoskeletal system, than patients with the diffuse and limited form of SSc. Besides that, they interestingly developed lung fibrosis and heart involvement significantly earlier and more often than lcSSc patients, but still less frequent and later than dcSSc patients [18] (see Fig. 6.1).

Therefore the identification of these patients is essential for clarifying prognosis and facilitating therapeutic options. The clinical signs include both cutaneous and extracutaneous features, depending on the overlapping connective tissue disease (CTD) and often overlap between the different overlap forms, especially regarding vasculopathy, gastrointestinal and cardiopulmonary involvement.

Raynaud phenomenon appears in more than 90 % of SSc patients and is also a very common feature in patients with SSc overlap syndromes (SS 20–50 %, myositis 20–40 %, SLE 20–30 %, RA <5 %) [2]. It is usually caused by coldness and/or emotional stress and classically occurs as episodic pallor of the digits followed by cyanosis, suffusion and/or

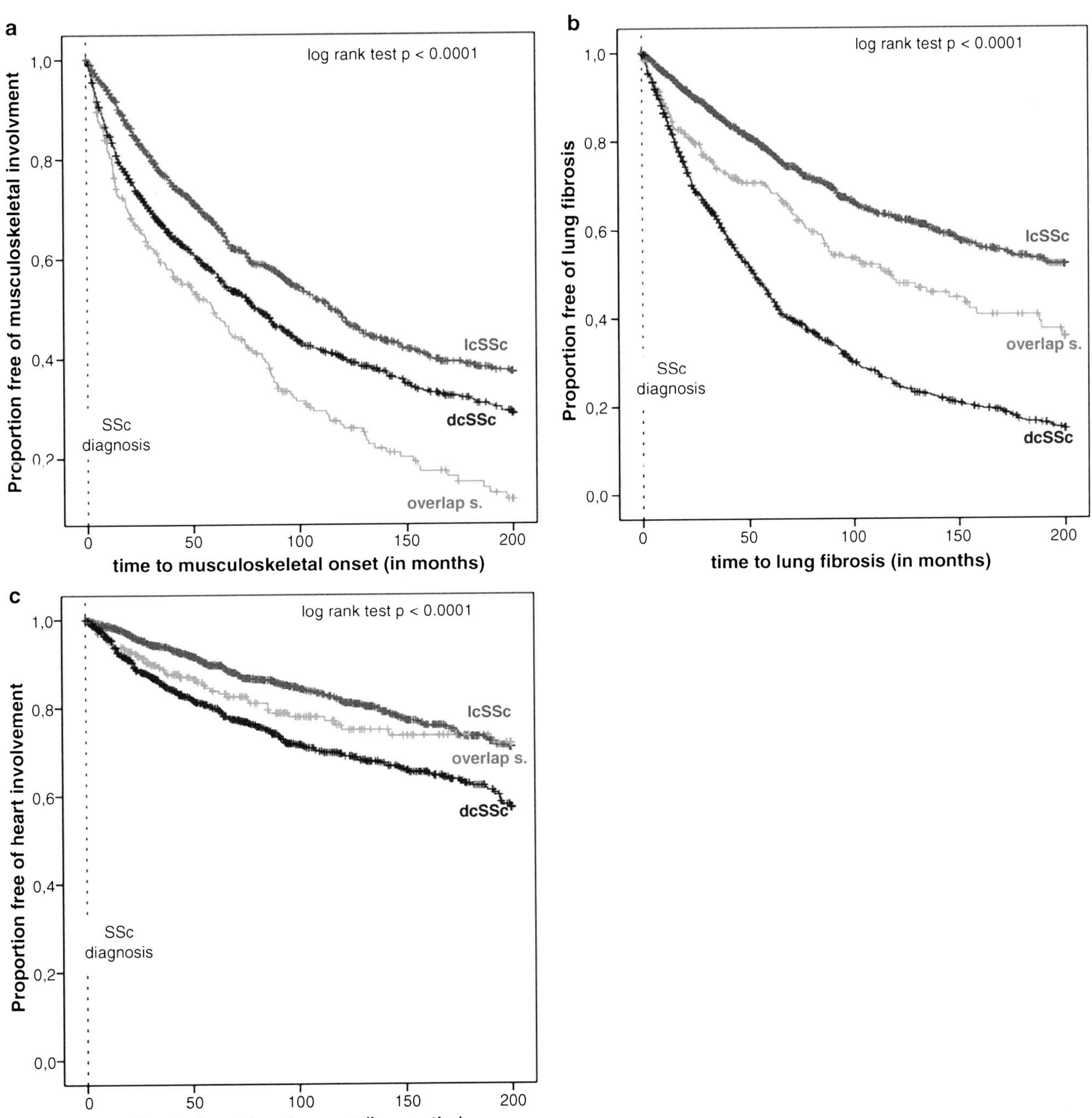

Fig. 6.1 Kaplan-Meier *curves* indicate a clear difference between SSc overlap syndrome patients and patients with lcSSc or dcSSc, especially for musculoskeletal involvement (**a**), lung fibrosis (**b**) and heart involvement (**c**) [18]

pain and tingling. Some SSc overlap patients also develop digital ulcerations but significantly less often, compared to limited and diffuse SSc patients [18].

The skin sclerosis in patients with SSc overlap syndromes can be generalized, similar to the diffuse SSc, but more frequently, it is only located below the elbow and knee joints, similar to the limited SSc form [4, 18]. The severity of the skin sclerosis, depending on the extension of thickened skin as well as the affected anatomic region, can cause all together a restricted mobility of extremities and especially joints (dermatogenous contractures).

Calcinosis cutis can be also observed in patients with SSc overlap syndromes and occurs usually over pressure points (acral or next to joints). Nevertheless, patients with SSc overlap syndromes, although having a limited skin sclerosis, have still a higher risk to develop severe internal organ manifestations [18]. Therefore these patients should be seen as a separate SSc subset.

The *involvement of the gastrointestinal tract* is probably the most commonly internal organ system involved in patients suffering from SSc and SSc overlap syndromes (around 50–60 %) [18, 22]. The clinical features include dysphagia, retrosternal discomfort due to reflux/oesophagitis and bowel disease with hypomotility. This all might lead to weight loss, cachexia, diarrhoea, pseudo-obstruction and malabsorption.

Lung fibrosis and myocardial involvement is significantly less frequent in patients with diffuse SSc but significantly more frequent in patients diagnosed with the limited form of SSc [18]. The clinical features of cardiac and pulmonary involvement are very similar and overlapping. To distinguish clinical features such as dyspnoea, nonproductive cough, disturbed diffusion-capacity and cyanoses to a specific organ manifestation might be sometimes a challenge.

Pulmonary arterial hypertension (PAH) occurs less frequent in patients with SSc overlap syndromes, while lung fibrosis occurs less frequent in SSc overlap syndromes, than in patients with diffuse SSc, but clearly more often than in patients with limited SSc [18].

Further Organ Manifestation Depending on SSc Overlap Syndromes

Systemic Sclerosis and Myositis

Myositis is the most frequent systemic involvement in patients with SSc overlap syndromes (frequency ranging between 5.3 and 60.1 %).

In some SSc patients, muscle weakness, pain and atrophy results from disuse secondary to joint contractures, dermatogenous contractures or chronic disease. However, significantly more patients with SSc overlap syndromes present with musculoskeletal involvement, associated with poly- or dermatomyositis, characterized by myalgia, muscle weakness and atrophy of muscles. Patients suffering from SSc/myositis overlap syndrome may develop myositis simultaneously, before or in already established SSc [3]. Additional main clinical features beside muscle involvement are arthralgia, RP and sclerotic skin thickening [2].

Raynaud phenomenon is present in 20–40 % of SSc/myositis overlap patients [2]. A generalized extent of skin thickening is interestingly more often prevalent in patients with the SSc/myositis overlap syndrome, compared to other overlap forms [3, 4]. Comparing the limited and diffuse skin sclerosis within each overlap syndrome demonstrates that the limited extent of skin thickening is still the most frequent form [3, 4].

Recent studies have shown, that an increased proportion of patients develop also lung fibrosis [18, 24]. Patients with SSc/myositis overlap syndromes have a higher risk to develop a diffuse interstitial myocardial fibrosis, which may lead to diastolic dysfunctions as well as restricted contractibility of the myocard. These patients typically present symptoms, such as cardiac arrhythmia, paroxysmal tachycardia and incomplete or complete right heart blocks, finally leading to heart insufficiency. The frequency of lung and gastrointestinal involvement varies among studies, ranging between 32.0 and 78.1 % [1]. It is well established that patients suffering from the SSc/polymyositis overlap have a worse prognosis due to an increased risk of myocardial involvement, compared to patients with only SSc [24].

SSc myositis overlap syndromes may be associated with specific autoantibodies, including PmScl, anti-Ku, anti-U2RNP and anti-U5snRNP [3, 25]. Patients, carrying the antibody to PmScl usually are younger, have limited skin involvement and suffer from arthritis and a benign course of interstitial lung disease (ILD) [3], which is also the reason for their better survival [15]. Positive antibodies against Ku are more characteristic for patients suffering from muscle involvement as well as severe ILD [26] (see Table 6.1).

Systemic Sclerosis and Rheumatoid Arthritis (RA)

Inflammatory joint involvement is reported to be the second most frequent manifestation in patients with musculoskeletal involvement and overlap syndromes [4]. These patients often present with typical clinical symptoms (usually limited skin involvement) together with high titers of anti-cyclic citrullinated peptides (CCP/ACPA) and/or higher rheumatoid factors (RF). It is often very difficult to distinguish between SSc patients with mild, seronegative arthralgia and significant arthritis associated with SSc/RA overlap syndrome. In 2012, Gheita TA and Hussein H have found significantly increased COMP levels in SSc patients with arthritis, indicating that COMP levels may become a marker for joint involvement in SSc patients [17].

Systemic Sclerosis and Systemic Lupus Erythematosus (SLE)

This subtype is a very rare condition [27]. Patients often have a fatal course of the disease due to a higher risk to develop polyserositis, pancreatitis, avascular bone necrosis,

PAH, lung involvement, lupus glomerulonephritis, skin rashes and leukoencephalopathy [3]. It is also difficult to distinguish whether the patient suffers from a lupus nephritis or a scleroderma renal crisis. Depending on the reason for renal failure, patients need a different therapeutic strategy to improve renal function. Skin lesions can be a major aesthetic disturbing factor, because of the predilection area, the face. Also enoral lesions may reduce the quality of life, due to the pain of ulcerations and the difficulties to eat. Usually, these patients have a combination of SSc-associated antibodies and double-stranded DNA antibodies.

Systemic Sclerosis and Sjogren's Syndrome (SS)

This SSc overlap syndrome has been firstly described in 1965 by Bloch et al. [28]. Enoral (xerostomia) and ocular sicca symptoms (xerophthalmia) are very common in patients suffering from SSc (68–83 %), but only 14–20 % of SSc patients really fulfil the criteria of Sjogren's syndrome [29], so that the diagnosis of SSc/SS overlap syndromes is always a challenge [30]. It is defined by a lymphocytic infiltration of the salivary glands. Patients with SSc/SS overlap syndrome show a limited form of skin involvement (83.6 % versus 16.4 %) and a very low frequency of lung involvement [3]. Antibodies against Ro are very likely in SSc/SS overlap syndromes, often together with ACA antibodies [4]. Anti-Ro and anti-La antibodies have been present in 38.8 % of cases, but unfortunately none of these antibodies can be used as a serological marker. One recent study has shown that ACA positivity allows the identification of SS overlap syndromes (not limited to SSc) [31].

Mixed Connective Tissue Disease (MCTD)

Mixed connective tissue disease (MCTD) was firstly described by Sharp and colleagues in 1972 [32]. These patients present clinical symptoms typically found in patients with polymyositis/dermatomyositis, SLE, inflammatory arthritis (RA) and scleroderma (SSc). Typical for this condition are puffy fingers (50 %), polyarthritis (65 %), RP (53 %), sclerodactyly (35 %), muscle involvement and oesophageal involvement [14, 33] and the occurrence of high ANA titers with high levels of U1snRNP antibodies, helping to differentiate the MCTD from other connective tissue diseases. Arthralgia occurs in approximately 60 % of patients, while muscle disease is present in 80–90 % of cases with proximal muscle involvement and elevation of serum creatine kinase (CK) levels [33]. Cardiovascular involvement (lung fibrosis and especially PAH) is less frequent but is the major contributor to a poor outcome/prognosis [14]. Immunogenetic studies have shown an association between the major histocompatibility complex (MHC), HLA-DR4 and -DR2 and the presence of U1snRNP antibodies [2, 34]. Paradowska-Gorycka A et al. have shown in their study of 66 MCTD patients that Il-10 gene variants may be considered as a genetic risk factor for MCTD susceptibility [35]. These patients also develop frequently sicca syndrome. Many patients suffer from oesophagus and lung involvement (Table 6.4).

Diagnostics (See Also Chapter for Systemic Sclerosis)

Vasculopathy (Raynaud Phenomenon)

To identify a secondary Raynaud phenomenon (RP) and predict the further course of the disease, two simple and noninvasive procedures are essential, namely, the assessment of serum autoantibodies and the nailfold capillaroscopy [38, 39].

Skin Sclerosis

Careful mapping of the degree and extent of skin involvement is the single best clinical technique. This helps to suggest/predict the risk for further organ manifestations. The most widely used technique is the modified Rodnan skin score (mRSS), consisting of a 0–3 grading at 17 skin sites (maximum score 51) [40, 41].

Muscle Involvement (Myositis/Myopathy)

Elevation of serum creatine phosphokinase, ESR, possible changes on electromyography (EMG) and histological assessment of a muscle biopsy as well as a MRI of the affected muscles are helpful to identify muscle inflammation and/or atrophy [42, 43]. Typical histopathological features are perivascular inflammatory infiltrates with focal replacement of myofibrils with collagen and perimysial and epimysial fibrosis.

Involvement of the Gastrointestinal Tract

The presence of oesophagitis can be determined by upper GI endoscopy with histological evaluations. Hypomotility can usually be diagnosed by oesophagus scintigraphy oesophagogastroscopy [43, 44].

Cardiopulmonary Involvement

All patients with systemic sclerosis and SSc overlap syndromes should be followed up by using pulmonary function test, echocardiography, 6-min walk test and high-resolution computerized tomography (HRCT), to determine a possible cardiopulmonary involvement. To detect fibrotic changes in the myocardium, noninvasive imaging techniques such as MRI or spiral CT scanning may be indicated, besides indirect clues of cardiac involvement, which may be deduced from ECG or

Table 6.4 Autoantibodies associated with SSc overlap syndromes

Autoantibodies	Definition
U1snRNP	Hallmark antibody for MCTD in high titres [33]
	Patients with high titres evolve into MCTD usually over 2 years [33]
	Positive in 75–90 % of MCTD cases, compared to just 20–50 % of SLE cases [14]
	Seem to interact with lung tissue, contributing to disease features [14]
PmScl	Serological marker for SSc/polymyositis overlap syndrome [25]
	Also found in other connective tissue diseases [25]
	Directed predominantly against two molecules of 100 kDa and 75 kDa [36]
	Strongly associated with HLA-DQA1*0501, HLA-DQB1*02 – DRB1*0301 [25]
	Patients were younger and showed more frequently limited cutaneous involvement [15]
	Overall survival was significantly better in PmScl positive patients [15]
	33.1 % of SSc/PM overlap syndrome carry this antibody [4]
Jo1	
Ku	Heterodimer, including a 70 kDa and 80 kDa peptide bound to a 350 kDa DNA-dependent protein kinase [36]
	2.3–55 % of patients with SSc/PM OS were positive for Ku antibodies
	Also found in other connective tissue diseases [36]
	Not predictive for prognosis of the disease and also not associated with cancer risk
dsDNA	In 70 % of SLE patients but very rare in SSc patients [27]
	In two cases, patients with Scl70 and dsDNA antibodies have been reported [27, 37]
RuvBL1/RuvBL2	Novel SSc-associated antibody [16]
	Associated with diffuse skin sclerosis and musculoskeletal involvement (myositis overlap) [16]

echocardiographic studies [43]. Conduction defect is the most frequently observed disturbances, up to complete heart block necessitating pacemaker implantation. Also the use of N-terminal brain natriuretic peptide (NTproBNP) in patient serum is helpful to detect right ventricular impairment [45].

Kidney Involvement

Creatinine clearance, urine sediments to control proteinuria and haematuria as well as regular blood pressure tests are necessary for the early identification of a renal involvement [43, 46]. In case of SSc-SLE overlap syndromes, it is sometimes necessary to take a kidney biopsy to distinguish between renal failures due to lupus nephritis [47] or scleroderma renal crisis [46].

Sicca Symptoms

Due to a reduced glandular function, especially patients with SSc-Sjogren's syndrome suffer from dry mouth (xerostomia) and dry eyes (xerophthalmia). Medical history, the assessment of ANAs (anti-Ro and anti-La antibodies) and the Schirmer test for ocular sicca symptoms together with a glandular biopsy can be helpful to define a possible Sjogren's syndrome [48].

Joint Involvement

Joint involvement might be due to dermatogenous contractures but also due to inflammation. It is recommendable to examine the rheumatoid factor and CCP antibodies in the serum of affected patients. X-ray of affected joints as well as MRI scans is helpful to identify inflammation areas and damage of the joints [43].

Management of SSc Overlap Syndromes

There have been major advances in treating many of the organ-specific complications of systemic sclerosis and overlapping diseases. Most of the patients are treated with standard drugs, which are usually used in the specific rheumatic disorder. Sometimes shared clinical symptoms between SSc and the other connective tissue diseases complicate the decision of treatment strategy.

Systemic Glucocorticoids

Systemic glucocorticoids can be used for musculoskeletal involvement together with other immunosuppressive agents. It can be combined with other drugs or just as monotherapy. The use of high-dose corticosteroids has to be used with cautious due to the increased risk in patients with diffuse extent of skin involvement to induce a renal crisis [1].

Methotrexate

Methotrexate is a well-known immunosuppressive agent, which has been used in adults and children, with long experience of well-documented side effects. MTX is still a first-line therapy in many autoimmune diseases. It is the treatment of choice in patients with SSc/myositis and SSc/RA overlap syndromes [49, 50] but has to be used with cautious in patients with alveolitis or in patients with liver damage or alcohol use.

Mycophenolate Mofetil

MMF is a well-tolerated immunosuppressive agent, which is increasingly used for many autoimmune diseases. It is recommended as long-term therapy in scleroderma and has successfully been applied in several overlap syndromes, which respond well.

Azathioprine

This immunosuppressive agent is usually well tolerated and has been used successfully in patients with MCTD as well as patients with SSc/SLE overlap. However, compared to MMF side effects seem to be more pronounced and the response to the therapy more limited.

Cyclophosphamide

Cyclophosphamide is often used for lung involvement in patients with SSc [51] and also SSc/myositis overlap or SSc/SLE overlap syndromes, in case of lupus nephritis. Cyclophosphamide should be used as a second-line immunosuppressive therapy after the others (MTX, MMF) have failed or cannot be used due to defined side effects. Similar to other autoimmune diseases, it can be used as i.v. pulse or oral treatment.

Specific Immunomodulatory Agents

For IVIG and anti-TNF therapy, only limited information is available for overlap syndromes. B-cell depletion by rituximab was initially described to be of only limited benefit in patients with scleroderma. More recent studies, however, have demonstrated better results and there are several case reports demonstrating that rituximab can be successfully used in patient with overlap syndromes, especially if these are characterized by inflammatory muscle involvement. Certainly long-term follow-ups of these patients are still missing, and no data are yet available for more potent B-cell-depleting agents. However, a clear clinical classification of this heterogeneous group of patients is required to allow the appropriate clinical studies.

Systemic Sclerosis and Myositis

In this group of patients, treatment is mainly directed against alveolitis, muscle inflammation and skin sclerosis. Intravenous pulsed glucocorticoid therapy (not in patients with a higher risk for renal crisis), methotrexate (not in case of alveolitis), azathioprine, IVIG and rituximab (in patients with uncontrolled myositis) may be helpful agents. Especially in patients with PmScl-positive overlap syndrome, the mild form of myositis responds very well to low dosages of corticosteroids. Mycophenolate mofetil can be used in patients, in whom the skin sclerosis is the predominant clinical feature, and cyclophosphamide is usually used in patients, in whom the alveolitis causes the most severe symptoms. IVIG has also shown a clear benefit in patients with myositis and interestingly has also shown an improvement in skin and gastrointestinal involvement [3, 52]. Some case reports have shown that Rituximab was effective in patients with uncontrolled myositis and also helped to improve alveolitis and skin involvement [53, 54].

Systemic Sclerosis and Rheumatoid Arthritis

These patients are usually treated with methotrexate, anti-TNF agents as well as with tocilizumab. All these treatments have to be used with caution especially regarding serious infections, tuberculosis and fibrosis. Infliximab and etanercept has shown controversial results, partly improving and partly causing more problems, like lupus-like disease [3]. Due to increased Il6 levels in serum of patients with rheumatoid arthritis and also in patients with SSc, tocilizumab has been approved for patients with rheumatoid arthritis and has been used in clinical trials of SSc.

Systemic Sclerosis and Systemic Lupus Erythematosus

The treatment of renal involvement differs between a lupus and a scleroderma-associated renal failure (cyclophosphamide versus vasoactive treatment with iloprost and ace inhibitors). SLE-driven PAH has to be treated with immunosuppressive agents, corticosteroids or cytotoxic drugs, such as cyclophosphamide. Vasodilators, such as iloprost, endothelin receptor antagonists or phosphodiesterase 5 inhibitors, are necessary to reduce the pulmonary hypertension. Especially in patients with diffuse extent of skin involvement, the use and dosage of corticosteroids have to be considered very carefully due to the increased risk to trigger SSc-related renal crisis.

Case studies have shown a positive effect of rituximab and MMF in SLE patients and should be considered for SSc-SLE overlap patients [3].

Mixed Connective Tissue Disease (MCTD)

Patients with MCTD usually respond well to systemic corticosteroid and immunosuppressive therapy with several classical agents. But some long-term studies have shown that a group of patients with MCTD develop more severe organ manifestations and need a more aggressive therapeutic strategy. Inflammatory features (elevated temperature, serositis, pleuritis, myositis and arthritis) respond well to steroid treatment, while symptoms, such as sclerotic skin changes and cardiopulmonary involvement, need immunosuppressive/cytotoxic drugs [33, 55]. The most frequently used drugs are cyclophosphamide and methotrexate as well as hydroxychloroquines [33].

Systemic Sclerosis and Sjogren's Overlap Syndrome

Usually clinical features, such as the xerostomia, can be improved by using various antiseptic mouth rinse as well as saliva substitutes. Also the xerophthalmia can be improved by using artificial tear drops [56]. Furthermore, it has been reported that especially in patients with primary SS, nonsteroidal antirheumatic drugs or low dosages of corticosteroids, as well as immunomodulatory drugs, such as hydroxychloroquine, azathioprine, methotrexate and rituximab, have been effective in open-label studies, but data about Sc/SS overlap syndromes are lacking [56] (Table 6.5).

Table 6.5 SSc-associated therapeutic strategies, including disease-modifying drugs

Clinical feature	Therapeutic strategies
Raynaud phenomenon	General recommendations: avoid coldness, keep body warm, paraffin bath, heatable soles and gloves
	Vitamins and supplements: fish oil capsules, antioxidant vitamins, *Ginkgo biloba*
	Oral treatments: calcium channel blockers, angiotensin II receptor 1 blocker or phosphodiesterase type 5 inhibitor (not licensed, trial in severe cases)
	Topical treatment: GTN patches
	Intravenous treatment: prostacyclin infusion
	Surgical treatment: lumbar sympathectomy, radical microaretriolysis
Skin	
Skin thickening	General recommendations: skin care with moisturizing cream or ointments
	Physical treatments: lymphatic drainage/physiotherapy, phototherapy
	Topical treatment: steroids or calcineurin inhibitors
	Systemic treatment: steroids (just short dated due to side effects and risk of renal crisis), methotrexate, mycophenolate mofetil [56–59] or cyclophosphamide (trials have shown significant improvement in mRSS) CAVE: side effects have to be balanced
Calcinosis cutis	General recommendations: improve blood flow and keep hands warm
	Local corticosteroid injections, laser therapy, surgery, minocycline or bisphosphonate p.o.
Telangiectasia	Laser therapy and/or camouflage
Gastrointestinal involvement	
Reflux	General recommendations: bed head elevated during the night, small meals
	Oral treatments: proton pump inhibitors, prokinetics and/or H_2 receptor antagonists
Dysphagia	General recommendations: change habit of eating, small meals
	Oral treatments: prokinetics
Gastric antral vascular ectasia (GAVE)	Argon plasma coagulation
Diarrhoea Constipation	General recommendations: change habit of eating
	Oral treatments: prokinetics, antibiotics, laxative
Kidney system	
Scleroderma renal crisis	Systemic treatments: ACE inhibitors (high-dosed) under blood pressure monitoring, iloprost intravenous
Respiratory system	
Lung fibrosis	Systemic treatments: cyclophosphamide orally or intravenous, glucocorticosteroids (short dated), azathioprine orally, mycophenolate mofetil orally
	Oxygen (if needed)
PAH	Systemic treatments: bosentan orally, sildenafil orally, epoprostenol orally
	Oxygen (if needed)
Cardiac myopathy	Systemic treatments: cyclophosphamide orally or intravenous, glucocorticosteroids (short dated), azathioprine orally, mycophenolate mofetil orally
	Pacemaker (if needed)

References

1. Iaccarino L, Gatto M, Bettio S, et al. Overlap connective tissue disease syndromes. Autoimmun Rev. 2013;12:363–73. Epub 2012/06/30.
2. Jury EC, D'Cruz D, Morrow WJ. Autoantibodies and overlap syndromes in autoimmune rheumatic disease. J Clin Pathol. 2001;54:340–7. Epub 2001/05/01.
3. Balbir-Gurman A, Braun-Moscovici Y. Scleroderma overlap syndrome. Isr Med Assoc J. 2011;13:14–20. Epub 2011/03/31.
4. Pakozdi A, Nihtyanova S, Moinzadeh P, et al. Clinical and serological hallmarks of systemic sclerosis overlap syndromes. J Rheumatol. 2011;38:2406–9. Epub 2011/08/17.
5. Preliminary criteria for the classification of systemic sclerosis (scleroderma). Subcommittee for scleroderma criteria of the American Rheumatism Association Diagnostic and Therapeutic Criteria Committee. Arthritis Rheum 1980;23:581–90. Epub 1980/05/01.
6. van den Hoogen F, Khanna D, Fransen J, et al. 2013 classification criteria for systemic sclerosis: an American College of Rheumatology/European League against rheumatism collaborative initiative. Arthritis Rheum. 2013;65:2737–47. Epub 2013/10/15.
7. LeRoy EC, Black C, Fleischmajer R, et al. Scleroderma (systemic sclerosis): classification, subsets and pathogenesis. J Rheumatol. 1988;15:202–5. Epub 1988/02/01.
8. Galluccio F, Walker UA, Nihtyanova S, et al. Registries in systemic sclerosis: a worldwide experience. Rheumatology (Oxford). 2011;50:60–8. Epub 2010/12/15.
9. Tan EM, Cohen AS, Fries JF, et al. The 1982 revised criteria for the classification of systemic lupus erythematosus. Arthritis Rheum. 1982;25:1271–7. Epub 1982/11/01.
10. Kay J, Upchurch KS. ACR/EULAR 2010 rheumatoid arthritis classification criteria. Rheumatology (Oxford). 2012;51 Suppl 6:vi5–9. Epub 2012/12/19.
11. Arnett FC, Edworthy SM, Bloch DA, et al. The American Rheumatism Association 1987 revised criteria for the classification of rheumatoid arthritis. Arthritis Rheum. 1988;31:315–24. Epub 1988/03/01.
12. Johnson PJ, McFarlane IG. Meeting report: International Autoimmune Hepatitis Group. Hepatology. 1993;18:998–1005. Epub 1993/10/01.
13. Habets WJ, de Rooij DJ, Salden MH, et al. Antibodies against distinct nuclear matrix proteins are characteristic for mixed connective tissue disease. Clin Exp Immunol. 1983;54:265–76. Epub 1983/10/01.
14. Tani C, Carli L, Vagnani S, et al. The diagnosis and classification of mixed connective tissue disease. J Autoimmun. 2014;48–49:46–9. Epub 2014/01/28.
15. Koschik 2nd RW, Fertig N, Lucas MR, et al. Anti-PM-Scl antibody in patients with systemic sclerosis. Clin Exp Rheumatol. 2012;30:S12–6. Epub 2012/01/21.
16. Kaji K, Fertig N, Medsger Jr TA, et al. Autoantibodies to RuvBL1 and RuvBL2: a novel systemic sclerosis-related antibody associated with diffuse cutaneous and skeletal muscle involvement. Arthritis Care Res. 2014;66:575–84. Epub 2013/09/12.
17. Gheita TA, Hussein H. Cartilage Oligomeric Matrix Protein (COMP) in systemic sclerosis (SSc): role in disease severity and subclinical rheumatoid arthritis overlap. Joint Bone Spine: Rev Rhum. 2012;79:51–6. Epub 2011/04/19.
18. Moinzadeh P, Aberer E, Ahmadi-Simab K, et al. Disease progression in systemic sclerosis-overlap syndrome is significantly different from limited and diffuse cutaneous systemic sclerosis. Ann Rheum Dis. 2014. Epub 2014/01/07.
19. Elhai M, Avouac J, Kahan A, et al. Systemic sclerosis at the crossroad of polyautoimmunity. Autoimmun Rev. 2013;12:1052–7. Epub 2013/06/25.
20. Caramaschi P, Biasi D, Volpe A, et al. Coexistence of systemic sclerosis with other autoimmune diseases. Rheumatol Int. 2007;27:407–10. Epub 2006/10/19.
21. Hudson M, Rojas-Villarraga A, Coral-Alvarado P, et al. Polyautoimmunity and familial autoimmunity in systemic sclerosis. J Autoimmun. 2008;31:156–9. Epub 2008/07/23.
22. Hunzelmann N, Genth E, Krieg T, et al. The registry of the German Network for Systemic Scleroderma: frequency of disease subsets and patterns of organ involvement. Rheumatology (Oxford). 2008;47:1185–92. Epub 2008/06/03.
23. Koumakis E, Dieude P, Avouac J, et al. Familial autoimmunity in systemic sclerosis – results of a French-based case-control family study. J Rheumatol. 2012;39:532–8. Epub 2012/01/17.
24. Bhansing KJ, Lammens M, Knaapen HK, et al. Scleroderma-polymyositis overlap syndrome versus idiopathic polymyositis and systemic sclerosis: a descriptive study on clinical features and myopathology. Arthritis Res Ther. 2014;16:R111. Epub 2014/06/03.
25. Mahler M, Raijmakers R. Novel aspects of autoantibodies to the PM/Scl complex: clinical, genetic and diagnostic insights. Autoimmun Rev. 2007;6:432–7. Epub 2007/07/24.
26. Rigolet A, Musset L, Dubourg O, et al. Inflammatory myopathies with anti-Ku antibodies: a prognosis dependent on associated lung disease. Medicine. 2012;91:95–102. Epub 2012/03/07.
27. Lin HK, Wang JD, Fu LS. Juvenile diffuse systemic sclerosis/systemic lupus erythematosus overlap syndrome – a case report. Rheumatol Int. 2012;32:1809–11. Epub 2011/05/03.
28. Bloch KJ, Buchanan WW, Wohl MJ, et al. Sjoegren's syndrome. A clinical, pathological, and serological study of sixty-two cases. Medicine. 1965;44:187–231. Epub 1965/05/01.
29. Ramos-Casals M, Brito-Zeron P, Font J. The overlap of Sjogren's syndrome with other systemic autoimmune diseases. Semin Arthritis Rheum. 2007;36:246–55. Epub 2006/09/26.
30. Avouac J, Sordet C, Depinay C, et al. Systemic sclerosis-associated Sjogren's syndrome and relationship to the limited cutaneous subtype: results of a prospective study of sicca syndrome in 133 consecutive patients. Arthritis Rheum. 2006;54:2243–9. Epub 2006/06/28.
31. Salliot C, Gottenberg JE, Bengoufa D, et al. Anticentromere antibodies identify patients with Sjogren's syndrome and autoimmune overlap syndrome. J Rheumatol. 2007;34:2253–8. Epub 2007/10/17.
32. Sharp GC, Irvin WS, Tan EM, et al. Mixed connective tissue disease – an apparently distinct rheumatic disease syndrome associated with a specific antibody to an extractable nuclear antigen (ENA). Am J Med. 1972;52:148–59. Epub 1972/02/01.
33. Ortega-Hernandez OD, Shoenfeld Y. Mixed connective tissue disease: an overview of clinical manifestations, diagnosis and treatment. Best Pract Res Clin Rheumatol. 2012;26:61–72. Epub 2012/03/20.
34. Hoffman RW, Greidinger EL. Mixed connective tissue disease. Curr Opin Rheumatol. 2000;12:386–90. Epub 2000/09/16.
35. Paradowska-Gorycka A, Jurkowska M, Czuszynska Z, et al. IL-10, IL-12B and IL-17 gene polymorphisms in patients with mixed connective tissue disease. Mod Rheumatol/Jpn Rheum Assoc. 2014;25:1–3. Epub 2014/08/28.
36. Sordet C, Goetz J, Sibilia J. Contribution of autoantibodies to the diagnosis and nosology of inflammatory muscle disease. Joint Bone Spine (revue du rhumatisme). 2006;73:646–54. Epub 2006/11/18.
37. Mok CC, Cheung JC, Yee YK, et al. Unusual overlap of systemic lupus erythematosus and diffuse scleroderma. Clin Exp Rheumatol. 2001;19:113–4. Epub 2001/03/15.
38. Cutolo M, Matucci Cerinic M. Nailfold capillaroscopy and classification criteria for systemic sclerosis. Clin Exp Rheumatol. 2007;25:663–5. Epub 2007/12/15.
39. Cutolo M, Sulli A, Secchi ME, et al. The contribution of capillaroscopy to the differential diagnosis of connective autoimmune diseases. Best Pract Res Clin Rheumatol. 2007;21:1093–108. Epub 2007/12/11.
40. Valentini G, D'Angelo S, Della Rossa A, et al. European Scleroderma Study Group to define disease activity criteria for systemic sclerosis. IV. Assessment of skin thickening by modified

Rodnan skin score. Ann Rheum Dis. 2003;62:904–5. Epub 2003/08/19.
41. Czirjak L, Nagy Z, Aringer M, et al. The EUSTAR model for teaching and implementing the modified Rodnan skin score in systemic sclerosis. Ann Rheum Dis. 2007;66:966–9. Epub 2007/01/20.
42. Akesson A, Fiori G, Krieg T, et al. Assessment of skin, joint, tendon and muscle involvement. Clin Exp Rheumatol. 2003;21:S5–8. Epub 2003/08/02.
43. Hunzelmann N, Genth E, Krieg T, et al. Organ-specific diagnosis in patients with systemic sclerosis: recommendations of the German Network for Systemic Sclerosis (DNSS). Z Rheumatol. 2008;67:334–6. 7–40. Epub 2008/04/18. Organspezifische Diagnostik von Patienten mit systemischer Sklerodermie : Empfehlungen des Deutschen Netzwerkes fur Systemische Sklerodermie (DNSS).
44. Jaovisidha K, Csuka ME, Almagro UA, et al. Severe gastrointestinal involvement in systemic sclerosis: report of five cases and review of the literature. Semin Arthritis Rheum. 2005;34:689–702. Epub 2005/02/05.
45. Thakkar V, Stevens W, Prior D, et al. The inclusion of N-terminal pro-brain natriuretic peptide in a sensitive screening strategy for systemic sclerosis-related pulmonary arterial hypertension: a cohort study. Arthritis Res Ther. 2013;15:R193. Epub 2013/11/20.
46. Steen VD, Mayes MD, Merkel PA. Assessment of kidney involvement. Clin Exp Rheumatol. 2003;21:S29–31. Epub 2003/08/02.
47. Kistler AD. [In Process Citation]. Therapeutische Umschau Revue therapeutique. Lupusnephritis. 2015;72:171–7. Epub 2015/02/28.
48. Santiago ML, Seisdedos MR, Garcia Salinas RN, et al. Usefulness of antibodies and minor salivary gland biopsy in the study of sicca syndrome in daily clinical practice. Utilidad de los anticuerpos y de la biopsia de glandula salival menor en el estudio del complejo sicca en la practica diaria. Rheumatol Clin. 2015;11(3):156–60. Epub 2015/01/13.
49. Kowal-Bielecka O, Distler O. Use of methotrexate in patients with scleroderma and mixed connective tissue disease. Clin Exp Rheumatol. 2010;28:S160–3. Epub 2010/11/26.
50. Fendler C, Braun J. Use of methotrexate in inflammatory myopathies. Clin Exp Rheumatol. 2010;28:S164–7. Epub 2010/11/26.
51. Walker KM, Pope J. Expert agreement on EULAR/EUSTAR recommendations for the management of systemic sclerosis. J Rheumatol. 2011;38:1326–8. Epub 2011/04/05.
52. Levy Y, Amital H, Langevitz P, et al. Intravenous immunoglobulin modulates cutaneous involvement and reduces skin fibrosis in systemic sclerosis: an open-label study. Arthritis Rheum. 2004;50:1005–7. Epub 2004/03/17.
53. Levine TD. Rituximab in the treatment of dermatomyositis: an open-label pilot study. Arthritis Rheum. 2005;52:601–7. Epub 2005/02/05.
54. Mok CC, Ho LY, To CH. Rituximab for refractory polymyositis: an open-label prospective study. J Rheumatol. 2007;34:1864–8. Epub 2007/08/28.
55. Lundberg IE. The prognosis of mixed connective tissue disease. Rheum Dis Clin N Am. 2005;31:535–47. vii–viii. Epub 2005/08/09.
56. Feltsan T, Stanko P, Mracna J. Sjogren's syndrome in present. Bratisl Lek Listy. 2012;113:514–6. Epub 2012/08/18.
57. van den Hoogen FH, Boerbooms AM, Swaak AJ, et al. Comparison of methotrexate with placebo in the treatment of systemic sclerosis: a 24 week randomized double-blind trial, followed by a 24 week observational trial. Br J Rheumatol. 1996;35:364–72. Epub 1996/04/01.
58. Pope JE, Bellamy N, Seibold JR, et al. A randomized, controlled trial of methotrexate versus placebo in early diffuse scleroderma. Arthritis Rheum. 2001;44:1351–8. Epub 2001/06/16.
59. Das SN, Alam MR, Islam N, et al. Placebo controlled trial of methotrexate in systemic sclerosis. Mymensingh Med J. 2005;14:71–4. Epub 2005/02/08.

Juvenile Localized and Systemic Scleroderma

7

Lauren V. Graham, Amy S. Paller, and Ivan Foeldvari

Juvenile Localized Scleroderma

Pediatric localized scleroderma comprises a group of conditions in which the skin and subcutaneous tissues become fibrotic. Lesions range from very small plaques to extensive indurated lesions which cause significant functional impairment and cosmetic deformity. Localized scleroderma also is called morphea. Pediatric localized scleroderma has been divided into five subtypes: circumscribed morphea, linear scleroderma, generalized morphea, pansclerotic morphea, and a mixed subtype with a combination of two or more subtypes (15 % of patients) (Table 7.1) [1, 2].

Epidemiology

Although pediatric localized scleroderma is an orphan disease, it is at least ten times more common than systemic sclerosis in childhood [3]. Girls predominate with the female/male ratio estimated at 1.9–2.7:1 [1, 3, 4]. The mean age at disease onset is 7.3–8.3 years of age [5, 6]. Less than one percent of cases are present at birth (congenital localized scleroderma) [6]. Linear scleroderma is the most common subtype seen in children; in one recent study, the overall incidence of localized scleroderma was 3.4 cases per million children per year with 2.7 cases per million per year of linear scleroderma [3]. Early-onset disease and more severe forms (linear scleroderma, generalized morphea, pansclerotic morphea) are risk factors for extracutaneous manifestations [4, 7].

L.V. Graham, MD, PhD
Department of Dermatology, Northwestern University, McGraw Medical Center, Chicago, IL 60657, USA

A.S. Paller, MS, MD
Department of Dermatology, Northwestern University Feinberg School of Medicine, Chicago, IL 60611, USA

I. Foeldvari, MD (✉)
Hamburg Centre for Pediatric Rheumatology, Head of the Juvenile Scleroderma Working Group (JSScWG), Hamburger Zentrum Für Kinder- und Jugendrheumatologie, Hamburg 22081, Germany
e-mail: sprechstunde@kinderrheumatologie.de; foeldvari@t-online.de

Clinical Manifestations

Circumscribed morphea (CM) is characterized by oval or round circumscribed areas of induration surrounded by a violaceous halo (Fig. 7.1). Superficial circumscribed morphea is confined to the dermis with only occasional involvement of the superficial panniculus. Circumscribed morphea is most commonly seen on the trunk and includes 15–37 % of pediatric localized scleroderma [1, 4, 5]. Guttate morphea (numerous small plaques) and localized scleroderma that resembles atrophoderma of Pasini and Pierini or lichen sclerosus et atrophicus are included in the circumscribed morphea subset. Deep morphea is another subset of circumscribed morphea, which can extend to the fascia and muscle and is more recalcitrant to intervention.

The diagnosis is *generalized morphea* (GM) when there are four or more plaques, often with plaque confluence, that are larger than 3 cm and involve at least two of seven anatomic sites (head-neck, right upper extremity, left upper extremity, right lower extremity, left lower extremity, anterior trunk, posterior trunk) (Fig. 7.2). Overall, 7–9 % of children with localized scleroderma have the generalized type [1, 4, 5]. Unilateral GM has been proposed as an uncommon variant, usually beginning in childhood [8].

Linear scleroderma is the most common subtype in children and adolescents, representing 42–65 % of cases of pediatric localized scleroderma [1, 4, 5, 9]. Linear scleroderma occurs more often in children than adults [10]. Linear scleroderma is characterized by one or more linear streaks that can extend through the dermis, subcutaneous tissue, and muscle to the underlying bone, often causing significant deformity (Fig. 7.3). In one study, 25.6 % of patients with linear

J. Varga et al. (eds.), *Scleroderma*, DOI 10.1007/978-3-319-31407-5_7

Table 7.1 Proposed preliminary classification criteria for juvenile localized scleroderma (Consensus Conference, Padua (Italy) 2004) [2]

Main group	Subtype	Description
1. Circumscribed morphea	(a) Superficial	Oval or round circumscribed areas of induration limited to the epidermis and dermis, often with altered pigmentation and violaceous, erythematous halo (lilac ring). Lesions can be single or multiple
	(b) Deep	Oval or round circumscribed deep induration of the skin involving subcutaneous tissue extending to fascia and may involve underlying muscle. Lesions can be single or multiple
		Subcutaneous tissue may be the primary site of involvement without involvement of overlying skin
2. Linear scleroderma	(a) Trunk/limbs	Linear induration involving the dermis, the subcutaneous tissue, and, sometimes, underlying muscle and bone and affecting the limbs and/or trunk
	(b) Head	En coup de sabre (ECDS). Linear induration that affects the face and/or the scalp and sometimes underlying muscle and bone
		Parry-Romberg or progressive hemifacial atrophy. Loss of tissue on one side of the face that may involve the dermis, subcutaneous tissue, muscle, and bone. The skin is mobile
3. Generalized morphea		Induration of the skin starting as individual plaques (four or more and larger than 3 cm) that become confluent and involve at least two anatomic sites
4. Pansclerotic morphea		Circumferential involvement of limb(s) affecting the skin, subcutaneous tissue, muscle, and bone. Lesions may involve more than one body area, but do not affect internal organs
5. Mixed type morphea		Combination of two or more of the previous subtypes. The order of the concomitant subtypes, specified in brackets, will follow their predominant representation in the individual patient (i.e., mixed (linear circumscribed))

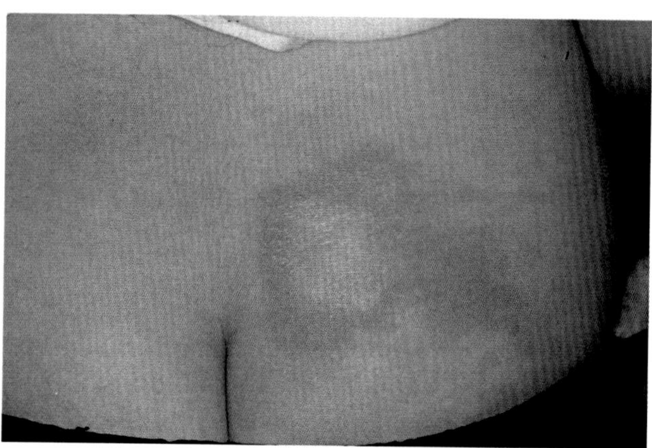

Fig. 7.1 Circumscribed localized scleroderma of the buttock area, characterized by an area of induration with waxy consistence (ivory color at center), surrounded by an inflammatory edge. Note the cutaneous atrophy, characterized by fine wrinkling and shininess

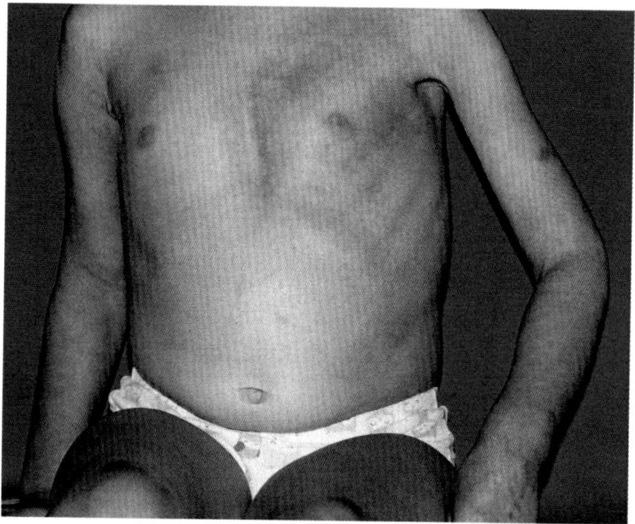

Fig. 7.2 Generalized morphea in this 4-year-old girl. Shown are sites of involvement on the left side of the trunk, left arm and hand, and right upper arm. The face, neck, and legs were also involved with circumscribed morphea lesions. Note increased visibility of veins on the left side of the chest because of cutaneous atrophy

morphea involving an extremity developed contractures and 32.6% developed limb undergrowth [4]. The *en coup de sabre* (ECDS) variety is linear localized scleroderma of the face and scalp. ECDS often affects the forehead unilaterally (Fig. 7.4) and can be associated with "white" anterior uveitis, alopecia, neurological, and/or ocular signs [7]. If involving the lower face, ECDS can be associated with dental and tongue abnormalities [11–14]. The presentation of ECDS of the forehead can be subtle and resemble a port-wine stain [15, 16]. The Parry-Romberg syndrome (PRS) is characterized by hemifacial atrophy with mild or absent involvement of the superficial skin and can involve the underlying fat, muscle, cartilage, or bone. It is considered the severe end of the spectrum of ECDS [11].

Pansclerotic morphea, an extremely rare but severe subtype, is characterized by generalized full-thickness involvement of the skin of the trunk, extremities, face, and/or scalp. It is more common in children than adults. Chronic ulcers may develop and evolve to squamous cell carcinoma [17–20]. Other complications are site specific: joint contractures, reduction of chest expansion, lagophthalmos and ectropion,

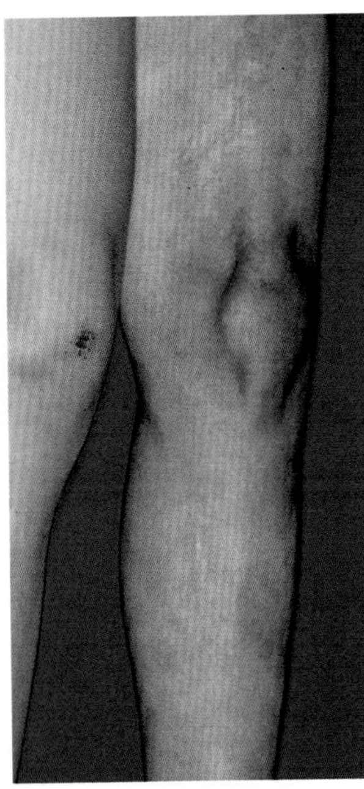

Fig. 7.3 Linear scleroderma. The lesion tracks down the anterior aspect of the left thigh to the lower leg. Not shown are involvement of the ankle and dorsal aspect of the foot. Note the irregular dyschromia (hypo- and hyperpigmentation) on the thigh and the prominent veins on the shin

gastrointestinal reflux, cicatricial alopecia, and thrombosis of the foot leading to amputation [21].

Up to 40 % of the patients have extracutaneous manifestations, most commonly individuals with linear scleroderma, generalized morphea, or pansclerotic morphea [4, 7, 22]. Arthralgias and arthritis are the most frequent finding (23 %) [4]. Children who develop arthritis often have a lesion that crosses over the joint, but some of them develop arthritis in joints without skin involvement. Gastroesophageal reflux is the only gastrointestinal complication reported so far in pediatric localized scleroderma [1, 23, 24], but it is not more common than expected in a pediatric population. Extracutaneous manifestations of ECDS are not uncommon. Migraine and non-migraine headaches can precede the development of cutaneous findings [25, 26], and seizures, behavioral changes, and learning disabilities have also been described [22, 27]. Abnormalities on magnetic resonance imaging (MRI), such as calcifications, white matter changes, vascular malformations, and vasculitis, may be associated, even without clinical evidence of neurological manifestations [28, 29]. Although most of the imaging abnormalities have little clinical relevance, biopsy findings have shown sclerosis, fibrosis, gliosis, as well as vasculitis [29, 30]. Ocular involvement has been found in 3.2–8.3 % of patients with ECDS linear scleroderma

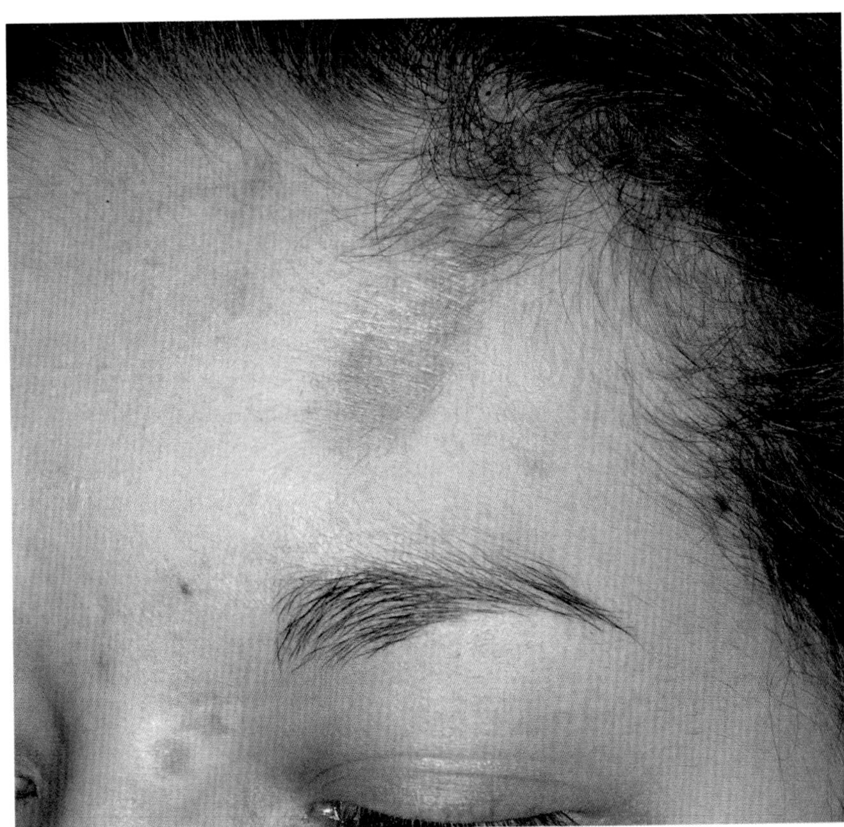

Fig. 7.4 En coup de sabre morphea. Note the old hyperpigmented streak on the left side of the forehead; the active, newer area on the left side of the upper nose; and the loss of medial eyebrow

[22, 31]. Ocular involvement most commonly includes a "white" anterior uveitis, eyelid and eyelash abnormalities, episcleritis, CNS abnormalities, glaucoma, papilledema, or xerophthalmia [22, 31]. Parry-Romberg syndrome can be associated with vascular changes (i.e., Raynaud's phenomenon and deep vein thrombosis), seizures, brain atrophy, and intracranial vascular malformation [32].

The concurrence of other autoimmune disorders is less common in children (3–10%) than in adults, although children with localized scleroderma are more likely to have a family history of autoimmune disease than adults with localized scleroderma [9]. These include juvenile idiopathic arthritis, systemic lupus erythematosus, autoimmune thyroid disease, Raynaud's syndrome, vitiligo, celiac disease, and alopecia areata [7, 22].

Autoantibodies

Antinuclear antibodies (ANA) have been reported in 30–40% of patients with pediatric localized scleroderma [1, 9]. This frequency is lower than in adults with localized scleroderma [33], but is significantly higher than in the normal population. Having a positive ANA does not correlate with any particular subtype or disease course [1, 34]. Rheumatoid factor (RF) has been detected at low titer in 16% of the patients with pediatric localized scleroderma [1]. Anti-histone antibodies (AHA) are detected in 47% of patients with pediatric localized scleroderma, most often in patients with generalized and linear localized scleroderma and rarely in circumscribed localized scleroderma [33, 34].

Diagnosis and Disease Assessment

There has been a recent validation of a clinical assessment tool for localized scleroderma, the modified localized scleroderma skin severity index (mLoSSI). The mLoSSI is easily applicable without any additional instruments beside clinical examination and is the summation of 18 anatomical sites evaluated for erythema, skin thickness, and new lesion/extension of lesions [35, 36]. The score changes with activity of disease. It does not assess extracutaneous manifestations. Additional objective measures such as ultrasound, infrared thermography, durometry, computerized skin score, and magnetic resonance imaging (MRI) promise to improve the clinical evaluation of localized scleroderma. However, all of these measures need validation to differentiate between activity and "scar" of the disease. In a pediatric population, the mLoSSI and physician's global assessment of disease activity were found to be sensitive to clinical change [37]. A validated quality-of-life assessment is not yet available.

The computerized skin score, which is only available in some centers, involves demarcation of hyperemic and indurated borders of the lesions onto an adhesive transparent film. The film is transferred over cardboard, scanned, and the affected area is calculated by computing software [38]. Although objective calculations increase reliability, the dyspigmentation of inactive lesions can be misinterpreted as disease activity.

High-frequency ultrasonography (18 MHz) has been used to detect clinical disease activity as assessed by dermal thickness, increased blood flow (inflammation), and increased echogenicity (atrophy, fibrosis) [39, 40]. Ultrasonography should be performed using a standardized protocol [41, 42]. Infrared thermography is able to detect disease activity based on increased temperature caused by the inflammatory process [43], but is rarely available. This noninvasive technique has shown high reproducibility, but yields false-positive results in assessing old lesions that are characterized by marked atrophy of the skin and subcutaneous tissues; the clinical examination can complement to distinguish old atrophic lesions. Durometry has been used for detecting induration/hardness of skin in systemic sclerosis and correlates with the modified Rodnan skin score and ultrasound thickness [44, 45]. MRI can be valuable in assessment of CNS abnormalities, limb discrepancies, arthritis, or eye involvement [46]. However, given the need for sedation in younger patients, cost, and the presence of possible artifacts, MRI is not a reasonable assessment tool for everyday practice.

Treatment

Treatment options are shown in Fig. 7.5. Localized scleroderma can lead to significant disability. Systemic treatment is suggested in cases of contractures or for lesions that (i) cross joint lines; (ii) are overlying the spine, which can cause severe scoliosis; (iii) affect the face because of the concern for cosmetic changes; (iv) course down the extremities, which can cause limb shortening and dysfunction of hands and feet; and (v) occur in other cosmetically sensitive areas. All of these can significantly influence the quality of life. The consensus meeting of the Pediatric Rheumatology European Society (PreS) made clear suggestions for the indications of systemic treatment (paper submitted).

Local treatment for circumscribed morphea is reserved for lesions small and not leading to any kind of disability. Local treatment is generally restricted to application of vitamin D analogues (calcipotriene or calcitriol) with or without topical corticosteroids. Calcipotriene and calcitriol are used twice daily, usually with the evening dose under occlusion [47, 48]. Newer studies have suggested that topical tacrolimus or imiquimod may be of benefit, but these are used less

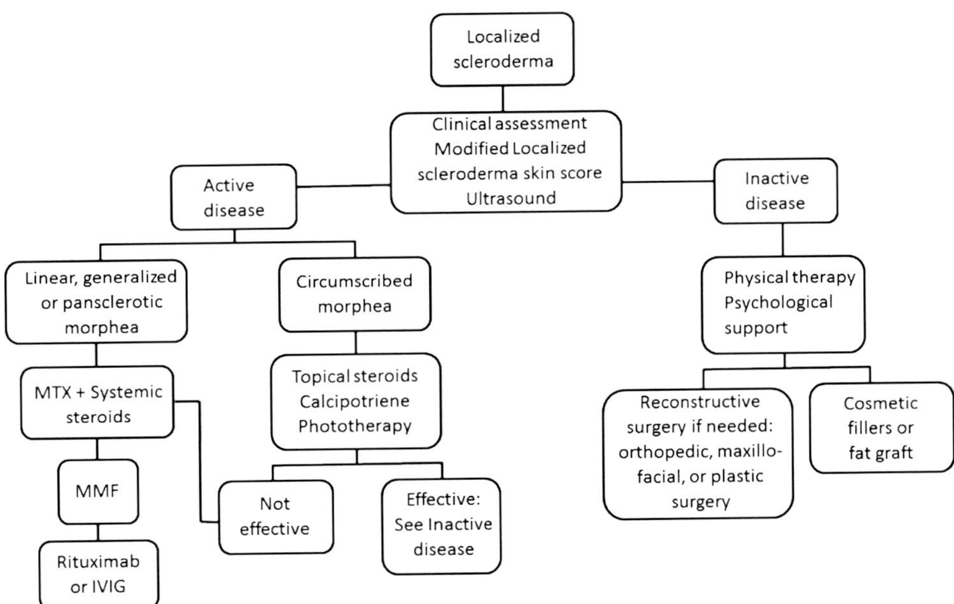

Fig. 7.5 Management of localized scleroderma

often. In a double-blind, placebo-controlled pilot study in adults, tacrolimus 0.1 % ointment twice daily was superior to placebo in decreasing skin hardness measured by durometer (not a validated measure) and improving clinical features (measuring erythema, induration, dyspigmentation, and atrophy) [49]. One case study described improvement of generalized morphea in an adult with tacrolimus 0.1 % ointment, applied twice daily for 8 weeks [50]. In a prospective, open-label, double-blind study of nine children, topical imiquimod 5 % cream, applied three times weekly for 1 month and then five times weekly for 32 weeks, led to improvement of induration/dermal thickness [51]. An open phase II clinical trial in adults suggests that topical pirfenidone, a molecule shown to have anti-fibrotic activity, led to improvement in the mLoSSI in 100 % of the patients after being used three times daily for 6 months [52].

Phototherapy with UVA1 represents another possible therapeutic choice for pediatric localized scleroderma [29, 30, 32], but requires long-term therapy. The relapse rate after UVA1 phototherapy in a study of both adults and children was 44 % and 48 %, respectively, by 2 and 3 years after discontinuation [53]. Recurrence was increased with older lesions, emphasizing the importance of early detection and treatment. Lack of long-term safety data with the use of UVA1 and adherence difficulties in young children (who need to sit in a light box for 20–30 min) are limitations. Given its potential long-term side effects, psoralen with UVA (PUVA) is not usually recommended for children.

In addition to topical vitamin D analogues, systemic vitamin D analogues have also been used. In an open prospective study, daily administration of oral calcitriol for 4–6 months improved skin induration, joint mobility, and skin extensibility [54]; however, oral calcitriol was not more effective than placebo in a controlled trial [55] and is associated with the risk of hypercalciuria and renal stones.

First-line systemic therapy is methotrexate, initiated with oral or pulsed intravenous corticosteroids [56–62], which has been found to be effective in 73.8 % of patients [63] (Table 7.2). The Childhood Arthritis and Rheumatology Research Alliance [5] recommended three treatment plans (without steroid, with oral steroid, with IV pulsed steroid), each with a dose of methotrexate of 1 mg/kg/week s.c. [64] based on 15 published studies with A ($n=1$) and B ($n=3$) levels of evidence. However, the suggested dose based on the only controlled trial [62] is 15 mg/m^2 body surface once a week (0.3 mg/kg/week) administered subcutaneously (maximum, 25 mg/week), and other reports suggest that 0.3–0.5 mg/kg/week given orally or subcutaneously is successful [4, 58]. During the first 2–3 months of therapy, a course of glucocorticoids may be used as adjunctive bridge therapy. The corticosteroid regimen can be (1) methylprednisolone IV 30 mg/kg/dose with a schedule of one dose/week × 12 weeks, (2) three consecutive daily doses/month × 3 months, or (3) oral prednisone 2 mg/kg/day (maximum dose of 60 mg) for a minimum of 2 weeks but maximum of 4 weeks. Success has also been described with oral prednisone at 1 mg/kg/day, either used for 1 month and then decreased to 0.5 mg/kg/day for 1–2 months or used continuously for 3 months and then tapered [4, 60, 62]. Weaning off methotrexate should be tried after 12–24 months of remission.

Side effects of methotrexate have been described in up to 48.3 % of children, but are generally mild and do not require discontinuation of therapy. Nausea is most common and can be mitigated by switching from oral to s.c. or manipulation of the folate dosing. All patients should receive folic acid supplementation, but whether to give folate 1 mg (most com-

Table 7.2 Treatment with methotrexate in localized scleroderma

Author (year)	Study design	Regimen	No. of patients (children)	Follow-up	Result	Assessment
Seyger (1998)	Retrospective	MTX 15 mg/week orally	9 (0)	24 weeks	Effective (67 %)	Skin score Durometer Patient's judgment (VAS)
Uziel (2000)	Retrospective	MTX 0.3–0.6 mg/kg/week orally or s.c. + MPDN 30 mg/kg/day pulse for 3 days/month for 3 months	10 (10)	8–30 weeks	Effective (90 %)	Clinical judgment
Kreuter (2005)	Pilot, uncontrolled	MTX 15 mg/week orally + MPDN 1,000 mg/day pulse for 3 days/month for 6 months	15 (0)	6–25 months	Effective (93 %)	Skin score Patient's judgment (VAS) USG, histopathology
Fitch (2006)	Retrospective	MTX 0.4–1.0 mg/kg/week os or sc ± PDN 1 mg/kg/day or every other day for 3–6 months	17 (17)	6–60 months	Effective (94 %)	Clinical judgment Telephone questionnaire
Wiebel (2006)	Retrospective	MTX 10 mg/m²/week ± PDN 1 mg/kg/day or every other day for 3–6 months	34 (34)	24 months	Effective (74 %)	Clinical judgment, thermography
Christen-Zaech (2008)	Retrospective chart review	MTX 0.3–0.5 mg/kg/week starting dose + PDN 1 mg/kg/day for 1 month and then decreased to 0.5 mg/kg/day		1 month–17 years	Effective	Clinical judgment
Zulian (2011)	Double-blind randomized controlled trial	MTX 15 mg/m²/week for 12 months + PDN 1 mg/kg/day for 3 months versus Placebo for 12 months + PDN 1 mg/kg/day for 3 months	70 (70)	12 months	Effective (MTX 67 %) (PLAC 29 %)	Clinical judgment Clinical judgment thermography Computerized skin score
Koch (2013)	Retrospective chart review	MTX 5–17.5 mg/week ± PDN 10–20 mg daily	17 (all subjects <25 years of age)	Average of 6.6 years	100 % had improvement but 54 % required second course of MTX	Clinical judgment

MPDN methylprednisolone, *MTX* methotrexate, *PDN* prednisolone, *USG* ultrasonography

However, the suggested dose based on the only controlled trial (62) is 15 mg/m2 body surface once a week (0.3 mg/kg/wk) administered subcutaneously (maximum, 25 mg/wk) and other reports suggest that 0.3-0.5 mg/kg/week given orally or subcutaneously is successful [4, 58]

mon dosing) daily or for 6 days, skipping the day of methotrexate administration, or whether a single dose of 5 mg folate (e.g., on the day after the methotrexate) remains controversial [65].

If a patient does not respond to methotrexate and corticosteroids, mycophenolate mofetil (MMF) can be added, although sometimes it is effective as a single agent. A retrospective review of ten patients with pediatric localized scleroderma who failed methotrexate and/or corticosteroids described clinical response to MMF [66]. Six of the patients who responded were concurrently administered methotrexate and corticosteroids, two patients were concurrently using corticosteroids, and two patients were administered only MMF. The CARRA consensus recommended treatment dosing with MMF 600 mg/m^2 twice daily for patients <1.25 m^2, 750 mg twice daily for 40–50 kg weight, and 1,000 mg twice daily for patients over 50 kg [64].

A 3-year-old girl with generalized morphea was successfully treated with MTX 0.5 mg/m^2/week, prednisolone 1 mg/kg/day (tapered after 3 months), and imatinib 235 mg/m^2/day with nearly complete resolution of her skin lesions after 1 year [67]. However, trials of imatinib in generalized morphea or systemic sclerosis have not shown changes in skin involvement as measured by modified Rodnan skin score or dermal thickness measured by skin biopsies [68, 69].

Rituximab, tocilizumab [70], abatacept [70, 71], and intravenous immunoglobulin (IVIG) are treatments that have been tried in refractory cases of adult systemic sclerosis and may be considered in severe cases of pediatric localized scleroderma. In adult patients, rituximab administration improved the skin score after two treatments given 6 months apart [72, 73]. An 11-year-old boy with ulcerating plaques of sclerotic skin and severe ankyloses improved with IVIG treatment [74].

Surgical reconstruction may be required if the disease has not been adequately controlled. Surgery should only be performed after the active phase of the disease has abated and when the child's growth is complete [75]. Facial recontouring is a surgical treatment option that may improve quality of life in adolescents with facial asymmetry due to en coup de sabre linear scleroderma [76]. A recent study in patients with Parry-Romberg syndrome found that fat graft assisted by bone marrow-derived mesenchymal stem cells required fewer injections to reach a satisfactory cosmetic outcome than fat graft treatment alone [77]. This technology requires larger studies but may be a viable treatment option in the future.

Quality of Life

There are no prospectively validated quality-of-life instruments for localized scleroderma. Localized scleroderma shows a moderate effect on quality of life [78]. Pain, itch, and tightness and especially cosmetic changes have been associated with a poorer quality of life in affected children [79].

Prognosis

Information on the long-term outcome of children with pediatric localized scleroderma is increasing. A retrospective review of 52 patients with linear scleroderma, seen over a span of 20 years, showed that 31 % of patients with disease duration of ≥10 years still had active disease [80]. A case of reactivation after 20 years was also reported. With an average of 5 years of follow-up time, 98 % of patients reported residual dyspigmentation, atrophy, or both [80]. A larger study of 344 patients showed disease recurrence in 27 % of pediatric-onset localized scleroderma as compared to 17 % recurrence for adult onset [81]. The median time between remission and first recurrence was similar in both groups (26–27 months). This new data confirms the importance of long-term follow-up in this patient population.

Juvenile Systemic Sclerosis

Juvenile systemic sclerosis (jSSc) is a rare multisystem connective tissue disease [82]. Approximately 5–10 % of all adults with systemic sclerosis (SSc) report the onset of the disease during childhood. It has a variety of clinical manifestation and the distribution of diffuse versus limited forms, and the proportion of patients with overlap features differs from the adult form. Mixed connective tissue disease (MCTD) and overlap syndromes have features of jSSc and sometimes even fulfill the criteria of jSSc [83]. Localized scleroderma is a separate disorder and does not evolve into systemic sclerosis, although some children develop some of the features of systemic disease, such as dysphagia or abnormal pulmonary function tests [4, 84].

jSSc is characterized by pathologic thickening and tethering of the skin. It is thought that the fibrosis is a consequence of a vasculopathy of the small vessel system, associated with altered endothelial cell function [85], which leads to fibrotic changes of the skin and other organs. Alterations of the immune system and genetic and environmental factors are part of the pathogenesis. Several recent publications review this topic extensively [85–89]. Triggers of the disease are still unclear. A positive family history of SSc is one of the strongest known risk factors for SSc [90, 91]. This chapter will be focused on clinical characteristics and outcome of jSSc in childhood and on the clinical presentation and outcome of jSSc patients in adult cohorts of SSc patients. The specific clinical features of jSSc will be compared to the adult-onset systemic sclerosis (aSSc). Unfortunately there is still no evidence-based data regarding treatment of jSSc patients. Most of the therapeutic suggestions are derived from the adult literature and the therapeutic recommendations of the EULAR/EUSTAR [92, 93], which summarizes the state of evidence-based expert opinion on SSc management.

Clinical Presentation of Patients with Juvenile Systemic Scleroderma

The first, large cross-sectional cohort based on a multinational survey of pediatric rheumatologists was published in 2000 [94]. A recently initiated prospective registry with standardized assessment of jSSc patients includes more than 70 patients to date (www.juvenile-scleroderma.com). In this prospective cohort, disease subset distribution differs from that of affected adults. The youngest patient enrolled is 2 years of age and the mean is 6.1 years of age; 77 % are female; and the mean age of onset of Raynaud's symptoms was 9.2 years old (range, 2–16 years). The mean age at the onset of symptoms other than Raynaud's was 9.7 years (range, 3–16 years). The diffuse subtype was recognized in 74 % and overlap symptoms in 38 % (submitted for publication, Foeldvari et al.); these data are consistent with previous survey data [10, 94].

In the large, multicenter cross-sectional case collection [94] of 135 jSSc patients followed for a mean of 5 years, the mean age of the disease onset was 8.8 years, significantly younger than previously expected. The male/female ratio of 1:2.85 showed less of a female preponderance than the adult cohort. In one other multicenter cross-sectional study of 153 patients [95], the mean age at disease onset was 8.1 years. Organ involvement in these patients is presented in Table 7.3. Taken together, these two studies showed that 63.5–79 % of patients have joint involvement, 65–69 % have gastrointestinal involvement, and 41.8–50 % have pulmonary involvement. Renal involvement is relatively infrequent (9.8–13 %). In the cohort of Foeldvari et al., 16 % of the patients had central nervous system involvement, which seems to be unique [94]. In the cohort of Martini et al., 90.8 % of the patients

Table 7.3 Organ involvement of the patients in the two pediatric multicenter cross-sectional studies

Organ involvement	Foeldvari et al. $n=135$ (%)	Martini et al. $n=153$ (%)
Skin	135 (100)	116 (75.8)[a]
Joints	106 (79)	97(63.5)
GI tract	88 (65)	106(69)
Only esophageal	63 (47)	47(31)
Pulmonary	68(50)	64(41.8)
Cardiovascular	60 (44)	44(28.8)
CNS	21 (16)	4 (3)
Renal	17 (13)	15 (9.8)
Muscular	13 (10)	37(24.2)
Raynaud's	97 (72)	128(83.7)
Calcinosis	36 (27)	28(18.3)
Sjögren's syndr.	7 (5)	?
CREST	1	?

[a]75.8 % skin induration; 66 % sclerodactyly; 44.1 % edema

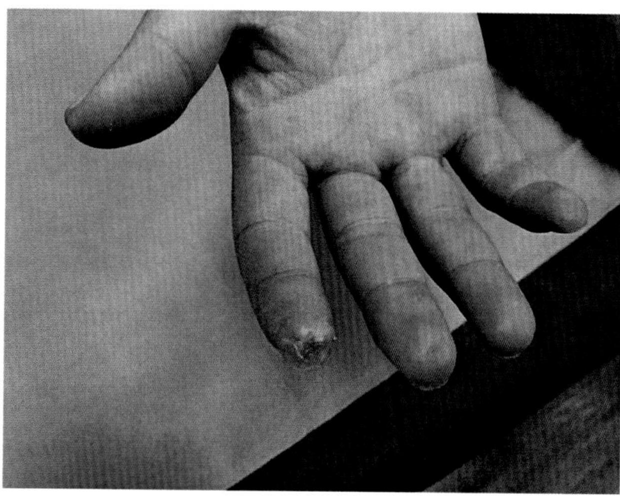

Fig. 7.6 Scarring on the fingertips associated with severe secondary Raynaud's in jSSc

showed a diffuse subtype, which was consistent with the few (7.1 %) patients with anti-centromere antibodies [95]. In the cohort of Foeldvari et al., no patient had anti-centromere antibodies, despite typical pitting fingertip scars that are reminiscent of a CREST pattern of limited scleroderma in adult patients (Fig. 7.6). Only one patient in either cohort had CREST syndrome, part of the limited subtype spectrum. In the prospective cohort, 68 % (34/50) of the patients have diffuse subset.

Of note, these studies represent retrospective multicenter data, with overlapping cohorts and evaluation of the organ involvement that was not standardized. However, results are comparable between the two, as well as with other published single-center case series from Japan (61 patients) [96], South America (23 cases) [97], and Asia (23 cases) [98]. Ethnic differences in the East Indian population may explain the 39 % of patients with the limited subtype [98]; in all other case series, the diffuse subtype affected 90.9–100 % of patients. The prevalence of the anti-centromere antibody positivity was from 0 to 7.1 %.

Incidence and Prevalence of Juvenile Systemic Sclerosis

Juvenile systemic sclerosis (jSSc) is an orphan autoimmune disease, and data regarding incidence and prevalence are rare. In a study from Finland in 1994 [91, 99], where nationwide, prospective, hospital-based assessments during a 4-year period were conducted and supplemented with data from the National Hospital Discharge Register, an annual incidence rate was found to be 0.05 per 100,000 with a population at risk of 1.02 million. According to a recent cross-sectional study from Herrick et al. [82], the incidence rate of patients younger than 16 years of age with abnormal skin thickening consistent with SSc or linear scleroderma was 0.27 (95 % confidence interval 0.1–0.5) per million children. The mean age of these patients was 12.1 years. No prevalence data has been published. In a German Pediatric Rheumatology Registry, 19 patients were recorded among 14 million children under the age of 18 years (1.36 cases per one million children; Dr. Kirsten Minden, personal communication).

Classification

The first classification criteria specific for jSSc were published in 2007 [83]. The patient has to fulfill one major and two minor criteria. Major criteria are proximal sclerosis and induration of the skin from the metacarpophalangeal joint or metatarsophalangeal joint. The established eight minor criteria domains are listed in Table 7.4 and are organ specific

Table 7.4 The provisional classification criteria for juvenile systemic sclerosis [83]

Major criteria	Minor criteria
Induration/sclerosis	Vascular changes
	Pulmonary involvement
	Gastrointestinal involvement
	Renal involvement
	Cardiovascular involvement
	Musculoskeletal involvement
	Neurologic involvement
	Serology

[83]. These proposed criteria have 90 % sensitivity and 96 % specificity, although prospective validation is pending.

Adult rheumatologists also have a consensus classification [100] with organ-specific scores. A score of 9 is required for the diagnosis of SSc. Skin involvement proximal to the metacarpophalangeal joint or metatarsophalangeal joint is sufficient to make the diagnosis. These criteria are currently in the process of validation testing in the adult SSc population. All children who meet pediatric criteria also meet the adult criteria.

Diagnosis and Assessment of the Patient

A key clinical goal is earlier detection and diagnosis of jSSc. The typical facial appearance of a child with juvenile-onset systemic scleroderma is shown in Fig. 7.7. Raynaud's phenomenon is the presenting symptom in 75 % of the patients at time of diagnosis [95], and sclerodactyly is another key feature at onset, but is present only in 37 % [95]. Capillaroscopy is not prospectively validated in jSSc patients, although it is used to diagnose SSc and specifically Raynaud's in adults. In the largest retrospective pediatric study [95], only 10 % of patients had capillary changes at disease onset and 25 % at diagnosis of jSSc. However, it is unclear how many reporting centers reviewed capillary changes routinely and what kind of capillaroscopy they used. Normal capillaries behave differently in children vs. adults, and capillary dimension needs to be age adjusted, since arterial and venous dimensions increase with age and tortuous capillaries can appear in healthy children [101–104]. Video capillaroscopy is the most sensitive for detecting changes. The handheld dermatoscope or ophthalmoscope can visualize changes, but these devices are inadequate to gauge quantitative change [105]. The Pediatric Rheumatology European Society (PreS) Juvenile Scleroderma Working Group recommends that patients with Raynaud's and pathologic nail fold capillary changes be followed at least every 6 months (paper submitted for publication).

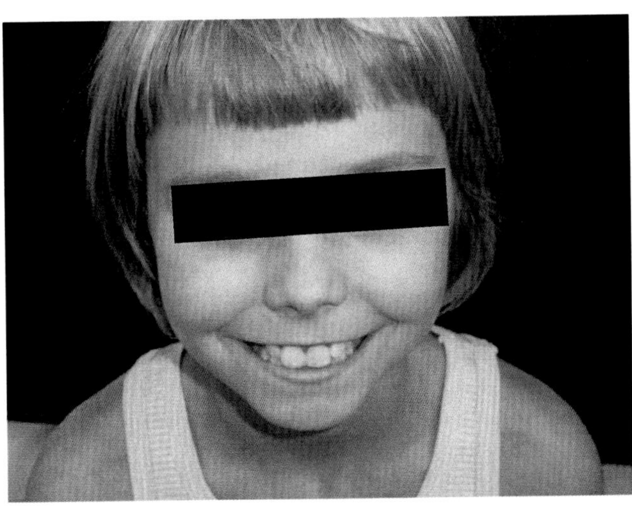

Fig. 7.7 Classical facial appearance of a child with juvenile-onset systemic scleroderma

The modified Rodnan skin score, which has been validated in adults, is not necessarily applicable to pediatric patients. The skin score in healthy children depends on Tanner stage and body mass index (BMI) [106]. The durometer, a handheld device, can differentiate between healthy and sclerotic skin but does not work well if a bony structure directly underlies the skin, like in the fingers, face, and dorsal foot.

The 6-min walk test (6MWT) is a well-established primary outcome measure in adult treatment studies for pulmonary hypertension but is not validated in jSSc patients. Two studies looked at normal values of 6MWT in children [107, 108], but the range for age groups in the two studies differs significantly, making analysis difficult. The length of the lap and the physical condition correlate with the distance that can be walked in 6 min and establish a percentile curve for normal values (paper submitted). Pulmonary function is one of the main dominators of the walk distance in jSSc patients. Pulmonary function tests in jSSc patients correlate well with the high-resolution computed tomography findings [109].

There is no specific antibody to prove the diagnosis. Because most pediatric patients have a diffuse subset, anti-Scl70 is more frequent, occurring in ~34 % [95]. Anti-centromere antibodies are detected in 0–7 % of children [94, 95, 110]. Inflammatory markers, such as sedimentation rate or CRP, are elevated in only 34–38 % and 12.6 % of patients, respectively.

Biologic markers of general disease or organ involvement may facilitate the diagnosis and serial evaluation of organ involvement or disease activity noninvasively [111–115]. In a pilot study, jSSc children with interstitial lung disease had higher levels of anti-KL6 than healthy children or children with jSSc without lung disease [116]. There are also studies regarding the prognostic value of B-type natriuretic peptide in children with pulmonary hypertension [117–119].

Differential Diagnosis

In scleroderma-like disorders, the distribution and characteristics of skin involvement seem to be "atypical" as compared to classic SSc, and the acral skin involvement and typical antibody pattern is usually missing. Exposure to certain chemicals or drugs may also suggest the presence of a scleroderma-like disease. These exposures are in the pediatric population less frequent as in the adult population. Lack of Raynaud's phenomenon, scleroderma-specific antinuclear antibodies, scleroderma capillary pattern on nail fold capillaroscopy, and typical internal organ manifestations may also indicate the presence of a scleroderma-like disorder. Skin biopsy may be valuable in considering the differential diagnosis.

Scleroderma-like disorders include diseases with mucin deposition (scleromyxedema, scleredema, etc.). Some disorders show papulonodular skin changes with or without dermal deposition of materials (amyloid, mucin deposition; fibroblastic rheumatism, etc.). Diseases with monoclonal gammopathy (scleromyxedema, POEMS syndrome, myeloma with scleroderma-like skin changes) also belong to the large group of scleroderma-like diseases. Some disorders are characterized by eosinophilia (diffuse fasciitis with eosinophilia, eosinophilia-myalgia syndrome, toxic oil syndrome), metabolic/biochemical abnormalities (IDDM, nephrogenic fibrosing dermopathy), and endocrine abnormalities (POEMS syndrome, hypo-/hyperthyroidism with mucin deposition, diabetes). Chronic graft-versus-host disease (cGVHD) may also show scleroderma-like skin changes.

Scleroderma-like disorders can be induced by drugs or chemicals (eosinophilia-myalgia syndrome, toxic oil syndrome, vinyl chloride disease; cytostatic agents (docetaxel, paclitaxel, gemcitabine, bleomycin, peplomycin, melphalan, capecitabine, and uracyl-tegafur); appetite suppressants; and physical injury (trauma, vibration stress, radiation injury). Inherited progeroid syndromes with early aging (e.g., Werner syndrome) and a large heterogeneous group of hereditary disorders with either skin thickening (porphyria, phenylketonuria) or skin atrophy/tightening (restrictive dermopathy, scleroatrophic and keratotic dermatosis of the limbs, etc.) should also be considered in the differential diagnosis of scleroderma-like disorders. These categories are not mutually exclusive, because the remarkably different scleroderma-like diseases show overlapping features.

Management

There are no controlled studies or specific recommendations for the treatment of pediatric disease. Therefore, therapeutic suggestions are based on publications in adult systemic sclerosis patients. Some of the medications used in adults are not available for children, there is no pediatric dosing for some drugs, and there is growing evidence that pediatric patients have higher or lower dosing requirements than adults. EULAR/EUSTAR, representing specialized centers for children, published its last therapeutic guidelines in 2009 [120].

There is no curative treatment for SSc. Autologous bone marrow transplantation is the most effective treatment with an effect on all organ systems if conducted early in the disease course in carefully selected, rapidly progressing patients [121]. If used as rescue therapy late in the disease course, transplantation has a high mortality rate [84]. There are only case reports regarding the effect of bone marrow transplantation in children.

Certain drugs have led to organ-specific improvement, such as the ameliorative effect of methotrexate on skin, joint, muscle, or interstitial lung disease. Most experts prefer methotrexate for pediatric SSc (15 mg/m^2) [122], but some prefer mycophenolate mofetil as first-line treatment. No comparative studies have been performed. Cyclophosphamide led to disease stabilization in two large adult studies [123, 124], but showed no significant effect after 12 months in a meta-analysis [125] and has higher toxicity. Several reports suggest some efficacy of biologics for the skin and organ involvement, including rituximab [126–128], tocilizumab [70], abatacept [70], and tumor necrosis factor (TNF) inhibitors. TNF inhibitors are particularly effective for the associated arthritis [129, 130]. Several controlled studies are currently underway in adults with SSc. Because they increase the risk of renal hypertension in adult SSc, medium to high-dose glucocorticoids are avoided, but to date there is no pediatric data regarding this increased risk.

Several "palliative" drugs influence the effect of disease without having a direct effect on the autoimmune process. Examples include proton pump inhibitors for reflux; calcium and anti-endothelin antagonists, phosphodiesterase blocking agents, and prostacyclins for Raynaud's phenomenon and associated ulceration; and prokinetics for obstipation. ACE inhibitors are the treatment of choice for renal crisis, but are not used prophylactically.

Comparison of the Largest Pediatric Cohort of jSSc with a Large Adult Cohort with Diffuse Subset jSSc

In comparison with the 1349 adult patients with diffuse aSSc from the EUSTAR cohort (Table 7.5) [131], jSSc patients had fewer digital infarcts, pulmonary involvement, gastrointestinal involvement, hypertension, muscle weakness, and tendon friction rub. It is unlikely that the difference in disease duration (mean 7.4 years in adults vs. 3.9 years in the pediatric cohort) accounted for these different features, since most new-onset organ involvement evolves during the first 4 years. The prevalence of anti-centromere antibodies was similar (6 % in the adult diffuse population).

There is scarce data regarding quality-of-life assessment in children with jSSc and no SSc-specific quality-of-life instrument has been validated in jSSc. A pilot study with four patients showed impairment of quality of life compared to a healthy population [78].

Table 7.5 Comparison of the largest pediatric cohort with the EUSTAR adult cohort

	Pediatric cohort [95]	EUSTAR-diffuse subtype [131]
Skin		
Edema	43.8	
Sclerodactyly	66.0	
Skin induration	75.8	100
Calcinosis	18.3	
Peripheral vascular system		
Raynaud's phenomenon	83.7	96
Digital infarcts	28.6	43
Digital pitting	37.9	
Abnormal nail fold capillaries	39.9	
Positive capillaroscopy	51.0	
Respiratory system		
Dyspnea	17.7	45
Abnormal chest X-rays	28.8	53
Abnormal chest HRCT	23.5	
Reduced DLCO	27.5	64
Reduced FVC	41.8	
Cardiac involvement		
Pericarditis/arrhythmias	9.8	13
Heart failure	7.2	17
Pulmonary hypertension	7.2	22
Musculoskeletal system		
Muscle weakness	24.2	37
Arthritis	27.5	21
Arthralgia	36.0	
Tendon friction rubs	10.5	22
Gastrointestinal system		
Dysphagia	24.2	68
Gastroesophageal reflux	30.1	68
Diarrhea	10.5	
Weight loss	27.5	
Renal system		
Raised creatinine/proteinuria	4.6	9
Renal crisis	0.7	4
Hypertension	2.6	19
Nervous system		
Seizures	2.6	
Peripheral neuropathy	1.3	
Abnormal brain MRI	2.6	

Outcome of the Patients in Two Pediatric Cohorts

In both the cohorts [95, 106], survival of the patients after 5 years of the disease was between 90 and 95 %. The eight deaths during the first 2 years of disease in the cohort of Foeldvari et al. [106] resulted from multisystem involvement with pulmonary (75 %), cardiovascular (100 %), central nervous system (38 %), and renal (50 %) involvement. The male-to-female ratio was 1:1 and the median age at disease onset was 10.5 years, but the ratio of fatality in the cohort of Martini et al. [95] was male/female 1:2.2 with a 10.4 years mean age of disease onset. Mean time until death was 4.6 years after diagnosis. Patients with fatal outcomes had higher rates of pulmonary, gastrointestinal, and cardiac involvement. All had the diffuse subtype of jSSc. The patients who died had a significantly shorter time interval to diagnosis (8.8 months vs. 23 months in patients who survived).

Special Issues in the Care for Children with jSSc

Patients and parents/caregivers can have different fears and hopes regarding the side effects of the treatment and side effects of the disease. Understanding of the treatment by the patient is essential.

Outcome of Pediatric-Onset Juvenile Systemic Sclerosis Patients into Adulthood

Three studies in adult SSc cohorts including patients with juvenile onset have evaluated long-term prognosis of jSSc [110, 132, 133]. In Table 7.6, the characteristics of adult patients with juvenile-onset SSc are compared to juvenile patients in a jSSc cohort. As noted above, the preponderance of females increases in the adult cohort (male/female ratio of 1:5–10 compared to 1:3.6 in the pediatric aged cohort), and the subset distribution at adult age of juvenile-onset patients changed to the adult pattern with 35–40 % the diffuse subtype and 46.7–61 % the limited subtype. In the Royal Free Cohort, a large percentage of the patients showed overlap features [132], which seemed to offer a survival advantage. The prevalence of anti-centromere antibodies remained low (5–6.5 %), consistent with better survival with more limited disease. The percentage of patients with pulmonary hypertension is lower than expected compared to the EUSTAR population (20 % in EUSTAR). Unfortunately, not all organ involvement is described in detail in the different populations, so it is not possible to have a complete comparison.

Summary

In summary, juvenile localized scleroderma and juvenile systemic sclerosis are a group of heterogeneous diseases. Both can cause significant morbidity in children. While there are treatment options for both disease groups, more research is needed to develop the best therapies for children.

Table 7.6 Comparison of characteristics in adults with SSc whose disease started during childhood vs. characteristics of children with jSSc (right column)

	jSSc in EUSTAR ($n=60$)	jSSc Royal Free ($n=57$)	jSSc Pittsburgh ($n=57$)	jSSc PRESS ($n=153$)
Mean age at disease onset	12.4 (2–15.9)	13.06 (5–16)	?	8.1 (0.4–15.6)
Disease duration	17.64 (1.8–54.8)	21.15 (3–58)	17.2	3.9 (0.2–18.1)
Sex (male/female)	5/55	11/35	19/92	33/120
Disease subtype diffuse (%)	40	39	35	90.9
Disease subtype limited (%)	46.7	61	40	9.1
Overlap features	NN	43.5	NN	NN
Outcome	59 (98 %)	97 %/15Y//93 %/20Y)//83%25Y	(89(5y)//74(20Y)	112/127(88) 15/127(12) 26
Lost to follow-up (%)	1 (2 %)	NN	NN	(17 %)
ANA positive	90 %		97	80.7 %
Anti-Scl 70 positive	40 %	26	23	34 %
Anti-centromere positive	5 %	6.5	0	7.1 %
Raynaud's phenomenon (%)	95	NN	96	83.7
Pulmonary hypertension (%)	13.3	15	3.6	7.2
Pulmonary fibrosis (%)	23.3	47	9	23.5
Renal crisis (%)	0	2	3.6	0.7

References

1. Zulian F, Athreya BH, Laxer R, Nelson AM, Feitosa de Oliveira SK, Punaro MG, et al. Juvenile localized scleroderma: clinical and epidemiological features in 750 children. An international study. Rheumatology. 2006;45(5):614–20.
2. Laxer R, Zulian F. Localized scleroderma. Curr Opin Rheumatol. 2006;18(6):606–13.
3. Herrick AL, Ennis H, Bhushan M, Silman AJ, Baildam EM. Incidence of childhood linear scleroderma and systemic sclerosis in the UK and Ireland. Arthritis Care Res. 2010;62(2):213–8.
4. Christen-Zaech S, Hakim MD, Afsar FS, Paller AS. Pediatric morphea (localized scleroderma): review of 136 patients. J Am Acad Dermatol. 2008;59(3):385–96.
5. Wu E, Li S, Torok K, Virkud Y, Fuhlbrigge R, Rabinovich C, et al. A28: description of the juvenile localized scleroderma subgroup of the CARRA registry. Arthritis Rheumatol. 2014;66(S3):S43–4.
6. Zulian F, Vallongo C, de Oliveira SKF, Punaro MG, Ros J, Mazur-Zielinska H, et al. Congenital localized scleroderma. J Pediatr. 2006;149(2):248–51.
7. Pequet MS, Holland KE, Zhao S, Drolet BA, Galbraith SS, Siegel DH, et al. Risk factors for morphoea disease severity: a retrospective review of 114 paediatric patients. Br J Dermatol. 2014;170(4):895–900.
8. Peterson LS, Nelson AM, Su WPD. Classification of morphea (localized scleroderma). Mayo Clin Proc. 1995;70(11):1068–76.
9. Leitenberger JJ, Cayce RL, Haley RW, Adams-Huet B, Bergstresser PR, Jacobe HT. Distinct autoimmune syndromes in morphea: a review of 245 adult and pediatric cases. Arch Dermatol. 2009;145(5):545–50.
10. Marzano A, Menni S, Parodi A, Borghi A, Fuligni A, Fabbri P, et al. Localized scleroderma in adults and children. Clinical and laboratory investigations on 239 cases. Eur J Dermatol. 2003;13(2):171–6.
11. Jablonska S, Blaszczyk M. Long-lasting follow-up favours a close relationship between progressive facial hemiatrophy and scleroderma en coup de sabre*. J Eur Acad Dermatol Venereol. 2005;19(4):403–4.
12. Menni S, Marzano A, Passoni E. Neurologic abnormalities in two patients with facial hemiatrophy and sclerosis coexisting with morphea. Pediatr Dermatol. 1997;14(2):113–6.
13. Blaszczyk M, Jablonska S. Linear scleroderma en Coup de Sabre. Relationship with progressive facial hemiatrophy. Adv Exp Med Biol. 1999;455:101–4.
14. Sommer A, Gambichler T, Bacharach-Buhles M, von Rothenburg T, Altmeyer P, Kreuter A. Clinical and serological characteristics of progressive facial hemiatrophy: a case series of 12 patients. J Am Acad Dermatol. 2006;54(2):227–33.
15. Kakimoto C, Ross V, Uebelhoer N. En Coup de Sabre presenting as a port-wine stain previously treated with pulsed dye laser. Dermatol Surg. 2009;35(1):165–7.
16. Kim HS, Lee JY, Kim HO, Park YM. En coup de sabre presenting as a port-wine stain initially treated with a pulsed dye laser. J Dermatol. 2011;38(2):209–10.
17. Petrov I, Gantcheva M, Miteva L, Vassileva S, Pramatarov K. Lower lip squamous cell carcinoma in disabling pansclerotic morphea of childhood. Pediatr Dermatol. 2009;26(1):59–61.
18. Wollina U, Buslau M, Weyers W. Squamous cell carcinoma in pansclerotic morphea of childhood. Pediatr Dermatol. 2002;19(2):151–4.
19. Parodi PC, Riberti C, Draganic Stinco D, Patrone P, Stinco G. Squamous cell carcinoma arising in a patient with long-standing pansclerotic morphea. Br J Dermatol. 2001; 144(2):417–9.
20. Maragh SH, Davis MDP, Bruce AJ, Nelson AM. Disabling pansclerotic morphea: clinical presentation in two adults. J Am Acad Dermatol. 2005;53(2, Supplement):S115–9.
21. Kura M, Jidai S. Disabling pansclerotic morphea of childhood with extracutaneous manifestations. Indian J Dermatol. 2013;58(2):159.
22. Zulian F, Vallongo C, Woo P, Russo R, Ruperto N, Harper J, et al. Localized scleroderma in childhood is not just a skin disease. Arthritis Rheum. 2005;52(9):2873–81.
23. Weber P, Ganser G, Frosch M, Roth J, Hulskamp G, Zimmer K. Twenty-four hour intraesophageal pH monitoring in children and adolescents with scleroderma and mixed connective tissue disease. J Rheumatol. 2000;27(11):2692–5.
24. Guariso G, Conte S, Galeazzi F, Vettorato M, Martini G, Zulian F. Esophageal involvement in juvenile localized scleroderma: a pilot study. Clin Exp Rheumatol. 2007;25(5):786–9.
25. Polcari I, Moon A, Mathes EF, Gilmore ES, Paller AS. Headaches as a presenting symptom of linear morphea en Coup de Sabre. Pediatrics. 2014;134(6):e1715–9.

26. Kraus V, Lawson EF, Scheven EV, Tihan T, Garza J, Nathan RG, et al. Atypical cases of scleroderma en Coup de Sabre. J Child Neurol. 2014;29(5):698–703.
27. Blaszczyk M, Królicki L, Krasu M, Glinska O, Jablonska S. Progressive facial hemiatrophy: central nervous system involvement and relationship with scleroderma en Coup de Sabre. J Rheumatol. 2003;30(9):1997–2004.
28. DeFelipe J, Segura T, Arellano JI, Merchán A, DeFelipe-Oroquieta J, Martín P, et al. Neuropathological findings in a patient with epilepsy and the Parry–Romberg syndrome. Epilepsia. 2001;42(9):1198–203.
29. Flores-Alvarado DE, Esquivel-Valerio JA, Garza-Elizondo M, Espinoza LR. Linear scleroderma en Coup de Sabre and brain calcification: is there a pathogenic relationship? J Rheumatol. 2003;30(1):193–5.
30. Holland KE, Steffes B, Nocton JJ, Schwabe MJ, Jacobson RD, Drolet BA. Linear scleroderma en Coup de Sabre with associated neurologic abnormalities. Pediatrics. 2006;117(1):e132–6.
31. Zannin ME, Martini G, Athreya BH, Russo R, Higgins G, Vittadello F, et al. Ocular involvement in children with localised scleroderma: a multi-centre study. Br J Ophthalmol. 2007;91(10):1311–4.
32. El-Kehdy J, Abbas O, Rubeiz N. A review of Parry-Romberg syndrome. J Am Acad Dermatol. 2012;67(4):769–84.
33. Takehara K, Sato S. Localized scleroderma is an autoimmune disorder. Rheumatology. 2005;44(3):274–9.
34. Warner Dharamsi J, Victor S, Aguwa N, et al. Morphea in adults and children cohort iii: nested case-control study—the clinical significance of autoantibodies in morphea. JAMA Dermatol. 2013;149(10):1159–65.
35. Arkachaisri T, Pino S. Localized scleroderma severity index and global assessments: a pilot study of outcome instruments. J Rheumatol. 2008;35(4):650–7.
36. Arkachaisri T, Vilaiyuk S, Li S, O'Neil KM, Pope E, Higgins GC, et al. The localized scleroderma skin severity index and physician global assessment of disease activity: a work in progress toward development of localized scleroderma outcome measures. J Rheumatol. 2009;36(12):2819–29.
37. Kelsey C, Torok K. The localized scleroderma assessment tool: responsiveness to change in a pediatric clinical population. JAAD. 2013;69(2):214–20.
38. Zulian F, Meneghesso D, Grisan E, Vittadello F, Belloni Fortina A, Pigozzi B, et al. A new computerized method for the assessment of skin lesions in localized scleroderma. Rheumatology. 2007;46(5):856–60.
39. Nezafati KA, Cayce RL, Susa JS, et al. 14-mhz ultrasonography as an outcome measure in morphea (localized scleroderma). Arch Dermatol. 2011;147(9):1112–5.
40. Porta F, Kaloudi O, Garzitto A, Prignano F, Nacci F, Falcini F, et al. High frequency ultrasound can detect improvement of lesions in juvenile localized scleroderma. Mod Rheumatol. 2014;24(5):869–73.
41. Li SC, Liebling MS, Haines KA, Weiss JE, Prann A. Initial evaluation of an ultrasound measure for assessing the activity of skin lesions in juvenile localized scleroderma. Arthritis Care Res (Hoboken). 2011;63(5):735–42.
42. Li SC, Liebling MS, Haines KA. Ultrasonography is a sensitive tool for monitoring localized scleroderma. Rheumatology. 2007;46(8):1316–9.
43. Martini G, Murray KJ, Howell KJ, Harper J, Atherton D, Woo P, et al. Juvenile-onset localized scleroderma activity detection by infrared thermography. Rheumatology. 2002;41(10):1178–82.
44. Kissin EY, Schiller AM, Gelbard RB, Anderson JJ, Falanga V, Simms RW, et al. Durometry for the assessment of skin disease in systemic sclerosis. Arthritis Care Res. 2006;55(4):603–9.
45. Kuwahara Y, Shima Y, Kawai M, Hagihara K, Hirano T, Arimitsu J, et al. What kind of durometer is best suited for the assessment of skin disease in systemic sclerosis? Comment on the article by Kissin et al. Arthritis Care Res. 2008;59(4):601.
46. Liu P, Uziel Y, Chuang S, Silverman E, Krakfchik B, Laxer R. Localized scleroderma: imaging features. Pediatr Radiol. 1994;24(3):207–9.
47. Dytoc MT, Kossintseva I, Ting PT. First case series on the use of calcipotriol–betamethasone dipropionate for morphoea. Br J Dermatol. 2007;157(3):615–8.
48. Cunningham BB, Landells IDR, Langman C, Sailer DE, Paller AS. Topical calcipotriene for morphea/linear scleroderma. J Am Acad Dermatol. 1998;39(2):211–5.
49. Kroft E, Groeneveld T, Seyger M, Jong ED. Efficacy of topical tacrolimus 0.1% in active plaque morphea. Am J Clin Dermatol. 2009;10(3):181–7.
50. Cantisani C, Miraglia E, Richetta A, Mattozzi C, Calvieri S. Generalized morphea successfully treated with tacrolimus 0.1% ointment. J Drugs Dermatol. 2013;12(1):14–5.
51. Pope E, Doria AS, Theriault M, Mohanta A, Laxer RM. Topical imiquimod 5% cream for pediatric plaque morphea: a prospective, multiple-baseline open-label pilot study. Dermatology. 2011;223(4):363–9.
52. Rodriquez-Castellanos M, Tlacuilo-Parra A, Sanchez-Enriquez S, Velez-Gomez E, Guevara-Gutierrez E. Pirfenidone gel in patients with localized scleroderma: a phase II study. Arthritis Res Ther. 2014;16(6):510.
53. Vasquez R, Jabbar A, Khan F, Buethe D, Ahn C, Jacobe H. Recurrence of morphea after successful ultraviolet A1 phototherapy: a cohort study. J Am Acad Dermatol. 2014;70(3):481–8.
54. Caca-Biljanovska N, Vickova-Laskoska M, Dervendi D, Pesic N, Laskoski D. Treatment of generalized morphea with oral 1,25-dihydroxyvitamin D3. Adv Exp Med Biol. 1999;455:299–304.
55. Hulshof M, Bavinck JB, Bergman W, Masclee A, Heickendorff L, Breedveld F, et al. Double-blind, placebo-controlled study of oral calcitriol for the treatment of localized and systemic scleroderma. J Am Acad Dermatol. 2000;43(6):1017–23.
56. Koch SB, Cerci FB, Jorizzo JL, Krowchuk DP. Linear morphea: a case series with long-term follow-up of young, methotrexate-treated patients. J Dermatol Treat. 2013;24(6):435–8.
57. Seyger MMB, van den Hoogen FHJ, de Boo T, de Jong EMGJ. Low-dose methotrexate in the treatment of widespread morphea. J Am Acad Dermatol. 1998;39(2):220–5.
58. Uziel Y, Feldman BM, Krafchik BR, Yeung RSM, Laxer RM. Methotrexate and corticosteroid therapy for pediatric localized scleroderma. J Pediatr. 2000;136(1):91–5.
59. Kreuter A, Gambichler T, Breuckmann F, et al. Pulsed high-dose corticosteroids combined with low-dose methotrexate in severe localized scleroderma. Arch Dermatol. 2005;141(7):847–52.
60. Fitch PG, Rettig P, Burnham JM, Finkel TH, Yan AC, Akin E, et al. Treatment of pediatric localized scleroderma with methotrexate. J Rheumatol. 2006;33(3):609–14.
61. Weibel L, Sampaio MC, Visentin MT, Howell KJ, Woo P, Harper JI. Evaluation of methotrexate and corticosteroids for the treatment of localized scleroderma (morphoea) in children. Br J Dermatol. 2006;155(5):1013–20.
62. Zulian F, Martini G, Vallongo C, Vittadello F, Falcini F, Patrizi A, et al. Methotrexate treatment in juvenile localized scleroderma: a randomized, double-blind, placebo-controlled trial. Arthritis Rheum. 2011;63(7):1998–2006.
63. Zulian F, Vallongo C, Patrizi A, Belloni-Fortina A, Cutrone M, Alessio M, et al. A long-term follow-up study of methotrexate in juvenile localized scleroderma (morphea). J Am Acad Dermatol. 2012;67(6):1151–6.
64. Li SC, Torok KS, Pope E, Dedeoglu F, Hong S, Jacobe HT, et al. Development of consensus treatment plans for juvenile localized

scleroderma: a roadmap toward comparative effectiveness studies in juvenile localized scleroderma. Arthritis Care Res. 2012; 64(8):1175–85.

65. Amarilyo G, Rullo OJ, McCurdy DK, Woo JM, Furst DE. Folate usage in MTX-treated juvenile idiopathic arthritis (JIA) patients is inconsistent and highly variable. Rheumatol Int. 2013; 33(9):2437–40.
66. Martini G, Ramanan AV, Falcini F, Girschick H, Goldsmith DP, Zulian F. Successful treatment of severe or methotrexate-resistant juvenile localized scleroderma with mycophenolate mofetil. Rheumatology. 2009;48(11):1410–3.
67. Inamo Y, Ochiai T. Successful combination treatment of a patient with progressive juvenile localized scleroderma (morphea) using imatinib, corticosteroids, and methotrexate. Pediatr Dermatol. 2013;30(6):e191–3.
68. Prey S, Ezzedine K, Doussau A, Grandoulier AS, Barcat D, Chatelus E, et al. Imatinib mesylate in scleroderma-associated diffuse skin fibrosis: a phase II multicentre randomized double-blinded controlled trial. Br J Dermatol. 2012;167(5):1138–44.
69. Fraticelli P, Gabrielli B, Pomponio G, Valentini G, Bosello S, Riboldi P, et al. Low-dose oral imatinib in the treatment of systemic sclerosis interstitial lung disease unresponsive to cyclophosphamide: a phase II pilot study. Arthritis Res Ther. 2014; 16(4):R144.
70. Elhai M, Meunier M, Matucci-Cerinic M, Maurer B, Riemekasten G, Leturcq T, et al. Outcomes of patients with systemic sclerosis-associated polyarthritis and myopathy treated with tocilizumab or abatacept: a EUSTAR observational study. Ann Rheum Dis. 2013;72(7):1217–20.
71. Stausbol-Gron B, Olesen AB, Deleuran B, Deleuran MS. Abatacept is a promising treatment for patients with disseminated morphea profunda: presentation of two cases. Acta Derm Venereol. 2011;91(6):686–8.
72. Smith V, Piette Y, van Praet JT, Decuman S, Deschepper E, Elewaut D, et al. Two-year results of an open pilot study of a 2-treatment course with rituximab in patients with early systemic sclerosis with diffuse skin involvement. J Rheumatol. 2013;40(1):52–7.
73. Jordan S, Distler JHW, Maurer B, Huscher D, van Laar JM, Allanore Y, et al. Effects and safety of rituximab in systemic sclerosis: an analysis from the European Scleroderma Trial and Research (EUSTAR) group. Ann Rheum Dis. 2015;74(6):1188–94.
74. Wollina U, Looks A, Schneider R, Maak B. Disabling morphoea of childhood—beneficial effect of intravenous immunoglobulin therapy. Clin Exp Dermatol. 1998;23(6):292–3.
75. Lapiere J-C, Aasi S, Cook B, Montalvo A. Successful correction of depressed scars of the forehead secondary to trauma and morphea en Coup de Sabre by en bloc autologous dermal fat graft. Dermatol Surg. 2000;26(8):793–7. doi:10.1046/j.524-4725.2000.00073.x.
76. Palmero MLH, Uziel Y, Laxer RM, Forrest CR, Pope E. En Coup de Sabre scleroderma and Parry-Romberg syndrome in adolescents: surgical options and patient-related outcomes. J Rheumatol. 2010;37(10):2174–9.
77. Zhao J, Chenggang Y, Binglun L, Yan H, Li Y, Xianjie M, et al. Autologous fat graft and bone marrow-derived mesenchymal stem cells assisted fat graft for treatment of Parry-Romberg syndrome. Ann Plast Surg. 2014;73 Suppl 1:S99–103.
78. Baildam EM, Ennis H, Foster HE, Shaw L, Chieng AS, Kelly J, et al. Influence of childhood scleroderma on physical function and quality of life. J Rheumatol. 2011;38(1):167–73.
79. Das S, Bernstein I, Jacobe H. Correlates of self-reported quality of life in adults and children with morphea. J Am Acad Dermatol. 2014;70(5):904–10.
80. Piram M, McCuaig CC, Saint-Cyr C, Marcoux D, Hatami A, Haddad E, et al. Short- and long-term outcome of linear morphoea in children. Br J Dermatol. 2013;169(6):1265–71.
81. Mertens JS, Seyger MMB, Kievit W, Hoppenreijs EPAH, Jansen TLTA, van de Kerkhof PCM, et al. Disease recurrence in localized scleroderma: a retrospective analysis of 344 patients with pediatric or adult-onset disease. Br J Dermatol. 2015;172(3):722–8.
82. Herrick AL, Ennis H, Bhushan M, Silman AJ, Baildam EM. Incidence of childhood linear scleroderma and systemic sclerosis in the UK and Ireland. Arthritis Care Res (Hoboken). 2010;62(2):213–8.
83. Zulian F, Woo P, Athreya BH, Laxer RM, Medsger Jr TA, Lehman TJ, et al. The Pediatric Rheumatology European Society/American College of Rheumatology/European league against rheumatism provisional classification criteria for juvenile systemic sclerosis. Arthritis Rheum. 2007;57(2):203–12.
84. Tyndall A, Furst D. Adult stem cell treatment of scleroderma. Curr Opin Rheumatol. 2007;19(6):604–10.
85. Matucci-Cerinic M, Kahaleh B, Wigley FM. Review: evidence that systemic sclerosis is a vascular disease. Arthritis Rheum. 2013;65(8):1953–62.
86. Reiff A, Weinberg KI, Triche T, Masinsin B, Mahadeo KM, Lin CH, et al. T lymphocyte abnormalities in juvenile systemic sclerosis patients. Clin Immunol. 2013;149(1):146–55.
87. Abraham DJ, Krieg T, Distler J, Distler O. Overview of pathogenesis of systemic sclerosis. Rheumatology (Oxford). 2009;48 Suppl 3:iii3–7.
88. Halper J, Kjaer M. Basic components of connective tissues and extracellular matrix: elastin, fibrillin, fibulins, fibrinogen, fibronectin, laminin, tenascins and thrombospondins. Adv Exp Med Biol. 2014;802:31–47.
89. Castelino FV, Varga J. Emerging cellular and molecular targets in fibrosis: implications for scleroderma pathogenesis and targeted therapy. Curr Opin Rheumatol. 2014;26(6):607–14.
90. Romano E, Manetti M, Guiducci S, Ceccarelli C, Allanore Y, Matucci-Cerinic M. The genetics of systemic sclerosis: an update. Clin Exp Rheumatol. 2011;29(2 Suppl 65):S75–86.
91. Mayes MD, Trojanowska M. Genetic factors in systemic sclerosis. Arthritis Res Ther. 2007;9 Suppl 2:S2–5.
92. Romano E, Manetti M, Guiducci S, Ceccarelli C, Allanore Y, Matucci-Cerinic M. The genetics of systemic sclerosis: an update. Clin Exp Dermatol. 2011;29(2 Suppl 65):S75–86.
93. Mayes M, Trojanowska M. Genetic factors in systemic sclerosis. Arthritis Res Ther. 2007;9 Suppl 2:S5.
94. Foeldvari I, Zhavania M, Birdi N, Cuttica RJ, de Oliveira SH, Dent PB, et al. Favourable outcome in 135 children with juvenile systemic sclerosis: results of a multi-national survey. Rheumatology (Oxford). 2000;39(5):556–9.
95. Martini G, Foeldvari I, Russo R, Cuttica R, Eberhard A, Ravelli A, et al. Systemic sclerosis in childhood: clinical and immunologic features of 153 patients in an international database. Arthritis Rheum. 2006;54(12):3971–8.
96. Aoyama K, Nagai Y, Endo Y, Ishikawa O. Juvenile systemic sclerosis: report of three cases and review of Japanese published work. J Dermatol. 2007;34(9):658–61.
97. Russo R, Katsicas M. Clinical characteristics of children with Juvenile Systemic Sclerosis: follow-up of 23 patients in a single tertiary center. Pediatr Rheumatol Online J. 2007;5:6.
98. Misra R, Singh G, Aggarwal P, Aggarwal A. Juvenile onset systemic sclerosis: a single center experience of 23 cases from Asia. Clin Rheumatol. 2007;26(8):1259–62.
99. Pelkonen PM, Jalanko HJ, Lantto RK, Makela AL, Pietikainen MA, Savolainen HA, et al. Incidence of systemic connective tissue diseases in children: a nationwide prospective study in Finland. J Rheumatol. 1994;21(11):2143–6.
100. van den Hoogen F, Khanna D, Fransen J, Johnson SR, Baron M, Tyndall A, et al. 2013 classification criteria for systemic sclerosis: an American college of rheumatology/European league against rheumatism collaborative initiative. Ann Rheum Dis. 2013;72(11):1747–55.

101. Terreri MT, Andrade LE, Puccinelli ML, Hilario MO, Goldenberg J. Nail fold capillaroscopy: normal findings in children and adolescents. Semin Arthritis Rheum. 1999;29(1):36–42.
102. Ingegnoli F, Herrick AL. Nailfold capillaroscopy in pediatrics. Arthritis Care Res (Hoboken). 2013;65(9):1393–400.
103. Herrick ML, Moore T, Hollis S, Jayson MIV. The influence of age on nailfold capillary dimension in childhood. J Rheumatol. 2000;27:797–800.
104. Dolezalova P, Young SP, Bacon PA, Southwood TR. Nailfold capillary microscopy in healthy children and in childhood rheumatic diseases: a prospective single blind observational study. Ann Rheum Dis. 2003;62:444–9.
105. Herrick AL, Cutolo M. Clinical implications from capillaroscopic analysis in patients with Raynaud's phenomenon and systemic sclerosis. Arthritis Rheum. 2010;62(9):2595–604.
106. Foeldvari I, Wierk A. Healthy children have a significantly increased skin score assessed with the modified Rodnan skin score. Rheumatology. 2006;45:76–8.
107. Li AM, Yin J, Au JT, So HK, Tsang T, Wong E, et al. Standard reference for the six-minute-walk test in healthy children aged 7 to 16 years. Am J Respir Crit Care Med. 2007;176(2):174–80.
108. Lammers AE, Hislop AA, Flynn Y, Haworth SG. The 6-minute walk test: normal values for children of 4–11 years of age. Arch Dis Child. 2008;93(6):464–8.
109. Panigada S, Ravelli A, Silvestri M, Granata C, Magni-Manzoni S, Cerveri I, et al. HRCT and pulmonary function tests in monitoring of lung involvement in juvenile systemic sclerosis. Pediatr Pulmonol. 2009;44(12):1226–34.
110. Scalapino K, Arkachaisri T, Lucas M, Fertig N, Helfrich DJ, Londino Jr AV, et al. Childhood onset systemic sclerosis: classification, clinical and serologic features, and survival in comparison with adult onset disease. J Rheumatol. 2006;33(5):1004–13.
111. Lanteri A, Sobanski V, Langlois C, Lefevre G, Hauspie C, Sanges S, et al. Serum free light chains of immunoglobulins as biomarkers for systemic sclerosis characteristics, activity and severity. Autoimmun Rev. 2014;13(9):974–80.
112. van Bon L, Affandi AJ, Broen J, Christmann RB, Marijnissen RJ, Stawski L, et al. Proteome-wide analysis and CXCL4 as a biomarker in systemic sclerosis. N Engl J Med. 2014;370(5):433–43.
113. Castelino FV, Varga J. Current status of systemic sclerosis biomarkers: applications for diagnosis, management and drug development. Expert Rev Clin Immunol. 2013;9(11):1077–90.
114. Kolto G, Vuolteenaho O, Szokodi I, Faludi R, Tornyos A, Ruskoaho H, et al. Prognostic value of N-terminal natriuretic peptides in systemic sclerosis: a single centre study. Clin Exp Rheumatol. 2014;32(Suppl 86 (6)):75–81.
115. Abignano G, Cuomo G, Buch MH, Rosenberg WM, Valentini G, Emery P, et al. The enhanced liver fibrosis test: a clinical grade, validated serum test, biomarker of overall fibrosis in systemic sclerosis. Ann Rheum Dis. 2014;73(2):420–7.
116. Vesely R, Vargova V, Ravelli A, et al. Serum level of KL-6 as a marker of interstitial lung disease in patients with juvenile systemic scleroderma. J Rheumatol. 2004;31:795–800.
117. Lammers AE, Hislop AA, Haworth SG. Prognostic value of B-type natriuretic peptide in children with pulmonary hypertension. Int J Cardiol. 2009;135(1):21–6.
118. Van Albada ME, Loot FG, Fokkema R, Roofthooft MT, Berger RM. Biological serum markers in the management of pediatric pulmonary arterial hypertension. Pediatr Res. 2008;63(3):321–7.
119. Bernus A, Wagner BD, Accurso F, Doran A, Kaess H, Ivy DD. Brain natriuretic peptide levels in managing pediatric patients with pulmonary arterial hypertension. Chest. 2009;135(3):745–51.
120. Kowal-Bielecka O, Landewé R, Avouac J, Chwiesko S, Miniati I, Czirjak L, et al. EULAR recommendations for the treatment of systemic sclerosis: a report from the EULAR Scleroderma Trials and Research group (EUSTAR). Ann Rheum Dis. 2009;68(5):620–8.
121. van Laar JM, Farge D, Sont JK, et al. Autologous hematopoietic stem cell transplantation vs intravenous pulse cyclophosphamide in diffuse cutaneous systemic sclerosis: a randomized clinical trial. JAMA. 2014;311(24):2490–8.
122. Lehman T. Methotrexate for the treatment of early diffuse scleroderma: comment on the article by Pope et al. Arthritis Rheum. 2002;46(3):845.
123. Tashkin DP, Elashoff R, Clements PJ, Roth MD, Furst DE, Silver RM, et al. Effects of 1-year treatment with cyclophosphamide on outcomes at 2 years in scleroderma lung disease. Am J Respir Crit Care Med. 2007;176(10):1026–34.
124. Clements PJ, Roth MD, Elashoff R, Tashkin DP, Goldin J, Silver RM, et al. Scleroderma lung study (SLS): differences in the presentation and course of patients with limited versus diffuse systemic sclerosis. Ann Rheum Dis. 2007;66(12):1641–7.
125. Poormoghim H, Moradi Lakeh M, Mohammadipour M, Sodagari F, Toofaninjed N. Cyclophosphamide for scleroderma lung disease: a systematic review and meta-analysis. Rheumatol Int. 2012;32(8):2431–44.
126. Smith V, Van Praet JT, Vandooren B, Van der Cruyssen B, Naeyaert JM, Decuman S, et al. Rituximab in diffuse cutaneous systemic sclerosis: an open-label clinical and histopathological study. Ann Rheum Dis. 2010;69(1):193–7.
127. Daoussis D, Liossis S, Tsamandas A, Kalogeropoulou C, Paliogianni F, Sirinian C, et al. Effect of long-term treatment with rituximab on pulmonary function and skin fibrosis in patients with diffuse systemic sclerosis. Clin Exp Dermatol. 2012;30(2 Suppl 71):S17–22.
128. Daoussis D, Liossis SN, Tsamandas AC, Kalogeropoulou C, Paliogianni F, Sirinian C, et al. Effect of long-term treatment with rituximab on pulmonary function and skin fibrosis in patients with diffuse systemic sclerosis. Clin Exp Rheumatol. 2012;30(2 Suppl 71):S17–22.
129. Distler J, Jordan S, Airo P, Alegre-Sancho J, Allanore Y, Gurman AB, et al. Is there a role for TNFalpha antagonists in the treatment of SSc? EUSTAR expert consensus development using the Delphi technique. Clin Exp Rheumatol. 2011;29(2 Suppl 65):S40–5.
130. Denton CP, Engelhart M, Tvede N, Wilson H, Khan K, Shiwen X, et al. An open-label pilot study of infliximab therapy in diffuse cutaneous systemic sclerosis. Ann Rheum Dis. 2009;68(9):1433–9.
131. Walker UA, Tyndall A, Czirják L, Denton C, Farge-Bancel D, Kowal-Bielecka O, et al. Clinical risk assessment of organ manifestations in systemic sclerosis: a report from the EULAR scleroderma trials and research group database. Ann Rheum Dis. 2007;66(6):754–63.
132. Foeldvari I, Nihtyanova SI, Wierk A, Denton CP. Characteristics of patients with juvenile onset systemic sclerosis in an adult single-center cohort. J Rheumatol. 2010;37:2422–6.
133. Foeldvari I, Tyndall A, Zulian F, Muller-Ladner U, Czirjak L, Denton C, et al. Juvenile and young adult-onset systemic sclerosis share the same organ involvement in adulthood: data from the EUSTAR database. Rheumatology (Oxford). 2012;51:1832–7.

Morphea (Localized Scleroderma)

8

Noelle M. Teske and Heidi T. Jacobe

Classification and Epidemiology of Morphea

Morphea, also called localized scleroderma, is a chronic autoimmune disease characterized by inflammation and sclerosis of the skin. Morphea, like scleroderma, is characterized as a sclerosing skin disorder, due to characteristic histological findings shared by both disorders, including sclerosis of the dermis and sometimes subcutis in the absence of fibroblast proliferation. However, morphea differs from scleroderma demographically and clinically. In contrast to scleroderma, involvement of internal organs in morphea is unusual and very different from that in scleroderma, and the diagnosis does not carry the same implications in terms of morbidity and increased mortality. Thus, it is the opinion of the authors that the term "localized scleroderma" should be avoided to limit unnecessary evaluation and anxiety for patients and confusion among providers. For the purposes of this chapter, we will exclusively use the term "morphea."

The clinical features of morphea are single or multiple sclerotic or indurated cutaneous plaques that are often dyspigmented (hypo- or hyperpigmented) and may have an erythematous border, depending on their stage of evolution. These plaques vary in appearance, depending on the subtype of morphea (Table 8.1) and activity of disease (see *Assessment of disease activity* and *Stages of morphea lesions*). Notably, cutaneous features of scleroderma, including Raynaud's phenomenon, mat-like telangiectasias, sclerodactyly, acrosclerosis, decreased oral aperture, and nailfold capillary changes, are not seen in morphea.

The major subtypes of morphea include circumscribed or plaque-type, linear, generalized, pansclerotic, and mixed forms. Clinical images of the morphea subtypes are presented in Fig. 8.1. The classification scheme presented herein was developed by the Committee on Classification Criteria for Juvenile Systemic Sclerosis, composed of members of the Pediatric Rheumatology European society (PRES), the American College of Rheumatology (ACR), and the European League Against Rheumatism (ELAR) [1] (Table 8.1). Although there are many reported classifications of morphea, the authors have found this to be the most clinically relevant. The classification of morphea is based on the morphology of the skin lesions, as histopathology is similar in all the forms of morphea, and there are no known biomarkers for morphea subtypes. Histology is useful, however, in excluding other entities in the differential diagnosis (see *Differential diagnosis of morphea*).

Variants and Related Entities When linear morphea occurs on the upper face, especially the paramedian forehead, it is often called en coup de sabre (ECDS) (Fig. 8.2a, b). When it involves the lower face or produces hemifacial atrophy of deeper tissues, it is called progressive hemifacial atrophy (PHA), also known as Parry-Romberg syndrome (PRS) (Fig. 8.2c–f). Whether these conditions represent an entity different from morphea has been a subject of considerable debate, but recent literature suggests that they are part of the morphea disease spectrum [2] in the sense that PHA represents deep involvement of the facial tissues with resultant residual atrophy.

Overlying lichen sclerosus, changes may be seen in morphea lesions of all subtypes (Fig. 8.3). This observation has led to controversy over whether these represent two independent processes or whether changes similar to lichen sclerosus occur in morphea. Eosinophilic fasciitis (EF) has also been considered by some to be a variant of morphea, as about a third of patients with EF have findings typical of classic plaque-type morphea [3].

Other entities such as bullous morphea and guttate morphea have been described in case reports and case series [4–13]. Examination of reports of bullous morphea reveals that bullae were largely present in areas of dense sclerosis in dependent areas [7]. This suggests that the bulla is a secondary

N.M. Teske, BA, MSc (✉) • H.T. Jacobe, MD, MSCS
Department of Dermatology, University of Texas Southwestern Medical Center, Dallas, TX 75093-9069, USA
e-mail: Noelle.Teske@UTSouthwestern.edu

J. Varga et al. (eds.), *Scleroderma*, DOI 10.1007/978-3-319-31407-5_8

Table 8.1 Classification of morphea

Morphea subtype	Modifiers	Clinical
Circumscribed	Superficial	Single or multiple oval/round lesions; pathology limited to the dermis
	Deep	Single or multiple oval/round lesions involving the dermis and subcutaneous tissue, fascia, or muscle
Linear	Trunk/limbs	Linear lesions; possible primary site of involvement in the subcutaneous tissue without involvement of the dermis; may involve the subcutaneous tissue, muscle, and/or bone
	Head	En coup de sabre (ECDS), progressive hemifacial atrophy (PHA), linear lesions of the face and scalp (may involve the underlying bone)
Generalized		
1. Coalescent plaque		≥4 plaques in at least 2 of 7 anatomic sites (head-neck, right/left upper extremity, right/left lower extremity, anterior/posterior trunk); Isomorphic pattern: coalescent plaques inframammary fold, waistline, lower abdomen, proximal thighs; symmetric pattern: symmetric plaque circumferential around the breasts, umbilicus, arms, and legs
2. Pansclerotic[a]		Circumferential involvement of majority of body surface area (sparing the fingertips and toes), affecting the skin, subcutaneous tissue, muscle, or bone; no internal organ involvement characteristic of scleroderma
Mixed		Combination of any above subtype:: linear – circumscribed

[a]While Zulian and Laxer categorized pansclerotic morphea separately, it is the opinion of the authors that this subtype can be classified under the broader heading of generalized morphea, as the features of pansclerotic morphea fulfill criteria for generalized morphea in terms of the extent of involvement. The classification was further modified by the authors from the original by clarifying the level of pathology of the various subtypes (Adapted with permission from Laxer and Zulian [110])

change related to edema in dependent areas or lymphatic obstruction due to sclerotic changes in the skin, rather than a primary process [7, 11, 14]. Therefore, it is the opinion of the authors that bullae should not warrant a designation as a separate subtype. Similarly, guttate lesions likely represent a variant of circumscribed morphea.

Epidemiology and Clinical Course Morphea has an estimated incidence of 2.7/10000 with a female to male ratio of 2–3:1 [15]. Existing studies suggest that morphea occurs most frequently in Caucasians, though population-based studies are needed to confirm this finding [16–18]. The reported frequency of different subtypes varies likely due to differing classification systems. However, linear morphea is more common in the pediatric population [15, 19], while the generalized and plaque subtypes predominate in adults. The clinical course is not well described, with periods of disease activity ranging from 3 to 6 years, and reactivation occurring after periods of remission in some patients [20]. Patients with pediatric-onset disease may also experience persistent disease and/or recurrences in adulthood [21, 22]. A retrospective evaluation of long-term outcomes of adults with pediatric-onset morphea from the Morphea in Adults and Children (MAC) cohort revealed that 89 % of patients (24/27) developed new or expanding lesions over time, suggesting that patients may need lifelong evaluation and repeated courses of treatment to prevent morbidity [21] (Fig. 8.4).

Studies examining recurrence rates after treatment with methotrexate and/or systemic steroids report recurrence 6–19 months after discontinuation of therapy in 10–44 % of patients [23–26]. Studies evaluating long-term outcomes after methotrexate therapy vary greatly in methods and duration of follow-up, so comparison of recurrence is difficult [23, 27]. Recurrence has also been described in patients after successful treatment with UVA-1 phototherapy at rates as high as 46 %, which may exceed those rates described with methotrexate. Median time to recurrence ranges from 10 months up to 20–30 months for those treated with UVA-1 and methotrexate, respectively [22, 23, 27–29]. These findings emphasize the need for regular monitoring of patients with morphea for signs of new disease activity even after successful treatment (see *Assessment of disease activity in morphea*).

Factors associated with recurrence in previous studies have included longer duration of disease before treatment

Fig. 8.1 (**a**) *Plaque-type morphea*. Circumscribed hyperpigmented plaques are present on the posterior legs of this patient with morphea. (**b**) *Generalized morphea on the trunk*. Hyperpigmented sclerotic plaques are present on the chest and abdomen. (**c**) *Generalized morphea on the extremities*. Symmetric, hypopigmented, sclerotic plaques are present on the legs of this patient with generalized morphea. (**d**) *Linear morphea*. Linear lesions of both the extremity and trunk are seen in this patient. Note that early linear lesions may not completely coalesce and may be confused with plaque-type morphea if not carefully examined. Note that on the trunk, linear lesions characteristically obey the midline. (**e**, **f**) *Pansclerotic morphea*. Note sheets of contiguous sclerosis, encompassing the majority of the body surface area (**e**) and characteristically sparing the fingertips, stopping at the metacarpophalangeal joints (**f**)

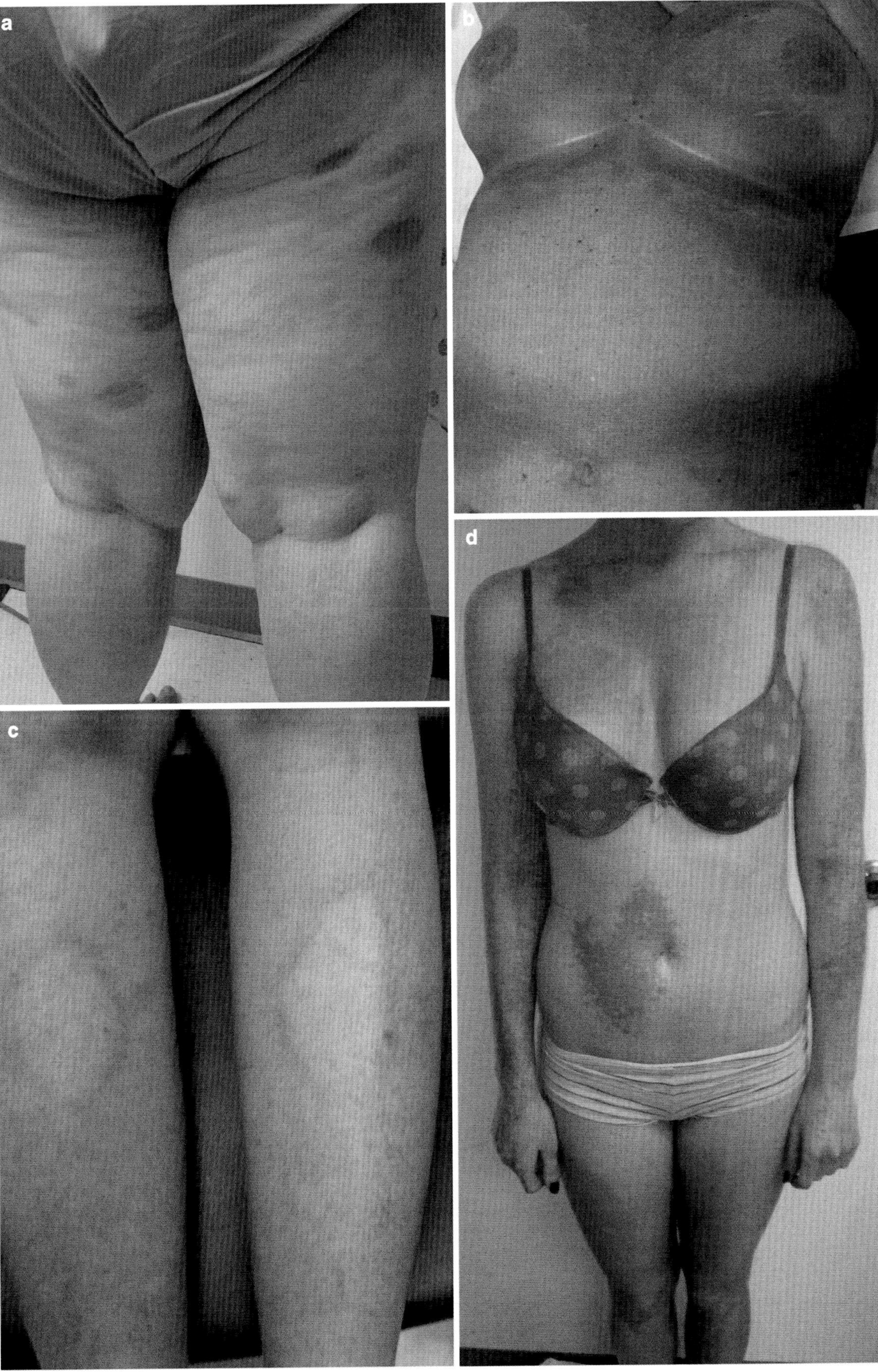
a
b
c
d

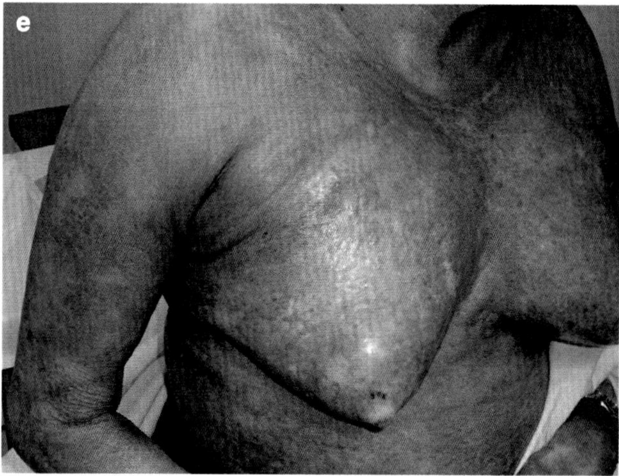

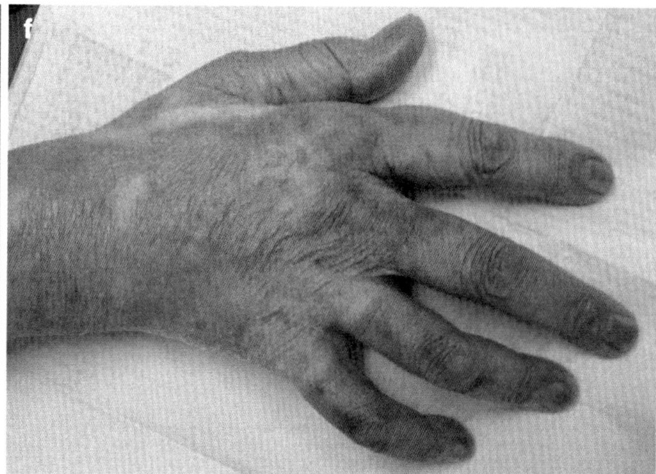

Fig.8.1 (continued)

[28], older age of onset in the pediatric population [25], and the presence of linear morphea of the limbs [25, 30]. However, these associations have not always been replicated across studies. Prognostic markers have not yet been identified for recurrent or chronic disease in the form of prospective longitudinal studies, but retrospective reviews and cross-sectional studies have implicated that increased duration of disease before treatment may be associated with increased likelihood of recurrent disease [28]. Preliminary analysis from the prospective MAC cohort has revealed similar recurrence rates between pediatric and adult patients and across subtypes of morphea. The only variable associated with recurrence in this cohort has been disease duration, in that patients with longer disease duration have been more likely to recur.

Etiology and Pathogenesis of Morphea

The etiology and pathogenesis of morphea is not well understood. Most pathological events ascribed to morphea have been extrapolated from research in scleroderma, as the two disorders are assumed to arise from a similar etiology [31]. Morphea, like other autoimmune disorders, likely arises from a genetic background of increased immune disease susceptibility, combined with other causative factors, such as trauma or environmental exposures, which modulate the expression of disease.

Genetics and Autoimmunity in Morphea Like many autoimmune connective tissue diseases, morphea is likely a complex genetic disease. Familial clustering has been reported, although rarely [18, 32, 33], and morphea is also associated with higher than expected rates of familial autoimmune disorders [18, 21, 34]. In retrospective studies, morphea patients have demonstrated concomitant autoimmune disease, including psoriasis, systemic lupus erythematosus, multiple sclerosis, and vitiligo, at higher than expected frequency when compared with published population-based prevalence estimates [18, 34–36]. A population-based study examining a rheumatoid arthritis population in Sweden reported a higher risk of morphea among these patients with a reported standardized incidence ratio (SIR) of 2.40 [35]. A similar population-based study in Sweden also reported a higher risk of morphea among siblings of patients with multiple sclerosis with an SIR of 1.72 [36]. Morphea has been reported, in case studies, to coexist with other autoimmune diseases, including inflammatory bowel disease [37], autoimmune thyroid disease [38, 39], alopecia areata, type I diabetes mellitus [37], antiphospholipid syndrome [40], and necrotizing vasculitis [68]. Other types of inflammatory skin disorders can also be associated with morphea, such as psoriasis [41] and lichen planopilaris [42].

Of interest, the risk for morphea has been associated with the presence of specific HLA class I and II alleles, further implicating a possible underlying genetic predisposition for the disease. A large case-control association study of patients from the MAC cohort revealed strong associations with specific HLA class I and II alleles, including, most significantly, HLA-B*37, as well as another, DRB1*04:04, in common with a risk allele previously identified for systemic sclerosis [43]. Alleles conferring the greatest risk included HLA DRB1*04:04 and HLAB37 [43]. Risk alleles identified in this case-control study have also been associated with the risk in rheumatoid arthritis and autoimmune thyroid disease [44, 45], implying that there may be a common genetic susceptibility to these disorders.

Increasing evidence supports immune dysregulation as an important pathogenic event early in the course of morphea.

Early morphea lesions are characterized by the influx of large amounts of mononuclear lymphocytes (usually activated T-lymphocytes), plasma cells, and eosinophils [31]. This is likely the result of autoimmunity, as there is widespread autoimmune reactivity in morphea patients including elevated ANAs (see *Laboratory findings in morphea*), cytokines, and adhesion molecules [18, 21, 46]. Vessel damage and upregulation of adhesion molecules (ICAM-1, VCAM 1, and E-selectin) occur related to the inflammatory cell infiltrate in morphea, which facilitates local monocyte recruitment [47]. These adhesion molecules also facilitate the recruitment of T-lymphocytes that are capable of producing pro-fibrotic cytokines (IL-4, IL-6, and TGF-beta) and may contribute to the development to sclerosis [31, 48]. Of note,

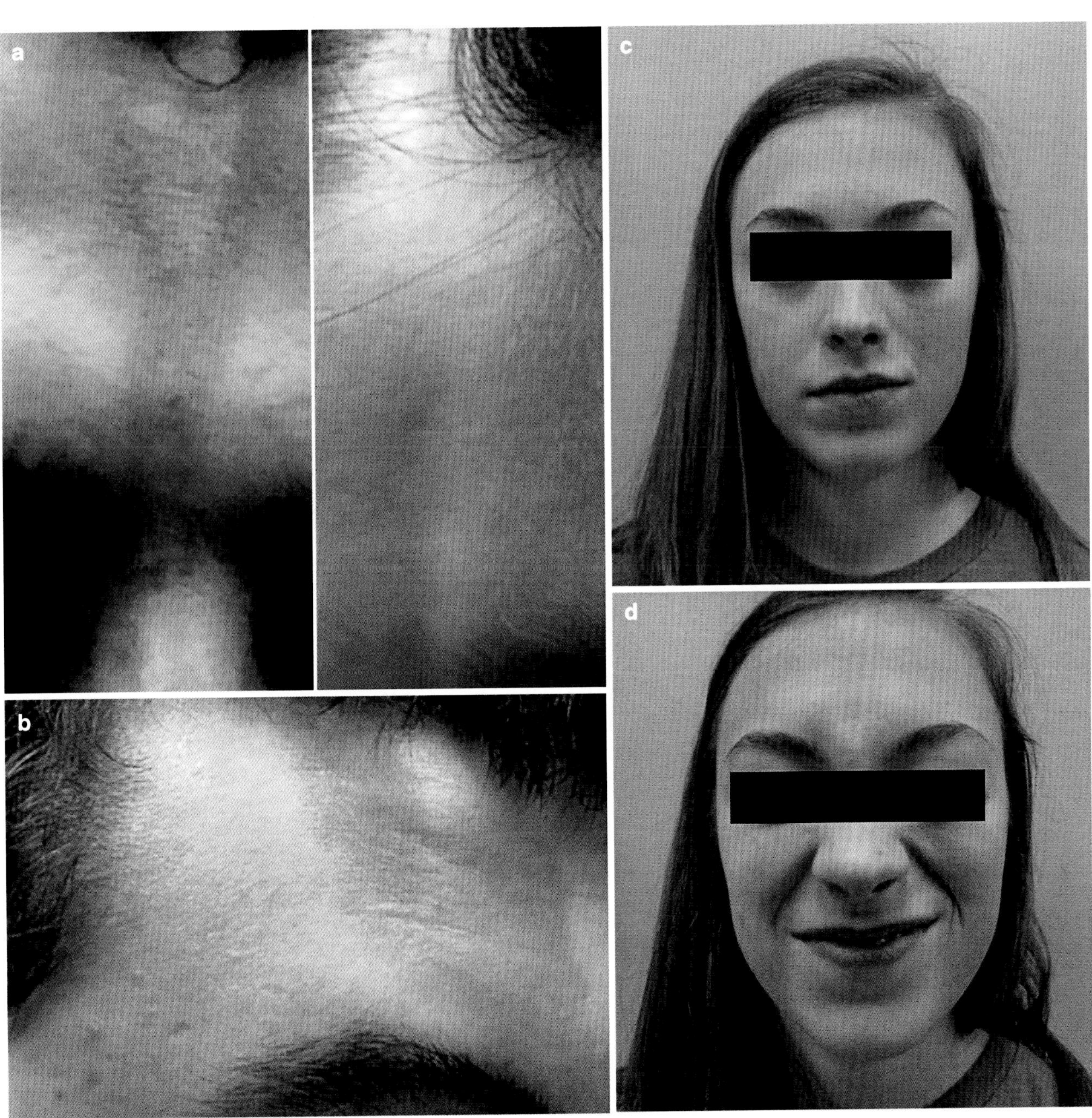

Fig. 8.2 (**a**, **b**) *En coup de sabre morphea*. Depressed linear plaques are present on the foreheads of these patients. These lesions are often dyspigmented and may have more obvious dermal changes (**a**) or change predominantly in the subcutis. Interestingly, years after his initial period of activity on the forehead, this patient (**b**) also developed tenosynovitis. (**c**–**f**) *Progressive hemifacial atrophy* also known as Parry-Romberg Syndrome may be subtle (**c**), requiring additional exam maneuvers to detect. Asymmetry can sometimes be better appreciated using different facial expressions (**d**). When progressive, hemifacial atrophy may lead to more obvious lesions, as seen here on the chin, mandible, neck and tongue (**e**–**f**)

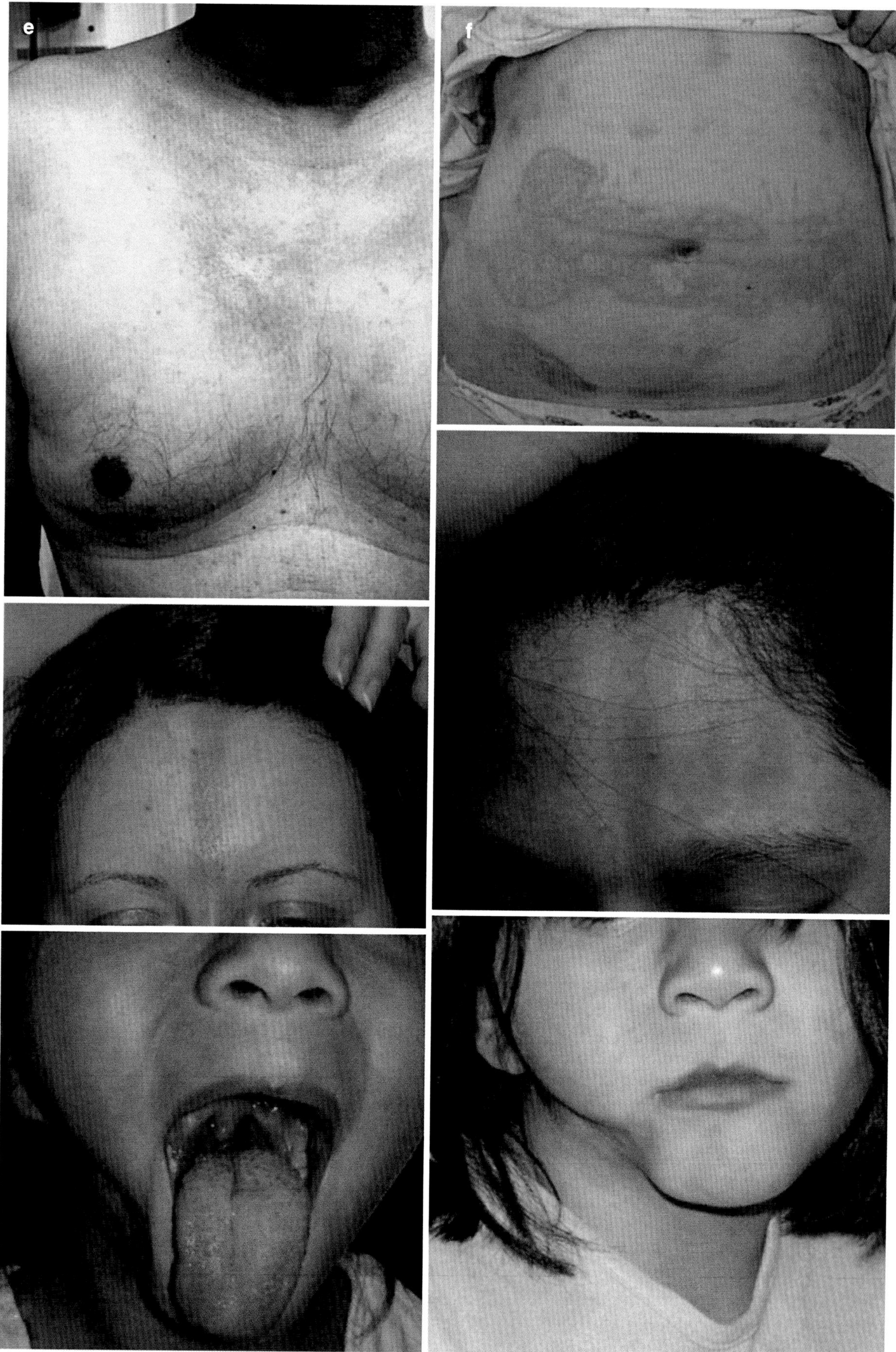

Fig. 8.2 (continued)

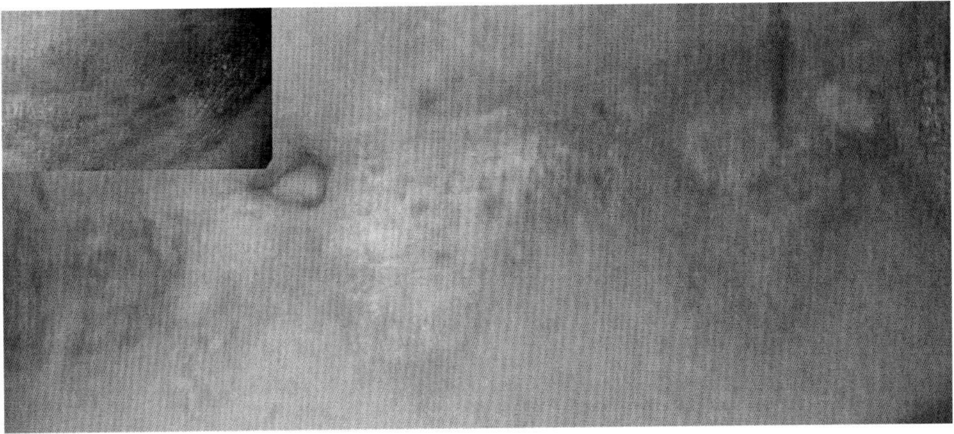

Fig. 8.3 *Morphea and lichen sclerosus*. Sclerotic lesions of morphea with overlying areas of fine, hypopigmented, wrinkled skin are present. This lesion also has features of active inflammatory morphea with an erythematous border

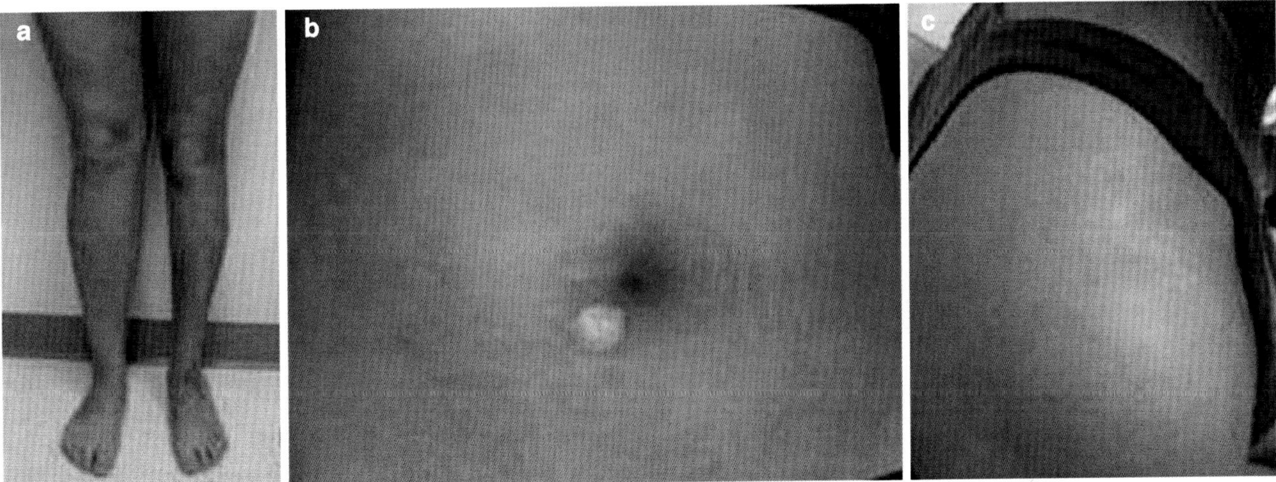

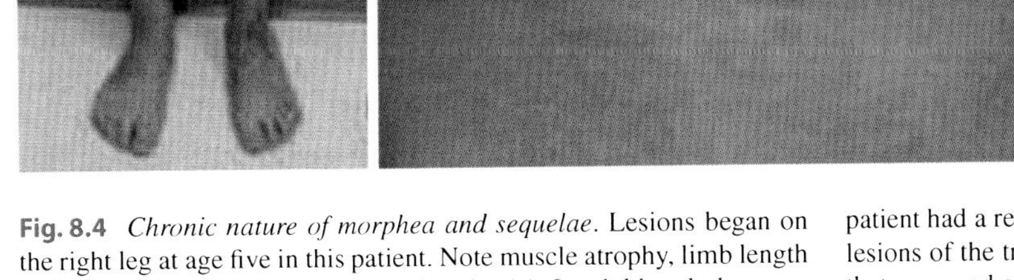

Fig. 8.4 *Chronic nature of morphea and sequelae*. Lesions began on the right leg at age five in this patient. Note muscle atrophy, limb length discrepancy, and pes planus foot deformity (**a**). In adulthood, the same patient had a recurrence of morphea in the form of active inflammatory lesions of the trunk, seen here on the abdomen (**b**), as well as a plaque that appeared on the shoulder (**c**)

increased levels of these vascular adhesion molecules have been detected in serum from patients with morphea [49]. These adhesion molecules are upregulated by cytokines classically associated with a Th2 immune response (IL-4, IL-1, and TNFs). Cytokines found in increased concentration in the sera and skin of morphea patients include IL-4, IL-6, and IL-8 [47, 50]. These cytokines, especially IL-4, upregulate TGF-beta, initiating a cascade of events that results in increased production of collagen and other extracellular matrix components via the induction of connective tissue growth factor, platelet-derived growth factor, and matrix metalloproteinases. Chimerism or nonself cells may also play a role in the pathogenesis of morphea by initiating a local inflammatory reaction [51].

In a recent study of 69 pediatric patients with morphea, interferon-gamma-inducible protein 10 (IP-10) levels were significantly elevated in the plasma of morphea patients when compared with healthy controls. Immunohistochemistry staining of IP-10 was also present in the dermal infiltrate of a subset of morphea patients who had available skin biopsies. IP-10 levels were significantly elevated in those with active versus inactive disease and correlated with standardized disease outcome measures of activity, further suggesting that IP-10 may be a potential biomarker for disease activity in morphea [52].

Although large-scale studies examining gene expression profiles in morphea are lacking, Milano et al. [53] have used gene expression array analysis to establish a gene expression signatures for scleroderma skin subsets as compared to unaffected skin of the same patient. In their first study, they included the skin from three patients with morphea. They identified five significantly different gene expression clusters: diffuse proliferation, inflammatory, limited, and normal-like in scleroderma. Gene expression profiles from all three biopsies of morphea skin fell into the inflammatory category, which was characterized by markers for an increase in immune response, response to pathogen, humoral defense, lymphocyte proliferation, chemokine binding, and chemokine receptor activity, and response to virus. These findings provide further evidence for an important role for immune dysregulation in morphea.

Taken together and extrapolating from research in scleroderma, these studies implicate an important role for interferons and Th1-skewed immune responses in early morphea, while Th2 cell lineages may become dominant in later disease as sclerosis predominates. Studies of this sort are necessary to identify pathways relevant to the pathogenesis of morphea and to pave the way for identification of biomarkers and therapeutic targets.

Histopathology of Morphea Histopathological changes in morphea evolve over the duration of individual lesions. The histopathological changes have been divided into indeterminate (early), inflammatory, mixed inflammatory and sclerotic, and sclerotic (late) stage morphea [54] (Figs. 8.5 and 8.6). Increased numbers of T-cells are present in the inflammatory stage compared with a normal skin. As in scleroderma, the inflammatory stage of morphea is characterized by dermal edema and by lymphocytic and histiocytic inflammatory cell infiltrates with plasma cells in a perivascular, periadnexal, and interstitial pattern. Eosinophils, mast cells, and macrophages may also be present. One finding particularly characteristic of morphea is the presence of an inflammatory cell infiltrate in the junction between the dermis and subcutaneous fat. From there, the inflammatory cell infiltrate may stream down the septa of the subcutaneous fat (Fig. 8.6c, d).

Recently, a cross-sectional study of the MAC cohort revealed a predilection for inflammatory cell infiltrate to occur in the border between the subcutis and the dermis. This was particularly true in cases where sclerosis followed a bottom-heavy pattern, characterized by hyalinized collagen bundles in the deep dermis and subcutis, sparing the papillary through the mid-dermis, a pattern which was typical of those with morphea profunda [55] (Fig. 8.6b). A biopsy with such changes, even in the absence of sclerosis, should alert providers to the possibility of early inflammatory morphea profunda. In contrast, in this the same study, a top-heavy pattern, characterized by collagen bundles exclusively in the papillary to superficial reticular dermis, was typical of those with lichen sclerosus overlap. Patterns of sclerosis varied equally in those with linear and plaque-type morphea between top-heavy, bottom-heavy, and full thickness patterns, with thickened collagen bundles throughout the dermis. Interestingly, among patients with generalized morphea, those with isomorphic pattern of distribution in patterns of chronic friction more often had top-heavy patterns of sclerosis, while bottom-heavy patterns predominated among those with symmetric patterns of distribution in generalized morphea. When inflammation was present, it consisted most often of lymphocytes (83/91, 91 %) and plasma cells (68/91, 75 %), but eosinophils were also noted with some frequency (17/91, 19 %).

The later sclerotic stage of morphea is characterized histopathologically by thickened, acellular, homogenized-appearing collagen bundles that may involve all levels of dermis and/or subcutis (where collagen bundles stream downward through the septa) (Fig. 8.6e, f). The adnexal structures (hair, eccrine glands) are surrounded by dense fibrosis with loss of fat around the eccrine glands in chronic disease (Fig. 8.6g). In specimens from morphea profunda, the deep reticular dermis, subcutis, and/or fascia also show sclerotic changes. It is not uncommon for inflammation and sclerosis to coexist (Fig. 8.6a). The atrophic stage is characterized by loss of inflammatory cell infiltrate, decreasing sclerosis, and an absence of appendageal structures. Telangiectasia may be evident.

Triggers and Precipitating Factors The emergence of morphea following exposure to environmental exposures is intriguing and may provide clues for the pathophysiology of morphea. While there are no definitive associations, the

Fig. 8.5 *Disease features in morphea.* (**a**) *Deep morphea.* The areas affected by deep morphea, also known as morphea profunda, may have a cobblestone appearance with subcutaneous atrophy. (**b–d**) *Inflammatory morphea.* An active plaque in the inflammatory stage is present on the left leg of this patient (**b**) note the violaceous border. There are also multiple early lesions present on the right. (**c**) Early morphea lesions may be subtle, as seen here on the patient's abdomen, where ill-defined indurated plaques with peripheral erythema indicate active inflammatory morphea. (**d**) This well-circumscribed plaque on the patient's breast exemplifies the erythematous border and central sclerosis typical of an early evolving morphea lesion. (**e**) *Sclerotic morphea.* This lesion demonstrates exuberant sclerosis centrally with surrounding hypopigmentation and erythema, likely indicating that the lesion is transitioning toward a more inactive state. Also note telangiectasias, which can occur in the surrounding atrophy and should not be mistaken for erythema indicating inflammation. (**f**) *Atrophoderma of Pasini and Pierini.* Preadolescent girl with several-year history of a large plaque and small patches of atrophy on the lumbar back. The lesions have a sharp drop-off with a "punched out" appearance and are not indurated clinically. (**g**) *Atrophy.* Severe subcutaneous atrophy is present in this patient with linear morphea in the atrophic stage, as well as postinflammatory hyperpigmentation changes and limb length discrepancy. (**h**, **i**) *Linear morphea of the extremity associated with disabling contractures.* Note contractures of the hands in children with long-standing linear morphea. Contractures can be a manifestation of damage occurring most commonly in linear lesions crossing joints, but may also be a component of other subtypes, including generalized morphea, when distributed over the joints

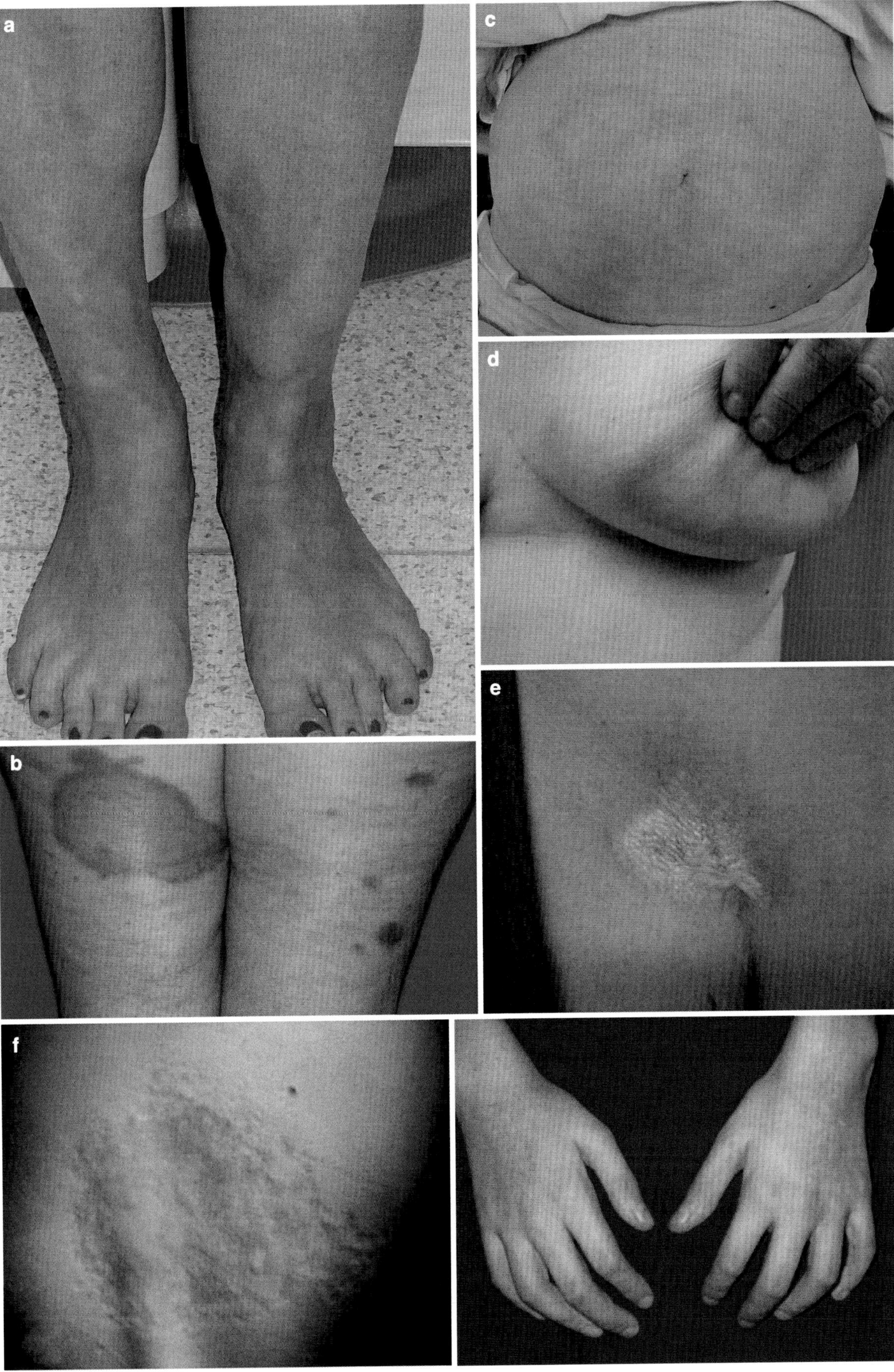
a
b
c
d
e
f

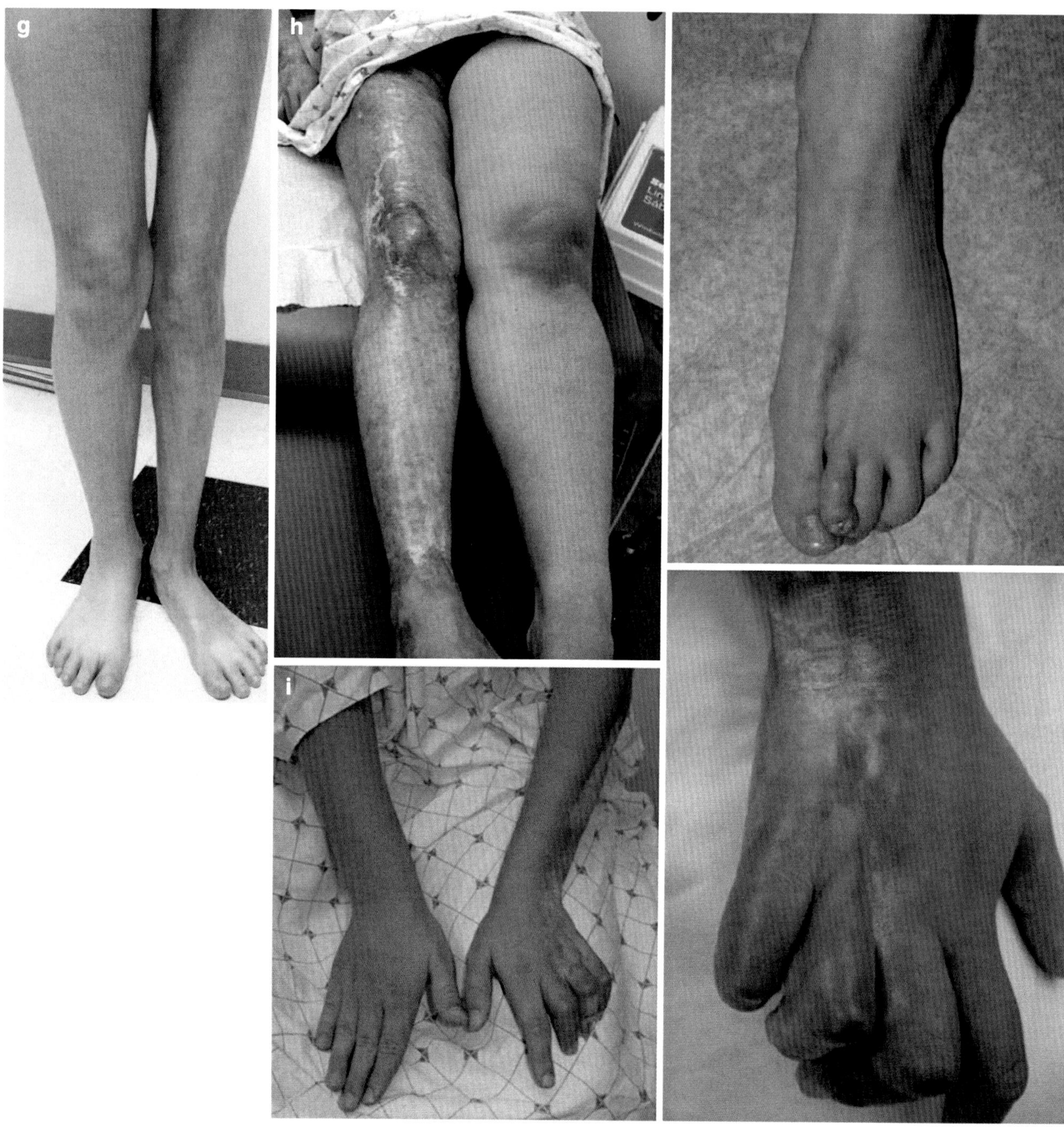

Fig. 8.5 (continued)

Fig. 8.6 (**a**) Skin biopsies of morphea have a characteristic "squared-off" shape because of the dense dermal sclerosis. There are patchy perivascular mononuclear cell infiltrates of lymphocytes, histiocytes, and occasional plasma cells, but otherwise the dermis is acellular compared with the normal skin. Flattening and atrophy of the epidermis are associated with underlying sclerosis. Hair follicles and sebaceous glands normally seen in a skin biopsy of hair-bearing skin are absent. (Magnification = 2.5×). (**b**) This specimen shows a pattern of "bottom-up" sclerosis that can be seen in morphea before the entire dermis is involved. The sclerotic collagen is in the *lower half* of dermis, while the normal collagen is in the *upper half*. Dense collagen has replaced normal collagen from the *arrow down*. The *left upper corner* of the image also shows the edge of an atrophic hair follicle. (Magnification = 5×). Sclerosis can also occur from the top down or may encompass the entire dermis, even extending into the subcutis and beyond in some cases. (**c**, **d**) Biopsies of active inflammatory morphea reveal perivascular, periadnexal, and interstitial inflammatory infiltrate. Also note the inflammatory cell infiltrate in the junction between the dermis and subcutaneous fat, streaming down through the septa of the subcutaneous fat. Though difficult to appreciate at this power, inflammatory infiltrate is typically composed of lymphocytes, plasma cells, and, occasionally, eosinophils. (**e**, **f**) Higher-power views of the non-sclerotic (**e**) and sclerotic (**f**) dermal areas show that the collagen in the sclerotic area has lost the fine fibrillar texture of normal collagen (Magnification = 40×). (**g**) Encasement of adnexal structures by dense collagen with loss of the fat around eccrine glands is shown. Eventually, atrophy of hair follicles, sebaceous glands, and eccrine glands (*arrow*) occurs in long-standing morphea (Magnification = 20×)

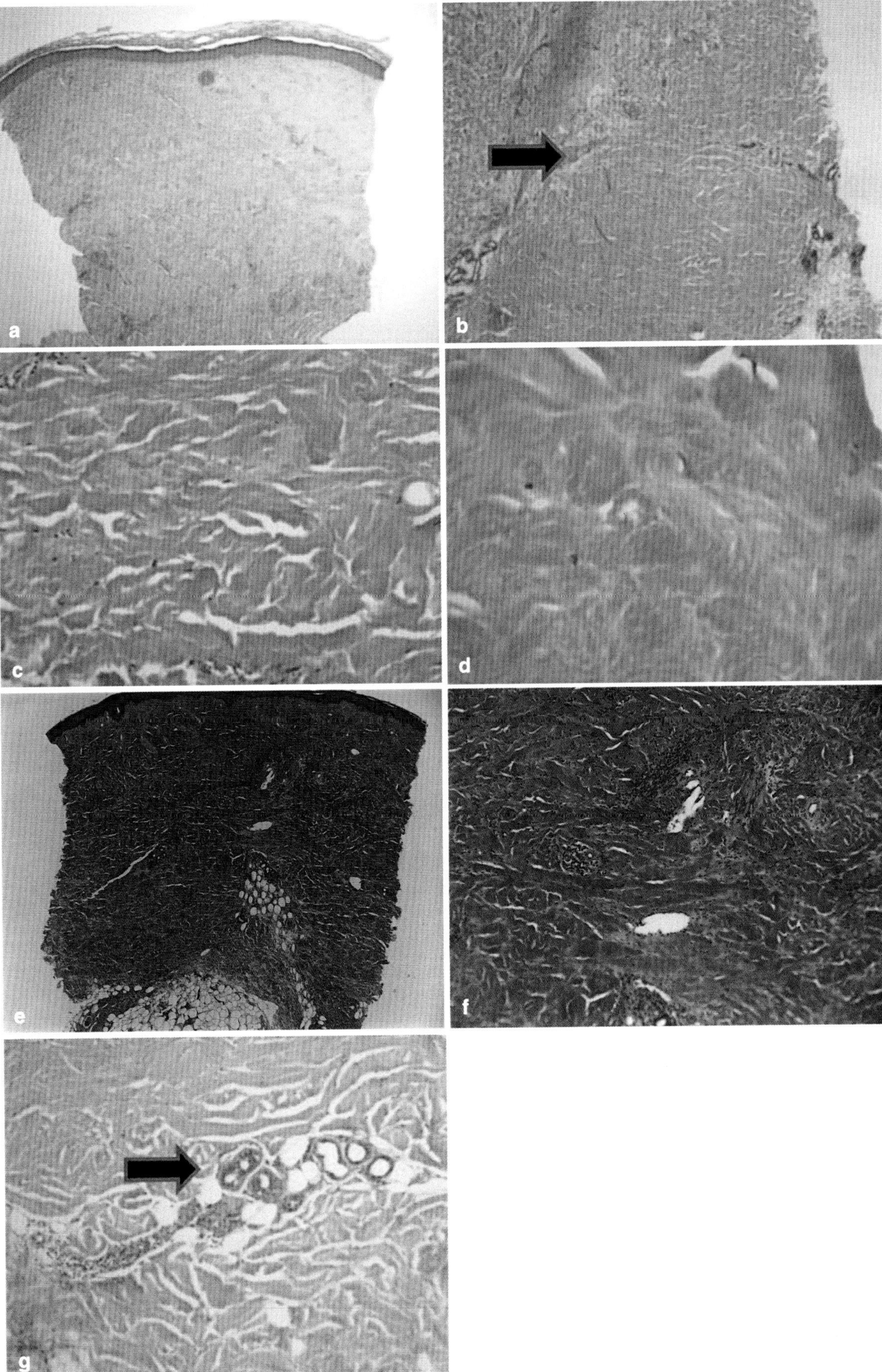

development of morphea lesions has been linked to local tissue trauma including radiation, surgery, insect bites, and intramuscular injections [56]. Although controversial, infectious agents have also been linked to pathogenesis. Studies in Europe had implicated a role for *Borrelia* infection in the pathogenesis of morphea, but this association has been largely discounted.

Increasing evidence, however, exists for the role of trauma in the development of morphea lesions. In a study of 26 patients with severe juvenile localized scleroderma, four (15 %) reported a history of trauma to the area, and one had a history of dental extraction ipsilateral to the area in which morphea developed [57]. There are many examples in the literature of injection-site morphea [56, 58], including the onset of morphea at the site of vaccinations as well as at the site of an insulin pump placement, observed by the authors. In a cross-sectional analysis of 329 patients in the MAC cohort, 52 (16 %) had trauma-associated lesions at the onset of disease, most commonly chronic friction (isomorphic) and surgery/isotopic triggers [59]. These findings, if confirmed in future studies, might suggest that elective procedures and skin trauma or friction be avoided in morphea patients. However, necessary and lifesaving surgery, radiation, or other procedures should not be avoided merely due to a diagnosis of morphea.

Clinical Features of Morphea

Assessment of Disease Activity in Morphea The assessment of disease activity in morphea is important to clinical decision-making, as most treatments with proven efficacy are directed at the inflammatory stage of disease and will not be effective in predominantly sclerotic or atrophic lesions. The risk-benefit assessment of pursuing treatment for morphea lesions depends on the potential for functional or cosmetic impairment and symptom burden due to active lesions. It is therefore important to make an accurate assessment of lesion activity in each clinical examination, including clinical photographs to compare lesions to prior visits, since active disease may warrant intervention, while inactive disease may be carefully observed over time (see Fig. 8.10). Though imaging modalities such as ultrasound can be useful for assessing disease activity (see *Imaging methods*), active morphea lesions can usually be distinguished from inactive lesions by clinical features. Signs of disease activity (which have been established by expert consensus and validated) include new lesions, lesions that have expanded in size from previous visits, the presence of an erythematous or violaceous border around lesions, and possibly increased patient symptomology such as pain or itch at the site of lesions [60, 61].

Stages of Morphea Lesions Morphea of all subtypes can begin as erythematous patches or plaques and may be preceded by pain or itch. Later, hypopigmentation with skin thickening, which is a manifestation of sclerosis, begins to develop at the center of lesions. These lesions typically have an erythematous/violaceous border indicative of active inflammation and expansion (inflammatory phase) (Fig. 8.5b–d). Sclerosis develops centrally and may lead to a shiny white-yellow color, with surrounding hyperpigmentation, as lesions stop expanding (sclerotic phase) (Fig. 8.5e). The loss of hair follicles can lead to alopecia in areas of morphea.

As activity subsides, these sclerotic plaques will soften over the course of months to years and become atrophic with hyper- or hypopigmentation (atrophic phase). Sclerosis can lead to contractures and limitations in range of motion and may impede growth in the pediatric population, leading to limb length discrepancies. Limitation in range of motion may actually improve as the lesions progress from sclerosis into atrophy.

Atrophy produces varying features depending on the level of skin involvement: cigarette-paper atrophy (papillary dermis), cliff-drop atrophy (dermis), or deep indentations that alter the contour of the affected site (subcutis). Atrophoderma of Pasini and Pierini (Fig. 8.5f) is thought to be the residua of plaque-type morphea involving dermal atrophy, as the borders of these lesions are characterized by the cliff-drop appearance. When morphea affects the subcutis or deeper, long-term sequelae may include limb length discrepancies, limitations in range of motion, and contractures (Fig. 8.5g–i).

Depth of Involvement Assessment of the level of involvement in morphea is important to recognize potential comorbidities as well as to guide treatment (see Fig. 8.10). Morphea involving the superficial to the mid-dermis may be amenable to topical or phototherapy. Deep morphea, or morphea profunda, on the other hand, which involves the deep dermis, subcutaneous tissue, fascia, and/or muscle, will require systemic therapy to suppress disease activity when lesions are widespread or threaten function or cosmesis.

Deep involvement can occur with any subtype of morphea. Hemifacial atrophy, previously known as Parry-Romberg syndrome, represents deep morphea (morphea profunda) of the face that may or may not be accompanied by a more dermal linear or en coup de sabre (ECDS) lesion. Similar changes are seen in other anatomic sites with deep involvement (morphea profunda). Lesions in which the pathology is predominantly located in the deep dermis/subcutis are poorly circumscribed and may be accompanied by changes such as cobblestoning and altered contour in the sclerotic phase, as the skin becomes tacked down by sclerosis to underlying fascia (Fig. 8.5a).

A "groove" sign or depression may be present at the site of tendons and ligaments, and deep tissue loss may result in the atrophic phase. However, as deep involvement can occur without obvious superficial changes, it may be more reliably detected with careful palpation, biopsy, and/or imaging than by visual exam alone (see Figs. 8.9 and 8.10).

Data is lacking on the correlation between depth and involvement and amount of damage in morphea. However, a preliminary analysis of the MAC cohort revealed that the vast majority of patients who had functional abnormalities (including limited range of motion, contractures, limb length discrepancies in morphea-involved areas) also had deep involvement of their disease (80/86, 93 %). These results imply a possible connection between the depth of disease and potential for damage and further emphasize the importance of assessment of the level of involvement as part of the clinical evaluation of the patient with morphea (Fig. 8.10) [62].

Morbidity in Morphea Quality-of-life assessments show that individuals with morphea have better outcomes than those with disabling severe atopic dermatitis, with the exception of children and adolescents with the more severe forms of morphea affecting the face and limbs [63]. However, large cross-sectional studies of the MAC cohort have demonstrated that morphea patients do experience impairment of health-related quality of life that is greater than those with nonmelanoma skin cancer, vitiligo, and alopecia [64]. Notably, symptoms of pruritus and pain have been significantly associated with impaired quality of life in morphea, contrary to conventional wisdom that morphea is an asymptomatic disorder [64, 65].

A variety of internal disorders are reported to occur in patients with morphea, more frequently in the linear [34] and generalized or mixed subtypes [18], though they are different than the internal organ manifestations of scleroderma. The most commonly associated disorders include musculoskeletal and deep soft tissue abnormalities and neurologic and ophthalmologic problems. Malignancy is a rarely associated morbidity and may include squamous cell carcinoma in long-standing pansclerotic morphea [66]. Few systematic studies have been performed because of the infrequency of morphea and even more infrequent coexisting morbidities, so relatively little is known about the course and treatment of these disorders in the context of morphea [57].

- *Musculoskeletal and soft tissue complications*. The most common extracutaneous finding in morphea patients is arthritis/arthralgias, which have been reported in 12 % of pediatric patients with morphea (Fig. 8.7a) [34]. Both articular and soft tissue/bony abnormalities are typically associated with linear morphea. Other musculoskeletal complications include joint swelling, myalgia, and limb contractures [18] (Fig. 8.4a). Individuals with facial linear

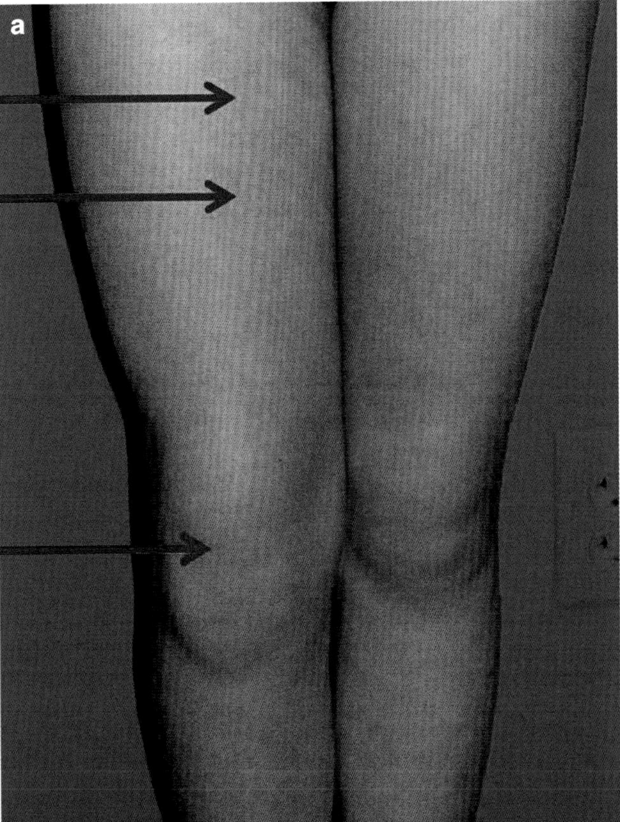

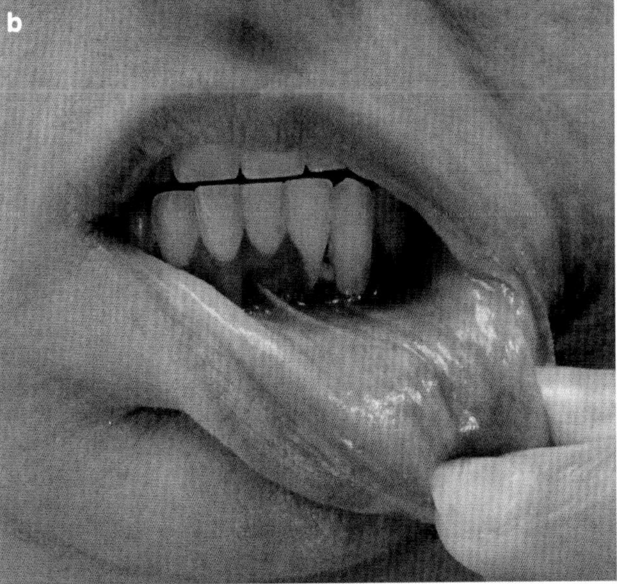

Fig. 8.7 *Morbidity in* morphea. (**a**) *Arthritis in morphea*. A swollen right knee with effusion (*lowest arrow*) is present in this patient with morphea (*upper areas*). Notably, this patient also had spondyloarthropathy. (**b**) *Gingival changes in morphea*. Gingival changes, in the form of a kind of destructive gingivitis, are seen in this patient with linear morphea of the face. Referral to oral maxillofacial surgery may be warranted to determine need for intervention once lesions are inactive

morphea can have dental abnormalities [66] including gingival involvement (Fig. 8.7b) and even ipsilateral tongue hypoplasia. Musculoskeletal changes including fascial thickening and enhancement, articular synovitis, tenosynovitis, perifascial enhancement, and myositis have been detected using MRI in morphea patients, particularly those with pansclerotic morphea, and have been observed in some cases even when involvement was not expected based on the exam [67]. However, the clinical significance of such findings has yet to be determined, and the authors would not recommend routine imaging in morphea patients without signs or symptoms of musculoskeletal involvement.

- *Neurologic complications*. Neurologic involvement was reported in 4 % of pediatric patients with morphea [34] and is more common in patients with linear morphea of the head. Complications include seizures, headache, and peripheral neuropathy among others. Intractable partial seizures [68], epileptic encephalopathy [69], status migrainosus [70], and central nervous system vasculitis [71, 72] have all been reported in association with morphea. Kistger et al. reviewed 54 patients with craniofacial scleroderma who also had neuroimaging (head CT or MRI) for neurologic symptoms. They found some common atypical features on imaging including atrophy, calcifications, and T2 hyperintensities. Others have described abnormal MRI results in patients with Parry-Romberg syndrome [73]. The clinical significance of such abnormal findings has yet to be determined, and at the current time, there is not sufficient evidence to recommend imaging in the morphea population in the absence of neurologic manifestations by history or physical examination.
- *Ophthalmologic complications*. Ocular involvement was reported in 2 % of pediatric patients with morphea [34]. Ocular involvement in morphea is also more common in patients with linear morphea that affects the face, although it has also been reported to occur in patients without facial lesions [74]. Associated ophthalmologic abnormalities may include enophthalmos, anterior uveitis, episcleritis, glaucoma, xerophthalmia, keratitis, and strabismus [74].
- *Other manifestations*. Genital involvement has been reported in association with morphea, particularly the generalized subtype, though to date, the frequency of such changes is not well described. Patients with genital involvement will often complain of pruritus, as well as dyspareunia, dysuria, and pain with defecation. Importantly, patients will not typically volunteer these symptoms without specific inquiry by providers [75, 76]. From the literature, the most common changes in the genital area include lichen sclerosus changes of porcelain-like polygonal macules, as well as more typical classical plaque-type morphea lesions with areas of waxy induration, and even labial fusion [75–78]. Patients with reported genital involvement have typically been postmenopausal women with the generalized subtype of morphea, though lichen sclerosus changes have also been reported with some frequency in plaque-type morphea [75, 78]. Review of the MAC cohort database revealed genital changes were present in 3.5 % of all participants (14/433), though this represented almost 10 % of patients with the generalized subtype of morphea (13/149, 8.7 %). Similar to reports in the literature, those affected were all women and were typically postmenopausal (13/14, 92.8 %). Similar to previous reports, genital involvement in the MAC cohort was primarily seen in patients with the generalized subtype of morphea, typically with features of lichen sclerosus overlap (13/14, 92.8 %).
- *Malignancy*. Rare cases of malignancy are reported in morphea lesions, such as squamous cell carcinoma of the lip that developed in an individual with pansclerotic disabling morphea [66]. The etiology is likely similar to carcinoma developing in chronic venous insufficiency ulcerations and burn scars. Providers should take care to exclude cutaneous metastasis in lesions of morphea involving the breast (see *Differential diagnosis of morphea*).

Laboratory Findings in Morphea Individuals with all subtypes of morphea, particularly those with deep involvement, may have peripheral eosinophilia and presence of markers of inflammation and autoimmunity (though this is relatively uncommon). The most common of these markers are positive antinuclear antibody (ANA) and/or rheumatoid factor and presence of anti-ssDNA and antihistone antibodies (AHAs), which suggest a predisposition to autoimmunity, but do not reliably correlate with disease activity or severity [16, 37, 38]. In one nested case-control study, morphea patients had a higher prevalence of ANA (63/187, 34 %) and AHA positivity (22/187, 22 %) as compared to matched healthy controls. There was a similar prevalence of ssDNA antibodies in cases (15/187, 8 %) and controls (10/149, 7 %). Of those morphea patients with positive ANA, most had speckled pattern (52/63, 81 %) at high titer (>1:1,280), though few patients with ANA positivity had extractable nuclear antigen (ENA) antibodies (7/63, 11 %), implying the possible presence of an unidentified antigen in morphea. The presence of these autoantibodies, however, has not reliably correlated with any measures of clinical activity. Thus ANAs and AHAs have limited clinical utility except in linear morphea, where their presence may be associated with greater disease burden and functional impairment [79].

There are no laboratory tests that confirm the diagnosis of morphea, which is made on clinical features with confirmatory histopathology. Biomarkers predictive of activity or prognosis are also lacking. Thus clinical assessment remains the mainstay of diagnosis and evaluation.

Differential Diagnosis of Morphea

Many morphea patients experience delay in diagnosis and treatment because providers fail to recognize this relatively rare disease [80]. The development of morphea can be insidious and subtle, and initial misdiagnosis, particularly by non-dermatologists, occurs frequently [80]. Morphea can mimic other cutaneous diseases, including atrophic conditions, vascular lesions, dyspigmenting disorders, and even more common skin lesions such as bruises and scars (see Table 8.2) [81–83]. Early morphea lesions have been periodically confused with port-wine stains in the pediatric population [83, 84], because early lesions may present as erythematous linear patches with minimal sclerosis. Histology can be useful to distinguish these entities, and lesions should also be monitored for changes over time, as induration, atrophy, and sclerosis may develop over time and reveal the correct diagnosis [83].

Providers should consider common entities in their differential diagnosis, including lipodermatosclerosis and trauma-induced fat necrosis. Steroid atrophy can mimic morphea, as subcutaneous atrophy may result at the site of steroid and other intramuscular injections, and injection of the scalp to treat other skin conditions can actually mimic linear morphea of the scalp. These entities can usually be differentiated from morphea by a careful history and physical examination, and, when necessary, a biopsy. Providers should also make sure to exclude more dangerous entities such as metastatic carcinoma in the appropriate settings (for instance, of lesions on the breast, overlying the site of known prior carcinoma). Post-radiation morphea can mimic radiation dermatitis, infection, or recurrent breast carcinoma (Fig. 8.8), and differentiating morphea from radiation dermatitis will depend on both clinical and histopathological features [85]. Special care should also be taken to distinguish morphea from scleroderma based on clinical features already described. Patients will often confuse the two entities, and misplaced concern over systemic disease damage to internal organs may impact negatively on patient quality of life [64].

The diagnosis of morphea is made clinically, but biopsy and histological examination may be useful to aid decision-making based on the depth of involvement (see Fig. 8.9). Biopsy should also be done to exclude potential malignancy

Table 8.2 Differential diagnosis of morphea

Most likely
1. Scleroderma (systemic sclerosis)
2. Lipodermatosclerosis
3. Eosinophilic fasciitis (may be a related process)
4. Trauma-induced fat necrosis (intramuscular injections)
5. Nephrogenic systemic fibrosis
6. Chronic graft-versus-host disease
7. Steroid atrophy
Consider
1. Lichen sclerosus (may be a related process)
2. Pretibial myxedema
3. Connective tissue nevi
4. Morpheaform basal cell carcinoma
5. Chemical-mediated sclerosing skin conditions (toxic oil syndrome, rapeseed oil)
6. Lyme disease (acrodermatitis atrophicans)
7. Phenylketonuria
8. Scleromyxedema
9. Pretibial myxedema
10. POEMS syndrome
11. Drug-induced sclerosing skin conditions: taxanes, IM injections, interferon-alpha
12. Lupus profundus
13. Port-wine stain
Always rule out
1. Carcinoma of the breast metastatic to the skin (*carcinoma en cuirase*)
2. Porphyria cutanea tarda
3. Dermatofibrosarcoma protuberans

POEMS polyneuropathy, *o*rganomegaly, *e*ndocrinopathy, *M* protein, and *s*kin changes (Reproduced with permission from: Saxton-Daniels and Jacobe [111])

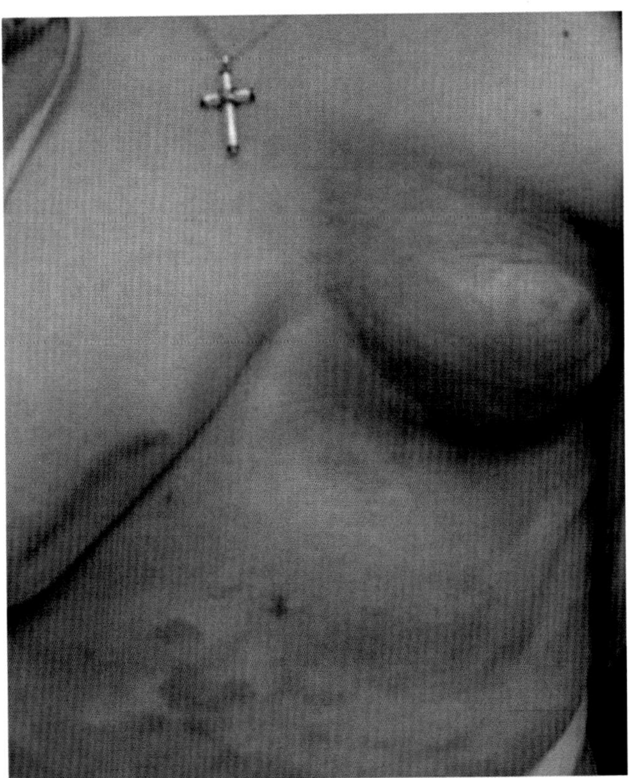

Fig. 8.8 *Postirradiation morphea on the breast*. Morpheaform changes occurred after breast reconstruction and radiation therapy in this patient with a history of breast cancer. Note the importance of a wider skin examination to differentiate this process from radiation dermatitis or recurrent carcinoma, as multiple morphea lesions are present on the trunk as well. Biopsy would be warranted in this case to rule out malignancy. Though postirradiation morphea has been reported, patients should not avoid necessary radiation or other lifesaving treatments due to a diagnosis of morphea

and in cases in which history and physical examination findings are not definitive, and pathology is needed to exclude disorders other than squamous cell carcinoma. Given the lack of accepted biomarkers, laboratory-based tests are not currently recommended for the evaluation of morphea in the absence of specific signs or symptoms that would otherwise prompt them (see *Laboratory findings in morphea*). Imaging is not recommended routinely for diagnosis, but may be useful to evaluate for depth of involvement or to monitor disease activity (see *Imaging methods* and Fig. 8.9).

Approach to the Evaluation of the Patient with Morphea

Approach to the patient with morphea depends on a number of factors, including disease subtype, disease activity, and depth of involvement, as well as patient symptomatology and the potential for cosmetic or functional impairment. Patients may benefit from a multidisciplinary approach to address functional and cosmetic issues as well as comorbidities when present (Fig. 8.9). As noted earlier, there are no widely accepted biomarkers for morphea, so laboratory-based tests are not routinely recommended for the evaluation of morphea in the absence of specific signs or symptoms that would otherwise warrant them. Depending on features found on clinical examination or on patient complaints (muscle pain, limited range of motion, neurologic symptoms or deficits, etc.), imaging may be warranted to evaluate the depth of lesions and involvement of underlying structures (see *Imaging methods*).

Imaging Methods

- *Ultrasound* [86–89]. The most reliable assessment uses 20–25 MHz ultrasound (US). Ultrasound at 10–15 MHz – which is more readily available in the United States – is also useful [86, 87]. This modality has been more extensively used in making the diagnosis of morphea, but has been used more recently for measuring disease activity based on increased cutaneous blood flow and increased subcutaneous tissue echogenicity, and has been found to be a sensitive tool for monitoring localized scleroderma in the pediatric population

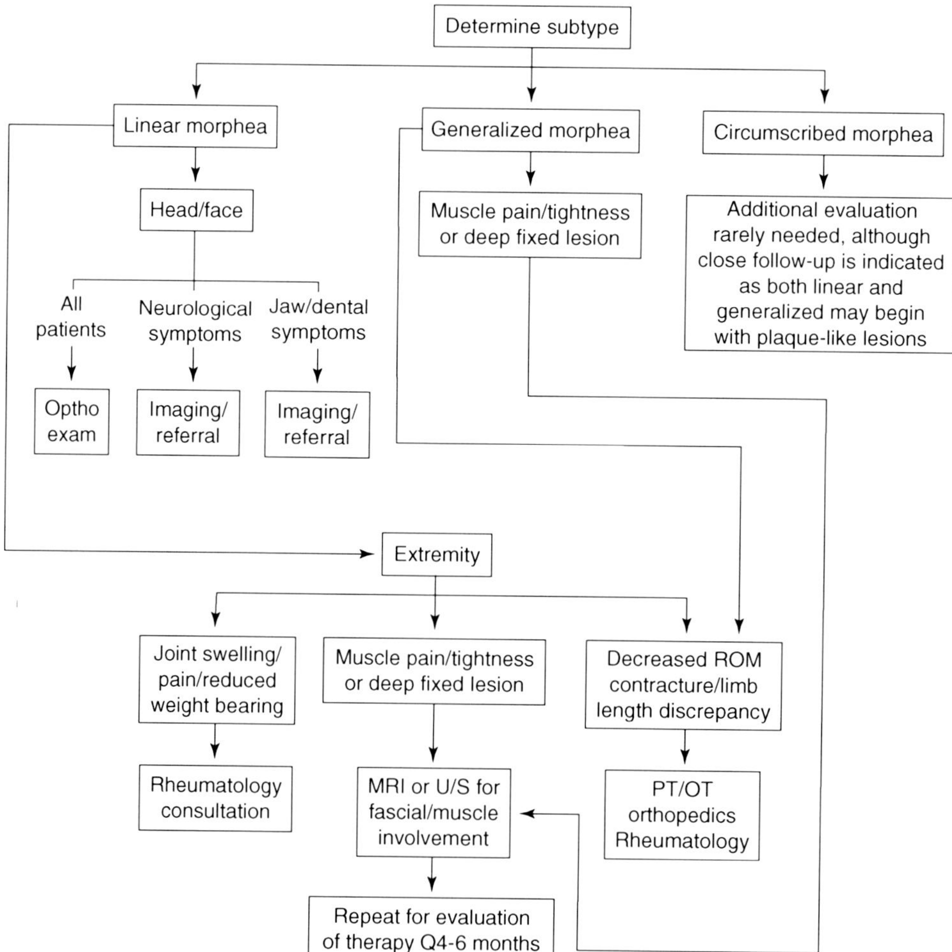

Fig. 8.9 Algorithm for the evaluation of patients with morphea (Reproduced with permission from: Jacobe H. Treatment of morphea (localized scleroderma) in adults. In: UpToDate, Post TW (Ed), UpToDate, Waltham, MA. (Accessed on 19 Dec 2014.) Copyright © 2014 UpToDate, Inc. For more information visit www.uptodate.com)

[86, 90, 91]. However, ultrasound assessment is operator dependent and lacks standardization.

- *Magnetic resonance imaging* (MRI) [67, 92]. Although the MRI findings in morphea can overlap with other soft tissue abnormalities such as fibromatoses and myofibromatoses, the experienced radiologist can distinguish features of morphea including thickening of the dermis and increased signal intensity during the inflammatory stages, as well as changes in signal in the bone marrow with deeper involvement. MRI is particularly useful for evaluation of the depth of infiltration in morphea and sequential analysis of disease activity [92]. MRI has also been used to detect musculoskeletal involvement, including fascial thickening and enhancement, articular synovitis, and tenosynovitis, in patients with morphea, even some in whom musculoskeletal involvement was not suspected based on the history and exam [67] However, the clinical significance of such findings has yet to be determined, and at this point there is no evidence for pan imaging in the patient diagnosed with morphea without signs or symptoms concerning for musculoskeletal involvement. Imaging is best done after conferring with a radiologist to optimize the methods in which the patient is imaged and to ensure attention to possible features of morphea.

Therapeutic Options for Morphea

A majority of morphea patients experience delay in diagnosis of greater than 6 months, as well as quite varied treatment that appears to depend more on provider specialty than on disease characteristics or evidence for treatment modalities [80]. However, there are a number of therapeutic options with proven efficacy in morphea (Table 8.3). Each of these may be considered depending on disease subtype, activity, depth of involvement, and other patient considerations. The authors recommend using the evidence-based algorithm below when considering therapeutic options for patients with morphea (Fig. 8.10).

It is important to note that, contrary to conventional wisdom, morphea can be successfully treated with proper therapy and patient selection. However, providers should remember, and emphasize to patients, that the therapeutic end point in morphea is not the complete resolution of lesions but rather the loss of features of activity (reduction of erythema, halting progression of lesions or development of new lesions). Disease damage may actually increase for a time with treatment as lesions transition from inflammatory to atrophic or sclerotic stages (though skin thickening is likely to soften over time, even after treatment cessation). Providers should make sure to distinguish features of damage, such as dyspigmentation or atrophy, which can result in more visible blood vessels and apparent erythema, from true erythema mediated by inflammation (this may be accomplished by examining areas of erythema with magnification and looking for the induration that accompanies inflammation).

The approach to the patient with morphea depends on the assessment of disease activity, depth of involvement, and the presence of other sequelae, which is typically based on clinical examination. Careful clinical photographs should be taken at each visit to monitor patient's lesions, as subtle changes indicative of disease activity may otherwise be missed. Clinical scoring measures, such as the LOSCAT, may also be useful for quantifying and monitoring progression of disease or efficacy of therapy [60, 93]. Histological examination may aid in initial therapeutic decision-making, as it can be difficult to determine the depth of involvement by clinical exam alone. In these cases, biopsy of the advancing edge of a lesion can be undertaken to provide insight into both activity and depth of morphea (see *Histopathology of morphea*).

Phototherapy There is substantial evidence for the efficacy of phototherapy in morphea, particularly for broadband UVA, narrowband UVB, and UVA-1 [94–99] (Table 8.3). UVB is more appropriate for lesions restricted to the superficial dermis, which are relatively thin on palpation and, on biopsy, have sclerosis and inflammation in the papillary and

Table 8.3 Treatments for morphea by the level of evidence

Treatment	Level of evidence
BB UVA	1,2
UVA-1	1,2
Calcitriol, oral (inefficacy 1)	1,2
MTX plus oral/IV corticosteroids	1,2
IFN-gamma (inefficacy 1)	1
PUVA bath	2
PUVA cream	2
ECP	2
Calcipotriene, topical	2
MTX monotherapy	2
PCMT	2
Tacrolimus, topical	2
Corticosteroids, oral	2
Hydroxychloroquine, mycophenolate mofetil, cyclosporine, bosentan, infliximab, imiquimod, antimicrobials, D-penicillamine, 585 nm long-pulse laser, wide surgical resection, orthopedic surgery, Apligraf	Minimal evidence (≥level 3)

BB broadband, *IFN* interferon, *ECP* extracorporeal photochemotherapy, *MTX* methotrexate

Level of evidence: *1*, indicates randomized controlled trial; 2, uncontrolled trial, *3*, case report, case series (Adapted from content in Jacobe H. Treatment of morphea (localized scleroderma) in adults. In: UpToDate, Post TW (Ed), UpToDate, Waltham, MA. (Accessed on 19 Dec 2014.) Copyright © 2014 UpToDate, Inc. For more information visit www.uptodate.com)

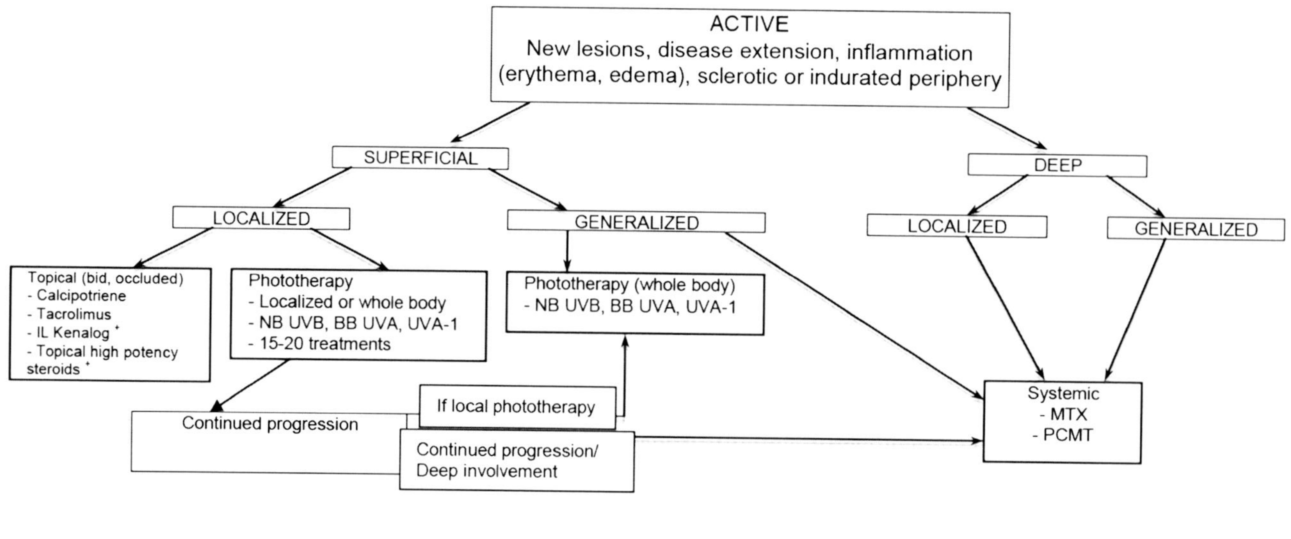

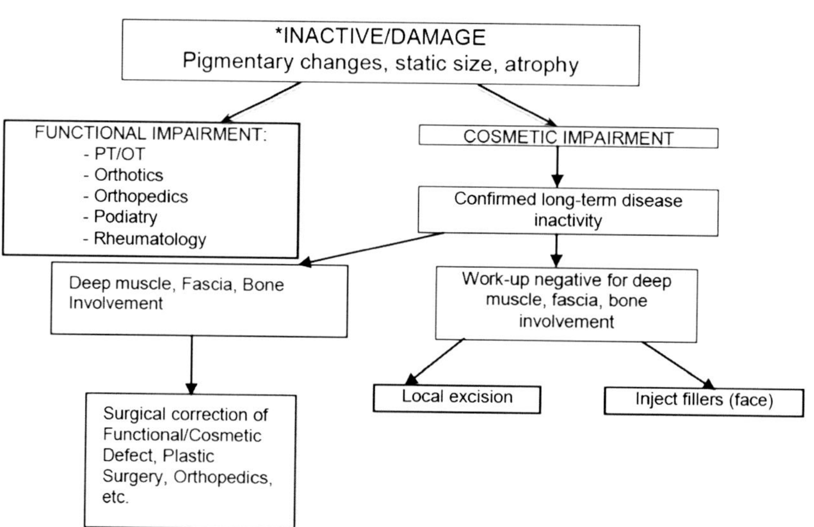

Fig. 8.10 Therapeutic algorithm for morphea based on existing evidence. Histological examination and/or MRI are encouraged to evaluate lesions for the depth of involvement and, likewise, determine appropriate treatment as well as evaluation of therapeutic efficacy. Superficial involvement is defined by histological evidence of papillary dermal involvement. Deep involvement is defined as sclerosis or inflammation of the deep dermis, subcutis, fascia, or muscle (Reproduced with permission from: Jacobe H. Treatment of morphea (localized scleroderma) in adults. In: UpToDate, Post TW (Ed), UpToDate, Waltham, MA. (Accessed on [19 Dec 2014].) Copyright © 2014 UpToDate, Inc. For more information visit www.uptodate.com). *There is very little evidence for any therapy addressing disease damage in morphea. The risk of disease reactivation is also unknown, but possible with the use of invasive procedures. Therefore, surgery and the like should only be undertaken after prolonged inactivity of disease. + There is no evidence for efficacy in the literature

superficial reticular dermis. UVA-based treatments can penetrate to a greater depth and are therefore more effective for deeper dermal lesions. UVA-1, in particular, has been shown to normalize dermal collagen and reduce inflammation in morphea and thus may be effective for disease in either inflammatory or sclerotic phase [95]. There is also evidence in the literature for the efficacy of broadband UVA phototherapy, which can be an appropriate alternative when UVA-1 is not available [94]. Improvement in disease, noted by the halting of lesion progression and the reduction of erythema, should be seen after 10–20 treatments. A trial can usually be stopped after 20–30 treatments if improvement is not seen in that period. Treatments are usually given three to five times weekly for a period of several weeks until this number of total treatments has been reached. Evidence suggests that patients may continue to improve even after the cessation of therapy, leading some to suggest an even greater number of treatments (30–50) for further therapeutic benefit. Optimum doses and regimen for UVA-1 phototherapy have yet to be determined; however, one randomized controlled trial has suggested that both low-dose (20 J per square centimeter) UVA-1 and medium-dose (50 J per square centimeter)

UVA-1 are equally effective, while medium-dose UVA-1 is more effective than narrowband UVB [96]. Phototherapy is not likely to be effective for lesions with deep involvement of the subcutis, fascia, or muscle and therefore should not be considered a primary therapy for such disease.

Vitamin D Derivatives Only one study provides level-1 evidence on the effect of vitamin D derivatives in morphea and actually showed no difference between oral calcitriol and placebo, with both groups improving equally [100] (Table 8.3). The authors also point out that this study was underpowered, making definitive conclusions about the efficacy of oral calcitriol difficult. Various uncontrolled trials and case reports have shown improvement in patients using topical vitamin D derivatives applied under occlusion. However, this improvement took place over a period of several months, during which time lesions might be expected to improve independently.

Immunomodulators

- *Methotrexate with or without corticosteroids*. The use of methotrexate monotherapy and methotrexate combined with systemic corticosteroids has been shown to be effective based on multiple prospective trials [2, 26, 29, 101–103] (Table 8.3). One double-blind randomized controlled trial has also shown that pediatric morphea patients treated with 15–20 mg weekly of methotrexate for 12 months, after induction with 1 mg/kg/day oral prednisone for 3 months, had lower clinical disease scores, decreased lesion temperature, and lower rates of relapse than those treated with prednisone induction alone (plus placebo) [29]. Relapse occurred within 12 months in 15 patients treated with methotrexate in addition to corticosteroids (32.6 %) versus 17 of those treated with placebo only after steroids (70.8 %). More specifically, new lesions developed in three methotrexate-treated patients (6.5 %) versus four placebo-treated patients (16.7 %) within 3–9 months. As the primary end point in the study was response to treatment within 12 months, it is difficult to determine the actual time for effect of this medication regimen. Similarly, optimum dose, route, and indications for the additions of corticosteroids to methotrexate, as well as duration of therapy, have not been definitively established. In most studies with combined therapy, including the randomized trial described, corticosteroids are used for induction therapy either orally or via intravenous pulse (IV methylprednisolone 30 mg/kg/day for 3 days per month or 1 mg/kg/day prednisone) over the first 3 months. Methotrexate is used as a steroid-sparing agent and initiated simultaneously (0.6 mg/kg/week in children or 15–25 mg/week for adults), then maintained for a prolonged period (1–2 years) and gradually tapered. Consensus treatment plans for pediatric morphea have recently been established that detail these monotherapy and combined therapy approaches [61]. As evidence to date has not suggested a difference in disease processes between pediatric and adult morphea, it is likely that adults will respond similarly to this regimen. From the literature, most patients will respond in a mean of 2–5 months with this approach, with patients early in their disease course typically responding best. Importantly, relapse has been noted frequently after cessation of therapy (see *Epidemiology and clinical course*), indicating that therapy suppresses disease activity but is not curative [27].
- *Other immunomodulators*. Level 2 evidence supports the use of topical tacrolimus 0.1 % ointment under occlusion for active, inflammatory superficial plaque-type morphea [104] (Table 8.3). Recent case series using oral mycophenolate mofetil indicate possible efficacy in patients who are refractory to methotrexate or have intolerable side effects [105]. Mycophenolate mofetil also may be effective as a treatment adjunct in children with morphea; in one retrospective analysis, ten patients with severe or methotrexate-resistant pediatric morphea experienced clinical improvement with mycophenolate mofetil that resulted in withdrawal or reduction of doses of corticosteroids and methotrexate [106]. Retrospective case reports on the use of oral cyclosporine, bosentan, infliximab, and topical imiquimod have reported some efficacy, but definitive studies are lacking (Table 8.3).

Antimicrobials Despite the widespread use of antimicrobials in morphea, including antibiotics and antimalarials, no published clinical trials of these agents exist [107]. Literature supporting the use of antimalarials is limited to a case series in which two patients improved with hydroxychloroquine, while simultaneously receiving methotrexate and corticosteroids [108]. In one retrospective review, 7 out of 11 patients had persistently active disease 3–153 months after initiating therapy with hydroxychloroquine [16]. At this time, the use of these agents in severe morphea is not indicated, pending more definitive evidence for their efficacy (Table 8.3).

Treatments Not Supported by Current Evidence The efficacy of the most commonly used treatment for morphea, topical corticosteroids, has never been formally evaluated [62, 80]. There have also been no studies investigating the use of intralesional steroids. In the authors' experience, intralesional steroids have been effective in treating circumscribed plaques of morphea or as an adjuvant for recalcitrant areas in patients receiving phototherapy or systemic treatment. Current evidence does not support the use of interferon-gamma in morphea [109], and the risks of penicillamine, including toxicities, outweigh its potential benefits, which have not been well established. At this time, there is no sufficient evidence to support the use of these agents, especially in moderate-to-severe morphea, when other agents have proven efficacy (unless contraindications exist to their use) (Table 8.3).

Adjunctive Therapy A significant number of patients with morphea suffer irreversible sequelae that persist even after disease activity has subsided. Patients should be carefully evaluated for limitations in range of motion, contractures, limb length discrepancies, or other functional impairments. Treatment modalities may include physical therapy techniques for improving range of motion of affected limbs, stretching exercises for contractures, orthotics or shoe inserts to adjust for limb length discrepancies and to compensate for loss of subcutaneous fat, or even tendon release in some cases [16]. Referral to specialists, such as rheumatologists, physical therapists, orthopedists, oral maxillofacial surgeons, or plastic surgeons, may be helpful to maximize cosmesis and function and to minimize further damage. Importantly, studies to date are completely lacking in addressing this type of damage due to morphea.

Surgical Therapies There is limited evidence to support the use of surgical therapies for morphea. Importantly, these therapies should only be considered when morphea has been inactive, and a patient has been off treatment for a number of years. Patients should be monitored closely with serial examinations for reactivation, and collaboration with an experienced plastic surgeon is vital.

Summary

Morphea is a relatively uncommon idiopathic inflammatory disorder that leads to the development of sclerotic plaques in the skin. Though morphea may share common histopathological features with scleroderma, the disease differs demographically and clinically. Involvement of internal organs in morphea is unusual and very different from that in scleroderma. Morphea occurs in adults and children and preferentially affects females. The pathogenesis of morphea is not well understood, but is likely to involve autoimmunity, as well as genetic and environmental factors. Lesions typically begin as inflammatory patches that evolve into firm, sclerotic plaques. Involvement may be limited to the dermis or may extend to underlying subcutaneous fat, muscle, or bone. Atrophic changes often remain after resolution of lesion activity.

Morphea has a variety of clinical presentations. Circumscribed and generalized morphea occurs more frequently in adults, while linear morphea predominates in children. The identification of characteristic clinical findings often is sufficient for the diagnosis of morphea, but biopsy may be performed to exclude other entities or to obtain information on the depth of disease. Antinuclear antibody (ANA) levels are elevated in some patients with morphea; however, routine testing for autoantibodies is not indicated. Magnetic resonance imaging (MRI) or ultrasound can be used to assess the extent of involvement, in those patients for whom clinical examination suggests involvement deeper than the dermis, and may be useful for following disease activity during treatment.

The assessment of disease activity and depth of involvement guides therapeutic decision-making in morphea. Because of the self-limited nature of morphea, patients with limited plaque disease may elect to defer therapy. For patients with superficial (dermal) circumscribed disease who desire treatment, but do not have access to or prefer to avoid the frequent visits required for phototherapy, treatment options include high-potency topical corticosteroids, intralesional corticosteroids, a topical vitamin D analogue, topical tacrolimus, or imiquimod. For patients with superficial (dermal) forms of morphea who are able to receive phototherapy, treatment with UVA-1 is preferred; alternatives include broadband UVA, narrowband UVB, or PUVA. Phototherapy is unlikely to be effective for morphea involving the subcutaneous tissue, muscle, or bone. Rapidly progressive, severe, disabling disease requires systemic therapy, involving a combination of methotrexate and systemic corticosteroids. Morphea may cause joint contractures and other functional impairments secondary to deep tissue sclerosis. All patients should be clinically assessed for the development of these findings. Physical therapy is essential for patients who are at risk for or who show evidence for functional impairments.

Acknowledgment The authors wish to thank Rose Ann Cannon for her support in the preparation of this manuscript.

References

1. Zulian F, Woo P, Athreya BH, Laxer RM, Medsger Jr TA, Lehman TJ, et al. The Pediatric Rheumatology European Society/American College of Rheumatology/European League against Rheumatism provisional classification criteria for juvenile systemic sclerosis. Arthritis Rheum. 2007;57(2):203–12.
2. Tollefson MM, Witman PM. En coup de sabre morphea and Parry-Romberg syndrome: a retrospective review of 54 patients. J Am Acad Dermatol. 2007;56(2):257–63.
3. Pinal-Fernandez I, Selva-O'Callaghan A, Grau JM. Diagnosis and classification of eosinophilic fasciitis. Autoimmun Rev. 2014;13(4–5):379–82.
4. Su WP, Greene SL. Bullous morphea profunda. Am J Dermatopathol. 1986;8(2):144–7.
5. Rencic A, Goyal S, Mofid M, Wigley F, Nousari HC. Bullous lesions in scleroderma. Int J Dermatol. 2002;41(6):335–9.
6. Trattner A, David M, Sandbank M. Bullous morphea: a distinct entity? Am J Dermatopathol. 1994;16(4):414–7.
7. Daoud MS, Su WP, Leiferman KM, Perniciaro C. Bullous morphea: clinical, pathologic, and immunopathologic evaluation of thirteen cases. J Am Acad Dermatol. 1994;30(6):937–43.
8. Kobayasi T, Willeberg A, Serup J, Ullman S. Generalized morphea with blisters. A case report. Acta Derm Venereol. 1990;70(5):454–6.

9. Blaya B, Gardeazabal J, de Lagran ZM, Diaz-Perez JL. Patient with generalized guttate morphea and lichen sclerosus et atrophicus. Actas Dermosifiliogr. 2008;99(10):808–11.
10. Yamanaka M, Ishikawa O. Guttate morphea in a scleroderma spectrum disorder patient with anticentromere antibody. Eur J Dermatol: EJD. 2009;19(6):630–1.
11. Synkowski DR, Lobitz Jr WC, Provost TT. Bullous scleroderma. Arch Dermatol. 1981;117(3):135–7.
12. Rencic A, Brinster N, Nousari CH. Keloid morphea and nodular scleroderma: two distinct clinical variants of scleroderma? J Cutan Med Surg. 2003;7(1):20–4.
13. Fernandez-Flores A, Gatica-Torres M, Tinoco-Fragoso F, Garcia-Hidalgo L, Monroy E, Saeb-Lima M. Three cases of bullous morphea: histopathologic findings with implications regarding pathogenesis. J Cutan Pathol. 2015;42(2):144–9.
14. Kavala M, Zindanci I, Demirkesen C, Beyhan EK, Turkoglu Z. Intertriginous bullous morphea: a clue for the pathogenesis? Indian J Dermatol Venereol Leprol. 2007;73(4):262–4.
15. Peterson LS, Nelson AM, Su WP, Mason T, O'Fallon WM, Gabriel SE. The epidemiology of morphea (localized scleroderma) in Olmsted County 1960–1993. J Rheumatol. 1997;24(1):73–80.
16. Christen-Zaech S, Hakim MD, Afsar FS, Paller AS. Pediatric morphea (localized scleroderma): review of 136 patients. J Am Acad Dermatol. 2008;59(3):385–96.
17. Sehgal VN, Srivastava G, Aggarwal AK, Behl PN, Choudhary M, Bajaj P. Localized scleroderma/morphea. Int J Dermatol. 2002;41(8):467–75.
18. Leitenberger JJ, Cayce RL, Haley RW, Adams-Huet B, Bergstresser PR, Jacobe HT. Distinct autoimmune syndromes in morphea: a review of 245 adult and pediatric cases. Arch Dermatol. 2009;145(5):545–50.
19. Vierra E, Cunningham BB. Morphea and localized scleroderma in children. Semin Cutan Med Surg. 1999;18(3):210–25.
20. Marzano AV, Menni S, Parodi A, Borghi A, Fuligni A, Fabbri P, et al. Localized scleroderma in adults and children. Clinical and laboratory investigations on 239 cases. Eur J Dermatol. 2003;13(2):171–6.
21. Saxton-Daniels S, Jacobe HT. An evaluation of long-term outcomes in adults with pediatric-onset morphea. Arch Dermatol. 2010;146(9):1044–5.
22. Condie D, Grabell D, Jacobe H. Comparison of outcomes in adults with pediatric-onset morphea and those with adult-onset morphea: a cross-sectional study from the morphea in adults and children cohort. Arthritis Rheum. 2014;66(12):3496–504.
23. Kroft EB, Creemers MC, van den Hoogen FH, Boezeman JB, de Jong EM. Effectiveness, side-effects and period of remission after treatment with methotrexate in localized scleroderma and related sclerotic skin diseases: an inception cohort study. Br J Dermatol. 2009;160(5):1075–82.
24. Cox D, OR G, Collins S, Byrne A, Irvine A, Watson R. Juvenile localised scleroderma: a retrospective review of response to systemic treatment. Ir J Med Sci. 2008;177(4):343–6.
25. Mirsky L, Chakkittakandiyil A, Laxer RM, O'Brien C, Pope E. Relapse after systemic treatment in paediatric morphoea. Br J Dermatol. 2012;166(2):443–5.
26. Weibel L, Sampaio MC, Visentin MT, Howell KJ, Woo P, Harper JI. Evaluation of methotrexate and corticosteroids for the treatment of localized scleroderma (morphoea) in children. Br J Dermatol. 2006;155(5):1013–20.
27. Zulian F, Vallongo C, Patrizi A, Belloni-Fortina A, Cutrone M, Alessio M, et al. A long-term follow-up study of methotrexate in juvenile localized scleroderma (morphea). J Am Acad Dermatol. 2012;67(6):1151–6.
28. Vasquez R, Jabbar A, Khan F, Buethe D, Ahn C, Jacobe H. Recurrence of morphea after successful ultraviolet A1 phototherapy: a cohort study. J Am Acad Dermatol. 2014;70(3):481–8.
29. Zulian F, Martini G, Vallongo C, Vittadello F, Falcini F, Patrizi A, et al. Methotrexate treatment in juvenile localized scleroderma: a randomized, double-blind, placebo-controlled trial. Arthritis Rheum. 2011;63(7):1998–2006.
30. Mertens JS, Seyger MM, Kievit W, Hoppenreijs EP, Jansen TL, van de Kerkhof PC, et al. Disease recurrence in localized scleroderma: a retrospective analysis of 344 patients with paediatric- or adult-onset disease. Br J Dermatol. 2015;172(3):722–8.
31. Badea I, Taylor M, Rosenberg A, Foldvari M. Pathogenesis and therapeutic approaches for improved topical treatment in localized scleroderma and systemic sclerosis. Rheumatology. 2009;48(3):213–21.
32. Wadud MA, Bose BK, Al Nasir T. Familial localised scleroderma from Bangladesh: two case reports. Bangladesh Med Res Counc Bull. 1989;15(1):15–9.
33. Rees RB, Bennett J. Localized scleroderma in father and daughter. AMA Arch Dermatol Syphilol. 1953;68(3):360.
34. Zulian F, Vallongo C, Woo P, Russo R, Ruperto N, Harper J, et al. Localized scleroderma in childhood is not just a skin disease. Arthritis Rheum. 2005;52(9):2873–81.
35. Hemminki K, Li X, Sundquist J, Sundquist K. Familial associations of rheumatoid arthritis with autoimmune diseases and related conditions. Arthritis Rheum. 2009;60(3):661–8.
36. Hemminki K, Li X, Sundquist J, Hillert J, Sundquist K. Risk for multiple sclerosis in relatives and spouses of patients diagnosed with autoimmune and related conditions. Neurogenetics. 2009;10(1):5–11.
37. Firoz EF, Kamino H, Lehman TJ, Orlow SJ. Morphea, diabetes mellitus type I, and celiac disease: case report and review of the literature. Pediatr Dermatol. 2010;27(1):48–52.
38. Dervis E, Acbay O, Barut G, Karaoglu A, Ersoy L. Association of vitiligo, morphea, and Hashimoto's thyroiditis. Int J Dermatol. 2004;43(3):236–7.
39. Hiremath NC, Madan Mohan NT, Srinivas C, Sangolli PM, Srinivas K, Vrushali VD. Juvenile localized scleroderma with autoimmune thyroid disorder. Indian J Dermatol. 2010;55(3):308–9.
40. Hasegawa M, Fujimoto M, Hayakawa I, Matsushita T, Nishijima C, Yamazaki M, et al. Anti-phosphatidylserine-prothrombin complex antibodies in patients with localized scleroderma. Clin Exp Rheumatol. 2006;24(1):19–24.
41. Slimani S, Hounas F, Ladjouze-Rezig A. Multiple linear sclerodermas with a diffuse Parry-Romberg syndrome. Joint Bone Spine: Rev Rhum. 2009;76(1):114–6.
42. Saleh Z, Arayssi T, Saleh Z, Ghosn S. Superficial morphea: 20-year follow up in a patient with concomitant psoriasis vulgaris. J Cutan Pathol. 2009;36(10):1105–8.
43. Jacobe H, Ahn C, Arnett FC, Reveille JD. Major histocompatibility complex class I and class II alleles may confer susceptibility to or protection against morphea: findings from the morphea in adults and children cohort. Arthritis Rheum. 2014;66(11):3170–7.
44. Simmonds MJ, Gough SC. Unravelling the genetic complexity of autoimmune thyroid disease: HLA, CTLA-4 and beyond. Clin Exp Immunol. 2004;136(1):1–10.
45. Weyand CM, Hicok KC, Conn DL, Goronzy JJ. The influence of HLA-DRB1 genes on disease severity in rheumatoid arthritis. Ann Intern Med. 1992;117(10):801–6.
46. Takehara K, Moroi Y, Nakabayashi Y, Ishibashi Y. Antinuclear antibodies in localized scleroderma. Arthritis Rheum. 1983;26(5):612–6.
47. Gruschwitz MS, Hornstein OP, von Den Driesch P. Correlation of soluble adhesion molecules in the peripheral blood of scleroderma patients with their in situ expression and with disease activity. Arthritis Rheum. 1995;38(2):184–9.
48. Fett N, Werth VP. Update on morphea: part I. Epidemiology, clinical presentation, and pathogenesis. J Am Acad Dermatol. 2011;64(2):217–28. quiz 29–30.

49. Yamane K, Ihn H, Kubo M, Yazawa N, Kikuchi K, Soma Y, et al. Increased serum levels of soluble vascular cell adhesion molecule 1 and E-selectin in patients with localized scleroderma. J Am Acad Dermatol. 2000;42(1 Pt 1):64–9.
50. Ihn H, Sato S, Fujimoto M, Kikuchi K, Takehara K. Demonstration of interleukin-2, interleukin-4 and interleukin-6 in sera from patients with localized scleroderma. Arch Dermatol Res. 1995;287(2):193–7.
51. McNallan KT, Aponte C, El-Azhary R, Mason T, Nelson AM, Paat JJ, et al. Immunophenotyping of chimeric cells in localized scleroderma. Rheumatology. 2007;46(3):398–402.
52. Magee KE, Kelsey CE, Kurzinski KL, Ho J, Mlakar LR, Feghali-Bostwick CA, et al. Interferon-gamma inducible protein-10 as a potential biomarker in localized scleroderma. Arthritis Res Ther. 2013;15(6):R188.
53. Milano A, Pendergrass SA, Sargent JL, George LK, McCalmont TH, Connolly MK, et al. Molecular subsets in the gene expression signatures of scleroderma skin. PLoS ONE. 2008;3(7):e2696.
54. Uziel Y, Feldman BM, Krafchik BR, Laxer RM, Yeung RS. Increased serum levels of TGFbeta1 in children with localized scleroderma. Pediatr Rheumatol Online J. 2007;5:22.
55. Walker D SJ, Karai L, Currimbhoy S, Jacobe H. Histopathological changes in morphea and their clinical correlates: results from the Morphea in Adults and Children Cohort (MAC) V. In preparation. 2015.
56. Torrelo A, Suarez J, Colmenero I, Azorin D, Perera A, Zambrano A. Deep morphea after vaccination in two young children. Pediatr Dermatol. 2006;23(5):484–7.
57. Beltramelli M, Vercellesi P, Frasin A, Gelmetti C, Corona F. Localized severe scleroderma: a retrospective study of 26 pediatric patients. Pediatr Dermatol. 2010;27(5):476–80.
58. Ueda T, Niiyama S, Amoh Y, Katsuoka K. Linear scleroderma after contusion and injection of mepivacaine hydrochloride. Dermatol Online J. 2010;16(5):11.
59. Grabell D, Hsieh C, Andrew R, Martires K, Kim A, Vasquez R, et al. The role of skin trauma in the distribution of morphea lesions: a cross-sectional survey of the Morphea in Adults and Children cohort IV. J Am Acad Dermatol. 2014;71(3):493–8.
60. Arkachaisri T, Vilaiyuk S, Torok KS, Medsger Jr TA. Development and initial validation of the localized scleroderma skin damage index and physician global assessment of disease damage: a proof-of-concept study. Rheumatology. 2010;49(2):373–81.
61. Li SC, Torok KS, Pope E, Dedeoglu F, Hong S, Jacobe HT, et al. Development of consensus treatment plans for juvenile localized scleroderma: a roadmap toward comparative effectiveness studies in juvenile localized scleroderma. Arthritis Care Res. 2012;64(8):1175–85.
62. Strickland NSA, Fett N, Connolly MK, Hansen C, Jacobe H. Current practices in the evaluation and treatment of morphea. in preparation. 2016.
63. Orzechowski NM, Davis DM, Mason 3rd TG, Crowson CS, Reed AM. Health-related quality of life in children and adolescents with juvenile localized scleroderma. Rheumatology. 2009;48(6):670–2.
64. Klimas NK, Shedd AD, Bernstein IH, Jacobe H. Health-related quality of life in morphea. Br J Dermatol. 2015;172(5):1329–37.
65. Das S, Bernstein I, Jacobe H. Correlates of self-reported quality of life in adults and children with morphea. J Am Acad Dermatol. 2014;70(5):904–10.
66. Petrov I, Gantcheva M, Miteva L, Vassileva S, Pramatarov K. Lower lip squamous cell carcinoma in disabling pansclerotic morphea of childhood. Pediatr Dermatol. 2009;26(1):59–61.
67. Schanz S, Fierlbeck G, Ulmer A, Schmalzing M, Kummerle-Deschner J, Claussen CD, et al. Localized scleroderma: MR findings and clinical features. Radiology. 2011;260(3):817–24.
68. Chiang KL, Chang KP, Wong TT, Hsu TR. Linear scleroderma "en coup de sabre": initial presentation as intractable partial seizures in a child. Pediatr Neonatol. 2009;50(6):294–8.
69. Rigante D, Battaglia D, Contaldo I, La Torraca I, Avallone L, Gaspari S, et al. Longstanding epileptic encephalopathy and linear localized scleroderma: two distinct pathologic processes in an adolescent. Rheumatol Int. 2008;28(9):925–9.
70. Menascu S, Padeh S, Hoffman C, Ben-Zeev B. Parry-Romberg syndrome presenting as status migrainosus. Pediatr Neurol. 2009;40(4):321–3.
71. Holl-Wieden A, Klink T, Klink J, Warmuth-Metz M, Girschick HJ. Linear scleroderma 'en coup de sabre' associated with cerebral and ocular vasculitis. Scand J Rheumatol. 2006;35(5):402–4.
72. Bonilla-Abadia F, Munoz-Buitron E, Ochoa CD, Carrascal E, Canas CA. A rare association of localized scleroderma type morphea, vitiligo, autoimmune hypothyroidism, pneumonitis, autoimmune thrombocytopenic purpura and central nervous system vasculitis. Case report. BMC Res Notes. 2012;5:689.
73. Moseley BD, Burrus TM, Mason TG, Shin C. Neurological picture. Contralateral cutaneous and MRI findings in a patient with Parry-Romberg syndrome. J Neurol Neurosurg Psychiatry. 2010;81(12):1400–1.
74. Zannin ME, Martini G, Athreya BH, Russo R, Higgins G, Vittadello F, et al. Ocular involvement in children with localised scleroderma: a multi-centre study. Br J Ophthalmol. 2007;91(10):1311–4.
75. Lutz V, Frances C, Bessis D, Cosnes A, Kluger N, Godet J, et al. High frequency of genital lichen sclerosus in a prospective series of 76 patients with morphea: toward a better understanding of the spectrum of morphea. Arch Dermatol. 2012;148(1):24–8.
76. Schlosser BJ. Practice gaps. Missing genital lichen sclerosus in patients with morphea: don't ask? Don't tell?: comment on "High frequency of genital lichen sclerosus in a prospective series of 76 patients with morphea". Arch Dermatol. 2012;148(1):28–9.
77. Farrell AM, Marren PM, Wojnarowska F. Genital lichen sclerosus associated with morphoea or systemic sclerosis: clinical and HLA characteristics. Br J Dermatol. 2000;143(3):598–603.
78. Kreuter A, Wischnewski J, Terras S, Altmeyer P, Stucker M, Gambichler T. Coexistence of lichen sclerosus and morphea: a retrospective analysis of 472 patients with localized scleroderma from a German tertiary referral center. J Am Acad Dermatol. 2012;67(6):1157–62.
79. Dharamsi JW, Victor S, Aguwa N, Ahn C, Arnett F, Mayes MD, et al. Morphea in adults and children cohort III: nested case-control study – the clinical significance of autoantibodies in morphea. JAMA Dermatol. 2013;149(10):1159–65.
80. Johnson W, Jacobe H. Morphea in adults and children cohort II: patients with morphea experience delay in diagnosis and large variation in treatment. J Am Acad Dermatol. 2012;67(5):881–9.
81. Sung JJ, Chen TS, Gilliam AC, McCalmont TH, Gilliam AE. Clinicohistopathological correlations in juvenile localized scleroderma: studies on a subset of children with hypopigmented juvenile localized scleroderma due to loss of epidermal melanocytes. J Am Acad Dermatol. 2011;65(2):364–73.
82. Kakimoto CV, Victor Ross E, Uebelhoer NS. En coup de sabre presenting as a port-wine stain previously treated with pulsed dye laser. Dermatol Surg Off Publ Am Soc Dermatol Surg. 2009;35(1):165–7.
83. Nijhawan RI, Bard S, Blyumin M, Smidt AC, Chamlin SL, Connelly EA. Early localized morphea mimicking an acquired port-wine stain. J Am Acad Dermatol. 2011;64(4):779–82.
84. Kim HS, Lee JY, Kim HO, Park YM. En coup de sabre presenting as a port-wine stain initially treated with a pulsed dye laser. J Dermatol. 2011;38(2):209–10.

85. Schaffer JV, Carroll C, Dvoretsky I, Huether MJ, Girardi M. Postirradiation morphea of the breast presentation of two cases and review of the literature. Dermatology. 2000;200(1):67–71.
86. Cosnes A, Anglade MC, Revuz J, Radier C. Thirteen-megahertz ultrasound probe: its role in diagnosing localized scleroderma. Br J Dermatol. 2003;148(4):724–9.
87. Bendeck SE, Jacobe HT. Ultrasound as an outcome measure to assess disease activity in disorders of skin thickening: an example of the use of radiologic techniques to assess skin disease. Dermatol Ther. 2007;20(2):86–92.
88. Li SC, Liebling MS. The use of Doppler ultrasound to evaluate lesions of localized scleroderma. Curr Rheumatol Rep. 2009;11(3):205–11.
89. Li SC, Feldman BM, Higgins GC, Haines KA, Punaro MG, O'Neil KM. Treatment of pediatric localized scleroderma: results of a survey of North American pediatric rheumatologists. J Rheumatol. 2010;37(1):175–81.
90. Wortsman X, Wortsman J, Sazunic I, Carreno L. Activity assessment in morphea using color Doppler ultrasound. J Am Acad Dermatol. 2011;65(5):942–8.
91. Li SC, Liebling MS, Haines KA. Ultrasonography is a sensitive tool for monitoring localized scleroderma. Rheumatology. 2007;46(8):1316–9.
92. Horger M, Fierlbeck G, Kuemmerle-Deschner J, Tzaribachev N, Wehrmann M, Claussen CD, et al. MRI findings in deep and generalized morphea (localized scleroderma). AJR Am J Roentgenol. 2008;190(1):32–9.
93. Kelsey CE, Torok KS. The localized scleroderma cutaneous assessment tool: responsiveness to change in a pediatric clinical population. J Am Acad Dermatol. 2013;69(2):214–20.
94. El-Mofty M, Mostafa W, Esmat S, Youssef R, Bousseila M, Nagi N, et al. Suggested mechanisms of action of UVA phototherapy in morphea: a molecular study. Photodermatol Photoimmunol Photomed. 2004;20(2):93–100.
95. El-Mofty M, Zaher H, Bosseila M, Yousef R, Saad B. Low-dose broad-band UVA in morphea using a new method for evaluation. Photodermatol Photoimmunol Photomed. 2000;16(2):43–9.
96. Kreuter A, Hyun J, Stucker M, Sommer A, Altmeyer P, Gambichler T. A randomized controlled study of low-dose UVA1, medium-dose UVA1, and narrowband UVB phototherapy in the treatment of localized scleroderma. J Am Acad Dermatol. 2006;54(3):440–7.
97. de Rie MA, Enomoto DN, de Vries HJ, Bos JD. Evaluation of medium-dose UVA1 phototherapy in localized scleroderma with the cutometer and fast Fourier transform method. Dermatology. 2003;207(3):298–301.
98. Kerscher M, Meurer M, Sander C, Volkenandt M, Lehmann P, Plewig G, et al. PUVA bath photochemotherapy for localized scleroderma. Evaluation of 17 consecutive patients. Arch Dermatol. 1996;132(11):1280–2.
99. Grundmann-Kollmann M, Behrens S, Gruss C, Gottlober P, Peter RU, Kerscher M. Chronic sclerodermic graft-versus-host disease refractory to immunosuppressive treatment responds to UVA1 phototherapy. J Am Acad Dermatol. 2000;42(1 Pt 1):134–6.
100. Hulshof MM, Bouwes Bavinck JN, Bergman W, Masclee AA, Heickendorff L, Breedveld FC, et al. Double-blind, placebo-controlled study of oral calcitriol for the treatment of localized and systemic scleroderma. J Am Acad Dermatol. 2000;43(6):1017–23.
101. Uziel Y, Feldman BM, Krafchik BR, Yeung RS, Laxer RM. Methotrexate and corticosteroid therapy for pediatric localized scleroderma. J Pediatr. 2000;136(1):91–5.
102. Seyger MM, van den Hoogen FH, de Boo T, de Jong EM. Low-dose methotrexate in the treatment of widespread morphea. J Am Acad Dermatol. 1998;39(2 Pt 1):220–5.
103. Kreuter A, Gambichler T, Breuckmann F, Rotterdam S, Freitag M, Stuecker M, et al. Pulsed high-dose corticosteroids combined with low-dose methotrexate in severe localized scleroderma. Arch Dermatol. 2005;141(7):847–52.
104. Mancuso G, Berdondini RM. Localized scleroderma: response to occlusive treatment with tacrolimus ointment. J Am Acad Dermatol. 2005;152(1):180–2.
105. Schlaak M, Friedlein H, Kauer F, Renner R, Rogalski C, Simon JC. Successful therapy of a patient with therapy recalcitrant generalized bullous scleroderma by extracorporeal photopheresis and mycophenolate mofetil. J Eur Acad Dermatol Venereol. 2008;22(5):631–3.
106. Martini G, Ramanan AV, Falcini F, Girschick H, Goldsmith DP, Zulian F. Successful treatment of severe or methotrexate-resistant juvenile localized scleroderma with mycophenolate mofetil. Rheumatology. 2009;48(11):1410–3.
107. Mohrenschlager M, Jung C, Ring J, Abeck D. Effect of penicillin G on corium thickness in linear morphea of childhood: an analysis using ultrasound technique. Pediatr Dermatol. 1999;16(4):314–6.
108. Maragh SH, Davis MD, Bruce AJ, Nelson AM. Disabling pansclerotic morphea: clinical presentation in two adults. J Am Acad Dermatol. 2005;53(2 Suppl 1):S115–9.
109. Hunzelmann N, Anders S, Fierlbeck G, Hein R, Herrmann K, Albrecht M, et al. Double-blind, placebo-controlled study of intralesional interferon gamma for the treatment of localized scleroderma. J Am Acad Dermatol. 1997;36(3 Pt 1):433–5.
110. Laxer R, Zulian F. Localized scleroderma. Curr Opin Rheumatol. 2006;18:606–3.
111. Saxton-Daniels S, Jacobe H. Morphea. In: Goldsmith L et al., editors. Fitzpatrick's dermatology in general medicine. 8th ed. Chicago: McGraw-Hill; 2012.

Scleroderma Mimics

9

Laura K. Hummers and Alan Tyndall

Differential Diagnosis of Raynaud Phenomenon

Cold sensitivity, color changes, and ischemic injury of the digits are cardinal features of scleroderma but may also be a presenting feature of other systemic, toxic, or infectious etiologies. When a patient presents with features typical of Raynaud phenomenon with or without ischemic digital lesions, one needs to consider the broad differential of potential etiologies that includes other rheumatic diseases, structural vessel abnormalities, embolic phenomena, or cold-precipitating circulating proteins.

Primary Raynaud phenomenon is common in the general population and presents without signs of structural vessel abnormalities or ischemic damage to tissues [2–5]. Primary Raynaud phenomenon typically begins in those younger than 30 and is more common in women (female/male ratio approximately 4:1). Primary Raynaud phenomenon is characterized by symmetric, episodic, cold-induced color changes in the fingers and/or toes and a normal physical examination and no signs of tissue damage such as ulceration of the skin or digital pitting. Blood vessel structure is normal as evidenced by nailfold capillaries that are thin, hairpin-like parallel vessels evenly distributed across the nailfold. Patients with primary Raynaud phenomenon should have normal lab values, no evidence of autoimmunity (antinuclear antibody (ANA) negative), and normal inflammatory markers. Treating physicians must determine whether the presence of Raynaud phenomenon is an early symptom of a secondary illness or is due to other causes such as medications, anatomic vessel changes, or other inflammatory conditions such as vasculitis (Table 9.1). There are several key points in the history and physical examination that should help clarify etiology. A history should explore vasoactive medications, toxins, trauma, or other associated medical issues that may point to a secondary cause. Physical examination should focus on several key findings including distal and proximal pulses, including provocative maneuvers for possible thoracic outlet syndrome (Adson's test), nailfold capillary examination, presence and location of ischemic injury, and other evidence of a systemic disease (rashes, synovitis, muscle weakness). Key history and exam features of some more common etiologies of Raynaud-like diseases are included in Table 9.1. Large prospective studies have demonstrated that abnormal nailfold capillaries or the presence of autoantibodies are each associated with a significant risk of future development of definite scleroderma and may be appropriately classified as early scleroderma when both nailfold capillaroscopy (NFC) abnormalities and scleroderma-specific autoantibodies are present [6]. However, the 2013 ACR/EULAR classification of systemic sclerosis would require one additional feature to support the diagnosis [1]. Alternatively, those patients with Raynaud alone and normal nailfold capillaries and negative serologies (including ANA) will only rarely progress to definite scleroderma [6]. While the majority of the 12 % of those patients with Raynaud phenomenon who went on to develop secondary disease do develop scleroderma, other connective tissue diseases may share Raynaud as a common feature. These would include particularly systemic lupus erythematosus (prevalence of 20 %, including infrequent cases of digital gangrene) [7], dermatomyositis (prevalence as high as 65 % in some subsets) [8], and mixed connective tissue disease (85 % prevalence, often with scleroderma-like nailfold capillary patterns), so a careful review of associated symptoms and appropriate serologic evaluation is warranted for patients exhibiting features of these diseases.

Other potential causes of Raynaud-like phenomenon include mechanical obstruction (thoracic outlet syndrome), neurovascular compression (carpal tunnel syndrome), and cold-precipitating agglutination processes (cold agglutinins, cryoglobulins). In addition, other circulating proteins may cause small vessel

L.K. Hummers, MD, ScM (✉)
Department of Medicine and Rheumatology, Johns Hopkins University, Baltimore, MD, USA
e-mail: lhummers@jhmi.edu

A. Tyndall, MBBS, FRACP, FRCP(Ed)
Department of Rheumatology, University Hospital Basel, Basel, Switzerland

J. Varga et al. (eds.), *Scleroderma*, DOI 10.1007/978-3-319-31407-5_9

Table 9.1 Differential diagnosis of Raynaud phenomenon

		History/physical examination	Laboratory findings
Small artery disease	Systemic lupus erythematosus	Arthritis, rash	+ANA, +Sm, +dsDNA, +RNP
	Dermatomyositis	Rash, muscle weakness	+Jo-1, +anti-synthetase antibodies
	Antiphospholipid antibody syndrome	Arterial/venous clots; splinter hemorrhage	Elevated PTT or RVTT; anticardiolipin or B2 glycoprotein-1 antibodies
	Small vessel vasculitis	Sinusitis, pulmonary hemorrhage, petechiae	ANCA, low C3/C4, HCV antibodies
	Cryoglobulinemia	Petechiae, distal ischemia	+ Cryoglobulins, C4, HCV antibodies
	Cryofibrinogenemia	Distal punctate lesions on toes	+ Cryofibrinogens
	Cold agglutinin disease	Recent infection; livedo reticularis	Anemia; (MGUS)
	Polycythemia	Pruritus; erythromelalgia; clots	Elevated WBC, RBC, platelets
	Thromboangiitis obliterans	Tobacco exposure; distal ischemia	None
Structural vasculopathy	Thoracic outlet syndrome	Positional symptoms; + Adson test	None
	Carpal tunnel syndrome	Positional symptoms; + Tinel test	None
	Atherosclerosis	Diminished distal pulses; claudication	Elevated lipids
Abnormal vasomotion	Primary Raynaud phenomenon	Normal nailfold capillaries; no ulcers	None
	Acrocyanosis	Painless persistent color changes	None
Medications/toxins	Sympathomimetics	Exposure to offending medication	None
	Polyvinyl chloride	Distal ischemia	None
	Nicotine	Tobacco exposure	None
	Cocaine	Exposure	+ Urinary toxin screening

occlusion such as antiphospholipid antibodies, paraproteinemias (IgM typically), and cryofibrinogenemia. Medications, particularly sympathomimetics, may induce Raynaud-like vasospasm and certain chemotherapeutic agents or toxins which may induce direct vascular injury (bleomycin, polyvinyl chloride, nicotine, levamisole) [9, 10]. Other forms of vascular damage may also lead to clinical syndromes including digital ischemia that may mimic Raynaud phenomenon (cutaneous polyarteritis nodosa, thromboangiitis obliterans, cryoglobulinemic vasculitis). These vasculitic syndromes often will be accompanied by tissue ischemia that is profound and threaten major distal tissue loss.

Differential Diagnosis of Skin Thickening

Scleroderma-like disorders often show features that are quite similar to systemic sclerosis, but the diagnostic evaluation, risk for internal organ complications, and treatment options are distinct, and a careful diagnostic evaluation is warranted when the diagnosis is unclear. A delay in diagnosis can impede access to potentially effective therapy or avoid toxic therapies that may not be needed. Several key clinical features early in presentation help distinguish these diseases and can prompt expedient screening for associated complications and facilitate treatment and appropriate referral to a specialty center.

Several diseases can present with thickening of the skin and mimic diffuse scleroderma. Such diseases include scleromyxedema, nephrogenic fibrosing dermopathy (NFD) or nephrogenic systemic fibrosis (NSF), eosinophilic fasciitis (EF), scleredema, toxic exposure-induced syndromes (eosinophilia-myalgia syndrome (EMS) and toxic oil syndrome (TOS)), and generalized subsets of localized scleroderma. These syndromes can be differentiated from systemic sclerosis by the pattern of distribution of skin changes, the texture and quality of the skin changes, and the presence and type of associated systemic manifestations, including Raynaud phenomenon and lab abnormalities (Table 9.2). These disorders have very diverse etiologies and often an unclear pathogenic mechanism. Distinct clinical characteristics, skin histology, and systemic and laboratory associations distinguish these conditions from scleroderma and from each other. A prompt diagnosis is important to spare the patients from ineffective treatments, to facilitate appropriate diagnostic

Table 9.2 Differentiating features of scleroderma-like disorders and scleroderma

Disorder	Distribution of the tight skin	Quality of the skin	Systemic features/associated conditions	Laboratory abnormalities	Raynaud phenomenon/nailfold capillaries
Eosinophilic fasciitis	Extremities and trunk; hands and feet spared	Woody induration deeper than superficial dermis	Can overlap with plaque morphea ; hematologic conditions; preceding intense exercise or trauma	Peripheral eosinophilia	Uncommon/normal
Nephrogenic fibrosing dermopathy	Extremities and trunk; face spared	Nodular, indurated plaques with brawny hyperpigmentation	Marked flexion contractures; renal failure and/or insufficiency; exposure to gadolinium	Renal failure/insufficiency (may be transient)	Rare/normal
Pansclerotic morphea	Extremities, the face, feet; hands spared	Thick induration similar to that of diffuse scleroderma; plaques	Contractures; no systemic features of scleroderma	None	Uncommon/normal
Scleredema	The neck, back and proximal arms, face	Doughy induration	Discomfort in areas of involvement Poorly controlled diabetes Recent streptococcal infection Monoclonal gammopathy (MGUS)	Hyperglycemia; MGUS	None
Scleroderma	Hands and face common; diffuse subset involves proximal extremities and trunk; mid-back spared	Thick, smooth, shiny induration	Gastroesophageal reflux; dysphagia; interstitial lung disease; pulmonary hypertension	Positive antinuclear antibody; scleroderma specific autoantibodies	Universal/Common
Scleromyxedema	Scleroderma distribution with prominent findings around the glabella, ears, and posterior neck	Cobblestone induration with 2–3 mm waxy papules	Dysphagia; musculoskeletal pain; neurologic involvement (seizures, coma)	MGUS	Uncommon/normal

evaluations, and to allow for accurate determination of prognosis.

There is a long list of disorders which may mimic scleroderma by having cutaneous fibrosis or mucin deposition and includes other immune-mediated diseases (eosinophilic fasciitis, graft-versus-host disease), deposition disorders (scleromyxedema, scleredema, nephrogenic systemic fibrosis, systemic amyloidosis), and toxic exposures including occupational and iatrogenic (aniline-denatured rapeseed oil, L-tryptophan, polyvinyl chloride, bleomycin, carbidopa) and genetic syndromes (progeroid disorders, stiff skin syndrome). A carefully performed clinical history and physical examination may distinguish these conditions from scleroderma and from each other. The distribution and the quality of skin involvement, the presence of Raynaud or abnormal nailfold capillary microscopy, and the association with particular concurrent diseases or specific laboratory parameters can be of substantial help in refining the diagnosis. In some cases a full-thickness skin biopsy is helpful to confirm the clinical suspicion. Effective therapies are available for some of these conditions, whereas others are more refractory. For this reason, a prompt diagnosis is important to guide treatment decisions wisely. We will discuss some of the conditions most often confused with scleroderma either by the nature of the skin involvement or the presence of systemic features which may also mimic scleroderma. We will not include some other conditions that resemble scleroderma, but where the diagnosis is clear based on other clinical features, such as graft-versus-host disease (in those posttransplant) or genetic conditions (progeroid syndromes which occur in the very young often with other complications).

Toxin-Associated Scleroderma-Like Disorders

We will only briefly review some scleroderma-like diseases that are mostly of historical interest (i.e., toxic oil syndrome, eosinophilia-myalgia syndrome). These conditions are a paradigm from which may arise suspicion for possible future similar outbreaks. There are infrequent instances where an exposure to agents such as aerosolized silica dust (as in coal miners and sandblasters) causes a syndrome indistinguishable from systemic sclerosis [11]. However, other clusters of a scleroderma-like diseases occurred in outbreaks that were linked to a specific toxic exposure. The two classic examples of this type of event are the epidemic of eosinophilia-myalgia syndrome associated with contaminated L-tryptophan supplements and toxic oil syndrome from tainted rapeseed oil in Spain in 1981. Eosinophilia-myalgia syndrome (EMS) was identified in 1989 and determined to be related to a single impurity by a single manufacturer of L-tryptophan, which was marketed as a sleep aid [12]. The syndrome consists of peripheral eosinophilia with prominent myalgias with induration of the skin in the upper and lower extremities. The skin involvement is distinct from scleroderma which spares the hands and feet, and the induration of the skin is deeper with a "woody" quality (similar to eosinophilic fasciitis). The muscles (myalgia and myoclonus) and peripheral nerves (axonal polyneuropathy) may be involved [13]. Toxic oil syndrome (TOS) was another acute epidemic which occurred in Spain in 1981 related to an adulterated rapeseed oil which had been denatured with aniline. The acute syndrome was manifested by interstitial pulmonary infiltrates and pleural effusions, myalgias, and peripheral eosinophilia. Associated features included skin itching and rash, peripheral sensory neuropathy, dysphagia, and pulmonary hypertension. Later manifestations included progressive fibrosing disease of the skin and lung [13, 14]. When the skin was involved, it seemed to have a clear progression from a more toxic-allergic presentation with distinct urticarial lesions to edema to fibrosis [15]. While we are unlikely to see new patients with these syndromes, there may be other similar outbreaks in the future related to yet-to-be-defined toxins, so having an appropriate level of awareness of these prior experiences is important.

Nephrogenic Systemic Fibrosis

A more recent exposure-associated scleroderma mimicker is nephrogenic fibrosing dermopathy (NFD) or nephrogenic systemic fibrosis (NSF) which was first reported in 2000 [16]. A new entity was initially described among patients receiving renal dialysis and ultimately linked to the use of high doses of linear-chelated gadolinium-based contrast agents (GBCA) for MRI studies among those with stage IV and V chronic kidney disease, although some patients are unaware of gadolinium exposure [17]. The connection with exposure to gadolinium-based contrast agents (GBCA) was recognized around 2006, and peak incidence of new cases occurred in 2005 and markedly dropped after 2007 and almost entirely eradicated by 2010 [18]. In the United States, an NSF registry has been established with more than 380 cases collected to date (http://www.icnsfr.org).

The illness is characterized by rapid development of fibrotic skin induration with associated nodular plaques, hyperpigmentation of the skin, and marked flexion contractures of the extremities. The skin lesions of NSF usually develop subacutely shortly after gadolinium exposure and subsequently assume a progressive course, rapidly developing joint contractures. The distribution is often symmetrical, commonly involving the extremities up to the knees and elbows. The hands and the trunk may be involved but typically spares the face. The texture of the skin is different than scleroderma in that the skin has a lumpy-nodular thickening with a tendency to form indurated irregular plaques with reticular discoloration varying from violaceous to brawny hyperpigmentation. A deeper subcutaneous fibrotic process leads to severe flexion contractures (particularly hands, wrists, ankles, and knees) which cause significant disability. Nerve conduction studies seem to confirm the presence of a true peripheral neuropathy, further complicating the management of the underlying pain syndrome, which is usually very difficult to control. NSF may be further distinguished from scleroderma by the absence of Raynaud phenomenon or nailfold capillary abnormalities. In addition antinuclear antibodies and scleroderma-specific autoantibodies are normal. Treatment has been largely unsatisfactory, although case reports highlight possible benefit with tyrosine kinase inhibitors (imatinib), thalidomide, phototherapy, and plasmapheresis.

Scleredema

Scleredema is a condition associated with deposition of collagen and mucin in the dermis and occurs in three specific conditions: (1) poorly controlled diabetes, (2) monoclonal gammopathies, and (3) postinfectious, particularly streptococcal pharyngitis. In a large case series of 44 patients, 30 were related to diabetes, 5 were related to monoclonal gammopathies, and the others were unclear [19]. Scleredema of any etiology causes scleroderma-like skin changes but in a distribution distinct from systemic sclerosis. It has been estimated that as many as 1–14 % of diabetics have scleredema in some cross-sectional studies, so it is thought that this subset may be underreported [20, 21]. Diabetic patients with scleredema are commonly poorly controlled and insulin requiring and have evidence of diabetic complications, specifically microangiopathy and retinopathy. There is an association with elevated hemoglobin A1C and the presence of scleredema [21]. The pathology of scleredema is notable for marked thickening of the upper and lower dermis, mucin deposition between thickened collagen bundles. Scleredema causes a non-pitting, doughy induration of the skin that characteristically involves the neck, back, interscapular region, face, and chest. Typically the fingers and feet are spared and, in contrast with scleroderma, the mid back is almost always involved (Fig. 9.1). Involvement of the face can cause ocular muscle palsy, diminished oral aperture, and periorbital edema. Systemic involvement has been only infrequently reported, but some case reports highlight involvement of the tongue, pharynx, and upper esophagus leading to dysphagia as a potentially reported systemic symptom [22]. Patients with infection-related disease are noted to have a rapid onset of symptoms days to months after the infection (often termed scleredema fulminans) with a course that typically resolves in several months to 2 years. Patients with diabetes and (MGUS)-associated scleredema have a very insidious onset with gradual progression of symptoms over many years. Treatment may be symptomatic only (with physical therapy), particularly in those with an expected self-limited course (postinfectious) [19]. Treatments for diabetes and monoclonal protein-associated scleredema include phototherapy, corticosteroids, bortezomib, and intravenous immunoglobulin (IVIG) (paraprotein-associated) [19, 23, 24].

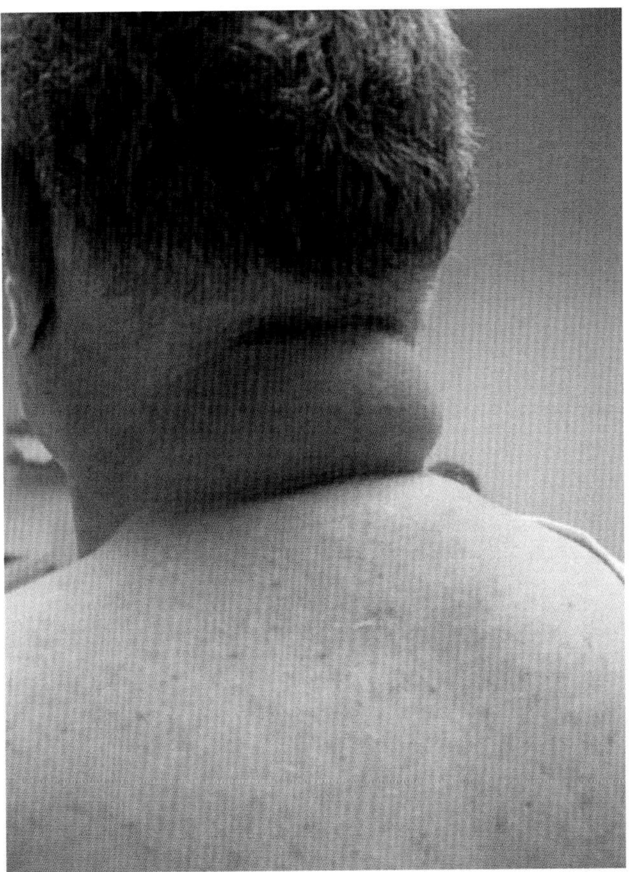

Fig. 9.1 Posterior neck in a patient with (MGUS)-associated scleredema

Scleromyxedema

Scleromyxedema (papular mucinosis) is a condition of mucinous deposition in the skin associated with a presence of a (MGUS) characterized by a diffuse, papular skin eruption. The average age of onset is around 50–55 years with a roughly equal gender distribution but has not been reported in children. Diagnosis requires the presence of a characteristic skin involvement, diagnostic biopsy (extensive interstitial mucin, thickened collagen bundles, and increased number of spindled fibroblast-like cells), and the presence of a monoclonal protein (typically IgG either kappa or lambda). More limited skin forms with restricted distribution may not be associated with monoclonal gammopathies. The skin in scleromyxedema is indurated and papular in quality with a cobblestone feel, and its involvement occurs in a characteristic distribution with the glabellum, posterior auricular area and neck being most commonly affected (Fig. 9.2). Other areas include the back and extremities but may be similar in distribution to scleroderma. Similar to scleredema, the mid-portion of the back is commonly affected in scleromyxedema and is almost never involved in scleroderma patients. Sclerodactyly is often present and appear identical to scleroderma, although it is papular in quality. In addition to skin findings, patients may have organ involvement that seems to mimic the pattern of scleroderma. Raynaud phenomenon, esophageal dysmotility, and myopathy have been reported [25, 26]. Less common but potentially life-threatening complications may involve the neurological system in the form of encephalopathy, seizures, coma, and psychosis [27, 28]. The natural history of this disease has not been well defined, but fatal cases have been reported, most commonly due to neurologic complications [29]. The most commonly reported treatment associated with benefit has been intravenous immunoglobulin (IVIG). Other treatments reported to be of benefit in some have included thalidomide, autologous hematopoetic stem cell transplant, and corticosteroids [30].

Eosinophilic Fasciitis

Eosinophilic fasciitis was first described in 1974 by Schulman who reported two patients with scleroderma-like skin changes, painful induration of subcutaneous tissues with marked peripheral eosinophilia, and histological evidence of a diffuse fasciitis [31]. EF has a slight male predominance and has been reported more in Caucasians than other groups with cases occurring across the age spectrum. Dominant laboratory features include peripheral blood and tissue eosinophilia, hypergammaglobulinemia, and elevated inflammatory markers [32]. The classic histopathologic changes in EF are dermal-hypodermic sclerosis associated with fibrotic thickening of the subcutaneous adipose lobular septa, superficial fascia, and perimysium, and there is no mucin. The epidermis is usually spared. Eosinophils can be enriched within affected tissues but are not likely to be present when biopsies are obtained after institution of corticosteroid therapy. Given the similar appearance of EF to the toxin-associated epidemic syndromes (TOS and EMS), exposure histories have been examined for EF. The only clear historical association has been with an antecedent history of vigorous exercise or trauma which is found in about half of the described cases [32]. In older series, there had been evidence of *Borrelia burgdorferi* infection, but this has not been replicated more recently [33]. There are reported associations between EF and immune-mediated cytopenias and localized forms of scleroderma (morphea profunda) [32]. The onset and distribution of EF is very similar to NSF which is usually subacute symmetric thickening predominantly over the distal extremities within a short period of time (typically weeks). The trunk or neck can be involved but typically spares the hands and face. Early on, the skin is edematous with a "peau de orange" appearance (Fig. 9.3). This is followed by a progressive "woody" induration of subcutaneous tissues leading to skin puckering and the "venous groove sign." Importantly, the superficial dermis is usually spared allowing an examiner to be able to pinch the skin, which may be a helpful distinguishing feature from scleroderma and other scleroderma-like disorders. Deeper involvement and fibrosis of periarticular structures can cause flexion contractures as well as disturbances secondary to peripheral nerve compression, such as carpal tunnel syndrome. Raynaud phenomenon is infrequently present, but the nailfold capillary microscopy examination is normal and systemic

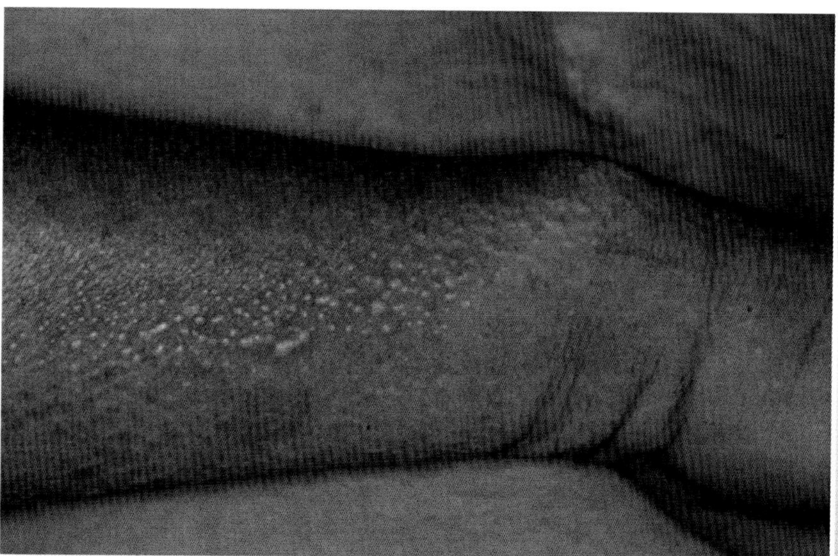
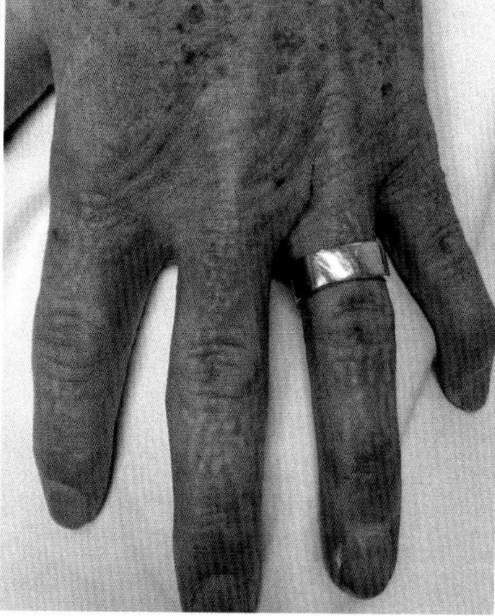

Fig. 9.2 The posterior forearm and hand in two patients with scleromyxedema

features are absent except in cases where the extensive fibrosis around the chest or neck may lead to chest wall restriction or dysphagia. Common laboratory features include peripheral eosinophilia, hypergammaglobulinemia, and elevated inflammatory markers but have low specificity to this condition compared with scleroderma and other scleroderma-like disorders. Monoclonal gammopathies and autoantibodies are typically absent however. The standard treatment for EF is corticosteroids, which are often intentionally avoided in scleroderma, making this diagnostic distinction particularly important. Pulse doses of steroids may be particularly beneficial and associated with higher rates of complete remission [34]. Refractory cases may be treated with methotrexate, mycophenolate mofetil of d-penicillamine [35]. In addition, the natural history is typically of remission with excellent prognosis. MRI (showing hyperintensity of the fascia on fluid sensitive and contrasted sequences) may be helpful in establishing the diagnosis and may help monitor disease activity and treatment response. Ultrasonography may also be useful and aldolase may be a possible biomarker [36, 37].

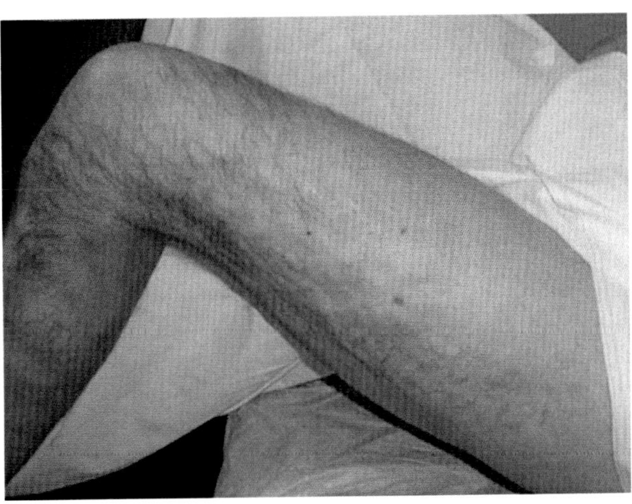

Fig. 9.3 The upper arm of a patient with eosinophilic fasciitis with "peau de orange" appearance and venous groove sign

Localized Scleroderma

Most forms of localized scleroderma are more prevalent in children and quite distinct in appearance from systemic disease. These include plaque morphea and linear (en coup de sabre) variants of localized scleroderma. However, some forms, such as generalized morphea and pansclerotic morphea, may be difficult to distinguish from diffuse cutaneous systemic sclerosis and require special mention. Generalized morphea refers to multiple patches of scleroderma skin involvement that evolves in discrete lesions. The lesions are typically circular with a violaceous or erythematosus border (when active) then often develop a white, fibrotic center. Some patients have extensive involvement of the skin which typically involves the trunk (back > chest) and may linearly extend down one or more extremities (linear morphea) but spares the fingers in all of these cases. Pansclerotic morphea (also known as disabling pansclerotic morphea of childhood) typically spreads homogeneously over large areas of the skin typically involving the whole trunk and proximal extremities almost always sparing of hands, fingers, and distal forearms; however the feet are often deeply and characteristically involved (Fig. 9.4). Histological examination reveals fibrosis that extends through all layers of the dermis and subcutaneous tissues and may extend deeper into muscles and around tendons. Occasionally patients with morphea have antinuclear antibodies but typically do not have scleroderma-specific autoantibodies, Raynaud phenomenon, or abnormal nailfold capillaries [38]. The distribution of skin involvement is differentiated from diffuse cutaneous systemic sclerosis, the typical sparing of the fingers and hands and the plaque-like dis-

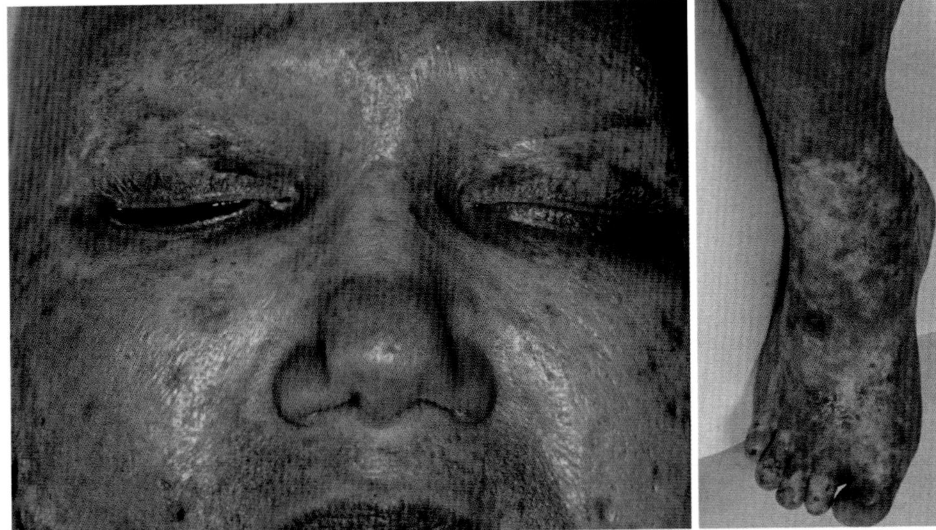

Fig. 9.4 The feet and face of a patient with severe pansclerotic morphea

Table 9.3 Screening algorithms and treatment options for scleroderma and related disorders

	Screening test in all patients	Treatment options
Scleroderma	Pulmonary function tests	Immunosuppression
	Echocardiogram	Vasodilators for Raynaud
	Ambulatory blood pressure monitoring	Acid suppression for gastroesophageal reflux disease (GERD)
		Vasodilators for pulmonary hypertension
Nephrogenic systemic fibrosis	None	Intravenous immunoglobulin
		Tyrosine kinase inhibitors
		Physical therapy
Eosinophilic fasciitis	Complete blood counts	Prednisone
Scleromyxedema	Serum protein electrophoresis with immunofixation	Intravenous immunoglobulin
		Thalidomide
Scleredema	Serum protein electrophoresis with immunofixation	UV light-based therapy
	Fasting blood glucose; hemoglobin A1C	Strict diabetes control
Pansclerotic morphea	ANA and scleroderma-specific antibodies	Immunosuppression (methotrexate, MMF)
		UV light-based therapy

tribution of skin lesions. This condition may or may not involve the back so the lack of back involvement may not be helpful in distinguishing it from systemic sclerosis as it is with scleredema, scleromyxedema, and generalized morphea. The most commonly utilized treatment modalities include phototherapy and methotrexate and other systemic immunosuppressants in more severe forms such as pansclerotic morphea where topical and UV-based therapy are unlikely to be effective.

Treatment Differences

There is no clinical trial data to guide therapy in any of the scleroderma mimics and very little in systemic sclerosis. These conditions are rare but need to be included in the differential when evaluating a patient with suspected scleroderma, so an internal organ disease screening may be performed, appropriate treatments may be suggested, and a more clear prognosis may be given. The therapeutic choices for someone with a "skin-only" disease may be markedly different than ones with potential for severe systemic involvement (scleroderma, scleromyxedema). Some conditions, such as infection-associated scleredema, eosinophilic fasciitis, and plaque morphea may be self-limited conditions that require short term or even no treatment, whereas others may require prolonged courses of immunosuppression and chronic management of complications (scleroderma, scleromyxedema, NFS). Table 9.3 includes common therapies and internal organ complication-screening strategies for each of the conditions discussed in this chapter.

References

1. van den Hoogen F, Khanna D, Fransen J, et al. 2013 classification criteria for systemic sclerosis: an American college of rheumatology/European league against rheumatism collaborative initiative. Ann Rheum Dis. 2013;72(11):1747–55.
2. Gelber AC, Wigley FM, Stallings RY, et al. Symptoms of Raynaud's phenomenon in an inner-city African-American community: prevalence and self-reported cardiovascular comorbidity. J Clin Epidemiol. 1999;52(5):441–6.
3. Jones GT, Herrick AL, Woodham SE, et al. Occurrence of Raynaud's phenomenon in children ages 12–15 years: prevalence and association with other common symptoms. Arthritis Rheum. 2003;48(12):3518–21.
4. Voulgari PV, Alamanos Y, Papazisi D, et al. Prevalence of Raynaud's phenomenon in a healthy Greek population. Ann Rheum Dis. 2000;59(3):206–10.
5. Maricq HR, Carpentier PH, Weinrich MC, et al. Geographic variation in the prevalence of Raynaud's phenomenon: a 5 region comparison. J Rheumatol. 1997;24(5):879–89.
6. Koenig M, Joyal F, Fritzler MJ, et al. Autoantibodies and microvascular damage are independent predictive factors for the progression of Raynaud's phenomenon to systemic sclerosis: a twenty-year prospective study of 586 patients, with validation of proposed criteria for early systemic sclerosis. Arthritis Rheum. 2008;58(12):3902–12. Epub 2008/11/28. eng.
7. Liu A, Zhang W, Tian X, et al. Prevalence, risk factors and outcome of digital gangrene in 2684 lupus patients. Lupus. 2009;18(12):1112–8. Epub 2009/09/19. eng.
8. Kalluri M, Sahn SA, Oddis CV, et al. Clinical profile of anti-PL-12 autoantibody. Cohort study and review of the literature. Chest. 2009;135(6):1550–6. Epub 2009/02/20. eng.
9. Glendenning JL, Barbachano Y, Norman AR, et al. Long-term neurologic and peripheral vascular toxicity after chemotherapy treatment of testicular cancer. Cancer. 2010;116(10):2322–31. Epub 2010/03/13. eng.
10. Maricq HR, Johnson MN, Whetstone CL, et al. Capillary abnormalities in polyvinyl chloride production workers. Examination by in vivo microscopy. JAMA. 1976;236(12):1368–71.
11. Rustin MH, Bull HA, Ziegler V, et al. Silica-associated systemic sclerosis is clinically, serologically and immunologically indistinguishable from idiopathic systemic sclerosis. Br J Dermatol. 1990;123(6):725–34.
12. Belongia EA, Hedberg CW, Gleich GJ, et al. An investigation of the cause of the eosinophilia-myalgia syndrome associated with tryptophan use. N Engl J Med. 1990;323(6):357–65. Epub 1990/08/09. eng.
13. Kaufman LD, Krupp LB. Eosinophilia-myalgia syndrome, toxic-oil syndrome, and diffuse fasciitis with eosinophilia. Curr Opin Rheumatol. 1995;7(6):560–7. Epub 1995/11/01. eng.
14. Kilbourne EM, Posada de la Paz M, Abaitua Borda I, et al. Toxic oil syndrome: a current clinical and epidemiologic summary, including

comparisons with the eosinophilia-myalgia syndrome. J Am Coll Cardiol. 1991;18(3):711–7. Epub 1991/09/01. eng.
15. Fonseca E, Contreras F. Cutaneous mucinosis in the toxic oil syndrome. J Am Acad Dermatol. 1987;16(1 Pt 1):139–40. Epub 1987/01/01. eng.
16. Cowper SE, Robin HS, Steinberg SM, et al. Scleromyxoedema-like cutaneous diseases in renal-dialysis patients. Lancet. 2000;356(9234):1000–1.
17. Bennett CL, Qureshi ZP, Sartor AO, et al. Gadolinium-induced nephrogenic systemic fibrosis: the rise and fall of an iatrogenic disease. Clin Kidney J. 2012;5(1):82–8. Pubmed Central PMCID: 3341839.
18. Bennett CL, Starko KM, Thomsen HS, et al. Linking drugs to obscure illnesses: lessons from pure red cell aplasia, nephrogenic systemic fibrosis, and Reye's syndrome. a report from the Southern Network on Adverse Reactions (SONAR). J Gen Intern Med. 2012;27(12):1697–703. Pubmed Central PMCID: 3509314.
19. Rongioletti F, Kaiser F, Cinotti E, et al. Scleredema. A multicentre study of characteristics, comorbidities, course and therapy in 44 patients. J Eur Acad Dermatol Venereol. 2015;29(12):2399–404.
20. Cole GW, Headley J, Skowsky R. Scleredema diabeticorum: a common and distinct cutaneous manifestation of diabetes mellitus. Diabetes Care. 1983;6(2):189–92. Epub 1983/03/01. eng.
21. Ghosh K, Das K, Ghosh S, et al. Prevalence of skin changes in diabetes mellitus and its correlation with internal diseases: a single center observational study. Indian J Dermatol. 2015;60(5):465–9. Pubmed Central PMCID: 4601413.
22. Wright RA, Bernie H. Scleredema adultorum of Buschke with upper esophageal involvement. Am J Gastroenterol. 1982;77(1):9–11. Epub 1982/01/01. eng.
23. Eastham AB, Femia AN, Velez NF, et al. Paraproteinemia-associated scleredema treated successfully with intravenous immunoglobulin. JAMA Dermatol. 2014;150(7):788–9.
24. Szturz P, Adam Z, Vasku V, et al. Complete remission of multiple myeloma associated scleredema after bortezomib-based treatment. Leuk Lymphoma. 2013;54(6):1324–6.
25. Dinneen AM, Dicken CH. Scleromyxedema. J Am Acad Dermatol. 1995;33(1):37–43.
26. Blum M, Wigley FM, Hummers LK. Scleromyxedema: a case series highlighting long-term outcomes of treatment with intravenous immunoglobulin (IVIG). Medicine (Baltimore). 2008;87(1):10–20.
27. Berger JR, Dobbs MR, Terhune MH, et al. The neurologic complications of scleromyxedema. Medicine (Baltimore). 2001;80(5):313–9.
28. Webster GF, Matsuoka LY, Burchmore D. The association of potentially lethal neurologic syndromes with scleromyxedema (papular mucinosis). J Am Acad Dermatol. 1993;28(1):105–8.
29. Godby A, Bergstresser PR, Chaker B, et al. Fatal scleromyxedema: report of a case and review of the literature. J Am Acad Dermatol. 1998;38(2 Pt 2):289–94.
30. Rongioletti F, Merlo G, Cinotti E, et al. Scleromyxedema: a multicenter study of characteristics, comorbidities, course, and therapy in 30 patients. J Am Acad Dermatol. 2013;69(1):66–72.
31. Shulman LE. Diffuse fasciitis with eosinophilia: a new syndrome? Trans Assoc Am Physicians. 1975;88:70–86. Epub 1975/01/01. eng.
32. Lakhanpal S, Ginsburg WW, Michet CJ, et al. Eosinophilic fasciitis: clinical spectrum and therapeutic response in 52 cases. Semin Arthritis Rheum. 1988;17(4):221–31. Epub 1988/05/01. eng.
33. Anton E. Failure to demonstrate Borrelia burgdorferi-specific DNA in lesions of eosinophilic fasciitis. Histopathology. 2006;49(1): 88–90.
34. Lebeaux D, Frances C, Barete S, et al. Eosinophilic fasciitis (Shulman disease): new insights into the therapeutic management from a series of 34 patients. Rheumatology (Oxford). 2012; 51(3):557–61.
35. Mendoza FA, Bai R, Kebede AG, et al. Severe eosinophilic fasciitis: comparison of treatment with d-penicillamine plus corticosteroids vs. corticosteroids alone. Scand J Rheumatol. 2015;3:1–6.
36. Mondal S, Goswami RP, Sinha D, et al. Ultrasound is a useful adjunct in diagnosis of eosinophilic fasciitis. Rheumatology (Oxford). 2015;54(11):2041.
37. Nashel J, Steen V. The use of an elevated aldolase in diagnosing and managing eosinophilic fasciitis. Clin Rheumatol. 2015;34(8):1481–4.
38. Kim A, Marinkovich N, Vasquez R, et al. Clinical features of patients with morphea and the pansclerotic subtype: a cross-sectional study from the morphea in adults and children cohort. J Rheumatol. 2014;41(1):106–12.

Systems Biology Approaches to Understanding the Pathogenesis of Systemic Sclerosis

10

J. Matthew Mahoney, Jaclyn N. Taroni, and Michael L. Whitfield

Introduction

Systemic sclerosis (SSc) is a heterogeneous disease with a widely varying clinical presentation and dynamic underlying molecular signature. SSc has a complex genetic risk, with many identified risk alleles having modest odds ratio for the disease or its various complications (for a recent review, see [1]). The most prominent clinical features of SSc are vascular and immunologic abnormalities, skin fibrosis, and variable internal organ involvement [2]. At the molecular level, there have been numerous studies demonstrating heterogeneity in gene expression in multiple tissues, including the skin [3–5], peripheral blood [6, 7], esophagus [8], and lung [9, 10]. A model of SSc pathogenesis has begun to emerge that suggests that SSc arises as the result of the complex interplay between multiple different cell types in end-target tissues, including resident fibroblasts, innate and adaptive immune cells, and potentially cells from other compartments [11]. These interactions involve the differential expression of thousands of genes in the genome that participate in many overlapping biochemical processes, implicating a broad, genome-wide dysregulation of gene expression in SSc tissues.

Interpreting the molecular data from the collection of published and publicly available SSc data sets is a more difficult and complicated task than one would predict from first inspection. First, biopsies from human patients are cell mixtures (e.g., a punch biopsy of SSc skin contains keratinocytes, fibroblasts, and immune infiltrates). The relative numbers of cells in the mixture determine the relative strength of a cell type-specific signal. Second, gene expression is a fundamentally dynamic process. Independent of measurement noise, the expression of a particular gene is determined through a complex network of interactions. The reliable signals within tissues are not necessarily single gene expression levels but the correlated expression of many genes within a process [12]. Many studies have made use of gene-gene correlations in expression data to infer these important processes. Systems biology augments this approach by considering the interconnectedness of biological processes as a fundamental organizing principle of biology.

Systems biology is a *paradigm* for the interpretation of biological data and the design of experiments that stresses the interactions between the constituent parts of organisms [13]. Biological systems are hierarchies of discrete, semi-autonomous parts; for example, cells make tissues, which make organs, which make organisms. These layers of organization feed back onto each other in complicated ways that preclude a complete understanding of a single part (e.g., a single human cell) from outside of its organismal context. Systems biology is often contrasted with the reductionist biological paradigm that seeks to describe biological systems by characterizing isolated components of systems (e.g., a culture of cancer cells, rather than a tumor in situ). Where a reductionist would describe a biological system by making specific, targeted perturbations, a systems biologist might gather a large collection of cross-sectional data under a variety of disease and normal conditions. Where a reductionist favors hypothesis testing in a clearly defined set of biological conditions and states, a systems biologist leans toward high-throughput observational data. It is important to stress that these points of view and approaches do not conflict. Biological systems function as the *interactions* between their component *parts*. The staggering complexity of biological systems often precludes strong predictions about how an

J.M. Mahoney, PhD
Department of Neurological Sciences, University of Vermont, Burlington, VT, USA

J. N. Taroni, PhD
Department of Genetics, Geisel School of Medicine at Dartmouth, Hanover, NH, USA

M.L. Whitfield, PhD (✉)
Department of Genetics, Geisel School of Medicine at Dartmouth, Hanover, NH, USA

Department of Genetics, Dartmouth Medical School, 7400 Remsen, Hanover, NH 03755, USA
e-mail: michael.whitfield@dartmouth.edu

J. Varga et al. (eds.), *Scleroderma*, DOI 10.1007/978-3-319-31407-5_10

isolated and well-understood biological component (e.g., a cultured dermal fibroblast) will function within an organism, much less a genetically diverse population. Systems biology embraces this complexity and seeks to develop tools to analyze data and generate testable hypotheses about the system as a whole. The development of high-throughput biological assays, modern information technology, and machine learning algorithms have allowed for unprecedented insights into biological systems, and this will only increase with more sophisticated approaches. Our ability to measure and analyze these systems has only recently begun to approach a scale that approximates the complexity of the human biological systems we wish to understand.

Anatomy of a Network

The goal of systems biology in medicine is to rigorously address the issue of molecular heterogeneity by extracting robust signatures of disease from high-throughput data and interpreting those signatures with the aid of bioinformatics databases, which encode information about known *molecular interactions* [14]. Some of the primary objects of study in systems biology are *molecular networks* that encode the relationships between genes, proteins, and other biomolecules.[1] Thus, the problem of interpreting molecular heterogeneity in terms of what genes or proteins are expressed across a set of conditions is transformed into the problem of characterizing the structure of a network.

Conceptually, a *network* is simply a set of objects called *nodes* and a set of connections between nodes called *links*. Thus, a network provides a formal way of encoding relationships. Molecular networks encode relationships between molecules or molecular units like genes. Molecular networks are highly structured and the mathematical theory of networks has developed many concepts and methods that can be used to characterize this network structure. Important among these are modularity, centrality, and bridgeness[2]. These concepts describe the local and global features of the network.

Centrality is a feature of the nodes of a network that describes how well connected a node is within the network. Many centrality measures have been proposed [15], but the most intuitive is the *degree*, which is the total number of connections a node has to other nodes in the network. In molecular networks, high degree nodes participate in many interactions and are thus likely to be important to the biological processes encoded by the network. Nodes with high degree are termed *hubs*. Centrality, however, is a "local" feature of the network. It describes how well connected a node is, but little about whom the connections are with.

Modularity describes the clustering of nodes in a network and is a "global" feature of the network. A modular network has connections that are not random but rather form groups of nodes, *modules* or *clusters*, with a high density of connections within groups and low density between groups. Molecular networks are highly modular; many biological processes require dedicated sets of genes to carry out the process. A variety of algorithms have been proposed to identify clusters within networks [15, 16], but in every case the goal is to identify subnetworks that are approximately decoupled from the rest of the network and can be analyzed as discrete entities in their own right. Clusters often represent distinct molecular processes.

However, clusters are rarely completely decoupled from the rest of the network. The connections between clusters encode the pathways through which modules can interact. Bridgeness is a feature of nodes that describes the extent to which a node sits between modules. Like centrality, bridgeness can be quantified in many ways [17, 18], but all measures have in common that they consider nodes to have high bridgeness if they connect disparate regions of the network, i.e., if they link different clusters. Nodes that connect different modules are called *bridges*. Bridges are likely to be important to the communication between molecular processes and potentially represent molecular bottlenecks between processes that can be targeted therapeutically (c.f. [19]).

The resolution of a network into modules, hubs, and bridges interpolates between the local structure of the network and the global structure; it is the "anatomy" of the network. The network integrates the raw molecular data (determining which genes are important) into a global picture of how a large number of dynamically interacting molecules fit into major processes (modules), the crucial molecules within those processes (hubs), and the connections between those processes (bridges).

Questions About SSc That Can Be Answered with Systems Biology

Systems biology can integrate disparate studies of multiple tissues with different molecular assays (gene expression, proteomic, interaction data) into a coherent global picture of

[1] The nature of the relationships used to build the network determines the appropriate interpretation of the network. For example, a protein-protein interaction network built from protein-binding data should be interpreted differently from a functional interaction network that encodes functional, but not necessarily physical, interactions between molecules.

[2] These concepts can be quantified in a number of different ways resulting in various measures of network properties. This is still a topic of active research in the complex networks community. The mathematical details of these measures are omitted here to allow for discussion of the intuition behind these concepts and to clarify their role in providing biological insight.

pathogenesis, disease progression, and response to therapy. This allows the identification of likely sources of clinical heterogeneity and possible pathways for therapeutic intervention. However, much work remains to be done. Several questions about SSc that are amenable to systems biology study include but are not limited to:

1. How do the molecular and cellular abnormalities observed in patient tissues interact to produce clinical pathophenotypes?
2. What are the functional roles of genetic risk loci in SSc? In particular, how might genetic polymorphisms contribute to clinical heterogeneity and influence the gene expression changes in end-target tissues?
3. Do genetic risk loci interact with each other to modify disease severity or risk?

These questions are fundamentally about the workings of a system because they are about interactions. Some attempts to address these questions have been made. For example, Berreta et al. [20, 21] report that there are interactions between single nucleotide polymorphisms in cytokine genes affecting SSc risk. Similarly, following epigenetic evidence in human tissue, Noda et al. [22] have reported on a synergistic interaction between Friend leukemia integration 1 (*Fli1*) and Krüppel-like factor 5 (*KLF5*) in mice. This is the first mouse model of SSc to simultaneously develop vasculopathy, skin and lung fibrosis, and autoantibodies. The role of genetic interactions and the optimization of mouse models of SSc is a large area to explore (see Future Directions).

Recently, the first systems-level meta-analysis of three SSc skin data sets was published [12]. The goal of this analysis was to address questions 1 and 2 above in SSc skin disease. The primary results of this study were that (1) there are reproducible sets of upregulated genes in the inflammatory and fibroproliferative intrinsic subsets (consensus genes), (2) that these gene sets take part in a complex network that includes most identified SSc risk polymorphisms, and (3) the network structure is likely to be highly relevant to SSc skin disease (Fig. 10.1). The molecular network used in the study was the publicly available integrated multispecies prediction (IMP) network developed by Wong et al. [23], which encodes the probability that a pair of genes is functionally related. The subset of the IMP network corresponding to the consensus genes has distinct clusters related to innate and adaptive immune processes, extracellular matrix processes, and cell proliferation (Fig. 10.1). Hub genes within these clusters include genes with known relationship to SSc (e.g., allograft inflammatory factor 1 (*AIF1*) and fibrillin 1 (*FBN1*)). Also, bridges between modules implicate particular molecular pathways of interaction between various processes; for example, TGF-β bridges process ECM deposition and proliferation (c.f. Fig. 6 in [12]).

In addition, the molecular network allows for inferences about the functional roles of SSc risk polymorphisms. Polymorphic genes either group with one cluster (e.g., *BANK1*, Fig. 10.1) or bridge multiple clusters (e.g., *PLAUR*, Fig. 10.1). Risk alleles in genes that group with a single cluster can be inferred to affect that cluster's processes directly, but the other clusters only indirectly. In contrast, polymorphic genes that bridge multiple clusters are inferred to be pleiotropic, affecting multiple molecular processes and possibly multiple clinical phenotypes simultaneously [24, 25].

Future Directions

Systems biology is a powerful tool for integrating large compendia of biological data. In recent years, many gene expression studies on multiple tissues from patients with SSc have become available. Likewise, proteomic, genetic, and epigenetic data have been collected. Concurrently, the publicly available data for developing updated and more nuanced networks (i.e., tissue-specific and disease-specific) are growing rapidly. In fact, a new, publicly accessible project from the developers of IMP has built networks on tissue- and cell type-specific bases [26]. These networks have demonstrated greater power to detect disease-related genes in multiple complex conditions by systematically incorporating information about gene-gene interactions based on tissue type. Furthermore, these tools have been extended to directly incorporate genetic data, without having to resort to ad hoc procedures as was done in Mahoney et al. [12]. Future work will focus on extracting robust signals from these new SSc data sets and then use the tissue-specific networks to determine the role of the microenvironment and tissue context in determining clinical outcome.

While Mahoney et al. focused on observational gene expression data from SSc skin, the use of molecular networks to analyze data is not limited to this case. Any rigorous procedure that selects a set of genes can be used. An important future application is the analysis of drug trials. High-throughput assays employed to measure molecular changes during drug trials can identify genes that respond to therapy and molecular network analysis can show the processes modified in response to therapy [27, 28]. It is highly likely that response genes will occupy "privileged" positions in the molecular network; for example, they may be hubs within a pro-inflammatory process or are bridges between inflammatory and fibrotic processes. Extracting these network-based signals is perhaps more urgent in SSc than other diseases because typical drug trial sizes are small due to the rarity of cases. The molecular networks could bolster a noisy signal from small trial data by placing them

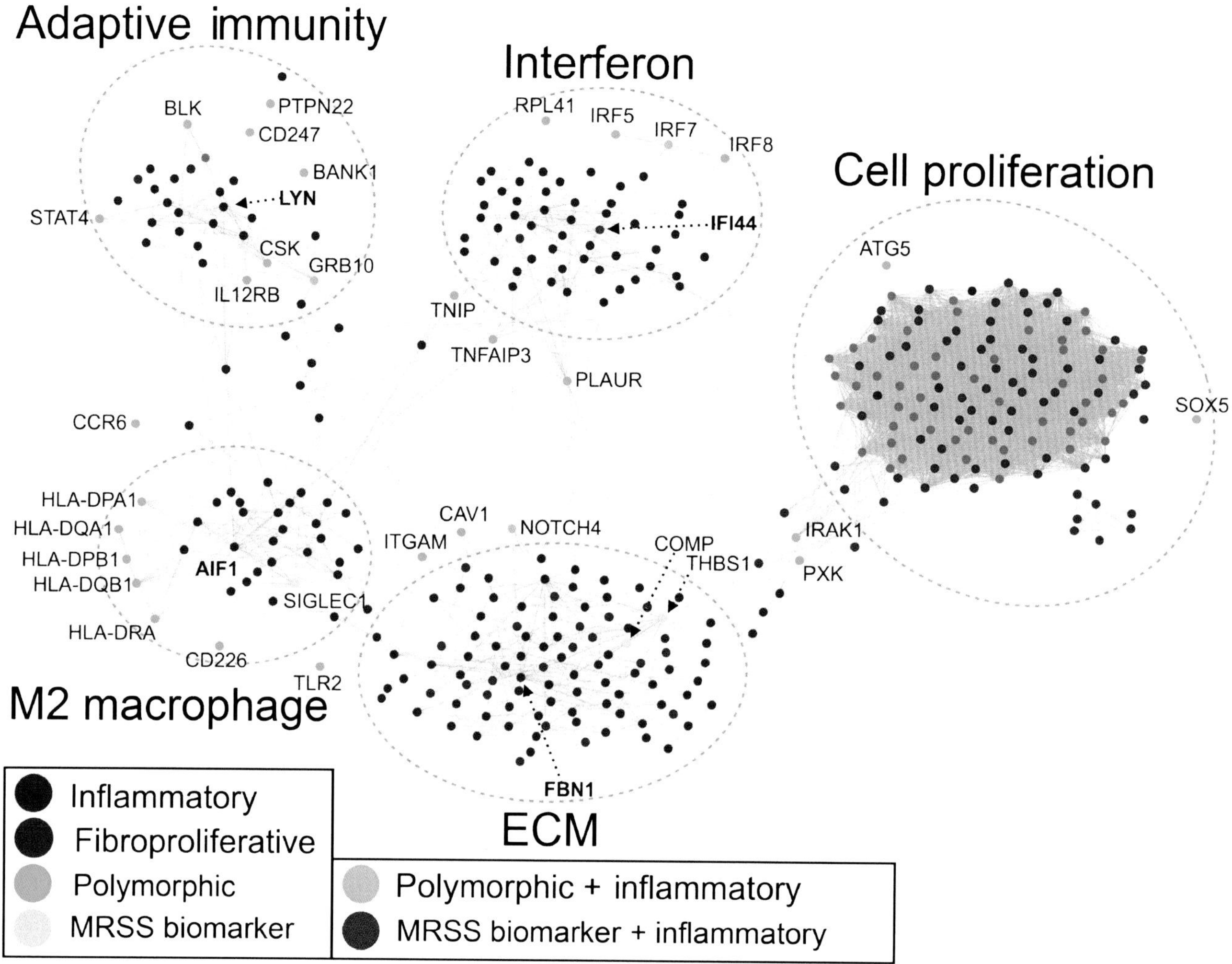

Fig. 10.1 Molecular network of upregulated genes in SSc skin disease. Molecular networks are highly structured. Genes form clusters representing biological processes (e.g., ECM deposition and interferon signaling). Highly connected genes (e.g., *AIF1* and *FBN1*) are called hubs. Genes that straddle multiple clusters (e.g., *PLAUR*) are called bridges. (Reprinted with permission from mahoney et al [15] PLoS Comp Biol)

within the context of other known biology. More ambitiously, by mining molecular networks for these "network privileged" genes, we might be able to extract novel targets for therapeutic intervention and drug repositioning. This strategy is in its early stages but has been successful in some cases [29–32].

SSc research relies heavily on preclinical animal models. There has been a long debate about the appropriate conclusions that can be drawn from the many mouse models of SSc. While many models capture important phenotypes, all have limitations as models of human disease. It is an open question how to generate mouse models that more accurately model the disease. As we learn more about genetic interactions in the human population, we might be able to construct more appropriate models. Likewise, as we develop complex hypotheses about the interactions between genes, we will need to test them in rigorous experiments in model organisms, analogous to the *Fli1-KLF5* mouse [22].

The role of systems biology is to collate large amounts of molecular data and to organize them into a coherent global picture to allow for the generation of hypotheses about disease mechanisms and the prediction of effective therapeutic interventions that can then be tested experimentally. This hypothesis-generating process is one that often identifies complex and nonobvious connections. The complexity of biological systems and the myriad ways that they can malfunction are likely the source of most of the difficult-to-treat clinical conditions like SSc. The advent of precision medicine in SSc will not occur solely from additional high-throughput data but also a conceptual framework that places those data in a context that clarifies why biological complexity results in clinical heterogeneity.

References

1. Assassi S, Radstake TRDJ, Mayes MD, Martin J. Genetics of scleroderma: implications for personalized medicine? BMC Med. BioMed Central Ltd; 2013;11(1):9.
2. Katsumoto TR, Whitfield ML, Connolly MK. The pathogenesis of systemic sclerosis. Annu Rev Pathol. 2011;6(1):509–37.
3. Milano A, Pendergrass SA, Sargent JL, George LK, McCalmont TH, Connolly MK, et al. Molecular subsets in the gene expression signatures of scleroderma skin. Butler G, editor. PLoS ONE. Public Library of Science; 2008;3(7):e2696.
4. Pendergrass SA, Lemaire R, Francis IP, Mahoney JM, Lafyatis R, Whitfield ML. Intrinsic gene expression subsets of diffuse cutaneous systemic sclerosis are stable in serial skin biopsies. J Invest Dermatol. Nature Publishing Group; 2012;132(5):1363–73.
5. Hinchcliff M, Huang C-C, Wood TA, Mahoney JM, Martyanov V, Bhattacharyya S, et al. Molecular Signatures in Skin Associated with ClinicalImprovement during Mycophenolate Treatment inSystemic Sclerosis. J Invest Dermatol. Nature Publishing Group; 2013;133(8):1979–89.
6. Pendergrass SA, Hayes E, Farina G, Lemaire R, Farber HW, Whitfield ML, et al. Limited systemic sclerosis patients with pulmonary arterial hypertension show biomarkers of inflammation and vascular injury. Morty RE, editor. PLoS ONE. Public Library of Science; 2010;5(8):e12106.
7. Risbano MG, Meadows CA, Coldren CD, Jenkins TJ, Edwards MG, Collier D, et al. Altered immune phenotype in peripheral blood cells of patients with scleroderma-associated pulmonary hypertension. Clin Transl Sci. Blackwell Publishing Inc; 2010;3(5):210–8.
8. Taroni JN, Martyanov V, Huang C-C, Mahoney JM, Hirano I, Shetuni B, et al. Molecular characterization of systemic sclerosis esophageal pathology identifies inflammatory and proliferative signatures. Arthritis Res Ther. 5th ed. BioMed Central Ltd; 2015;17(1):194.
9. Hsu E, Shi H, Jordan RM, Lyons-Weiler J, Pilewski JM, Feghali-Bostwick CA. Lung tissues in patients with systemic sclerosis have gene expression patterns unique to pulmonary fibrosis and pulmonary hypertension. Arthritis Rheum. Wiley Subscription Services, Inc., A Wiley Company; 2011;63(3):783–94.
10. Christmann RB, Sampaio-Barros P, Stifano G, Borges CL, de Carvalho CR, Kairalla R, et al. Association of Interferon- and transforming growth factor β-regulated genes and macrophage activation with systemic sclerosis-related progressive lung fibrosis. Arthritis Rheumatol. 2014;66(3):714–25.
11. Marangoni RG, Korman BD, Wei J, Wood TA, Graham LV, Whitfield ML, et al. Myofibroblasts in murine cutaneous fibrosis originate from adiponectin-positive intradermal progenitors. Arthritis Rheumatol. 2015;67(4):1062–73.
12. Mahoney JM, Taroni J, Martyanov V, Wood TA, Greene CS, Pioli PA, et al. Systems level analysis of systemic sclerosis shows a network of immune and profibrotic pathways connected with genetic polymorphisms. Assassi S, editor. PLoS Comp Biol. Public Library of Science; 2015;11(1):e1004005.
13. Chuang H-Y, Hofree M, Ideker T. A decade of systems biology. Annu Rev Cell Dev Biol. Annual Reviews; 2010;26(1):721–44.
14. Barabási A-L, Gulbahce N, Loscalzo J. Network medicine: a network-based approach to human disease. Nat Rev Genet. 2011;12(1):56–68.
15. Newman M. Networks: an introduction. New York City: OUP Oxford; 2010.
16. Fortunato S. Community detection in graphs. Physics Rep. 2010;486(3–5):75–174.
17. Nepusz T, Petróczi A, Négyessy L, Bazsó F. Fuzzy communities and the concept of bridgeness in complex networks. Phys Rev E. 2008;77(1):016107.
18. Hwang, W, Cho, Y. R, Zhang, A, and Ramanathan, M (2006). Bridging centrality: identifying bridging nodes in scale-free networks. In Proceedings of the 12th ACM SIGKDD international conference on Knowledge discovery and data mining. pp. 20–23.
19. Yu H, Kim PM, Sprecher E, Trifonov V, Gerstein M. The importance of bottlenecks in protein networks: correlation with gene essentiality and expression dynamics. PLoS Comp Biol. Public Library of Science; 2007;3(4):e59.
20. Beretta L, Cappiello F, Moore JH, Barili M, Greene CS, Scorza R. Ability of epistatic interactions of cytokine single-nucleotide polymorphisms to predict susceptibility to disease subsets in systemic sclerosis patients. Arthritis Rheum. Wiley Subscription Services, Inc., A Wiley Company; 2008;59(7):974–83.
21. Beretta L, Cappiello F, Moore JH, Scorza R. Interleukin-1 gene complex single nucleotide polymorphisms in systemic sclerosis: a further step ahead. Hum Immunol. 2008;69(3):187–92.
22. Noda S, Asano Y, Nishimura S, Taniguchi T, Fujiu K, Manabe I, et al. Simultaneous downregulation of KLF5 and Fli1 is a key feature underlying systemic sclerosis. Nat Commun. Nature Publishing Group; 2014;5:5797.
23. Wong AK, Park CY, Greene CS, Bongo LA, Guan Y, Troyanskaya OG. IMP: a multi-species functional genomics portal for integration, visualization and prediction of protein functions and networks. Nucleic Acids Res. Oxford University Press; 2012;40(Web Server issue):W484–90.
24. Tyler AL, Asselbergs FW, Williams SM, Moore JH. Shadows of complexity: what biological networks reveal about epistasis and pleiotropy. Bioessays. WILEY-VCH Verlag; 2009;31(2):220–7.
25. Tyler AL, Crawford DC, Pendergrass SA. The detection and characterization of pleiotropy: discovery, progress, and promise. Brief Bioinformatics. 2016;17(1):13–22.
26. Greene CS, Krishnan A, Wong AK, Ricciotti E, Zelaya RA, Himmelstein DS, et al. Understanding multicellular function and disease with human tissue-specific networks. Nat Genet. 2015;47(6):569–76.
27. Chakravarty EF, Martyanov V, Fiorentino D, Wood TA, Haddon DJ, Jarrell JA, et al. Gene expression changes reflect clinical response in a placebo-controlled randomized trial of abatacept in patients with diffuse cutaneous systemic sclerosis. Arthritis Res Ther. BioMed Central Ltd; 2015;17(1):159.
28. Gordon JK, Martyanov V, Magro C, Wildman HF, Wood TA, Huang W-T, et al. Nilotinib (Tasigna™) in the treatment of early diffuse systemic sclerosis: an open-label, pilot clinical trial. Arthritis Res Ther. BioMed Central Ltd; 2015;17(1):213.
29. Niepel M, Hafner M, Pace EA, Chung M, Chai DH, Zhou L, et al. Profiles of Basal and stimulated receptor signaling networks predict drug response in breast cancer lines. Sci Signal. American Association for the Advancement of Science; 2013;6(294):ra84–4.
30. Niepel M, Hafner M, Pace EA, Chung M, Chai DH, Zhou L, et al. Analysis of growth factor signaling in genetically diverse breast cancer lines. BMC Biol. BioMed Central Ltd; 2014;12(1):20.
31. Jahchan NS, Dudley JT, Mazur PK, Flores N, Yang D, Palmerton A, et al. A drug repositioning approach identifies tricyclic antidepressants as inhibitors of small cell lung cancer and other neuroendocrine tumors. Cancer Discov. American Association for Cancer Research; 2013;3(12):1364–77.
32. Kodama K, Toda K, Morinaga S, Yamada S, Butte AJ. Anti-CD44 antibody treatment lowers hyperglycemia and improves insulin resistance, adipose inflammation, and hepatic steatosis in diet-induced obese mice. Diabetes. American Diabetes Association; 2015;64(3):867–75.

Part III

The Biological Basis of Systemic Sclerosis

Introduction: The Etiopathogenesis of Systemic Sclerosis – An Integrated Overview

11

Carol Feghali-Bostwick and John Varga

Introduction

Systemic sclerosis (SSc) is a heterogeneous chronic multisystem disease of unknown etiology. It has global distribution and like other connective diseases, a strong female predominance. The onset of SSc shows age-dependence and modest familial clustering, but no compelling geographic or temporal clustering. Multiple genes are implicated in SSc susceptibility, and the genetic architecture, dominated by the HLA locus, shows considerable overlap with other autoimmune diseases. The variable disease course, its high burden of mortality and morbidity, and lack of effective therapies make SSc a top research priority in the field of rheumatic diseases. A bird's-eye view of SSc suggests the following paradigm for disease pathogenesis, supported by current data in the chapters that follow: initial injury in an individual with a permissive genetic background triggers complex and sustained interactions among immune and vascular cells in a variety of tissues. Oxidative stress ensues, and a range of soluble and matrix-associated signals are generated that trigger and maintain mesenchymal cell activation and survival, leading to matrix accumulation and culminating in progressive multi-organ fibrosis. Details of this process are described in the following chapters and are summarized in Fig. 11.1.

C. Feghali-Bostwick, PhD (✉)
Department of Medicine, Medical University of South Carolina, Charleston, SC, USA
e-mail: feghalib@musc.edu

J. Varga, MD
Northwestern Scleroderma Program, John and Nancy Hughes Professor, Feinberg School of Medicine Northwestern University, Chicago, IL, USA

Intermediate Pathophenotypes (the Triad), Disease Heterogeneity, and the Role of Heredity

The hallmarks of SSc are widespread microvascular abnormalities, immune dysregulation with inflammation and autoimmunity, and fibrosis of the skin and internal organs. These three distinct yet intricately linked dynamic processes, designated "intermediate pathophenotypes," constitute the characteristic triad of SSc and underlie its clinical picture or phenotype. The tissues affected by these processes, the relative impact and activity of these individual processes in a given patient, and their rates of progression or regression vary widely. This heterogeneity in the phenotypic expression of SSc, no doubt determined in part by individual host genetic factors and their epistatic interactions, accounts for the exceptional variability of SSc and the difficulty in accurately predicting its natural history and outcomes. The genetic basis of SSc is complex and incompletely understood [1]. A growing number of genetic loci are recognized to be associated with SSc and point to an important role for immunity in disease susceptibility. However, a great deal of the heritability of SSc remains unaccounted for, and the genetic associations recognized to date carry only a modest risk. The complex role of heredity in SSc is highlighted by a twin study, which reveals a low concordance rate for disease but a very high concordance rate for autoimmunity [2]. Environmental influences elicit both transient effects, as well as stable changes in the transcriptome due to epigenetic modifications (imprinting). The three primary epigenetic modifications, histone acetylation, DNA and histone methylation, and noncoding RNAs (microRNAs and long noncoding RNAs), together drive environmentally induced heritable changes in gene expression that are not due to changes in the DNA sequence. The epigenome, which represents a record of accrued environmental influences, has received scant attention in SSc to date, and its study, while likely to be highly informative, will require analysis at the

J. Varga et al. (eds.), *Scleroderma*, DOI 10.1007/978-3-319-31407-5_11

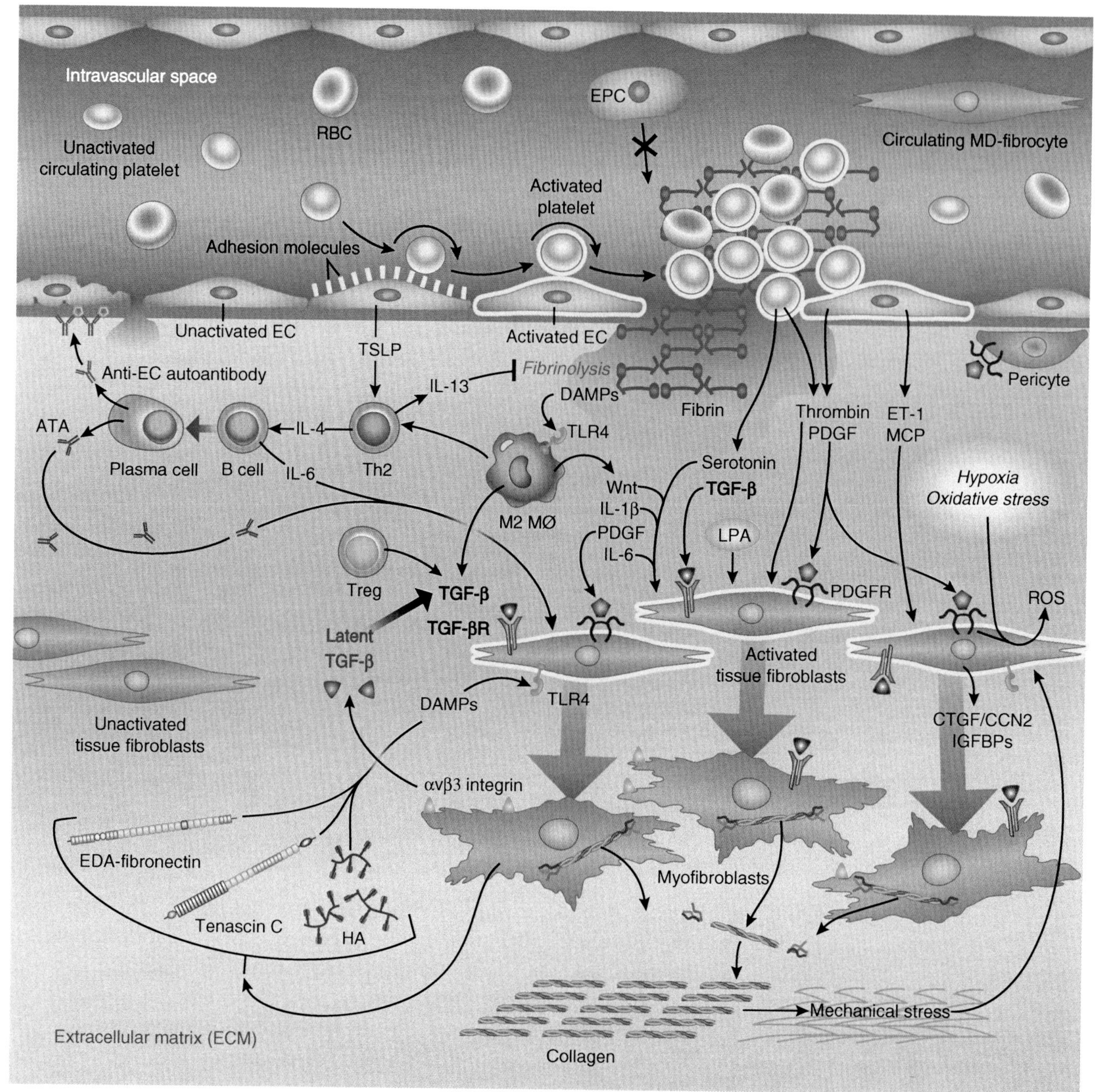

Fig. 11.1 Integrated view of SSc pathogenesis: key cellular players and molecular mediators at various stages of disease. In early disease, initial injury to vascular endothelial cells causes their activation, expression of adhesion molecules, production of chemokines, and endothelin-1 and platelet activation. Activated platelets release thrombin and thromboxane, promoting coagulation. In the inflammatory stage of SSc, chemokines recruit monocytes and macrophages from the circulation into the tissue. Activated T cells are polarized to a Th2 pattern and secrete TGF-ß and IL-13. Plasma cells secrete autoantibodies, and macrophages secrete TGF-ß and other M2-type cytokines. Dendritic cells stimulated via TLR4 secrete type I interferon. In the fibrotic phase of SSc, resident fibroblasts are activated by TGF-ß, IL-13, IL-6, thrombin, and PDGF, generate ROS, and undergo differentiation into myofibroblasts which produce ECM molecules that form the fibrotic matrix. Moreover, activated myofibroblasts secrete profibrotic growth factors such as TGF-ß and CTGF and activate latent TGF-ß. Surface TLR4 senses damage-associated endogenous TLR ligands such as tenascin C, driving persistence of myofibroblast activation. Structural cells including pericytes and adipocytes undergo dedifferentiation, further expanding the pool of activated profibrotic myofibroblasts. Over time, perhaps facilitated by cellular aging and senescence, both immune and fibrotic processes abate ("burn out"), and vascular and connective tissue atrophy results. Transcriptomic analysis of skin and lung biopsies shows the existence of distinct yet overlapping inflammatory, fibroproliferative, and "normal-like" intrinsic subsets. These subsets are likely to represent distinct stages of disease evolution. Late-stage atrophic skin is associated with a "normal-like" gene signature

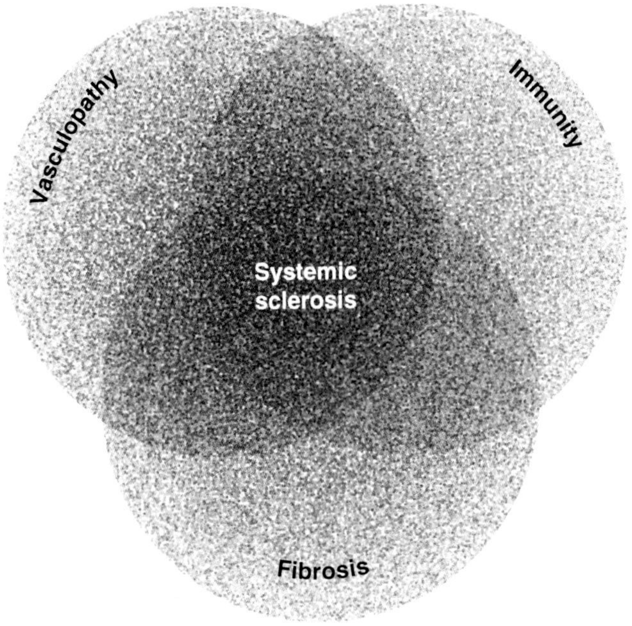

Fig. 11.2 The pathogenesis of SSc: triad of intermediate pathophenotypes. Illustrated are the three biological processes termed "intermediate pathophenotypes" that characterize SSc. The dynamic interplay of these intermediate pathophenotypes underlies the protean and fluctuating clinical manifestations of the disease. The three intermediate pathophenotypes of SSc share traits such as impaired autophagy, endoplasmic reticulum stress and oxidative stress, reduced cell-intrinsic cytoprotective mechanisms, loss of immune self-tolerance, disruption of circadian rhythms, and failure to replenish injured cells and regenerate damaged structures. It does not escape our attention that these same traits are hallmarks of biological aging, suggesting mechanistic parallels between biological aging and SSc (Illustration by Jacqi Schaffer)

single-cell level. Additionally, random (stochastic) events, together with biological aging, may cause somatic mutations and modulate the epigenome, particularly in cells of the immune system, resulting in break in immune tolerance. Gene-environment interactions therefore are likely to be of paramount significance in disease risk and progression, but the environmental and stochastic events contributing to the etiopathogenesis of SSc are virtually unknown [3].

Heterogeneity is a notable feature of SSc. Nevertheless, despite varying disease duration, clinical manifestations, internal organ involvement, and disease progression, patients with SSc share some key features. In particular, all patients with SSc display the triad of intermediate pathophenotypes (Fig. 11.2): vascular damage, immune abnormalities, and fibrosis. Consequently, a staggering diversity of cell types, progenitor cells, and lineages are known to play important roles in pathogenesis. These include immune cells, vascular cells, and stromal cells (Table 11.1), with many showing considerable plasticity in their capacity to differentiate into alternate cell types.

There is currently neither a cure nor effective disease-modifying therapies for SSc, and findings to date suggest that there may not be a "one-size-fits-all" therapy. Consequently, research in the field focuses on gaining a detailed understanding of the pathogenesis of SSc and its various subsets or "endophenotypes," the development and validation of animal models of disease, developing stratification tools to better identify patient subsets and disease variants, and identifying key mediators for the development of targeted therapies [4].

In this brief introductory chapter, we provide a bird's-eye view of the etiopathogenesis of SSc that attempts to synthesize current data. We highlight key themes that are discussed in detail in the chapters in the pathogenesis section that follows.

Table 11.1 Cell types prominently implicated in the pathogenesis of SSc

Immune	Monocytes/macrophages
	Dendritic cells
	B lymphocytes, plasma cells
	T lymphocytes, subsets
	Mast cells
Vascular	Endothelial cells
	Vascular smooth muscle cells
	Pericytes
	Platelets
Stromal cells	Mesenchymal stem cells
	Epithelial cells
	Fibroblasts/myofibroblasts
	Adipocytes

The Scleroderma Triad of Intermediate Pathophenotypes

The pathogenesis of SSc is complex, multifactorial, and incompletely understood. Evidence of a characteristic triad of so-called intermediate pathophenotypes – vascular damage, immune abnormalities, and fibrosis – can be detected in every patient with SSc. These processes are interwoven and dynamically modulate each other in a cascade of events that culminate in the overall clinical disease phenotype and endophenotype (Fig. 11.3). Research on SSc has been hampered by the lack of appropriate animal models, since no single animal model faithfully phenocopies all the cardinal features and temporal evolution and chronicity of the human disease.

Primacy of Vascular Injury and Damage

Vascular injury and consequent damage are a prominent, and perhaps primary, event in the pathogenesis of SSc [5]. Widespread vascular abnormalities in virtually all organs, a distinguishing hallmark of SSc, present clinically as

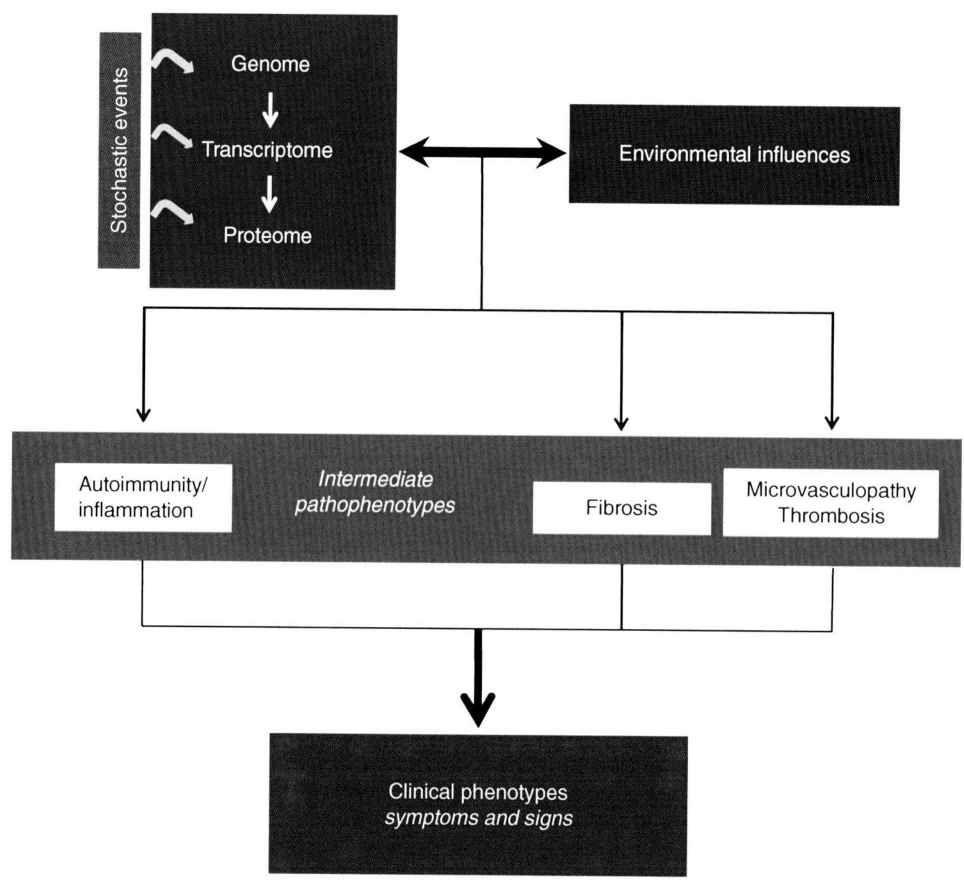

Fig. 11.3 The etiopathogenesis of SSc. Reciprocal interactions of genetic and environmental influences, impacted by random (stochastic) events, yield a triad of intermediate pathophenotypes in SSc. Variations in the timing and intensity of the intermediate pathophenotypes in affected tissues determine the unique clinical presentations of SSc among different individuals and different time points during the evolution of the disease (Modified after Barabasi and Loscalzo [14])

Raynaud phenomenon, abnormal nail fold capillaries, mucocutaneous telangiectasias, ischemic digital ulcers, gastric antral vascular ectasia, PAH, and scleroderma renal crisis [6]. Vascular abnormalities are commonly the earliest disease manifestations of SSc and typically precede immune abnormalities and fibrosis. Vascular injury triggered by toxic, autoimmune, metabolic, or infectious factors affects the endothelium and is initially associated with largely reversible functional changes in the blood vessels. Over time, progressive and irreversible structural vascular alterations accrue involving endothelial cells, vascular smooth muscle cells, adventitial cells, and perivascular supporting cells called pericytes. Progressive vascular damage leads to neointima formation, luminal narrowing, and obliteration of small- and medium-sized arteries in multiple vascular beds. Endothelial cells show increased oxidative stress and express a variety of cell adhesion molecules, facilitating the exit of inflammatory cells from the circulation into damaged tissues. Perivascular inflammation is common and plays an important role in vasculopathy, particularly that underlying pulmonary artery hypertension. Platelet aggregation and activation of thrombotic and coagulation cascades ensue. Compromised vascular supply leads to chronic tissue hypoxia, ischemic complications, and tissue necrosis.

Vascular dysfunction may be triggered by endothelial cell injury and release of reactive oxygen species, thromboxane, and antiangiogenic factors and generation of anti-endothelial cell antibodies, although the specific nature of the injurious agents remains elusive. Additional factors implicated in SSc vascular disease include a marked imbalance between factors promoting vasodilation versus vasoconstriction, including angiotensin, nitric oxide, and endothelin-1, as well as the development of functional autoantibodies directed against vascular receptors on endothelial cells. There is additionally evidence for impaired vasculogenesis, the formation of new blood vessels to replace lost and damaged ones, in SSc. Despite tissue ischemia and elevated levels of angiogenic factors that normally serve as potent stimuli for vasculogenesis, in SSc the number and function of endothelial progenitor cells is reduced. Pericytes, which help maintain the structural integrity of small blood vessels, are dysfunctional, further aggravating the loss of vasculature. Additionally, both pericytes and adventitial fibroblasts are activated and have the capacity to transdifferentiate into myofibroblasts, which contribute to perivascular and interstitial fibrosis. The sequence of microvascular injury, vascular damage, and fibrosis leading to capillary rarefaction in the skin and other organs is partially phenocopied in Fra-2 transgenic mice, as well as in Fli1 and uPAR

Table 11.2 Prominent mouse models for SSc

Primarily vasculopathy[a]	Fra-2 transgenic
	VEGF transgenic
	uPAR null
	Fli1 null
Primarily immune	Inducible: injection of bleomycin, hypochlorous acid
	Mouse cGVHD
	PSGL null (also develop vasculopathy)
Primarily fibrotic	TSK1 and TSK2 spontaneous mutants
	Wnt10 transgenic
	Fibrillin mutant transgenic (stiff skin)
	PDGFRα transgenic
	CTGF transgenic

cGVDH chronic graft-versus-host disease, *uPAR* urokinase-type plasminogen activator receptor, *PSGL* P-selectin glycoprotein ligand-1
[a]Each of these models is associated with prominent fibrotic features in the skin

knockout mice. In these genetically engineered mouse models, microangiopathy is prominently associated with tissue fibrosis (Table 11.2).

The Immune System: Autoimmunity, Adaptive Immunity, and Innate Immunity

SSc has been traditionally viewed as an autoimmune disease, but the relative inefficacy of many immunosuppressive therapies has led many to question the importance of immunity in pathogenesis. Whether immune dysregulation is a primary pathogenic event in SSc, or is secondary to vascular injury, remains a subject of debate. Nevertheless, recent insights from genetic studies unequivocally point to a fundamental role of altered immune responses in the disease, and, together with the presence of autoantibodies in the circulation and of inflammatory signatures in lesional tissue, justify the classification of SSc as an autoimmune disease. Abnormalities in the numbers, distribution, and function of cells of the immune system are prevalent in all forms of SSc. Local and systemic changes in cytokine, chemokine, and growth factor levels and activation, migration, and differentiation of T cells, B cells, monocytes, macrophages, NK cells, and dendritic cells have been documented [7]. T lymphocytes show a pronounced skewing toward a Th2 pattern, which creates a fibrosis-prone milieu. The cytokine thymic stromal lymphopoietin (TSLP) appears to be a major factor driving T-cell polarization in SSc. An important role for B cells in SSc in generating autoantibodies as well as IL-6 and other pathogenic cytokines is emerging and provides the therapeutic rationale for the use of B-cell depletion. Recent studies using genome-wide transcriptome analysis of SSc skin and lung reveal a robust and consistent inflammatory signature, indicating activation of immune signaling within lesional tissues. These observations lead to a plausible scenario for the development of autoimmunity and inflammation in SSc: innate immune responses in dendritic cells, NK cells, and monocytes/macrophages trigger adaptive immunity, including skewing the T-cell response toward a Th2 predominant pattern. Since immune cells must exit the circulation in order to accumulate within lesional tissue, leukocyte interaction with the damaged endothelium mediated via endothelial and leukocyte adhesion molecules plays an important role in SSc, a notion supported by the observation that mice deficient in the leukocyte adhesion receptor PSGL-1 spontaneously develop age-dependent skin fibrosis.

Highlighting the role of immune mechanisms in the pathogenesis of SSc is the profound effect of immune cells and their secreted factors on other cells and tissues including endothelial cells and fibroblasts. Innate immunity is increasingly recognized as having a key role in pathogenesis. Type I interferon, produced in response to activation of toll-like receptors (TLRs) and other pattern recognition receptors, contributes to systemic inflammation and tissue damage. TLRs are expressed on both immune cells, such as dendritic cells and monocytes, as well as nonimmune cells including endothelial cells and fibroblasts. A key arm of innate immunity is the inflammasome, which by generating active IL-1, contributes to the pro-inflammatory and profibrotic cellular milieu in SSc. Multiple studies in mice have established an indispensible role for both TLRs and the inflammasome in experimental fibrosis.

Autoantibodies in SSc: Markers of Autoimmunity and Drivers of Disease?

The presence of one of the nine SSc-associated autoantibodies correlates with internal organ involvement. SSc-associated autoantibodies are typically mutually exclusive and while their direct role (if any) in disease pathogenesis remains to be demonstrated, they can serve as tools for patient stratification. These antibodies target self-antigens including Scl-70 (topoisomerase I), centromere, RNA polymerase, U1 RNP, U3 RNP, U11/U12 RNP, Th/To, Ku, and PM-Scl. In addition to their usefulness in diagnosis, prognosis, and patient stratification, SSc-associated autoantibodies may potentiate immune responses and TLR activation, amplifying pathological immune responses. The mechanisms responsible for generating a highly specific immune response to self-antigens in SSc remain elusive. One intriguing clue has recently emerged from the study of cancer associated with SSc. This study revealed an association between oncogenic mutations in the gene encoding RNA polymerase III, anti-RNA polymerase III antibodies, and the near-contemporaneous onset of cancer and SSc in a group of patients [8]. These observations suggest that the origin of (at least some) SSc-associated autoantibodies might lie in an antitumor immune response targeting oncogenic tumor mutations. In addition to these SSc-associated autoantibodies, an increasing number of functional antibodies with agonistic activity for vascular receptors have been described in SSc. Targets include the endothelin-1 receptor and the angiotensin II receptor which are activated by these antibodies. The pathogenic role of functional autoantibodies in SSc is being elucidated.

Multisystem Fibrosis: The Distinguishing Hallmark of SSc

Fibrosis as a predominant pathophenotype distinguishes SSc from other autoimmune diseases. A truly remarkable and unique feature of SSc is that fibrosis invariably affects multiple organs in addition to the skin, most commonly the lungs, heart, gastrointestinal tract, and kidneys [9]. Within affected organs, fibrosis due to SSc is no different from organ-specific forms of fibrosis such as idiopathic pulmonary fibrosis (IPF). Nevertheless the genetic loci implicated in SSc-associated versus idiopathic lung fibrosis show no overlap, suggesting that diverse etiopathogenic processes may converge on a generic intermediate pathophenotype such as fibrosis [10].

Fibrosis results when extracellular matrix (ECM) homeostasis is disrupted, and the dynamic balance between ECM synthesis and turnover is perturbed. Numerous soluble factors, mechanical forces, and cell lineages have been implicated in the process. Cytokines, chemokines, growth factors, bioactive lipids, coagulation factors, hypoxia, reactive oxygen species (ROS), and biomechanical forces generated within a stiff matrix provide signals triggering fibroblast activation. Transforming growth factor-ß is the master regulator of fibrogenesis, and much evidence implicates it in the pathogenesis of SSc. The source of excessive TGF-ß is not well established, but activated platelets, tissue macrophages, and T lymphocytes might contribute to its production. In addition, aberrant activation of tissue-sequestered latent TGF-ß by fibroblasts expressing surface integrins such as αvß3 and αvß8 has been documented in SSc; moreover, this process is accentuated in a mechanically stressed microenvironment. A variety of developmental morphogen pathways are deregulated in patients with SSc and are increasingly implicated in the pathogenesis of fibrosis. Bone morphogenetic proteins, Wnt, Notch, and sonic hedgehog regulate embryonic development and are tightly regulated in healthy adults but become aberrantly expressed during sustained injury. In the case of Wnt signaling, deregulation of the pathway in SSc reflects epigenetic silencing of Wnt repressors such as DKK1. Mice with overexpression of Wnt ligand and other developmental pathways spontaneously develop age-dependent organ fibrosis. While targeting morphogen pathways in experimental animal models of fibrosis is associated with amelioration of the process, translation of these successful strategies into clinical therapies for SSc remains a major challenge.

Increasingly recognized for their role in triggering and maintaining the fibrotic process are endogenous TLR ligands collectively termed DAMPs (damage-associated molecular patterns). These molecules, including proteins, peptides, glycoproteins, and lipids, as well as nucleic acids, are generated at sites of tissue injury and cell death. Fibronectin-EDA and tenascin C are endogenous ECM-related TLR ligands that act as "danger signals" alerting the host to tissue damage. In response, TLRs on resident stromal cells initiate a self-limited tissue repair process. While beneficial under normal conditions, deregulated TLR activation by uncontrolled accumulation of DAMPs, as can be seen in the skin and lungs in patients with SSc, is deleterious and is responsible for maintaining sustained fibroblast activation [11].

Cellular Mediators of Fibrosis

The key effector cell of fibrosis is the fibroblast and its activated progeny the myofibroblast. These intermediate cells display features of both fibroblasts and smooth muscle cells, contributing to both the biochemical and biomechanical attributes of tissue fibrosis by copious collagen and other ECM protein production as well as tissue contraction. Myofibroblasts within the lesional tissue are a hallmark of SSc and distinguish affected versus unaffected skin. Numerous cell types exhibit plasticity that allows them to undergo phenotypic transitions called "epithelial mesenchymal transition" and "endothelial mesenchymal transition." These processes may contribute to expansion of the myofibroblast pool in SSc. Additional sources for activated myofibroblasts in the lesional dermis include Sox2-expressing skin progenitor cells and intradermal preadipocytes, which undergo transdifferentiation under the influence of TGF-ß, PDGF, Wnts, and other profibrotic ligands. There is also evidence that bone marrow-derived monocytes and fibrocytes differentiate into myofibroblasts in SSc. However, despite experimental support for the role of such processes in fibrosis, primarily from studies in mice, the occurrence, extent, and pathogenic significance of such cell fate changes in patients with SSc remain to be validated.

The "scleroderma fibroblast" exhibits a variety of prominent cell-autonomous abnormalities. These include constitutive ECM production, spontaneous generation of both mitochondrial and cytosolic ROS, focal adhesion assembly, and FAK activation. Moreover, these cells show diminished autophagic flux that is reminiscent of aged fibroblasts. Relative resistance to apoptosis, inherent adhesive and contractile properties, impaired cytoprotective mechanisms, altered miR29 expression, and other epigenomic changes, along with a variety of other abnormalities, persist even when SSc fibroblasts are removed from their *in vivo* milieu.

This suggests that fibroblast activators in SSc induce sustained and heritable cellular changes driving fibrosis. Such changes are likely to involve epigenetic mechanisms that modulate the transcription of genes encoding key transcription factors and signaling molecules.

The Interplay of the Triad of Intermediate Pathophenotypes in the Pathogenesis of SSc

The dynamic interplay between the vascular, immune, and fibrosis-promoting processes illustrated in Fig. 11.2 underlies the protean and fluctuating manifestations of SSc and their evolution during the course of the disease. It is difficult to ascertain which of these processes are primary; however, the observation that Raynaud phenomenon is very commonly the initial disease manifestation of SSc suggests that vascular changes precede, and may be responsible for, other disease manifestations. Furthermore, based on current data, vascular changes are likely to be responsible for triggering inflammation, innate immunity, and ischemic responses that might be linked to the initiation and maintenance of the deregulated wound repair process underlying fibrosis. Nevertheless, in a given individual with SSc, the vascular, immune, and fibrotic processes coexist, and their activity and impact fluctuate during the course of the disease. The coexistence of inflammatory and fibrotic processes within the same tissue is highlighted by transcriptomic analyses of skin biopsies in longitudinally followed patient cohorts [12]. Accordingly, effective therapies will need to address the predominant pathomechanism driving the disease at a given point in time, which will vary from one patient to another, and within the same patient with temporal evolution of the disease. The modern tools of precision medicine hold the promise of therapeutic interventions that selectively target the process or processes most prominent in a given patient at a specific point along their disease trajectory. Biomarkers, and in particular tissue-based genomic and epigenomic analyses and peripheral blood proteomics and cell type analyses, are likely to emerge as powerful precision weapons in the fight against SSc [13].

References

1. Korman BD, Criswell LA. Recent advances in the genetics of systemic sclerosis: toward biological and clinical significance. Curr Rheumatol Rep. 2015;17:21.
2. Feghali-Bostwick C, Medsger Jr TA, Wright TM. Analysis of systemic sclerosis in twins reveals low concordance for disease and high concordance for the presence of antinuclear antibodies. Arthritis Rheum. 2003;48:1956–63.
3. Roberts-Thomson PJ, Walker JG. Stochastic processes in the aetiopathogenesis of scleroderma. Intern Med J. 2012;42:235–42.
4. Varga J, Hinchcliff M. Connective tissue diseases: systemic sclerosis: beyond limited and diffuse subsets? Nat Rev Rheumatol. 2014;10:200–2.
5. Matucci-Cerinic M, Kahaleh B, Wigley FM. Review: evidence that systemic sclerosis is a vascular disease. Arthritis Rheum. 2013;65:1953–62.
6. Trojanowska M. Cellular and molecular aspects of vascular dysfunction in systemic sclerosis. Nat Rev Rheumatol. 2010;6: 453–60.
7. Greenblatt MB, Aliprantis AO. The immune pathogenesis of scleroderma: context is everything. Curr Rheumatol Rep. 2013; 15:297.
8. Joseph CG, Darrah E, Shah AA, Skora AD, Casciola-Rosen LA, Wigley FM, Boin F, Fava A, Thoburn C, Kinde I, Jiao Y, Papadopoulos N, Kinzler KW, Vogelstein B, Rosen A. Association of the autoimmune disease scleroderma with an immunologic response to cancer. Science. 2014;343:152–7.
9. Varga J, Abraham D. Systemic sclerosis: a prototypic multisystem fibrotic disorder. J Clin Invest. 2007;117:557–67.
10. Herzog EL, Mathur A, Tager AM, Feghali-Bostwick C, Schneider F, Varga J. Review: interstitial lung disease associated with systemic sclerosis and idiopathic pulmonary fibrosis: how similar and distinct? Arthritis Rheumatol. 2014;66:1967–78.
11. Bhattacharyya S, Tamaki Z, Wang W, Hinchcliff M, Hoover P, Getsios S, White ES, Varga J. Fibronectineda promotes chronic cutaneous fibrosis through toll-like receptor signaling. Sci Transl Med. 2014;6:232ra250.
12. Mahoney JM, Taroni J, Martyanov V, Wood TA, Greene CS, Pioli PA, Hinchcliff ME, Whitfield ML. Systems level analysis of systemic sclerosis shows a network of immune and profibrotic pathways connected with genetic polymorphisms. PLoS Comput Biol. 2015;11:e1004005.
13. Castelino FV, Varga J. Current status of systemic sclerosis biomarkers: applications for diagnosis, management and drug development. Expert Rev Clin Immunol. 2013;9:1077–90.
14. Loscalzo J, Kohane I, Barabasi AL. Human disease classification in the postgenomic era: a complex systems approach to human pathobiology. Mol Syst Biol. 2007;3:124.

Pathology of Systemic Sclerosis

12

Lisa M. Rooper and Frederic B. Askin

Introduction

Although the clinical syndrome of systemic sclerosis (SSc) was described as early as the seventeenth century, a detailed characterization of its associated pathologic findings was not published until the middle of the twentieth century [1]. Autopsy studies played a vital role in initially characterizing the many visceral manifestations of this disease [2–5]. Despite recent advances in imaging and laboratory diagnosis of SSc, pathologic examination remains essential to the diagnosis and management of affected patients today. Skin biopsy is frequently employed in the initial evaluation of SSc patients, lung and kidney biopsies are utilized to diagnose its most deadly visceral manifestations, and GI biopsy aids in the investigation of many disabling complications. Moreover, autopsy of SSc patients still may be the most comprehensive way to directly visualize the protean manifestations of this devastating disease.

While the specific pathologic manifestations of SSc vary widely across anatomic sites, several common features can be identified irrespective of organ system. Indeed, the hallmark pathophysiologic triad of vascular damage, immune dysfunction, and tissue remodeling with fibrosis discussed elsewhere in this book is reflected in the pathologic findings in SSc [6]. Most obviously, vascular pathology, including thrombotic microangiopathy and luminal obliteration, can be recognized in virtually every organ affected by SSc, especially the skin, lungs, kidneys, gastrointestinal tract, and placenta. Tissue remodeling, represented histologically as fibrosis, also is a key finding, particularly in the skin, cardiovascular, gastrointestinal, and musculoskeletal systems. Lastly, inflammation serves as a direct microscopic correlate for immune dysregulation, being most consistently seen in the lungs and cardiovascular system. This chapter will describe the most common and distinctive pathologic findings in SSc across these organ systems.

L.M. Rooper, MD
Department of Pathology, Johns Hopkins Hospital, Baltimore, MD, USA
e-mail: rooper@jhmi.edu

F.B. Askin, MD (✉)
Department of Pathology, Johns Hopkins University School of Medicine, Baltimore, MD, USA
e-mail: faskin@jhmi.edu

Skin

The namesake skin thickening was the first reported clinical manifestation of SSc, and the pathological findings in the skin remain one of this disease's most characteristic histologic features. Although the 2013 American College of Rheumatology/European League Against Rheumatism (ACR/EULAR) criteria do not require skin biopsy for diagnosis of SSc [7], it is often performed to support the diagnosis in seronegative patients or to differentiate SSc from other skin thickening disorders, including stiff skin syndrome, eosinophilic fasciitis, graft versus host disease, scleromyxedema, amyloidosis, nephrogenic systemic fibrosis, and overlap syndromes with other collagen vascular diseases [8]. Moreover, histologic examination of skin specimens also helps characterize the many other skin lesions associated with SSc. Skin in SSc commonly demonstrates morpheaform thickening, telangiectasias, ulceration, and calcinosis cutis. Less commonly, livedoid vasculopathy and lipodystrophy can also be seen.

Even though the clinical appearance of skin thickening in SSc is so classic that biopsy is rarely performed, the equally distinctive histologic appearance can go far to resolve any diagnostic uncertainty [9]. At low power, skin biopsies demonstrate characteristic squared-off edges, in contrast to the irregular borders seen in most conditions. The dermis is thickened by broad, elongated bundles of homogenized collagen that are oriented parallel to the surface epithelium (Fig. 12.1a). Adnexal glands appear atrophic with loss of periadnexal adipose tissue (Fig. 12.1b). This appearance contrasts sharply to the irregular collagen bundles and abundant periadnexal adipose tissue in normal skin (Fig. 12.1c, d). In rare cases of nodular SSc, the abnormal collagen can

J. Varga et al. (eds.), *Scleroderma*, DOI 10.1007/978-3-319-31407-5_12

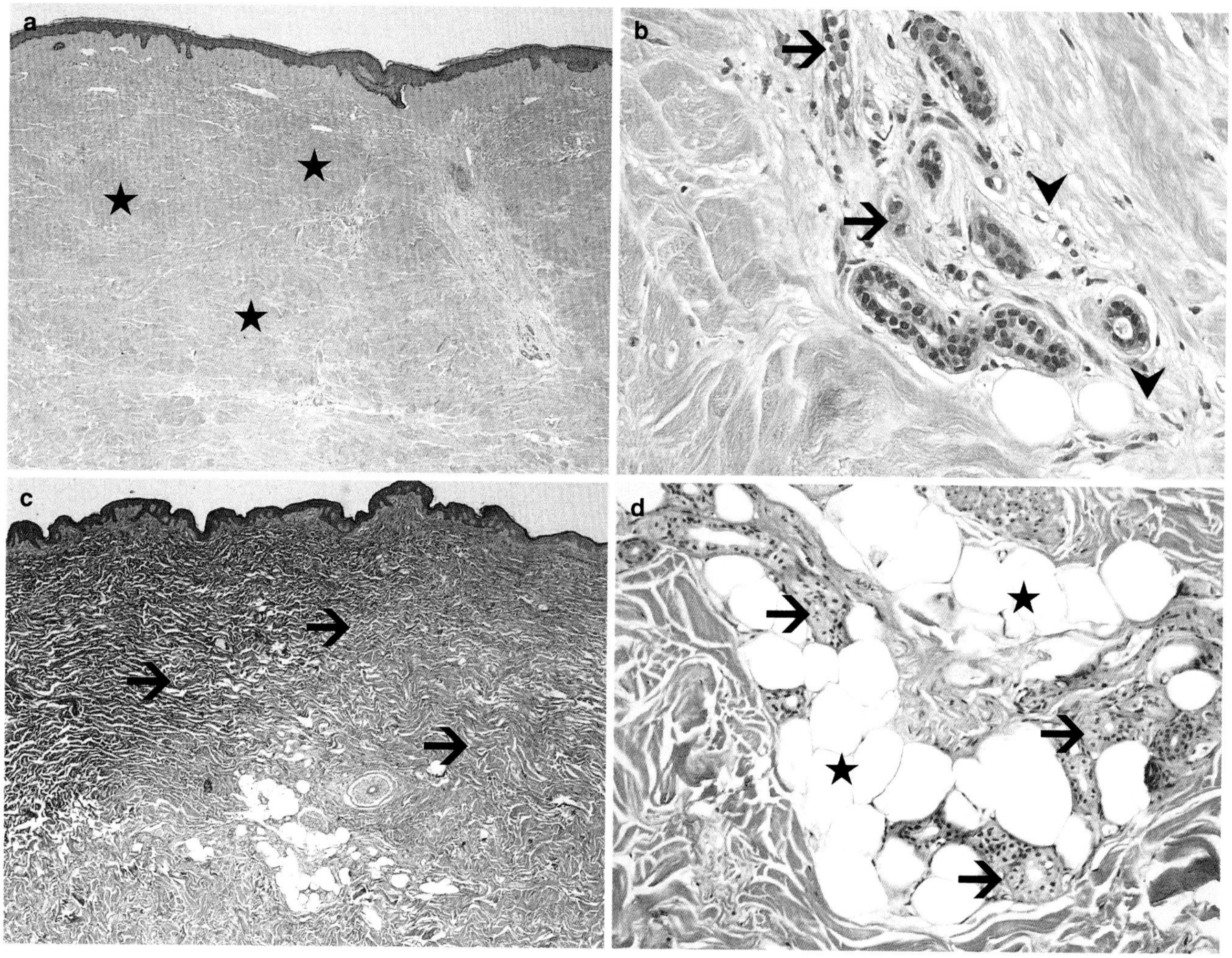

Fig. 12.1 Comparison of skin in SSc to normal. Skin in SSc has broad bundles of homogenized collagen (★) running parallel to the epidermis (**a**). Adnexal glands are atrophic (→) and show loss of periadnexal adipose tissue (▼) (**b**). In contrast, normal skin demonstrates irregular collagen bundles (→) (**c**) and abundant adipose tissue (★) surrounding plump apocrine glands (→) (**d**)

also appear as keloidal nodules [10] (Fig. 12.2). Arteries in the dermis and subcutis demonstrate intimal thickening and medial hypertrophy with occasional complete occlusion (Fig. 12.3a, b). A mononuclear cell infiltrate can be seen around blood vessels in early disease, but established lesions tend to lack chronic inflammation. While histologic skin thickening correlates closely with the clinical modified Rodnan skin score [11], it is rarely quantitated in clinical practice. The findings in SSc are histologically indistinguishable from those of localized SSc, or morphea, and are thus frequently described as morpheaform [12].

Beyond the diagnostic skin thickening, several other characteristic skin lesions are frequently seen in SSc. Telangiectasias are one common finding that are present in almost all SSc patients and are included in the ACR/EULAR 2013 criteria for diagnosis of SSc [7]. While they are also rarely biopsied, telangiectasias can easily be identified histologically as dilated blood vessels in the superficial dermis (Fig. 12.4a). In contrast

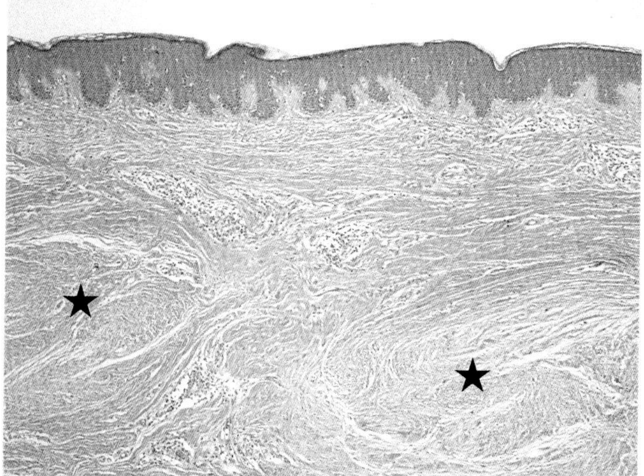

Fig. 12.2 Nodular scleroderma. In this rare variant of SSc, the collagen maintains a morpheaform homogenized appearance but is organized in keloidal nodules (★)

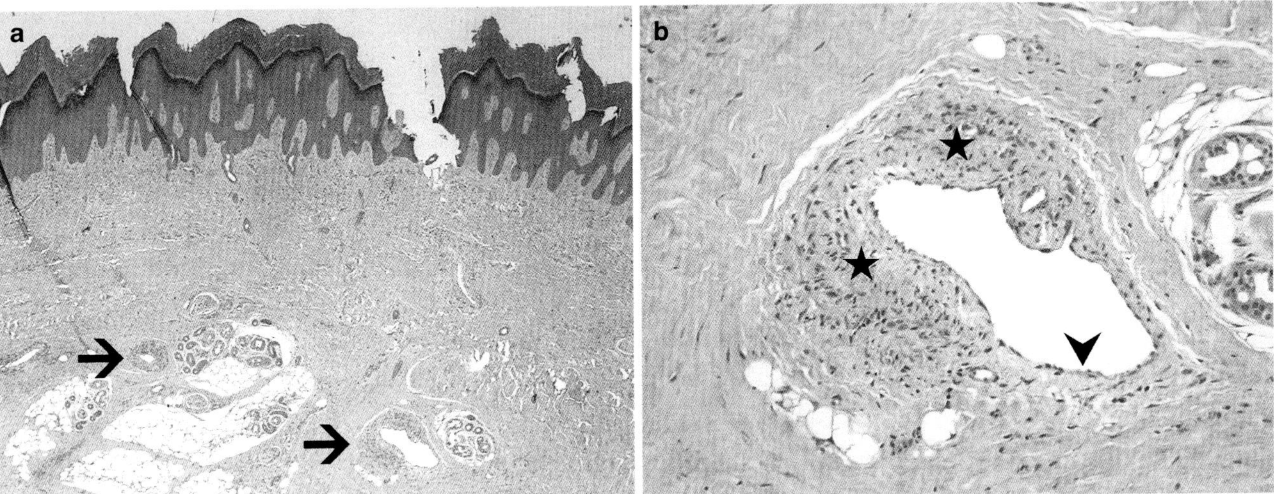

Fig. 12.3 Cutaneous blood vessel remodeling. Blood vessels in the dermis and subcutis of SSc patients show marked intimal and medial hypertrophy (→) with resultant luminal narrowing (**a**). A partially affected vessel allows direct comparison of normal wall thickness (▼) to that seen after remodeling (★) (**b**)

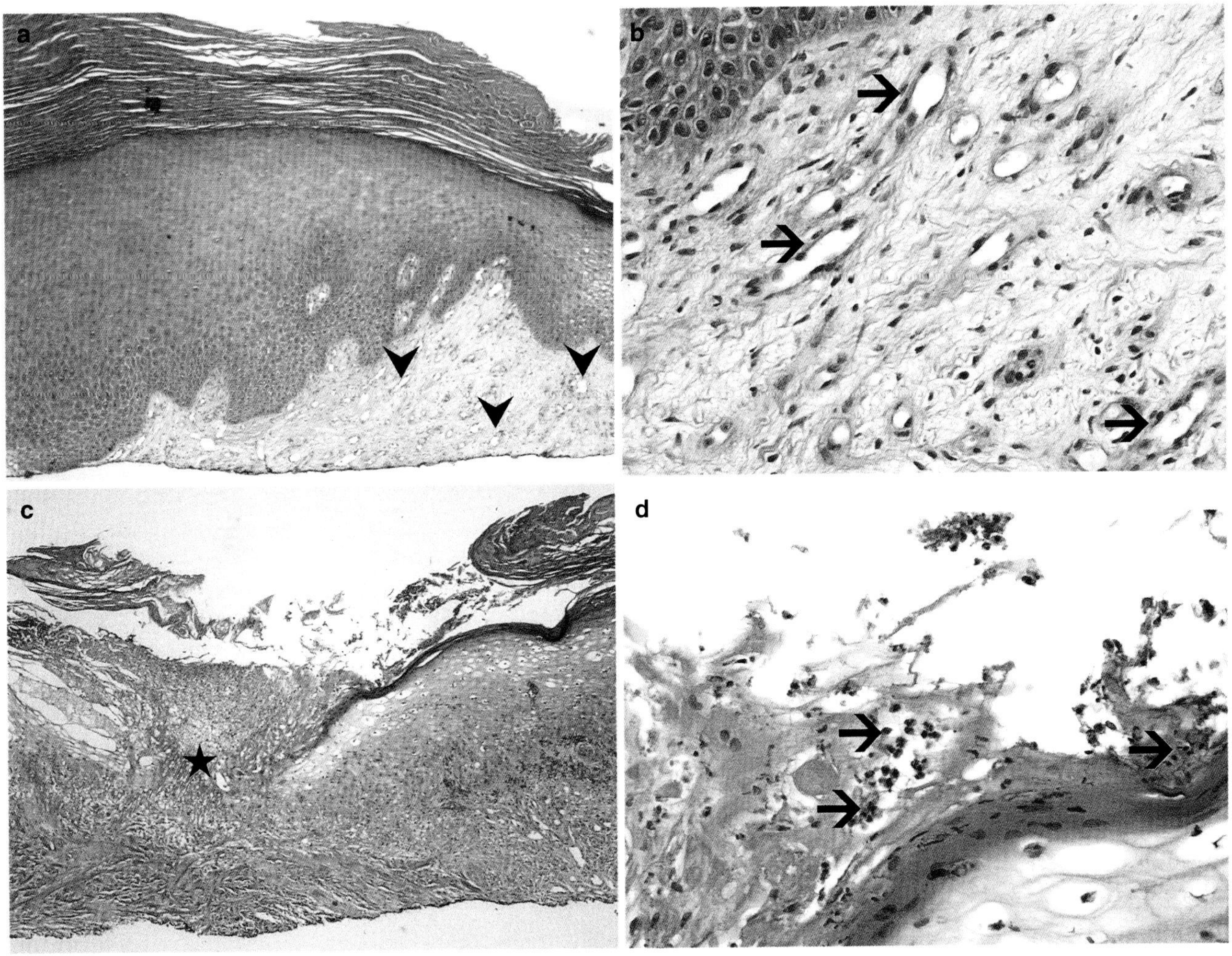

Fig. 12.4 Common dermatologic findings. SSc patients almost universally have telangiectasias with diffusely dilated dermal blood vessels (▼) (**a**). These blood vessels are thin-walled (→), without endothelial proliferation (**b**). In digital ulceration, the skin shows erosion of the epidermis (★) and underlying dermal tissue (**c**). Many neutrophils (→) can be seen in the associated fibrinopurulent inflammatory infiltrate (**d**). Deep subcutaneous arterioles in an amputation specimen demonstrate intimal and medial proliferation and fibrosis (▼) (**e**). The blood vessel shows complete luminal occlusion with associated hemosiderin deposition (→) (**f**). Calcinosis cutis demonstrates acellular deposition of purple calcified material (★) in the dermis and subcutis (**g**). Calcinosis cutis can have associated fibrosis and foreign body giant cell reaction (▼) (**h**)

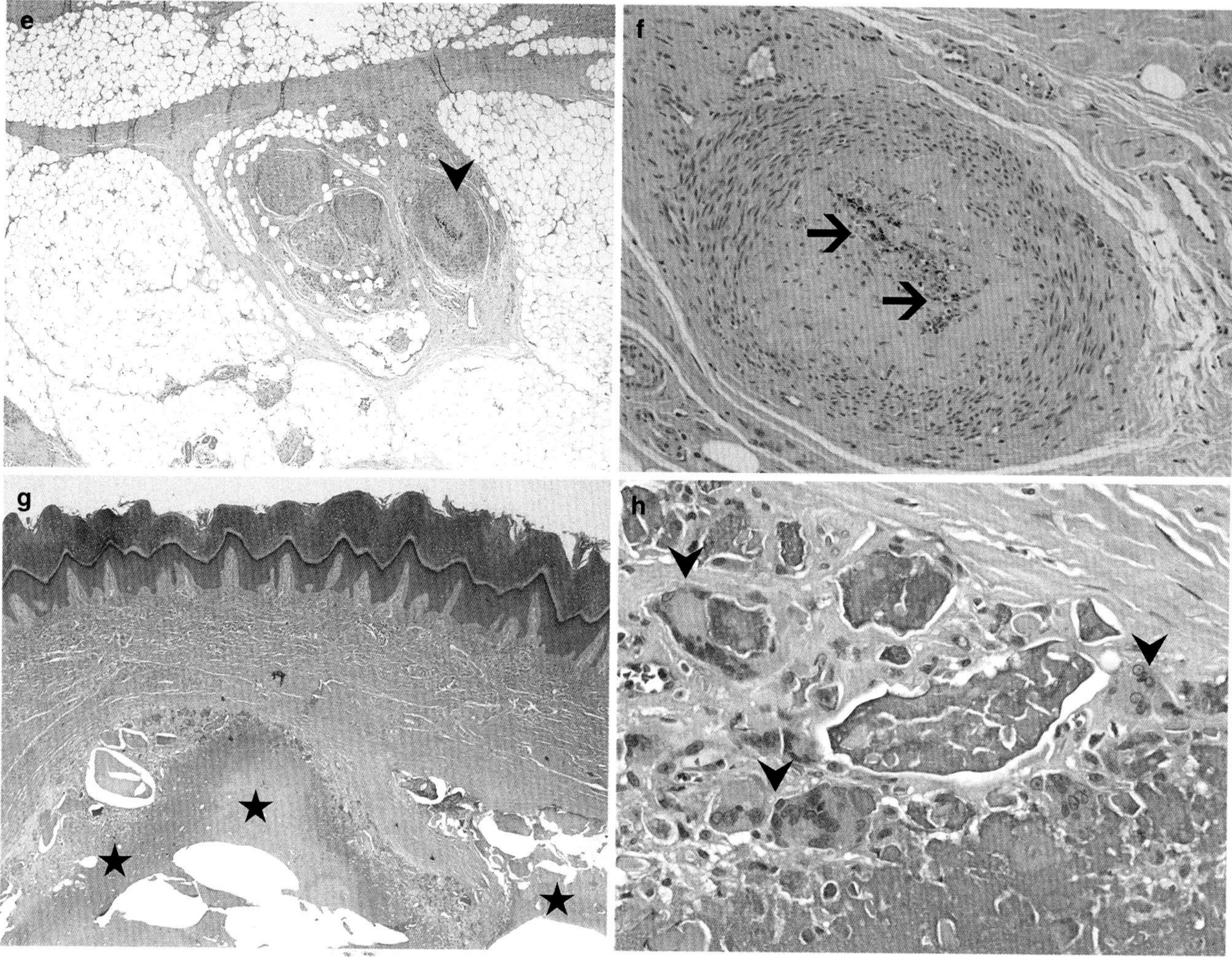

Fig. 12.4 (continued)

to vascular abnormalities seen in other diseases, telangiectasias in SSc do not represent vascular malformation or neovascularization but instead are simple dilations of the postcapillary venules of the upper dermal plexus [13]. As such, they lack endothelial proliferation or an organized growth pattern (Fig. 12.4b). They likely occur secondary to abnormalities in downstream blood flow [14].

Fingertip ulceration is another skin lesion that occurs frequently in SSc; it also counts toward the ACR/EULAR 2013 criteria for diagnosis [7]. Digital ulcers are more likely to occur in patients who present at a younger age and have more extensive skin involvement, and they are linked to earlier development of visceral organ involvement [14, 15]. Histologic sections show erosion of the epidermis and superficial dermis (Fig. 12.4c) with an overlying fibrinopurulent exudate (Fig. 12.4d). Ultimately, ulceration reflects tissue ischemia due to underlying vasculopathy. Affected vessels demonstrate intimal thickening, medial hypertrophy, and luminal occlusion (Fig. 12.4e, f). In 5.9 % of cases, resultant ischemia progresses beyond ulceration and culminates in digital amputation [16]. Gross examination of such fingers show black discoloration; gangrenous necrosis can be confirmed microscopically.

Approximately 25 % of limited cutaneous SSc patients develop calcinosis cutis, which frequently occurs 10 years or more after their diagnosis [17]. Although the exact mechanism is still unknown, calcinosis cutis is thought to arise when cellular injury provides a nidus for ectopic calcification in a setting of altered extracellular proteins [18]. Histologic sections show large mass-like deposits as well as smaller irregular accumulations of extracellular calcium in the dermis and subcutaneous tissue (Fig. 12.4g). Ulceration of the overlying epidermis and surrounding foreign body giant cell reaction, inflammation, or fibrosis may be seen in association with these lesions (Fig. 12.4h). Calcinosis cutis must be differentiated from other syndromes of aberrant calcification, including tumoral calcinosis, metastatic calcification, and calciphylaxis. While calcinosis cutis is classically associated with limited cutaneous SSc, it also occurs in the setting of diffuse cutaneous disease as well as several other autoimmune diseases [19].

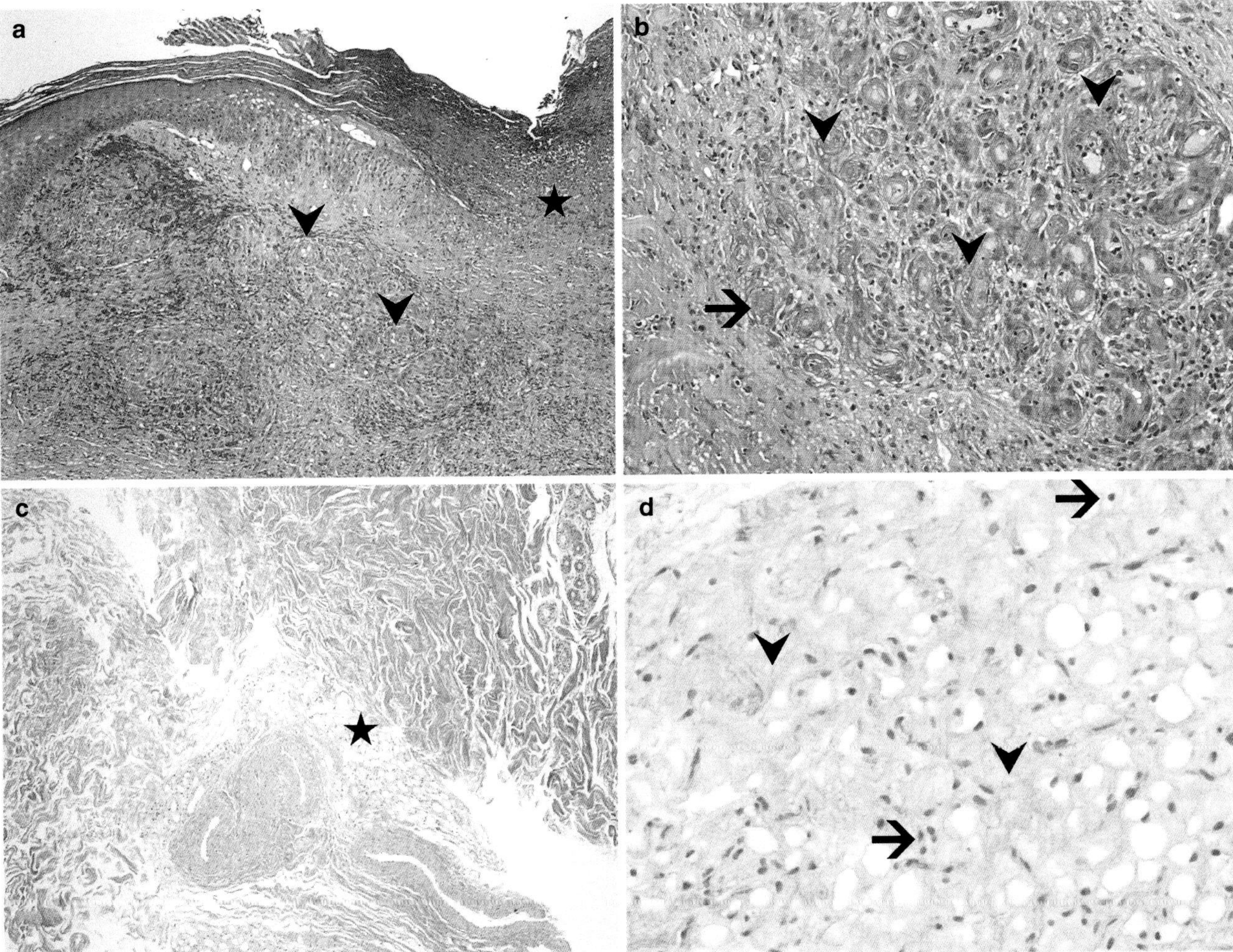

Fig. 12.5 Uncommon dermatologic complications. Livedoid vasculopathy is characterized by thickened and damaged dermal blood vessels (▼); it frequently leads to ulceration (★) of the overlying epithelium (**a**). A Periodic-Acid Schiff (PAS) stain highlights the fibrin deposition in the blood vessel walls (▼) and focal fibrin thrombi (→) (**b**). In lipodystrophy, the lipid mass (★) is decreased in the subcutaneous adipose tissue (**c**). There is hyalinization of the adipose cells (▼) with rare interspersed lymphocytes (→) (**d**)

In addition to the common skin findings described above, several rarer skin lesions have been associated with SSc. Livedoid vasculopathy, with resultant development of atrophie blanche, is one such uncommon complication [20]. Although early livedoid vasculopathy can have various clinical appearances, the histologic appearance is distinct with fibrin deposition within the lumens and walls of dermal blood vessels in the absence of inflammatory cells (Fig. 12.5a, b). As lesions progress, segmental infarction and hyalinization of the vessel walls develop. Older lesions are labeled atrophie blanche because of the distinctive ivory-white plaques seen on physical examination and microscopically show dermal sclerosis, scarring, epidermal atrophy, and dilated lymphatics. Livedoid vasculopathy is not unique to SSc and has been linked with a wide range of diseases that cause endothelial injury, including other autoimmune diseases and coagulopathies [21].

A final uncommon and nonspecific skin finding associated with SSc is lipodystrophy, which is thought to arise because of the local mechanical effects of fibrosis [22]. In a small series of SSc patients with limb ischemia, the prevalence of lipodystrophy was 50 % [23]. In this condition, the subcutaneous adipose tissue becomes atrophic (Fig. 12.5c), with loss of lipid volume, hyalinization of fibrous septae, and occasional mononuclear cell infiltrates (Fig. 12.5d). Other cases can demonstrate cystic structures lined by amorphous PAS-positive, diastase-resistant eosinophilic membranes [24]. Lipodystrophy can also be seen in isolation as a rare genetic disease, in various collagen vascular diseases, and as a consequence of chronic circulatory disturbance.

Pulmonary

Pulmonary complications currently represent the predominant cause of death among SSc patients, accounting for 33–60 % of disease-specific mortality [25–28]. Clinically, pulmonary disease in SSc tends to be classified as either interstitial fibrosis or pulmonary arterial hypertension (PAH), both of which are included in the ACR/EULAR 2013 criteria for diagnosis of SSc [7]. However, three distinct patterns of lung damage can be identified histologically: interstitial pneumonitis, pulmonary vascular damage, and bronchiolitis. All of these patterns of damage are thought to have their origins in similar pathways of inflammatory injury and microvascular remodeling [29, 30]. Although open lung biopsy is not always carried out in SSc patients because of high surgical risk and acceptable surrogate clinical studies, pathological evaluation can be useful to help evaluate the extent of disease and presence of overlapping histologic patterns [31].

Early autopsy studies found evidence of pulmonary fibrosis in 100 % of SSc patients [5, 32], while more recent series using high-resolution CT scans demonstrate some changes in 90 % (Solomon 2013). Overall, interstitial lung disease appears to be responsible for 19 % of SSc deaths [28]. Many of these end-stage lesions are best diagnosed as honeycomb change, which is characterized grossly and microscopically by extensive interstitial fibrosis with peripheral cyst formation. However, more distinctive pathologic findings can be seen in early lesions. On pathologic evaluation, between 50 % and 77 % of interstitial pneumonitis cases in SSc demonstrate a nonspecific interstitial pneumonia (NSIP) pattern [33–35]. Histologically, NSIP is characterized by temporally uniform lung damage with minimal to moderate interstitial fibrosis and interspersed chronic inflammation (Fig. 12.6a, c, e). It lacks the heterogeneity of the usual interstitial pneumonia (UIP) pattern described below. A minority of cases can be classified within the fibrotic subtype of NSIP, which demonstrates fibrosis with only minimal inflammation.

SSc-associated interstitial lung disease can also manifest in a UIP pattern, although these findings are seen in less than 10 % of cases [35]. UIP is a nonspecific but distinctive pattern of lung damage characterized by spatial and temporal heterogeneity (Fig. 12.6b). Histologic sections demonstrate simultaneous areas of acute lung injury with inflammation or diffuse alveolar damage, fibroblast foci reflecting ongoing subacute organizing injury, and old fibrosis (Fig. 12.6d, f). In contrast to patients with a clinical diagnosis of idiopathic pulmonary fibrosis, UIP that occurs in the setting of SSc tends to have more germinal centers and inflammation and fewer fibroblast foci [36, 37]. While patients with UIP have worse outcomes than NSIP in the general population and in some series of SSc patients [38], other investigators have observed that the outcome in SSc interstitial lung disease is more closely linked to disease severity at presentation than histologic pattern [35].

The estimated prevalence of PAH in SSc ranges from 8 % at cardiac catheterization to 49 % using echocardiography [39]. PAH is responsible for approximately 14 % of deaths in SSc [28]. In pathologic material, lesions of pulmonary hypertension can show a spectrum of histologic changes that are graded from least (grade I) to most severe (grade VI) using the modified Heath and Edwards classification [40]. Early lesions show medial then intimal hypertrophy, subsequent subintimal fibrosis in an onion-skin pattern, and eventual reduplication of the internal elastic lamina (Fig. 12.7a). Later disease demonstrates plexiform and glomeruloid nodules in small arteries with fibrin thrombi formation (Fig. 12.7b). Rarely, acute necrotizing arteritis with fibrinoid necrosis can be seen. It may be difficult to separate PAH in SSc from pulmonary hypertension associated with vascular and alveolar remodeling (honeycomb change) in patients with advanced interstitial lung disease; the latter patients have a markedly worse prognosis [41]. Nevertheless, there is clearly a subset of patients, mostly with limited SSc, who have pulmonary artery disease without interstitial lung disease [42].

Interestingly, patients with systemic sclerosis-associated PAH have also been shown to have a worse prognosis than idiopathic PAH [39]. Recent pathological studies have linked such outcomes to the almost uniform additional presence of veno-occlusive disease in SSc patients [43,44]. Histologically, such venous pathology can be identified as fibrosis and intimal proliferation of preseptal venules and veins (Fig. 12.7c). Systemic sclerosis patients also can have coexisting interstitial pneumonitis and PAH, which not only complicates the diagnosis as described above, but also contributes to worse outcomes by decreasing pulmonary reserve [44]. Moreover, SSc patients also have a high risk of pulmonary thromboembolism, which can still further compound vascular disease (Fig. 12.8).

Finally, perhaps the least well-recognized pulmonary manifestation of SSc is constrictive and/or lymphocytic bronchiolitis. Between 13 % and 25 % of SSc patients are estimated to demonstrate small airway disease [45]. Although most patients are asymptomatic, the resultant decrease in the maximal mid-expiratory flow rate can come to clinical attention in patients with other pulmonary pathology [45]. Histologic sections of SSc-associated bronchiolitis show a chronic inflammatory infiltrate involving the submucosa of terminal and respiratory bronchioles. Affected airways may demonstrate luminal constriction, fibrosis, and smooth muscle proliferation (Fig. 12.9a, b). Similar microscopic findings can be seen in other autoimmune diseases, particularly Sjogren syndrome, as well as in drug reactions [45].

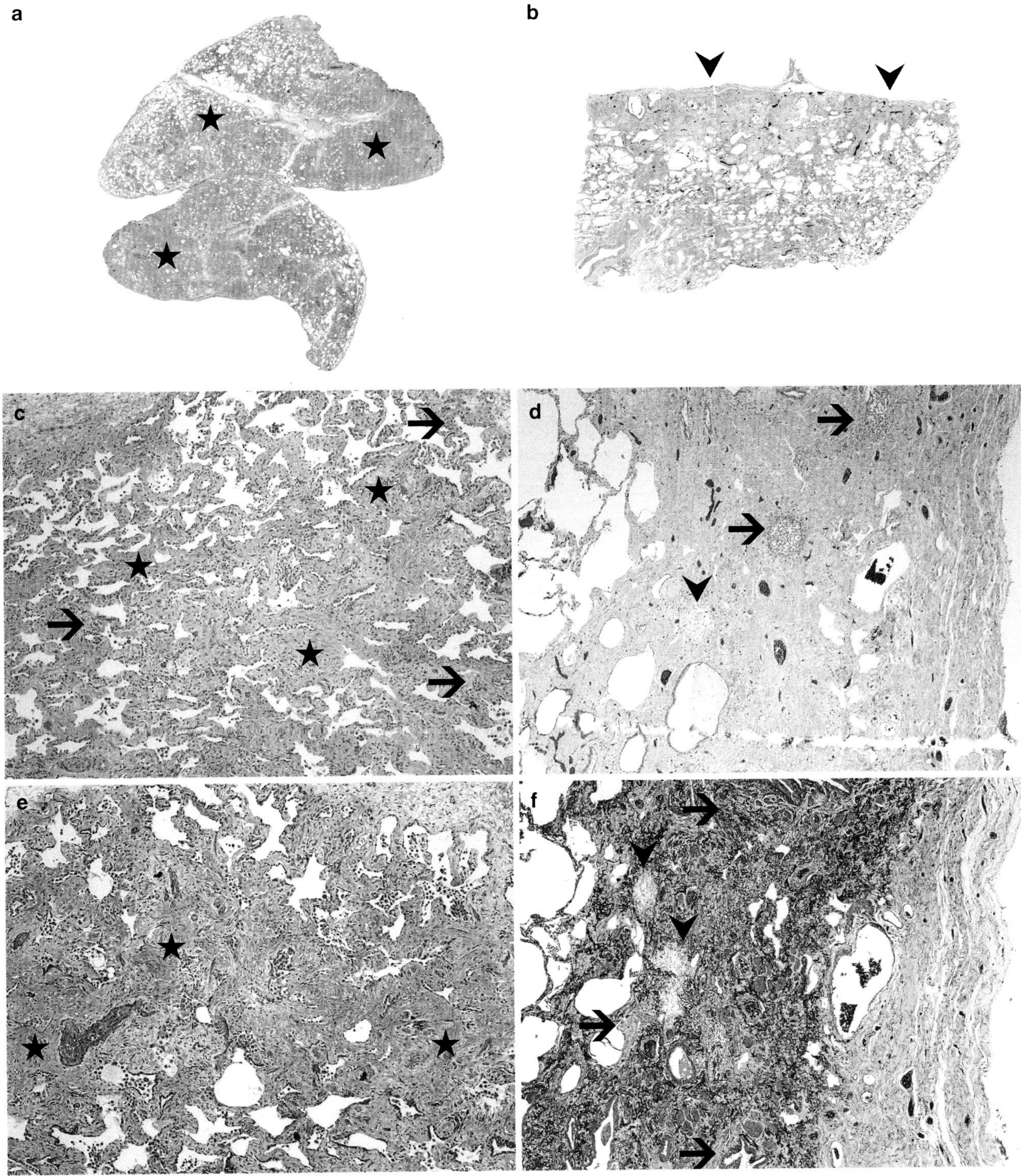

Fig. 12.6 Interstitial lung disease. At low power, non-specific interstitial fibrosis (NSIP) shows homogenous involvement with similar degrees of fibrosis in most areas (★) of the lung (**a**) while usual interstitial pneumonitis (UIP) has subpleural (▼) accentuation (**b**). At higher power, NSIP demonstrates moderate interstitial fibrosis (★) with interspersed chronic inflammatory cells (→) (**c**). A Masson trichrome (Masson) stain highlights the fibrosis in blue (★) (**e**). UIP demonstrates more lymphoid aggregates (→) and fewer fibroblast foci (▼) in SSc than would be expected in idiopathic pulmonary fibrosis (**d**). A Movat pentachrome stain emphasizes the temporal and spatial heterogeneity, with fibroblast foci staining light blue (▼) and old fibrosis staining yellow (→) (**f**)

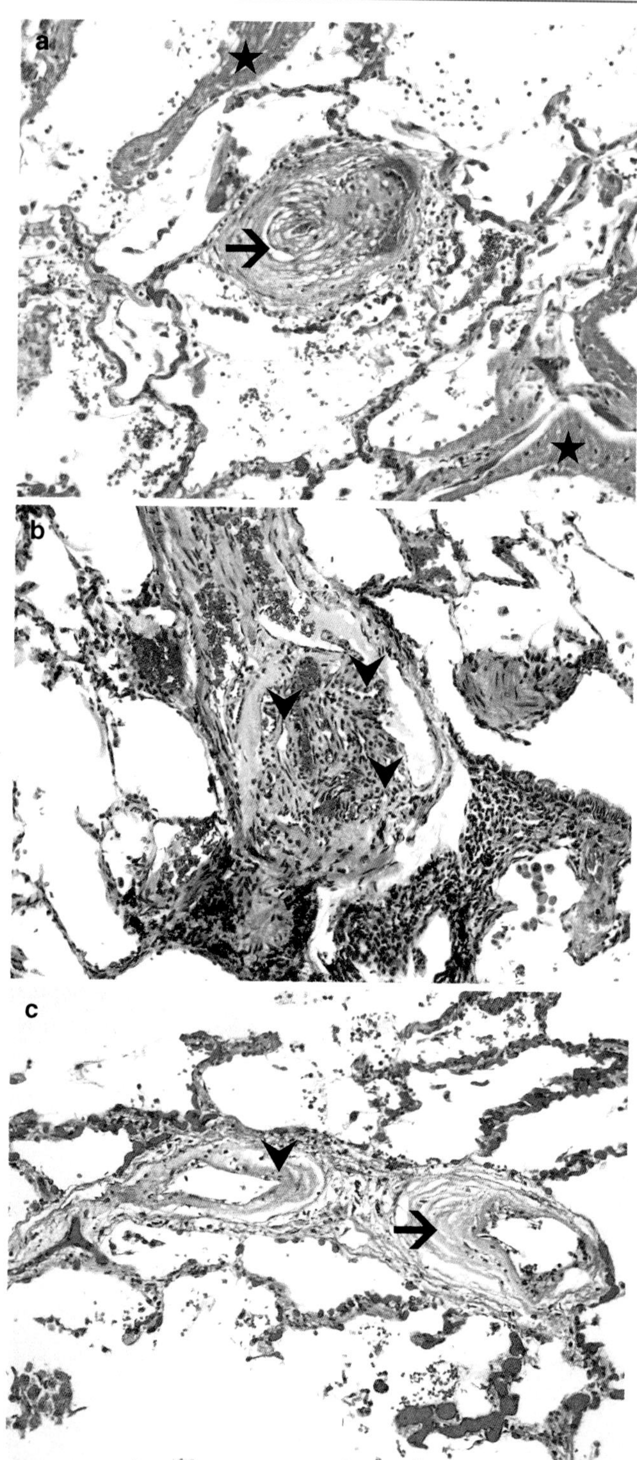

Fig. 12.7 Pulmonary vascular disease. Early lesions of pulmonary artery hypertension (PAH) in SSc demonstrate intimal hypertrophy with onion-skin fibrosis (→) of the vessel wall. In this case, the surrounding lung also demonstrates diffuse alveolar damage with hyaline membranes (★) (**a**). Later lesions of PAH have plexiform vascular proliferation with many small vascular channels (▼) in a previously obstructed vessel (**b**). PAH in SSc also shows veno-occlusive disease with intimal proliferation (→) and fibrosis (▼) of preseptal venules (**c**).

Such constrictive or obliterative bronchiolitis must be separated both morphologically and semantically from the intraluminal fibrosis seen in bronchiolitis obliterans organizing pneumonia (BOOP) [46].

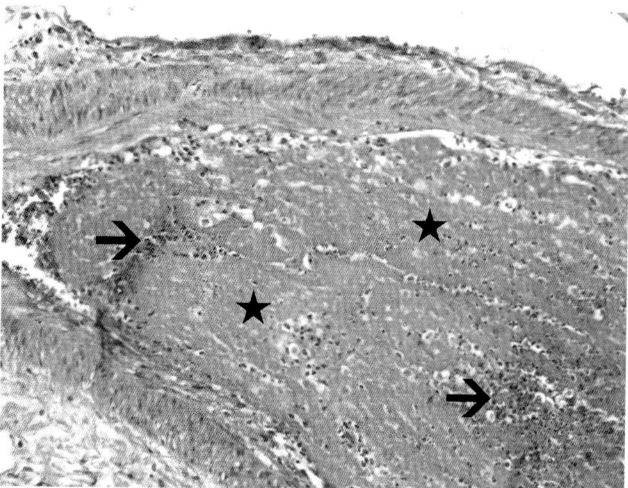

Fig. 12.8 Organizing thromboembolus with intermixed fibrin (★) and inflammatory cells (→). Pulmonary thromboembolism can complicate PAH in SSc patients

Renal

While the historically high mortality rate of scleroderma renal crisis meant that renal disease was once responsible for 42 % of deaths in SSc patients, the use of angiotensin converting enzyme inhibitors have decreased the death rate from renal complications to less than 6 % in recent years [25, 47, 48]. However, the existence of highly effective treatments makes it all the more essential to diagnose this condition in an accurate and timely manner. Although appropriate clinical findings can strongly favor scleroderma renal crisis, kidney biopsy is required to definitively differentiate it from overlap syndromes or other unrelated conditions; it also can provide important prognostic information. Moreover, histological examination is essential in the 10 % of renal crisis patients who are normotensive at presentation [49]. It is also important to note that scleroderma renal crisis is not the only manifestation of SSc in the kidneys; chronic kidney disease and inflammatory conditions are also seen histologically.

Scleroderma renal crisis occurs in up to 15 % of SSc patients [49]. If examined grossly, affected kidneys demonstrate multiple surface petechial hemorrhages and wedge-shaped cortical infarcts. In early disease, histologic sections show accumulation of myxoid material in the intima of interlobular arteries (Fig. 12.10a, b), while afferent arterioles demonstrate fibrinoid necrosis (Fig. 12.10c, d). Later on, vessels undergo intimal proliferation in an onion-skin pattern (Fig. 12.10e, f), while glomeruli develop ischemic changes with collapse and wall thickening (Fig. 12.10g, h). These findings are identical to those seen in malignant hypertension but are distinguishable from other thrombotic microangiopathies because of the predominance of small vessel involvement over glomerular changes [50]. Patients with extensive vascular thrombosis, severe glomerular ischemic collapse, and peritubular capillary C4d deposits at biopsy have been

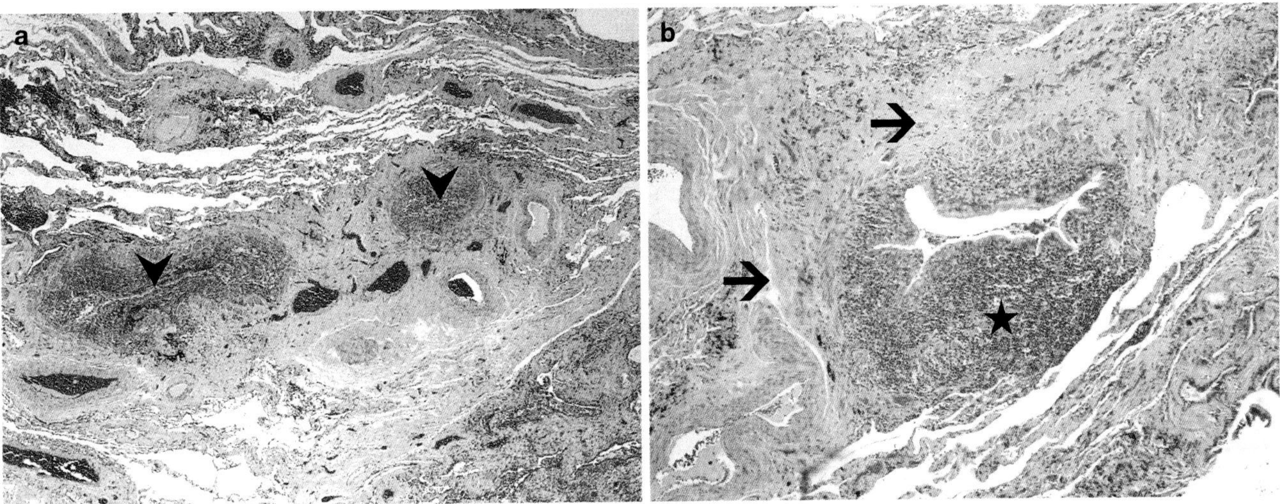

Fig. 12.9 Follicular and constrictive bronchiolitis. At low power, the bronchial lumen (▼) is largely obliterated (**a**). Peribronchial fibrosis (→) and a prominent lymphoid aggregate (★) are highlighted at higher power (**b**)

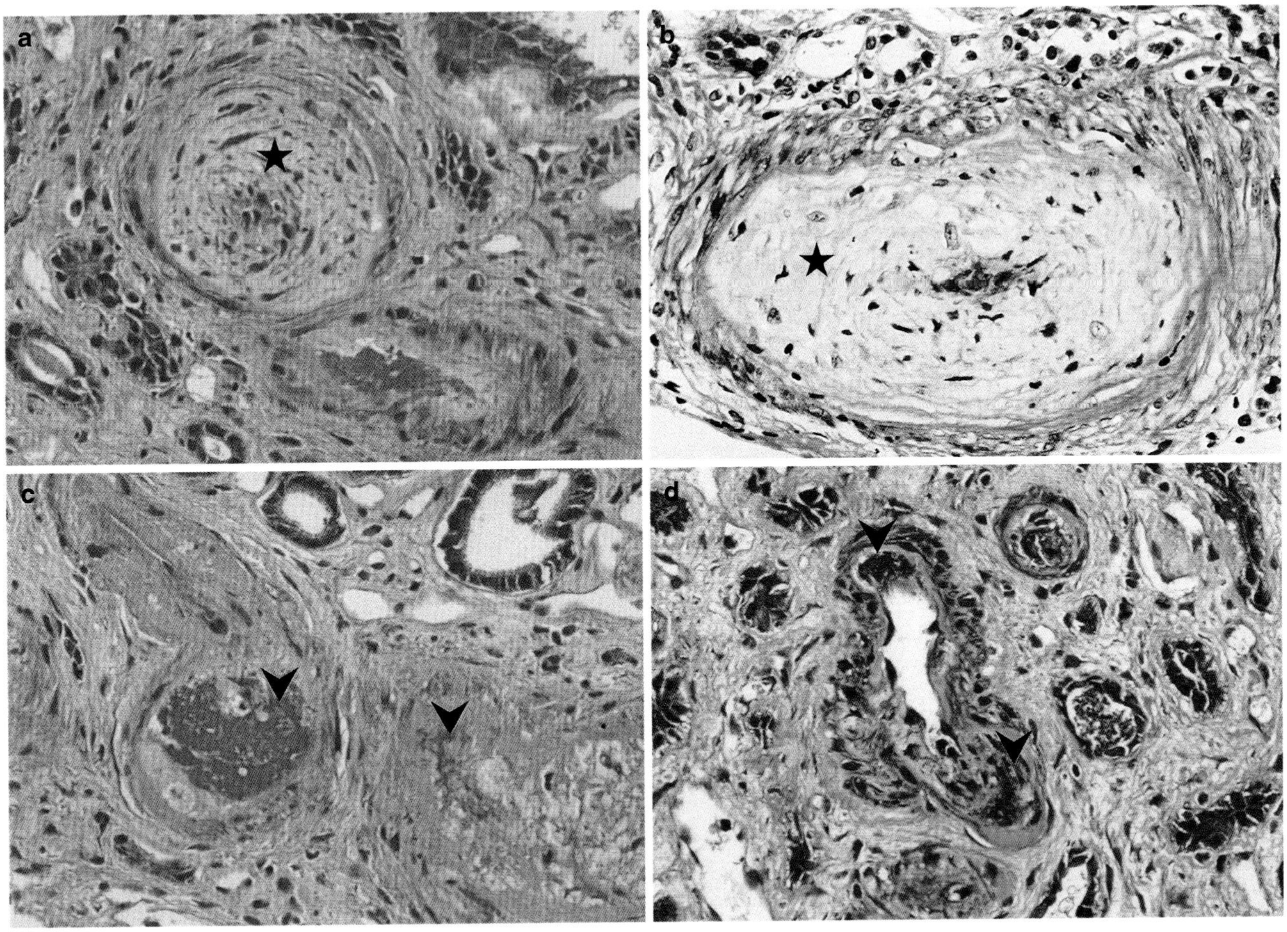

Fig. 12.10 Scleroderma renal crisis. In early scleroderma renal crisis, myxoid material is deposited in the intima (★) of interlobular arteries (**a**). A Masson stain highlights the grey-blue myxoid material (★) in the intima surrounded by red muscle fibers in the media (**b**). Fibrinoid necrosis of afferent arterioles with red blood cells in vessel walls (▼) is also characteristic of early changes in scleroderma renal crisis (**c**). On trichrome, the fibrinoid necrosis appears bright red (▼) (**d**). Chronic changes in scleroderma renal crisis include onion-skin change (→) in renal blood vessels (**e**). A VVG emphasizes the reduplication of elastic fibers (→) in the vessel media (**f**). A PAS stain highlights thickening (▼) and wrinkling (→) of glomerular capillary loops (→) (**g**). Capillary wall collapse and thickening (→) is emphasized on a PAS-Methamine Silver stain (**h**).

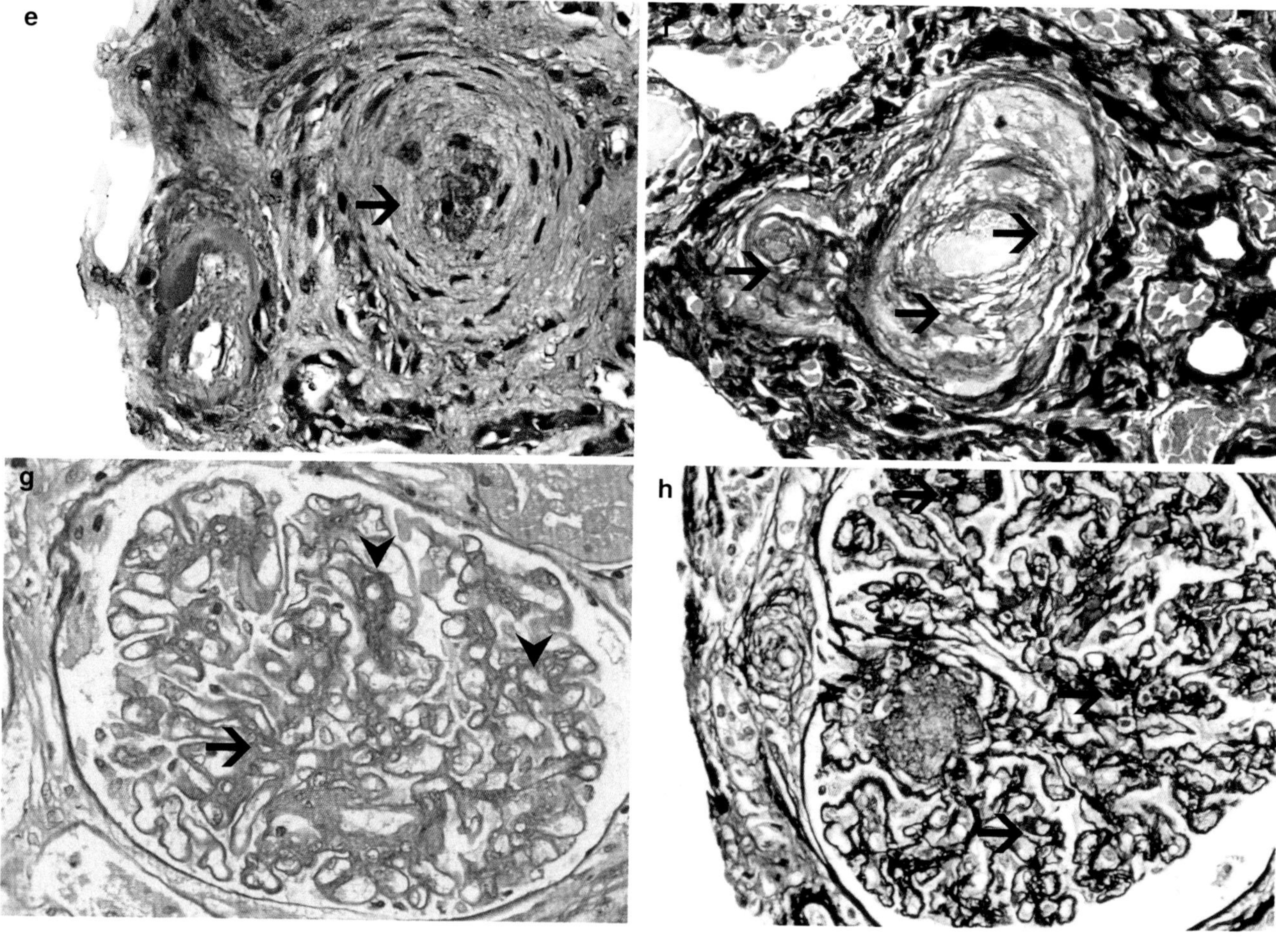

Fig. 12.10 (continued)

shown to have an increased risk of irreversible renal failure and death [51].

Other evidence of chronic kidney disease can also be identified histologically in SSc patients. Even patients who never demonstrated symptoms of scleroderma renal crisis can show some of the characteristic vascular changes, particularly vascular fibrosis and accumulation of extracellular matrix material [5, 50] (Fig. 12.11a, b). Less specific evidence of chronic vasculopathy and surrounding renal parenchymal damage is frequently seen as well, including intimal fibrosis, tubulointerstitial fibrosis, tubular atrophy, and interstitial chronic inflammation [52] (Fig. 12.11c, d). In contrast to most other autoimmune diseases, underlying chronic renal disease does not correlate with prognosis in scleroderma renal crisis, and some investigators postulate that it is somehow protective against the more damaging acute injury [53].

Finally, inflammatory renal disease is another rare complication of SSc. Parenchymal inflammation is not classically associated with scleroderma renal crisis but is not uncommon in acute episodes. A wide range of different inflammatory findings have also been reported in SSc outside of renal crisis, including focal segmental glomerulonephritis, mesangioproliferative glomerulonephritis, and diffuse membranous glomerulonephritis [54]. Several cases of ANCA-associated vasculitis, including granulomatosis with polyangiitis, microscopic polyangiitis, and Churg-Strauss syndrome have been reported in association with SSc and may represent an uncommon overlap syndrome [55, 56]. Histologic findings in these cases include crescentic glomerulonephritis.

Cardiovascular

Cardiovascular disease is the cause of death in 14–36 % of all SSc cases [28, 47, 48, 57], a proportion that is similar to the recognized incidence of clinically symptomatic cardiovascular disease in these patients [58]. However, both radiologic and autopsy studies have reported much higher rates of cardiac involvement, with subclinical disease identified in up to 100 % of patients in some series [5, 59, 60]. Although myocardial biopsy is occasionally performed on these patients, the heart is rarely assessed

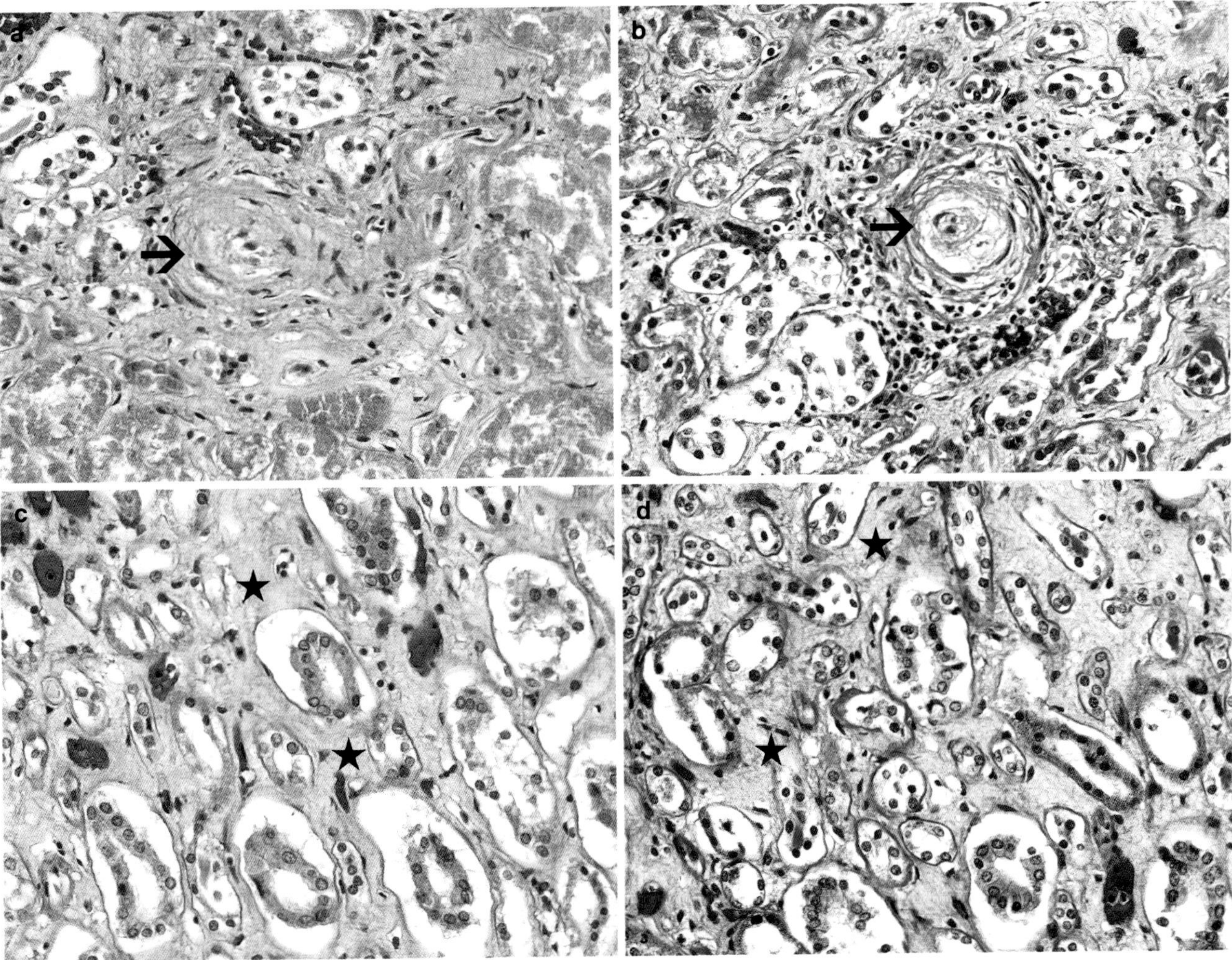

Fig. 12.11 Chronic kidney disease. Even patients with no history of scleroderma renal crisis can show onion-skin changes (→) in renal vessel walls (**a**). A Masson stain emphasizes accompanying fibrosis (→) of the vessel walls (**b**). Kidneys also demonstrate interstitial scarring (★) (**c**). A Masson stain highlights the interstitial fibrosis (★) (**d**)

pathologically in SSc outside the autopsy setting. Nevertheless, a wide range of cardiac manifestations can be identified in pathologic material from SSc patients, including myocardial fibrosis, microvascular disease, atherosclerotic coronary artery disease, pericarditis, and secondary cor pulmonale.

The hallmark histologic lesion of SSc is patchy myocardial fibrosis, which contributes to the cardiac arrhythmias and impaired contractility that are appreciated clinically. As in other organ systems affected by SSc, this fibrosis is thought to arise secondary to microvascular abnormalities [61]. At autopsy, scarring is grossly visible within the myocardium of SSc patients in only a few cases. However, patchy replacement of cardiac myocytes with acellular collagenous material can be seen microscopically throughout the heart (Fig. 12.12a, b). Unlike the myocardial fibrosis characteristic of atherosclerotic cardiovascular disease, that seen in SSc can affect the immediate subendocardial layer and tends to lack associated hemosiderin deposition [5, 60]. Rarely, fibrosis extends directly into the endocardium and even involves cardiac valves (Fig. 12.13).

Despite the central role of microvascular pathology in precipitating the aforementioned fibrosis, it is uncommon to see histologic evidence of actual microcirculatory obstruction in SSc patients. Instead, autopsy studies have documented a wide range of underlying vascular abnormalities in coronary arteries of <1 mm in size, including fibrinoid necrosis, mural fibrosis, intimal proliferation, and medial hyperplasia, with rare identification of luminal obstruction by platelet-fibrin clots (Fig. 12.14) [62]. The more frequently reported indication of microvascular obstruction is contraction band necrosis in the absence of atherosclerotic coronary vascular disease [5, 63]. Overall, these changes reflect decreased reserve capacity in the cardiac microvasculature, precipitating intermittent ischemia, and eventually fibrosis [64].

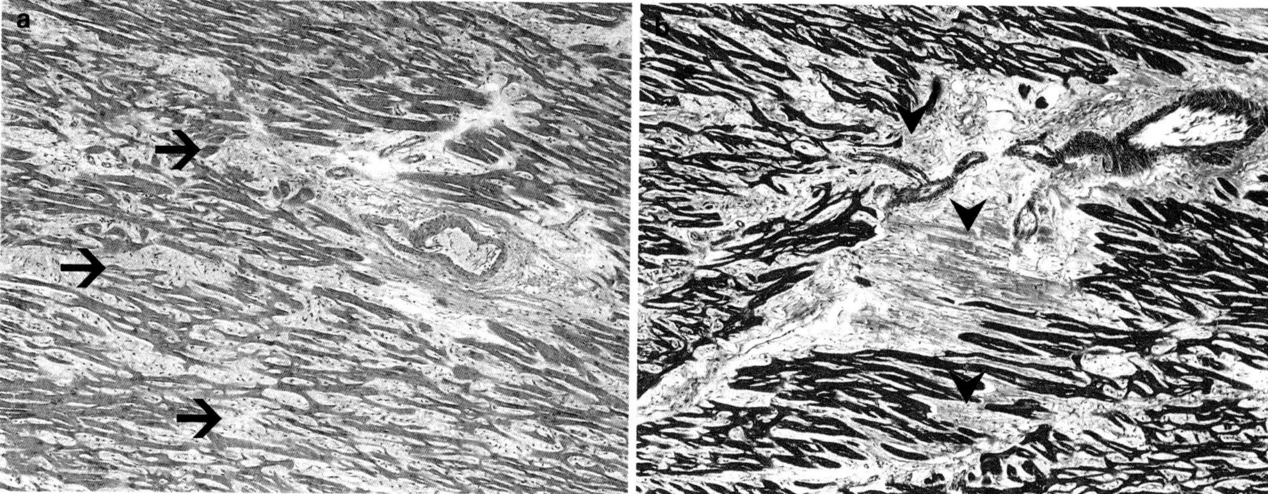

Fig. 12.12 Myocardial fibrosis. Patients with SSc demonstrate patchy myocardial fibrosis (→) throughout the heart (**a**). A Masson stain highlights the replacement of red cardiac myocytes with blue-staining fibrosis (▼) (**b**)

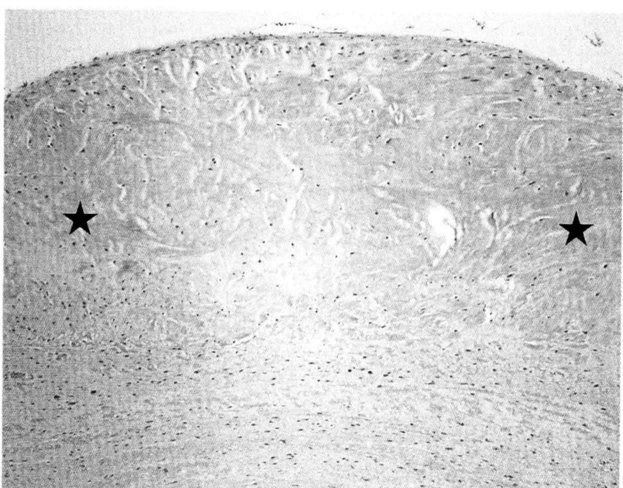

Fig. 12.13 Valve fibrosis. The aortic valve from a scleroderma patient shows increased fibrosis (★)

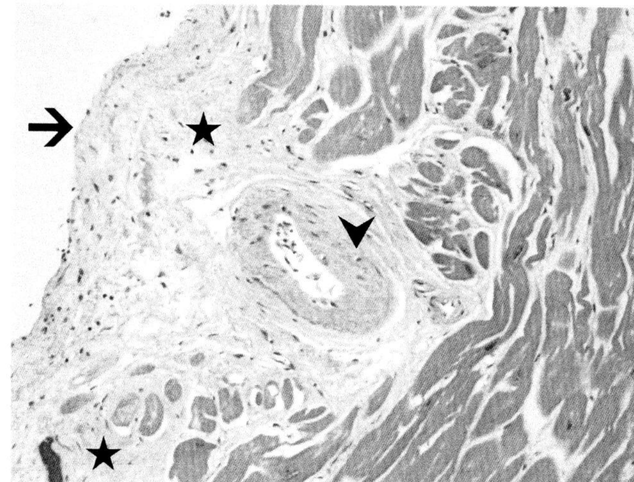

Fig. 12.14 Myocardial blood vessel remodeling. The cardiac microcirculation in SSc can demonstrate thickening of the tunica media (▼). Surrounding fibrosis (▼), which can extend into the endothelium (→) as well as the myocardium, suggests periodic ischemia

The question of systemic large-vessel involvement in SSc is also not entirely resolved. While older autopsy studies reported that the rates of atherosclerotic cardiovascular disease in SSc was no higher than that in the unaffected population [5, 60], more recent imaging studies have demonstrated that some SSc patients do experience accelerated atherosclerosis, similar to that seen in other systemic inflammatory disease [61, 65]. Regardless of specific etiology, the atherosclerosis seen in SSc patients appears identical to that arising from more frequent causes. Affected arteries have thickened intima and occlusion by atheromatous plaques containing abundant foamy macrophages and cholesterol clefts with an overlying fibrous cap.

Pericardial disease is another common pathologic finding in systemic sclerosis. Large autopsy studies have suggested that up to 62 % of SSc patients show evidence of acute pericarditis [5, 60, 63], even though reviews identify clinical symptoms in only 5–16 % of patients [65]. Grossly, the affected pericardium appears dull and roughened. Microscopic sections demonstrate a fibrinous exudate on the pericardial surface with intermixed acute and chronic inflammatory cells (Fig. 12.15). Patients frequently develop a pericardial effusion in association with pericarditis, although pericardial tamponade is rare. Cytologic examination of the pericardial fluid generally demonstrates reactive mesothelial cells, histiocytes, and variable numbers of acute and chronic inflammatory cells.

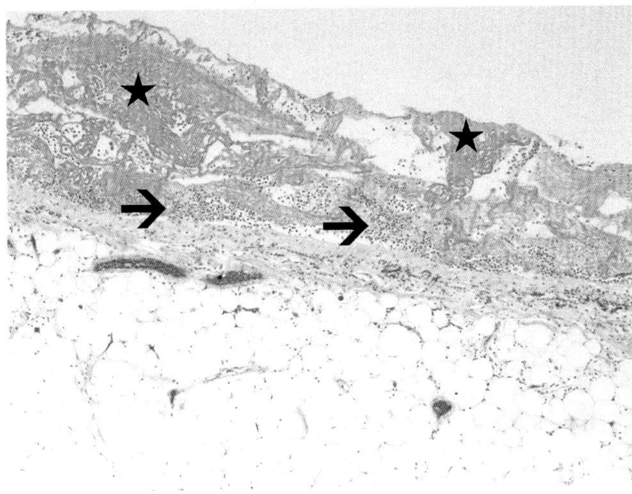

Fig. 12.15 Fibrinous pericarditis. SSc patients commonly have a pericardial exudate with fibrin deposition (★) and a prominent acute inflammatory infiltrate (→)

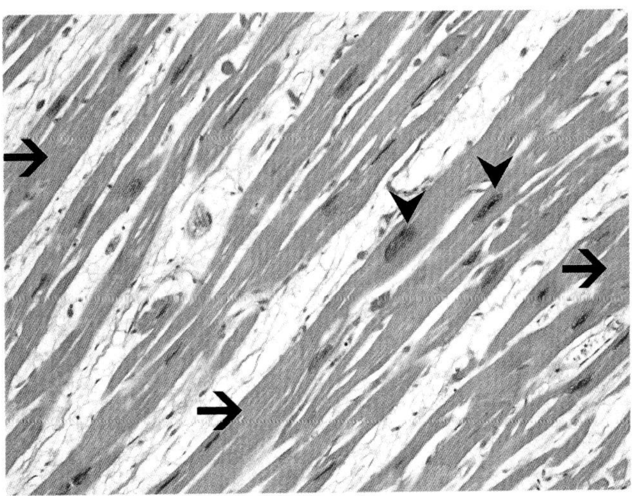

Fig. 12.16 Myocyte hypertrophy. The right ventricle shows marked hypertrophy with nuclear (▼) and cytoplasmic (→) enlargement secondary to pulmonary hypertension

Finally, cardiovascular pathology can also arise secondary to the aforementioned pulmonary complications of SSc. Most notably, heart failure is a common consequence of pulmonary arterial hypertension and is thought to be a determining factor in the prognosis of affected patients [66]. Pathologically, the findings in cor pulmonale in SSc are indistinguishable from those in patients without underlying autoimmune disease. At gross examination, the heart demonstrates hypertrophy and dilation of both the right atrium and ventricle, with normal to increased wall thickness and enlarged cardiac chambers. Microscopically, individual cardiac myocytes also demonstrate marked hypertrophy, with simultaneous nuclear and cytoplasmic enlargement (Fig. 12.16).

Gastrointestinal

Although gastrointestinal (GI) complications are responsible for fewer than 10 % of SSc-related deaths, they affect more than 90 % of SSc patients and represent a considerable source of morbidity and decreased quality of life [67, 68]. GI biopsy can be very helpful in SSc patients to differentiate complications of the disease from more treatable conditions such as *Helicobacter pylori* infection or drug reactions. Other GI manifestations of SSc can be seen pathologically when surgical resection is employed in management. While many of the GI complications of SSc have similar appearances throughout the GI tract, other manifestations are site specific. Findings include fibrosis of the muscularis propria, gastroesophageal reflux, mucosal ulceration, thermal injury, telangiectasias, and gastric antral vascular ectasia.

As in the myocardium, muscular fibrosis is the pathognomonic lesion of SSc in the GI tract. In one large autopsy series, 74 % of patients with SSc demonstrated fibrosis or atrophy of the esophageal muscularis propria, while 48 % and 39 %, respectively, demonstrated such changes in the small and large bowel [5]. Grossly, these organs are characterized by stiff, thin walls and can have wide-mouthed diverticula [69]. Microscopic sections demonstrate collagenous replacement of the muscularis propria, often with associated wall thinning and flattening of the overlying epithelium (Fig. 12.17a–d). Perforation is a common complication of this process. As in other organ systems, vasculopathy is thought to be the underlying cause of fibrosis [70], and intimal thickening of muscularis propria vessels is frequently observed histologically (Fig. 12.18).

The impaired smooth muscle motility that results from such fibrosis can lead to additional complications for SSc patients. While obstruction, malabsorption, delayed gastric emptying, and constipation are primarily clinical diagnoses [71], defects in motility often lead to direct mucosal injury that can be appreciated pathologically. The most common such injury is gastroesophageal reflux. On biopsy, the esophageal mucosa demonstrates basal cell hyperplasia, elongation of the lamina propria into the upper third of the epithelium, and scattered intraepithelial eosinophils (Fig. 12.19a). Prolonged reflux underlies the propensity to develop Barrett esophagus in SSc patients, with an estimated incidence of 6.8–12.7 % and an attendant increased risk of esophageal adenocarcinoma [71]. Biopsy of Barrett lesions shows distinctive incomplete intestinal metaplasia of the esophageal mucosa. Reflux also has a strong association with the development of interstitial lung disease [72].

Other forms of mucosal injury can also be seen in SSc patients. Mucosal erosion and ulceration can result from a number of causes throughout the GI tract, including bacterial

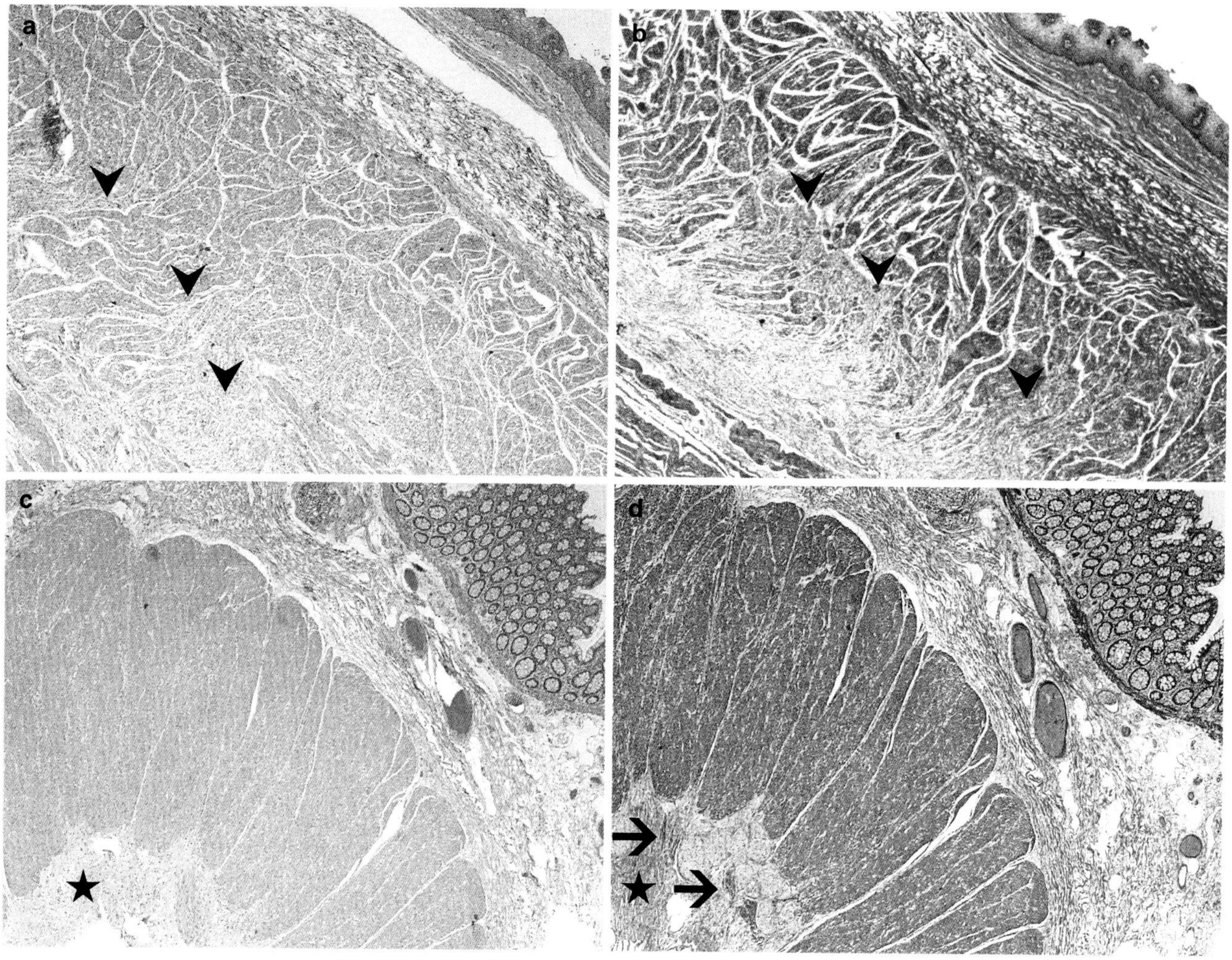

Fig. 12.17 Gastrointestinal smooth muscle fibrosis. A section of esophagus demonstrates partial fibrosis of the inner circular layer of the muscularis propria, barely visible as areas of pale pink collagen on H&E (▼) (**a**). A Masson stain highlights the fibrils of collagen in blue (▼) interdigitating between red muscle fibers. Likewise, there is almost complete replacement of the outer longitudinal muscle of this colon with pale pink fibrosis (★) (**c**). A Masson stain highlights the complete fibrosis in blue (★) with only rare remaining red muscle fibers (→) (**d**)

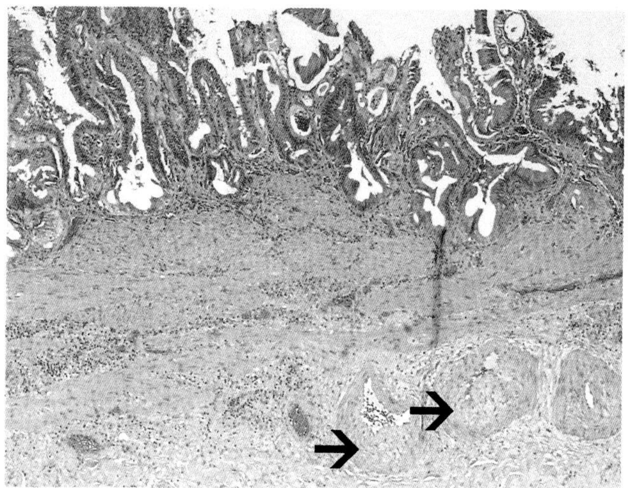

Fig. 12.18 Gastrointestinal blood vessel remodeling. Asymmetric intimal and medial hypertrophy (→) is seen in blood vessels within the gallbladder muscularis propria of an SSc patient

overgrowth, obstruction, and mechanical trauma [69]. Similar to sampling of skin ulcerations, biopsies of these lesions demonstrate a loss of surface epithelium with associated fibrinopurulent inflammatory exudate (Fig. 12.19b). A more specific injury pattern occurs in the esophagus when impaired esophageal peristalsis allows hot substances to have prolonged contact with the mucosal surfaces, leading to thermal damage. Histologically, this appears as mummification of the upper third of the epithelium with coagulative necrosis, loss of nuclear basophilia, and separation from the underlying layers of cells (Fig. 12.19c).

Vascular pathology is also common within the GI mucosa in SSc. Indeed, 15 % of SSc patients experience GI hemorrhage at some point during their illness [69]. Telangiectasias are the most common source of GI bleeding but are rarely biopsied. Histologically, they appear as dilated blood vessels in the lamina propria, similar to those seen in the skin. Another rare source of GI bleeding frequently linked to SSc is gastric antral vascular ectasia (GAVE) [73]. This condition

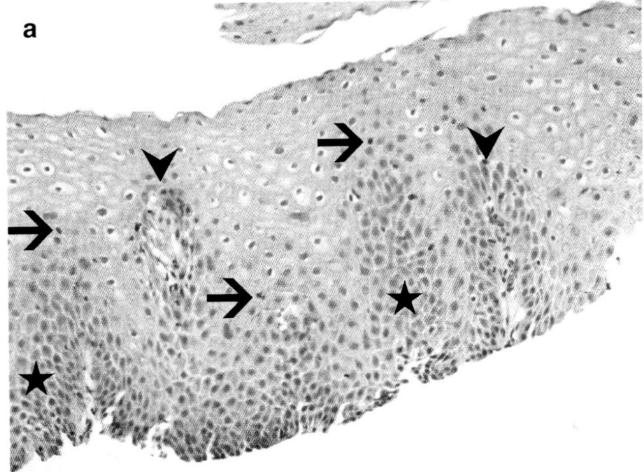

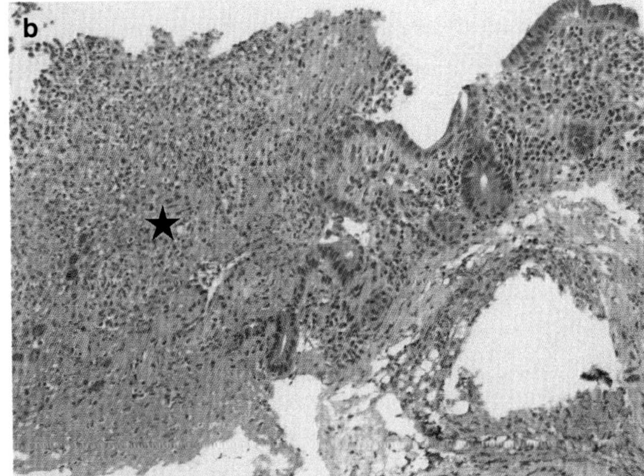

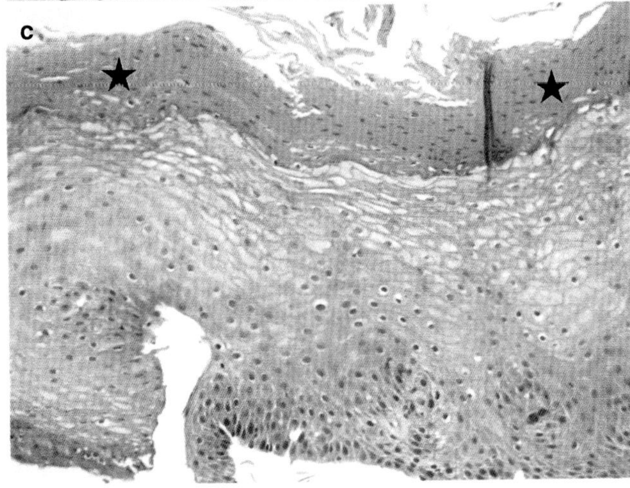

Fig. 12.19 Gastrointestinal mucosal injury. In reflux esophagitis, the epithelium displays basal cell hyperplasia (★), elongation of the rete ridges into the upper third of the epithelium (→), and intraepithelial eosinophils (→) (**a**). Colonic ulceration results in loss of surface epithelium and lamina propria with associated fibrinopurulent exudate (★) (**b**). Thermal injury in the esophagus demonstrates coagulative necrosis of the upper third of the epithelium (→) (**c**).

is colloquially known as watermelon stomach because dilated blood vessels in the antrum grossly appear as parallel red stripes, similar to a watermelon rind. Biopsies show dilated vessels in the lamina propria plugged by fibrin thrombi, reactive changes in surrounding epithelial cells, and smooth muscle hyperplasia of the lamina propria (Fig. 12.20).

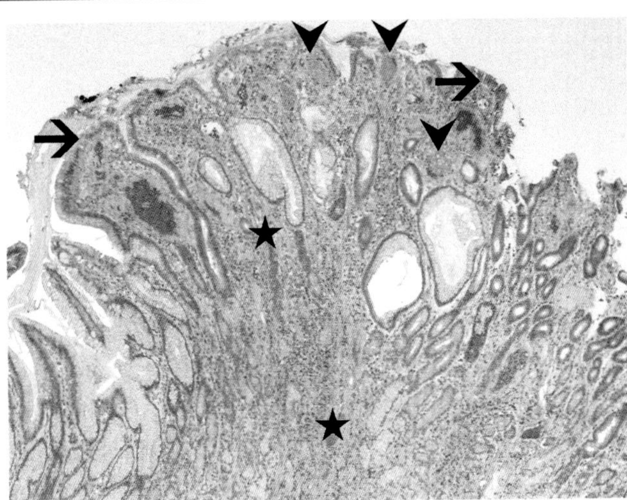

Fig. 12.20 Gastric antral vascular ectasia. There are fibrin thrombi in lamina propria vessels (▼), reactive epithelial changes (→), and foveolar hyperplasia with prominent smooth muscle bundles (★)

Musculoskeletal

Although musculoskeletal involvement is not as widely recognized in SSc as in other autoimmune diseases, it also represents a significant source of disability and decreased quality of life for affected patients [68]. Approximately 24 % of SSc patients demonstrate proximal limb weakness [16], and 20–86 % report muscle or joint pain [74]. Although histologic assessment of muscle and joint tissue is rarely made in clinical practice, these tissues do demonstrate characteristic pathologic findings. Musculoskeletal involvement includes skeletal muscle inflammation and fibrosis, tendon fibrosis, and synovitis.

Muscular involvement in SSc has two main manifestations: atrophy and inflammation. Histologically, 41 % of SSc patients demonstrate skeletal muscular atrophy at autopsy, while 8 % show myositis with chronic inflammation [5]. Sections of skeletal muscle demonstrate a wide range of nonspecific findings. Myocyte atrophy can be identified with loss of contractile fibers, perimysial and epimysial fibrosis, fibrous replacement of muscle cells, rare necrosis, and variable degrees of regeneration (Fig. 12.21). Inflammation tends to consist of a mild mononuclear cell infiltrate involving the muscle parenchyma. Overall, the muscular findings in SSc are indistinguishable from patients with polymyositis and dermatomyositis [74].

In addition to direct involvement of skeletal muscle, SSc also can affect tendons. Clinically, tendon disease is measured by the presence of tendon friction rubs, defined as a rubbing sensation upon movement of the tendon. Such rubs

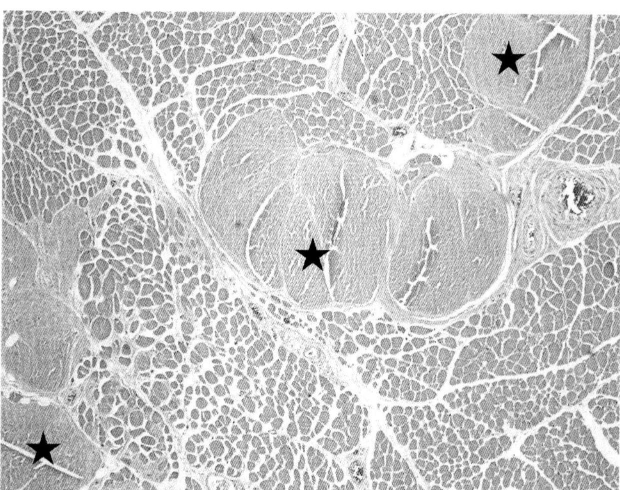

Fig. 12.21 Skeletal muscle fibrosis. At autopsy, a section of skeletal muscle demonstrates loss of myocytes with fibrous replacement (★)

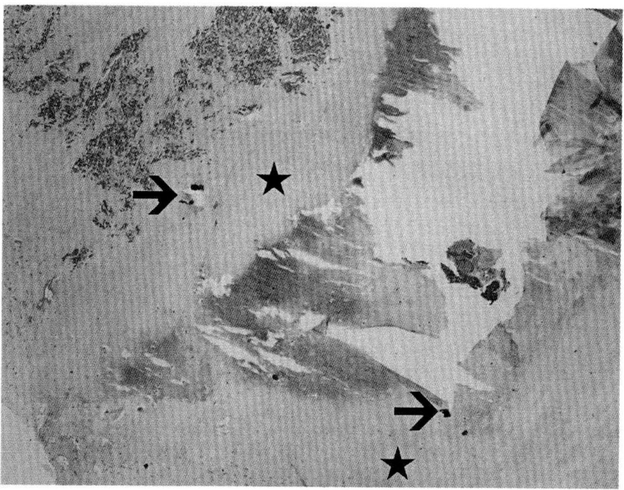

Fig. 12.22 Tendon rupture. A biceps tendon from a scleroderma patient shows fibrosis (★), calcification (→), and disruption

have a strong association with visceral involvement and disease progression [75]. Imaging studies have suggested that tendon friction rubs reflect fibrous remodeling of the tendon rather than an active inflammatory process [76]. Histologically, tendons from SSc confirm the presence of fibrosis with occasional calcifications (Fig. 12.22). Blood vessels with intimal proliferation and luminal obliteration can occasionally be noted in the tendon sheath [1]. Tendon rupture is a rare late complication of this finding.

Joint synovitis is another common finding in SSc that has been reported in anywhere between 18 % and 60 % of patients [1, 75]. This finding seems to be independent from tendon involvement but is also a strong predictor of disease progression [75]. Most studies of synovitis rely on imaging findings, but a few cases have been studied histologically [77]. Cases of acute synovitis demonstrate focal to diffuse lymphoplasmacytic inflammation in the synovium with variable associated fibrin deposition. In contrast to rheumatoid arthritis, SSc joint disease is not associated with pannus formation or bone resorption. Chronic synovitis histologically is characterized by vascular obliteration and synovial atrophy.

Placenta

While careful clinical monitoring can allow for successful pregnancies in SSc, an overall higher rate of adverse pregnancy outcomes is well documented in these patients [78]. Although studies have differed regarding whether the rate of miscarriage in SSc patients is significantly higher than that of normal controls, they do highlight a uniformly elevated frequency of preterm births of up to 29 % in pregnancies of affected mothers [78, 79]. Women with SSc also have a higher rate of delivering low-birth weight infants even at term [80]. Pathologic examination of the placenta is frequently carried out in cases with such pregnancy complications, and several histologic abnormalities strongly correlate with the aforementioned clinical findings.

The most significant lesion identified in placentas from SSc pregnancies is decidual vasculopathy, which has been identified in up to 38 % of placentas and associated with poor perinatal outcomes and fetal death [81]. Decidual vasculopathy is a broad term that encompasses several abnormalities of the placental vasculature, including fibrinoid necrosis of the vascular wall, subendothelial and intramural accumulation of macrophages, and thickening of the muscular wall of small blood vessels (Fig. 12.23a). These findings can occur focally or may diffusely involve the decidual blood vessels. Decidual vasculopathy is not specific for SSc and, indeed, is most commonly seen in preeclampsia; it has also been documented in a wide range of autoimmune diseases [81].

Placentas from SSc pregnancies have also been shown to demonstrate several other abnormalities which arise secondary to the previously described vascular compromise. Placental infarcts can be visible both grossly and microscopically [81] (Fig. 12.23b), reflecting complete loss of blood flow to all or part of the placenta. Gross examination reveals pale induration of the placental parenchyma with a granular cut surface, corresponding histologically to an area of coagulative necrosis with architectural collapse of villi, increased fibrin deposition, villous agglutination, and loss of nuclear basophilia. The placental villi can also show abnormal growth patterns for gestational age, including fibrosis; distal villous hypoplasia with long, avascular villi; and increased syncytial knotting (Fig. 12.23c) [82]. Placental mesenchymal dysplasia, including stem villi with mesenchymal proliferation, foci of myxoid degeneration, and large stromal macrophages, has also been rarely reported [83].

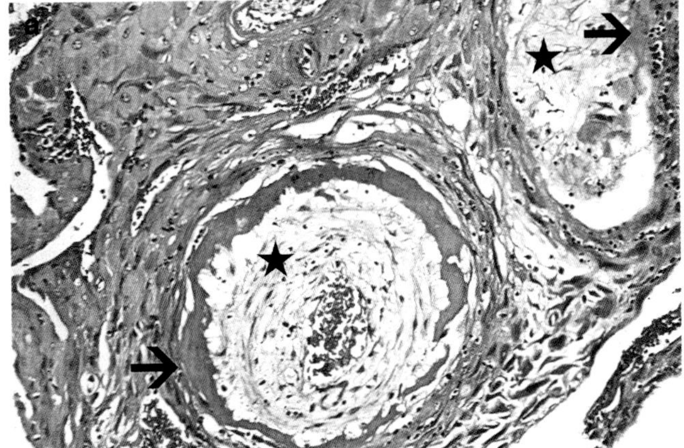

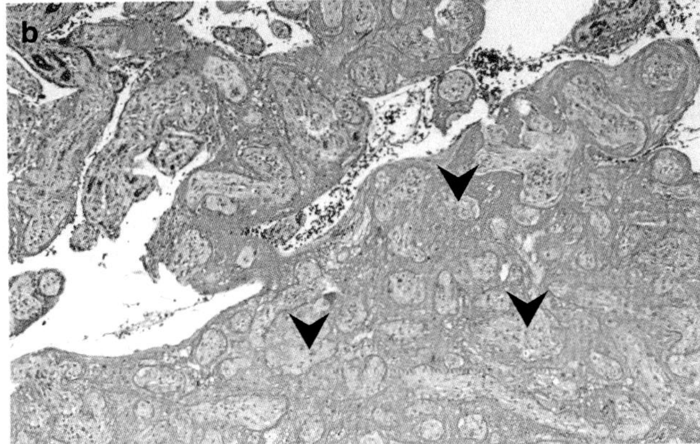

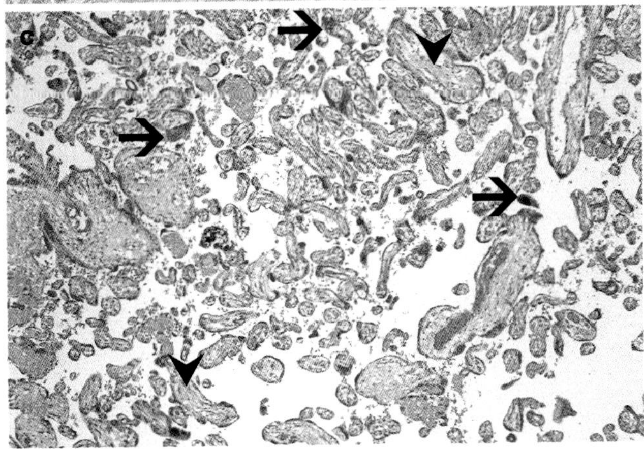

Fig. 12.23 Placental changes. In decidual vasculopathy, maternal decidual blood vessels undergo acute atherosis with accumulation of foamy macrophages (★) and associated fibrinoid necrosis of the vessel walls (→) (**a**). This vascular compromise often leads to placental infarct, with condensation of villi and complete loss of nuclear basophilia (▼) (**b**). Viable placental tissue can demonstrate distal villous hypoplasia with elongated, avascular villi (▼) and increased numbers of syncytial knots (→) for gestational age (**c**)

References

1. Gardner DL. In: Gardner DL, editor. Pathological basis of the connective tissue diseases. 2nd ed. Philadelphia: Lea & Febiger; 1992.
2. Piper WN, Helwig EB. Progressive systemic sclerosis; visceral manifestations in generalized scleroderma. AMA Arch Dermatol. 1955;72(6):535–46.
3. Klemperer P, Pollack AD, Baehr G. Landmark article May 23, 1942: Diffuse collagen disease. Acute disseminated lupus erythematosus and diffuse scleroderma. By Paul Klemperer, Abou D. Pollack and George Baehr. JAMA. 1984;251(12):1593–4.
4. Kinder RR, Fleischmajer R. Systemic scleroderma: a review of organ systems. Int J Dermatol. 1974;13(6):382–95.
5. D'Angelo WA, Fries JF, Masi AT, Shulman LE. Pathologic observations in systemic sclerosis (scleroderma). A study of fifty-eight autopsy cases and fifty-eight matched controls. Am J Med. 1969;46(3):428–40.
6. Rockey DC, Bell PD, Hill JA. Fibrosis–a common pathway to organ injury and failure. N Engl J Med. [Comment Letter]. 2015;373(1):96.
7. van den Hoogen F, Khanna D, Fransen J, Johnson SR, Baron M, Tyndall A, et al. 2013 classification criteria for systemic sclerosis: an American College of Rheumatology/European League against Rheumatism collaborative initiative. Arthritis Rheum. 2013;65(11):2737–47.
8. Tyndall A, Fistarol S. The differential diagnosis of systemic sclerosis. Curr Opin Rheumatol. [Review]. 2013;25(6):692–9.
9. Calonje JE. In: Brenn T, Lazar A, McKee PH, editors. McKee's pathology of the skin with clinical correlations. 4th ed. Saint Louis: Elsevier/Saunders; 2012.
10. Wriston CC, Rubin AI, Elenitsas R, Crawford GH. Nodular scleroderma: a report of 2 cases. Am J Dermatopathol. 2008;30(4):385–8.
11. Verrecchia F, Laboureau J, Verola O, Roos N, Porcher R, Bruneval P, et al. Skin involvement in scleroderma – where histological and clinical scores meet. Rheumatology (Oxford). 2007;46(5):833–41.
12. Fett N, Werth VP. Update on morphea: part I. Epidemiology, clinical presentation, and pathogenesis. J Am Acad Dermatol. 2011;64(2):217–28; quiz 29–30.
13. Braverman IM. Ultrastructure and organization of the cutaneous microvasculature in normal and pathologic states. J Invest Dermatol. 1989;93(2 Suppl):2S–9.
14. Sticherling M. Systemic sclerosis-dermatological aspects. Part 1: pathogenesis, epidemiology, clinical findings. J Dtsch Dermatol Ges. 2012;10(10):705–18; quiz 16.
15. Sunderkötter C, Herrgott I, Brückner C, Moinzadeh P, Pfeiffer C, Gerss J, et al. Comparison of patients with and without digital ulcers in systemic sclerosis: detection of possible risk factors. Br J Dermatol. 2009;160(4):835–43.
16. Muangchan C, Baron M, Pope J, Canadian Scleroderma Research G. The 15% rule in scleroderma: the frequency of severe organ complications in systemic sclerosis. A systematic review. J Rheumatol. 2013;40(9):1545–56.
17. Gutierrez Jr A, Wetter DA. Calcinosis cutis in autoimmune connective tissue diseases. Dermatol Ther. 2012;25(2):195–206.
18. Reiter N, El-Shabrawi L, Leinweber B, Berghold A, Aberer E. Calcinosis cutis: part I. Diagnostic pathway. J Am Acad Dermatol. 2011;65(1):1–12; quiz 3–4.
19. Boulman N, Slobodin G, Rozenbaum M, Rosner I. Calcinosis in rheumatic diseases. Semin Arthritis Rheum. 2005;34(6):805–12.
20. Alavi A, Hafner J, Dutz JP, Mayer D, Sibbald RG, Criado PR, et al. Atrophie blanche: is it associated with venous disease or livedoid vasculopathy? Adv Skin Wound Care. 2014;27(11):518–24.
21. Criado PR, Rivitti EA, Sotto MN, de Carvalho JF. Livedoid vasculopathy as a coagulation disorder. Autoimmun Rev. 2011;10(6):353–60.
22. Varga J. In: Denton CP, Wigley FM, editors. Scleroderma from pathogenesis to comprehensive management. 1st ed. Boston: Springer US; 2012.
23. Machinami R. Incidence of membranous lipodystrophy-like change among patients with limb necrosis caused by chronic arterial obstruction. Arch Pathol Lab Med. 1984;108(10):823–6.
24. Snow JL, Su WP, Gibson LE. Lipomembranous (membranocystic) changes associated with morphea: a clinicopathologic review of three cases. J Am Acad Dermatol. 1994;31(2 Pt 1):246–50.

25. Steen VD, Medsger TA. Changes in causes of death in systemic sclerosis, 1972–2002. Ann Rheum Dis. 2007;66(7):940–4.
26. Akter T, Silver RM, Bogatkevich GS. Recent advances in understanding the pathogenesis of scleroderma-interstitial lung disease. Curr Rheumatol Rep. [Research Support, N.I.H., Extramural Review]. 2014;16(4):411.
27. Solomon JJ, Olson AL, Fischer A, Bull T, Brown KK, Raghu G. Scleroderma lung disease. Eur Respir Rev. 2013;22(127):6–19.
28. Nikpour M, Baron M. Mortality in systemic sclerosis: lessons learned from population-based and observational cohort studies. Curr Opin Rheumatol. 2014;26(2):131–7.
29. du Bois RM. Mechanisms of scleroderma-induced lung disease. Proc Am Thorac Soc. 2007;4(5):434–8.
30. Farkas L, Kolb M. Pulmonary microcirculation in interstitial lung disease. Proc Am Thoracic Soc. [Research Support, Non-U.S. Gov't Review]. 2011;8(6):516–21.
31. Wagenvoort CA. Lung biopsy specimens in the evaluation of pulmonary vascular disease. Chest. 1980;77(5):614–25.
32. Weaver AL, Divertie MB, Titus JL. Pulmonary scleroderma. Dis Chest. 1968;54(6):490–8.
33. Fujita J, Yoshinouchi T, Ohtsuki Y, Tokuda M, Yang Y, Yamadori I, et al. Non-specific interstitial pneumonia as pulmonary involvement of systemic sclerosis. Ann Rheum Dis. 2001;60(3):281–3.
34. Fischer A, Meehan RT, Feghali-Bostwick CA, West SG, Brown KK. Unique characteristics of systemic sclerosis sine scleroderma-associated interstitial lung disease. Chest. 2006;130(4):976–81.
35. Bouros D, Wells A, Nicholson A, Colby T, Polychronopoulos V, Pantelidis P, et al. Histopathologic subsets of fibrosing alveolitis in patients with systemic sclerosis and their relationship to outcome. Am J Respir Crit Care Med. [Article|Proceedings Paper]. 20022002;165(12):1581–6.
36. Song JW, Do KH, Kim MY, Jang SJ, Colby TV, Kim DS. Pathologic and radiologic differences between idiopathic and collagen vascular disease-related usual interstitial pneumonia. Chest. 2009;136(1):23–30.
37. Herzog EL, Mathur A, Tager AM, Feghali-Bostwick C, Schneider F, Varga J. Review: interstitial lung disease associated with systemic sclerosis and idiopathic pulmonary fibrosis: how similar and distinct? Arthritis Rheumatol. [Comparative Study Research Support, N.I.H., Extramural Review]. 2014;66(8):1967–78.
38. Fischer A, Swigris JJ, Groshong SD, Cool CD, Sahin H, Lynch DA, et al. Clinically significant interstitial lung disease in limited scleroderma: histopathology, clinical features, and survival. Chest. 2008;134(3):601–5.
39. Hassoun PM. Lung involvement in systemic sclerosis. Presse Med. 2011;40(1 Pt 2):e3–17.
40. Heath D, Edwards JE. The pathology of hypertensive pulmonary vascular disease; a description of six grades of structural changes in the pulmonary arteries with special reference to congenital cardiac septal defects. Circulation. 1958;18(4 Part 1):533–47.
41. Launay D, Humbert M, Berezne A, Cottin V, Allanore Y, Couderc LJ, et al. Clinical characteristics and survival in systemic sclerosis-related pulmonary hypertension associated with interstitial lung disease. Chest. [Comparative Study Research Support, Non--U.S. Gov't]. 2011;140(4):1016–24.
42. Yousem SA. The pulmonary pathologic manifestations of the CREST syndrome. Hum Pathol. [Research Support, Non-U.S. Gov't Review]. 1990;21(5):467–74.
43. Overbeek MJ, Vonk MC, Boonstra A, Voskuyl AE, Vonk-Noordegraaf A, Smit EF, et al. Pulmonary arterial hypertension in limited cutaneous systemic sclerosis: a distinctive vasculopathy. Eur Respir J. 2009;34(2):371–9.
44. Dorfmüller P, Humbert M, Perros F, Sanchez O, Simonneau G, Müller KM, et al. Fibrous remodeling of the pulmonary venous system in pulmonary arterial hypertension associated with connective tissue diseases. Hum Pathol. 2007;38(6):893–902.
45. Breit SN, Thornton SC, Penny R. Lung involvement in scleroderma. Clin Dermatol. 1994;12(2):243–52.
46. Urisman A, Jones KD. Pulmonary pathology in connective tissue disease. Semin Respirat Crit Care Med. [Review]. 2014;35(2):201–12.
47. Steen VD, Medsger Jr TA. Severe organ involvement in systemic sclerosis with diffuse scleroderma. Arthritis Rheum. 2000;43(11):2437–44.
48. Ferri C, Sebastiani M, Lo Monaco A, Iudici M, Giuggioli D, Furini F, et al. Systemic sclerosis evolution of disease pathomorphosis and survival. Our experience on Italian patients' population and review of the literature. Autoimmun Rev. 2014;13(10):1026–34.
49. Bose N, Chiesa-Vottero A, Chatterjee S. Scleroderma renal crisis. Semin Arthritis Rheum. 2005;44(6):687–94.
50. Batal I, Domsic RT, Medsger TA, Bastacky S. Scleroderma renal crisis: a pathology perspective. Int J Rheumatol. 2010;2010:543704.
51. Batal I, Domsic RT, Shafer A, Medsger Jr TA, Kiss LP, Randhawa P, et al. Renal biopsy findings predicting outcome in scleroderma renal crisis. Hum Pathol. 2009;40(3):332–40.
52. Lee S, Sharma K. The pathogenesis of fibrosis and renal disease in scleroderma: recent insights from glomerulosclerosis. Curr Rheumatol Rep. 2004;6(2):141–8.
53. Penn H, Howie AJ, Kingdon EJ, Bunn CC, Stratton RJ, Black CM, et al. Scleroderma renal crisis: patient characteristics and long-term outcomes. Qjm-Int J Med. 2007;100(8):485–94.
54. Scheja A, Bartosik I, Wuttge DM, Hesselstrand R. Renal function is mostly preserved in patients with systemic sclerosis. Scand J Rheumatol. 2009;38(4):295–8.
55. Shanmugam VK, Steen VD. Renal disease in scleroderma: an update on evaluation, risk stratification, pathogenesis and management. Curr Opin Rheumatol. 2012;24(6):669–76.
56. Kao L, Weyand C. Vasculitis in systemic sclerosis. Int J Rheumatol. 2010;2010:385938.
57. Elhai M, Meune C, Avouac J, Kahan A, Allanore Y. Trends in mortality in patients with systemic sclerosis over 40 years: a systematic review and meta-analysis of cohort studies. Rheumatology (Oxford). 2012;51(6):1017–26.
58. Kahan A, Coghlan G, McLaughlin V. Cardiac complications of systemic sclerosis. Rheumatology (Oxford). 2009;48 Suppl 3:iii45–8.
59. Rodriguez-Reyna TS, Morelos-Guzman M, Hernandez-Reyes P, Montero-Duarte K, Martinez-Reyes C, Reyes-Utrera C, et al. Assessment of myocardial fibrosis and microvascular damage in systemic sclerosis by magnetic resonance imaging and coronary angiotomography. Rheumatology (Oxford). 2015;54(4):647–54.
60. Bulkley BH, Ridolfi RL, Salyer WR, Hutchins GM. Myocardial lesions of progressive systemic sclerosis. A cause of cardiac dysfunction. Circulation. 1976;53(3):483–90.
61. Allanore Y, Meune C. Primary myocardial involvement in systemic sclerosis: evidence for a microvascular origin. Clin Exp Rheumatol. 2010;28(5 Suppl 62):S48–53.
62. James TN. De subitaneis mortibus. VIII. Coronary arteries and conduction system in scleroderma heart disease. Circulation. 1974;50(4):844–56.
63. McWhorter JE, LeRoy EC. Pericardial disease in scleroderma (systemic sclerosis). Am J Med. 1974;57(4):566–75.
64. Parks JL, Taylor MH, Parks LP, Silver RM. Systemic sclerosis and the heart. Rheum Dis Clin North Am. 2014;40(1):87–102.
65. Lambova S. Cardiac manifestations in systemic sclerosis. World J Cardiol. 2014;6(9):993–1005.
66. Lefevre G, Dauchet L, Hachulla E, Montani D, Sobanski V, Lambert M, et al. Survival and prognostic factors in systemic sclerosis-associated pulmonary hypertension: a systematic review and meta-analysis. Arthritis Rheum. 2013;65(9):2412–23.
67. Klein-Weigel P, Opitz C, Riemekasten G. Systemic sclerosis – a systematic overview: part 1 – disease characteristics and classification, pathophysiologic concepts, and recommendations for diagnosis and surveillance. Vasa. 2011;40(1):6–19.
68. Johnson SR, Glaman DD, Schentag CT, Lee P. Quality of life and functional status in systemic sclerosis compared to other rheumatic diseases. J Rheumatol. 2006;33(6):1117–22.

69. Ebert EC. Gastric and enteric involvement in progressive systemic sclerosis. J Clin Gastroenterol. 2008;42(1):5–12.
70. Di Ciaula A, Covelli M, Berardino M, Wang DQ, Lapadula G, Palasciano G, et al. Gastrointestinal symptoms and motility disorders in patients with systemic scleroderma. BMC Gastroenterol. 2008;8:7.
71. Forbes A, Marie I. Gastrointestinal complications: the most frequent internal complications of systemic sclerosis. Rheumatology. 2009;48:36–9.
72. Christmann RB, Wells AU, Capelozzi VL, Silver RM. Gastroesophageal reflux incites interstitial lung disease in systemic sclerosis: clinical, radiologic, histopathologic, and treatment evidence. Semin Arthritis Rheumatism. [Research Support, Non--U.S. Gov't Review]. 2010;40(3):241–9.
73. Watson M, Hally RJ, McCue PA, Varga J, Jimenez SA. Gastric antral vascular ectasia (watermelon stomach) in patients with systemic sclerosis. Arthritis Rheum. 1996;39(2):341–6.
74. Lóránd V, Czirják L, Minier T. Musculoskeletal involvement in systemic sclerosis. Presse Med. 2014;43(10 Pt 2):e315–28.
75. Avouac J, Walker UA, Hachulla E, Riemekasten G, Cuomo G, Carreira PE, et al. Joint and tendon involvement predict disease progression in systemic sclerosis: a EUSTAR prospective study. Ann Rheum Dis. 2016;75(1):103–9.
76. Elhai M, Guerini H, Bazeli R, Avouac J, Freire V, Drapé JL, et al. Ultrasonographic hand features in systemic sclerosis and correlates with clinical, biologic, and radiographic findings. Arthritis Care Res (Hoboken). 2012;64(8):1244–9.
77. Rodnan GP. The nature of joint involvement in progressive systemic sclerosis (diffuse scleroderma). Ann Intern Med. 1962;56:422–39.
78. Steen VD. Pregnancy in scleroderma. Rheum Dis Clin North Am. 2007;33(2):345–58. vii.
79. Steen VD. Pregnancy in women with systemic sclerosis. Obstet Gynecol. 1999;94(1):15–20.
80. Steen VD, Conte C, Day N, Ramsey-Goldman R, Medsger Jr TA. Pregnancy in women with systemic sclerosis. Arthritis Rheum. 1989;32(2):151–7.
81. Doss BJ, Jacques SM, Mayes MD, Qureshi F. Maternal scleroderma: placental findings and perinatal outcome. Hum Pathol. 1998;29(12):1524–30.
82. Ibba-Manneschi L, Manetti M, Milia AF, Miniati I, Benelli G, Guiducci S, et al. Severe fibrotic changes and altered expression of angiogenic factors in maternal scleroderma: placental findings. Ann Rheum Dis. 2010;69(2):458–61.
83. Papakonstantinou K, Hasiakos D, Kondi-Paphiti A. Clinicopathology of maternal scleroderma. Int J Gynaecol Obstet. 2007;99(3):248–9.

13 Inflammation and Immunity

Francesco Boin and Carlo Chizzolini

Introduction

Systemic sclerosis (SSc) is classically included within the spectrum of autoimmune systemic disorders. Two are the main historical reasons. One is the high prevalence of antinuclear autoantibodies (ANA) in the sera of individuals suffering from SSc, which for several decades has been taken per se as a proof of autoimmunity. The second is that clinical features characteristically present in SSc are shared with other autoimmune systemic conditions such as systemic lupus erythematosus (SLE), rheumatoid arthritis (RA), or overlapping syndromes including mixed connective tissue disease and overlaps with myositis. It should be noted though that there is no established animal model able to reproduce convincingly the clinical phenotype of SSc upon immunization or passive transfer of immune cells or antibodies. Thus, SSc falls short of satisfying the postulates that allow a nosology entity to be definitively classified within the disorders having an autoimmune origin. Nonetheless, during the last several decades, an enormous amount of work has provided evidence indicating that different cells and soluble mediators belonging to the immune system present abnormalities that correlate with distinct SSc phenotypes and may be pathologically linked to disease development and progression. It remains however challenging to reconstruct the sequence of events leading to the perturbed state in SSc and attributing them a causal rather than a consequential role.

There are four major types of observations supporting a direct involvement of the immune system in the pathogenesis of SSc. First, the presence of autoantibodies (autoAbs) is directed against ubiquitous but also non-ubiquitous autoantigens in the sera of SSc individuals. Second, the presence within SSc target organs of T cells expressing oligoclonal antigen-receptors (TcR) provides indirect evidence that T cell proliferation and tissue localization may be driven by specific antigens and possibly distinct autoantigens [1–4]. Third, data from studies investigating the genetic susceptibility to SSc have shown through hypothesis-driven as well as unbiased approaches that the strongest genetic variability associated with SSc involves molecules pivotal to the function of the immune system and in particular of the adaptive immune response, and not those more directly linked to fibrosis. Fourth, while no cure is available for the fibrotic component of the disease, immunosuppressive agents and in particular aggressive immunosuppressive strategies seem to positively impact fibrosis in SSc patients. This is the case for cyclophosphamide, which has been proven to be efficacious in reducing progression of SSc-associated ILD after daily oral administration or in reversing severe diffuse skin fibrosis when given at immuno- or myeloablative regimens with or without autologous hematopoietic stem cell transplantation [4–8]. As cyclophosphamide does not have a known direct impact on fibroblast proliferation and extracellular matrix (ECM) deposition, the evidence generated by these clinical studies indirectly indicates that components of the immune system targeted by this drug, namely, T and B cells, may be causally involved in sustaining fibrosis in SSc.

As a general rule, which particularly applies to autoimmune diseases, an adaptive immune response initiates only when cells of the innate immune system become activated and express molecules indicating danger. Thus, it is important to consider also in the context of SSc that the activation of the innate immune system chronologically precedes the activation of the adaptive system and that the close interrelationship between these two systems clearly plays an essential role to initiate and amplify the disease process.

In this chapter we will review the evidence generated through experimental approaches and clinical observations indicating involvement of the immune system and the

F. Boin, MD (✉)
Division of Rheumatology, Department of Medicine, University of California San Francisco, 513 Parnassus Avenue, Med Sci, S-847, Box 0500, San Francisco, CA 94143, USA
e-mail: francesco.boin@ucsf.edu

C. Chizzolini, MD
Immunology and Allergy, Department of Medical Specialties, Geneva University Hospital and School of Medicine, Rue Gabrielle Perret-Gentil, 4, Geneva 14 1211, Switzerland
e-mail: carlo.chizzolini@unige.ch

J. Varga et al. (eds.), *Scleroderma*, DOI 10.1007/978-3-319-31407-5_13

inflammatory response in SSc pathogenesis. The first part will address the role of innate immunity in relationship with SSc. This will cover TLR (Table 13.1), monocytes/macrophages, dendritic cells, NK cells, interferons, pro-inflammatory cytokines of the IL-1 family, TNF, IL-6, and the inflammasomes. The second part will focus on molecular and cellular effectors of the adaptive immune response. This will cover T and B cells and the related cytokines. Additional information on cytokines and chemokines is condensed in Tables 13.2, 13.3, and 13.4.

Table 13.1 TLR in systemic sclerosis and animal models of fibrosis

TLR4	FN^{EDA}, induced by TGF-β, binds to TLR4 and enhances collagen production	[9]
TLR4	TLR4 enhanced expression in SSc skin and lung Enhanced expression of FN^{EDA}, tenascin, hyaluronan, in SSc skin LPS enhances fibroblast responses to LPS with increased collagen C3H/HeJ (TLR4 nonfunctional) mice have attenuated bleomycin-induced SSc	[10]
TLR4	TLR4 enhanced expression in bleomycin-induced mouse skin TLR4–/– mice resistant to bleomycin-induced skin and lung fibrosis, with decreased skin inflammation, reduced numbers of Th2 and Th177 cells, decreased titers of anti-Topo-1 Ab TLR4–/– in TSK-1+ mice attenuate hypodermal fibrosis	[11]
TLR4	S100A8/A9 putative TLR4 ligand is increased in SSc serum	[12]
TLR4	S100A9 is produced by keratinocytes and increased in SSc skin	[13]
TLR7/8 TLR9	IFN-alpha is produced by SSc pDC activated by R848 and CpG via CXCL4	[14]
TLR7 TLR9	Upregulated in fibroblasts by EBV infection and induce IRF5, IRF7, CXCL9, TNF, SMAD, collagen, myofibroblasts	[15]
TLR3	TLR3 is upregulated in a subset of SSc	[16]
MDA5	Poly (I:C) enhances IFN-beta production by fibroblasts	
RIG1	Poly (I:C) inhibits spontaneous and TGF-stimulated collagen production in fibroblasts via MDA5 and RIG1 by inducing Smad7	
TLR3	Poly (I:C) enhances the production of TSLP in fibroblasts TSLP is upregulated in SSc skin and lung TSLP–/– mice develop less bleomycin-induced scleroderma in parallel with less IL-13	[17]
TLR8	SSc monocytes activated with ssRNA produce more TIMP than CTRL (similarly when stimulated with Pam3CSK4 and LPS)	[18]
(TLR1/2)	Monocytes cultured in SSc serum produced more TIMP	
(TLR4)	MyD88 dependent, IRAK-4 dependent	
TLR4	TLR4 is overexpressed in SSc skin Chronic LPS challenge in mice induces inflammation and TGF-β signature	[19]
TLR2	Rare functional polymorphism in TLR2 (Pro631His) is associated with Scl-70, dSSc, and PAH This polymorphism increases the responses (IL-6 and TNF) to the ligand Pam3CSK4	[20]
TLR3	TLR3 upregulated by IFN-alpha2a in SSc and CTRL fibroblasts with enhanced prod of IL-6	[21]
TLR3	Poly (I:C) enhances the production of ET-1 and ICAM-1 by EC and fibroblasts. ET-1 induction depends on IFNAR signaling	[22]
HA (TLR4)	IL-27 production is high in SSc and correlates with disease subset and inversely with disease duration Stimulated by HA in monocytes more in SSc than controls IL-27 stimulates collagen prod by fibroblasts	[23]
Poly(I:C) TLR3	Poly(I:C) in fibroblasts induces IFN-I and TGF-β signatures	[24]
Stimulated mDC (human)	LPS (TLR4), R848 (TLR7/8), Pam3CSK4 (TLR2), poly(I:C) (TLR3) induce high IL-10, somewhat augmented IL-6 and TNF, mostly in response to LPS in early diffuse SSc compared to HD	[25]
Mono and mDC (LPS)	SSc sera induce responses in CHO expressing TLR4, LPS induces CCL18 prod via IL-10 in SSc monocytes and mDC	[26]
TLR4	Anti-fibroblast antibodies induce pro-fibrotic chemokines partially using TLR4	[27]
SSc sera	IFN-I production by Scl-70 sera> than others, pDC and FcγRII dependent	[28]
SSc sera	IFN-I prod by SSc sera containing anti-RNP and anti-SSA, pDC and FcγRII dependent	[29]
HA, (TLR2), TLR4 mouse	Bleomycin enhances HA production and fibrosis in a CD19-dependent manner	[30]
TLR5	Upregulated by TGF/SMAD in SSc fibroblasts	[31]
TLR10	Flagellin downregulates collagen production	
TLR4	Required for the resolution of pulmonary inflammation and fibrosis after acute and chronic lung injury	[32]

FN^{EDA} fibronectin extracellular domain A, *HA* hyaluronan, *IFN* interferon, *PAH* pulmonary artery hypertension, *TLR* Toll-like receptor, *TSLP* thymic stromal lymphopoietin

Table 13.2 Cytokines in systemic sclerosis

Name	Source/cell type/animal model	Relevant aspects	References
Intracellular IL-1 alpha	Fibroblasts	Constitutively upregulated in SSc fibroblasts, nuclear localization, enhances IL-6 and PDGF-A and procollagen synthesis	[33]
Pre-IL-1 alpha	Fibroblasts	Intranuclear localization dependent on HAX-1 induces IL-6 and procollagen	[34] [35]
Intracellular IL-1Ra	Fibroblasts	Hyper-expression induces alpha-smooth actin, plasminogen activator inhibitor and reduces MMP-1	[36]
IL-1 alpha	Endothelial cells	Higher sensitivity in SSc fibroblasts, increased expression of ICAM-1	[37]
IL-1 alpha	Keratinocytes	Contractility and CTGF production	[38]
IL-1 beta	Mouse model	Essential for bleomycin-induced lung fibrosis	[39]
IL-2	Serum	Increased in SSc Correlates with disease progression	[40] [41, 42] [43]
IL-4	Serum	Increased in SSc	[43] [44] [45]
	SSc skin	Enhanced expression in SSc skin	[46]
IL-4	CD8 T cells in BALF; CD4 and CD8 PBT cells; CD4 T cells in SSc skin; microchimeric alloreactive CD4+ T cells; CD4+CD8+ double positive T cells in SSc skin	IL-4 production I BALF correlates with greater decline in lung function	[47, 48] [3, 49, 50]
IL-4	Fibroblasts	Enhances collagen production by fibroblasts	[51] [52]
	TSK-1/+ mice	In fibroblasts reduces miRNA-29, thus enhancing type I and III collagen production Similar effects with TGF-b, PDGF-B Involved in fibrosis development	[53]
IL-6	Serum	Increased in SSc, correlate with mRSS and disease duration	[43] [54] [55–57] [58] [59]
		Independent predictor of DLCO decline in both IPF and SSc-ILD	[60]
	Serum		[61]
	BALF	Decreased after B cell depletion therapy	[62] [63]
	Fibroblast	Increased	[33] [64] [65]
		High spontaneous	
	PBMC	Production in SSc	[66]
	Skin	Induced by AFA, IL-1a, PDGF Spontaneous enhanced production Increased mRNA in skin fibroblasts and EC	[67]
	Bleomycin-induced scleroderma	IL-6 blockade protects	[68, 69]
	Sclerodermatous GVHD in mice	IL-6 blockade protects	[70]
IL-8	Serum	Increased in SSc (Gro-a also)	[71] [72] [73]
	BALF		[61]
		Increased in SSc-ILD	[74]
	Skin		[67]
	Fibroblasts	Increased mRNA in skin Induced by AFA	[27]

(continued)

Table 13.2 (continued)

Name	Source/cell type/animal model	Relevant aspects	References
IL-9	Transgenic overexpression	Increases subepithelial fibrosis in an asthma	[75]
		Model	[76]
	Transgenic overexpression in vivo	Decreases lung fibrosis in a silica model	
IL-10	Serum	Increased in SSc, correlate with mRSS and ILD	[77] [45, 56]
	DC	TLR4 agonist induces higher production of IL-10 in SSc	[26] [25]
	DC	Higher production in response to various TLR ligands	
IL-11	Transgenic overexpression in vivo	Increases subepithelial accumulation of myofibroblasts and fibrosis in the airways	[78]
IL-12	Serum	Increased in SSc, increases with disease duration	[79] [45, 56]
	DC	Increases concomitantly to reduced skin fibrosis Decreased production upon TLR stimulation in SSc	[25]
IL-13	Serum	Increased in SSc	[44] [45]
	CD8+ T cells	Increased production correlates with MRSS	[80]
IL-15	Serum	Increased in SSc	[81]
IL-17	Serum	Increased in SSc	[82] [83]
		Not increased in SSc	[58]
	Recombinant IL-17	Enhances fibroblast production of IL-6, IL-8, MCP-1, MMPs, and surface expression of ICAM-1	[84] [82, 85]
		Reduces type I collagen in human dermal fibroblasts and α-SMA-positive fibroblasts	[86, 87]
	PBMC	Enhances fibroblast proliferation	[58] [88]
		Increased frequency of Th17 in SSc peripheral blood, BAL, skin	[58, 89–93]
	SSc skin	High IL-17A, high IL-17F, low IL-17C, high IL-17E	[94, 95]
IL-18	Serum	Similar levels in SSc and Ctrl	[55] [96]
		Decreases collagen production by fibroblasts	
IL-21	Skin	Increased expression of IL-21R in SSc epidermis	[95, 97]
IL-22	γ/δ T cells	Protects from lung fibrosis in bleomycin model	[98] [84]
	PBMC	Increased frequency of IL-22 producing CD4+ T cells in SSC	
IL-23	Serum	Increased in SSc	[99] [58]
IL-27	Serum	Increased in SSc Increased fibroblast proliferation and increased collagen synthesis Correlate with MRSS and lung function tests	[23]
IL-33		Induces IL-13-dependent (produced by eosinophils) fibrosis in vivo	[100]
IL-35	SSc serum	Increased in early disease	[101]
	SSc skin	Increased in SSc compared to HD	
	Dermal fibroblasts	Induced in response to TGF-β	
EBI3 (β-chain of IL-35)	Dermal fibroblasts	Downregulates collagen production	[102]
	SSc skin	Decreased expression compared to HD	
	Bleomycin-induced mouse scleroderma	Reduces fibrosis	

Table 13.2 (continued)

Name	Source/cell type/animal model	Relevant aspects	References
AIF	SSc skin and lung	Expressed in EC, T cells, macrophages	[103]
	AIF-transfected Jurkat T cells	Enhanced chemotaxis and collagen deposition	[104]
APRIL	Serum	Elevated in SSc, associated with ILD	[105]
BAFF	Serum	Elevated in SSc, correlated with skin involvement	[106] [105]
	SSc skin	Increased BAFF mRNA	
	SSc B cells	Increased response to BAFF	[107]
	TSK-1	BAFF-antagonist attenuates TSK-1 phenotype	
	Human B cell/fibroblast cocultures	Enhanced production of IL-6, TGF-β, CCL2, and collagen secretion	[108]
HGF		Attenuates fibrosis, IL-4, and TGF-b production in TSK-1 mice	[109]
IFN-α	Serum	Increased levels correlated with ILD	[28] [29]
		Increased levels correlated with ILD and DU	[96] [29]
	pDC	Scl70/Ab IC-induced IFN-a production Anti-nucleoprotein Ab-induced IFN-a production	
IFN-α	Th1 cells	Serum levels lower in SSc than Ctrl	[43] [49]
		Decreases type I collagen production more in healthy than SSc fibroblasts	[55] [110] [111] [112]
		Produced by T cells infiltrating the skin	[113, 114] [115]
		mRNA present in ILD	
		Induces MHC-II ad ICAM-1 in fibroblasts and EC	
TNFα	Serum	Increased in SSc	[77] [45, 55, 61]
	BALF	Increased In SSc Induces MHC-II and ICAM-1 in fibroblasts and EC	[115]
TNFα	Th1 and Th2 cells	Decreases type I collagen production by healthy but not SSc fibroblasts	[116]
CD40/CD40L	CD4+ T cells	Increased expression of	[117]
	Serum	CD40L in SSc Increased levels of soluble CD40 in SSc	[118] [119]
	Fibroblast	Increased levels of soluble CD40L in SSc	[120]
	Bleomycin mouse model	SSc fibroblasts express high levels of CD40 Soluble CD40L induces the production of CCL2 and IL-6 Blockade of CD40/CD40L interaction reduced fibrosis	[121]
CTGF	Serum	Increased in SSc	[45]
Multiplex analysis	Serum levels in 444 SSc and 216 HC	TNFα, IL-6, IFN-g higher in SSc IL-17, IL-23 lower in SSc	[122]
Multiplex analysis	BALF, 32 SSc (27 with ILD, 5 w/o ILD), 26 CTRL	Higher IL-4, IL-6, IL-8, CCL2 in SSc BALF with ILD than w/o ILD, High IL-17 in SSc compared to CTRL TNFα and IL-2 predictors of progressive disease	[123]

AIF allograft inflammatory factor, *AFA* anti-fibroblast antibodies, *APRIL* a proliferation-inducing ligand, *BAFF* B cell activating factor, *BALF* bronchoalveolar lavage fluid, *CTGF* connective tissue growth factor, *Ctrl* controls, *DU* digital ulcers, *HAX-1* HCLS1-associated protein X-1, *DC* dendritic cells, *EC* endothelial cell, *HS1* associated protein-1, *Gro-a* growth-related oncogene a, *HGF* hepatocyte growth factor, *ICAM* intercellular adhesion molecule, *IFN* interferon, *ILD* interstitial lung disease, *MHC* major histocompatibility complex, *miRNA* microRNA, *MMP* matrix metalloproteinase, *mRSS* modified Rodnan skin score, *PDGF* platelet-derived growth factor, *SSc* systemic sclerosis, *TGF* transforming growth factor, *TLR* Toll-like receptor, *TSK* tight skin

Table 13.3 Evidence indicating a preferential Th2 response in SSc and relevant animal models

IL-4	Increased levels in the serum of SSc individuals Enhanced expression in SSc skin Enhanced production in BALF correlates with greater decline in lung functions Presence of CD8+ T cells producing IL-4 in BALF Presence of CD8+ and CD4+CD8+ double positive T cells producing IL-4 in SSc skin Presence of microchimeric alloreactive CD4+ T cells producing IL-4 in blood and skin Presence in SSc skin of Treg producing IL-4 and expressing high levels of the receptor for IL-33 Involved in skin fibrosis in TSK-1/+ mice
IL-13	Increased levels in the serum of SSc individuals, correlates with MRSS Presence of CD8+ T cells with enhanced expression of GATA-3 and production of IL-13 in the peripheral blood and skin of SSc which correlate with skin score and lung involvement IL-13 inhibition attenuates bleomycin-induced lung fibrosis IL-13 overexpression causes lung fibrosis IL-13 deficiency protects against FITC-induced lung fibrosis IL-13 mediates fibrosis induced by bleomycin in T bet null mice
IL-33	High serum levels early in disease course, high levels of ST2 (IL-33 receptor) expression in EC
TSLP	Increased expression in SSc, induces the expression of IL-13 and TGF-β upon stimulation with TLR3 ligands TSLP receptor deficiency, partially protects against bleomycin-induced skin fibrosis

BALF bronchoalveolar lavage fluid, TLR Toll-like receptor, *TSLP* thymic stroma lymphopoietin, *TSK* tight-skin mouse

Table 13.4 Chemokines and chemokine receptors in systemic sclerosis

Old name	New name	Receptor	Source	Function	Findings in SSc patients	References
MCP-1	CCL2	CCR2	Mononuclear cells, macrophages, fibroblasts, epithelium, endothelium, VSMCs	Chemotaxis monocytes, T cells, and eosinophils	Higher serum levels associated with early disease (dcSSC phenotype) and ILD Higher BAL levels in SSc patients with ILD; associated with worse lung function and CT score for lung fibrosis Higher (constitutive) expression in SSc skin fibroblasts Increased expression in lesional SSc skin Stimulation of collagen and MMP-1 secretion from human fibroblasts	[29, 74, 123–131]
MCP-3	CCL7	CCR1 CCR2 CCR3	Fibroblasts	Chemotaxis monocytes, DCs, NK cells, stimulate fibroblast activation and secretion of ECM	Overexpression in human fibroblasts from early dcSSc skin disease High serum levels and association with extent of skin disease (higher in dcSSc)	[132] [133]
MCP-4	CCL13	CCR1 CCR2 CCR3	Fibroblasts	Chemotaxis eosinophils, monocytes and T cells	High serum levels	[134]
MIP-1α	CCL3	CCR5 CCR1	Lymphocytes, monocytes, mast cells	Chemotaxis monocytes, T and B lymphocyte eosinophils	Higher serum levels and skin expression Higher serum levels	[61, 66] [135]
MIP-1β	CCL4	CCR5 CCR1			Higher BAL levels in patients with active alveolitis Higher PBMC gene expression in patients with severe PAH	[136] [137]
RANTES	CCL5	CCR1 CCR3 CCR5	Lymphocytes, keratinocytes, endothelium	Chemotaxis T and B cells, stimulate expression of ET-1	Higher BAL levels Higher skin expression (lesional and uninvolved) Gene-gene interaction with CXCL8	[138] [61, 139] [140]

Table 13.4 (continued)

Old name	New name	Receptor	Source	Function	Findings in SSc patients	References
MPIF-1 MIP-3	CCL23	CCR1	Monocytes	Chemotaxis mononuclear cells, DCs, endothelial cells	High serum levels, association with shorter disease duration and the presence of PAH	[141]
TARC	CCL17	CCR4	Thymus DCs Keratinocytes Macrophages	T cell chemotaxis, pro-fibrotic	Higher serum levels Association with anti-topoisomerase 1 antibody positivity and titer	[142]
MDC	CCL22	CCR4	Lymphocytes Macrophages Keratinocytes DCs	Pro-fibrotic, chemotaxis activated T cells, NK, eosinophils, monocytes	Higher serum levels	[142]
CTACK	CCL27	CCR10	Epithelium Keratinocytes	Chemotaxis T cells T cell-mediated inflammation of the skin	High serum levels Higher expression in SSc skin	[143]
PARC	CCL18	Unknown	Monocytes Macrophages DCs	T cell chemotaxis Stimulate collagen fibroblast secretion	High serum and BAL levels High serum levels correlate with active ILD and declining lung volumes Induce collagen production in SSc lung fibroblasts	[144, 145] [146] [147] [148]
ELC	CCL19	CCR7	Thymus Lymphocytes Epithelium Endothelium	DCs, macrophages, B cell and T cell chemotaxis	High expression in dcSSc skin, association with vascular inflammation	[149]
LARC	CCL20	CCR6	Lymphocytes Epithelium Endothelium Neurons	Lymphocytes, DC chemotaxis	Higher expression in SSc skin	[150]
IL-8`	CXCL8	CXCR1 CXCR2	Macrophages, fibroblasts Epithelial Endothelium	Neutrophil and T cell chemotaxis, pro-angiogenic	Higher levels in serum, BAL, skin, and cultured SSc fibroblasts or alveolar macrophages Association with the presence of active ILD, worse lung fibrosis, and lower FVC or DLCO SNPs of CXCL8 and CXCR2 genes associated with increased SSc risk	[72, 89, 123] [61, 138, 151–154]
GROα	CXCL1	CXCR2	Macrophages Neutrophils, epithelium, endothelium fibroblasts	Granulocyte chemotaxis	Higher levels in serum; association with lower VC and DLCO Higher PBMC gene expression in patients with severe PAH	[72, 137]
PF4	CXCL4	CXCR2	Platelets pDCs	Neutrophil and fibroblast chemotaxis, pro-coagulant, pro-fibrotic, antiangiogenic	High serum and BAL levels (in SSc-ILD) High serum level associated with more severe disease, predict progression	[155, 156] [14]
ENA-78	CXCL5	CXCR2	Macrophages Fibroblasts Epithelial cells	Neutrophil and T cell chemotaxis, pro-angiogenic	Higher serum and BAL levels, associated with presence of ILD Decreased levels in early SSc	[157] [153] [158]
IP-10	CXCL10	CXCR3	Neutrophils, monocytes, endothelium, epithelium, keratinocytes	Chemotaxis T cells (Th1), NK cells, monocytes; Pro-inflammatory, anti-fibrotic, angiostatic	High serum levels, association with PAH, vascular manifestations High serum level and skin involvement	[29, 159, 160] [124, 142, 161]

(continued)

Table 13.4 (continued)

Old name	New name	Receptor	Source	Function	Findings in SSc patients	References
Mig	CXCL9	CXCR3	Monocytes, macrophages, endothelium	Th1 T cell chemotaxis, pro-inflammatory, angiostatic	High serum levels	[142, 161]
I-TAC	CXCL11	CXCR3	Leukocytes, endothelium	Th1 T cell chemotaxis, pro-inflammatory, angiostatic	Higher serum levels, worse lung disease. BAL levels predict FVC decline	[160] [162]
SDF-1α/β	CXCL12	CXCR4	Stromal cells, epithelium, endothelium, DCs	Chemotaxis lymphocytes, monocytes, hematopoietic and mesenchymal progenitors (endothelial precursors, fibrocytes)	Increased expression in skin and ECs of patients with early active dcSSc SNPs associated with vascular disease manifestations	[163, 164]
	CXCL16	CXCR6	Macrophages, DCs, lymphocytes Endothelium, keratinocytes	Chemotaxis effector/ memory T cells and natural killer cells	High serum levels, correlation with degree of skin fibrosis	[165]
Fractalkine	CX3CL1	CX3R1	Endothelium, epithelial cells	Monocytes, NK cells, effector T cell chemotaxis, and adhesion	Higher serum levels and increased expression in fibrotic skin and ILD lungs of dcSSc patients Higher frequency of CX3CR1-positive circulating T cells and monocytes SNPs associated with PAH in lcSSc patients	[166] [167] [168]

BAL bronchoalveolar lavage, *CT* computed tomography, *DC* dendritic cell, *dcSSc* diffuse cutaneous SSc, *DLCO* carbon monoxide diffusing capacity, *ECM* extracellular matrix, *EC* endothelial cell, *ET* endothelin, *FVC* forced vital capacity, *ILD* interstitial lung disease, *lcSSc* limited cutaneous SSc, *MMP* matrix metalloproteinases, *NK* natural killer, *PAH* pulmonary arterial hypertension, *SNP* single nucleotide polymorphism, *SSc* systemic sclerosis, *Th* T helper, *VSMC* vascular smooth muscle cell

Innate Immunity

Toll-Like Receptors and Other Pattern Recognition Receptors

The cells of the innate immune system and in particular monocytes/macrophages and dendritic cells (DCs) are equipped with receptors that sense danger whether derived from pathogen-associated molecular patterns (PAMP) or from endogenous molecules released by cells under stress (damage-associated molecular patterns: DAMP). Engagement of these receptors initiates inflammatory responses and participates to the antigenic priming of naïve T cells. The most studied family of receptors, named Toll-like receptor (TLR) family, encompasses several members (9 in humans) expressed at the cell surface (TLR 1/2, 2, 4, 5, 6) or in cytoplasmic vacuoles (TLR 3, 7, 8, 9). These receptors recruit MyD88 or TRIF and activate the NFkB or interferon regulatory factor (IRF) signaling cascades, thus initiating the production, among others, of inflammatory cytokines and interferons (IFN). A further important event linked to activation of TLR on professional antigen-presenting cells (APCs) is the upregulation on the cell surface of co-stimulatory molecules like B7 (CD80) which provide the second signal mandatory for naïve T cell activation upon antigen encounter. Further sensors of danger exist in the cytoplasm and include the RIG-I-like receptors (RLR), the NOD-like receptors (NLR), as well as additional sensors of nucleic acids [169, 170]. The contribution of TLRs to SSc pathogenesis (Table 13.1) has received increasing attention in the last few years in two distinct directions. The first concerns the contribution of TLRs to the production of type I interferons (IFN-I) or other cytokines by cells of the innate immune system and the second the contribution of TLRs in activating mesenchymal cells, in particular fibroblasts. Sera from SSc patients, particularly those containing anti-topoisomerase-1 or other anti-ribonucleoprotein autoantibodies (autoAbs), induce the production of IFN-I when added to peripheral blood mononuclear cells (PBMCs) in a plasmacytoid dendritic cell (pDC) and FcgammaRII-dependent manner [28, 29]. The digestion of nucleic acids abrogates the response and the addition of necrotic/apoptotic cells increases the response, indirectly suggesting a role for TLRs in IFN-I production. IFN-I levels are indeed elevated in the sera of SSc individuals and gene array profiles indicate that an IFN-induced gene signature is present in approximately half of the SSc patients [171–174].

A direct role for TLR4 has also been proposed. SSc myeloid DC (mDC) activated by lipopolysaccharide (LPS) produces higher amounts of IL-10 compared to controls, and SSc sera are capable of activating CHO cells transfected with human TLR4 [25, 26]. Furthermore, the same group, by using a proteomic approach, has identified CXCL4 (also known as platelet factor 4) as a serum biomarker of SSc, particularly of early active diffuse SSc. In their hands, CXCL4 enhances the production of IFN-I by pDC activated by ligands of TLR7/8 (R848) and TLR9 (CpG) and appears to be present in skin-resident pDC [14].

Several papers have addressed the role of TLR expressed on fibroblasts. Thus, fibronectin extracellular domain A (FN^{EDA}), expressed in high amounts in involved skin, was shown to bind TLR4 and enhance collagen production in an in vivo murine model of scleroderma. FN^{EDA} production is induced by TGF-β and simultaneously enhances TGF-β production by fibroblasts, thus providing a positive feedback loop potentially able to maintain in an autonomous manner sustained fibroblast activation [9, 10]. TLR4 was shown to be hyper-expressed in SSc skin and consistently chronic LPS challenge in mice induced inflammation and TGF-gene signature [19]. Hyaluronan (HA), a putative TLR4 ligand, was shown to be involved in bleomycin-induced murine fibrosis in a CD19-dependent manner, and in humans, HA enhanced the production of IL-27 by monocytes [30]. IL-27 was high in the sera from early SSc and stimulated collagen production by human dermal fibroblasts [23]. In contrast with these results, however, TLR4 activity has been shown to be required for resolving pulmonary fibrosis in murine models of acute and chronic lung injury [32].

Human SSc monocytes activated by the TLR8 ligand ssRNA (and to a lesser extent by LPS/TLR4) produce enhanced levels of TIMP-1 (tissue inhibitor of matrix metalloproteinases) [18]. Furthermore, chronic EBV infection, specifically demonstrated in human SSc fibroblasts, results in TLR7 and TLR9 enhanced expression leading to interferon-releasing factor (IRF) signaling and enhanced collagen production [15]. Somehow controversial is the role of TLR3 which has been explored through fibroblast responses to poly(I:C). Stimulation with poly(I:C) can induce IFN and TGF signatures and enhance the production of endothelin-1 as well as ICAM-1 in human fibroblasts and endothelial cells [22, 24]. TLR3 is upregulated by IFN-alpha2a in SSc and control fibroblasts with enhanced production of IL-6 [21]. Finally, poly(I:C) induces the production of thymic stromal lymphopoietin (TSLP) in fibroblasts which may participate to skin fibrosis in response to bleomycin [17]. In contrast with these results, poly(I:C) has been shown to inhibit spontaneous and TGF-induced collagen production in fibroblasts via the intracellular sensors MDA5 and RIG1 [16]. Overall, accumulating evidence strongly support the contention that molecules belonging to the innate immune system, particularly TLRs, are involved in SSc development. Further studies are however needed to pinpoint their exact role.

Dendritic Cells

Dendritic cells (DCs) are specialized innate immune cells present throughout the body that collect information from the external environment and transfer it to effectors of the adaptive immune system such as T and B cells. DCs comprise several subsets of which two are easily detected in humans: one in the lymphoid (plasmacytoid DC or pDC) and the other in the myeloid (myeloid DC or mDC) lineage [175, 176]. The recognition of PAMPs or DAMPs through different types of receptors, including TLRs, Fc gamma receptors, and lectins, among others, prompts DC activation and maturation with upregulation of chemokine receptors, secretion of cytokines, expression of co-stimulatory molecules, and ultimately enhancement of their function as antigen-presenting cells (APCs). In response to viral products, pDCs secrete abundant type I interferons (IFN-α/β), which further favor their own differentiation into mature DC and initiation of T cell-dependent immune responses [177, 178]. pDCs can also promote differentiation of naïve T cells into Th2 effectors with production of IL-10 and pro-fibrotic mediators such as IL-13 and TGFβ [179]. Activation of mDC by PAMPs or CD40L results in the secretion of IL-12 and several other cytokines (including TNFα and TGFβ), together with the expression of T cell co-stimulatory molecules such as CD80 (B7.1) and CD86 (B7.2) [180, 181]. Antigen-specific T cells primed by mDC differentiate into Th1 IFNγ-secreting effectors.

While their function is essential for host protection against external pathogens, DCs can also exert a crucial role in promoting peripheral tolerance to self-antigens. Processing and presentation of endogenous molecules deriving from damaged tissues or apoptotic cells by immature DCs result in anergy or deletion of autoreactive T cells [180]. Failure of this function may lead to insufficient self-tolerance and induction of autoimmunity. Based on the type of secreted cytokines and expression of surface molecules, DCs can drive T cells toward different polarized subsets (i.e., Th1/Th2, Th17, or Tregs). Interestingly, both monocyte-derived and freshly isolated mDC from SSc patients with early (<2 years) limited and diffuse disease show higher secretion of pro-inflammatory cytokines (i.e., IL-6 and TNFα) upon stimulation with several TLRs (2,3,4, 7/8), compared to late SSc or control subjects [25]. In contrast, TLR4 stimulation of DCs from early SSc patients induces lower IL-12 and higher IL-10 secretion compared to healthy subjects, which is consistent with a Th2-skewed pro-inflammatory function. This activation may happen in vivo and drive further secretion of cytokines relevant for the fibrotic process observed in SSc. Other mechanisms may contribute to this imbalanced immune response. For example, DCs activated by thymic stromal lymphopoietin (TSLP) have the ability to drive a Th2 T cell differentiation and to maintain survival of Th2 polarized memory T cells [182]. The interaction between OX40 ligand (OX40L) on the surface of DCs with OX40 expressed on activated T cells is critical for this function [183]. An association between several SNPs in the gene encoding for OX40L (tumor necrosis factor ligand superfamily member 4 or TNFSF4) and susceptibility for SSc has been reported [184]. In addition, higher serum levels of soluble OX40 are found in SSc patients compared to healthy controls and associate with shorter disease duration [185].

Monocytes/Macrophages

Monocyte-derived cells and macrophages are essential mediators of chronic inflammation and are an important component of the cellular infiltrates present in early SSc skin lesions or lung tissues in active SSc-ILD [186–188]. Depending on the microenvironment, macrophage activation can be quite heterogeneous and acquire a diversified functional phenotype and polarization. Two main subsets have been used in the past to characterize opposite macrophage function: the "classical" (M1) activation phenotype, which can be induced by IFNγ, LPS, or TNFα and is associated with secretion of pro-inflammatory cytokines (i.e., IL-6, TNFα, IL-1β), tumor resistance, and strong anti-microbial activity, and the "alternatively" activated (M2) phenotype, which can be induced by type 2 cytokines such as IL-4 and IL-13 and is characterized by the secretion of specific cytokines and chemokines (IL-1RA, IL-10, CCL1, CCL17, CCL18, CCL22) and by the expression of distinct membrane receptors including scavenger receptor 1 (CD204), mannose receptor (CD206), c-type mannose receptor-1 (CD163), and chemokine receptors CXCR1, CXCR2, and CCR2 [189, 190]. This subset is involved in immune-regulatory functions, angiogenesis, and tissue remodeling. In particular, M2 macrophages have shown the ability to contribute to fibrogenesis by secreting TGFβ and induction of myofibroblast differentiation [191, 192]. Recently, a new nomenclature has been proposed to recognize macrophage plasticity and to reflect that activation of macrophages by specific cytokine mediators can generate a spectrum of subsets rather than two main groups [193]. Macrophages at the M1 end of the spectrum which are activated by IFNγ have been called M(IFNγ). Conversely, macrophages with M2 characteristics, activated by IL-4, have been defined as M(IL-4).

In patients with pulmonary fibrosis, alveolar macrophages exhibit an enhanced M2/M(IL-4) phenotype and secrete pro-fibrotic chemokines [194]. Activated macrophages exhibiting an M2 phenotype (CD204+) are increased in the skin of SSc patients [195]. Soluble CD163 levels are elevated in the serum of SSc patients and SSc-PBMCs secrete higher amounts of CD163 compared to controls, which supports an "alternative" macrophage activation [196–198]. In addition, circulating PBMCs in subjects with limited SSc exhibit increased expression of CD206 in association with PAH and worse clinical outcome [199]. Mathai et al. showed that circulating monocytes from SSc patients exhibit a pro-fibrotic phenotype and unexpectedly acquire an M2 activation upon stimulation with the TLR4 agonist LPS, which normally induces an M1 phenotype [200]. A similar M2-skewed response to LPS has been demonstrated for SSC monocyte-derived DCs [26].

Interestingly, several IFN-regulated genes are overexpressed in PBMC from SSc patients [201]. In particular, sialic acid-binding Ig-like lectin-1 (Siglec-1) is upregulated on circulating CD14+ monocytes and skin macrophages, suggesting that type I IFN stimulation may also be implicated in the activation of these cells in SSc. Other abnormalities have been detected in monocytes from SSc patients that may be associated with disease pathogenesis. In particular, levels of caveolin-1, a negative modulator of TGFβ signaling and function, are decreased in monocytes from SSc patients [202, 203]. The enhanced pro-fibrotic phenotype detected in these cells and their ability to differentiate into fibrocytes is abrogated by restoring normal expression of caveolin-1 [203, 204]. In keeping with these data, the expression caveolin-1 has been also found to be significantly lower in affected lung tissues and skin of SSc patients [205]. Taken together, these findings suggest that monocytes are likely to play crucial roles in the pathogenesis of SSc by linking activation of the innate immunity to inflammation and fibrogenesis. In particular, it is likely that M2(IL-4) macrophages are tightly linked with fibro-proliferation.

NK Cells

Natural killers (NKs) are cellular effectors of the innate immunity mediating non-MHC-restricted cytotoxic functions also named innate lymphoid cells-1 (ILC-1). A study from Horikawa et al. reports that circulating CD16 + CD56+ NK cells are increased in patients with dcSSc compared to lcSSc or healthy controls and that NKs in dcSSc exhibit an activated phenotype [206]. This finding is not consistent with previous studies, which have shown normal or even decreased NK cell counts in SSc patients [207–210]. Indeed, almost uniformly it is reported that SSc NK cells present decreased cytotoxicity and killer function compared to normal controls [206, 211, 212]. The increased frequency of solid malignancies reported in SSc patients may indirectly confirm a general defect in cell-mediated immunity in this disease.

An additional, poorly characterized, cellular subset named NKT cells expresses CD3 and alpha/beta TcR with limited usage of the alpha- and beta-chains (in humans Valpha24 and Vbeta11, respectively) and recognizes glycolipid antigens presented by the MHC-like molecule CD1d. NKT cells exert important regulatory properties either by direct cell-cell interaction with other immune cells or through secretion of cytokines [118]. Their dysfunction has been linked to several autoimmune diseases. Riccieri et al. report a significant decrease of NKT cell frequency in the blood of SSc patients. Similar abnormalities (decreased NKT cells or function) have been reported in other autoimmune conditions (i.e., SLE, RA, MS) [213–215]. It is plausible that a deficit in NKT suppressive/regulatory function may favor the amplification of pro-inflammatory pathways or the loss of immune tolerance thus contributing to autoimmunity.

Interferons

Recent studies have addressed the role of interferons (IFNs) in SSc. Candidate gene and genome-wide association studies have shown that single nucleotide polymorphisms (SNPs) in genes coding for regulators of IFN-mediated pathways such as *STAT4*, *IRF5*, *IRF7*, *IRF8*, and TBX21 confer susceptibility for SSc or its clinical outcomes [171, 216–221]. An increased expression of type I IFN genes has been detected in the peripheral blood and the skin of patients with SSc [24, 171, 172, 174]. The serum of anti-topoisomerase 1 (Scl70)-positive SSc patients has shown ability to induce IFNα production in vitro significantly more than seronegative patients, and the presence of an IFN signature has been described in association with anti-Scl70 and anti-U1 RNP antibodies, suggesting that RNA-containing immune complexes may be implicated in triggering IFNα secretion in SSc [28, 173]. Concordantly, SSc patients with early diffuse disease have been reported to have higher numbers of CD123+ plasmacytoid dendritic cells (pDCs) in the dermis which is associated with high levels of IFNα mRNA by in situ hybridization [222]. Interestingly, Eloranta et al. have confirmed that SSc sera can activate pDCs in the presence of necrotic or apoptotic cell material, boosting their secretion of IFNα possibly through the formation of interferogenic immune complexes [29].

Importantly, the set of genes upregulated in response to IFN is similar across SSc and other rheumatic diseases including systemic lupus erythematosus, primary Sjögren's syndrome, and dermatomyositis, and many genes thought to be specifically induced by type I IFN can also be effectively induced by IFNγ (type II IFN) [223–225].

IFNγ is generally considered to exert anti-fibrotic functions [110]. Accordingly, several studies have shown its ability to block in vitro collagen synthesis in normal and SSc fibroblasts, and its serum levels have been found to be lower in SSc patients compared to healthy controls [43, 55, 111, 112, 226]. In addition, studies conducted on the peripheral blood or bronchoalveolar lavage fluid obtained from SSc patients have shown a skewing of the T cell repertoire toward a Th2/Tc2 phenotype, suggesting an overall deficit of IFNγ function which normally drives a predominant Th1/Tc1 immune response [47, 227].

In contrast with these observations, other experimental data have demonstrated enrichment of IFNγ secreting T cells in the skin of SSc patients, and increased levels of IFNγ mRNA have been found in the lung tissues from patients with fibrosing alveolitis associated with SSc as opposed to those with cryptogenic fibrosing alveolitis exhibiting a predominant Th2 gene expression profile [113–115]. Moreover, chemoattractants induced by IFNγ such as IP-10/CXCL10, MIG/CXCL9, MIP-1α/CCL3, and MIP-1β/CCL4 are elevated in SSc patients compared to normal controls and are highly expressed in SSc skin [29, 124, 142, 161, 228, 229]. IFNγ can also trigger secretion of MCP-1/CCL2 by different cells types including monocytes and endothelial cells [230–232]. This chemokine is widely recognized as a key player in SSc pathogenesis and has been identified as a reliable marker for disease activity [123, 233, 234]. While overall these data provide evidence for the presence of an IFN-driven immune activation in the blood and skin of SSc patients, the main role of IFNs in SSc pathogenesis and the magnitude of their effect at different stages of the disease process remain still unclear.

Pro-inflammatory Cytokines (IL-1 Family, TNF, IL-6) and Inflammasome

The presence of aberrant expression of nuclear IL-1α has been associated in SSc with higher IL-6, platelet-derived growth factor (PDGF), and procollagen levels [33–35]. SSc fibroblasts spontaneously overexpress IL-1α within the nucleus in a manner that depends on IL-1α-binding protein homologous to HS1-associated protein-1 (HAX-1) [35]. Interestingly, intracellular levels of the natural IL-1 inhibitor named IL-1 receptor antagonist (icIL-1RA) have been found increased in SSc fibroblasts. Transfection of normal fibroblasts with icIL-1Rα results in increased a-smooth muscle actin and decreased MMP-1 expression [36]. IL-1α expression on the surface of endothelial cells or keratinocytes have shown to enhance expression of ICAM-1, connective tissue growth factor (CTGF), and increased contractility in SSc fibroblasts [37, 38]. Finally, IL-1β was shown to play a major role in a mouse model of bleomycin-induced lung fibrosis [39]. These findings make IL-1 a privileged target for immuno-intervention in SSc, but no clinical data are available to date for such a therapeutic strategy.

TNFα is increased in the serum and BALF of SSc patients, and high TNF mRNA expression has been documented in involved skin [45, 55, 61, 77, 115]. Since agents capable of blocking its biological activity are widely available for clinical use, the possible function of TNFα in SSc has attracted considerable interest. However, TNFα has been considered an anti-fibrotic cytokine and there have been some case reports describing the onset or exacerbation of fibrosing alveolitis in patients using anti-TNF agents [235–238]. TNFα is a powerful inducer of matrix metalloproteinases involved in collagen degradation and inhibits in a dose-dependent manner collagen production by inhibiting the transcription of type I and type III procollagen mRNA [239, 240]. In addition, molecular studies have shown that TNFα inhibits TGF-β signaling in human fibroblasts by a variety of additional mechanisms (AP-1 activation, downregulation of TGF-β RII, and CBP/p300 sequestration) [241]. However, SSc T cells co-stimulated with TNF produce more pro-fibrotic cytokines and enhance collagen production by fibroblasts [242]. In addition, some animal models have provided evidence also for a pro-fibrotic function of TNFα [243, 244]. For example, TNF blockade prevents development of lung fibrosis after bleomycin inhalation in mice [134]. The discrepancy between findings obtained in vitro (in which TNFα decreases collagen production) and in vivo (in which TNFα blockade prevents fibrosis) may be related to the function of the inflammatory components preceding bleomycin-induced fibrosis. Nonetheless, it may be safer not to use TNF-blockers in SSc.

The role of IL-6 in fibrosis development has attracted enormous attention. High serum levels of IL-6 have been described in SSc by several authors, with some reporting a positive correlation with skin scores [43, 45, 54–56]. Similarly, increased levels of IL-6 have been found in SSc BALF [61]. Furthermore, serum IL-6 was an independent predictor of DLCO decline in both IPF and SSc-ILD [60]. These data are corroborated by an increased IL-6 production by SSc fibroblasts or PBMCs under basal conditions or after stimulation [33, 62–66]. Of interest, decreased IL-6 serum levels and decreased skin scores have been reported in SSc patients treated with B cell depletion therapy in an uncontrolled study [59]. Furthermore, IL-6 blockade has a protective role in bleomycin-induced skin fibrosis but not in TSK-1+ mice [68, 69].

While controlled studies using tocilizumab, a IL-6 blocking agent, are currently underway with promising results, Japanese investigators have reported decreased skin thickness in two SSc patients receiving this drug for 6 months, while no effect on lung fibrosis was detected in one of them [245].

Overall, the pro-inflammatory cytokines IL-1, TNF, and IL-6 appear to be dysregulated in SSc. Further investigations are needed in order to define the extent of their involvement in SSc disease development and progression.

IL-33, a novel member of the IL-1 family that promotes Th2 responses and inflammation through the ST2 receptor, appears to be increased in the serum of SSc patients and correlated with the extent of skin fibrosis and the severity of pulmonary involvement [246]. Histological analysis reveals that ECs, but also perivascular infiltrating mast cells, CD68-positive macrophages, CD3-positive T cells, CD20-positive B cells, and activated fibroblasts/myofibroblasts, exhibited strong ST2 expression early in the disease course. Consistently, IL-33 raised levels are characteristic of early SSc in association with elevated tissue expression of its receptor, ST2, on endothelial cells (EC) [247, 248]. In contrast, the soluble form of the ST2 receptor is increased late in the disease course, which may indicate a distinct involvement of IL-33 and ST2 early and late in disease course [249]. Finally, it should be stressed that T regulatory cells resident in SSc skin expressed high levels of ST2 receptor and produce large amounts of IL-4, a finding not present in healthy Treg [250]. These data are highly suggestive of an important role of IL-33 and its receptor ST2 in the pathogenesis of SSc, implicating EC in its production and providing a mechanistic link between vascular dysfunction and immune-inflammatory responses.

Inflammasomes are multi-protein scaffolds, which upon assembly of their components activate caspase-1 resulting in the cleavage of pro-IL-1 and IL-18 into their biologically active forms. Dysregulated activation of the inflammasome machinery is responsible for various inflammatory disorders [251]. Since IL-1 has been implicated in the pathogenesis of SSc, a few studies have addressed the potential role of inflammasome components in SSc. Thus, NLRP1 has been found to be a genetic susceptibility factor for SSc-related pulmonary fibrosis and anti-topoisomerase-positive SSc phenotypes [252]. Furthermore, inhibition of caspase-1 in SSc dermal and lung fibroblasts abrogated the secretion of collagens, IL-1β, and IL-18 resulting in decreased expression of the myofibroblast protein α-SMA in SSc dermal fibroblasts. Consistently, NLRP3(−/−) mice and ASC(−/−) mice are resistant to bleomycin-induced skin fibrosis [253]. Compared to healthy individuals, the SSc skin shows a significant increase in NLRP3, caspase-1, IL-1β, and IL-18 mRNA, and dermal thickness significantly correlates with their levels. It should be noted, however, that immunohistochemical analysis identified staining of NLRP3 and IL-1β in the keratinizing squamous epithelium of skin [254]. Therefore, combined genetic, functional, and histological evidence suggests a possible involvement of inflammasomes in SSc pathogenesis, resulting in excessive production of IL-1 and IL-18.

Adaptive Immune Response and Scleroderma T Cells

Histological examination of early SSc skin lesions has demonstrated that an inflammatory infiltrate precedes fibrosis and development of vascular disease, including ultrastructural changes affecting endothelial cells (Fig. 13.1) [257]. Of interest, collagen synthesis determined by in situ localization of procollagen I mRNA appears to be higher in fibroblasts adjacent to inflammatory cells [255, 256]. These findings have led to the hypothesis that inflammatory cells and in particular T cells could provide important stimuli that drive collagen synthesis in fibroblasts, in addition to the development of abnormalities involving endothelial cells. Cutaneous mononuclear cell infiltrates are notably pronounced early on, during the edematous-inflammatory phase of the disease, and then tend to disappear with transition to the sclerotic phase. Consistently, the majority of infiltrating T cells in SSc skin lesions express activation markers and secrete products of activated T cells such as soluble CD25 (the soluble form of the high-affinity IL-2 receptor chain), which have been found in fluid obtained from suction skin blister of SSc patients with early cutaneous disease [258].

Polarized T Cell Subsets (Th1, Th2, Th17, Th22)

T cells are tremendously heterogeneous in terms of T cell receptor (TcR) expression, function, and usage of accessory molecules. While in previous decades the research enquiry was devoted to the study of the CD4+ helper and CD8+ cytolytic T cellular subsets, as well as to the characterization of T cells bearing the α/β or γ/δ TcR in the peripheral blood and affected tissues, most of the recent attention has been focused on the identification of the pattern of cytokines produced by the T cells in SSc [259]. It is indeed felt that the cytokine produced by T cells may have a major impact on endothelial cells and fibroblast function and can yield effects favoring or inhibiting vascular disease and development of fibrosis. Classically, CD4+ T helper cells have been categorized into the Th1 and Th2 subsets. In the last few years, additional subsets have been identified in humans, which include Th17, Th22, and T regulatory cells (Tregs). Of major importance for the fate determination of CD4+ T helper cells is the cytokine milieu where T cell activation takes place. Thus, in the presence of IL-12 and interferons, T helper precursor cells become Th1 and high producers of IFNγ, while in the presence of IL-4 and IL-2, they become Th2 and high producers of IL-4, IL-5, and IL-13. The simultaneous presence of TGFβ and pro-inflammatory cytokines such as IL-1 or IL-6 favors the production of IL-17A and IL-17F by T cells, which are thus defined as Th17 cells. These can further differentiate and proliferate in the presence of IL-23 or IL-21, while TGFβ in conjunction with IL-2 favors the polarization toward cells with regulatory function (Tregs) and producing TGF-β and IL-10 [260]. In humans, but not in mice, an additional terminally differentiated subset characterized by the production of IL-22 in the absence of the other prototypic cytokines exists (Fig. 13.2) [261, 262].

Transcriptome analysis in animal models performed before the discovery of Th17 cells has shown that genes involved in wound healing and fibrosis are associated with Th2 polarized responses and are characterized by the production of IL-4, IL-5, IL-13, and IL-21 as opposed to IFNγ which is typical of a Th1 polarization [263, 264]. Considerable evidence indicates that indeed type 2 polarized responses are important for fibrosis development [265, 266]. Interestingly, IFNγ inhibits collagen synthesis, while IL-4 and IL-13 enhance it [110, 226, 267, 268]. The in vivo relevance of IL-4 in fibrogenesis has been documented in several animal models including among others the tight-skin-1 (Tsk-1) mice, where a targeted mutation of the IL-4 receptor α-chain

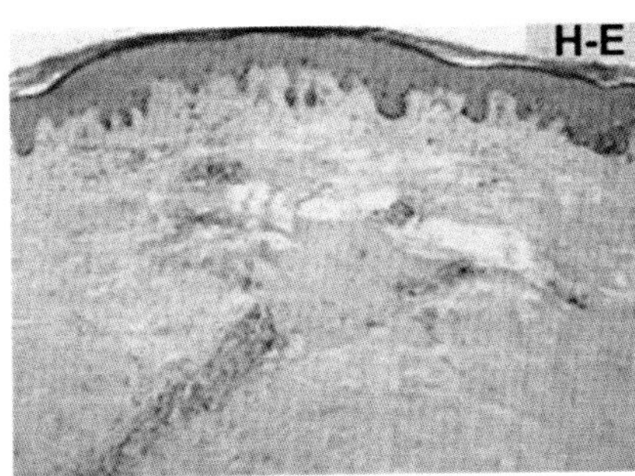

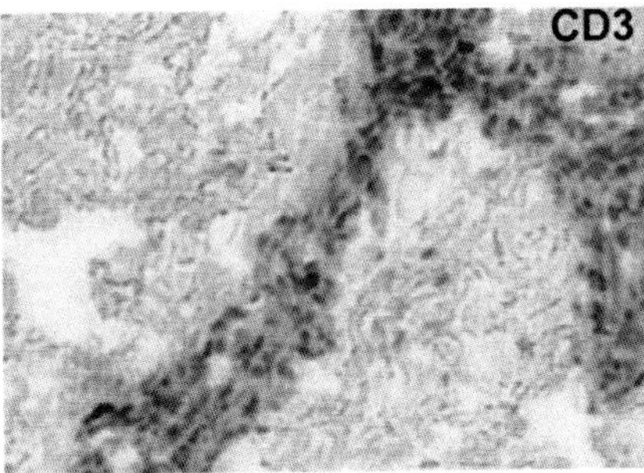

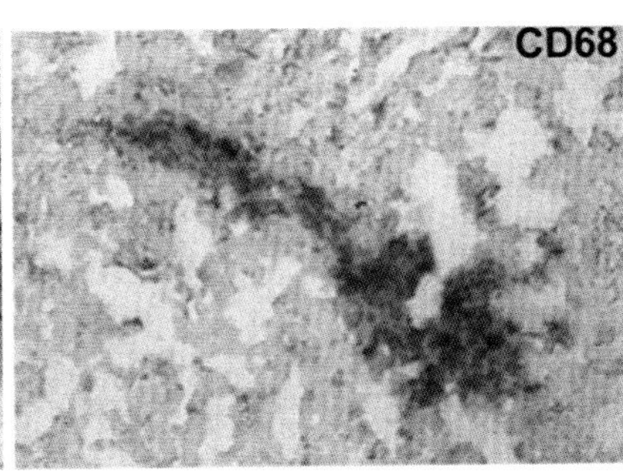

Fig. 13.1 Representative immunohistological analysis of the inflammatory infiltrate characteristic of early skin involvement in SSc. *Left panel*: (low-magnification) hematoxylin-eosin staining showing thickened dermis with increased collagen deposition and perivascular inflammatory infiltrate. *Middle panel*: (high-power magnification) T cell infiltrates identified by anti-CD3 monoclonal antibody. *Right panel*: (high-power magnification) macrophages are identified by anti-CD68 monoclonal antibody. Of note, some studies have shown by in situ hybridization that type I collagen mRNA is abundantly expressed by fibroblasts present in the dermal region adjacent to the inflammatory infiltrate [255, 256]. This suggests an important pro-fibrotic role of the cells present in the inflammatory infiltrate, including T cells

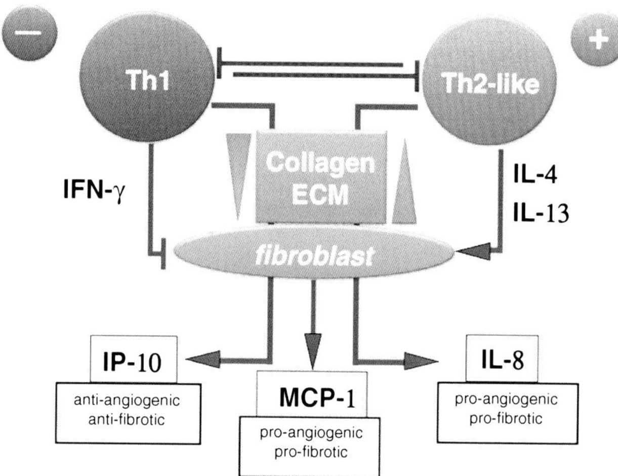

Fig. 13.2 Opposing roles of Th1 and Th2-like cells in respect of ECM deposition and fibroblast inflammatory responses. *Arrows* and *arrowheads* indicate stimulation; blunted ends indicate inhibition. IFNγ produced by Th1 cells directly inhibits collagen production by fibroblasts. IL-4 and IL-13 produced by Th2 cells directly favors collagen production by fibroblasts. Illustrated the capacity of fibroblasts to differentially produce chemokines under polarized stimulation. IFNγ favors the production of the anti-fibrotic CXCL10; IL4/IL13 favors the production of the pro-fibrotic IL-8. MCP-1 is induced by both Th1 and Th2 cells

or IL-4 gene can prevent development of fibrosis [269, 270]. Additional data indicate that IL-13 interaction with the IL-13Rα2 receptor induces in macrophages the production of TGFβ and drives enhanced collagen synthesis and fibrosis [271, 272]. Therefore, the dichotomous view of the adaptive immune response condensed in the Th1 and Th2 paradigm can appropriately be translated in the field of fibrosis as Th2/Tc2 cells being pro-fibrotic and Th1/Tc1 cells anti-fibrotic [266]. The major findings supporting a role of Th2-like responses in SSc pathogenesis are summarized in Table 13.3.

Most of the studies performed in SSc patients have investigated the characteristics of T cells present in the peripheral blood. While this is justified by an easier access, it is noteworthy to remind that the peripheral compartment may not reflect the ongoing inflammatory process present in different target organs such as the skin or the lungs, and it may imperfectly represent the complexity associated with T cell responses in SSc. In addition, it has not been demonstrated that the mechanisms leading to fibrosis in different tissues and organs or in different SSc clinical subsets (i.e., lcSSc vs dcSSc) are uniformly the same.

Not surprisingly, there is a functional heterogeneity among T cells present in the peripheral blood and those infiltrating the skin or the lungs in SSc patients. Some studies suggest the predominance in SSc of polarized T cells preferentially producing IFNγ and therefore belonging to the Th1 subset, while others report a preferential expansion of T cells producing high levels of IL-4 and therefore belonging to the Th2 subset, particularly in subjects with early active or severe disease [3, 47, 49, 50, 113, 115]. Accordingly, in SSc patients IL-4 and IL-13 serum levels are increased, inflammatory skin infiltrates exhibit high IL-4 and low IFN-g mRNA expression, and the number of CD30+ T cells in the skin and the levels of serum soluble CD30 are higher (CD30 being preferentially expressed by Th2 cells) (Table 13.3) [39, 49]. Furthermore, the frequency of IL-13-producing CD8+ T cells in the peripheral blood is associated with severity of skin fibrosis, while that of IL-4-producing CD8+ T cells quantitatively predicts a faster decline in lung function, and the presence of CD4 + CD8+ double positive T cells with very high IL-4 production potential clearly distinguishes SSc skin from controls [3, 47, 80]. Finally, microchimeric T cells of male origin recovered from the peripheral blood and skin of SSc-affected woman preferentially produce IL-4 [50]. While Th2 cytokines directly favor collagen production by fibroblasts (Fig. 13.2) and consequently the presence of Th2-like cells may be directly linked to fibrosis development, the reality appears more complex. For instance, a higher frequency of Th1 cells in the peripheral blood and increased serum levels of IL-12, a cytokine favoring Th1 cell differentiation, have been reported in SSc patients [45, 79, 273]. Interestingly, this was detected especially in subjects with later stages of the disease, when fibrosis tends to regress [56, 273].

Adding to the complexity of our knowledge about T cell function in SSc, recent findings indicate a role for IL-17 and the cytokines promoting Th17 cellular subset differentiation and expansion. Increased levels of IL-17 have been detected in the sera of SSc patients, and intriguingly IL-17 appears to be overproduced during early stages of the disease [82, 83]. Th17 cells produce high levels of IL-17A, IL-17F, IL-21, IL-22, and CCL20, express the master transcription factors retinoic acid nuclear orphan receptor (ROR)γT and RORα, and depend on signal transducer and activator of transcription-3 (STAT-3). Th17 cells are involved in protection against extracellular bacteria and fungi. Their role in inflammatory disorders has been amply investigated in recent years [274]. Concerning animal models of fibrosis, IL-17A was shown to be involved in bleomycin-induced lung and skin fibrosis [39, 275–277]. Furthermore, Th17-polarized responses mediate lung fibrosis in a model of chronic hypersensitivity and IL-17A deficiency attenuates skin thickness in tight-skin-1 (TSK-1/$^{+}$) mice [98, 277]. Consistently, IL-17 increases TGF-β, CTGF, and collagen production by mouse skin fibroblasts and promotes collagen production and epithelial-mesenchymal transition in mouse alveolar epithelial cells in a TGF-β-dependent manner [275, 277].

In humans, IL-17 enhances proliferation, IL-6 and IL-8 production, and ICAM-1 expression by fibroblasts and endothelial cells [82, 84]. However, Nakashima et al. report that IL-17A possesses direct anti-fibrogenic properties in normal human fibroblasts by upregulating miR-129-5p and down-regulating connective tissue growth factor and type I collagen [86]. SSc fibroblasts may escape this repressive effect of IL-17A because of reduced expression of the IL-17RA subunit. Others have found that IL-17A failed to increase type I and type III procollagen mRNA expression in fibroblasts from healthy controls and SSc patients [82]. Our findings support the contention that IL-17A does not favor type I collagen production at both mRNA and protein levels by control and SSc fibroblasts but rather limits the transdifferentiation of fibroblast into pro-fibrotic myofibroblasts, simultaneously favoring the production of IL-8, IL-6, MCP-1, and MMP-1 [85, 87, 94]. Nonetheless, there is ample agreement that Th17 cell numbers are increased in SSc peripheral blood as well as in involved lungs and skin [58, 89–92]. An increased frequency of Th22 cells has also been reported [278, 279].

Regarding the question whether IL-17A-producing cells are also present in the skin, it has been reported that IL-17A+ cells are significantly more numerous in SSc skin than in healthy controls. Both T cells and mast cells stain positive for IL-17A. Interestingly, the frequency of IL-17A+ cells is higher in the skin of SSc patients with less severe skin fibrosis [87]. Furthermore, the frequency of IL-17A+ cells increases significantly with disease duration when the skin becomes less fibrotic and more atrophic, further stressing the potential for IL-17A in reducing rather than enhancing fibrosis [94]. In in vitro cultures, IL-17A induces the production of inflammatory mediators and MMPs by healthy and SSc fibroblasts but fails to upregulate collagen production [85]. These data are in agreement with those obtained by others in vitro on human fibroblasts indicating that IL-17 represses rather than enhances ECM deposition and clear discrepancy with regard to the pro-fibrotic role by IL-17A demonstrated in mice [82, 86]. To further appreciate the role of the IL-17 family members in human dermal fibrosis, the presence of cells expressing IL-17A, IL-17F, IL-17C, and IL-17E (also known as IL-25) was searched in systemic sclerosis and morphea (a condition characterized by skin fibrosis with no internal organ involvement) allowing the identification of a molecular motif characterized by high IL-17E and low IL-17C distinctly present in morphea and SSc and not in healthy skin, suggestive of a pro-fibrotic cytokine pattern [94]. It should be further emphasized that iloprost, a PGI2 analog used to control Raynaud's phenomenon and digital ulcers, has the capacity to increase IL-17 production by Th17 in an IL-23-dependent manner [280, 281]. These data, together with the evidence that iloprost has the potential ability to reduce skin fibrosis in SSc, provide further support to a predominantly anti-fibrotic effect of IL-17A in humans [282]. An integrated view of IL-17 function and its modulatory effect on the fibrotic process is shown in Fig. 13.3. Clearly, further investigations are required to better understand the relevance of this cytokine and other members of the IL-17 family in fibrotic disorders.

Fibroblasts carry CD40 on their surface and can respond upon engagement with its ligand CD40L (CD154) expressed on activated T cells. Interestingly, CD40 is upregulated on SSc fibroblasts, and T cells from SSc patients exhibit a higher expression of CD40L. In addition, serum levels of both soluble CD40 and CD40L molecules are increased in SSc [118–120]. All these findings, together with the fact that blockade of the CD40-CD40L interaction attenuates fibrosis in the TSK-1 mouse model, indicate a possible role for this biologic axis in fibrogenesis [121, 283]. The interaction of T cells with fibroblasts may occur also through membrane-bound cytokines. T cell membranes from activated Th1 and Th2 cells have been shown to inhibit fibroblast collagen I production through different molecular mechanisms. In fact, Th1-mediated inhibition was shown to depend on IFNγ function, while Th2 cell-dependent inhibition was essentially mediated by TNFα. In addition, T cell contact inhibition was

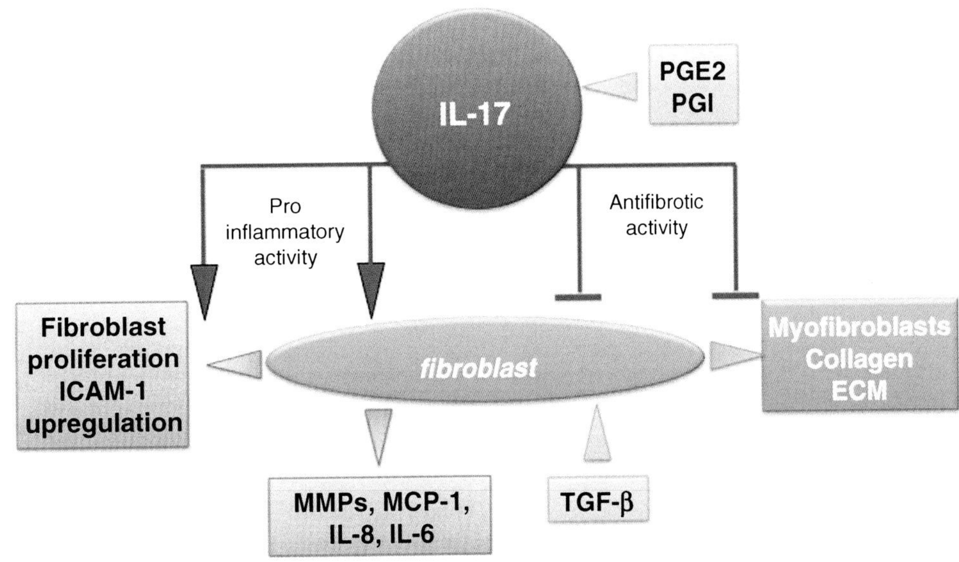

Fig. 13.3 IL-17 exerts a wide array of different functions on human fibroblasts, which may vary according to the context in which they take place. *Arrows* and *arrowheads* indicate stimulation; blunted ends indicate inhibition. *Green boxes*: endogenous and exogenous mediators that modify the context. Thus, PGE2 and PGI enhance IL-17 production by Th17. The anti-fibrotic potential of IL-17A is illustrated by the capacity of this cytokine to inhibit the pro-fibrotic activity of TGF-β

dominant over pro-fibrotic IL-4 and TGFβ cytokines and was specific for collagen I, since mRNA levels of COL1A1 were decreased, while mRNA levels of MMP-1 were strongly increased [112, 116].

IL-12 Family Members

IL-12 family members are heterodimeric cytokines that encompass IL-12, IL-23, IL-27, and IL-35 (Table 13.2). Despite sharing many structural features and molecular partners, cytokines of the IL-12 family mediate surprisingly diverse functional effects [284]. From a T cell point of view, IL-12 promotes Th1 differentiation and IL-23 participates in conjunction with IL-1, IL-6, and TGF-β to the differentiation of Th17 cells. This diversity is becoming clear also in the context of SSc.

The importance of IL-12 in SSc is underscored by genetic polymorphisms of TYK2, an IL-12 signaling element associated with SSc and of the IL-12 receptor β-chain [285, 286]. Furthermore, the concentration of serum IL-12 increases in SSc with disease duration concomitantly with reduced skin fibrosis and its production is decreased upon TLR stimulation in SSc. This is consistent with a potentially protective role of Th1 responses in SSc (see below).

IL-23 receptor polymorphisms associated with the presence of anti-Topo-1 and PAH in SSc have been reported in one study but no association was found in two others [216, 287, 288]. IL-23 serum levels are increased in SSc serum and modulated positively by prostacyclin therapeutic infusions [280, 281].

As reported in Table 13.2, a single paper indicates that IL-27 serum levels are increased in SSc and correlated positively with the extent of skin and pulmonary fibrosis and immunological abnormalities. Interestingly IL-27 serum levels tended to decrease with disease duration, which is the opposite of what was reported for IL-12. Furthermore, IL-27 stimulation increased IgG production of B cells, IL-17 production of CD4 T cells, and proliferation and collagen synthesis of fibroblasts in patients with SSc compared with those in healthy controls [23].

While relatively little is known about IL-35 in SSc, two recent publications have reported discordant results. On the one hand, IL-35 and in particular its EBI3 chain expression was reported decreased in keratinocytes and dermal regulatory T cells in SSc compared to normal skin [102]. Consistently with an anti-fibrotic potential of IL-35, IL-35 decreases type I collagen production irrespective of the presence of TGFβ and exerts protective effects when injected in bleomycin-induced mouse skin fibrosis. On the other hand, serum levels of IL-35 were reported elevated in SSc, particularly in early disease, and its expression increased in affected SSc skin. Consistently with a pro-fibrotic potential of IL-35, IL-35 induced by TGFβ enhances collagen production by dermal fibroblasts [101]. Future studies clearly are needed to reconcile these findings.

Collectively, available data support a dysregulated expression and function of the cytokines of the IL-12 family in SSc. It is likely that distinct roles are played during different phases of the disease course, with IL-27 levels being higher early on and IL-12 expression increasing at later stages. However, the interaction between these cytokines and their role in the SSc disease process remain complex, as highlighted by the fact that IL-23 production is upregulated by therapeutic agents beneficial on Raynaud's phenomenon and digital ulcers.

Regulatory T Cells

Regulatory T cells (Tregs) play a pivotal role in maintaining immunologic self-tolerance and preventing autoimmunity. Their ability to limit potentially dangerous immune responses and to regulate the function of other T cells is exerted by a variety of mechanisms including the production of immunosuppressive cytokines (TGF-β, IL-10), the inhibition by contact of effector T cells or antigen-presenting cells via surface molecules such as CTLA-4, or the expression of enzymes such as indoleamine 2,3-dioxygenase, which, by reducing the availability of the essential amino acid tryptophan, drives potent anti-proliferative effects [289]. At least two main subsets of Tregs are recognized: the natural Tregs (nTreg) and the inducible Tregs (iTreg). nTregs are CD4+ T cells generated in the thymus during the process of negative selection which allows retention of cells bearing TcR with an intermediate affinity for self-antigens associated with a developmental program leading to a regulatory phenotype [290]. iTregs develop from naïve, mature CD4+ T cells after encountering their nominal antigen within secondary lymphoid organs in the presence of TGF-β and high levels of IL-2 [291]. Markers used for their identification include the intracellular expression of the transcription factor FOXP3, the surface high expression of CD25, the combination of CD45 isoforms with the above molecules, and the expression of CD127 [292]. The not uniform use of these cell markers may explain why the literature concerning Tregs in SSc does not provide homogenous data and a uniformed view regarding their role and function. Some authors have reported that the number of Tregs is markedly increased in all clinical SSc phenotypes, but these Tregs exhibit a diminished capacity to control CD4 effector T cells [293–295]. Furthermore, this defective function seems to correlate with lower expression of CD69 and TGF-β. Others have found a quantitative reduction of Tregs in the skin and peripheral blood of affected patients [279, 293]. In particular, Mathian et al. have reported that "activated" Treg (CD4 CD45RA–FOXP3brightCD25bright) is decreased in SSc patients at any disease stage, while "resting" Treg (CD4 CD45RA+FOXP3+CD25+) frequency declines in late phases of SSc [279]. Their data also show that both subsets retain an intact suppressive function and support the possibility that the quantitative deficit of Tregs may drive activation and proliferation of effector T cells. Another study has shown that the proportion of Treg is lower than in controls within affected tissues but not in the peripheral blood [296]. A small prospective study conducted in seven SSc patients with diffuse skin phenotype found that the depressed Treg number and function were restored after autologous hematopoietic stem cell transplantation [297]. Aberrant epigenetic modifications such as hypermethylation of FOXP3 gene have also been detected in Tregs from SSc patients and indicated as a possible cause for decreased FOXP3 expression and lower circulating levels of this cell type [298]. It has been reported that X-chromosome inactivation is more skewed in SSc than in the general population and that this is not related to age. Skewed X-chromosome usage correlates with lower FOXP3 expression in the CD25+ high Treg cells [299]. An intriguing twist to this topic has been brought about by the demonstration that FOXP3-positive cells with high IL-4 and IL-13 production are enriched in the skin of SSc patients compared to normal controls [250]. The authors of this investigation concluded that these FOXP3+ T cells may indeed be Tregs with a functional Th2-like phenotype, which could contribute to enhance pro-fibrotic responses in dermal fibroblasts. Of interest, this study also found that skin-infiltrating FOXP3+ T cells express high levels of the IL-33 receptor ST2 and that the number of IL-13-producing FOXP3+ T cells is increased by culturing SSc skin biopsies in the presence of IL-33. This, together with the fact that only the skin but not peripheral blood FOXP3+ T cells manifested this aberrant Th2-like behavior, further supports the possibility that the skin of SSc patients provides the appropriate environment for transdifferentiation of Tregs (CD4+FOXP3+ T cells) toward a Th2-like phenotype with the consequent amplification of a pro-fibrotic loop.

Autoantigen-Specific T Cell Response

The detection of expanded oligoclonal T cell subsets in affected skin or lungs (BALF) of SSc patients supports the notion that an antigen-driven, T cell-dependent process may be involved in SSc pathogenesis [1–4, 300]. While T cells recognizing SSc-specific autoantigens such as topoisomerase-1 (topo-1) or RNA polymerase III (RNApol3) have been documented in humans, the detection of autoantigen-specific T cells in the peripheral blood of SSc patients has been difficult due to technical limitations and their very low frequency, particularly in patients under immunosuppression [301–304]. In addition, the identification of autoreactive T cells has shown poor specificity as they have been found also in anti-topo-1-negative patients as well as in healthy controls [300, 305–307]. More recently, a close temporal association between the onset of SSc and the detection of cancer has been described in a subset of patients positive for anti-RNA polymerase III antibodies [308]. This observation has lead to the discovery that mutated autoantigens (RNApol3) are present in the tumors obtained from these patients and result in mutant-specific T cell immune responses as well as in the generation cross-reactive autoantibodies [303]. These findings support the possibility that, at least in some patients, an abnormal (mutated) cancer antigen may be the initial trigger for an autoimmune T cell activation in SSc. Animal models have also been used to test whether the generation of autoimmune responses against topo-1 could drive a pathological phenotype resembling SSc. The immunization of mice prone to autoimmunity with the human recombinant protein induced T cell responses and antibodies against topo-1 but did not drive any pathologic features resembling SSc [309]. In contrast, when C57BL/6 mice were repeatedly immunized with human topo-1 in the presence of complete Freund's adjuvant, skin and lung fibroses in addition to autoimmune manifestations were generated [310]. Of interest, pathologic manifestations were associated with the increased production of IL-6 and IL-17 as well as higher levels of circulating IL-17-secreting T cells (Th17). This landmark report, which is still awaiting confirmation, indicates that besides an autoimmune background, a second trigger may be needed, such as the one provided by repeated stimulation of the innate immune system by complete Freund's adjuvant, to direct the immune response toward a permissive pro-fibrotic milieu.

The observation that a higher proportion of SSc women compared to healthy controls have circulating male cells, which can be found in tissues undergoing fibrosis, suggests the possibility that alloantigens may also drive the immune response in SSc and play a possible pathogenetic role [311, 312]. The hypothesis that microchimerism may be mechanistically relevant in SSc has been supported by the close similarity between fibrotic skin lesions observed in SSc and chronic graft-versus-host disease (GVHD) after allogeneic bone marrow transplantation. In fact, murine models of fibrosis have been developed based on chimerism and GVHD [313].

Overall, these data support the concept that T cells upon nominal antigen recognition may initiate an inflammatory process ultimately resulting in tissue fibrosis. It remains however possible that T cells may be only activated bystanders with functional characteristics depending on and not causing the underlying disease process. Furthermore, the possibility that T cells, at least in certain phases of the disease, may restrain rather than favor fibrosis cannot be fully disregarded.

B Cells

Antinuclear antibodies are characteristically present in SSc. A full spectrum of autoAbs directed against distinct ubiquitous autoantigens (centromeric protein B, topoisomerase-1, RNA polymerase III, etc.) are detected in patients with specific clinical manifestations. Anti-centromere autoAbs are associated with limited cutaneous SSc (lcSSc) and more intense vascular disease, anti-topoisomerase-1 (Scl70) with diffuse cutaneous SSc (dcSSc) and pulmonary fibrosis, anti-RNA polymerase III with scleroderma renal crisis, and anti-fibrillin with pulmonary arterial hypertension (PAH). These associations have been consistently verified across individuals with different ethnic origin and justify the hypothesis of a causative link between a specific autoAbs and the corresponding clinical phenotype. However, to date this legitimate question has eluded the investigation enquire.

The participation of B cells to the immune response is not exclusively mediated by the production of antibodies but includes key activities such as antigen presentation, cytokine secretion, modulation of T cell, and dendritic cell activation (Fig. 13.4) [314]. B cell responses are mainly determined by signaling thresholds through the B cell receptor (BcR) complex and are regulated by specific cell surface and cytoplasmic molecules. These "response regulators" concurrently contribute to the amplification (i.e., CD19, CD21, CD45) or suppression (i.e., CD22, CD72, FcγRIIB) of the BcR signal and modulate the resulting B cell activity. Abnormal B cell function and homeostasis have been implicated in the onset and progression of different systemic autoimmune disorders. In SSc patients, lesional skin and lung tissues from subjects with ILD demonstrate prominent B cell infiltration [315, 316]. Gene expression studies have shown significant upregulation of B cell-related genes in affected SSc skin [316]. By using a signature array, plasma cells have been found increased in the skin of SSc patients compared to healthy donors [317]. Analysis of circulating B cell repertoire in SSc has shown expansion of the ($CD27^-$) naïve B cell subset and the concurrent decline of memory B cell and plasmacellular components [318]. Interestingly, these memory B cells retain a strong immunoglobulin secretory function and exhibit upregulation of co-stimulatory molecules (CD80 and CD86) and CD95, suggesting a chronic activation state and an increased sensitivity to proapoptotic stimuli [318, 319]. Accordingly, the expression of positive response regulators such as CD19 and the associated molecule CD21 (complement receptor type 2) are increased in naïve as well as memory B cells of SSc patients compared to healthy controls [57, 318]. A single nucleotide polymorphism (SNP) in the upstream region of CD19 gene has been associated with higher expression of this molecule in circulating B cells and susceptibility to SSc [320]k. Loss of CD19 expression attenuates skin and lung fibrosis in the bleomycin-induced SSc mouse model [30]. Furthermore, over the recent past, several genome-wide association studies (GWAS) have identified multiple B cell genes associated with increased susceptibility for SSc, including BANK1, BLK, CSK, PTPN22, and IRF8 [321].

Few studies have addressed the ability of B cells to activate dermal fibroblasts. Francois et al. demonstrated that

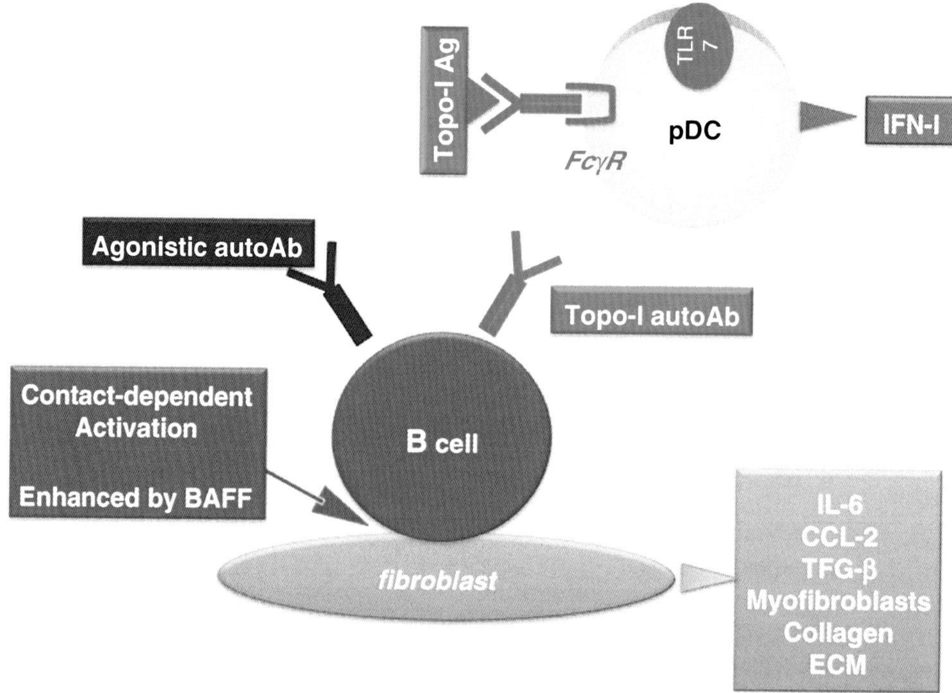

Fig. 13.4 B cells play multiple roles in systemic sclerosis. Autoantibody directed against ubiquitous autoantigens (*green*) may form immune complexes, which may be captured by pDC trough Fcg-receptors, internalized in endosomal compartments where they may interact with TLR and induce an interferon response. Autoantibodies (*red*) against surface receptors such as TLR, endothelin-1 receptors, and angiotensin-receptors may display agonistic activity resulting in the activation of cells bearing such receptors. B cells may directly interact with fibroblasts in a cell-cell-dependent manner and favor pro-fibrotic responses augmented by BAFF. The capacity of B cells to produce regulatory IL-10, a property decreased in SSc, is not here represented

peripheral blood B cells can stimulate IL-6, TGFβ, CCL2, and collagen secretion, as well as α-SMA, TIMP1, and MMP9 expression in dermal fibroblasts isolated from SSc patient [108]. Importantly, this induction was dependent on cell-cell contact and the addition of BAFF to these cocultures enhanced fibroblast activation. The role of BAFF, in conjunction with IL-17, in favoring fibrosis development, has been documented also in a model of bleomycin-induced SSc lung disease [108].

A novel B cell subset producing high levels of IL-10 has been identified and found capable of regulating immune responses, therefore named Breg [322]. In SSc, high-IL-10-producing Breg cells are decreased compared to healthy controls and their suppressive function appears to be impaired. Breg levels correlate negatively with anti-topo I and anti-centromere antibody titers. In addition, Breg counts increase significantly in dcSSc patients after treatment [323, 324].

A proliferation-inducing ligand (APRIL) and B cell activating factor (BAFF) are members of the tumor necrosis factor (TNF) superfamily exerting important homeostatic functions on B cells such as maturation, activation, and survival (anti-apoptotic) [325]. Serum levels of BAFF and APRIL are increased in SSc patients compared to controls and are associated with specific clinical manifestations such as extent of skin involvement (BAFF) and the presence of pulmonary fibrosis (APRIL) [105, 106]. Secretion of APRIL from PBMCs is significantly higher in SSc patients compared to controls and is associated with diffuse skin phenotype, the presence of ILD, and anti-Topo-1 positivity among other SSc clinical features [326]. Interestingly, BAFF serum levels are increased in the tight-skin (TSK/+) mouse, and blockade of the BAFF/BAFF-receptor interaction can prevent the development of skin fibrosis, inhibit autoantibody generation, and increase the production of anti-fibrotic cytokines (i.e., IFNγ) [105].

All these data indicate that B cell activation and overactivity are important features of the immune response in SSc and that an imbalance of B cell homeostasis and function may contribute to the amplification of the inflammatory as well as fibrotic process in this disease. This hypothesis is further supported by recent data indicating beneficial results from the use of therapeutic interventions aimed at depleting CD20+ B cell (rituximab) in SSc patients [327, 328].

Chemokines and Chemokine Receptors

A dysregulated expression of chemokines and their receptors may be pivotal during SSc pathogenesis, modulating leukocytes chemotaxis and migration through the endothelium into target tissues and promoting pathological interactions between immune effectors and fibroblasts. In particular, fibroblasts express chemokine receptors and have shown the ability to impart chemotactic stimuli, which contribute to the amplification of local inflammation as well as of their own activation and secretive function. Moreover, chemokines may be relevant in the SSc disease process for their ability to modulate angiogenesis, endothelial function, and blood vessel homeostasis.

Chemokines are a family of more than 50 small molecules (8–14 kDa) released by different cell types in response to injury or homeostatic stimuli. There are 20 chemokine receptors characterized by a seven-transmembrane domain coupled to heterodimeric G-proteins [329].

Chemokines are segregated into four groups based on the position of the N-terminal two cysteine residues [330]. The CC chemokines (adjacent cysteine residues) primarily mediate chemotactic function toward mononuclear cells and also mediate inflammation. The CXC (cysteine residues separated by a variable single amino acid) chemokines exert regulatory function on angiogenesis. In particular, the CXC chemokines with a typical N-terminal glutamate-leucine-arginine or ELR motif are pro-angiogenic and promote wound healing, while ELR-negative chemokines tend to inhibit neovascularization [331]. The other minor groups are the CX3C (cysteine residues separated by three amino acids) and the C chemokines (missing one cysteine residue). Table 13.4 summarizes the chemokines and chemokine receptors associated with the SSc disease process or with specific SSc clinical manifestations in humans.

CC Chemokines

CCL2 (monocyte chemoattractant protein 1 or MCP-1) has been repeatedly linked to the pathogenesis of SSc. A single nucleotide polymorphism (–2,518 G) in the promoter region of the CCL2 gene has been associated with SSc, but this finding has not been confirmed by subsequent studies [220, 332, 333]. Several reports have shown that CCL2 is increased in the serum of SSc patients and is associated with early active disease, diffuse SSc phenotype, and the presence of pulmonary fibrosis [124, 130, 228]. Higher CCL2 bronchoalveolar lavage fluid (BALF) levels are associated with worsening lung function and more severe pulmonary fibrosis by lung CT score [123]. The role of CCL2 in mediating pro-fibrotic immune responses is supported by solid evidence [334]. CCL2 has been shown to promote Th2 T cell differentiation and secretion of IL-4, an important mediator of fibrosis [127]. Mice knocked out for its receptor (CCR2–/–) are protected from bleomycin-induced lung fibrosis and CCL2-blocking antibodies can prevent skin fibrosis in the same SSc animal model [335–337]. CCL2 expression in lesional skin and its serum levels in SSc patients have shown correlation with the extent of cutaneous fibrosis (mRSS) [126, 131]. A direct pro-fibrotic role is also supported by the findings that CCL2 promotes collagen and matrix metalloproteinase-1 synthesis in human fibroblasts and that is upregulated in tissues undergoing fibrosis [128, 129]. CCL2 exhibits a higher constitutive expression in human skin fibroblasts from SSc patients, and SSc fibroblast-conditioned medium is chemotactic for leukocytes [125, 338]. Whether the effect of CCL2 on fibroblasts is direct or secondary to the recruitment and activation of pro-fibrotic immune effectors remains still unclear, as the ability of CCL2 to stimulate collagen secretion by fibroblast has not been uniformly reported [130]. The CCL2 receptor (CCR2) has been found only on fibroblasts from early lesions or on myofibroblasts, suggesting that CCL2 function may be restricted to certain phases of the disease process or to specific cell types [234]. It is possible that in early skin disease the monocytes represent the main source of CCL2 while, at later stages, the fibroblasts become the main suppliers, thus contributing to the chronic activation of fibrogenesis in target tissues.

Other chemokines of the MCP family have been associated with SSc pathogenesis. These molecules regulate monocyte recruitment during inflammation to sites of trauma, infection, or ischemia and are also chemotactic for eosinophils and T cells. Ong et al. detected overexpression of CCL7 (MCP-3) in fibroblasts obtained from type 1 tight-skin (Tsk1) mice as well as from the skin of SSc patients with early-stage diffuse cutaneous involvement [133]. Others have shown that serum levels of CCL7 and CCL13 (MCP-4) are higher in SSc patients compared to healthy controls, particularly in subjects with the diffuse cutaneous phenotype [132, 339]. CCL13 expression was also increased in lesional skin from SSc subjects.

CCL3 (macrophage inflammatory protein 1α or MIP-1α) and CCL4 (MIP-1β) are secreted by activated lymphocytes, monocytes, and mast cells and favor selective recruitment of mononuclear cells to the sites of inflammation. Together with CCL5 (regulated upon activation, normal T cell expressed and secreted or RANTES), CCL3 and CCL4 mediate a strong pro-inflammatory function through their main receptor CCR5. This results predominantly in a Th1/Tc1 T cell effector response, which may be important during early phases of the disease or initial organ involvement, and may precede the establishment of a chronic pro-fibrotic inflammatory milieu. CCR5 and its ligands play an important role in SSc fibrogenesis. $CCR5^{-/-}$ knockout mice are resistant to bleomycin-induced lung fibrosis [340]. In addition, chemotaxis of pro-fibrotic monocytes toward target tissues are mediated in a bleomycin SSc animal model by CCR5 [341].

CCL3 and CCL4 have been found elevated in the serum of SSc patients and have shown higher expression in SSc-affected skin [135, 136, 228]. They are also increased in the BAL of SSc subjects and are associated with the presence of active interstitial lung disease (alveolitis) [61, 123]. Interestingly, an increased CCL3 and CCL5 expression precedes the development of skin and lung fibrosis in a murine GVHD model of SSc [313]. In addition, mice knocked out for CCL3 or its receptor CCR1 do not develop radiation-induced lung inflammation and fibrosis, suggesting its possible contribution to the pathogenesis of pulmonary fibrosis [342].

The expression of CCL5 is increased in lesional as well as uninvolved skin of SSc patients [139, 140]. This may indicate a role for this chemokine during early phases of SSc pathogenesis before the fibrotic loop takes over the disease process.

Interestingly, this group of chemokines has also been implicated in SSc vasculopathy. Their gene expression is higher in PBMCs (CCL3 and CCL4) and lung biopsies (CCL5) of SSC patients with severe PAH [137, 343]. In particular, CCL5 has been selectively detected at higher levels in pulmonary endothelial cells, suggesting a possible role of this chemokine in the recruitment of perivascular cellular infiltrates in the plexiform lesions of PAH [344]. CCL5 may also play an indirect role in pulmonary vascular disease through the induction of factors with vasoconstrictive and mitogenic function for pulmonary artery smooth muscle cells such as endothelin-1 and endothelin-converting enzyme-1 [345]. A significant gene-gene interaction in SSc has been reported by Lee et al. between the polymorphisms in the CCL5 and CXCL8 genes [138].

CCL23 (myeloid progenitor inhibitory factor 1 or MPIF-1) is expressed predominantly in the lung tissue and is chemotactic for resting mononuclear cells, DCs, and also endothelial cells [346]. Its levels have been found elevated in the serum of SSc patients compared to healthy controls or other CTDs and were associated with shorter disease duration and the presence of PAH [141]. Since CCL23 secretion by monocytes is triggered by IL-4, it is possible that this chemokine may contribute to T cell recruitment in a Th2/Tc2 polarized environment [347].

CCL17 (thymus- and activation-regulated chemokine or TARC) and CCL22 (macrophage-derived chemokine or MDC) are recognized as Th2/Tc2-type chemokines and bind to the chemokine receptor CCR4. Elevated levels of CCL17 and CCL22 have been detected in the BAL fluid of IPF patients, particularly in those with more severe disease, and the expression of CCR4 has been found higher in CD4 T cells from BAL of subjects with pulmonary fibrosis [348–350]. Alveolar macrophages from ILD patients exhibit a pro-fibrotic M2 phenotype and spontaneously secrete CCL17 and CCL22, which therefore may be relevant in the pathogenesis of fibrotic lung injury [248]. Similarly, mice lacking CCR4 are protected from bleomycin-induced lung fibrosis, and neutralization of CCL17 (but not CCL22) reduces pulmonary scarring in this animal model [351, 352]. Interestingly, CCR4 is expressed by virtually all cutaneous memory T cells, and the ligand CCL17 is displayed on the luminal surface of cutaneous venules [353]. In addition,

CCL17 together with CCL27 (CTACK) is also secreted by keratinocytes, suggesting their possible role in promoting T cells homing to inflamed skin [354]. In SSc patients, serum CCL17 and CCL22 are increased compared to controls, and CCL17 is positively associated with anti-topoisomerase 1 antibody [142]. Similarly, serum levels of CCL27, a chemokine directing T cell homing to the skin, and its cutaneous expression are higher in dcSSc subjects in association with more elevated inflammatory markers [143].

The chemokine CCL18 (pulmonary and activation-regulated chemokine or PARC) has sparked significant interest for its pro-fibrotic function and its value as a novel biomarker for disease activity in pulmonary fibrosis. CCL18 is actively secreted by alveolar macrophages, in particular following stimulation ("alternative activation") with Th2 cytokines, and can induce direct collagen production by lung fibroblasts [147, 355, 356]. CCL18 expression and spontaneous production by BAL fluid cells is pronounced in patients with SSc [145, 357]. BAL and serum levels of CCL18 are increased compared to healthy controls or SSc patients without lung fibrosis and exhibit a negative correlation with lung volumes (VC and TLC) and carbon monoxide diffusing capacity (DLCO) [26, 145, 146]. CCL18 serum levels were significantly associated with the presence of active ILD, and they declined following immunosuppressive treatment and stabilization of lung volumes [146]. A prospective study has confirmed a robust association between baseline serum CCL18 level and subsequent worsening of the lung function over time [148]. In addition, gene expression data on the skin of dcSSc patients have shown a significant upregulation of CCL18, CCL19, and CXCL13 [149]. In particular, CCL19 expression was associated with vascular inflammation and macrophage activation. In another report, CCL20 expression was increased in SSc skin compared to controls [150].

CXC Chemokines

Chemokines carrying the glutamyl-leucyl-arginyl (ELR) motif share common receptors (mainly CXCR1 and CXCR2) as well as the ability to attract neutrophils into sites of inflammation and to provide neo-angiogenetic stimuli during tissue repair [358]. Their induction by IL-1 and TNFα suggests a relevant function during the initial stages of the inflammatory response [359]. CXCL8 (IL-8), CXCL1 (growth-regulated oncogene-alpha or GROα), and CXCL5 (epithelial-derived neutrophil-activating peptide 78 or ENA-78) are ELR + chemokines with a possible role in SSc pathogenesis.

A significant gene-gene interaction involving CXCL8 and two SNPs of one of its receptors (CXCR2) has been associated with increased risk for SSc [138, 152]. These findings have been recently confirmed [154]. Skin specimens derived from early (<1 year) SSc cutaneous involvement exhibit overexpression of CXCL8 [67]. High levels of CXCL8 have been detected in the serum and the BAL of SSc patients, particularly in those with active ILD (presence of alveolitis), more extensive fibrosis, and declining lung volumes [72, 123, 153, 360]. Interestingly, alveolar macrophages and fibroblasts of patients with fibrosing alveolitis secrete higher amounts of CXCL8 [361, 362]. Considering that BAL neutrophilia and eosinophilia have been associated with activity and progression of SSc-ILD, it is plausible that CXCL8 may in part contribute to the damage/repair processes leading to lung fibrosis by recruiting granulocytes into inflamed tissues [363]. Higher serum levels of CXCL1 have also been associated with compromised lung function (lower VC and DLCO) in SSc patients [72].

The expression and secretion of CXCL8, CXCL1, and CCL2 (all cytokines with pro-fibrotic potential) can be triggered in fibroblasts after exposure to SSc IgG containing anti-fibroblast antibodies or in response to IL-1 and TNFα bound to the T cell membranes [27, 364]. These findings further confirm that these chemokines may represent important links between the humoral or cellular immune response in SSc and the progression of the fibrotic damage in target tissues.

SSc vasculopathy is characterized by endothelial dysfunction and microvascular injury leading to chronic platelet activation [155, 365]. CXCL4 (platelet factor 4 or PF4) is a protein stored in platelet α granules and secreted during activation. It exerts chemotactic stimuli for neutrophils and fibroblasts and mediates pro-coagulable functions. CXCL4 has been implicated during inflammation and wound repair, acting as a local pro-fibrotic mediator during the associated scarring response. Increased serum levels of CXCL4 have been previously reported in SSc patients, and concentrations in the lungs (BAL) were found higher in subjects with established ILD [155, 156]. A recent study has reported that CXCL4 is one of the main molecules secreted by plasmacytoid DCs isolated from SSc patients. In addition, CXCL4 serum levels are significantly elevated in SSc patients compared to healthy controls (particularly in subjects with early disease) and exhibit a robust association with the clinical phenotype, including severity of skin involvement and presence of ILD as well as PAH [14]. Remarkably, higher baseline CXCL4 levels also predicted progression of skin and lung disease. CXCL4 exerts potent antiangiogenic properties and upregulate pro-fibrotic cytokines. Thus, these findings support an integrated view of SSc pathogenesis where the secretion of CXCL4 by pDCs can link the activation of the innate immune system to abnormal adaptive immune responses driving fibrosis and vascular damage in SSc.

CXCL5, another chemokine secreted by activated platelets and exerting pro-angiogenic properties, has been reported elevated in the serum as well as BAL fluid of SSc patients compared to normal controls and has shown an association with the presence of ILD [153, 157]. In contrast, Ichimura et al. have reported that CXCL5 serum levels as well as its expression in cutaneous blood vessels are decreased in SSc patients, particularly during early phases of the disease, possibly in relationship with aberrant angiogenesis [158].

CXCL10 (interferon gamma-induced protein 10 or IP-10) and CXCL9 (monokine induced by gamma interferon or Mig) are ELR-negative CXC chemokines induced by interferon gamma during early inflammatory responses and differ from other CXC chemokines in that they exert dominant chemotaxis on NK and T cells and inhibit angiogenesis. Their receptor CXCR3 is expressed preferentially on activated CD4+ T lymphocytes (preTh1 or effector memory Th1), but not on resting cells. CXCR3 appears to be crucial for the recruitment of activated T cells into sites of inflammation, such as synovial tissues in RA, brain lesions in experimental autoimmune encephalomyelitis or multiple sclerosis, and solid organ transplants undergoing acute allograft rejection [366–370]. In addition to their proinflammatory effect, CXCL10 and CXCL9 have also shown the ability to mediate anti-fibrotic and angiostatic functions [331]. Administration of exogenous CXCL10 attenuates bleomycin-induced pulmonary fibrosis, and blockage of its receptor CXCR3 results in progressive interstitial disease and increased mortality in animal models of pulmonary fibrosis [371, 372]. CXCL10 has been found to be elevated in the serum of SSc patients, particularly during early phases of the disease [124, 142, 161].

Antonelli et al. showed that CXCL10 serum titers tend to decline over time with longer disease duration, suggesting that this chemokine may be relevant during early stages of SSc when it may be involved in triggering and amplifying the inflammatory process leading to tissue injury, before the profibrotic pathways are ignited. Interestingly, CXCR3-associated cytokines have been associated with inflammation and tissue injury preceding fibrosis in the liver of patients with hepatitis C, or during renal interstitial scarring [373, 374].

CXCL10 may also contribute to progression of SSc vasculopathy in virtue of its angiostatic potential and negative effects on blood vessels homeostasis. An association between CXCL10 serum levels and vascular disease (i.e., PAH) has been reported in SSc patients [29]. In particular, serum levels of CXCL10 exhibited a strong correlation with the severity of PAH, measured by hemodynamic parameters, serum BNP, and 6-min walk test [159]. In addition, CXCR3 expression has been shown to be low in endothelial cells from the dermal microvasculature of SSc individuals compared to controls, which may suggest a compensatory mechanism in the attempt to restore neoangiogenesis [229]. Higher CXCL10 and CXCL11 serum levels have also been reported in SSc patients compared to controls with positive association with skin (CXCL10) and lung (CXCL11) disease severity [160]. High BAL CXCL11 levels predicted subsequent FVC decline in SSc patients without established ILD [162].

CXCL12 (stromal cell-derived factors 1 or SDF-1) is a pleiotropic chemokine constitutively expressed in two splice variants by several tissues and cell types including stromal cells, endothelium, and DCs. The biologic axis involving CXCL12 and its receptor CXCR4 plays important homeostatic roles in hematopoiesis, leukocyte chemotaxis, lymphocytes homing to sites of inflammation, and mobilization from the bone marrow of hematopoietic and mesenchymal progenitor cells (including fibrocytes and endothelial precursors) [375]. CXCL12 levels are elevated in the lungs and plasma of the patients with pulmonary fibrosis, and its neutralization by anti-CXCL12 antibodies results in a marked reduction of fibrocyte extravasation into the lungs as well as attenuation of the consequent pulmonary fibrosis in the bleomycin mouse model [375–379]. CXCL12 has also shown important roles in promoting angiogenesis by amplifying secretion of other mediators (i.e., VEGF) and by mobilizing to sites of ischemia endothelial progenitors [380, 381]. CXCL12 and CXCR4 are upregulated in the skin as well as in isolated cutaneous microvascular endothelial cells of SSc patients with early active disease [164]. In addition, a CXCL12 gene polymorphism has been significantly associated with the presence of PAH and history of digital ulceration in SSc subjects [163]. It is therefore plausible that an abnormal regulation of this chemokine may be involved in the pathogenesis of SSc vascular disease.

CXCL16 is a chemokine induced by inflammatory cytokines such as IFN-gamma and TNFα providing important chemotactic stimuli to CXCR6-expressing cells (effector/memory T cells and natural killer cells) and recruiting them into sites of active inflammation [382]. Higher serum levels of CXCL16 have been detected in SSc patients and have shown a correlation with the degree of skin fibrosis [165].

CX3C Chemokine

CX3CL1 (fractalkine) is a unique membrane-bound chemokine expressed mostly on the surface of endothelial cells acting as an adhesion molecule for leukocyte trafficking. After proteolytic cleavage, it can be released as a soluble mediator and exert chemotactic functions on mononuclear cells. Expression of CX3CL1 is low in physiologic conditions, but it can be strongly upregulated in response to type 1 inflammatory stimuli (i.e., IFNγ and TNFα) [383, 384].

Higher serum levels of CX3CL1 have been detected in SSc patients [166, 168]. Hasegawa et al. have also shown that CX3CL1 is upregulated on endothelial cells of lesional skin and lung biopsies and that the expression of the receptor CX3R1 is increased in circulating T cells and monocytes of diffuse SSc patients [101]. The CX3CL1/CX3CR1-mediated recruitment of leukocytes into sites of inflammation through an activated endothelium may be relevant during early inflammatory phases of SSc, when a type 1 immune response may be prevalent, or may drive specific disease manifestations such as the SSc vasculopathy. Interestingly, the number of circulating CX3R1-positive T cells and the expression of CX3CL1 on pulmonary artery endothelial cells from patients with PAH were increased [385]. In addition, two CX3CL1 SNPs were associated with echocardiographic evidence of PAH in limited SSc patients [167]. CXCR1-mediated recruitment of inflammatory cells may also play a role in driving skin disease in SSc, as cutaneous fibrosis is greatly attenuated in CX3CR1$^{-/-}$ mice compared to WT after serial TGF-β and CTGF injections [386].

Concluding Remarks

The immune system and its tightly intertwined inflammatory response are clearly deeply involved in the pathophysiological processes underlying SSc (Fig. 13.5). An abnormal immune activation involving humoral as well as cellular events appears to be a fundamental step for disease initiation and amplification. We have learned that T helper cells have a skewed functional repertoire, which may vary along disease progression. Autoantibodies have agonistic activities on fibroblasts and endothelial cells, which by far exceed their role as markers of disease. Increasing evidence indicates that the innate immune system participates in many ways in shaping the SSc-specific adaptive immune response as well as the aberrant fibroblast activation involved in SSc pathogenesis. Secretion of IFN-α appears to be very important, tipping the balance of the internal milieu in favor of autoimmunity. New data have been provided suggesting a possible important role for TLRs in virtue of their ability to bind autoantigens or modified self-antigens as well as their expression on mesenchymal cells and in particular in fibroblasts. We have learned that the cytokine network has SSc-specific characteristics shared only in part by other autoimmune disorders. We started to recognize how cytokine with synergistic and antagonistic activities fine-tune fibroblast and endothelial cells' metabolic activities and how the interplay with receptors and modulation of intracellular signaling results in long-lasting imprinting in fibroblast dysfunction.

Despite all the advances achieved over the past few decades, the understanding of how the immune response can drive such different clinical phenotypes, like those existing in patients with the limited or the diffuse form of SSc, and determine such diverse patterns of organ involvement remains largely unsatisfactory. The answer to the important question of the relationship between the vasculopathic and fibrotic processes and the possible role of the immune response in linking these two pathogenetic hallmarks also is still very speculative. Further studies elucidating the close temporal as well as biological relationship existing between the abnormal immune activation and the other SSc pathogenetic events are much needed. Along the same line, it remains unclear why the SSc fibrotic process after initiation and substantial amplification (particularly at the skin level) tends in many cases to stop or to enter into a

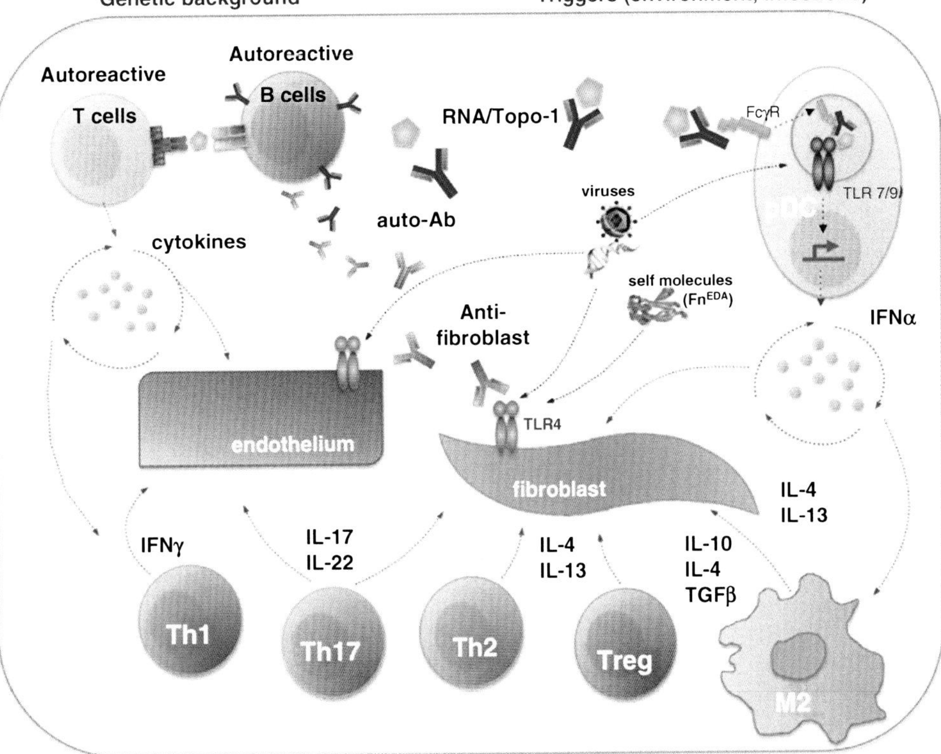

Fig. 13.5 Integrated view of the immuno-pathogenesis of systemic sclerosis. The innate immune systems and in particular Toll-like receptors (TLRs) contribute to the initiation of the inflammatory response and may contribute directly to activate fibroblast function. Macrophage undergoes "alternative" activation and promotes a pro-fibrotic microenvironment. Autoreactive T and B cells cooperate with autoantigen recognition and amplify the unfolding immune response through secretion of cytokines and autoantibodies. Polarized T helper cellular subsets such as Th1 and Th2 become activated at different stages of the disease and exert unique functions on different targets and body compartments. The role of other T cell subsets such as Th17, Th22, or Tregs is emerging and currently is under intense investigation

very low-grade progression loop. Furthermore, even if it is widely accepted that type 2 responses may contribute to the development of fibrosis in SSc, it remains unclear what drives the Th2/Tc2 cell differentiation. The emerging role of other T cell subsets such as Th17, Th22, or Tregs is under intense investigation. Finally, while it has been possible to demonstrate a restricted usage of the T cell receptor (TcR), indicating an antigen-driven T cell expansion in SSc skin and lungs, no progress has been made in identifying the responsible antigen(s). The complex and pleiotropic nature of the immune response in SSc constitutes a great challenge. The identification of SSc-specific cellular and molecular immune effectors will not only provide a new understanding of SSc pathogenesis but also offer the rationale to develop more selective and effective therapeutic strategies. Avenues for future understanding are clearly linked to our capacity to integrate knowledge acquired analyzing SSc-specific biological responses with the swift deciphering of the genetic contribution to the disease. Functional genomic studies conducted in large cohorts should thoroughly take into consideration the various clinical phenotypes of SSc and compare data with other systemic autoimmune disorders in order to distinguish common biological processes from disease-specific characteristics. Through this process we may learn with greater precision the distinct immunological abnormalities underlying specific disease manifestations and identify more targeted therapeutic interventions.

References

1. Yurovsky VV, Wigley FM, Wise RA, White B. Skewing of the CD8+ T-cell repertoire in the lungs of patients with systemic sclerosis. Hum Immunol. 1996;48:84–97.
2. Sakkas LI, Xu B, Artlett CM, Lu S, Jimenez SA, Platsoucas CD. Oligoclonal T cell expansion in the skin of patients with systemic sclerosis. J Immunol. 2002;168:3649–59.
3. Parel Y, Aurrand-Lions M, Scheja A, Dayer JM, Roosnek E, Chizzolini C. Presence of CD4+CD8+ double-positive T cells with very high interleukin-4 production potential in lesional skin of patients with systemic sclerosis. Arthritis Rheum. 2007;56:3459–67.
4. Farge D, Henegar C, Carmagnat M, Daneshpouy M, Marjanovic Z, Rabian C, et al. Analysis of immune reconstitution after autologous bone marrow transplantation in systemic sclerosis. Arthritis Rheum. 2005;52:1555–63.
5. McSweeney PA, Nash RA, Sullivan KM, Storek J, Crofford LJ, Dansey R, et al. High-dose immunosuppressive therapy for severe systemic sclerosis: initial outcomes. Blood. 2002;100:1602–10.
6. Oyama Y, Barr WG, Statkute L, Corbridge T, Gonda EA, Jovanovic B, et al. Autologous non-myeloablative hematopoietic stem cell transplantation in patients with systemic sclerosis. Bone Marrow Transplant. 2007;40:549–55.
7. van Laar JM, Farge D, Sont JK, Naraghi K, Marjanovic Z, Larghero J, et al. Autologous hematopoietic stem cell transplantation vs intravenous pulse cyclophosphamide in diffuse cutaneous systemic sclerosis. JAMA. 2014;311:2490.
8. Burt RK, Shah SJ, Dill K, Grant T, Gheorghiade M, Schroeder J, et al. Autologous non-myeloablative haemopoietic stem-cell transplantation compared with pulse cyclophosphamide once per month for systemic sclerosis (ASSIST): an open-label, randomised phase 2 trial. Lancet (London, England). 2011;378:498–506.
9. Bhattacharyya S, Tamaki Z, Wang W, Hinchcliff M, Hoover P, Getsios S, et al. FibronectinEDA promotes chronic cutaneous fibrosis through Toll-like receptor signaling. Sci Transl Med. 2014;6:232ra50.
10. Bhattacharyya S, Kelley K, Melichian DS, Tamaki Z, Fang F, Su Y, et al. Toll-like receptor 4 signaling augments transforming growth factor-beta responses: a novel mechanism for maintaining and amplifying fibrosis in scleroderma. Am J Pathol. 2013;182:192–205.
11. Takahashi T, Asano Y, Ichimura Y, Toyama T, Taniguchi T, Noda S, et al. Amelioration of tissue fibrosis by toll-like receptor 4 knockout in murine models of systemic sclerosis. Arthritis Rheumatol. 2015;67:254–65.
12. van Bon L, Cossu M, Loof A, Gohar F, Wittkowski H, Vonk M, et al. Proteomic analysis of plasma identifies the Toll-like receptor agonists S100A8/A9 as a novel possible marker for systemic sclerosis phenotype. Ann Rheum Dis. 2014;73:1585–9.
13. Nikitorowicz-Buniak J, Shiwen X, Denton CP, Abraham D, Stratton R. Abnormally differentiating keratinocytes in the epidermis of systemic sclerosis patients show enhanced secretion of CCN2 and S100A9. J Invest Dermatol. 2014;134(11):2693–702.
14. van Bon L, Affandi AJ, Broen J, Christmann RB, Marijnissen RJ, Stawski L, et al. Proteome-wide analysis and CXCL4 as a biomarker in systemic sclerosis. N Engl J Med. 2014;370:433–43.
15. Farina A, Cirone M, York M, Lenna S, Padilla C, McLaughlin S, et al. Epstein-Barr virus infection induces aberrant TLR activation pathway and fibroblast-myofibroblast conversion in scleroderma. J Invest Dermatol. 2014;134:954–64.
16. Fang F, Ooka K, Sun X, Shah R, Bhattacharyya S, Wei J, et al. A synthetic TLR3 ligand mitigates profibrotic fibroblast responses by inducing autocrine IFN signaling. J Immunol. 2013;191:2956–66.
17. Usategui A, Criado G, Izquierdo E, Del Rey MJ, Carreira PE, Ortiz P, et al. A profibrotic role for thymic stromal lymphopoietin in systemic sclerosis. Ann Rheum Dis. 2013;72:2018–23.
18. Ciechomska M, Huigens CA, Hugle T, Stanly T, Gessner A, Griffiths B, et al. Toll-like receptor-mediated, enhanced production of profibrotic TIMP-1 in monocytes from patients with systemic sclerosis: role of serum factors. Ann Rheum Dis. 2013;72:1382–9.
19. Stifano G, Affandi AJ, Mathes AL, Rice LM, Nakerakanti S, Nazari B, et al. Chronic Toll-like receptor 4 stimulation in skin induces inflammation, macrophage activation, transforming growth factor beta signature gene expression, and fibrosis. Arthritis Res Ther. 2014;16:R136.
20. Broen JC, Bossini-Castillo L, van Bon L, Vonk MC, Knaapen H, Beretta L, et al. A rare polymorphism in the gene for Toll-like receptor 2 is associated with systemic sclerosis phenotype and increases the production of inflammatory mediators. Arthritis Rheum. 2012;64:264–71.
21. Agarwal SK, Wu M, Livingston CK, Parks DH, Mayes MD, Arnett FC, et al. Toll-like receptor 3 upregulation by type I interferon in healthy and scleroderma dermal fibroblasts. Arthritis Res Ther. 2011;13:R3.
22. Farina G, York M, Collins C, Lafyatis R. dsRNA activation of endothelin-1 and markers of vascular activation in endothelial cells and fibroblasts. Ann Rheum Dis. 2011;70:544–50.
23. Yoshizaki A, Yanaba K, Iwata Y, Komura K, Ogawa A, Muroi E, et al. Elevated serum interleukin-27 levels in patients with systemic sclerosis: association with T cell, B cell and fibroblast activation. Ann Rheum Dis. 2011;70:194–200.
24. Farina GA, York MR, Di Marzio M, Collins CA, Meller S, Homey B, et al. Poly(I:C) drives type I IFN- and TGFbeta-mediated

inflammation and dermal fibrosis simulating altered gene expression in systemic sclerosis. J Invest Dermatol. 2010;130:2583–93.
25. van Bon L, Popa C, Huijbens R, Vonk M, York M, Simms R, et al. Distinct evolution of TLR-mediated dendritic cell cytokine secretion in patients with limited and diffuse cutaneous systemic sclerosis. Ann Rheum Dis. 2010;69:1539–47.
26. van Lieshout AW, Vonk MC, Bredie SJ, Joosten LB, Netea MG, van Riel PL, et al. Enhanced interleukin-10 production by dendritic cells upon stimulation with Toll-like receptor 4 agonists in systemic sclerosis that is possibly implicated in CCL18 secretion. Scand J Rheumatol. 2009;38:282–90.
27. Fineschi S, Goffin L, Rezzonico R, Cozzi F, Dayer JM, Meroni PL, et al. Antifibroblast antibodies in systemic sclerosis induce fibroblasts to produce profibrotic chemokines, with partial exploitation of toll-like receptor 4. Arthritis Rheum. 2008;58:3913–23.
28. Kim D, Peck A, Santer D, Patole P, Schwartz SM, Molitor JA, et al. Induction of interferon-alpha by scleroderma sera containing autoantibodies to topoisomerase I: association of higher interferon-alpha activity with lung fibrosis. Arthritis Rheum. 2008;58:2163–73.
29. Eloranta ML, Franck-Larsson K, Lovgren T, Kalamajski S, Ronnblom A, Rubin K, et al. Type I interferon system activation and association with disease manifestations in systemic sclerosis. Ann Rheum Dis. 2010;69:1396–402.
30. Yoshizaki A, Iwata Y, Komura K, Ogawa F, Hara T, Muroi E, et al. CD19 regulates skin and lung fibrosis via Toll-like receptor signaling in a model of bleomycin-induced scleroderma. Am J Pathol. 2008;172:1650–63.
31. Sakoguchi A, Nakayama W, Jinnin M, Wang Z, Yamane K, Aoi J, et al. The expression profile of the toll-like receptor family in scleroderma dermal fibroblasts. Clin Exp Rheumatol. 2014;32(6 Suppl 86):S-4–9.
32. Yang HZ, Wang JP, Mi S, Liu HZ, Cui B, Yan HM, et al. TLR4 activity is required in the resolution of pulmonary inflammation and fibrosis after acute and chronic lung injury. Am J Pathol. 2012;180:275–92.
33. Kawaguchi Y, Hara M, Wright TM. Endogenous IL-1alpha from systemic sclerosis fibroblasts induces IL-6 and PDGF-A. J Clin Invest. 1999;103:1253–60.
34. Kawaguchi Y, McCarthy SA, Watkins SC, Wright TM. Autocrine activation by interleukin 1alpha induces the fibrogenic phenotype of systemic sclerosis fibroblasts. J Rheumatol. 2004;31:1946–54.
35. Kawaguchi Y, Nishimagi E, Tochimoto A, Kawamoto M, Katsumata Y, Soejima M, et al. Intracellular IL-1alpha-binding proteins contribute to biological functions of endogenous IL-1alpha in systemic sclerosis fibroblasts. Proc Natl Acad Sci U S A. 2006;103:14501–6.
36. Kanangat S, Postlethwaite AE, Higgins GC, Hasty KA. Novel functions of intracellular IL-1ra in human dermal fibroblasts: implications in the pathogenesis of fibrosis. J Invest Dermatol. 2006;126:756–65.
37. Denton CP, Xu S, Black CM, Pearson JD. Scleroderma fibroblasts show increased responsiveness to endothelial cell-derived IL-1 and bFGF. J Invest Dermatol. 1997;108:269–74.
38. Aden N, Nuttall A, Shiwen X, de Winter P, Leask A, Black CM, et al. Epithelial cells promote fibroblast activation via IL-1alpha in systemic sclerosis. J Invest Dermatol. 2010;130:2191–200.
39. Wilson MS, Madala SK, Ramalingam TR, Gochuico BR, Rosas IO, Cheever AW, et al. Bleomycin and IL-1beta-mediated pulmonary fibrosis is IL-17A dependent. J Exp Med. 2010;207:535–52.
40. Kahaleh MB, LeRoy EC. Interleukin-2 in scleroderma: correlation of serum level with extent of skin involvement and disease duration. Ann Intern Med. 1989;110:446–50.
41. Clements PJ, Peter JB, Agopian MS, Telian NS, Furst DE. Elevated serum levels of soluble interleukin 2 receptor, interleukin 2 and neopterin in diffuse and limited scleroderma: effects of chlorambucil. J Rheumatol. 1990;17:908–10.
42. Famularo G, Procopio A, Giacomelli R, Danese C, Sacchetti S, Perego MA, et al. Soluble interleukin-2 receptor, interleukin-2 and interleukin-4 in sera and supernatants from patients with progressive systemic sclerosis. Clin Exp Immunol. 1990;81:368–72.
43. Needleman BW, Wigley FM, Stair RW. Interleukin-1, interleukin-2, interleukin-4, interleukin-6, tumor necrosis factor alpha, and interferon-gamma levels in sera from patients with scleroderma. Arthritis Rheum. 1992;35:67–72.
44. Hasegawa M, Fujimoto M, Kikuchi K, Takehara K. Elevated serum levels of interleukin 4 (IL-4), IL-10, and IL-13 in patients with systemic sclerosis. J Rheumatol. 1997;24:328–32.
45. Sato S, Hasegawa M, Takehara K. Serum levels of interleukin-6 and interleukin-10 correlate with total skin thickness score in patients with systemic sclerosis. J Dermatol Sci. 2001;27:140–6.
46. Salmon-Ehr V, Serpier H, Nawrocki B, Gillery P, Clavel C, Kalis B, et al. Expression of interleukin-4 in scleroderma skin specimens and scleroderma fibroblast cultures. Potential role in fibrosis. Arch Dermatol. 1996;132:802–6.
47. Atamas SP, Yurovsky VV, Wise R, Wigley FM, Goter Robinson CJ, Henry P, et al. Production of type 2 cytokines by CD8+ lung cells is associated with greater decline in pulmonary function in patients with systemic sclerosis. Arthritis Rheum. 1999;42:1168–78.
48. Tsuji-Yamada J, Nakazawa M, Minami M, Sasaki T. Increased frequency of interleukin 4 producing CD4+ and CD8+ cells in peripheral blood from patients with systemic sclerosis. J Rheumatol. 2001;28:1252–8.
49. Mavalia C, Scaletti C, Romagnani P, Carossino AM, Pignone A, Emmi L, et al. Type 2 helper T-cell predominance and high CD30 expression in systemic sclerosis. Am J Pathol. 1997;151:1751–8.
50. Scaletti C, Vultaggio A, Bonifacio S, Emmi L, Torricelli F, Maggi E, et al. Th2-oriented profile of male offspring T cells present in women with systemic sclerosis and reactive with maternal major histocompatibility complex antigens. Arthritis Rheum. 2002;46:445–50.
51. Fertin C, Nicolas JF, Gillery P, Kalis B, Banchereau J, Maquart FX. Interleukin-4 stimulates collagen synthesis by normal and scleroderma fibroblasts in dermal equivalents. Cell Mol Biol. 1991;37:823–9.
52. Lee KS, Ro YJ, Ryoo YW, Kwon HJ, Song JY. Regulation of interleukin-4 on collagen gene expression by systemic sclerosis fibroblasts in culture. J Dermatol Sci. 1996;12:110–7.
53. Maurer B, Stanczyk J, Jungel A, Akhmetshina A, Trenkmann M, Brock M, et al. MicroRNA-29, a key regulator of collagen expression in systemic sclerosis. Arthritis Rheum. 2010;62:1733–43.
54. Hasegawa M, Sato S, Fujimoto M, Ihn H, Kikuchi K, Takehara K. Serum levels of interleukin 6 (IL-6), oncostatin M, soluble IL-6 receptor, and soluble gp130 in patients with systemic sclerosis. J Rheumatol. 1998;25:308–13.
55. Scala E, Pallotta S, Frezzolini A, Abeni D, Barbieri C, Sampogna F, et al. Cytokine and chemokine levels in systemic sclerosis: relationship with cutaneous and internal organ involvement. Clin Exp Immunol. 2004;138:540–6.
56. Matsushita T, Hasegawa M, Hamaguchi Y, Takehara K, Sato S. Longitudinal analysis of serum cytokine concentrations in systemic sclerosis: association of interleukin 12 elevation with spontaneous regression of skin sclerosis. J Rheumatol. 2006;33:275–84.
57. Sato S, Hasegawa M, Fujimoto M, Tedder TF, Takehara K. Quantitative genetic variation in CD19 expression correlates with autoimmunity. J Immunol (Baltimore, Md 1950). 2000;165:6635–43.
58. Radstake TR, van Bon L, Broen J, Hussiani A, Hesselstrand R, Wuttge DM, et al. The pronounced Th17 profile in systemic sclerosis (SSc) together with intracellular expression of TGFbeta and IFNgamma distinguishes SSc phenotypes. PLoS One. 2009;4:e5903.

59. Bosello S, De Santis M, Lama G, Spano C, Angelucci C, Tolusso B, et al. B cell depletion in diffuse progressive systemic sclerosis: safety, skin score modification and IL-6 modulation in an up to thirty-six months follow-up open-label trial. Arthritis Res Ther. 2010;12:R54.
60. De Lauretis A, Sestini P, Pantelidis P, Hoyles R, Hansell DM, Goh NS, et al. Serum interleukin 6 is predictive of early functional decline and mortality in interstitial lung disease associated with systemic sclerosis. J Rheumatol. 2013;40:435–46.
61. Bolster MB, Ludwicka A, Sutherland SE, Strange C, Silver RM. Cytokine concentrations in bronchoalveolar lavage fluid of patients with systemic sclerosis. Arthritis Rheum. 1997;40: 743–51.
62. Feghali CA, Bost KL, Boulware DW, Levy LS. Control of IL-6 expression and response in fibroblasts from patients with systemic sclerosis. Autoimmunity. 1994;17:309–18.
63. Chizzolini C, Raschi E, Rezzonico R, Testoni C, Mallone R, Gabrielli A, et al. Autoantibodies to fibroblasts induce a proadhesive and proinflammatory fibroblast phenotype in patients with systemic sclerosis. Arthritis Rheum. 2002;46:1602–13.
64. Takemura H, Suzuki H, Fujisawa H, Yuhara T, Akama T, Yamane K, et al. Enhanced interleukin 6 production by cultured fibroblasts from patients with systemic sclerosis in response to platelet derived growth factor. J Rheumatol. 1998;25:1534–9.
65. Giacomelli R, Cipriani P, Danese C, Pizzuto F, Lattanzio R, Parzanese I, et al. Peripheral blood mononuclear cells of patients with systemic sclerosis produce increased amounts of interleukin 6, but not transforming growth factor beta 1. J Rheumatol. 1996;23:291–6.
66. Hasegawa M, Sato S, Ihn H, Takehara K. Enhanced production of interleukin-6 (IL-6), oncostatin M and soluble IL-6 receptor by cultured peripheral blood mononuclear cells from patients with systemic sclerosis. Rheumatology (Oxford). 1999;38:612–7.
67. Koch AE, Kronfeld-Harrington LB, Szekanecz Z, Cho MM, Haines GK, Harlow LA, et al. In situ expression of cytokines and cellular adhesion molecules in the skin of patients with systemic sclerosis. Their role in early and late disease. Pathobiology. 1993;61:239–46.
68. Kitaba S, Murota H, Terao M, Azukizawa H, Terabe F, Shima Y, et al. Blockade of interleukin-6 receptor alleviates disease in mouse model of scleroderma. Am J Pathol. 2012;180:165–76.
69. Desallais L, Avouac J, Frechet M, Elhai M, Ratsimandresy R, Montes M, et al. Targeting IL-6 by both passive or active immunization strategies prevents bleomycin-induced skin fibrosis. Arthritis Res Ther. 2014;16:R157.
70. Le Huu D, Matsushita T, Jin G, Hamaguchi Y, Hasegawa M, Takehara K, et al. IL-6 blockade attenuates the development of murine sclerodermatous chronic graft-versus-host disease. J Invest Dermatol. 2012;132:2752–61.
71. Reitamo S, Remitz A, Varga J, Ceska M, Effenberger F, Jimenez S, et al. Demonstration of interleukin 8 and autoantibodies to interleukin 8 in the serum of patients with systemic sclerosis and related disorders. Arch Dermatol. 1993;129:189–93.
72. Furuse S, Fujii H, Kaburagi Y, Fujimoto M, Hasegawa M, Takehara K, et al. Serum concentrations of the CXC chemokines interleukin 8 and growth-regulated oncogene-alpha are elevated in patients with systemic sclerosis. J Rheumatol. 2003;30: 1524–8.
73. Southcott AM, Jones KP, Li D, Majumdar S, Cambrey AD, Pantelidis P, et al. Interleukin-8. Differential expression in lone fibrosing alveolitis and systemic sclerosis. Am J Respir Crit Care Med. 1995;151:1604–12.
74. Meloni F, Caporali R, Marone Bianco A, Paschetto E, Morosini M, Fietta AM, et al. BAL cytokine profile in different interstitial lung diseases: a focus on systemic sclerosis. Sarcoidosis Vasc Diffuse Lung Dis. 2004;21:111–8.
75. van den Brule S, Heymans J, Havaux X, Renauld JC, Lison D, Huaux F, et al. Profibrotic effect of IL-9 overexpression in a model of airway remodeling. Am J Respir Cell Mol Biol. 2007;37:202–9.
76. Arras M, Louahed J, Simoen V, Barbarin V, Misson P, van den Brule S, et al. B lymphocytes are critical for lung fibrosis control and prostaglandin E2 regulation in IL-9 transgenic mice. Am J Respir Cell Mol Biol. 2006;34:573–80.
77. Hasegawa M, Fujimoto M, Kikuchi K, Takehara K. Elevated serum tumor necrosis factor-alpha levels in patients with systemic sclerosis: association with pulmonary fibrosis. J Rheumatol. 1997;24:663–5.
78. Zhu Z, Lee CG, Zheng T, Chupp G, Wang J, Homer RJ, et al. Airway inflammation and remodeling in asthma. Lessons from interleukin 11 and interleukin 13 transgenic mice. Am J Respir Crit Care Med. 2001;164:S67–70.
79. Sato S, Hanakawa H, Hasegawa M, Nagaoka T, Hamaguchi Y, Nishijima C, et al. Levels of interleukin 12, a cytokine of type 1 helper T cells, are elevated in sera from patients with systemic sclerosis. J Rheumatol. 2000;27:2838–42.
80. Fuschiotti P, Jr Medsger TA, Morel PA. Effector CD8+ T cells in systemic sclerosis patients produce abnormally high levels of interleukin-13 associated with increased skin fibrosis. Arthritis Rheum. 2009;60:1119–28.
81. Wuttge DM, Wildt M, Geborek P, Wollheim FA, Scheja A, Akesson A. Serum IL-15 in patients with early systemic sclerosis: a potential novel marker of lung disease. Arthritis Res Ther. 2007;9:R85.
82. Kurasawa K, Hirose K, Sano H, Endo H, Shinkai H, Nawata Y, et al. Increased interleukin-17 production in patients with systemic sclerosis. Arthritis Rheum. 2000;43:2455–63.
83. Murata M, Fujimoto M, Matsushita T, Hamaguchi Y, Hasegawa M, Takehara K, et al. Clinical association of serum interleukin-17 levels in systemic sclerosis: is systemic sclerosis a Th17 disease? J Dermatol Sci. 2008;50:240–2.
84. Fossiez F, Djossou O, Chomarat P, Flores-Romo L, Ait-Yahia S, Maat C, et al. T cell interleukin-17 induces stromal cells to produce proinflammatory and hematopoietic cytokines. J Exp Med. 1996;183:2593–603.
85. Brembilla NC, Montanari E, Truchetet ME, Raschi E, Meroni P, Chizzolini C. Th17 cells favor inflammatory responses while inhibiting type I collagen deposition by dermal fibroblasts: differential effects in healthy and systemic sclerosis fibroblasts. Arthritis Res Ther. 2013;15:R151.
86. Nakashima T, Jinnin M, Yamane K, Honda N, Kajihara I, Makino T, et al. Impaired IL-17 signaling pathway contributes to the increased collagen expression in scleroderma fibroblasts. J Immunol. 2012;188:3573–83.
87. Truchetet ME, Brembilla NC, Montanari E, Lonati P, Raschi E, Zeni S, et al. Interleukin-17A+ cell counts are increased in systemic sclerosis skin and their number is inversely correlated with the extent of skin involvement. Arthritis Rheum. 2013;65:1347–56.
88. Brembilla NC, Truchetet ME, Montanari E, Allanore Y, Chizzolini C. Enhanced IL-17A and IL-22 production by peripheral blood mononuclear cells distinguish systemic sclerosis from healthy individuals. Submitted 2010.
89. Meloni F, Solari N, Cavagna L, Morosini M, Montecucco CM, Fietta AM. Frequency of Th1, Th2 and Th17 producing T lymphocytes in bronchoalveolar lavage of patients with systemic sclerosis. Clin Exp Rheumatol. 2009;27:765–72.
90. Rodriguez-Reyna TS, Furuzawa-Carballeda J, Cabiedes J, Fajardo-Hermosillo LD, Martinez-Reyes C, Diaz-Zamudio M, et al. Th17 peripheral cells are increased in diffuse cutaneous systemic sclerosis compared with limited illness: a cross-sectional study. Rheumatol Int. 2011;32:2653–60.
91. Fenoglio D, Battaglia F, Parodi A, Stringara S, Negrini S, Panico N, et al. Alteration of Th17 and Treg cell subpopulations co-exist

in patients affected with systemic sclerosis. Clin Immunol. 2011;139:249–57.
92. Yang X, Yang J, Xing X, Wan L, Li M. Increased frequency of Th17 cells in systemic sclerosis is related to disease activity and collagen overproduction. Arthritis Res Ther. 2014;16:R4.
93. Truchetet ME, Raschi E, Lubatti C, Fontao L, Meroni PL, Chizzolini C, editors. T helper 17 cells are increased in the skin of systemic sclerosis individuals [abstract]. Scleroderma Res – 12th Int Work. 2011.
94. Lonati PA, Brembilla NC, Montanari E, Fontao L, Gabrielli A, Vettori S, et al. High IL-17E and low IL-17C dermal expression identifies a fibrosis-specific motif common to morphea and systemic sclerosis. PLoS One. 2014;9:e105008.
95. Zhou Y, Hou W, Xu K, Han D, Jiang C, Mou K, et al. The elevated expression of Th17-related cytokines and receptors is associated with skin lesion severity in early systemic sclerosis. Hum Immunol. 2015;76:22–9.
96. Kim HJ, Song SB, Choi JM, Kim KM, Cho BK, Cho DH, et al. IL-18 downregulates collagen production in human dermal fibroblasts via the ERK pathway. J Invest Dermatol. 2010;130:706–15.
97. Distler JH, Jungel A, Kowal-Bielecka O, Michel BA, Gay RE, Sprott H, et al. Expression of interleukin-21 receptor in epidermis from patients with systemic sclerosis. Arthritis Rheum. 2005;52:856–64.
98. Simonian PL, Roark CL, Born WK, O'Brien RL, Fontenot AP. Gammadelta T cells and Th17 cytokines in hypersensitivity pneumonitis and lung fibrosis. Transl Res. 2009;154:222–7.
99. Komura K, Fujimoto M, Hasegawa M, Ogawa F, Hara T, Muroi E, et al. Increased serum interleukin 23 in patients with systemic sclerosis. J Rheumatol. 2008;35:120–5.
100. Rankin AL, Mumm JB, Murphy E, Turner S, Yu N, McClanahan TK, et al. IL-33 induces IL-13-dependent cutaneous fibrosis. J Immunol (Baltimore, Md 1950). 2010;184:1526–35.
101. Tomcik M, Zerr P, Palumbo-Zerr K, Storkanova H, Hulejova H, Spiritovic M, et al. Interleukin-35 is upregulated in systemic sclerosis and its serum levels are associated with early disease. Rheumatology. 2015;54(12):2273–82.
102. Kudo H, Wang Z, Jinnin M, Nakayama W, Inoue K, Honda N, et al. EBI3 downregulation contributes to type I collagen overexpression in scleroderma skin. J Immunol. 2015;195(8):3565–73.
103. Del Galdo F, Maul GG, Jimenez SA, Artlett CM. Expression of allograft inflammatory factor 1 in tissues from patients with systemic sclerosis and in vitro differential expression of its isoforms in response to transforming growth factor beta. Arthritis Rheum. 2006;54:2616–25.
104. Del Galdo F, Jimenez SA. T cells expressing allograft inflammatory factor 1 display increased chemotaxis and induce a profibrotic phenotype in normal fibroblasts in vitro. Arthritis Rheum. 2007;56:3478–88.
105. Matsushita T, Fujimoto M, Hasegawa M, Tanaka C, Kumada S, Ogawa F, et al. Elevated serum APRIL levels in patients with systemic sclerosis: distinct profiles of systemic sclerosis categorized by APRIL and BAFF. J Rheumatol. 2007;34:2056–62.
106. Matsushita T, Hasegawa M, Yanaba K, Kodera M, Takehara K, Sato S. Elevated serum BAFF levels in patients with systemic sclerosis: enhanced BAFF signaling in systemic sclerosis B lymphocytes. Arthritis Rheum. 2006;54:192–201.
107. Matsushita T, Fujimoto M, Hasegawa M, Matsushita Y, Komura K, Ogawa F, et al. BAFF antagonist attenuates the development of skin fibrosis in tight-skin mice. J Invest Dermatol. 2007;127:2772–80.
108. François A, Chatelus E, Wachsmann D, Sibilia J, Bahram S, Alsaleh G, et al. B lymphocytes and B-cell activating factor promote collagen and profibrotic markers expression by dermal fibroblasts in systemic sclerosis. Arthritis Res Ther. 2013;15:R168.
109. Iwasaki T, Imado T, Kitano S, Sano H. Hepatocyte growth factor ameliorates dermal sclerosis in the tight-skin mouse model of scleroderma. Arthritis Res Ther. 2006;8:R161.
110. Rosenbloom J, Feldman G, Freundlich B, Jimenez SA. Inhibition of excessive scleroderma fibroblast collagen production by recombinant gamma-interferon. Association with a coordinate decrease in types I and III procollagen messenger RNA levels. Arthritis Rheum. 1986;29:851–6.
111. Gillery P, Serpier H, Polette M, Bellon G, Clavel C, Wegrowski Y, et al. Gamma-interferon inhibits extracellular matrix synthesis and remodeling in collagen lattice cultures of normal and scleroderma skin fibroblasts. Eur J Cell Biol. 1992;57:244–53.
112. Chizzolini C, Rezzonico R, Ribbens C, Burger D, Wollheim FA, Dayer JM. Inhibition of type I collagen production by dermal fibroblasts upon contact with activated T cells: different sensitivity to inhibition between systemic sclerosis and control fibroblasts. Arthritis Rheum. 1998;41:2039–47.
113. Ferrarini M, Steen V, Jr Medsger TA, JR Whiteside TL. Functional and phenotypic analysis of T lymphocytes cloned from the skin of patients with systemic sclerosis. Clin Exp Immunol. 1990;79:346–52.
114. Majumdar S, Li D, Ansari T, Pantelidis P, Black CM, Gizycki M, et al. Different cytokine profiles in cryptogenic fibrosing alveolitis and fibrosing alveolitis associated with systemic sclerosis: a quantitative study of open lung biopsies. Eur Respir J Off J Eur Soc Clin Respir Physiol. 1999;14:251–7.
115. Gruschwitz MS, Vieth G. Up-regulation of class II major histocompatibility complex and intercellular adhesion molecule 1 expression on scleroderma fibroblasts and endothelial cells by interferon-gamma and tumor necrosis factor alpha in the early disease stage. Arthritis Rheum. 1997;40:540–50.
116. Chizzolini C, Parel Y, De Luca C, Tyndall A, Akesson A, Scheja A, et al. Systemic sclerosis Th2 cells inhibit collagen production by dermal fibroblasts via membrane-associated tumor necrosis factor alpha. Arthritis Rheum. 2003;48:2593–604.
117. Valentini G, Romano MF, Naclerio C, Bisogni R, Lamberti A, Turco MC, et al. Increased expression of CD40 ligand in activated CD4+ T lymphocytes of systemic sclerosis patients. J Autoimmun. 2000;15:61–6.
118. Komura K, Fujimoto M, Matsushita T, Yanaba K, Kodera M, Kawasuji A, et al. Increased serum soluble CD40 levels in patients with systemic sclerosis. J Rheumatol. 2007;34:353–8.
119. Komura K, Sato S, Hasegawa M, Fujimoto M, Takehara K. Elevated circulating CD40L concentrations in patients with systemic sclerosis. J Rheumatol. 2004;31:514–9.
120. Fukasawa C, Kawaguchi Y, Harigai M, Sugiura T, Takagi K, Kawamoto M, et al. Increased CD40 expression in skin fibroblasts from patients with systemic sclerosis (SSc): role of CD40-CD154 in the phenotype of SSc fibroblasts. Eur J Immunol. 2003;33:2792–800.
121. Kawai M, Masuda A, Kuwana M. A CD40-CD154 interaction in tissue fibrosis. Arthritis Rheum. 2008;58:3562–73.
122. Gourh P, Arnett FC, Assassi S, Tan FK, Huang M, Diekman L, et al. Plasma cytokine profiles in systemic sclerosis: associations with autoantibody subsets and clinical manifestations. Arthritis Res Ther. 2009;11:R147.
123. Schmidt K, Martinez-Gamboa L, Meier S, Witt C, Meisel C, Hanitsch LG, et al. Bronchoalveolar lavage fluid cytokines and chemokines as markers and predictors for the outcome of interstitial lung disease in systemic sclerosis patients. Arthritis Res Ther. 2009;11:R111.
124. Antonelli A, Ferri C, Fallahi P, Ferrari SM, Giuggioli D, Colaci M, et al. CXCL10 (alpha) and CCL2 (beta) chemokines in systemic sclerosis – a longitudinal study. Rheumatology (Oxford). 2008;47:45–9.
125. Galindo M, Santiago B, Rivero M, Rullas J, Alcami J, Pablos JL. Chemokine expression by systemic sclerosis fibroblasts: abnormal regulation of monocyte chemoattractant protein 1 expression. Arthritis Rheum. 2001;44:1382–6.

126. Bandinelli F, Del Rosso A, Gabrielli A, Giacomelli R, Bartoli F, Guiducci S, et al. CCL2, CCL3 and CCL5 chemokines in systemic sclerosis: the correlation with SSc clinical features and the effect of prostaglandin E1 treatment. Clin Exp Rheumatol. 2012;30:S44–9.
127. Distler JH, Jungel A, Caretto D, Schulze-Horsel U, Kowal-Bielecka O, Gay RE, et al. Monocyte chemoattractant protein 1 released from glycosaminoglycans mediates its profibrotic effects in systemic sclerosis via the release of interleukin-4 from T cells. Arthritis Rheum. 2006;54:214–25.
128. Distler O, Pap T, Kowal-Bielecka O, Meyringer R, Guiducci S, Landthaler M, et al. Overexpression of monocyte chemoattractant protein 1 in systemic sclerosis: role of platelet-derived growth factor and effects on monocyte chemotaxis and collagen synthesis. Arthritis Rheum. 2001;44:2665–78.
129. Yamamoto T, Eckes B, Mauch C, Hartmann K, Krieg T. Monocyte chemoattractant protein-1 enhances gene expression and synthesis of matrix metalloproteinase-1 in human fibroblasts by an autocrine IL-1 alpha loop. J Immunol. 2000;164:6174–9.
130. Carulli MT, Handler C, Coghlan JG, Black CM, Denton CP. Can CCL2 serum levels be used in risk stratification or to monitor treatment response in systemic sclerosis? Ann Rheum Dis. 2008;67:105–9.
131. Greenblatt MB, Sargent JL, Farina G, Tsang K, Lafyatis R, Glimcher LH, et al. Interspecies comparison of human and murine scleroderma reveals IL-13 and CCL2 as disease subset-specific targets. Am J Pathol. 2012;180:1080–94.
132. Yanaba K, Komura K, Kodera M, Matsushita T, Hasegawa M, Takehara K, et al. Serum levels of monocyte chemotactic protein-3/CCL7 are raised in patients with systemic sclerosis: association with extent of skin sclerosis and severity of pulmonary fibrosis. Ann Rheum Dis. 2006;65:124–6.
133. Ong VH, Evans LA, Shiwen X, Fisher IB, Rajkumar V, Abraham DJ, et al. Monocyte chemoattractant protein 3 as a mediator of fibrosis: overexpression in systemic sclerosis and the type 1 tight-skin mouse. Arthritis Rheum. 2003;48:1979–91.
134. Piguet PF, Collart MA, Grau GE, Kapanci Y, Vassalli P. Tumor necrosis factor/cachectin plays a key role in bleomycin-induced pneumopathy and fibrosis. J Exp Med. 1989;170:655–63.
135. Codullo V, Baldwin HM, Singh MD, Fraser AR, Wilson C, Gilmour A, et al. An investigation of the inflammatory cytokine and chemokine network in systemic sclerosis. Ann Rheum Dis. 2011;70:1115–21.
136. Hasegawa M, Asano Y, Endo H, Fujimoto M, Goto D, Ihn H, et al. Serum chemokine levels as prognostic markers in patients with early systemic sclerosis: a multicenter, prospective, observational study. Mod Rheumatol. 2013;23:1076–84.
137. Grigoryev DN, Mathai SC, Fisher MR, Girgis RE, Zaiman AL, Housten-Harris T, et al. Identification of candidate genes in scleroderma-related pulmonary arterial hypertension. Transl Res. 2008;151:197–207.
138. Lee EB, Zhao J, Kim JY, Xiong M, Song YW. Evidence of potential interaction of chemokine genes in susceptibility to systemic sclerosis. Arthritis Rheum. 2007;56:2443–8.
139. Distler O, Rinkes B, Hohenleutner U, Scholmerich J, Landthaler M, Lang B, et al. Expression of RANTES in biopsies of skin and upper gastrointestinal tract from patients with systemic sclerosis. Rheumatol Int. 1999;19:39–46.
140. Anderegg U, Saalbach A, Haustein UF. Chemokine release from activated human dermal microvascular endothelial cells – implications for the pathophysiology of scleroderma? Arch Dermatol Res. 2000;292:341–7.
141. Yanaba K, Yoshizaki A, Muroi E, Ogawa F, Asano Y, Kadono T, et al. Serum CCL23 levels are increased in patients with systemic sclerosis. Arch Dermatol Res. 2011;303:29–34.
142. Fujii H, Shimada Y, Hasegawa M, Takehara K, Sato S. Serum levels of a Th1 chemoattractant IP-10 and Th2 chemoattractants, TARC and MDC, are elevated in patients with systemic sclerosis. J Dermatol Sci. 2004;35:43–51.
143. Hayakawa I, Hasegawa M, Matsushita T, Yanaba K, Kodera M, Komura K, et al. Increased cutaneous T-cell-attracting chemokine levels in sera from patients with systemic sclerosis. Rheumatology (Oxford). 2005;44:873–8.
144. van Lieshout AW, Vonk MC, Bredie SJ, Joosten LAB, Netea MG, van Riel PL, et al. Elevated serum interleukin-27 levels in patients with systemic sclerosis: association with T cell, B cell and fibroblast activation. Arthritis Rheum. 2011;27:535–52.
145. Prasse A, Pechkovsky DV, Toews GB, Schafer M, Eggeling S, Ludwig C, et al. CCL18 as an indicator of pulmonary fibrotic activity in idiopathic interstitial pneumonias and systemic sclerosis. Arthritis Rheum. 2007;56:1685–93.
146. Kodera M, Hasegawa M, Komura K, Yanaba K, Takehara K, Sato S. Serum pulmonary and activation-regulated chemokine/CCL18 levels in patients with systemic sclerosis: a sensitive indicator of active pulmonary fibrosis. Arthritis Rheum. 2005;52:2889–96.
147. Atamas SP, Luzina IG, Choi J, Tsymbalyuk N, Carbonetti NH, Singh IS, et al. Pulmonary and activation-regulated chemokine stimulates collagen production in lung fibroblasts. Am J Respir Cell Mol Biol. 2003;29:743–9.
148. Tiev KP, Hua-Huy T, Kettaneh A, Gain M, Duong-Quy S, Tolédano C, et al. Serum CC chemokine ligand-18 predicts lung disease worsening in systemic sclerosis. Eur Respir J. 2011;38:1355–60.
149. Mathes AL, Christmann RB, Stifano G, Affandi AJ, Radstake TRDJ, Farina GA, et al. Global chemokine expression in systemic sclerosis (SSc): CCL19 expression correlates with vascular inflammation in SSc skin. Ann Rheum Dis. 2014;73:1864–72.
150. Tao J, Li L, Tan Z, Li Y, Yang J, Tian F, et al. Up-regulation of CC chemokine ligand 20 and its receptor CCR6 in the lesional skin of early systemic sclerosis. Eur J Dermatol. 2011;21:731–6.
151. Kadono T, Kikuchi K, Ihn H, Takehara K, Tamaki K. Increased production of interleukin 6 and interleukin 8 in scleroderma fibroblasts. J Rheumatol. 1998;25:296–301.
152. Renzoni E, Lympany P, Sestini P, Pantelidis P, Wells A, Black C, et al. Distribution of novel polymorphisms of the interleukin-8 and CXC receptor 1 and 2 genes in systemic sclerosis and cryptogenic fibrosing alveolitis. Arthritis Rheum. 2000;43:1633–40.
153. Hesselstrand R, Wildt M, Bozovic G, Andersson-Sjöland A, Andréasson K, Scheja A, et al. Biomarkers from bronchoalveolar lavage fluid in systemic sclerosis patients with interstitial lung disease relate to severity of lung fibrosis. Respir Med. 2013;107:1079–86.
154. Salim PH, Jobim M, Bredemeier M, Chies JAB, Brenol JCT, Jobim LF, et al. Combined effects of CXCL8 and CXCR2 gene polymorphisms on susceptibility to systemic sclerosis. Cytokine. 2012;60:473–7.
155. Macko RF, Gelber AC, Young BA, Lowitt MH, White B, Wigley FM, et al. Increased circulating concentrations of the counteradhesive proteins SPARC and thrombospondin-1 in systemic sclerosis (scleroderma). Relationship to platelet and endothelial cell activation. J Rheumatol. 2002;29:2565–70.
156. Kowal-Bielecka O, Kowal K, Lewszuk A, Bodzenta-Lukaszyk A, Walecki J, Sierakowski S. Beta thromboglobulin and platelet factor 4 in bronchoalveolar lavage fluid of patients with systemic sclerosis. Ann Rheum Dis. 2005;64:484–6.
157. Nomura S, Inami N, Ozaki Y, Kagawa H, Fukuhara S. Significance of microparticles in progressive systemic sclerosis with interstitial pneumonia. Platelets. 2008;19:192–8.
158. Ichimura Y, Asano Y, Akamata K, Takahashi T, Noda S, Taniguchi T, et al. Fli1 deficiency contributes to the suppression of endothelial CXCL5 expression in systemic sclerosis. Arch Dermatol Res. 2014;306:331–8.
159. George PM, Oliver E, Dorfmuller P, Dubois OD, Reed DM, Kirkby NS, et al. Evidence for the involvement of type I interferon in pulmonary arterial hypertension. Circ Res. 2014;114:677–88.

160. Liu X, Mayes MD, Tan FK, Wu M, Reveille JD, Harper BE, et al. Correlation of interferon-inducible chemokine plasma levels with disease severity in systemic sclerosis. Arthritis Rheum. 2013;65:226–35.
161. Hasegawa M, Fujimoto M, Matsushita T, Hamaguchi Y, Takehara K, Sato S. Serum chemokine and cytokine levels as indicators of disease activity in patients with systemic sclerosis. Clin Rheumatol. 2011;30:231–7.
162. Sfriso P, Cozzi F, Oliviero F, Caso F, Cardarelli S, Facco M, et al. CXCL11 in bronchoalveolar lavage fluid and pulmonary function decline in systemic sclerosis. Clin Exp Rheumatol. 2012;30:S71–5.
163. Manetti M, Liakouli V, Fatini C, Cipriani P, Bonino C, Vettori S, et al. Association between a stromal cell-derived factor 1 (SDF-1/CXCL12) gene polymorphism and microvascular disease in systemic sclerosis. Ann Rheum Dis. 2009;68:408–11.
164. Cipriani P, Franca Milia A, Liakouli V, Pacini A, Manetti M, Marrelli A, et al. Differential expression of stromal cell-derived factor 1 and its receptor CXCR4 in the skin and endothelial cells of systemic sclerosis patients: Pathogenetic implications. Arthritis Rheum. 2006;54:3022–33.
165. Yanaba K, Muroi E, Yoshizaki A, Hara T, Ogawa F, Shimizu K, et al. Serum CXCL16 concentrations correlate with the extent of skin sclerosis in patients with systemic sclerosis. J Rheumatol. 2009;36:1917–23.
166. Hasegawa M. Up regulated expression of fractalkine/CX3CL1 and CX3CR1 in patients with systemic sclerosis. Ann Rheum Dis. 2005;64:21–8.
167. Marasini B, Cossutta R, Selmi C, Pozzi MR, Gardinali M, Massarotti M, et al. Polymorphism of the fractalkine receptor CX3CR1 and systemic sclerosis-associated pulmonary arterial hypertension. Clin Dev Immunol. 2005;12:275–9.
168. Sicinska J, Gorska E, Cicha M, Kuklo-Kowalska A, Hamze V, Stepien K, et al. Increased serum fractalkine in systemic sclerosis. Down-regulation by prostaglandin E1. Clin Exp Rheumatol. 2008;26:527–33.
169. Kumar H, Kawai T, Akira S. Pathogen recognition by the innate immune system. Int Rev Immunol. 2011;30:16–34.
170. Kawasaki T, Kawai T, Akira S. Recognition of nucleic acids by pattern-recognition receptors and its relevance in autoimmunity. Immunol Rev. 2011;243:61–73.
171. Tan FK, Zhou X, Mayes MD, Gourh P, Guo X, Marcum C, et al. Signatures of differentially regulated interferon gene expression and vasculotrophism in the peripheral blood cells of systemic sclerosis patients. Rheumatology. 2006;45:694–702.
172. Duan H, Fleming J, Pritchard DK, Amon LM, Xue J, Arnett HA, et al. Combined analysis of monocyte and lymphocyte messenger RNA expression with serum protein profiles in patients with scleroderma. Arthritis Rheum. 2008;58:1465–74.
173. Assassi S, Mayes MD, Arnett FC, Gourh P, Agarwal SK, McNearney TA, et al. Systemic sclerosis and lupus: points in an interferon-mediated continuum. Arthritis Rheum. 2010;62:589–98.
174. Higgs BW, Liu Z, White B, Zhu W, White WI, Morehouse C, et al. Patients with systemic lupus erythematosus, myositis, rheumatoid arthritis and scleroderma share activation of a common type I interferon pathway. Ann Rheum Dis. 2011;70:2029.
175. Liu YJ. Dendritic cell subsets and lineages, and their functions in innate and adaptive immunity. Cell. 2001;106:259–62.
176. Banchereau J, Briere F, Caux C, Davoust J, Lebecque S, Liu YJ, et al. Immunobiology of dendritic cells. Annu Rev Immunol. 2000;18:767–811.
177. Siegal FP, Kadowaki N, Shodell M, Fitzgerald-Bocarsly PA, Shah K, Ho S, et al. The nature of the principal type 1 interferon-producing cells in human blood. Science. 1999;284:1835–7.
178. Cella M, Jarrossay D, Facchetti F, Alebardi O, Nakajima H, Lanzavecchia A, et al. Plasmacytoid monocytes migrate to inflamed lymph nodes and produce large amounts of type I interferon. Nat Med. 1999;5:919–23.
179. Kadowaki N, Antonenko S, Lau JY, Liu YJ. Natural interferon alpha/beta-producing cells link innate and adaptive immunity. J Exp Med. 2000;192:219–26.
180. Banchereau J, Steinman RM. Dendritic cells and the control of immunity. Nature. 1998;392:245–52.
181. de Saint-Vis B, Fugier-Vivier I, Massacrier C, Gaillard C, Vanbervliet B, Ait-Yahia S, et al. The cytokine profile expressed by human dendritic cells is dependent on cell subtype and mode of activation. J Immunol (Baltimore, Md 1950). 1998;160:1666–76.
182. Ziegler SF, Artis D. Sensing the outside world: TSLP regulates barrier immunity. Nat Immunol. 2010;11:289–93.
183. Ito T, Wang YH, Duramad O, Hori T, Delespesse GJ, Watanabe N, et al. TSLP-activated dendritic cells induce an inflammatory T helper type 2 cell response through OX40 ligand. J Exp Med. 2005;202:1213–23.
184. Gourh P, Arnett FC, Tan FK, Assassi S, Divecha D, Paz G, et al. Association of TNFSF4 (OX40L) polymorphisms with susceptibility to systemic sclerosis. Ann Rheum Dis. 2010;69:550–5.
185. Komura K, Yoshizaki A, Kodera M, Iwata Y, Ogawa F, Shimizu K, et al. Increased serum soluble OX40 in patients with systemic sclerosis. J Rheumatol. 2008;35:2359–62.
186. Ishikawa O, Ishikawa H. Macrophage infiltration in the skin of patients with systemic sclerosis. J Rheumatol. 1992;19:1202–6.
187. Kraling BM, Maul GG, Jimenez SA. Mononuclear cellular infiltrates in clinically involved skin from patients with systemic sclerosis of recent onset predominantly consist of monocytes/macrophages. Pathobiology. 1995;63:48–56.
188. Taylor ML, Noble PW, White B, Wise R, Liu MC, Bochner BS. Extensive surface phenotyping of alveolar macrophages in interstitial lung disease. Clin Immunol. 2000;94:33–41.
189. Gordon S. Alternative activation of macrophages. Nat Rev. 2003;3:23–35.
190. Mantovani A, Sica A, Sozzani S, Allavena P, Vecchi A, Locati M. The chemokine system in diverse forms of macrophage activation and polarization. Trends Immunol. 2004;25:677–86.
191. Fadok VA, Bratton DL, Konowal A, Freed PW, Westcott JY, Henson PM. Macrophages that have ingested apoptotic cells in vitro inhibit proinflammatory cytokine production through autocrine/paracrine mechanisms involving TGF-beta, PGE2, and PAF. J Clin Invest. 1998;101:890–8.
192. Song E, Ouyang N, Horbelt M, Antus B, Wang M, Exton MS. Influence of alternatively and classically activated macrophages on fibrogenic activities of human fibroblasts. Cell Immunol. 2000;204:19–28.
193. Murray PJ, Allen JE, Biswas SK, Fisher EA, Gilroy DW, Goerdt S, et al. Macrophage activation and polarization: nomenclature and experimental guidelines. Immunity. 2014;41:14–20.
194. Pechkovsky DV, Prasse A, Kollert F, Engel KM, Dentler J, Luttmann W, et al. Alternatively activated alveolar macrophages in pulmonary fibrosis-mediator production and intracellular signal transduction. Clin Immunol. 2010;137:89–101.
195. Higashi-Kuwata N, Jinnin M, Makino T, Fukushima S, Inoue Y, Muchemwa FC, et al. Characterization of monocyte/macrophage subsets in the skin and peripheral blood derived from patients with systemic sclerosis. Arthritis Res Ther. 2010;12:R128.
196. Shimizu K, Ogawa F, Yoshizaki A, Akiyama Y, Kuwatsuka Y, Okazaki S, et al. Increased serum levels of soluble CD163 in patients with scleroderma. Clin Rheumatol. 2012;31:1059–64.
197. Nakayama W, Jinnin M, Makino K, Kajihara I, Makino T, Fukushima S, et al. Serum levels of soluble CD163 in patients with systemic sclerosis. Rheumatol Int. 2012;32:403–7.
198. Bielecki M, Kowal K, Lapinska A, Chyczewski L, Kowal-Bielecka O. Increased release of soluble CD163 by the peripheral

blood mononuclear cells is associated with worse prognosis in patients with systemic sclerosis. Adv Med Sci. 2013;58:126–33.

199. Christmann RB, Hayes E, Pendergrass S, Padilla C, Farina G, Affandi AJ, et al. Interferon and alternative activation of monocyte/macrophages in systemic sclerosis-associated pulmonary arterial hypertension. Arthritis Rheum. 2011;63:1718–28.

200. Mathai SK, Gulati M, Peng X, Russell TR, Shaw AC, Rubinowitz AN, et al. Circulating monocytes from systemic sclerosis patients with interstitial lung disease show an enhanced profibrotic phenotype. Lab Invest. 2010;90:812–23.

201. York MR, Nagai T, Mangini AJ, Lemaire R, van Seventer JM, Lafyatis R. A macrophage marker, Siglec-1, is increased on circulating monocytes in patients with systemic sclerosis and induced by type I interferons and toll-like receptor agonists. Arthritis Rheum. 2007;56:1010–20.

202. Tourkina E, Richard M, Oates J, Hofbauer A, Bonner M, Gööz P, et al. Caveolin-1 regulates leucocyte behaviour in fibrotic lung disease. Ann Rheum Dis. 2010;69:1220–6.

203. Reese C, Perry B, Heywood J, Bonner M, Visconti RP, Lee R, et al. Caveolin-1 deficiency may predispose African Americans to systemic sclerosis-related interstitial lung disease. Arthritis Rheumatol (Hoboken, NJ). 2014;66:1909–19.

204. Lee R, Reese C, Perry B, Heywood J, Bonner M, Zemskova M, et al. Enhanced chemokine-receptor expression, function, and signaling in healthy African American and scleroderma-patient monocytes are regulated by caveolin-1. Fibrogenesis Tissue Repair. 2015;8:11.

205. Del Galdo F, Sotgia F, de Almeida CJ, Jasmin J-F, Musick M, Lisanti MP, et al. Decreased expression of caveolin 1 in patients with systemic sclerosis: crucial role in the pathogenesis of tissue fibrosis. Arthritis Rheum. 2008;58:2854–65.

206. Horikawa M, Hasegawa M, Komura K, Hayakawa I, Yanaba K, Matsushita T, et al. Abnormal natural killer cell function in systemic sclerosis: altered cytokine production and defective killing activity. J Invest Dermatol. 2005;125:731–7.

207. Holcombe RF, Baethge BA, Wolf RE, Betzing KW, Stewart RM. Natural killer cells and gamma delta T cells in scleroderma: relationship to disease duration and anti-Scl-70 antibodies. Ann Rheum Dis. 1995;54:69–72.

208. Riccieri V, Spadaro A, Parisi G, Taccari E, Moretti T, Bernardini G, et al. Down-regulation of natural killer cells and of gamma/delta T cells in systemic lupus erythematosus. Does it correlate to autoimmunity and to laboratory indices of disease activity? Lupus. 2000;9:333–7.

209. Frieri M, Angadi C, Paolano A, Oster N, Blau SP, Yang S, et al. Altered T cell subpopulations and lymphocytes expressing natural killer cell phenotypes in patients with progressive systemic sclerosis. J Allergy Clin Immunol. 1991;87:773–9.

210. Miller EB, Hiserodt JC, Hunt LE, Steen VD, Medsger Jr TA. Reduced natural killer cell activity in patients with systemic sclerosis. Correlation with clinical disease type. Arthritis Rheum. 1988;31:1515–23.

211. Kantor TV, Whiteside TL, Friberg D, Buckingham RB, Medsger Jr TA. Lymphokine-activated killer cell and natural killer cell activities in patients with systemic sclerosis. Arthritis Rheum. 1992;35:694–9.

212. Wright JK, Hughes P, Rowell NR. Spontaneous lymphocyte-mediated (NK cell) cytotoxicity in systemic sclerosis: a comparison with antibody-dependent lymphocyte (K cell) cytotoxicity. Ann Rheum Dis. 1982;41:409–13.

213. Kojo S, Adachi Y, Keino H, Taniguchi M, Sumida T. Dysfunction of T cell receptor AV24AJ18+, BV11+ double-negative regulatory natural killer T cells in autoimmune diseases. Arthritis Rheum. 2001;44:1127–38.

214. van der Vliet HJ, von Blomberg BM, Nishi N, Reijm M, Voskuyl AE, van Bodegraven AA, et al. Circulating V(alpha24+) Vbeta11+ NKT cell numbers are decreased in a wide variety of diseases that are characterized by autoreactive tissue damage. Clin Immunol. 2001;100:144–8.

215. Illes Z, Kondo T, Newcombe J, Oka N, Tabira T, Yamamura T. Differential expression of NK T cell V alpha 24J alpha Q invariant TCR chain in the lesions of multiple sclerosis and chronic inflammatory demyelinating polyneuropathy. J Immunol (Baltimore, Md 1950). 2000;164:4375–81.

216. Rueda B, Broen J, Simeon C, Hesselstrand R, Diaz B, Suárez H, et al. The STAT4 gene influences the genetic predisposition to systemic sclerosis phenotype. Hum Mol Genet. 2009;18:2071–7.

217. Dieude P, Guedj M, Wipff J, Avouac J, Fajardy I, Diot E, et al. Association between the IRF5 rs2004640 functional polymorphism and systemic sclerosis: a new perspective for pulmonary fibrosis. Arthritis Rheum. 2009;60:225–33.

218. Gorlova O, Martin JE, Rueda B, Koeleman BP, Ying J, Teruel M, et al. Identification of novel genetic markers associated with clinical phenotypes of systemic sclerosis through a genome-wide association strategy. PLoS Genet. 2011;7:e1002178.

219. Carmona FD, Gutala R, Simeón CP, Carreira P, Ortego-Centeno N, Vicente-Rabaneda E, et al. Novel identification of the IRF7 region as an anticentromere autoantibody propensity locus in systemic sclerosis. Ann Rheum Dis. 2012;71:114–9.

220. Radstake TR, Gorlova O, Rueda B, Martin JE, Alizadeh BZ, Palomino-Morales R, et al. Genome-wide association study of systemic sclerosis identifies CD247 as a new susceptibility locus. Nat Genet. 2010;42:426–9.

221. Gourh P, Agarwal SK, Divecha D, Assassi S, Paz G, Arora-Singh RK, et al. Polymorphisms in TBX21 and STAT4 increase the risk of systemic sclerosis: evidence of possible gene-gene interaction and alterations in Th1/Th2 cytokines. Arthritis Rheum. 2009;60:3794–806.

222. Fleming JN, Nash RA, McLeod DO, Fiorentino DF, Shulman HM, Connolly MK, et al. Capillary regeneration in scleroderma: stem cell therapy reverses phenotype? PLoS One. 2008;3:e1452.

223. Kirou KA, Lee C, George S, Louca K, Papagiannis IG, Peterson MGE, et al. Coordinate overexpression of interferon-alpha-induced genes in systemic lupus erythematosus. Arthritis Rheum. 2004;50:3958–67.

224. Sanda C, Weitzel P, Tsukahara T, Schaley J, Edenberg HJ, Stephens MA, et al. Differential gene induction by type I and type II interferons and their combination. J Interf Cytokine Res. 2006;26:462–72.

225. Wong D, Kea B, Pesich R, Higgs BW, Zhu W, Brown P, et al. Interferon and biologic signatures in dermatomyositis skin: specificity and heterogeneity across diseases. Nataf S, ed. PLoS One. 2012;7:e29161.

226. Serpier H, Gillery P, Salmon-Ehr V, Garnotel R, Georges N, Kalis B, et al. Antagonistic effects of interferon-gamma and interleukin-4 on fibroblast cultures. J Invest Dermatol. 1997;109:158–62.

227. Boin F, De Fanis U, Bartlett SJ, Wigley FM, Rosen A, Casolaro V. T cell polarization identifies distinct clinical phenotypes in scleroderma lung disease. Arthritis Rheum. 2008;58:1165–74.

228. Hasegawa M, Sato S, Takehara K. Augmented production of chemokines (monocyte chemotactic protein-1 (MCP-1), macrophage inflammatory protein-1alpha (MIP-1alpha) and MIP-1beta) in patients with systemic sclerosis: MCP-1 and MIP-1alpha may be involved in the development of pulmonary fibrosis. Clin Exp Immunol. 1999;117:159–65.

229. Rabquer BJ, Tsou PS, Hou Y, Thirunavukkarasu E, Haines 3rd GK, Impens AJ, et al. Dysregulated expression of MIG/CXCL9, IP-10/CXCL10 and CXCL16 and their receptors in systemic sclerosis. Arthritis Res Ther. 2011;13:R18.

230. Venkatesan BA, Mahimainathan L, Ghosh-Choudhury N, Gorin Y, Bhandari B, Valente AJ, et al. PI 3 kinase-dependent Akt kinase and PKCepsilon independently regulate interferon-gamma-induced

STAT1alpha serine phosphorylation to induce monocyte chemotactic protein-1 expression. Cell Signal. 2006;18:508–18.
231. Rimbach G, Valacchi G, Canali R, Virgili F. Macrophages stimulated with IFN-gamma activate NF-kappa B and induce MCP-1 gene expression in primary human endothelial cells. Mol Cell Biol Res Commun. 2000;3:238–42.
232. Liebler JM, Kunkel SL, Allen RM, Burdick MD, Strieter RM. Interferon-gamma stimulates monocyte chemotactic protein-1 expression by monocytes. Mediators Inflamm. 1994;3:27–31.
233. Distler JHW, Akhmetshina A, Schett G, Distler O. Monocyte chemoattractant proteins in the pathogenesis of systemic sclerosis. Rheumatology (Oxford). 2009;48:98–103.
234. Carulli MT, Ong VH, Ponticos M, Shiwen X, Abraham DJ, Black CM, et al. Chemokine receptor CCR2 expression by systemic sclerosis fibroblasts: evidence for autocrine regulation of myofibroblast differentiation. Arthritis Rheum. 2005;52:3772–82.
235. Mauviel A, Daireaux M, Redini F, Galera P, Loyau G, Pujol JP. Tumor necrosis factor inhibits collagen and fibronectin synthesis in human dermal fibroblasts. FEBS Lett. 1988;236:47–52.
236. Chizzolini C, Parel Y, Scheja A, Dayer JM. Polarized subsets of human T helper cells induce distinct patterns of chemokine production by normal and systemic sclerosis dermal fibroblasts (Abstract). Clin Exp Rheumatol. 2005;23:739.
237. Ostor AJ, Crisp AJ, Somerville MF, Scott DG. Fatal exacerbation of rheumatoid arthritis associated fibrosing alveolitis in patients given infliximab. BMJ. 2004;329:1266.
238. Allanore Y, Devos-Francois G, Caramella C, Boumier P, Jounieaux V, Kahan A. Fatal exacerbation of fibrosing alveolitis associated with systemic sclerosis in a patient treated with adalimumab. Ann Rheum Dis. 2006;65:834–5.
239. Mauviel A, Heino J, Kahari VM, Hartmann DJ, Loyau G, Pujol JP, et al. Comparative effects of interleukin-1 and tumor necrosis factor-alpha on collagen production and corresponding procollagen mRNA levels in human dermal fibroblasts. J Invest Dermatol. 1991;96:243–9.
240. Solis-Herruzo JA, Brenner DA, Chojkier M. Tumor necrosis factor alpha inhibits collagen gene transcription and collagen synthesis in cultured human fibroblasts. J Biol Chem. 1988;263:5841–5.
241. Verrecchia F, Mauviel A. TGF-beta and TNF-alpha: antagonistic cytokines controlling type I collagen gene expression. Cell Signal. 2004;16:873–80.
242. Hugle T, O'Reilly S, Simpson R, Kraaij MD, Bigley V, Collin M, et al. Tumor necrosis factor-costimulated T lymphocytes from patients with systemic sclerosis trigger collagen production in fibroblasts. Arthritis Rheum. 2013;65:481–91.
243. Sime PJ, Marr RA, Gauldie D, Xing Z, Hewlett BR, Graham FL, et al. Transfer of tumor necrosis factor-alpha to rat lung induces severe pulmonary inflammation and patchy interstitial fibrogenesis with induction of transforming growth factor-beta1 and myofibroblasts. Am J Pathol. 1998;153:825–32.
244. Sullivan DE, Ferris M, Pociask D, Brody AR. Tumor necrosis factor-alpha induces transforming growth factor-beta1 expression in lung fibroblasts through the extracellular signal-regulated kinase pathway. Am J Respir Cell Mol Biol. 2005;32:342–9.
245. Shima Y, Kuwahara Y, Murota H, Kitaba S, Kawai M, Hirano T, et al. The skin of patients with systemic sclerosis softened during the treatment with anti-IL-6 receptor antibody tocilizumab. Rheumatology (Oxford). 2010;49:2408–12.
246. Yanaba K, Yoshizaki A, Asano Y, Kadono T, Sato S. Serum IL-33 levels are raised in patients with systemic sclerosis: association with extent of skin sclerosis and severity of pulmonary fibrosis. Clin Rheumatol. 2011;30:825–30.
247. Manetti M, Ibba-Manneschi L, Liakouli V, Guiducci S, Milia AF, Benelli G, et al. The IL1-like cytokine IL33 and its receptor ST2 are abnormally expressed in the affected skin and visceral organs of patients with systemic sclerosis. Ann Rheum Dis. 2010;69:598–605.
248. Vettori S, Cuomo G, Iudici M, D'Abrosca V, Giacco V, Barra G, et al. Early systemic sclerosis: serum profiling of factors involved in endothelial, T-cell, and fibroblast interplay is marked by elevated interleukin-33 levels. J Clin Immunol. 2014;34:663–8.
249. Wagner A, Kohm M, Nordin A, Svenungsson E, Pfeilschifter JM, Radeke HH. Increased serum levels of the IL-33 neutralizing sST2 in limited cutaneous systemic sclerosis. Scand J Immunol. 2015;82:269–74.
250. MacDonald KG, Dawson NA, Huang Q, Dunne JV, Levings MK, Broady R. Regulatory T cells produce profibrotic cytokines in the skin of patients with systemic sclerosis. J Allergy Clin Immunol. 2015;135:946–955.e9.
251. Martinon F, Mayor A, Tschopp J. The inflammasomes: guardians of the body. Annu Rev Immunol. 2009;27:229–65.
252. Dieude P, Guedj M, Wipff J, Ruiz B, Riemekasten G, Airo P, et al. NLRP1 influences the systemic sclerosis phenotype: a new clue for the contribution of innate immunity in systemic sclerosis-related fibrosing alveolitis pathogenesis. Ann Rheum Dis. 2011;70:668–74.
253. Artlett CM, Sassi-Gaha S, Rieger JL, Boesteanu AC, Feghali-Bostwick CA, Katsikis PD. The inflammasome activating caspase 1 mediates fibrosis and myofibroblast differentiation in systemic sclerosis. Arthritis Rheum. 2011;63:3563–74.
254. Martinez-Godinez MA, Cruz-Dominguez MP, Jara LJ, Dominguez-Lopez A, Jarillo-Luna RA, Vera-Lastra O, et al. Expression of NLRP3 inflammasome, cytokines and vascular mediators in the skin of systemic sclerosis patients. Isr Med Assoc J. 2015;17:5–10.
255. Kahari VM, Sandberg M, Kalimo H, Vuorio T, Vuorio E. Identification of fibroblasts responsible for increased collagen production in localized scleroderma by in situ hybridization. J Invest Dermatol. 1988;90:664–70.
256. Scharffetter K, Lankat-Buttgereit B, Krieg T. Localization of collagen mRNA in normal and scleroderma skin by in-situ hybridization. Eur J Clin Invest. 1988;18:9–17.
257. Prescott RJ, Freemont AJ, Jones CJ, Hoyland J, Fielding P. Sequential dermal microvascular and perivascular changes in the development of scleroderma. J Pathol. 1992;166:255–63.
258. Sondergaard K, Stengaard-Pedersen K, Zachariae H, Heickendorff L, Deleuran M, Deleuran B. Soluble intercellular adhesion molecule 1 (sICAM-1) and soluble interleukin-2 receptors (sIL-2R) in scleroderma skin. Br J Rheumatol. 1998;37:304–10.
259. Truchetet ME, Brembilla NC, Montanari E, Chizzolini C. T-cell subsets in scleroderma patients. Expert Rev Dermatol. 2010;5:403–15; 403.
260. Zhu J, Paul WE. CD4 T cells: fates, functions, and faults. Blood. 2008;112:1557–69.
261. Annunziato F, Romagnani S. Do studies in humans better depict Th17 cells? Blood. 2009;114(11):2213–9.
262. Annunziato F, Romagnani S. Heterogeneity of human effector CD4+ T cells. Arthritis Res Ther. 2009;11:257.
263. Hoffmann KF, McCarty TC, Segal DH, Chiaramonte M, Hesse M, Davis EM, et al. Disease fingerprinting with cDNA microarrays reveals distinct gene expression profiles in lethal type 1 and type 2 cytokine-mediated inflammatory reactions. Faseb J. 2001;15:2545–7.
264. Sandler NG, Mentink-Kane MM, Cheever AW, Wynn TA. Global gene expression profiles during acute pathogen-induced pulmonary inflammation reveal divergent roles for Th1 and Th2 responses in tissue repair. J Immunol. 2003;171:3655–67.
265. Wynn TA. Cellular and molecular mechanisms of fibrosis. J Pathol. 2008;214:199–210.
266. Wynn TA. Fibrotic disease and the T(H)1/T(H)2 paradigm. Nat Rev Immunol. 2004;4:583–94.
267. Postlethwaite AE, Holness MA, Katai H, Raghow R. Human fibroblasts synthesize elevated levels of extracellular matrix proteins in response to interleukin 4. J Clin Invest. 1992;90:1479–85.

268. Oriente A, Fedarko NS, Pacocha SE, Huang SK, Lichtenstein LM, Essayan DM. Interleukin-13 modulates collagen homeostasis in human skin and keloid fibroblasts. J Pharmacol Exp Ther. 2000;292:988–94.
269. McGaha T, Saito S, Phelps RG, Gordon R, Noben-Trauth N, Paul WE, et al. Lack of skin fibrosis in tight skin (TSK) mice with targeted mutation in the interleukin-4R alpha and transforming growth factor-beta genes. J Invest Dermatol. 2001;116:136–43.
270. Kodera T, McGaha TL, Phelps R, Paul WE, Bona CA. Disrupting the IL-4 gene rescues mice homozygous for the tight-skin mutation from embryonic death and diminishes TGF-beta production by fibroblasts. Proc Natl Acad Sci U S A. 2002;99:3800–5.
271. Lee CG, Homer RJ, Zhu Z, Lanone S, Wang X, Koteliansky V, et al. Interleukin-13 induces tissue fibrosis by selectively stimulating and activating transforming growth factor beta(1). J Exp Med. 2001;194:809–21.
272. Fichtner-Feigl S, Strober W, Kawakami K, Puri RK, Kitani A. IL-13 signaling through the IL-13alpha2 receptor is involved in induction of TGF-beta1 production and fibrosis. Nat Med. 2006;12:99–106.
273. Valentini G, Baroni A, Esposito K, Naclerio C, Buommino E, Farzati A, et al. Peripheral blood T lymphocytes from systemic sclerosis patients show both Th1 and Th2 activation. J Clin Immunol. 2001;21:210–7.
274. Korn T, Bettelli E, Oukka M, Kuchroo VK. IL-17 and Th17 cells. Annu Rev Immunol. 2009;27:485–517.
275. Mi S, Li Z, Yang HZ, Liu HZ, Wang JP, Ma YG, et al. Blocking IL-17A promotes the resolution of pulmonary inflammation and fibrosis via TGF-beta1-dependent and -independent mechanisms. J Immunol. 2011;187:3003–14.
276. Gasse P, Riteau N, Vacher R, Michel ML, Fautrel A, di Padova F, et al. IL-1 and IL-23 mediate early IL-17A production in pulmonary inflammation leading to late fibrosis. PLoS One. 2011;6:e23185.
277. Okamoto Y, Hasegawa M, Matsushita T, Hamaguchi Y, Huu DL, Iwakura Y, et al. Potential roles of interleukin-17A in the development of skin fibrosis in mice. Arthritis Rheum. 2012;64:3726–35.
278. Truchetet ME, Brembilla NC, Montanari E, Allanore Y, Chizzolini C. Increased frequency of circulating Th22 in addition to Th17 and Th2 lymphocytes in systemic sclerosis: association with interstitial lung disease. Arthritis Res Ther. 2011;13:R166.
279. Mathian A, Parizot C, Dorgham K, Trad S, Arnaud L, Larsen M, et al. Activated and resting regulatory T cell exhaustion concurs with high levels of interleukin-22 expression in systemic sclerosis lesions. Ann Rheum Dis. 2012;71:1227–34.
280. Truchetet ME, Allanore Y, Montanari E, Chizzolini C, Brembilla NC. Prostaglandin I2 analogues enhance already exuberant Th17 cell responses in systemic sclerosis. Ann Rheum Dis. 2012;71:2044–50.
281. Auriemma M, Vianale G, Reale M, Costantini E, Di Nicola M, Romani GL, et al. Iloprost treatment summer-suspension: effects on skin thermal properties and cytokine profile in systemic sclerosis patients. G Ital Dermatol Venereol. 2013;148:209–16.
282. Kawald A, Burmester GR, Huscher D, Sunderkotter C, Riemekasten G. Low versus high-dose iloprost therapy over 21 days in patients with secondary Raynaud's phenomenon and systemic sclerosis: a randomized, open, single-center study. J Rheumatol. 2008;35(9):1830–7.
283. Komura K, Fujimoto M, Yanaba K, Matsushita T, Matsushita Y, Horikawa M, et al. Blockade of CD40/CD40 ligand interactions attenuates skin fibrosis and autoimmunity in the tight-skin mouse. Ann Rheum Dis. 2008;67:867–72.
284. Vignali DA, Kuchroo VK. IL-12 family cytokines: immunological playmakers. Nat Immunol. 2012;13:722–8.
285. Lopez-Isac E, Campillo-Davo D, Bossini-Castillo L, Guerra SG, Assassi S, Simeon CP, et al. Influence of TYK2 in systemic sclerosis susceptibility: a new locus in the IL-12 pathway. Ann Rheum Dis. 2015 [Epub ahead of print].
286. Bossini-Castillo L, Martin JE, Broen J, Gorlova O, Simeon CP, Beretta L, et al. A GWAS follow-up study reveals the association of the IL12RB2 gene with systemic sclerosis in Caucasian populations. Hum Mol Genet. 2012;21:926–33.
287. Agarwal SK, Gourh P, Shete S, Paz G, Divecha D, Reveille JD, et al. Association of interleukin 23 receptor polymorphisms with anti-topoisomerase-I positivity and pulmonary hypertension in systemic sclerosis. J Rheumatol. 2009;36:2715–23.
288. Farago B, Magyari L, Safrany E, Csongei V, Jaromi L, Horvatovich K, et al. Functional variants of interleukin-23 receptor gene confer risk for rheumatoid arthritis but not for systemic sclerosis. Ann Rheum Dis. 2008;67:248–50.
289. Sakaguchi S, Miyara M, Costantino CM, Hafler DA. FOXP3+ regulatory T cells in the human immune system. Nat Rev Immunol. 2010;10:490–500.
290. Ohkura N, Kitagawa Y, Sakaguchi S. Development and maintenance of regulatory T cells. Immunity. 2013;38:414–23.
291. Zhu J, Yamane H, Paul WE. Differentiation of effector CD4 T cell populations (*). Annu Rev Immunol. 2010;28:445–89.
292. Miyara M, Yoshioka Y, Kitoh A, Shima T, Wing K, Niwa A, et al. Functional delineation and differentiation dynamics of human CD4+ T cells expressing the FoxP3 transcription factor. Immunity. 2009;30:899–911.
293. Antiga E, Quaglino P, Bellandi S, Volpi W, Del Bianco E, Comessatti A, et al. Regulatory T cells in the skin lesions and blood of patients with systemic sclerosis and morphoea. Br J Dermatol. 2010;162:1056–63; 1056.
294. Radstake TR, van Bon L, Broen J, Wenink M, Santegoets K, Deng Y, et al. Increased frequency and compromised function of T regulatory cells in systemic sclerosis (SSc) is related to a diminished CD69 and TGFbeta expression. PLoS One. 2009;4:e5981.
295. Slobodin G, Ahmad MS, Rosner I, Peri R, Rozenbaum M, Kessel A, et al. Regulatory T cells (CD4(+)CD25(bright)FoxP3(+)) expansion in systemic sclerosis correlates with disease activity and severity. Cell Immunol. 2010;261:77–80.
296. Klein S, Kretz CC, Ruland V, Stumpf C, Haust M, Hartschuh W, et al. Reduction of regulatory T cells in skin lesions but not in peripheral blood of patients with systemic scleroderma. Ann Rheum Dis. 2010;70:1475–81.
297. Baraut J, Grigore EI, Jean-Louis F, Khelifa SH, Durand C, Verrecchia F, et al. Peripheral blood regulatory T cells in patients with diffuse systemic sclerosis (SSc) before and after autologous hematopoietic SCT: a pilot study. Bone Marrow Transpl. 2014;49:349–54.
298. Wang YY, Wang Q, Sun XH, Liu RZ, Shu Y, Kanekura T, et al. DNA hypermethylation of the forkhead box protein 3 (FOXP3) promoter in CD4+ T cells of patients with systemic sclerosis. Br J Dermatol. 2014;171:39–47.
299. Broen JC, Wolvers-Tettero IL, Geurts-van Bon L, Vonk MC, Coenen MJ, Lafyatis R, et al. Skewed X chromosomal inactivation impacts T regulatory cell function in systemic sclerosis. Ann Rheum Dis. 2010;69(12):2213–6.
300. Kuwana M, Medsger TA, Wright TM. T cell proliferative response induced by DNA topoisomerase I in patients with systemic sclerosis and healthy donors. J Clin Invest. 1995;96:586–96.
301. Boin F, Wigley FM, Schneck JP, Oelke M, Rosen A. Evaluation of topoisomerase-1-specific CD8+ T-cell response in systemic sclerosis. Ann N Y Acad Sci. 2005;1062:137–45.
302. Hu PQ, Oppenheim JJ, Jr. Medsger A, Wright TM. T cell lines from systemic sclerosis patients and healthy controls recognize multiple epitopes on DNA topoisomerase I. J Autoimmun. 2006;26:258–67.
303. Joseph CG, Darrah E, Shah AA, Skora AD, Casciola-Rosen LA, Wigley FM, et al. Association of the autoimmune disease

scleroderma with an immunologic response to cancer. Science. 2014;343:152–7.
304. Kuwana M, Feghali CA, Medsger TA, Wright TM. Autoreactive T cells to topoisomerase I in monozygotic twins discordant for systemic sclerosis. Arthritis Rheum. 2001;44:1654–9.
305. Oriss TB, Hu PQ, Wright TM. Distinct autoreactive T cell responses to native and fragmented DNA topoisomerase I: influence of APC type and IL-2. J Immunol. 2001;166:5456–63.
306. Rands AL, Whyte J, Cox B, Hall ND, McHugh NJ. MHC class II associations with autoantibody and T cell immune responses to the scleroderma autoantigen topoisomerase I. J Autoimmun. 2000;15:451–8.
307. Veeraraghavan S, Renzoni EA, Jeal H, Jones M, Hammer J, Wells AU, et al. Mapping of the immunodominant T cell epitopes of the protein topoisomerase I. Ann Rheum Dis. 2004;63:982–7.
308. Shah AA, Rosen A, Hummers L, Wigley F, Casciola-Rosen L. Close temporal relationship between onset of cancer and scleroderma in patients with RNA polymerase I/III antibodies. Arthritis Rheum. 2010;62:2787–95.
309. Hu PQ, Hurwitz AA, Oppenheim JJ. Immunization with DNA topoisomerase I induces autoimmune responses but not scleroderma-like pathologies in mice. J Rheumatol. 2007;34:2243–52.
310. Yoshizaki A, Yanaba K, Ogawa A, Asano Y, Kadono T, Sato S. Immunization with DNA topoisomerase I and complete Freund's adjuvant induces skin and lung fibrosis and autoimmunity via interleukin-6 signaling. Arthritis Rheum. 2011;63:3575–85.
311. Artlett CM, Smith JB, Jimenez SA. Identification of fetal DNA and cells in skin lesions from women with systemic sclerosis. N Engl J Med. 1998;338:1186–91.
312. Nelson JL, Furst DE, Maloney S, Gooley T, Evans PC, Smith A, et al. Microchimerism and HLA-compatible relationships of pregnancy in scleroderma. Lancet. 1998;351:559–62.
313. Zhang Y, McCormick LL, Desai SR, Wu C, Gilliam AC. Murine sclerodermatous graft-versus-host disease, a model for human scleroderma: cutaneous cytokines, chemokines, and immune cell activation. J Immunol. 2002;168:3088–98.
314. Lipsky PE. Systemic lupus erythematosus: an autoimmune disease of B cell hyperactivity. Nat Immunol. 2001;2:764–6.
315. Lafyatis R, O'Hara C, Feghali-Bostwick CA, Matteson E. B cell infiltration in systemic sclerosis-associated interstitial lung disease. Arthritis Rheum. 2007;56:3167–8.
316. Whitfield ML, Finlay DR, Murray JI, Troyanskaya OG, Chi JT, Pergamenschikov A, et al. Systemic and cell type-specific gene expression patterns in scleroderma skin. Proc Natl Acad Sci U S A. 2003;100:12319–24.
317. Streicher K, Morehouse CA, Groves CJ, Rajan B, Pilataxi F, Lehmann KP, et al. The plasma cell signature in autoimmune disease. Arthritis Rheumatol. 2014;66:173–84.
318. Sato S, Fujimoto M, Hasegawa M, Takehara K. Altered blood B lymphocyte homeostasis in systemic sclerosis: expanded naive B cells and diminished but activated memory B cells. Arthritis Rheum. 2004;50:1918–27.
319. Wang J, Watanabe T. Expression and function of Fas during differentiation and activation of B cells. Int Rev Immunol. 1999;18:367–79.
320. Tsuchiya N, Kuroki K, Fujimoto M, Murakami Y, Tedder TF, Tokunaga K, et al. Association of a functional CD19 polymorphism with susceptibility to systemic sclerosis. Arthritis Rheum. 2004;50:4002–7.
321. Wu M, Mohan C. B-cells in systemic sclerosis: emerging evidence from genetics to phenotypes. Curr Opin Rheumatol. 2015;27:537–41.
322. Rosser EC, Mauri C. Regulatory B cells: origin, phenotype, and function. Immunity. 2015;42:607–12.
323. Matsushita T, Hamaguchi Y, Hasegawa M, Takehara K, Fujimoto M. Decreased levels of regulatory B cells in patients with systemic sclerosis: association with autoantibody production and disease activity. Rheumatology. 2015 [Epub ahead of print].
324. Mavropoulos A, Simopoulou T, Varna A, Liaskos C, Katsiari C, Bogdanos DP, et al. B regulatory cells are decreased and functionally impaired in patients with systemic sclerosis. Arthritis Rheumatol. 2016;68:494–504.
325. Mackay F, Browning JL. BAFF: a fundamental survival factor for B cells. Nat Rev Immunol. 2002;2:465–75.
326. Bielecki M, Kowal K, Lapinska A, Bernatowicz P, Chyczewski L, Kowal-Bielecka O. Increased production of a proliferation-inducing ligand (APRIL) by peripheral blood mononuclear cells is associated with antitopoisomerase I antibody and more severe disease in systemic sclerosis. J Rheumatol. 2010;37:2286–9.
327. Jordan S, Distler JH, Maurer B, Huscher D, van Laar JM, Allanore Y, et al. Effects and safety of rituximab in systemic sclerosis: an analysis from the European Scleroderma Trial and Research (EUSTAR) group. Ann Rheum Dis. 2015;74:1188–94.
328. Bosello SL, De Luca G, Rucco M, Berardi G, Falcione M, Danza FM, et al. Long-term efficacy of B cell depletion therapy on lung and skin involvement in diffuse systemic sclerosis. Semin Arthritis Rheum. 2015;44:428–36.
329. Allen SJ, Crown SE, Handel TM. Chemokine: receptor structure, interactions, and antagonism. Annu Rev Immunol. 2007;25:787–820.
330. Bacon K, Baggiolini M, Broxmeyer H, Horuk R, Lindley I, Mantovani A, et al. Chemokine/chemokine receptor nomenclature. J Interferon Cytokine Res. 2002;22:1067–8.
331. Strieter RM, Belperio JA, Keane MP. CXC chemokines in angiogenesis related to pulmonary fibrosis. Chest. 2002;122:298S–301.
332. Karrer S, Bosserhoff AK, Weiderer P, Distler O, Landthaler M, Szeimies RM, et al. The -2518 promoter polymorphism in the MCP-1 gene is associated with systemic sclerosis. J Invest Dermatol. 2005;124:92–8.
333. Carulli MT, Spagnolo P, Fonseca C, Welsh KI, duBois RM, Black CM, et al. Single-nucleotide polymorphisms in CCL2 gene are not associated with susceptibility to systemic sclerosis. J Rheumatol. 2008;35:839–44.
334. Gu L, Tseng S, Horner RM, Tam C, Loda M, Rollins BJ. Control of TH2 polarization by the chemokine monocyte chemoattractant protein 1. Nature. 2000;404:407–11.
335. Gharaee-Kermani M, McCullumsmith RE, Charo IF, Kunkel SL, Phan SH. CC-chemokine receptor 2 required for bleomycin-induced pulmonary fibrosis. Cytokine. 2003;24:266–76.
336. Yamamoto T, Nishioka K. Role of monocyte chemoattractant protein-1 and its receptor, CCR-2, in the pathogenesis of bleomycin-induced scleroderma. J Invest Dermatol. 2003;121:510–6.
337. Kimura M, Kawahito Y, Hamaguchi M, Nakamura T, Okamoto M, Matsumoto Y, et al. SKL-2841, a dual antagonist of MCP-1 and MIP-1 beta, prevents bleomycin-induced skin sclerosis in mice. Biomed Pharmacother. 2007;61:222–8.
338. Denton CP, Shi-Wen X, Sutton A, Abraham DJ, Black CM, Pearson JD. Scleroderma fibroblasts promote migration of mononuclear leucocytes across endothelial cell monolayers. Clin Exp Immunol. 1998;114:293–300.
339. Yanaba K, Yoshizaki A, Muroi E, Hara T, Ogawa F, Shimizu K, et al. CCL13 is a promising diagnostic marker for systemic sclerosis. Br J Dermatol. 2010;162:332–6.
340. Ishida Y, Kimura A, Kondo T, Hayashi T, Ueno M, Takakura N, et al. Essential roles of the CC chemokine ligand 3-CC chemokine receptor 5 axis in bleomycin-induced pulmonary fibrosis through regulation of macrophage and fibrocyte infiltration. Am J Pathol. 2007;170:843–54.
341. Lee R, Perry B, Heywood J, Reese C, Bonner M, Hatfield CM, et al. Caveolin-1 regulates chemokine receptor 5-mediated contribution of bone marrow-derived cells to dermal fibrosis. Front Pharmacol. 2014;5:140.

342. Yang X, Walton WW, Cook DN, Hua X, Tilley S, Haskell CA, et al. The chemokine, CCL3, and its receptor, CCR1, mediate thoracic radiation-induced pulmonary fibrosis. Am J Respir Cell Mol Biol. 2011;45:127–35.
343. Dorfmuller P, Zarka V, Durand-Gasselin I, Monti G, Balabanian K, Garcia G, et al. Chemokine RANTES in severe pulmonary arterial hypertension. Am J Respir Crit Care Med. 2002;165:534–9.
344. Tuder RM, Groves B, Badesch DB, Voelkel NF. Exuberant endothelial cell growth and elements of inflammation are present in plexiform lesions of pulmonary hypertension. Am J Pathol. 1994;144:275–85.
345. Molet S, Furukawa K, Maghazechi A, Hamid Q, Giaid A. Chemokine- and cytokine-induced expression of endothelin 1 and endothelin-converting enzyme 1 in endothelial cells. J Allergy Clin Immunol. 2000;105:333–8.
346. Patel VP, Kreider BL, Li Y, Li H, Leung K, Salcedo T, et al. Molecular and functional characterization of two novel human C-C chemokines as inhibitors of two distinct classes of myeloid progenitors. J Exp Med. 1997;185:1163–72.
347. Novak H, Muller A, Harrer N, Gunther C, Carballido JM, Woisetschlager M. CCL23 expression is induced by IL-4 in a STAT6-dependent fashion. J Immunol (Baltimore, Md 1950). 2007;178:4335–41.
348. Yogo Y, Fujishima S, Inoue T, Saito F, Shiomi T, Yamaguchi K, et al. Macrophage derived chemokine (CCL22), thymus and activation-regulated chemokine (CCL17), and CCR4 in idiopathic pulmonary fibrosis. Respir Res. 2009;10:80.
349. Shinoda H, Tasaka S, Fujishima S, Yamasawa W, Miyamoto K, Nakano Y, et al. Elevated CC chemokine level in bronchoalveolar lavage fluid is predictive of a poor outcome of idiopathic pulmonary fibrosis. Respiration. 2009;78:285–92.
350. Pignatti P, Brunetti G, Moretto D, Yacoub MR, Fiori M, Balbi B, et al. Role of the chemokine receptors CXCR3 and CCR4 in human pulmonary fibrosis. Am J Respir Crit Care Med. 2006;173:310–7.
351. Trujillo G, O'Connor EC, Kunkel SL, Hogaboam CM. A novel mechanism for CCR4 in the regulation of macrophage activation in bleomycin-induced pulmonary fibrosis. Am J Pathol. 2008;172:1209–21.
352. Belperio JA, Dy M, Murray L, Burdick MD, Xue YY, Strieter RM, et al. The role of the Th2 CC chemokine ligand CCL17 in pulmonary fibrosis. J Immunol (Baltimore, Md 1950). 2004;173:4692–8.
353. Campbell JJ, Haraldsen G, Pan J, Rottman J, Qin S, Ponath P, et al. The chemokine receptor CCR4 in vascular recognition by cutaneous but not intestinal memory T cells. Nature. 1999;400:776–80.
354. Reiss Y, Proudfoot AE, Power CA, Campbell JJ, Butcher EC. CC chemokine receptor (CCR)4 and the CCR10 ligand cutaneous T cell-attracting chemokine (CTACK) in lymphocyte trafficking to inflamed skin. J Exp Med. 2001;194:1541–7.
355. Prasse A, Pechkovsky DV, Toews GB, Jungraithmayr W, Kollert F, Goldmann T, et al. A vicious circle of alveolar macrophages and fibroblasts perpetuates pulmonary fibrosis via CCL18. Am J Respir Crit Care Med. 2006;173:781–92.
356. Luzina IG, Todd NW, Nacu N, Lockatell V, Choi J, Hummers LK, et al. Regulation of pulmonary inflammation and fibrosis through expression of integrins alphaVbeta3 and alphaVbeta5 on pulmonary T lymphocytes. Arthritis Rheum. 2009;60:1530–9.
357. Luzina IG, Atamas SP, Wise R, Wigley FM, Xiao HQ, White B. Gene expression in bronchoalveolar lavage cells from scleroderma patients. Am J Respir Cell Mol Biol. 2002;26:549–57.
358. Strieter RM, Belperio JA, Phillips RJ, Keane MP. CXC chemokines in angiogenesis of cancer. Semin Cancer Biol. 2004;14:195–200.
359. Chang MS, McNinch J, Basu R, Simonet S. Cloning and characterization of the human neutrophil-activating peptide (ENA-78) gene. J Biol Chem. 1994;269:25277–82.
360. Meloni F, Caporali R, Marone Bianco A, Paschetto E, Morosini M, Fietta AM, et al. Cytokine profile of bronchoalveolar lavage in systemic sclerosis with interstitial lung disease: comparison with usual interstitial pneumonia. Ann Rheum Dis. 2004;63:892–4.
361. Pantelidis P, Southcott AM, Black CM, Du Bois RM. Up-regulation of IL-8 secretion by alveolar macrophages from patients with fibrosing alveolitis: a subpopulation analysis. Clin Exp Immunol. 1997;108:95–104.
362. Ludwicka-Bradley A, Tourkina E, Suzuki S, Tyson E, Bonner M, Fenton 2nd JW, et al. Thrombin upregulates interleukin-8 in lung fibroblasts via cleavage of proteolytically activated receptor-I and protein kinase C-gamma activation. Am J Respir Cell Mol Biol. 2000;22:235–43.
363. Silver RM, Metcalf JF, Stanley JH, LeRoy EC. Interstitial lung disease in scleroderma. Analysis by bronchoalveolar lavage. Arthritis Rheum. 1984;27:1254–62.
364. Chizzolini C, Parel Y, Scheja A, Dayer JM. Polarized subsets of human T-helper cells induce distinct patterns of chemokine production by normal and systemic sclerosis dermal fibroblasts. Arthritis Res Ther. 2006;8:R10.
365. Postlethwaite AE, Chiang TM. Platelet contributions to the pathogenesis of systemic sclerosis. Curr Opin Rheumatol. 2007;19:574–9.
366. Ruth JH, Rottman JB, Katschke Jr KJ, Qin S, Wu L, LaRosa G, et al. Selective lymphocyte chemokine receptor expression in the rheumatoid joint. Arthritis Rheum. 2001;44:2750–60.
367. Balashov KE, Rottman JB, Weiner HL, Hancock WW. CCR5(+) and CXCR3(+) T cells are increased in multiple sclerosis and their ligands MIP-1alpha and IP-10 are expressed in demyelinating brain lesions. Proc Natl Acad Sci U S A. 1999;96:6873–8.
368. Sorensen TL, Tani M, Jensen J, Pierce V, Lucchinetti C, Folcik VA, et al. Expression of specific chemokines and chemokine receptors in the central nervous system of multiple sclerosis patients. J Clin Invest. 1999;103:807–15.
369. Hancock WW, Lu B, Gao W, Csizmadia V, Faia K, King JA, et al. Requirement of the chemokine receptor CXCR3 for acute allograft rejection. J Exp Med. 2000;192:1515–20.
370. Belperio JA, Keane MP, Burdick MD, Lynch JP, Zisman DA, Xue YY, et al. Role of CXCL9/CXCR3 chemokine biology during pathogenesis of acute lung allograft rejection. J Immunol (Baltimore, Md 1950). 2003;171:4844–52.
371. Jiang D, Liang J, Hodge J, Lu B, Zhu Z, Yu S, et al. Regulation of pulmonary fibrosis by chemokine receptor CXCR3. J Clin Invest. 2004;114:291–9.
372. Keane MP, Belperio JA, Arenberg DA, Burdick MD, Xu ZJ, Xue YY, et al. IFN-gamma-inducible protein-10 attenuates bleomycin-induced pulmonary fibrosis via inhibition of angiogenesis. J Immunol (Baltimore, Md 1950). 1999;163:5686–92.
373. Zeremski M, Dimova R, Brown Q, Jacobson IM, Markatou M, Talal AH. Peripheral CXCR3-associated chemokines as biomarkers of fibrosis in chronic hepatitis C virus infection. J Infect Dis. 2009;200:1774–80.
374. Ho J, Rush DN, Gibson IW, Karpinski M, Storsley L, Bestland J, et al. Early urinary CCL2 is associated with the later development of interstitial fibrosis and tubular atrophy in renal allografts. Transplantation. 2010;90:394–400.
375. Murdoch C. CXCR4: chemokine receptor extraordinaire. Immunol Rev. 2000;177:175–84.
376. Phillips RJ, Burdick MD, Hong K, Lutz MA, Murray LA, Xue YY, et al. Circulating fibrocytes traffic to the lungs in response to CXCL12 and mediate fibrosis. J Clin Invest. 2004;114:438–46.
377. Mehrad B, Burdick MD, Zisman DA, Keane MP, Belperio JA, Strieter RM. Circulating peripheral blood fibrocytes in human fibrotic interstitial lung disease. Biochem Biophys Res Commun. 2007;353:104–8.
378. Moeller A, Gilpin SE, Ask K, Cox G, Cook D, Gauldie J, et al. Circulating fibrocytes are an indicator of poor prognosis in idiopathic pulmonary fibrosis. Am J Respir Crit Care Med. 2009;179:588–94.

379. Strieter RM, Keeley EC, Hughes MA, Burdick MD, Mehrad B. The role of circulating mesenchymal progenitor cells (fibrocytes) in the pathogenesis of pulmonary fibrosis. J Leukoc Biol. 2009;86:1111–8.
380. Mohle R, Bautz F, Rafii S, Moore MA, Brugger W, Kanz L. The chemokine receptor CXCR-4 is expressed on CD34+ hematopoietic progenitors and leukemic cells and mediates transendothelial migration induced by stromal cell-derived factor-1. Blood. 1998;91:4523–30.
381. Asahara T, Murohara T, Sullivan A, Silver M, van der Zee R, Li T, et al. Isolation of putative progenitor endothelial cells for angiogenesis. Science. 1997;275:964–7.
382. Abel S, Hundhausen C, Mentlein R, Schulte A, Berkhout TA, Broadway N, et al. The transmembrane CXC-chemokine ligand 16 is induced by IFN-gamma and TNF-alpha and shed by the activity of the disintegrin-like metalloproteinase ADAM10. J Immunol (Baltimore, Md 1950). 2004;172:6362–72.
383. Umehara H, Bloom ET, Okazaki T, Nagano Y, Yoshie O, Imai T. Fractalkine in vascular biology: from basic research to clinical disease. Arterioscler Thromb Vasc Biol. 2004;24:34–40.
384. Fraticelli P, Sironi M, Bianchi G, D'Ambrosio D, Albanesi C, Stoppacciaro A, et al. Fractalkine (CX3CL1) as an amplification circuit of polarized Th1 responses. J Clin Invest. 2001;107:1173–81.
385. Balabanian K, Foussat A, Dorfmuller P, Durand-Gasselin I, Capel F, Bouchet-Delbos L, et al. CX(3)C chemokine fractalkine in pulmonary arterial hypertension. Am J Respir Crit Care Med. 2002;165:1419–25.
386. Arai M, Ikawa Y, Chujo S, Hamaguchi Y, Ishida W, Shirasaki F, et al. Chemokine receptors CCR2 and CX3CR1 regulate skin fibrosis in the mouse model of cytokine-induced systemic sclerosis. J Dermatol Sci. 2013;69:250–8.

Autoantibodies as Markers and Possible Mediators of Scleroderma Pathogenesis

14

Kimberly Doering Maurer and Antony Rosen

Introduction

Scleroderma or systemic sclerosis (SSc) is a systemic autoimmune disease characterized by a distinct, proliferative vasculopathy associated with skin thickening and fibrosis within internal organs and is associated with a unique autoimmune response. While vascular damage is almost universal in scleroderma, disease expression is heterogeneous in terms of phenotypic characteristics and disease course. Nevertheless, clear clinical subtypes can be discerned. The limited cutaneous form of scleroderma (lcSSc) is characterized by skin thickening on the distal limbs, face, and neck and an increased prevalence of isolated pulmonary hypertension and ischemic digital loss. In contrast, the diffuse form of the disease also involves more proximal skin and affects visceral organs, including the lung, heart, gastrointestinal tract, skeletal muscle, and kidneys, with attendant negative effects on mortality. There are striking associations between specific autoantibodies and the distinct phenotypic subsets of scleroderma. These associations are clinically useful, suggesting, at a minimum, that the different autoantibodies are reporting on specific circumstances which underlie disease propagation in different tissues. It is also possible that specific autoantibodies play a direct pathogenic role in the propagation and amplification of autoimmune reactions and pathology in SSc. This chapter reviews some of the interesting insights which autoantibodies and their specificity provide into scleroderma pathogenesis.

K.D. Maurer, PhD (✉)
Undergraduate Medical Education, University of California, San Francisco, CA, USA
e-mail: kimberly.maurer@ucsf.edu

A. Rosen, MB ChB, BSc
Division of Rheumatology, The Johns Hopkins Hospital, Baltimore, MD, USA

Autoantibody Profiles as Markers of Pathogenic Events

Although the role of disease-specific autoantibodies in the systemic autoimmune diseases remains controversial, the specificity of these antibodies provides a critical clue to understanding their origin. Each systemic autoimmune disease (e.g., scleroderma, systemic lupus erythematosus (SLE), rheumatoid arthritis, autoimmune myositis, Sjögren's syndrome) is characterized by the elaboration of a distinct group of autoantibodies that target a limited number of ubiquitously expressed autoantigens. Within the scleroderma spectrum, autoantibody profiles are associated with specific disease phenotypes, making serological tests helpful in diagnosis and prognosis. The major clinical subsets of scleroderma have distinct serological associations, with topoisomerase-1 and RNA polymerase antibodies associated with the diffuse form of the disease, and centromere autoantibodies enriched in the limited form. Many of these SSc-specific autoantibodies are mutually exclusive, a finding that has been conclusively established over the past 25 years [25, 43, 52]. In one study of 5,423 patients, only 26 (0.52 %) had coexistence of anti-topoisomerase-1 and anti-centromere antibodies [9].

The existence of significant phenotypic differences between limited and diffuse forms of scleroderma has led some to propose that these are discrete disease processes, and thus the distinct autoantibody profiles in the two subsets are not surprising. However, distinct autoantibody patterns with specific target tissue involvement, even within the diffuse disease spectrum, suggest that autoantibody specificity might reflect unique amplification pathways within specific tissues. For example, while antibodies to topoisomerase-1 and RNA polymerases are both associated with a more aggressive form of diffuse skin disease in scleroderma, anti-topoisomerase is associated with interstitial lung disease and RNA polymerase I/III antibodies are not. The latter autoantibodies occur in patients with rapidly progressive, severe skin

J. Varga et al. (eds.), *Scleroderma*, DOI 10.1007/978-3-319-31407-5_14

disease, as well as renal crisis [12, 33]. Additionally, patients with scleroderma in overlap with other autoimmune diseases express antibodies to "overlap"' antigens, including anti-PM-Scl antibodies with myositis [27] or anti-U1-RNP antibodies with SLE [12, 33]. Taken together, the observation of specific autoantibody associations with distinct tissue injury patterns, and the tendency for autoantibody subsets to be non-overlapping, suggests that target tissue and immune response interact and both participate in antigen selection, tissue damage, and disease manifestations.

Although there is widespread agreement that autoimmunity is an important participant in scleroderma pathogenesis, there is a subgroup of patients (~10 %) with classical scleroderma phenotypes who do not have either ANAs or scleroderma-specific autoantibodies. This patient subgroup is extremely interesting, as they may shed light on critical mechanisms of tissue damage which are not evident from studying the autoantibodies to ubiquitously expressed antigens (see below).

Some Autoantibody Titers Can Change Over Time: Association with Disease Severity and Activity

Since the autoantibody response in various autoimmune rheumatic diseases has been noted to be antigen driven and T cell dependent, there have been numerous attempts to define whether autoantibody titers and disease activity/severity in SSc are related [15, 22, 35]. This is a particularly difficult task in SSc, where quantitation of disease activity and severity are insensitive compared to other rheumatic processes like RA. In some studies, topoisomerase-1 autoantibody titers in SSc appear to be positively correlated with total skin score measurements [17]. Additionally, the rate of deterioration in lung function tests (forced vital capacity and carbon monoxide diffusing capacity) was greater in patients whose anti-topoisomerase antibodies were sustained over time [22]. However, the dynamic range of changes of anti-toposiomerase-1 titers is quite limited, and changes in titers of other autoantibodies (CENP or RNA polymerase) do not appear to be associated with clinically significant variation in disease activity. Therefore, the available data suggests that the levels of defined autoantibody specificities in scleroderma do not vary in clinically meaningful ways. The implications of this conclusion may include the following scenarios, depicted in Fig. 14.1. (1) Although the generation of autoantibodies might be initiated after exposure of these specific antigens during early events in the disease, they may be driven by events not directly on the pathogenic pathway. The specific autoantigens themselves may be released in a disease-nonspecific way during homeostasis, becoming markers of damage, or possibly other antigens, unrelated to the disease, may be present and continue to drive a cross-reactive antibody response. (2) There have been recent studies showing that antibody effector function can be modified by Fc posttranslational modification like sialylation, where antibody titers do not reflect inflammatory properties [2]. (3) All of the autoantigens discussed above are intracellular and ubiquitously expressed, making it less likely that autoantibodies to these antigens have easy access to the relevant antigens. Using the antibodies to identify important antigen specificities, and then prospectively quantifying antigen-specific T cells recognizing these scleroderma autoantigens over time, may better allow associations to be defined

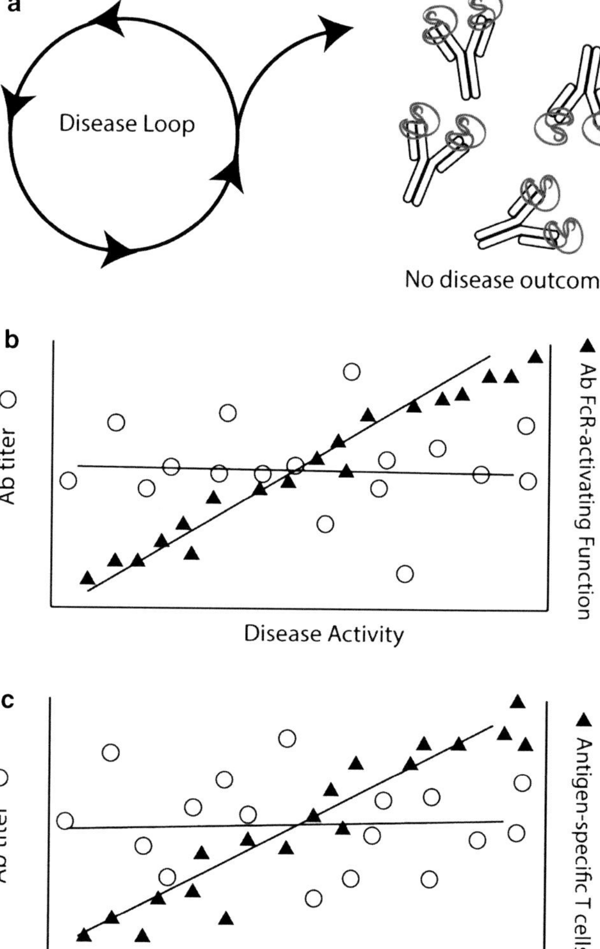

Fig. 14.1 Possible reasons that autoantibody titers do not correlate with disease activity. (**a**) Autoantibodies may simply be markers of tissue damage and not play a role in disease propagation. (**b**) Total antibody titers may not correlate with disease activity because only a subset of autoantibodies bind to activating FcRs and therefore mediate effector functions (e.g., non-sialylated Fc sugars). The extent of Ig sialylation, therefore, may correlate with disease activity or severity. (**c**) Autoantibody specificity may be significantly impacted by intra- and intermolecular epitope spreading and therefore be driven by the specific disease-associated epitopes as well as cross-reactive antigens

between magnitude of immune response to specific antigens and rate of phenotypic changes. (4) The fact that anti-topoisomerase antibodies do change in association with severity and activity suggests that disease activity in some organs may be associated with antigen exposure or release, contributing to the autoimmune response. This would suggest the existence of a potentially auto-amplifying loop, where antigen expression, immune response, and tissue damage are all components of the mechanism driving the increased autoantibody titers. Defining the components of such a loop and the sites at which this occurs is of great importance and can only be accomplished in vivo in scleroderma patients.

Autoantigen in Target Tissue: Partner in Propagation

The frequently targeted autoantigens in scleroderma are all ubiquitously expressed molecules, participating in numerous important cellular processes. In spite of ubiquitous expression, the immune response to these autoantigens is associated with specific phenotypes, often enriching for damage of a specific tissue. For example, interstitial lung disease is associated with anti-topoisomerase-1 antibodies. This association of specificity of immune response and phenotype has the potential to greatly clarify pathogenesis. One possible explanation that has been advanced is that unique features of autoantigens in specific microenvironments participate in their selection as autoantigens (Fig. 14.2). These features could include novel autoantigen forms which alter autoantigen structure and processing (e.g., novel isoforms, proteolytic cleavage, posttranslational modifications; see below), increased antigen expression levels [6, 55], and microenvironment-specific modifications which allow autoantigens themselves to activate the innate immune system [16, 19].

Although studies of autoantigen levels and conformation in target tissues would really be optimal, data from such studies is not yet available. However, multiple studies have shown that scleroderma autoantigens are particularly susceptible to structural modifications by pathways induced during scleroderma tissue damage. For example, numerous data have shown that cytotoxic T lymphocyte (CTL) granule-mediated killing results in the generation of altered forms of self-antigens (Fig. 14.2d). Granzyme B (GrB), a protease contained within the cytotoxic granules released by CTLs and NK cells, cleaves 80 % of autoantigens targeted in systemic autoimmune diseases to generate novel fragments [1, 5]. Several scleroderma autoantigens (including topoisomerase-1, CENPs B and C, RNA polymerases, U1-RNP, PM-Scl, fibrillarin, and B23) are all cleaved by granzyme B [5, 50]. Interestingly, sera from 84.2 % of patients with ischemic digital loss (IDL) recognized granzyme B-cleaved antigens [38]. This was in contrast to only 40 % of patients without IDL. Some IDL sera preferentially recognize the cleaved fragment of the centromere protein

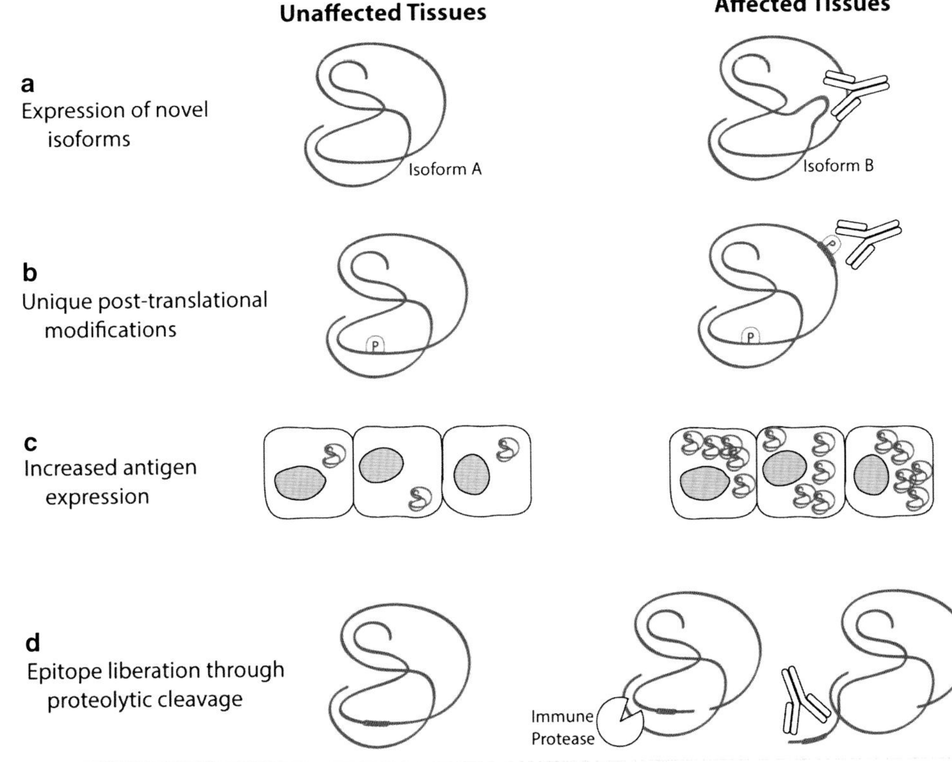

Fig. 14.2 Possible mechanisms underlying association of specific immune responses with distinct patterns of tissue damage in scleroderma. (**a**) Autoantibodies may recognize a polypeptide sequence expressed in protein isoforms restricted to a particular tissue. (**b**) Affected tissue may express an antigen with a unique posttranslational modification. (**c**) Affected tissue may express higher amounts of antigen. (**d**) Proteolytic cleavage may reveal an autoantibody epitope typically hidden within the molecule

CENP-C, but not the intact CENP-C molecule, suggesting that granzyme B might unmask a cryptic B-cell epitope in this molecule and potentially play a pathogenic role in the IDL process [38].

The state of the cell being killed by CTLs may also play an important role in providing altered forms of autoantigens. Indeed, scleroderma autoantigens are not all equally susceptible to cleavage by GrB during cytotoxic killing of all cells. Although B23 is a sensitive substrate for GrB in vitro, it was poorly cleaved in numerous intact cells. Since the immune response to B23 is associated with pulmonary hypertension, Ulanet et al. examined B23 cleavage in vascular smooth muscle (VSM) cells in distinct differentiation states. They found that B23 was poorly cleaved in undifferentiated vascular smooth muscle cells, but was exquisitely sensitive to cleavage when these cells are differentiated toward the contractile phenotype, suggesting the presence of a unique form of B23 in this cell population [49]. The proposed association between scleroderma and cancer [31, 32] is intriguing. Shah et al. have made several observations which suggest that cancers might express scleroderma autoantigens at high levels and serve as an initiating stimulus for autoimmunity in patients who develop scleroderma. In studies examining whether autoantibody status was associated with the temporal relationship between cancer and scleroderma, they examined autoantibody responses in patients that had both scleroderma and cancer. Interestingly, while the mean duration of scleroderma at cancer diagnosis among 23 scleroderma patients was 7.2 ± 10.4 years, patients positive for anti-RNA polymerase I/III antibodies had a significantly lower duration of -1.2 years. The investigators then addressed the expression of RNA polymerases in tumor specimens isolated from these patients. Most of the cancer sections from RNA polymerase III antibody-positive patients showed distinct, nucleolar staining with the anti-RNA polymerase III antibody. In contrast, this pattern was not seen in the cancer specimens from patients negative for this antibody. These observations suggested that the form of RNA polymerase III in cancer tissue might be distinctly immunogenic, capable of initiating an antitumor immune response, and potentially cross-reacting with RNA polymerase III in other tissues (e.g., blood vessels, skin), generating tissue damage characteristic of scleroderma [41]. Evidence in this regard was recently provided by Joseph et al. Characterization of tumors from patients with RNA polymerase III-antibody-positive scleroderma and cancer identified somatic mutations in the *POLR3A* gene. Mutations in the *POLR3A* gene were not present in cancers from scleroderma patients with any other autoantibody specificity. Interestingly, patients with antibodies recognizing RNA polymerase III also had striking loss of heterozygosity (LOH) at the *POLR3A* locus. In these patients, LOH was not evident at chromosomal regions containing either the *TOP1* or *CENP-B* genes, demonstrating a striking association between the target of the immune response and the target of LOH and indicating that these two phenomena are likely mechanistically related. Interestingly in this regard, in two of three patients with somatic mutations in their tumors, the mutations generated peptides predicted to bind with high affinity to one of the patient's MHC class II alleles. Studies directly showed specific CD4 T cell responses recognizing the mutated epitope. There was also evidence in one patient of a distinct population of CD4 T cells responding specifically to the wild-type antigen, suggesting that the mutant-specific immune response spreads to recognize the wild-type version and cross-reacts with normal tissue, possibly through a B-cell-dependent mechanism (Fig. 14.2a). Interestingly, the accompanying autoantibody response was cross-reactive and could not distinguish between mutant and WT antigen. The reason that specific normal tissues might be targeted by the antigen-specific immune response may relate to tissue-specific expression of autoantigens either in the baseline or the damaged state. Understanding what antigen expression in vivo in different tissues under different perturbed states will shed important insights on to this matter. The observation that only 20 % of scleroderma patients with RNA polymerase III antibodies have a malignancy diagnosed, together with the observations of RNA polymerase-specific T cells and frequent LOH at the POLR3A locus, strongly suggests the existence of immunoediting of cancers in scleroderma patients. The authors proposed that scleroderma patients with RNA polymerase III autoantibodies may have successfully cleared an occult malignancy [19].

Autoantibodies as Possible Mediators of SSc Pathogenesis

The data demonstrating that autoantibodies are serological markers of a specific disease phenotype in SSc is extremely strong, but the mechanistic implications of such observations remain uncertain. The use of transformed cell lines as an antigen source to identify all intracellular autoantigens defined to date raises important cautions about whether all relevant autoantibodies have been identified. Two major outstanding questions remain: (1) Do phenotype-specific antibodies themselves play a role in the generation of that phenotype? (2) Are there antibodies which might participate directly in generating the phenotype, potentially through ligation of antigens which are extracellularly exposed? Potential pathogenic roles for autoantibodies in scleroderma can be divided into several categories, amplification of the immune response and direct pathogenicity, which will each be addressed below. A summary of antibodies discussed in this chapter can be found in Table 14.1.

Table 14.1 Summary of autoantibodies with pathogenic potential

I. Amplification of immune responses		
Anti-topoisomerase-1	Recruitment and activation of immune cells	[24, 25]
	Induction of type I IFN secretion from pDCs	[26]
II. Direct pathogenicity		
A. Antibodies against unidentified cell surface molecules		
Anti-endothelial cell antibodies (specific antigens unknown)	Endothelial cell apoptosis	[33, 34]
Anti-fibroblast antibodies (specific antigens unknown)	Pro-adhesive phenotype in fibroblasts and cytokine modulation	[35]
	Upregulation of pro-fibrotic and pro-angiogenic transcriptional programs in fibroblasts	[36]
B. Antibodies against extracellular matrix components		
Anti-fibrillin	Regulation of extracellular matrix components and TGFβ signaling (controversial; see text)	[43–44]
Anti-matrix metalloproteinases 1 and 3	Inhibition of ECM turnover	[49, 50]
C. Antibodies stimulating receptor signaling		
Antiplatelet-derived growth factor receptor	Generation of cellular smooth muscle and fibroblast lesions and upregulation of collagen production (highly controversial; see text)	[51]
Anti-M3 muscarinic receptor	Inhibition of muscle contraction	[54]

Amplification of Immune Responses

Although many of the defined autoantigens in scleroderma are intracellular, such antigens may become re-localized during cell damage or death and potentially during other physiological processes. Such re-localization may allow autoantibodies to access these antigens, with pro-inflammatory consequences. Cells that have a special tendency to bind the antigen may therefore become targets of a redirected immune effector pathway. Antibodies to topoisomerase-1 appear to be relevant in this regard. Henault et al. demonstrated that anti-topoisomerase 1 antibodies bind the surface of fibroblasts, but not smooth muscle or endothelial cells. In a tissue culture-based cell adhesion assay, they showed that the binding of anti-topoisomerase-1 antibodies to fibroblasts was dose dependent and saturable [14]. This phenomenon was facilitated by purified topoisomerase protein or topoisomerase protein released from apoptotic endothelial cells. Bound anti-topoisomerase-1 antibodies enhanced the adhesion and activation of THP1 human monocytes [13]. It is important to note the limited power of such a "redirected" effector pathway to explain self-sustaining, amplifying, tissue-specific phenotypes. Additional parameters still to be defined include whether topoisomerase-1 binding to the surface of a bystander cell induces damage of the bystander, thus supplying additional autoantigen to further drive immune response and bystander injury, as well as whether the specificity of surface binding directs the amplifying effects to particular cells and tissues.

The recent description of the ability of CENP-B, an autoantigen whose targeting of the immune system is associated with limited cutaneous scleroderma, to ligate and activate signaling through CCR3, supports this general mechanism [29].

The "trans" effects of anti-topoisomerase-1 on inflammatory signaling in the setting of released nuclear topoisomerase-1 antigen have also recently been demonstrated. Kim et al. showed that anti-topoisomerase-1-positive sera, but not sera containing autoantibodies to other well-characterized SSc antigens, could induce the secretion of high levels of interferon α (IFNα) in PBMC preparations when supplied with nuclear cell extracts [20]. This group when on to show that the observed production of IFNα was as a result of suspected immune complexes (containing likely anti-topoisomerase-1 IgG antibodies, nuclear cell extracts of protein and nucleic acids) which are able to bind FCγ receptor and TLRs in plasmacytoid dendritic cells (pDCs), potent producers of type I interferons. Interestingly, the induction of IFNα was more prominent in patients with diffuse disease as compared to limited scleroderma (multivariate analysis, however, was not performed to determine whether this was accounted for by increased titers of topoisomerase-1 antibodies). Perhaps even more interesting was the observation that increased IFNα secretion was associated with interstitial lung disease, with a median IFN secretion almost threefold higher in those with lung fibrosis [20]. It is important to recognize that the number of patients studied in this way to date is very small, and these observations and their clinical associations need to be confirmed. However, the potential of association of increased activation of the IFN pathway with clinical phenotype is very intriguing, as it implies that specific autoantibodies might exert feedforward properties which do not require binding to autoantigen within unperturbed cells.

Additionally, aberrant regulation of B lymphocytes is also a suspected driving force of the SSc phenotype. SSc patients have somewhat higher levels of CD19 on their peripheral blood B cells [36]. Similarly, B cells from the tight skin mouse (TSK/+), which develops a scleroderma-like, fibrotic disease [18, 39], are hyperactive and display enhanced signaling through the CD19-associated pathway [34]. Although it is not clear how faithful this model of human scleroderma is, the similarity of findings in CD19 makes it a reasonable model for interrogating the role of B cells in driving fibrosis. On the TSK/+ background, CD19 deficiency reduced B-cell activity, decreased serum autoantibody titers, and attenuated but did not prevent fibrotic skin changes [34]. This suggests that B cells play an amplifying role in skin fibrosis, although the mechanisms whereby they may be contributing remain unclear. Their contributions certainly include increasing autoantibody titers, antigen presentation, and providing help to T cells. Any of these functions could contribute to the self-reinforcing nature of T- and B-cell interactions, which Schlomchik et al. have proposed could be a major driving force behind systemic autoimmune disease [42]. The role of cellular immunity in the development of skin fibrosis within the TSK/+ mouse model is, however, still controversial [18], but may be influenced by the different genetic backgrounds of the animals used in these studies [34].

Direct Pathogenicity

A major requirement for antibodies to exert direct pathogenic effects on intact cells, not through binding of intracellular antigens on the surface of bystander cells, is availability of antigen at an accessible site on the surface of the target cell. One of the major challenges in this area is careful molecular definition of these autoantigens, which are, with some exceptions, poorly defined. Defining membrane and extracellular autoantigens is a notoriously difficult task, with challenges of solubility, affinity, and posttranslational modifications. Nevertheless, it is likely that directly pathogenic autoantibodies do exist in this disease and can contribute to ongoing tissue damage and dysfunction. Defining the key antigens is critical.

Antibodies Recognizing Unidentified Cell Surface Molecules

Anti-endothelial cell antibodies (AECA), although not specific for SSc, are observed in 25–85 % of SSc patients and may define a subgroup of patients that have a high incidence of vascular involvement [28]. These antibodies are thought to induce endothelial apoptosis in SSc [53]. Endothelial cell death and dysfunction might play direct roles in thwarting normal vessel function in SSc [40]. Dying cells might also constitute a source of autoantigens, which, through binding to bystander cells, might contribute to pathogenicity [13]. A proposed model about how some of these antibodies may contribute to an auto-amplifying loop of immune activation, vasculopathy, and fibrosis is shown in Fig. 14.3. It is important to note that this pathway is not a documented one; it is merely a hypothetical model to show potential ways that antibodies with proposed pathogenic roles in scleroderma could collaborate to sustain disease processes.

Antibodies recognizing fibroblasts have also been identified by many groups of investigators. Reported frequency of these so-called anti-fibroblast antibodies (AFA) range from 26.3 % to 58 % of screened scleroderma patients [7, 10, 14, 30, 44, 48]. In one study, 58 % of 69 patients were found to be positive for AFA, and these sera promoted a pro-adhesive phenotype in fibroblasts, induced upregulation of the adhesion molecule, ICAM-1, and enhanced mRNA expression of the cytokines IL-1α, IL-1β, and IL-6 [7]. Further evidence for the presence and effects of anti-fibroblast antibodies continue to accumulate. For example, in a study where 40 % of patients with SSc were positive for AFA, microarrays containing probes for 112 human chemokines and receptors were used to interrogate the transcriptional program triggered by incubation of fibroblasts with AFA [10]. Compared to control sera, AFA+ sera upregulated the expression of a number of genes considered to be pro-fibrotic and pro-angiogenic, such as CCL2 and CXCL8. This response was partially dependent on signaling through TLR4 as shown by use of selective inhibitors, TLR4-deficient mouse cells, and an antagonistic anti-TLR4 antibody. The specific molecular targets of these antibodies, the cell type-specific expression of such molecules, and the in vivo effects of such antibodies in scleroderma remain to be defined. If pathologic in nature, such antibodies could initiate and/or amplify vascular inflammation and fibrosis in SSc.

Autoantibodies Affecting Extracellular Matrix and Its Components

Several components of the extracellular matrix (ECM) have been shown to be targets of autoantibodies in patients with SSc. There are reports of autoantibodies against fibrillin-1 in the TSK/+ mouse model and in some SSc patient cohorts [18, 21, 45–47]. Demonstration of anti-fibrillin-1 antibodies in SSc has not, however, been broadly confirmed [4]. The reasons for these differences are not clear, but fibrillin-1 is a very difficult molecule to assay in numerous formats, being a large molecule whose recognition by antibodies is influenced by whether it is in the disulfide-bonded or reduced state, and the presence of posttranslational modifications [51, 54]. Although fibrillin-1 may be controversial in terms of the presence and role of autoantibodies, the fibrillin family is very interesting in terms of its role in fibrosis and TGFβ binding. Studies of families with multiple members afflicted with stiff skin syndrome (SSS) have shed interesting insights into the role of ECM components in SSc. SSS is an autosomal dominant, noninflammatory disorder characterized by hard, thick skin and subsequent limited joint mobility. Recently, SSS was ascribed to mutations in fibrillin [23].

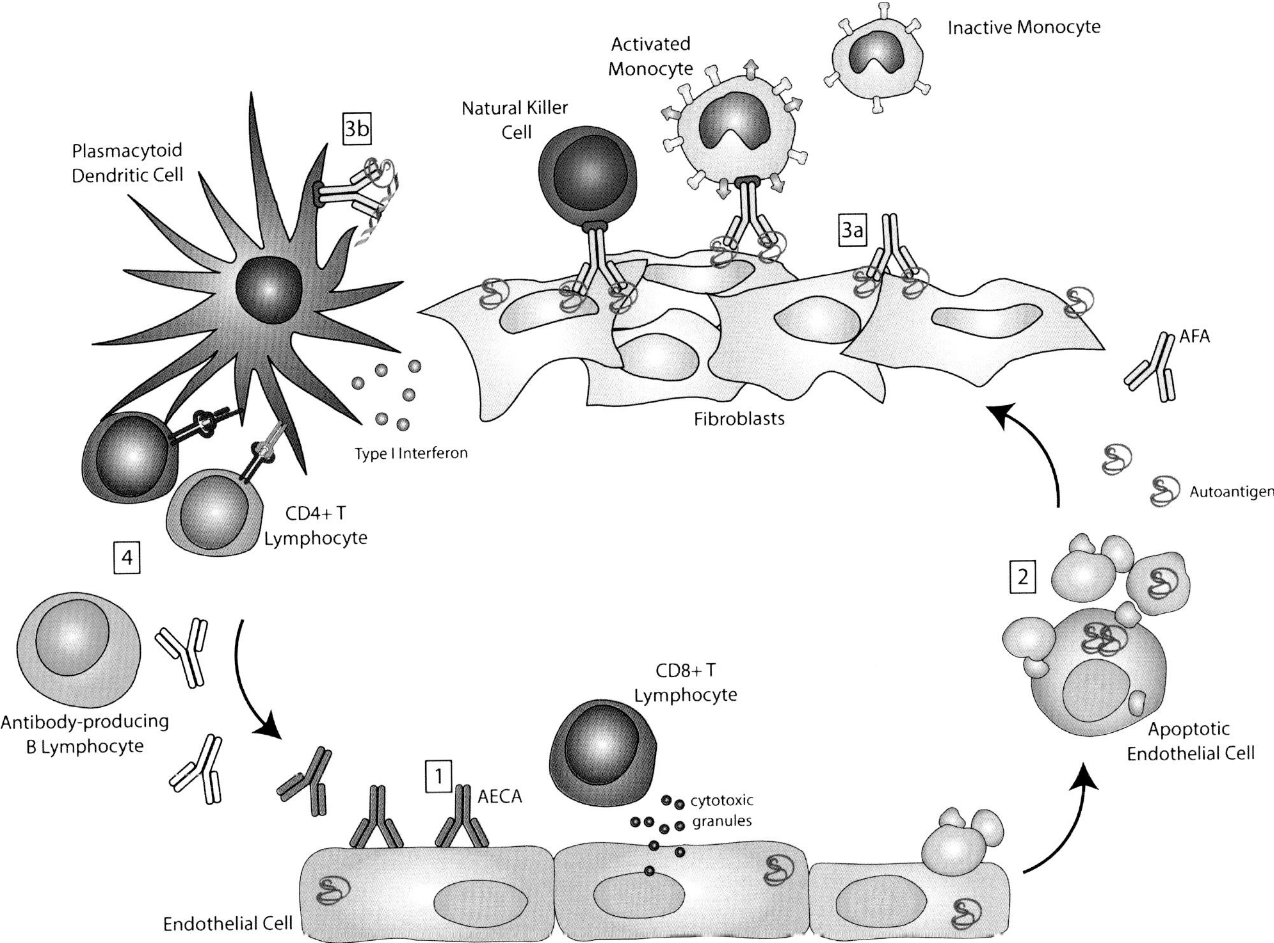

Fig. 14.3 Hypothetical model of immune-mediated vascular damage, highlighting potential opportunities of antibody-assisted disease propagation. *1* AECA and likely cytotoxic T cells can cause endothelial cell apoptosis. *2* Apoptotic endothelial cells may be a cause of vascular dysfunction and a source of ongoing antigen to drive the immune response. *3* Since it has been proposed that antigen (e.g., topoisomerase-1) can preferentially bind to fibroblasts, anti-topoisomerase-1 antibodies might recruit immune effector cells (such as monocytes and NK cells) to sites of tissue damage and amplify the destruction (*3a*). Additionally, immune complexes containing anti-topoisomerase-1 antibodies may contribute to pathogenesis via their ability to stimulate IFN production from pDCs (*3b*). *4* Activation and stimulation of the adaptive immune response perpetuates these cycles through further augmenting antibody, T cell, cytokine, and tissue damage pathways

Loeys and colleagues recently provided important evidence suggesting that the fibrosis in SSS and SSc may share similar mechanisms. Mutations in fibrillin decreased binding to integrins, caused aberrant ECM accumulation and TGFβ signaling, and increased numbers of cells expressing α-smooth muscle cell actin, indicative of cells recruited to assist in tissue remodeling. Whether autoimmunity to matrix components can have similar consequences to those observed in SSS skin is of significant interest.

Autoantibodies against matrix metalloproteinase-1 (MMP-1), an enzyme that degrades collagen types I and III, have been found in sera of up to 75 % of patients with diffuse SSc [37]. Anti-MMP-1 IgG titers were higher in patients with diffuse disease than in those with limited disease ($P<0.001$) and correlated with the extent of fibrosis in the lung (vital capacity, $r=0.36$, $P<0.01$ and diffusion capacity for carbon monoxide, $r=0.43$, $P<0.005$), skin (total skin score, $r=0.06$, $P<0.002$), and renal blood vessels (pulsatility index, $r=0.52$, $P<0.001$). Serum IgG fractions were also able to inhibit MMP-1 collagenase activity by 77 % as compared to normal control IgG ($P<0.001$). Similar findings have been presented for autoantibodies targeting MMP-3 [26]. The authors speculate that anti-MMP antibodies might disrupt the balance between collagen synthesis and degradation, ultimately promoting excessive extracellular matrix deposition and fibrosis in SSc.

Autoantibodies Stimulating Receptor Signaling

The recent identification of platelet-derived growth factor receptor (PDGFR) as a target of the autoimmune response in scleroderma patients has also generated significant interest and discussion. The investigators found anti-PDGFR antibodies capable of stimulating cells specifically through ligation of this receptor and initiating a series of downstream effects including increased reactive oxygen species (ROS) generation, Ras activation, collagen production, and myofibroblast conversion [3]. The presence of autoantibodies appeared to be a very frequent finding in scleroderma patients and did not associate with the disease phenotype. An attractive aspect of the model presented was that such antibodies could participate directly in generating cellular smooth muscle and fibroblast lesions. PDGFR autoantibodies have not been found in other studies, using different techniques for identification and functional activity [8, 24]. Additional studies to resolve these different findings and define whether scleroderma autoantibodies have the capacity to bind extracellular antigens and affect the function of cells relevant to connective tissue structure and function are critical.

Another study [11] showed that the immunoglobulin fractions from sera of SSc and Sjögren's syndrome patients (but not healthy controls) could inhibit M3-muscarinic receptor (M3R)-mediated contractions in mouse colon longitudinal muscle. This result is of interest because a significant number of SSc patients have gastrointestinal dysmotility, and some SSc patients experience prominent sicca symptoms. Although no direct binding of antibodies to M3R was demonstrated, autoantibody binding to membrane receptors is frequently difficult to demonstrate by standard assays. Further work to define the prevalence, phenotypic associations, and functional consequences of such antibodies is a priority, both in terms of identifying novel pathogenic mechanisms and potentially therapeutically amenable pathways.

Conclusions

Autoimmunity in scleroderma may play important pathogenic roles in the disease. The striking specificity of this immune response and association with distinct clinical phenotypes has provided important diagnostic and predictive markers in this disease. The value of these specific immune responses as markers (and potentially mediators) of disease initiation and propagation in SSc cannot be overstated. With time, such immune responses may well become useful for monitoring and eventually for specific therapies.

References

1. Andrade F, Roy S, Nicholson D, Thornberry N, Rosen A, Casciola-Rosen L. Granzyme B directly and efficiently cleaves several downstream caspase substrates: implications for CTL-induced apoptosis. Immunity. 1998;8(4):451–60.
2. Anthony RM, Ravetch JV. A novel role for the IgG fc glycan: the anti-inflammatory activity of sialylated IgG fcs. J Clin Immunol. 2010;30 Suppl 1:S9–14.
3. Baroni SS, Santillo M, Bevilacqua F, Luchetti M, Spadoni T, Mancini M, et al. Stimulatory autoantibodies to the PDGF receptor in systemic sclerosis. N Engl J Med. 2006;354(25):2667–76.
4. Brinckmann J, Hunzelmann N, El-Hallous E, Krieg T, Sakai LY, Krengel S, et al. Absence of autoantibodies against correctly folded recombinant fibrillin-1 protein in systemic sclerosis patients. Arthritis Res Ther. 2005;7(6):R1221–6.
5. Casciola-Rosen L, Andrade F, Ulanet D, Wong WB, Rosen A. Cleavage by granzyme B is strongly predictive of autoantigen status: implications for initiation of autoimmunity. J Exp Med. 1999;190(6):815–26.
6. Casciola-Rosen L, Nagaraju K, Plotz P, Wang K, Levine S, Gabrielson E, et al. Enhanced autoantigen expression in regenerating muscle cells in idiopathic inflammatory myopathy. J Exp Med. 2005;201(4):591–601.
7. Chizzolini C, Raschi E, Rezzonico R, Testoni C, Mallone R, Gabrielli A, et al. Autoantibodies to fibroblasts induce a proadhesive and proinflammatory fibroblast phenotype in patients with systemic sclerosis. Arthritis Rheum. 2002;46(6):1602–13.
8. Classen JF, Henrohn D, Rorsman F, Lennartsson J, Lauwerys BR, Wikstrom G, et al. Lack of evidence of stimulatory autoantibodies to platelet-derived growth factor receptor in patients with systemic sclerosis. Arthritis Rheum. 2009;60(4):1137–44.
9. Dick T, Mierau R, Bartz-Bazzanella P, Alavi M, Stoyanova-Scholz M, Kindler J, et al. Coexistence of antitopoisomerase I and anticentromere antibodies in patients with systemic sclerosis. Ann Rheum Dis. 2002;61(2):121–7.
10. Fineschi S, Goffin L, Rezzonico R, Cozzi F, Dayer JM, Meroni PL, et al. Antifibroblast antibodies in systemic sclerosis induce fibroblasts to produce profibrotic chemokines, with partial exploitation of toll-like receptor 4. Arthritis Rheum. 2008;58(12):3913–23.
11. Goldblatt F, Gordon TP, Waterman SA. Antibody-mediated gastrointestinal dysmotility in scleroderma. Gastroenterology. 2002;123(4):1144–50.
12. Harvey GR, McHugh NJ. Serologic abnormalities in systemic sclerosis. Curr Opin Rheumatol. 1999;11(6):495–502.
13. Henault J, Robitaille G, Senecal JL, Raymond Y. DNA topoisomerase I binding to fibroblasts induces monocyte adhesion and activation in the presence of anti-topoisomerase I autoantibodies from systemic sclerosis patients. Arthritis Rheum. 2006;54(3):963–73.
14. Henault J, Tremblay M, Clement I, Raymond Y, Senecal JL. Direct binding of anti-DNA topoisomerase I autoantibodies to the cell surface of fibroblasts in patients with systemic sclerosis. Arthritis Rheum. 2004;50(10):3265–74.
15. Henry PA, Atamas SP, Yurovsky VV, Luzina I, Wigley FM, White B. Diversity and plasticity of the anti-DNA topoisomerase I autoantibody response in scleroderma. Arthritis Rheum. 2000;43(12):2733–42.
16. Howard OM, Dong HF, Yang D, Raben N, Nagaraju K, Rosen A, et al. Histidyl-tRNA synthetase and asparaginyl-tRNA synthetase, autoantigens in myositis, activate chemokine receptors on T lymphocytes and immature dendritic cells. J Exp Med. 2002;196(6):781–91.
17. Hu PQ, Fertig N, Medsger Jr TA, Wright TM. Correlation of serum anti-DNA topoisomerase I antibody levels with disease severity and activity in systemic sclerosis. Arthritis Rheum. 2003;| 48(5):1363–73.
18. Jimenez SA, Christner PJ. Murine animal models of systemic sclerosis. Curr Opin Rheumatol. 2002;14(6):671–80.
19. Joseph CG, Darrah E, Shah AA, Skora AD, Casciola-Rosen LA, Wigley FM, Boin F, Fava A, Thoburn C, Kindle I, Jiao Y, Papadopoulos N, Kinzler KW, Vogelstein B, Rosen A. Association of the autoimmune disease scleroderma with an immunological response to cancer. Science. 2014;343:152–7.
20. Kim D, Peck A, Santer D, Patole P, Schwartz SM, Molitor JA, et al. Induction of interferon-alpha by scleroderma sera containing auto-

antibodies to topoisomerase I: association of higher interferon-alpha activity with lung fibrosis. Arthritis Rheum. 2008; 58(7):2163–73.

21. Kodera T, Tan FK, Sasaki T, Arnett FC, Bona CA. Association of 5′-untranslated region of the fibrillin-1 gene with Japanese scleroderma. Gene. 2002;297(1–2):61–7.
22. Kuwana M, Kaburaki J, Mimori T, Kawakami Y, Tojo T. Longitudinal analysis of autoantibody response to topoisomerase I in systemic sclerosis. Arthritis Rheum. 2000;43(5):1074–84.
23. Loeys BL, Gerber EE, Riegert-Johnson D, Iqbal S, Whiteman P, McConnell V, et al. Mutations in fibrillin-1 cause congenital scleroderma: stiff skin syndrome. Sci Transl Med. 2010;2(23):23ra20.
24. Loizos N, Lariccia L, Weiner J, Griffith H, Boin F, Hummers L, et al. Lack of detection of agonist activity by antibodies to platelet-derived growth factor receptor alpha in a subset of normal and systemic sclerosis patient sera. Arthritis Rheum. 2009;60(4):1145–51.
25. Maes L, Blockmans D, Verschueren P, Westhovens R, De Beeck KO, Vermeersch P, et al. Anti-PM/Scl-100 and anti-RNA-polymerase III antibodies in scleroderma. Clin Chim Acta; Int J Clin Chem. 2010;411(13–14):965–71.
26. Nishijima C, Hayakawa I, Matsushita T, Komura K, Hasegawa M, Takehara K, et al. Autoantibody against matrix metalloproteinase-3 in patients with systemic sclerosis. Clin Exp Immunol. 2004;138(2):357–63.
27. Reimer G, Steen VD, Penning CA, Medsger Jr TA, Tan EM. Correlates between autoantibodies to nucleolar antigens and clinical features in patients with systemic sclerosis (scleroderma). Arthritis Rheum. 1988;31(4):525–32.
28. Renaudineau Y, Revelen R, Levy Y, Salojin K, Gilburg B, Shoenfeld Y, et al. Anti-endothelial cell antibodies in systemic sclerosis. Clin Diagn Lab Immunol. 1999;6(2):156–60.
29. Robitaille G, Christin MS, Clement I, Senecal JL, Raymond Y. Nuclear autoantigen CENP-B transactivation of the epidermal growth factor receptor via chemokine receptor 3 in vascular smooth muscle cells. Arthritis Rheum. 2009;60(9):2805–16.
30. Ronda N, Raschi E, Testoni C, Borghi MO, Gatti R, Dayer JM, et al. Anti-fibroblast antibodies in systemic sclerosis. Israel Med Assoc J: IMAJ. 2002;4(11 Suppl):858–64.
31. Rosenthal AK, McLaughlin JK, Gridley G, Nyren O. Incidence of cancer among patients with systemic sclerosis. Cancer. 1995;76(5):910–4.
32. Rosenthal AK, McLaughlin JK, Linet MS, Persson I. Scleroderma and malignancy: an epidemiological study. Ann Rheum Dis. 1993;52(7):531–3.
33. Rothfield NF. Autoantibodies in scleroderma. Rheum Dis Clin North Am. 1992;18(2):483–98.
34. Saito E, Fujimoto M, Hasegawa M, Komura K, Hamaguchi Y, Kaburagi Y, et al. CD19-dependent B lymphocyte signaling thresholds influence skin fibrosis and autoimmunity in the tight-skin mouse. J Clin Invest. 2002;109(11):1453–62.
35. Sato S, Hamaguchi Y, Hasegawa M, Takehara K. Clinical significance of anti-topoisomerase I antibody levels determined by ELISA in systemic sclerosis. Rheumatology (Oxford, England). 2001; 40(10):1135–40.
36. Sato S, Hasegawa M, Fujimoto M, Tedder TF, Takehara K. Quantitative genetic variation in CD19 expression correlates with autoimmunity. J Immunol (Baltimore, Md: 1950). 2000;165(11):6635–43.
37. Sato S, Hayakawa I, Hasegawa M, Fujimoto M, Takehara K. Function blocking autoantibodies against matrix metalloproteinase-1 in patients with systemic sclerosis. J Invest Dermatol. 2003;120(4):542–7.
38. Schachna L, Wigley FM, Morris S, Gelber AC, Rosen A, Casciola-Rosen L. Recognition of granzyme B-generated autoantigen fragments in scleroderma patients with ischemic digital loss. Arthritis Rheum. 2002;46(7):1873–84.
39. Sgonc R. The vascular perspective of systemic sclerosis: of chickens, mice and men. Int Arch Allergy Immunol. 1999;120(3):169–76.
40. Sgonc R, Gruschwitz MS, Dietrich H, Recheis H, Gershwin ME, Wick G. Endothelial cell apoptosis is a primary pathogenetic event underlying skin lesions in avian and human scleroderma. J Clin Invest. 1996;98(3):785–92.
41. Shah AA, Rosen A, Hummers L, Wigley F, Casciola-Rosen L. Close temporal relationship between onset of cancer and scleroderma in patients with RNA polymerase I/III antibodies. Arthritis Rheum. 2010;62(9):2787–95.
42. Shlomchik MJ, Craft JE, Mamula MJ. From T to B and back again: positive feedback in systemic autoimmune disease. Nat Rev Immunology. 2001;1(2):147–53.
43. Steen VD, Powell DL, Medsger Jr TA. Clinical correlations and prognosis based on serum autoantibodies in patients with systemic sclerosis. Arthritis Rheum. 1988;31(2):196–203.
44. Tamby MC, Humbert M, Guilpain P, Servettaz A, Dupin N, Christner JJ, et al. Antibodies to fibroblasts in idiopathic and scleroderma-associated pulmonary hypertension. Eur Respir J: Off J Eur Soc Clin Respir Physiol. 2006;28(4):799–807.
45. Tan FK, Arnett FC, Antohi S, Saito S, Mirarchi A, Spiera H, et al. Autoantibodies to the extracellular matrix microfibrillar protein, fibrillin-1, in patients with scleroderma and other connective tissue diseases. J Immunol (Baltimore, Md: 1950). 1999;163(2):1066–72.
46. Tan FK, Arnett FC, Reveille JD, Ahn C, Antohi S, Sasaki T, et al. Autoantibodies to fibrillin 1 in systemic sclerosis: ethnic differences in antigen recognition and lack of correlation with specific clinical features or HLA alleles. Arthritis Rheum. 2000;43(11): 2464–71.
47. Tan FK, Wang N, Kuwana M, Chakraborty R, Bona CA, Milewicz DM, et al. Association of fibrillin 1 single-nucleotide polymorphism haplotypes with systemic sclerosis in choctaw and japanese populations. Arthritis Rheum. 2001;44(4):893–901.
48. Terrier B, Tamby MC, Camoin L, Guilpain P, Broussard C, Bussone G, et al. Identification of target antigens of antifibroblast antibodies in pulmonary arterial hypertension. Am J Respir Crit Care Med. 2008;177(10):1128–34.
49. Ulanet DB, Flavahan NA, Casciola-Rosen L, Rosen A. Selective cleavage of nucleolar autoantigen B23 by granzyme B in differentiated vascular smooth muscle cells: insights into the association of specific autoantibodies with distinct disease phenotypes. Arthritis Rheum. 2004;50(1):233–41.
50. Ulanet DB, Torbenson M, Dang CV, Casciola-Rosen L, Rosen A. Unique conformation of cancer autoantigen B23 in hepatoma: a mechanism for specificity in the autoimmune response. Proc Natl Acad Sci U S A. 2003;100(21):12361–6.
51. Wallis DD, Tan FK, Kielty CM, Kimball MD, Arnett FC, Milewicz DM. Abnormalities in fibrillin 1-containing microfibrils in dermal fibroblast cultures from patients with systemic sclerosis (scleroderma). Arthritis Rheum. 2001;44(8):1855–64.
52. Weiner ES, Earnshaw WC, Senecal JL, Bordwell B, Johnson P, Rothfield NF. Clinical associations of anticentromere antibodies and antibodies to topoisomerase I. A study of 355 patients. Arthritis Rheum. 1988;31(3):378–85.
53. Worda M, Sgonc R, Dietrich H, Niederegger H, Sundick RS, Gershwin ME, et al. In vivo analysis of the apoptosis-inducing effect of anti-endothelial cell antibodies in systemic sclerosis by the chorio-allantoic membrane assay. Arthritis Rheum. 2003;48(9):2605–14.
54. Yuan X, Downing AK, Knott V, Handford PA. Solution structure of the transforming growth factor beta-binding protein-like module, a domain associated with matrix fibrils. EMBO J. 1997; 16(22):6659–66.
55. Zhou X, Tan FK, Xiong M, Milewicz DM, Feghali CA, Fritzler MJ, et al. Systemic sclerosis (scleroderma): specific autoantigen genes are selectively overexpressed in scleroderma fibroblasts. J Immunol (Baltimore, Md: 1950). 2001;167(12):7126–33.

15 The Clinical Aspects of Autoantibodies

Masataka Kuwana and Thomas A. Medsger Jr.

Introduction

Since clinical presentation in patients with systemic sclerosis (SSc) is highly heterogeneous, disease subgrouping and prediction of future organ involvement and prognosis are extremely important in the clinical setting. Another distinctive feature of SSc is the presence of circulating autoantibodies reactive with various cellular components. Autoimmune targets include a variety of nuclear antigens that are present in cells with nuclei. In this case, they are termed antinuclear antibodies (ANAs). It has been shown that distinct ANA specificities are detected in SSc patients and are associated with unique disease manifestations. Therefore, SSc-related ANAs are attractive biomarkers in routine rheumatology practice, owing to their high specificity, mutual exclusivity, persistence for the duration of illness, and, most importantly, strong associations with characteristic constellations of clinical features [1–3]. In addition, a new group of autoantibodies reactive with functional proteins, such as cell surface receptors and extracellular matrix (ECM) proteins, have been identified in SSc patients. They seem to directly activate pathways that may contribute to the pathophysiology of SSc. This chapter covers the spectrum of autoantibody specificities reported in SSc patients, their detection methods, and their clinical utility.

SSc-Related ANAs

ANAs detected by the indirect immunofluorescence (IIF) technique are a hallmark of SSc and are found in >95 % of the patients. The majority of nuclear autoantigens specifically recognized by SSc sera have been already identified. As of this writing, ten ANA specificities associated with SSc have been reported and well characterized, and >80 % of SSc patients have one of these SSc-related ANAs. Two classic autoantibodies discovered in the late 1970s are anti-Scl-70 or anti-topoisomerase I (topo I) antibody and anti-centromere antibody (ACA). Another group of antibodies, including anti-U1 ribonucleoprotein (RNP), anti-Ku, and anti-PM-Scl antibodies, were first identified using the double immunodiffusion (DID) technique. The remaining ANA specificities were discovered using immunoprecipitation (IP). SSc-related ANAs target various nuclear components involved in essential cellular processes, such as cell division and transcription (Table 15.1). These autoantibodies are rarely seen in patients with other connective tissue diseases without SSc features and thus are important diagnostic markers. In addition, detection of SSc-related ANAs is clinically useful in classifying SSc patients into subtypes that are almost exclusively associated with characteristic clinical phenotypes (Table 15.2). SSc-related ANAs are usually present at the onset of SSc symptoms and do not switch from one antibody to another during the course of the disease. These autoantibodies typically remain detectable throughout the course of the disease, regardless of whether patients receive treatment or not. Patients rarely have two or more SSc-related ANAs together, indicating mutual exclusiveness.

ACA

Moroi and colleagues were the first investigators to describe the presence of ACA originally associated with the CREST (calcinosis, Raynaud's phenomenon, esophageal dysmotility, sclerodactyly, and telangiectasia) variant of SSc [4]. ACA is directed against centromere proteins, CENP-A, CENP-B, and CENP-C. The frequency of ACA in SSc patients has been reported to be 20–30 % in many ethnic groups. ACA produces discrete speckled staining on

M. Kuwana, MD, PhD (✉)
Department of Allergy and Rheumatology, Nippon Medical School Graduate School of Medicine, Tokyo, Japan
e-mail: kuwanam@nms.ac.jp

T.A. Medsger Jr., MD
Division of Rheumatology, Department of Medicine, University of Pittsburgh, Pittsburgh, PA, USA

J. Varga et al. (eds.), *Scleroderma*, DOI 10.1007/978-3-319-31407-5_15

Table 15.1 Structure and function of molecules targeted by SSc-related ANAs

ANA specificity	Structure	Cellular localization	Main cellular function
Anticentromere (ACA)	CENP-A, CENP-B, and CENP-C	Chromatin	Separation of chromosome
Anti-topo I (Scl-70)	DNA topoisomerase I	Chromatin	Relaxation of supercoiled DNA
Anti-RNAP III	Multi-subunit components of RNA polymerase III, including RPC155	Nucleoplasm	Transcription of small nuclear RNAs
Anti-U3 RNP	U3 RNA and related components including fibrillarin	Nucleoli	Processing of pre-ribosomal RNAs
Anti-Th/To	RNase P/RNase MRP	Nucleoli	Processing of transfer RNAs and other small RNAs
Anti-U11/U12 RNP	U11/U12 RNA and related components	Nucleoplasm	Regulation of mRNA splicing
Anti-PM-Scl	Exosome complex containing PM-Scl-100 and PM-Scl-75	Nucleoli	Processing and degradation of RNAs
Anti-Ku	Ku80 and Ku70	Nucleoplasm	DNA repair
Anti-RuvBL1/2	Double hexamer consisting RuvBL1 and RuvBL2	Nucleoplasm	DNA repair and chromatin remodeling
Anti-U1 RNP	U1 RNA and related components including 70 K, A, and C proteins	Nucleoplasm	mRNA splicing

Table 15.2 Methods for detection and clinical associations with SSc-related ANAs

ANA specificity	Staining pattern on IF (ANA test)	Assay for detection	Disease subset	Clinical phenotype
Anticentromere (ACA)	Discrete speckled	IIF, EIA	lcSSc	PAH; severe peripheral vascular disease
Anti-topo I	Speckled (with or without nucleolar)	EIA, DID, IP	dcSSc	ILD; severe peripheral vascular disease
Anti-RNA polymerase III	Speckled (with or without nucleolar)	EIA, IP	dcSSc	Rapid progression of skin thickening; SRC; malignancy
Anti-U3 RNP/fibrillarin	Nucleolar	IP	dcSSc/lcSSc	ILD, PAH, SRC, GI
Anti-Th/To	Nucleolar	IP	lcSSc	ILD, PAH
Anti-U11/U12 RNP	Speckled	IP	dcSSc/lcSSc	ILD
Anti-PM-Scl	Nucleolar	DID, IP	lcSSc (myositis overlap)	Myositis (DM rash)
Anti-Ku	Speckled	DID, IP	lcSSc (myositis overlap)	Myositis
Anti-RuvBL1/2	Speckled	IP	dcSSc (myositis overlap)	Myositis
Anti-U1 RNP	Speckled	EIA, DID, IP	lcSSc (“MCTD”)	Inflammatory arthritis, myositis, PAH

DID double immunodiffusion, *EIA* enzyme immunoassay, *IIF* indirect immunofluorescence, *IP* immunoprecipitation, *MCTD* mixed connective tissue disease, *PAH* pulmonary arterial hypertension, *ILD* interstitial lung disease, *SRC* scleroderma renal crisis, *GI* gastrointestinal tract involvement, *DM* dermatomyositis

IIF. The recognition of kinetochore proteins located at the centromeric regions of individual metaphase chromosomes is highly specific to ACA. However, IIF using chromosomal spreads as the substrate is necessary to confirm the presence of ACA, especially when other high-titer ANA specificities coexist. ACA is sometimes detected in patients with primary Sjögren’s syndrome or primary biliary cirrhosis as well as in individuals without an apparent connective tissue disease, who are almost always elderly [5]. The natural history of ACA-positive SSc patients includes long-standing Raynaud’s phenomenon followed by appearance of puffy fingers after a variable period of time (months to ten or more years). The presence of ACA in patients with Raynaud’s phenomenon and/or nailfold capillary abnormalities is predictive of future development of SSc [6]. Patients with ACA are often classified as having limited cutaneous SSc (lcSSc) [7, 8], a term which has now replaced CREST. Severe interstitial lung disease (ILD), cardiomyopathy, or scleroderma renal crisis (SRC) almost never occurs in ACA-positive patients, but 10–20% of them develop pulmonary arterial hypertension (PAH) later in the course of the disease.

Anti-topo I Antibody

The Scl-70 antigen was originally isolated from rat liver extracts as a basic nonhistone chromosome protein [9], which was later identified as an enzyme that catalyzes relaxation of supercoiled double-stranded DNA, termed topo I [10]. Anti-topo I antibody is detected in 20–30 % of SSc patients in many ethnic groups, but in Europe the proportion is higher (40–69 %). The coexistence of anti-topo I and other SSc-related ANAs including ACA is rare (~0.5 %). The majority of anti-topo I-positive patients have diffuse cutaneous SSc (dcSSc), but progression of skin thickening is slower than those with anti-RNA polymerase (RNAP) III antibody [11]. Anti-topo I antibody is associated with a high risk for severe ILD, cardiomyopathy, and peripheral vascular complications, such as digital ulcer (DU) and gangrene, particularly early in the disease course [7, 8]. This antibody is associated with myocardial involvement in patients with dcSSc and rapidly progressive skin thickening [12]. Anti-topo I antibody is considered to be a marker for poor prognosis, and patients with severe ILD die of this complication at an average of 10 years after onset of SSc.

Anti-RNAP III Antibody

SSc sera contain autoantibodies directed to the three forms of RNAPs [13]. Anti-RNAP antibodies detected in SSc patients fall into four groups: those reactive with RNAP I, II, and III; those with RNAP I and III; those with RNAP III alone; and those with RNAP II alone [14]. Since antibodies to RNAP II alone are often found in association with anti-topo I antibody in SSc patients and are also detected in patients without SSc [15], they are not considered the primary antibody subset. Instead, antibodies reactive with RNAP III, which are recognized commonly by the remaining three specificities, are most often regarded as the SSc-related ANA. Sera positive for anti-RNAP III antibody produce a speckled staining pattern on IIF but also produce nucleolar staining if anti-RNAP I antibody coexists. Anti-RNAP III is mutually exclusive to anti-topo I and ACA and highly specific to SSc. The frequency of anti-RNAP III antibody in SSc patients varies among ethnic groups. There is a higher frequency in North American Caucasian and UK patients (20–25 %) in comparison with French or Japanese patients (5 %) [16, 17]. Nearly all patients with this antibody have dcSSc with rapidly progressive skin thickening. Patients with anti-RNAP III antibody have the highest risk for developing SRC, but they seldom develop severe ILD [13, 18]. In many patients, skin thickening regresses over time even without treatment. In recent cohorts, survival in patients with anti-RNAP III is better than those with anti-topo I, since SRC is more easily treated with angiotensin-converting enzyme inhibitors than ILD [19]. Several reports indicate that patients with anti-RNAP III antibody have better long-term survival rates compared with those with ACA or anti-Th/To antibody. Recently, it has been reported that there is an association with cancer among SSc patients with anti-RNAP III in close temporal relationship to onset of SSc, which suggests that SSc is a paraneoplastic phenomenon in this subset [20, 21].

Anti-U3 RNP Antibody

Anti-U3 RNP antibody reacts with 34-kD fibrillarin complexed with U3 RNA [22]. This antibody produces bright nucleolar staining on IIF. Anti-U3 RNP antibody is found in 4–10 % of patients with SSc and is most frequent in African-Americans [23]. Two-thirds of the patients have dcSSc. A noninflammatory skeletal myopathy is a distinctive feature. Severe internal organ involvement, including ILD, PAH, cardiomyopathy, SRC, and small bowel involvement with pseudo-obstruction and malabsorption, is common. Prognosis in this subset is comparable to that in patients with anti-topo I antibody. An unusual combination of SRC followed later by PAH is occasionally found in patients with dcSSc and anti-U3 RNP antibody [24].

Anti-Th/To Antibody

Anti-Th/To autoantibodies are directed against subunits of mitochondrial RNA processing and ribonuclease P RNP complexes [25]. Anti-Th/To antibody occurs in patients with lcSSc, although its frequency overall in SSc patients is only 2–5 %. Like ACA-positive patients, anti-Th/To-positive patients are predominantly Caucasians, but tend to have a shorter duration of Raynaud's phenomenon before onset of other symptoms such as puffy fingers. DU and digital gangrene are infrequent, but patients with anti-Th/To antibody can have significant ILD or PAH, the latter often independent of ILD, which often occurs early in the disease course [26]. This increased frequency and severity of pulmonary complications result in a decreased survival compared with lcSSc patients without this antibody.

Anti-U11/U12 RNP Antibody

Anti-U11/U12 RNP antibody is a rare antibody specificity found in 1–3 % of patients with SSc [27]. This antibody produces speckled nuclear staining on IIF and sometimes is associated with low-titer anti-U1 RNP antibodies. Patients with this antibody are classified as having either dcSSc or lcSSc. A characteristic feature of patients with anti-U11/U12 RNP antibody is a high frequency of ILD (~80 %), which is often severe and rapidly progressive, and associated with a 2.25-fold greater risk of death in comparison with anti-U11/U12 RNP-negative patients with ILD.

Anti-PM-Scl Antibody

The PM-Scl complex is composed of several subunits, of which the 100-kD and 75-kD proteins are the main autoantigenic determinants. Anti-PM-Scl antibody produces a homogenous nucleolar pattern and is rarely found in non-Caucasian patients [28]. Anti-PM-Scl-positive patients often present with the subacute myositis but also have typical Raynaud's phenomenon and scleroderma skin changes, usually lcSSc [29, 30]. They are most frequently diagnosed as having SSc-polymyositis (PM) overlap, but a significant proportion of the patients have rashes consistent with dermatomyositis (DM). This antibody is found in more than 25 % of SSc patients with myositis overlap, but in only 2 % of SSc patients overall. Serious internal organ involvement is rare, leading to a favorable prognosis. Myositis is usually mild and shows a good response to moderate-dose corticosteroids. In a recent large cross-sectional study of patients with idiopathic inflammatory myopathies, 9 % had anti-PM-Scl antibody in the absence of any skin changes [31].

Anti-Ku Antibody

The Ku autoantigen is a heterodimer of 70-kD and 80-kD subunits that is recognized by autoantibodies in a small percentage of sera from SSc patients (~2 %) [32]. Anti-Ku antibody is primarily detected in patients with SSc in overlap. The majority of patients have typical Raynaud's phenomenon and scleroderma skin changes, usually lcSSc. Concomitant myositis is common, but some have additional features of lupus. Anti-Ku antibody is rarely detected in patients with systemic lupus erythematosus (SLE) or PM/DM without SSc features, but additional lupus-associated autoantibodies such as anti-DNA are always positive in the patients with SLE alone [33]. Disease onset in these patients is usually younger than age 50. Internal organ involvement is infrequent and usually mild if present, but arthritis is common. Anti-Ku antibody is associated with fewer vascular manifestations such as DU or telangiectasia [34]. Myositis is usually mild and shows a good response to moderate-dose corticosteroids, leading to favorable prognosis.

Anti-RuvBL1/2 Antibody

This newly identified antibody recognizes a double hexamer consisting of RuvBL1 and RuvBL2, which is located in the nucleoplasm [35]. Anti-RuvBL1/2 antibody is a rare antibody specificity detected in 1–2 % of patients with SSc. This antibody produces speckled nuclear staining with a high antibody titer on IIF. Patients with this antibody are mostly males and have a unique combination of clinical features, including diffuse cutaneous involvement and myositis overlap. Internal organ involvement is mild in general, but some develop significant myocardial dysfunction.

Anti-U1 RNP Antibody

Anti-U1 RNP antibodies are directed against the 70 K, A, and C proteins associated with U1 RNA, while anti-Sm antibodies are directed against the B/B′ and D proteins that are core components of the U series small nuclear RNAs involved in pre-messenger RNA splicing [36]. Anti-U1 RNP antibody, which produces a pure speckled pattern with a high antibody titer, is primarily detected in patients with SSc in overlap. This antibody is preferentially found in African-Americans and Orientals. Anti-U1 RNP antibody was first described as a serological marker for mixed connective tissue disease (MCTD) [37] but is also found in sera from patients with SSc, SLE, PM/DM, or Sjögren's syndrome alone. Disease onset is at a relatively young age in these patients. SSc patients with this antibody usually present with inflammatory symptoms, such as myositis and arthritis. Raynaud's phenomenon and puffy fingers occur early in the disease, but later these patients develop typical manifestations of SSc. Most of them have lcSSc, although approximately 20 % develop dcSSc. Serious complications are relatively uncommon, but pulmonary complications, including PAH and ILD, are sometimes life-threatening [38]. Prognosis is favorable, but PAH is the most common cause of death.

Other ANAs Related to SSc

Other anti-nucleolar antibodies reported in SSc patients include anti-nucleolar organizing region 90 (NOR-90) and anti-B23 antibodies. NOR-90, also termed the human upstream binding factor (hUBF) of RNAP I, is composed of two isoforms, which are derived from the same gene by alternative splicing. Anti-NOR-90 antibody was first reported in patients with malignancy, but later in individuals with connective tissue diseases, including SSc, Sjögren's syndrome, and rheumatoid arthritis [39]. Nearly all SSc patients with this antibody have lcSSc, but detailed clinical characteristics have not been assessed [40]. B23 is a nucleolar phosphoprotein which is overexpressed in many cancer cells. In contrast to the well-characterized targeting of B23 as an autoantigen in some patients with malignancy, anti-B23 antibody also occurs in ~11 % of sera from SSc patients [41]. Anti-B23 reactivity is associated with PAH and often coexists with anti-U3 RNP or anti-U1 RNP antibodies. Other autoantibodies, such as anti-SSA/Ro and anti-SSB/La, can occur in SSc patients, but are usually associated with concomitant Sjögren's syndrome. The SSA/Ro autoantigen has two isoforms, Ro60 and Ro52. The latter has recently been termed the tripartite motif-containing protein 21 (TRIM21), which may be targeted separately by sera from patients with connective tissue diseases. A recent multicenter cohort study from the Canadian Scleroderma Research Group (CSRG) involving 963 patients with SSc has found that anti-Ro52/TRIM21 antibodies are present in 20 % of SSc patients and coexist with other SSc-related ANAs, including ACA, anti-topo I, anti-RNAP III, and anti-PM-Scl antibodies [42]. Anti-Ro52/TRIM21 antibodies are strongly associated with ILD and overlap syndrome. Antibodies to interferon-inducible genes designated HIN-200, which encode evolutionarily related nuclear phosphoproteins (IFI16), are also detected in 30 % of SSc patients in conjunction with anti-topo I or ACA [43]. Autoantibodies to cytoplasmic mitochondrial proteins are found in patients with SSc and coexist with ACA and are associated with concomitant primary biliary cirrhosis [44].

ANA-Negative SSc

There is a small proportion of SSc patients who are negative for ANA by IIF. In a recent cohort study involving 3,249 patients with SSc from a multicenter registry in North America, 6.4 % were negative for ANA [45]. ANA-negative SSc patients constitute a distinct subset with a greater proportion of males, less vasculopathy (PAH, DU, and telangiectasia), and more frequent lower GI involvement.

Screening of SSc-Related ANAs

A conventional method for ANA detection is IIF on cultured HEp-2 cell slides. This technique is recommended as the first ANA screening test because it is highly sensitive and provides additional information on the antibody titer and staining pattern. Speckled staining is often detected in patients with dcSSc and suggests the presence of anti-topo I in case of a high ANA titer (≥1:320) or anti- RNAP III in case of a low ANA titer (<1:160). Anti-U1 RNP and anti-RuvBL1/2 antibodies, which are associated with SSc in overlap, also produce a high-titer speckled pattern, while titers of anti-U11/U12 RNP antibody vary among the positive sera. A nucleolar pattern is fairly specific to SSc, and the three major SSc-related anti-nucleolar antibodies are anti-U3 RNP, anti-Th/To, and anti-PM-Scl antibodies. Anti-RNAP III antibody also produces a nucleolar pattern when anti-RNAP I antibody coexists, but a concomitant speckled pattern is always present. A discrete speckled pattern is often detected in patients with lcSSc and suggests the presence of ACA, which recognizes a pair of dots located at the centromeric lesion of individual metaphase chromosomes.

Solid-phase ANA assays have been commercially available since the early 1990s and might be viable alternatives to ANA detection on HEp-2 cells. This method has considerable potential, but it is of note that many SSc-related ANAs, including anti-RNAP III antibody and anti-nucleolar antibodies, are not identified by these assays and thus are reported as "a negative ANA." This is because the sensitivity ultimately depends on the choice of autoantigens used. In fact, one retrospective study of 238 SSc patients which compared ANA by IIF with multiplex bead assay from two commercial laboratories concluded that the bead testing failed to identify 50 % of the SSc patients, particularly those with anti-RNAP III or anti-nucleolar staining on IIF [46]. Therefore, it is our strong recommendation to use the conventional IIF for screening SSc-related ANAs.

Methods for Detection of Individual SSc-Related ANAs

Identification of individual SSc-related ANAs requires additional techniques, such as DID, IP assay, and specific immunoassays including enzyme immunoassay (EIA) (Table 15.2). DID technique (Ouchterlony or counter-immune electrophoresis) has been used for more than 50 years and is still used in clinical laboratories because it is inexpensive and specific. Immunoblots either in-house or commercially available may provide advantages in determining detailed specificity of autoantigen recognition, e.g., the antigen recognition profile within a complex autoantigen. Multianalyte line-blot assay is commercially available for simultaneous detection of a series of SSc-related ANAs [47]. IP assay of either protein or RNA components is a valuable detection method that is able to detect all SSc-related ANAs except ACA. However, these conventional techniques are of limited use in routine clinical practice because they are labor-intensive, time-consuming, and limited in throughput.

The solid-phase immunoassays have several advantages over other traditional techniques in terms of simplicity, reproducibility, speed, and ability to handle many samples at the same time. In addition they provide semiquantitative results, and thus, there is the potential for more close investigation of how autoantibody levels relate to disease activity and severity. The majority of commercially available immunoassays utilize recombinant autoantigens, which are expressed in the bacterial or eukaryotic system, while some assays still use native proteins purified from cellular extracts. However, solid-phase assay requires the availability of highly purified autoantigens that contain the major epitopes recognized by virtually all sera positive for given SSc-related ANAs. This is a critical limitation for developing immunoassays. For example, it is easy to prepare topo I as an antigenic source for immunoassays because the autoimmune

Table 15.3 Putative pathogenetic molecules targeted by autoantibodies in SSc patients

Autoantibody targets	Frequency in SSc patients, n/n (%)	Clinical correlations	References
Platelet-derived growth factor receptor	46/46 (100 %)	ND	[50]
Muscarinic-3 receptor	7/7 (100 %)	ND	[51]
	11/76 (14 %)	Lower GI	[52]
Angiotensin II type 1 receptor	253/298 (85 %)	PAH, SRC, DU	[53]
Endothelin-1 type A receptor	249/198 (84 %)	PAH, SRC, DU	[53]
Fibrillin-1	107/225 (48 %)		[54]
Matrix metalloproteinase-1	28/57 (49 %)	dcSSc, ILD	[55]
Matrix metalloproteinase-3	30/58 (52 %)	dcSSc, ILD	[56]
Peroxiredoxin 1	23/70 (33 %)	ILD, cardiac	[57]
Methionine sulfoxide reductase A	23/69 (33 %)	ILD, cardiac	[58]
4-Sulfated N-acetyl-lactosamine	27/181 (15 %)	PAH	[59]
Estrogen receptor-α	30/71 (42 %)	EScSG activity index	[60]

ND not determined, *GI* gastrointestinal involvement, *PAH* pulmonary arterial hypertension, *SRC* scleroderma renal crisis, *DU* digital ulcer, *dcSSc* diffuse cutaneous systemic sclerosis, *ILD* interstitial lung disease, *EScSG* European Scleroderma Study Group

target is a single molecule. However, the majority of autoantigens recognized by SSc-related ANAs are multiprotein complexes consisting of many constituents and, in some cases, small RNAs. In this case, it is necessary to determine the antigenic subunit that is most commonly recognized by autoantibodies. For example, RNAP III exists as a multiprotein complex consisting of >12 subunits, requiring identification of the antigenic subunit recognized by all anti-RNAP III-positive sera. A series of experiments using individual subunits successfully identified the largest subunit (RPC155) as the antigenic subunit, facilitating development of a sensitive immunoassay [48]. Multiplex technologies, such as multibead arrays in combination with flow cytometry techniques, have been developed and used for detection of multiple SSc-related ANAs at the same time [49].

Autoantibodies to Functional Molecules

There has been considerable interest in autoantibodies directed to cell surface or ECM proteins in SSc patients (Table 15.3). However, reproducibility of the published data is poor, probably because of difficulty in reproducing antigenicity of the autoantigens with highly complicated conformation in the assays. This results in lack of reliable commercial assay kits for detection of these autoantibodies. Nevertheless, these autoantibodies are potentially relevant to the pathophysiology of SSc by modulating disease-related pathways, including those mediated by platelet-derived growth factor receptor [50], muscarinic-3 receptor [51, 52], angiotensin II type 1 receptor [53], and endothelin-1 type A receptor [53]. In addition, antibodies directed to fibrillin 1 may act to release active transforming growth factor (TGF)-β by blocking binding sites for the latent form [54], and antibodies to matrix metalloproteinases may dysregulate ECM turnover [55, 56]. Antibodies against enzymes of the oxidative stress cascade are also found in a subset of SSc patients [57, 58]. A recent study has identified autoantibodies to glycosylated structures expressed on endothelium and ECMs in SSc patients [59]. Serum autoantibodies against intracellular estrogen receptor-α were also reported in SSc patients with an increased proportion of activated regulatory T cells in the circulation [60]. Lack of commercially available kits that have been validated by multicenter studies results in difficulty in assessing clinical significance. Pathogenic potentials of these autoantibodies are discussed in detail in another chapter.

Utility in SSc Diagnosis

The majority of SSc-related ANAs are useful in support of the diagnosis of SSc because of their highly specific nature. In cohorts of patients with established SSc and those with other connective tissue diseases, the specificity of anti-topo I and anti-RNAP III antibodies for SSc is >95 %. ACA, anti-U3 RNP, anti-Th/To, and anti-U11/U12 RNP have specificity for SSc of approximately 90 %, but are sometimes found in patients with Raynaud's phenomenon alone, Sjögren's syndrome, or even in persons without apparent connective tissue disease. In contrast, anti-PM-Scl, anti-Ku, and anti-U1 RNP can be detected in patients with SLE or PM/DM without SSc features. No patient with anti-RuvBL1/2 antibody has been reported yet to have PM alone. In this regard, the presence of ACA, anti-topo I, or anti-RNAP III antibody is included in one of the criterion domains of a new set of classification criteria for SSc, which has been proposed by the American College of Rheumatology (ACR) and the

European League against Rheumatism (EULAR) [61]. Inclusion of these three antibodies was based on their high specificity for SSc and the availability of reliable assay kits worldwide.

In a prospective study involving a large cohort of patients who were referred for evaluation of Raynaud's phenomenon, nailfold capillary abnormalities, the presence of SSc-related ANAs, including ACA, anti- topo I, anti-RNAP III, and anti-Th/To, was found to be an independent predictor for developing SSc during long-term follow-up [62]. To promote early detection and diagnosis of SSc, the EULAR Scleroderma Trials and Research group (EUSTAR) has proposed the term very early diagnosis of SSc (VEDOSS) in patients with Raynaud's phenomenon who also have one of the following: a SSc-related ANA, nailfold capillary abnormality, or puffy fingers [63].

Epidemiological Characteristics

Age at Onset

The distribution of SSc-related ANAs varies according to age. In a series of 111 cases of childhood-onset SSc, there was a greater frequency of antibodies to anti-PM-Scl and anti-U1 RNP in comparison to adult-onset SSc [64, 65]. Accordingly, childhood SSc is associated with a much greater prevalence of myositis overlap. Anti-topo I antibody is commonly found in patients with childhood-onset and adult-onset SSc, but ACA and anti-RNAP III are almost lacking in childhood-onset SSc. Even in the adult SSc population, age at onset is older in patients with anti-RNAP III and anti-RuvBL1/2, while anti-Ku, resulting in abti-U3 RNP, anti-PM-Scl, anti-Ku, and anti-U1 RNP are more common in younger patients.

Gender

The majority of patients with SSc are female, and hence, all antibodies are found more commonly in females than males. There are, however, gender-related differences in SSc-related ANA specificities. ACA is particularly prominent in females (>95% of ACA-positive SSc patients are female). In contrast, proportion of males tends to be higher in SSc patients with anti-RNAP III, anti-U3RNP, or anti-RuvBL1/2 antibodies than in those without.

Ethnicity

There are significant differences in the distribution of SSc-related ANAs among ethnic groups (Table 15.4) [16, 17, 66–68]. Interestingly, even in the United States, differences are observed between cohorts from the University of Pittsburgh, University of Texas at Houston, and University of Florida, likely owing to ethnic diversity. In this regard, there are also major differences in the antibody profile among SSc patients in European countries when compared to UK, French, Italian, and Swedish cohorts. ACA is frequent in Caucasians, but are found far less frequently in African-American and Thai patients with SSc [69]. Anti-RNAP III is more common in North American Caucasians and UK cohort, compared with Japanese, French, and Italian cohorts [70], although anti-topo I is commonly detected in many ethnic groups. A notable exception is that >80% of Oklahoma Choctaw Native Americans (an inbred population) with SSc have anti-topo I antibody [71]. A greater frequency of anti-U3 RNP has been identified in African-Americans with SSc compared with Caucasian populations. Anti-PM-Scl antibody has never been reported in Japanese patients with SSc. Anti-U1RNP antibody is more prevalent in African-American and Japanese SSc patients compared with Caucasians.

Table 15.4 Frequencies (percent) of SSc-related ANAs in various ethnic groups

	North American Caucasian			Hispanic	North American-African			French	Italian	Japanese
ANA specificity	Pittsburgh (*n*=416)	Texas (*n*=191)	Florida (*n*=75)	Texas (*n*=77)	Pittsburgh (*n*=22)	Texas (*n*=77)	Florida (*n*=23)	Paris (*n*=127)	Brescia (*n*=216)	Tokyo (*n*=275)
References	[15]	[65]	[66]	[65]	[15]	[65]	[66]	[16]	[67]	[15]
ACA	19	32	17	18	8	4	0	18	31	15
Anti-topo I	21	13	15	19	13	16	35	35	38	26
Anti-RNAP III	23	ND	19	ND	13	ND	9	4	7	4
Anti-U3 RNP	4	4	3	7	42	17	30	2	0	3
Anti-Th/To	4	ND	9	ND	0	ND	4	1	4	3
Anti-PM-Scl	3	ND	6	ND	0	ND	0	6	ND	0
Anti-Ku	1	ND	ND	ND	8	ND	ND	2	ND	2
Anti-U1 RNP	8	5	13	11	33	29	30	9	ND	34

Some patients have more than one SSc-related ANA
ND not determined

Disease Subset Classification

Classification of patients into dcSSc and lcSSc subsets is useful in predicting future organ involvement and prognosis, and more precise subgrouping is possible by also considering SSc-related ANAs. The large-scale database of the German Network for Systemic Scleroderma has found that SSc in overlap is a separate SSc subset, distinct from lcSSc and dcSSc, due to a different progression of the disease, different proportional distribution of specific autoantibodies, and different organ involvement [72]. In addition, it is often difficult to classify patients into dcSSc or lcSSc early in the course of the disease when skin thickness is restricted to the distal portion of extremities. In this case, information on SSc-related ANAs is useful in predicting the future extent of skin involvement. Figure 15.1 illustrates distribution of SSc-related ANAs in association with disease classification.

lcSSc

ACA is the most common SSc-related ANA in patients with lcSSc (~50 %). Approximately 93 % of patients with ACA are classified as having lcSSc [73]. Anti-Th/To is another antibody associated with lcSSc. Compared with ACA-positive patients with lcSSc, anti-Th/To-positive patients have more subtle cutaneous, vascular, and gastrointestinal involvement, but more often have PAH and ILD [26, 68].

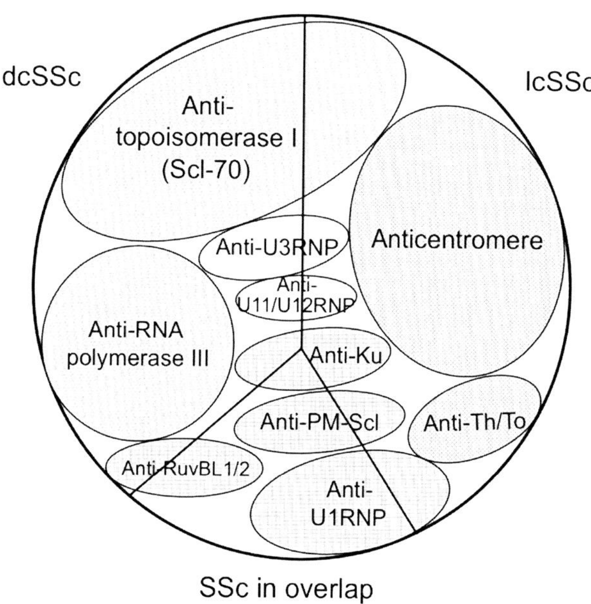

Fig. 15.1 Diagram showing SSc subsets stratified by SSc-related ANAs. Areas of individual circles represent approximate proportions in the entire SSc patients

Other antibodies typically found in patients with lcSSc include anti-U3 RNP, anti-PM-Scl, and anti-U1 RNP.

dcSSc

Almost two-thirds of patients with anti-topo I are classified as having dcSSc [74]. French patients with anti-topo I antibody, however, are less likely to have dcSSc when compared with their US counterparts (38 % versus 65 %) [17]. Likewise only 14 % of French Canadians with dcSSc carry anti-topo I [75]. Anti-RNAP III antibody is also associated with dcSSc; over 80 % of patients with this antibody have dcSSc [13, 18, 76]. Compared to patients with anti-topo I, those with anti-RNAP III have a significantly higher modified Rodnan total skin thickness score (MRSS) [18]. The rate of progression of skin involvement also differs dependent on antibody specificity [11]. In a recent series, all patients with anti-RNAP III had developed skin fibrosis within 6 months of the appearance of Raynaud's phenomenon in contrast to only 34 % of those with anti-topo I [77]. Anti-U3 RNP is typically associated with dcSSc, particularly in African-American patients. However, patients with dcSSc who carry anti-U3 RNP antibody have been found to have a lower MRSS when compared with patients with dcSSc and other SSc-related ANAs [23].

SSc in Overlap

Up to 20 % of SSc patients have overlapping features of other connective tissue diseases. The most common SSc in overlap is SSc-PM/DM, often termed sclerodermatomyositis. In this group, anti-PM-Scl, anti-Ku, anti-RuvBL1/2, or anti-U1 RNP antibodies cover >70 % of the patients. Of these, patients with anti-PM-Scl, anti-Ku, or anti-U1 RNP usually show limited cutaneous involvement, but those with anti-RuvBL1/2 frequently have diffuse cutaneous involvement [34]. Patients with anti-U1 RNP often have additional lupus features, consistent with MCTD.

SSc Sine Scleroderma

It has been shown that SSc sine scleroderma should not be considered clinically distinct from SSc because organ manifestations and natural history of disease are similar to those with lcSSc [78]. ACA was the most prevalent SSc-related ANA in patients with SSc sine scleroderma, although 44 % were positive for ANA but negative for known SSc-related ANAs [78]. In another series, anti-topo I was identified in 28 % of such cases [79]. Anti-Th/To has also been identified in patients with a diagnosis of idiopathic pulmonary fibrosis in the absence of any skin involvement [80, 81].

Prediction of Organ Manifestations

Clinical features in SSc patients are remarkably heterogeneous and grouping patients based on autoantibody profiles is a useful approach in the clinical setting. The main organ-specific manifestations associated with SSc-related ANAs are summarized in Table 15.2.

Peripheral Vascular Manifestations

Raynaud's phenomenon is seen in virtually all patients with SSc although the degree of peripheral vascular dysfunction varies considerably between subgroups stratified by SSc-related ANAs. Specifically, prevalence of DU differs according to autoantibody specificity. Digital ischemia is most prevalent in patients with ACA and anti-topo I with similar proportions experiencing DU. The lowest prevalence of DU is found in patients with either anti-Th/To or anti-RNAP III. High levels of antibodies against angiotensin II type 1 receptor and endothelin-1 type A receptor are shown to be useful in predicting development of DU [53].

Joint Involvement

Up to two-thirds of patients with SSc experience joint pain, although a much smaller proportion have physical examination evidence of true polyarthritis. Arthritis is seen commonly in SSc patients who carry antibodies associated with overlap features, such as anti-PM-Scl, anti-Ku, and anti-U1RNP. The majority of such patients have nonerosive arthritis [34]. In contrast, joint involvement is less frequent in patients with ACA or anti-Th/To antibody when compared with other SSc-related ANAs [82]. When erosive arthritis is present, a diagnosis of SSc in overlap with rheumatoid arthritis should be considered. These patients frequently have anti-cyclic citrullinated peptide antibodies [83].

GI Involvement

In terms of upper GI involvement, there is virtually no difference among patients stratified by SSc-related ANAs, but anti-Th/To and anti-PM-Scl antibodies are associated with somewhat lower frequency of esophageal dysfunction [26, 30]. It has been reported that severe GI involvement, including small bowel malabsorption, is associated with anti-U3 RNP antibody, especially in early the course of the disease (<2 years) [84, 85], although the largest study to specifically characterize patients with anti-U3 RNP did not identify an overall greater prevalence of GI involvement compared with patients with other SSc-related ANAs [23]. A case-control study using the EUSTAR database identified anti-RNAP III as one of risk factors for gastric antral vascular ectasia (GAVE; "watermelon stomach") [86], but this correlation was not replicated in a North American cohort of patients with early and severe dcSSc [87]. However, in this study, of the 16 patients with anti-RNAP III, 5 (31 %) had GAVE, while only 3 of 20 (15 %) with anti-topo I had this complication [87]. In SSc patients, autoantibodies to muscarinic-3 acetylcholine receptor are associated with severe GI dysmotility [51].

Renal Crisis

In Northern Europe and North America, approximately 60 % of all patients experiencing SRC carry anti-RNAP III [88]. SRC can also occur in the context of other SSc-related ANAs, including anti-topo I and anti-U3 RNP, and antibody status has not been shown to influence outcomes following SRC in such patients [88]. In SSc patients with anti-RNAP III antibody, coexistence of anti-RNAP II and a higher EIA index is associated with SRC [89]. Lower incidence of SRC in Japan, French, and Mediterranean countries is thought to reflect the lower prevalence of anti-RNAP III antibody within these populations when compared with the UK, Demark, and North America [70]. Despite the lower prevalence of anti-RNAP III in French SSc patients, this antibody remains the most common serological marker for SRC [76]. In contrast, a recent study from Italy identified a much greater proportion of anti-topo I in patients with SRC [90]. SRC is rarely seen in the context of ACA or anti-PM-Scl. Interesting patients who survived SRC and then later developed PAH have been reported in the context of anti-RNAP III, anti-Th/To, and anti-U3 RNP [24]. Anti-RNAP III antibody has been detected in patients complicating acute renal failure mimicking SRC in the absence of sclerotic skin disease [91]. These patients eventually develop rapidly progressive skin thickening. The presence of anti-RNAP III antibody should alert the managing physician to the increased risk of SRC and appropriate monitoring of blood pressure for early detection of this complication since the prompt introduction of angiotensin-converting enzyme inhibitor can be lifesaving.

Cardiac Involvement

Diastolic and systolic cardiac involvement potentially due to patchy fibrosis in the myocardium is relatively common in SSc patients, particularly in those with long-standing disease.

There is one report describing a potential association between anti-RNAP III and cardiac involvement [16], but others found that the overall frequency of serious cardiac abnormalities in patients with anti-RNAP III is lower than that observed with anti-topo I [18]. There is no definitive association of cardiac involvement with SSc-related ANAs, probably owing to heterogeneous nature of the cardiac involvement, and the difficulty in distinguishing SSc-associated from other causes of myocardial and conduction system abnormalities, such as ischemic and nonischemic disease, particularly in older adults.

PAH

PAH affects approximately 10 % of patients with SSc and has now become a leading cause of SSc-related mortality. PAH can occur in the context of several SSc-related ANAs, including ACA, anti-U3 RNP, anti-Th/To, anti-Ku, and anti-U1 RNP antibodies. Around 20 % of patients with ACA develop PAH later in the course of the disease, although large case-control studies have failed to identify ACA as an independent risk factor for PAH [92]. Despite these findings, the evidence-based DETECT algorithm for PAH identification of SSc patients at high risk for PAH includes ACA as one of the useful characteristics [93], likely reflecting the fact that the majority of SSc patients with PAH have ACA. A high prevalence of PAH is also found in patients with anti-nucleolar antibodies, including anti-U3 RNP and anti-Th/To. Anti-U3 RNP was the only SSc antibody identified as an independent risk factor for the development of PAH in the large case-control study [92]. When comparing anti-U3 RNP with other antibody specificities, PAH was the most common cause of death, leading to an increased mortality in this group of patients [23], and this may explain poor survival in patients with African-American patients with SSc and PAH [94]. Coexistence with autoantibodies to another nucleolar protein, B23, further increases the PAH risk in patients with anti-U3 RNP [41]. The overall prevalence of PAH in anti-Th/To positivity is similar to that seen with ACA [26]. In addition, patients with anti-Th/To also develop pulmonary hypertension in the context of ILD. Patients with MCTD have an increased risk of PAH, and all such patients have anti-U1 RNP antibodies [38]. Patients with anti-topo I rarely develop PAH, but have pulmonary hypertension secondary to ILD and chronic hypoxia [95]. PAH can occur in some patients with anti-RNAP III, another antibody associated with dcSSc. Anti-angiotensin receptor type 1 and anti-endothelin receptor type A autoantibodies are associated with PAH and serve as poor prognostic markers in SSc patients [96]. Antibodies reactive with 4-sulfated N-acetyl-lactosamine are detected in SSc patients and are associated with a higher prevalence of PAH [59].

ILD

More than 70 % of patients with anti-topo I have ILD, and ~25 % develop severe disease which requires oxygen supplementation [73, 74]. A novel autoantibody targeting U11/U12 RNP is associated with severe ILD and decreased survival [27]. Other antibodies associated with ILD include anti-nucleolar antibodies, including anti-U3 RNP and anti-Th/To antibodies [23, 26, 95]. In the context of lcSSc with severe ILD, anti-U11/U12 RNP and anti-Th/To are the most common autoantibodies. In contrast, fewer than 1 % of patients with ACA develop severe ILD and the presence of ACA is an independent protective factor for restrictive lung disease [97]. Likewise, severe ILD is only rarely associated with anti-RNAP III despite the high prevalence of dcSSc within this group [14, 18]. Indeed, SSc patients who survive SRC are less likely to die of SSc-related complications due, in part, to the high prevalence of anti-RNAP III and relatively low frequency of severe ILD in such patients. Anti-Th/To is sometimes detected in patients with idiopathic pulmonary fibrosis or SSc sine scleroderma [80, 81].

Cancer

A potential association between the development of cancer in SSc and the presence of ACA or anti-topo I has been reported [98, 99], although a large case-control study failed to support this relationship. A more recent prospective study has identified a similar prevalence of anti-RNAP III, ACA, and anti-topo I among patients with SSc and cancer [20]. However, the temporal relationship between cancer and SSc differed according to antibody status, with a median disease duration of 13.4 and 11.1 years for anti-topo I and ACA, respectively, in comparison to a nearly contemporaneous association between cancer and anti-RNAP III (median disease duration of 1.2 years). Recently, it has been reported that there is an association with cancer among SSc patients with anti-RNAP III antibody in close temporal relationship to onset of SSc, which suggests that SSc is a paraneoplastic disorder in this patient subset [21]. Another large-scale cohort including 1,044 patients with SSc found anti-RNAP III is an independent marker of coincident cancer [100].

Survival

Associations between SSc-related antibodies and mortality have also been investigated. The presence of anti-topo I in subjects with dcSSc carries independent prognostic information with regard to SSc-related survival [101]. Other studies have identified an association between anti-topo I and a greater risk of mortality [7, 8]. Anti-RNAP III has also been associated with increased mortality, primarily due to an increased prevalence of cardiac and renal involvement in these patients [8], but with improvement in the management of SRC, such associations may not be replicated in the future. In fact, anti-RNAP III has been shown to be protective for 2-year mortality in one cohort enrolled after the introduction of angiotensin-converting enzyme inhibitor therapy [11]. Anti-U3 RNP is another SSc-specific antibody associated with increased mortality, particularly in relation to PAH [23]. In the largest study to date, using the Pittsburgh Scleroderma Databank of 1,432 patients, anti-Th/To predicted the lowest 10-year survival among lcSSc (65 % versus 88 % and 75 % with U1 RNP and ACA, respectively) [19]. In dcSSc, the best 10-year survival was identified in those carrying anti-RNAP III (75 %) and the lowest survival with anti-U3 RNP (61 %) [19].

Autoantibody Titer and Disease Activity

There have been relatively few studies that have investigated whether autoantibody levels are useful in monitoring disease activity in SSc. The task is challenging, because the course of SSc is more indolent, and indices or biomarkers of disease activity are less developed. Most evidence for an association of autoantibody level with disease activity comes from studies of anti-topo I, where changing levels may correlate with progression of skin thickness [102, 103]. In contrast, patients who lose anti-topo I antibody over time may have a more favorable outcome [103]. Anti-RNAP III antibody levels may also correlate with MRSS and onset of SRC [104, 105] and more recently have been reported to show temporal clustering with onset of cancer [20]. Now that quantitative and semiquantitative laboratory tests are available, additional reports will help to clarify whether antibody levels will be helpful biomarkers in clinical practice or clinical trials.

Conclusions

In summary, autoantibodies are the best biomarkers for diagnosis and clinical subgrouping of SSc patients. Characterization of autoantibody status is an essential tool in clinical practice in the evaluation of patients who have SSc or are suspected to have this disease. Because of their specificity, they are highly useful in the diagnosis of SSc as well as in predicting future development to definite SSc in patients with Raynaud's phenomenon without any sclerodermatous skin changes. In addition, because of their strong clinical associations, they allow clinicians to predict future disease manifestations. It is important to note, however, that these major clinical associations are not absolute, and organ-specific manifestations can occur in the presence of any autoantibody reactivity. Novel antibodies which have their own clinical associations continue to be discovered.

References

1. Okano Y. Antinuclear antibody in systemic sclerosis (scleroderma). Rheum Dis Clin North Am. 1996;22(4):709–35.
2. Hamaguchi Y. Autoantibody profiles in systemic sclerosis: predictive value for clinical evaluation and prognosis. J Dermatol. 2010;37(1):42–53.
3. Mehra S, Walker J, Patterson K, Fritzler MJ. Autoantibodies in systemic sclerosis. Autoimmun Rev. 2013;12(3):340–54.
4. Moroi Y, Peebles C, Fritzler MJ, Steigerwald J, Tan EM. Autoantibody to centromere (kinetochore) in scleroderma sera. Proc Natl Acad Sci U S A. 1980;77(3):1627–31.
5. Gelber AC, Pillemer SR, Baum BJ, Wigley FM, Hummers LK, Morris S, et al. Distinct recognition of antibodies to centromere proteins in primary Sjogren's syndrome compared with limited scleroderma. Ann Rheum Dis. 2006;65(8):1028–32.
6. Senecal JL, Dieudé M, Koenig M. Predictive value of antinuclear autoantibodies: the lessons of the systemic sclerosis autoantibodies. Autoimmun Rev. 2008;7(8):588–93.
7. Steen VD, Powell DL, Medsger Jr TA. Clinical correlations and prognosis based on serum autoantibodies in patients with systemic sclerosis. Arthritis Rheum. 1988;31(2):196–203.
8. Kuwana M, Kaburaki J, Okano Y, Tojo T, Homma M. Clinical and prognostic associations based on serum antinuclear antibodies in Japanese patients with systemic sclerosis. Arthritis Rheum. 1994;37(1):75–83.
9. Douvas AS, Achten M, Tan EM. Identification of a nuclear protein (Scl-70) as a unique target of human antinuclear antibodies in scleroderma. J Biol Chem. 1979;254(20):10514–22.
10. Shero JH, Bordwell B, Rothfield NF, Earnshaw WC. High titers of autoantibodies to topoisomerase I (Scl-70) in sera from scleroderma patients. Science. 1986;231(4739):737–40.
11. Domsic RT, Rodriguez-Reyna T, Lucas M, Fertig N, Medsger Jr TA. Skin thickness progression rate: a predictor of mortality and early internal organ involvement in diffuse scleroderma. Ann Rheum Dis. 2011;70(1):104–9.
12. Perera A, Fertig N, Lucas M, Rodriguez-Reyna TS, Hu P, Steen VD, Medsger Jr TA. Clinical subsets, skin thickness progression rate, and serum antibody levels in systemic sclerosis patients with anti-topoisomerase I antibody. Arthritis Rheum. 2007;56(8):2740–6.
13. Kuwana M, Kaburaki J, Mimori T, Tojo T, Homma M. Autoantibody reactive with three classes of RNA polymerases in sera from patients with systemic sclerosis. J Clin Invest. 1993;91(4):1399–404.
14. Kuwana M, Okano Y, Kaburaki J, Medsger Jr TA, Wright TM. Autoantibodies to RNA polymerases recognize multiple subunits and demonstrate cross-reactivity with RNA polymerase complexes. Arthritis Rheum. 1999;42(2):275–84.
15. Satoh M, Kuwana M, Ogasawara T, Ajmani AK, Langdon JJ, Kimpel D, et al. Association of autoantibodies to topoisomerase I and the phosphorylated (IIO) form of RNA polymerase II in Japanese scleroderma patients. J Immunol. 1994;153(12):5838–48.
16. Kuwana M, Okano Y, Kaburaki J, Tojo T, Medsger Jr TA. Racial differences in the distribution of systemic sclerosis-related serum antinuclear antibodies. Arthritis Rheum. 1994;37(6):902–6.
17. Meyer OC, Fertig N, Lucas M, Somogyi N, Medsger Jr TA. Disease subsets, antinuclear antibody profile, and clinical features in 127 French and 247 US adult patients with systemic sclerosis. J Rheumatol. 2007;34(1):104–9.
18. Okano Y, Steen VD, Medsger Jr TA. Autoantibody reactive with RNA polymerase III in systemic sclerosis. Ann Intern Med. 1993;119(10):1005–13.
19. Steen VD. Autoantibodies in systemic sclerosis. Semin Arthritis Rheum. 2005;35(1):35–42.
20. Shah AA, Rosen A, Hummers L, Wigley F, Casciola-Rosen L. Close temporal relationship between onset of cancer and

scleroderma in patients with RNA polymerase I/III antibodies. Arthritis Rheum. 2010;62(9):2787–95.

21. Moinzadeh P, Fonseca C, Hellmich M, Shah AA, Chighizola C, Denton CP, Ong VH. Association of anti-RNA polymerase III autoantibodies and cancer in scleroderma. Arthritis Res Ther. 2014;16(1):R53.
22. Lischwe MA, Ochs RL, Reddy R, Cook RG, Yeoman LC, Tan EM, et al. Purification and partial characterization of a nucleolar scleroderma antigen (Mr = 34,000; pI, 8.5) rich in NG, NG-dimethylarginine. J Biol Chem. 1985;260(26):14304–10.
23. Aggarwal R, Lucas M, Fertig N, Oddis CV, Medsger Jr TA. Anti-U3 RNP autoantibodies in systemic sclerosis. Arthritis Rheum. 2009;60(4):1112–8.
24. Gündüz OH, Fertig N, Lucas M, Medsger Jr TA. Systemic sclerosis with renal crisis and pulmonary hypertension: a report of eleven cases. Arthritis Rheum. 2001;44(7):1663–6.
25. Van Eenennaam H, Vogelzangs JH, Lugtenberg D, Van Den Hoogen FH, Van Venrooij WJ, Pruijn GJ. Identity of the RNase MRP- and RNase P-associated Th/To autoantigen. Arthritis Rheum. 2002;46(12):3266–72.
26. Mitri GM, Lucas M, Fertig N, Steen VD, Medsger Jr TA. A comparison between anti-Th/To-and anticentromere antibody-positive systemic sclerosis patients with limited cutaneous involvement. Arthritis Rheum. 2003;48(1):203–9.
27. Fertig N, Domsic RT, Rodriguez-Reyna T, Kuwana M, Lucas M, Medsger Jr TA, et al. Anti-U11/U12 RNP antibodies in systemic sclerosis: a new serologic marker associated with pulmonary fibrosis. Arthritis Rheum. 2009;61(7):958–65.
28. Reimer G, Scheer U, Peters JM, Tan EM. Immunolocalization and partial characterization of a nucleolar autoantigen (PM-Scl) associated with polymyositis/scleroderma overlap syndromes. J Immunol. 1986;137(12):3802–8.
29. Koschik 2nd RW, Fertig N, Lucas MR, Domsic RT, Medsger Jr TA. Anti-PM-Scl antibody in patients with systemic sclerosis. Clin Exp Rheumatol. 2012;30(2 Suppl 71):S12–6.
30. D'Aoust J, Hudson M, Tatibouet S, Wick J, Mahler M, Baron M, Fritzler MJ, Canadian Scleroderma Research Group. Clinical and serologic correlates of anti-PM/Scl antibodies in systemic sclerosis: a multicenter study of 763 patients. Arthritis Rheumatol. 2014;66(6):1608–15.
31. Brouwer R, Hengstman GJ, Vree Egberts W, Ehrfeld H, Bozic B, Ghirardello A, et al. Autoantibody profiles in the sera of European patients with myositis. Ann Rheum Dis. 2001;60(2):116–23.
32. Mimori T, Akizuki M, Yamagata H, Inada S, Yoshida S, Homma M. Characterization of a high molecular weight acidic nuclear protein recognized by autoantibodies in sera from patients with polymyositis-scleroderma overlap. J Clin Invest. 1981;68(3):611–20.
33. Cavazzana I, Fredi M, Taraborelli M, Quinzanini M, Tincani A, Franceschini F. A subset of systemic sclerosis but not of systemic lupus erythematosus is defined by isolated anti-Ku autoantibodies. Clin Exp Rheumatol. 2013;31(2 Suppl 76):118–21.
34. Rozman B, Cucnik S, Sodin-Semrl S, Czirjak L, Varju C, Distler O, et al. Prevalence and clinical associations of anti-Ku antibodies in patients with systemic sclerosis: a European EUSTAR-initiated multi-centre case-control study. Ann Rheum Dis. 2008;67(9): 1282–6.
35. Kaji K, Fertig N, Medsger Jr TA, Satoh T, Hoshino K, Hamaguchi Y, et al. Autoantibodies to RuvBL1 and RuvBL2: a novel systemic sclerosis-related antibody associated with diffuse cutaneous and skeletal muscle involvement. Arthritis Care Res (Hoboken). 2014;66(4):575–84.
36. Pettersson I, Hinterberger M, Mimori T, Gottlieb E, Steitz JA. The structure of mammalian small nuclear ribonucleoproteins. Identification of multiple protein components reactive with anti-(U1)ribonucleoprotein and anti-Sm autoantibodies. J Biol Chem. 1984;259(9):5907–14.
37. Sharp GC, Irvin WS, Tan EM, Gould RG, Holman HR. Mixed connective tissue disease-an apparently distinct rheumatic disease syndrome associated with a specific antibody to an extractable nuclear antigen (ENA). Am J Med. 1972;52(2):148–59.
38. Gunnarsson R, Andreassen AK, Molberg Ø, Lexberg ÅS, Time K, Dhainaut AS, et al. Prevalence of pulmonary hypertension in an unselected, mixed connective tissue disease cohort: results of a nationwide, Norwegian cross-sectional multicentre study and review of current literature. Rheumatology (Oxford). 2013;52(7): 1208–13.
39. Rodriguez-Sanchez JL, Gelpi C, Juarez C, Hardin JA. A new autoantibody in scleroderma that recognizes a 90-kDa component of the nucleolus-organizing region of chromatin. J Immunol. 1987;139(8):2579–84.
40. Dagher JH, Scheer U, Voit R, Grummt I, Lonzetti L, Raymond Y, et al. Autoantibodies to NOR 90/hUBF: longterm clinical and serological followup in a patient with limited systemic sclerosis suggests an antigen driven immune response. J Rheumatol. 2002;29(7):1543–7.
41. Ulanet DB, Wigley FM, Gelber AC, Rosen A. Autoantibodies against B23, a nucleolar phosphoprotein, occur in scleroderma and are associated with pulmonary hypertension. Arthritis Rheum. 2003;49(1):85–92.
42. Hudson M, Pope J, Mahler M, Tatibouet S, Steele R, Baron M, et al. Clinical significance of antibodies to Ro52/TRIM21 in systemic sclerosis. Arthritis Res Ther. 2012;14(2):R50.
43. Costa S, Mondini M, Caneparo V, Afeltra A, Airò P, Bellisai F, et al. Detection of anti-IFI16 antibodies by ELISA: clinical and serological associations in systemic sclerosis. Rheumatology (Oxford). 2011;50(4):674–81.
44. Cavazzana I, Ceribelli A, Taraborelli M, Fredi M, Norman G, Tincani A, et al. Primary biliary cirrhosis-related autoantibodies in a large cohort of Italian patients with systemic sclerosis. J Rheumatol. 2011;38(10):2180–5.
45. Salazar GA, Assassi S, Wigley F, Hummers L, Varga J, Hinchcliff M, et al. Antinuclear antibody-negative systemic sclerosis. Semin Arthritis Rheum. 2014. doi:10.1016/j.semarthrit.2014.11.006 [Epub ahead of print].
46. Shanmugam VK, Swistowski DR, Saddic N, Wang H, Steen VD. Comparison of indirect immunofluorescence and multiplex antinuclear antibody screening in systemic sclerosis. Clin Rheumatol. 2011;30(10):1363–8.
47. Damoiseaux J, Boesten K, Giesen J, Austen J, Tervaert JW. Evaluation of a novel line-blot immunoassay for the detection of antibodies to extractable nuclear antigens. Ann N Y Acad Sci. 2005;1050(6):340–7.
48. Kuwana M, Kimura K, Kawakami Y. Identification of an immunodominant epitope on RNA polymerase III recognized by systemic sclerosis sera: application to enzyme-linked immunosorbent assay. Arthritis Rheum. 2002;46(10):2742–7.
49. Op De Beéck K, Vermeersch P, Verschueren P, Westhovens R, Mariën G, Blockmans D, et al. Antinuclear antibody detection by automated multiplex immunoassay in untreated patients at the time of diagnosis. Autoimmun Rev. 2012;12(2):137–43.
50. Baroni SS, Santillo M, Bevilacqua F, Luchetti M, Spadoni T, Mancini M, et al. Stimulatory autoantibodies to the PDGF receptor in systemic sclerosis. N Engl J Med. 2006;354(25): 2667–76.
51. Singh J, Mehendiratta V, Del Galdo F, Jimenez SA, Cohen S, et al. Immunoglobulins from scleroderma patients inhibit the muscarinic receptor activation in internal anal sphincter smooth muscle cells. Am J Physiol Gastrointest Liver Physiol. 2009;297(6): G1206–13.

52. Kawaguchi Y, Nakamura Y, Matsumoto I, Nishimagi E, Satoh T, Kuwana M, et al. Muscarinic-3 acetylcholine receptor autoantibody in patients with systemic sclerosis: contribution to severe gastrointestinal tract dysmotility. Ann Rheum Dis. 2009;68(5): 710–4.
53. Riemekasten G, Philippe A, Näther M, Slowinski T, Müller DN, Heidecke H, et al. Involvement of functional autoantibodies against vascular receptors in systemic sclerosis. Ann Rheum Dis. 2011;70(3):530–6.
54. Tan FK, Arnett FC, Antohi S, Saito S, Mirarchi A, Spiera H, et al. Autoantibodies to the extracellular matrix microfibrillar protein, fibrillin-1, in patients with scleroderma and other connective tissue diseases. J Immunol. 1999;163(2):1066–72.
55. Sato S, Hayakawa M, Hasegawa M, Fujimoto M, Takehara K. Function blocking autoantibodies against matrix metalloproteinase-1 patients with systemic sclerosis. J Invest Dermatol. 2003;120(4):542–7.
56. Nishijima C, Hayakawa I, Matsushita T, Komura K, Hasegawa M, Takehara K. Autoantibody against matrix metalloproteinase-3 patients with systemic sclerosis. Clin Exp Immunol. 2004;138(2): 357–63.
57. Iwata Y, Ogawa F, Komura K, Muroi E, Hara T, Shimizu K, et al. Autoantibody against peroxiredoxin I, an antioxidant enzyme, in patients with systemic sclerosis: possible association with oxidative stress. Rheumatology (Oxford). 2007;46(5):790–5.
58. Ogawa F, Shimizu K, Hara T, Muroi E, Komura K, Takenaka M, et al. Autoantibody against one of the antioxidant repair enzymes, methionine sulfoxide reductase A, in systemic sclerosis: association with pulmonary fibrosis and vascular damage. Arch Dermatol Res. 2010;302(1):27–35.
59. Grader-Beck T, Boin F, von Gunten S, Smith D, Rosen A, Bochner BS. Antibodies recognising sulfated carbohydrates are prevalent in systemic sclerosis and associated with pulmonary vascular disease. Ann Rheum Dis. 2011;70(12):2218–24.
60. Giovannetti A, Maselli A, Colasanti T, Rosato E, Salsano F, Pisarri S, et al. Autoantibodies to estrogen receptor α in systemic sclerosis (SSc) as pathogenetic determinants and markers of progression. PLoS One. 2013;8(9):e74332.
61. van den Hoogen F, Khanna D, Fransen J, Johnson SR, Baron M, Tyndall A, et al. 2013 classification criteria for systemic sclerosis: an American College of Rheumatology/European League against Rheumatism collaborative initiative. Arthritis Rheum. 2013; 65(11):2734–47.
62. Koenig M, Joyal F, Fritzler MJ, Roussin A, Abrahamowicz M, Boire G, et al. Autoantibodies and microvascular damage are independent predictive factors for the progression of Raynaud's phenomenon to systemic sclerosis: a twenty-year prospective study of 586 patients, with validation of proposed criteria for early systemic sclerosis. Arthritis Rheum. 2008;58(12):3902–12.
63. Matucci-Cerinic M, Allanore Y, Czirják L, Tyndall A, Müller-Ladner U, Denton C, et al. The challenge of early systemic sclerosis for the EULAR Scleroderma Trial and Research group (EUSTAR) community. It is time to cut the Gordian knot and develop a prevention or rescue strategy. Ann Rheum Dis. 2009 68(9):1377–80.
64. Scalapino K, Arkachaisri T, Lucas M, Fertig N, Helfrich DJ, Londino Jr AV, et al. Childhood onset systemic sclerosis: classification, clinical and serologic features, and survival in comparison with adult onset disease. J Rheumatol. 2006;33(5):1004–13.
65. Martini G, Foeldvari I, Russo R, Cuttica R, Eberhard A, Ravelli A, et al. Systemic sclerosis in childhood: clinical and immunologic features of 153 patients in an international database. Arthritis Rheum. 2006;54(12):3971–8.
66. Reveille JD, Fischbach M, McNearney T, Friedman AW, Aguilar MB, Lisse J, et al. Systemic sclerosis in 3 US ethnic groups: a comparison of clinical, sociodemographic, serologic, and immunogenetic determinants. Semin Arthritis Rheum. 2001;30(5): 332–46.
67. Krzyszczak ME, Li Y, Ross SJ, Ceribelli A, Chan EK, Bubb MR, et al. Gender and ethnicity differences in the prevalence of scleroderma-related autoantibodies. Clin Rheumatol. 2011;30 (10):1333–9.
68. Ceribelli A, Cavazzana I, Franceschini F, Airò P, Tincani A, Cattaneo R, et al. Anti-Th/To are common antinucleolar autoantibodies in Italian patients with scleroderma. J Rheumatol. 2010; 37(10):2071–5.
69. Panicheewa S, Chitrabamrung S, Verasertniyom O, Vanichaphantu M, Kraisit SO, Chiewsilp P, et al. Diffuse systemic sclerosis and related diseases in Thailand. Clin Rheumatol. 1991;10(2):124–9.
70. Sobanski V, Dauchet L, Lefèvre G, Lambert M, Morell-Dubois S, Sy T, et al. Prevalence of anti-RNA polymerase III antibodies in systemic sclerosis: new data from a French cohort and a systematic review and meta-analysis. Arthritis Rheumatol. 2014;66(2):407–17.
71. Arnett FC, Howard RF, Tan F, Moulds JM, Bias WB, Durban E, et al. Increased prevalence of systemic sclerosis in a Native American tribe in Oklahoma Association with an Amerindian HLA haplotype. Arthritis Rheum. 1996;39(8):1362–70.
72. Moinzadeh P, Aberer E, Ahmadi-Simab K, Blank N, Distler JH, Fierlbeck G, et al. Disease progression in systemic sclerosis-overlap syndrome is significantly different from limited and diffuse cutaneous systemic sclerosis. Ann Rheum Dis. 2015; 74(4):730–7.
73. Reveille JD, Solomon DH. Evidence-based guidelines for the use of immunologic tests: anticentromere, Scl-70, and nucleolar antibodies. Arthritis Rheum. 2003;49(3):399–412.
74. Hanke K, Dahnrich C, Bruckner CS, Huscher D, Becker M, Jansen A, et al. Diagnostic value of anti-topoisomerase I antibodies in a large monocentric cohort. Arthritis Res Ther. 2009; 11(1):R28.
75. Scussel-Lonzetti L, Joyal F, Raynauld JP, Roussin A, Rich E, Goulet JR, et al. Predicting mortality in systemic sclerosis: analysis of a cohort of 309 French Canadian patients with emphasis on features at diagnosis as predictive factors for survival. Medicine (Baltimore). 2002;81(2):154–67.
76. Meyer O, De Chaisemartin L, Nicaise-Roland P, Cabane J, Tubach F, Dieude P, Allanore Y, et al. Anti-RNA polymerase III antibody prevalence and associated clinical manifestations in a large series of French patients with systemic sclerosis: a cross-sectional study. J Rheumatol. 2010;37(1):125–30.
77. Cavazzana I, Angela C, Paolo A, Stefania Z, Angela T, Franco F. Anti-RNA polymerase III antibodies: a marker of systemic sclerosis with rapid onset and skin thickening progression. Autoimmun Rev. 2009;8(7):580–4.
78. Poormoghim H, Lucas M, Fertig N, Medsger Jr TA. Systemic sclerosis sine scleroderma: demographic, clinical, and serologic features and survival in forty-eight patients. Arthritis Rheum. 2000;43(2):444–51.
79. Toya SP, Tzelepis GE. The many faces of scleroderma sine scleroderma: a literature review focusing on cardiopulmonary complications. Rheumatol Int. 2009;29(8):861–8.
80. Fischer A, Pfalzgraf FJ, Feghali-Bostwick CA, Wright TM, Curran-Everett D, West SG, et al. Anti-th/to-positivity in a cohort of patients with idiopathic pulmonary fibrosis. J Rheumatol. 2006;33(8):1600–5.
81. Fischer A, Meehan RT, Feghali-Bostwick CA, West SG, Brown KK. Unique characteristics of systemic sclerosis sine scleroderma-associated interstitial lung disease. Chest. 2006;130(4):976–81.
82. Okano Y, Medsger Jr TA. Autoantibody to Th ribonucleoprotein (nucleolar 7–2 RNA protein particle) in patients with systemic sclerosis. Arthritis Rheum. 1990;33(12):1822–8.
83. Generini S, Steiner G, Miniati I, Conforti ML, Guiducci S, Skriner K, et al. Anti-hnRNP and other autoantibodies in systemic sclero-

sis with joint involvement. Rheumatology (Oxford). 2009;48 (8):920–5.
84. Sharif R, Fritzler MJ, Mayes MD, Gonzalez EB, McNearney TA, Draeger H, et al. Anti-fibrillarin antibody in African American patients with systemic sclerosis: immunogenetics, clinical features, and survival analysis. J Rheumatol. 2011;38(8):1622–30.
85. Nishimagi E, Tochimoto A, Kawaguchi Y, Satoh T, Kuwana M, Takagi K, et al. Characteristics of patients with early systemic sclerosis and severe gastrointestinal tract involvement. J Rheumatol. 2007;34(10):2050–5.
86. Ghrénassia E, Avouac J, Khanna D, Derk CT, Distler O, Suliman YA, et al. Prevalence, correlates and outcomes of gastric antral vascular ectasia in systemic sclerosis: a EUSTAR case-control study. J Rheumatol. 2014;41(1):99–105.
87. Hung EW, Mayes MD, Sharif R, Assassi S, Machicao VI, Hosing C, et al. Gastric antral vascular ectasia and its clinical correlates in patients with early diffuse systemic sclerosis in the SCOT trial. J Rheumatol. 2013;40(4):455–60.
88. Penn H, Howie AJ, Kingdon EJ, Bunn CC, Stratton RJ, Black CM, et al. Scleroderma renal crisis: patient characteristics and long-term outcomes. QJM. 2007;100(8):485–94.
89. Hamaguchi Y, Kodera M, Matsushita T, Hasegawa M, Inaba Y, Usuda T, et al. Clinical and immunological predictors of scleroderma renal crisis for Japanese systemic sclerosis patients with anti-RNA polymerase III autoantibodies. Arthritis Rheumatol. 2014. doi:10.1002/art.38994 [Epub ahead of print].
90. Codullo V, Cavazzana I, Bonino C, Alpini C, Cavagna L, Cozzi F, et al. Serologic profile and mortality rates of scleroderma renal crisis in Italy. J Rheumatol. 2009;36(7):1464–9.
91. Bhavsar SV, Carmona R. Anti-RNA polymerase III antibodies in the diagnosis of scleroderma renal crisis in the absence of skin disease. J Clin Rheumatol. 2014;20(7):379–82.
92. Steen V, Medsger Jr TA. Predictors of isolated pulmonary hypertension in patients with systemic sclerosis and limited cutaneous involvement. Arthritis Rheum. 2003;48(2):516–22.
93. Coghlan JG, Denton CP, Grünig E, Bonderman D, Distler O, Khanna D, et al. Evidence-based detection of pulmonary arterial hypertension in systemic sclerosis: the DETECT study. Ann Rheum Dis. 2014;73(7):1340–9.
94. Blanco I, Mathai S, Shafiq M, Boyce D, Kolb TM, Chami H, et al. Severity of systemic sclerosis-associated pulmonary arterial hypertension in African Americans. Medicine (Baltimore). 2014;93(5):177–85.
95. Steen VD, Lucas M, Fertig N, Medsger Jr TA. Pulmonary arterial hypertension and severe pulmonary fibrosis in systemic sclerosis patients with a nucleolar antibody. J Rheumatol. 2007;34(11): 2230–5.
96. Becker MO, Kill A, Kutsche M, Guenther J, Rose A, Tabeling C, et al. Vascular receptor autoantibodies in pulmonary arterial hypertension associated with systemic sclerosis. Am J Respir Crit Care Med. 2014;190(7):808–17.
97. McNearney TA, Reveille JD, Fischbach M, Friedman AW, Lisse JR, Goel N, et al. Pulmonary involvement in systemic sclerosis: associations with genetic, serologic, sociodemographic, and behavioral factors. Arthritis Rheum. 2007;57(2):318–26.
98. Higuchi M, Horiuchi T, Ishibashi N, Yoshizawa S, Niho Y, Nagasawa K. Anticentromere antibody as a risk factor for cancer in patients with systemic sclerosis. Clin Rheumatol. 2000;19(2):123–6.
99. Rothfield N, Kurtzman S, Vazques-Abad D, Charron C, Daniels L, Greenberg B. Association of anti-topoisomerase I with cancer. Arthritis Rheum. 1992;35(6):724.
100. Shah AA, Hummers LK, Casciola-Rosen L, Visvanathan K, Rosen A, Wigley FM. Examination of autoantibody status and clinical features that associate with cancer risk and cancer-associated scleroderma. Arthritis Rheumatol. 2015. doi:10.1002/art.39022 [Epub ahead of print].
101. Jacobsen S, Ullman S, Shen GQ, Wiik A, Halberg P. Influence of clinical features, serum antinuclear antibodies, and lung function on survival of patients with systemic sclerosis. J Rheumatol. 2001;28(11):2454–9.
102. Hu PQ, Fertig N, Medsger Jr TA, Wright TM. Correlation of serum anti-DNA topoisomerase I antibody levels with disease severity and activity in systemic sclerosis. Arthritis Rheum. 2003; 48(5):1363–73.
103. Kuwana M, Kaburaki J, Mimori T, Kawakami Y, Tojo T. Longitudinal analysis of autoantibody response to topoisomerase I in systemic sclerosis. Arthritis Rheum. 2000;43(5):1074–84.
104. Kuwana M, Okano Y, Pandey JP, Silver RM, Fertig N, Medsger Jr TA. Enzyme-linked immunosorbent assay for detection of anti-RNA polymerase III antibody: analytical accuracy and clinical associations in systemic sclerosis. Arthritis Rheum. 2005;52 (8):2425–32.
105. Nihtyanova SI, Parker JC, Black CM, Bunn CC, Denton CP. A longitudinal study of anti-RNA polymerase III antibody levels in systemic sclerosis. Rheumatology (Oxford). 2009;48(10): 1218–21.

Mechanisms of Vascular Disease

16

Mirko Manetti and Bashar Kahaleh

Introduction

Scleroderma (systemic sclerosis (SSc)) is to a large degree identified by the vascular features which may precede the onset of fibrosis by months or even years. Abnormalities in microvessel morphology and vascular dysfunction occur early during the disease course and evolve into a distinctive vasculopathy that relentlessly advances in nearly all affected organs. This evidence suggests that endothelial cells (ECs) are the primary target in SSc and that multiple interactions of ECs with other cells and pathways, including cells of both the innate and adaptive immune systems, platelets and coagulation factors, vascular smooth muscle cells (VSMCs), and fibroblasts, position ECs in center stage of disease pathogenesis. In SSc, vascular injury includes persistent EC activation/damage and apoptosis, intimal thickening, vessel narrowing, and obliteration. These profound vascular changes lead to vascular tone dysfunction and reduced capillary blood flow, with consequent chronic tissue ischemia. The resulting tissue hypoxia induces complex cellular and molecular mechanisms in the attempt to recover EC functions including adequate tissue perfusion. Nonetheless, there is no evidence of significant compensatory angiogenesis in SSc, and the disease evolves toward irreversible structural changes in multiple vascular beds culminating in the loss of the peripheral capillary network. A critical imbalance between proangiogenic and antiangiogenic factors may be largely responsible for the lack of vascular regeneration in SSc. Besides insufficient angiogenesis, increasing evidence indicates that defective vasculogenesis with altered numbers and functional defects of bone marrow-derived endothelial progenitor cells (EPCs) may contribute to the pathogenesis of SSc vasculopathy.

Clinically, the vascular manifestations in SSc include Raynaud's phenomenon (RP), the early edematous puffy hands, telangiectasias, digital ulcers, gastric antral vascular ectasia (GAVE), pulmonary arterial hypertension (PAH), myocardial dysfunction, and scleroderma renal crisis. Therapeutically, the use of angiotensin-converting enzyme inhibitors for scleroderma renal crisis, endothelin receptor antagonists for PAH, and phosphodiesterase inhibitors for PAH, RP, and digital ulcers have significantly improved the care of SSc patients. However, despite this symptomatic improvement, regression of the vascular lesions has been difficult to achieve.

The Vascular Problem

Vascular involvement in SSc includes a spectrum of changes that affect predominantly the microcirculation, mainly the capillaries and the small arterioles. The pathologic changes in the vascular tree range from EC activation with increased expression of adhesion molecules to EC apoptosis, capillary necrosis, intimal proliferation, and luminal occlusion that result in tissue ischemia and contribute to organ failure together with concomitant fibrosis. The current hypotheses in SSc vascular pathogenesis implicate a possible, yet unidentified, microbial trigger and an immune-mediated mechanism that results in vascular injury possibly through recognition of a putative vascular or perivascular autoantigen and the induction of autoantibodies. This chapter will review the morphologic and functional features of SSc vasculopathy with special emphasis on the mechanisms and pathologic sequences of vascular injury.

M. Manetti, PhD (✉)
Section of Anatomy and Histology,
Department of Experimental and Clinical Medicine,
University of Florence, Florence, Italy
e-mail: mirkomanetti@yahoo.it

B. Kahaleh, MD
Division of Rheumatology and Immunology,
University of Toledo Medical Center, Toledo, OH, USA

J. Varga et al. (eds.), *Scleroderma*, DOI 10.1007/978-3-319-31407-5_16

The Vascular Lesion

The prominent vascular abnormalities in SSc are typically observed in the capillaries and the small blood vessels [1]. Swelling and proliferation of the intima with mononuclear cell infiltration are seen in the small arterioles. In the capillary network, the vascular disease is characterized by distorted and irregular capillary loops in all involved organs including the skin, kidneys, lungs, heart, and muscles, reflecting the diffuse nature of the microvascular disorder in SSc, even in sites not affected by fibrosis [1, 2]. At the ultrastructural level, the earliest vascular changes in the edematous stage of the disease consist of opening of EC tight junctions, vacuolization of cytoplasm with increase in the number of basal lamina-like layers, and occasional entrapment of lymphocytes and cellular vesicles in the vessel wall [1]. Further signs of nuclear injury in association with EC membrane disruption occur in more advanced disease. Ghost vessels consisting of an intact basal lamina with remnants of ECs are occasionally noted in association with perivascular cellular infiltrates that consist of macrophages and T and B cells, with predominance of $CD4^+$ T cells [3]. EC apoptosis was first described on ultrastructural examination of SSc skin biopsies in the early inflammatory stages of the disease, suggesting a causal association [3]. It was later noted in the University of California at Davis (UCD) lines 200/206 chickens that spontaneously develop a systemic disease that closely resembles human SSc [4]. Apoptosis of ECs is not unique to SSc vasculopathy and is frequently observed in diseases with prominent vascular involvement, such as early atherosclerotic lesions, graft rejection, thrombotic thrombocytopenic purpura, and the hemolytic uremic syndrome, suggesting that EC apoptosis may be a common prerequisite for a variety of vascular disorders [5, 6]. The fate of apoptotic ECs in SSc is not well examined. A possible defect in the orderly removal of apoptotic cells may lead to phagocytosis by dendritic cells and macrophages and subsequent presentation of cellular antigens to $CD8^+$ T cells [7], leading to immune recognition of vascular antigens. Moreover, apoptotic ECs can activate the alternative complement and coagulation cascades leading to vascular microthrombosis and further tissue compromise [8, 9]. Typical ultrastructural SSc microvascular changes are shown in Fig. 16.1.

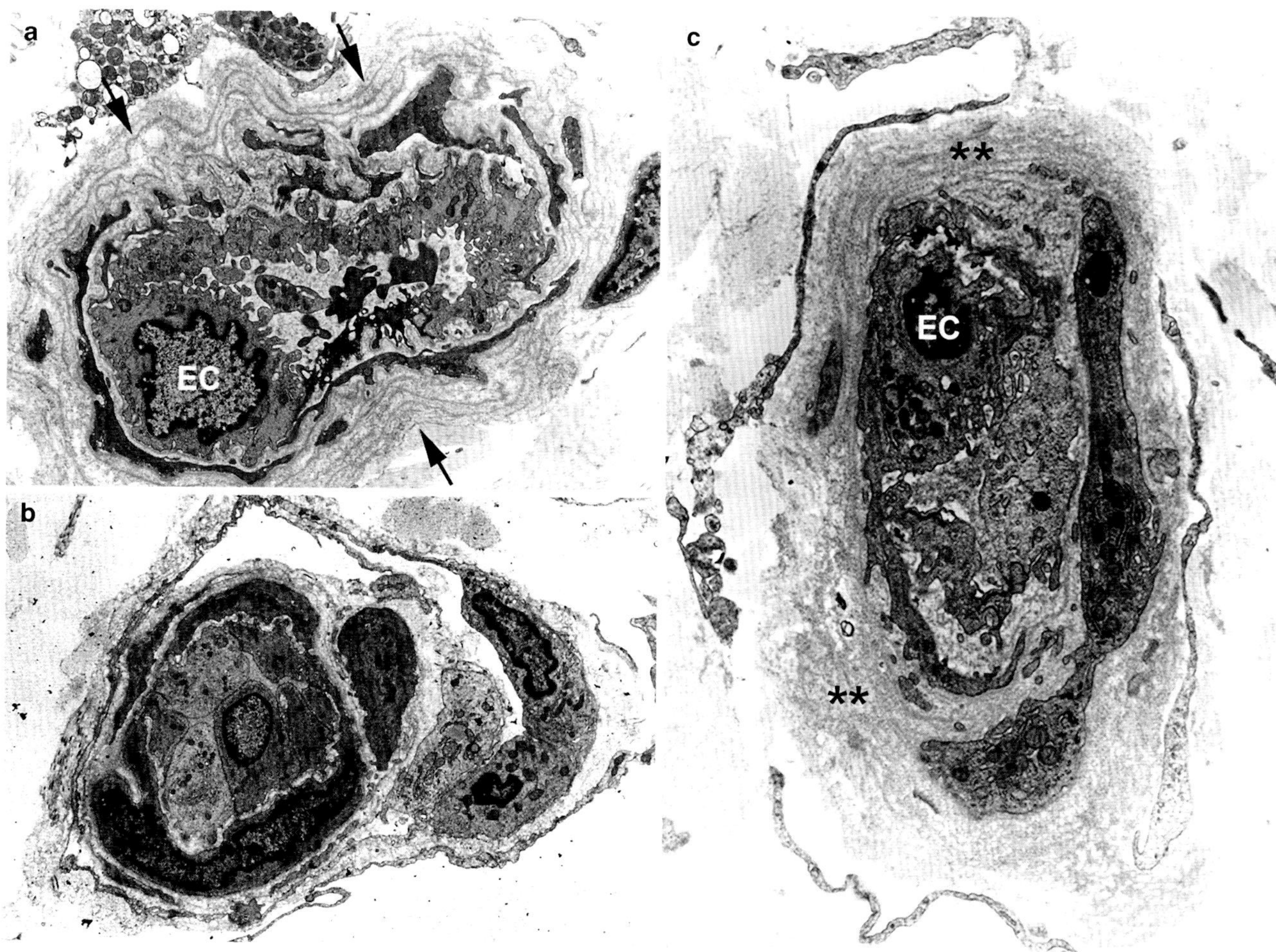

Fig. 16.1 (**a**–**c**) Representative transmission electron microscopy (TEM) photomicrographs of SSc dermal microvessels. (**a**) Microvessel shows apoptosis of ECs and delaminated basal lamina (*arrows*). Apoptotic ECs display plasma membrane blebbing with release of apoptotic bodies. (**b**) Swollen ECs occluding microvessel's lumen. (**c**) Microvessel with an occluded lumen shows thickened basal lamina (*asterisks*). *EC endothelial cell*. TEM; original magnification: ×6000

Increased EC thymidine labeling has been reported in SSc, particularly in the indurated phase of the disease [10]. EC thymidine labeling is seen only in the involved "fibrotic" skin, suggesting that EC changes in the uninvolved skin represent cellular activation but not true injury. Significant intimal proliferation and accumulation of proteoglycans in the arterioles and small-sized arteries are common in SSc [11]. Moreover, abnormality of the vessel wall is likely to result from increased synthesis of extracellular matrix (ECM) by intimal and adventitial fibroblasts. Transdifferentiation of ECs into profibrotic myofibroblasts via the process of endothelial–mesenchymal transition (EndoMT) may contribute further to vascular wall fibrosis [12].

The presence of vascular pathology at one site does not necessarily indicate similar pathology at other sites; for instance, the presence of vascular pulmonary pathology clinically manifesting as PAH may not be associated with vascular pathology in the kidneys nor is there any relationship between vascular changes in the gastrointestinal tract (GAVE) and vascular changes in either the lungs or the kidneys. Milder degrees of vascular changes can be seen in clinically uninvolved skin, mainly in the papillary dermal layer in association with platelets adhering to the vessel walls of the dermal microvasculature [3]. It is not known if these changes precede the development of tissue fibrosis or are independent of it. In contrast to small arterioles, large-sized vessel occlusion in SSc is unusual; however, it can occur particularly in the ulnar arteries in patients with the limited form of SSc in association with anticentromere antibodies [13]. In the arteries, intimal proliferation of a uniform and symmetrical nature leads to the formation of a neointima indistinguishable from that seen in other autoimmune diseases, chronic homograft rejection, and accelerated atherosclerosis such as restenosis after coronary bypass [14]. The medial layers are usually thinned, except in hypertensive patients where medial hypertrophy and fibrinoid deposition can be seen [15]. The capillary changes in SSc are most visible in the nail folds.

Nailfold Capillaroscopy The first description of capillary abnormalities in SSc was published in 1925 by Brown and O'Leary who employed a simple technique to describe capillary changes typical of the microvasculature involvement in SSc [16]. In the 1970s–1980s, the seminal work by Maricq and colleagues popularized the use of wide-field capillary microscopy and described specific "SSc patterns" of capillary changes [17–22] (Fig. 16.2).

Nailfold capillaroscopy has great diagnostic value in the early stages of the disease. It is the technique of choice for the identification of patients with RP who are at risk for developing SSc [23–25].

Vascular Dysfunction in Scleroderma

The normal vascular endothelium is a single-cell thick layer that is endowed with remarkably diverse functions. ECs regulate coagulation and fibrinolysis, vascular permeability, vascular tone, and metabolism and nutrition of surrounding cells. Injury to the endothelium in SSc leads to profound vascular dysfunction that is prominent in the early stages of the disease and progressively worsens over time [3, 26]. ECs also regulate vascular tone by producing vasoconstrictive and vasodilatory molecules. Vascular dysfunction can cause an imbalance favoring the production of vasoconstrictors. Impaired endothelial-dependent vasodilation in SSc may be due both to overexpression of the potent vasoconstrictor endothelin-1 (ET-1) and reduced production of the vasodilators nitric oxide (NO) and prostacyclin.

Endothelin-1

ET-1 is a powerful dose-dependent vasoconstrictor. At low concentrations, ET-1 is vasodilator, while at higher concentrations, it mediates vasoconstriction and reduction of blood flow [27]. ET-1 is overexpressed in the skin of SSc patients [28, 29]. Moreover, the circulating levels of ET-1 and tissue concentrations of ET-1 in the lungs, kidneys, and liver are elevated in SSc [30–33].

Early studies showed that ET-1 induces fibroblast proliferation and collagen synthesis in a dose-dependent manner, potentially linking ET-1 to vascular dysfunction and fibrosis. ET-1 acts through the endothelin receptors type A (ET_A) and type B (ET_B) that are expressed on various cell types. An imbalanced expression of ET_A and ET_B receptors has been reported in SSc patients [34, 35]. The role of endogenous ET-1 in EC dysfunction was examined in tight-skin mice (TSK1), a mouse model of SSc [36]. The mesenteric arteries of TSK1 mice showed decrease responses to acetylcholine, suggesting impaired NO-independent, prostaglandin-mediated relaxation that was partially restored by the dual endothelin receptor antagonist (ERA) bosentan [37], suggesting a role for ET1 in the impaired vasodilation.

ET-1 also stimulates VSMC proliferation and contraction, possibly contributing to remodeling of the vascular wall and vasculopathic manifestations characteristic of SSc, such as PAH and digital ulcers. Indeed, clinical studies have shown that ERAs may be effective in the treatment of SSc-related PAH and in the prevention of digital ulcers [38, 39]. Treatment with the ERA bosentan may also improve peripheral microcirculation in SSc patients, as demonstrated by the shifting from the "late" to the "active" nailfold videocapillaroscopy pattern after therapy [40]. In another study, long-term treatment with bosentan in combination with iloprost reduced the progression of nailfold microvascular damage in SSc patients over a 3-year follow-up period [41].

Nitric Oxide

NO can play a dual role in the endothelium, depending on which NO synthase (NOS) catalyzes its synthesis from

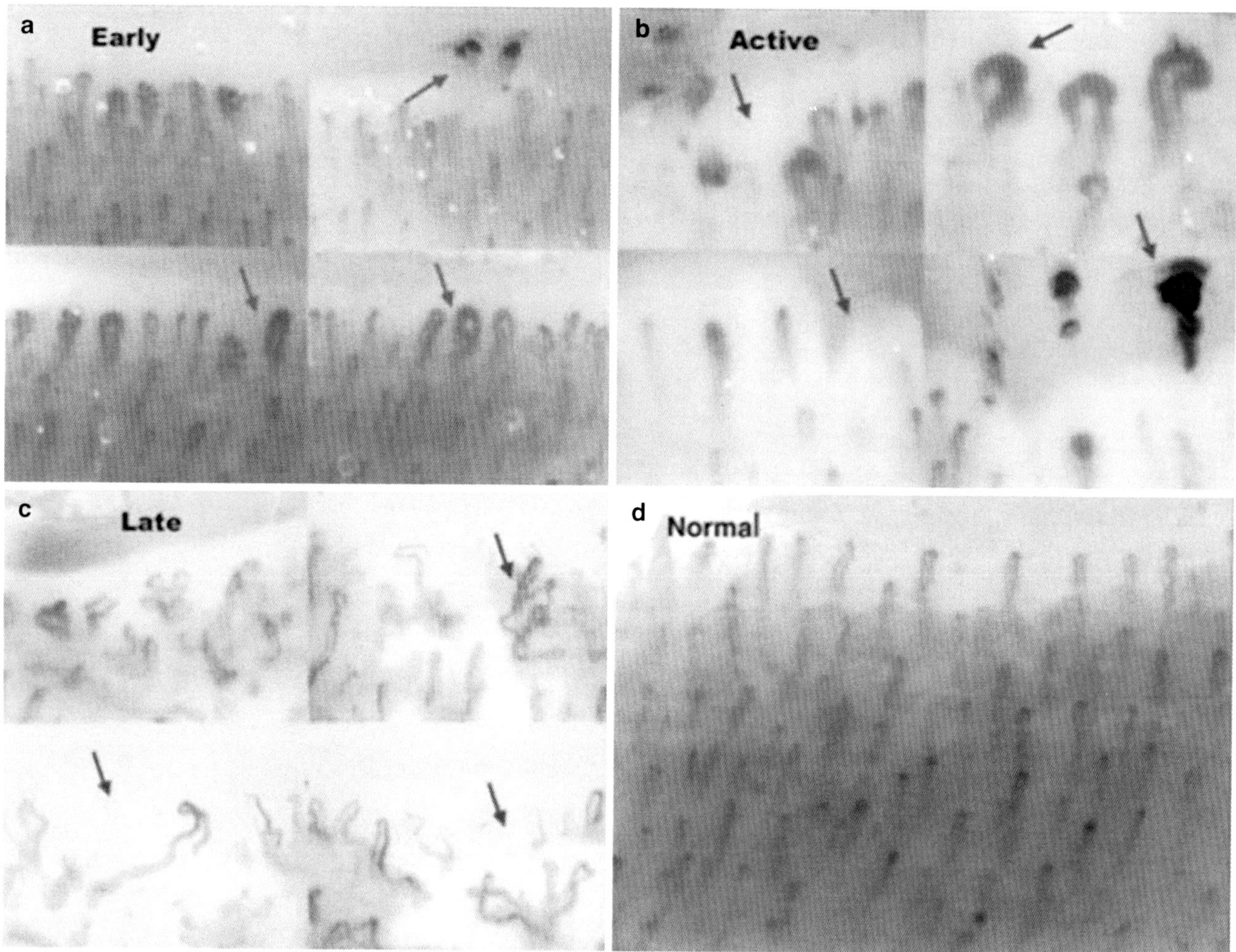

Fig. 16.2 Nailfold capillaroscopy. (**a**) Early scleroderma pattern shows well-preserved capillary architecture and density and presence of dilated and giant capillaries. (**b**) Active scleroderma pattern shows frequent giant capillaries and hemorrhages, moderate loss of capillaries, and disorganization of capillary architecture. (**c**) Late scleroderma pattern shows severe capillary architecture disorganization with dropouts, presence of arborized capillaries, and absence of giant capillaries. (**d**) Normal nailfold capillaroscopic pattern (Courtesy of Cutolo et al. [22], published by Oxford University Press. With permission)

L-arginine. Mammals produce three NOS isoforms. Two are expressed in the endothelium; endothelial NO synthase (eNOS) is expressed in ECs, whereas inducible NO synthase (iNOS) is expressed in ECs, VSMCs, fibroblasts, macrophages, and other cell types [42]. Endothelial NOS plays an important role in maintaining vasorelaxation and in controlling vascular tone, blood pressure, and thrombosis [43]. Disruption of the endothelium reduces NO synthesis and release with significant consequences to the vasculature. Deficient endothelial-dependent relaxation in SSc is suggested by impaired maximal responses to endothelial-dependent vasodilators and normal responses to endothelial-independent dilators [44–47].

Despite the expectation that NO production would be reduced in a dysfunctional endothelium, NOx (NO and NO_2) levels appear to be elevated in SSc patients, as shown by immunohistochemical studies on skin biopsies [48]. This is probably related to the upregulation of iNOS expression in association with increased levels of immunodetectable nitrotyrosine, a marker of NO-mediated free radical injury [49]. Thus, endothelial dysfunction in SSc may be in part attributable to abnormal regulation of the NO pathway.

Nature of the Endothelial Injury

The triggers for vascular injury and dysfunction in SSc are largely unknown. However, infectious agents, EC cytotoxicity, activation and apoptosis, autoantibodies, shear stress, and ischemia/reperfusion are among the potential contributors. Current hypotheses in the pathogenesis of SSc vascular disease implicate a possible, yet unidentified, microbial trigger and an immune-mediated activation that lead to vascular injury and the generation of progressive occlusive arteriolar disease (Fig. 16.3).

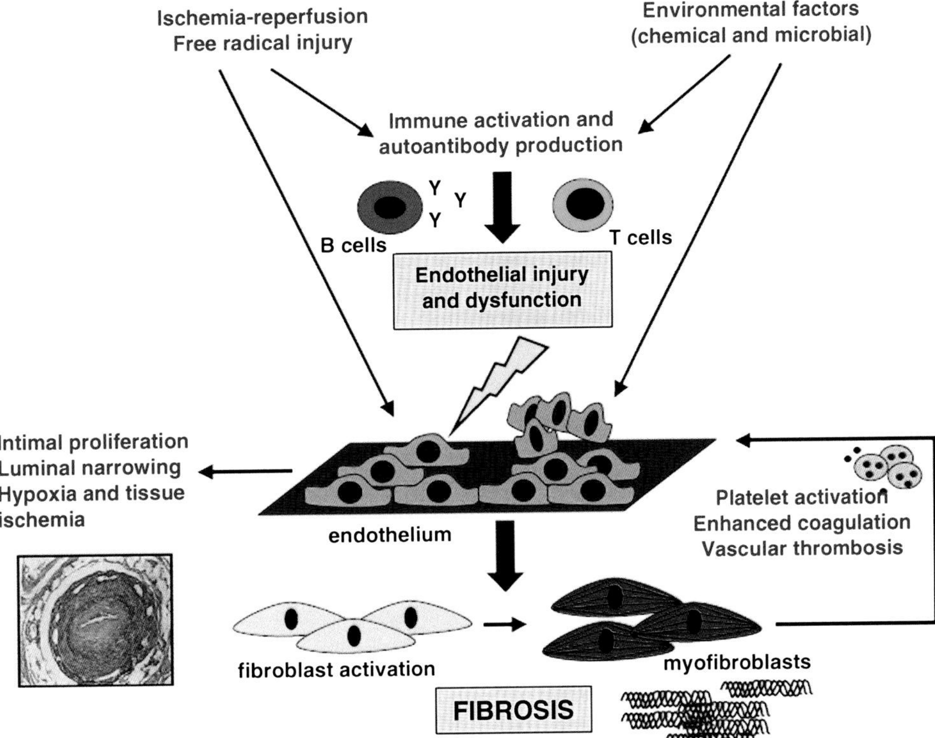

Fig. 16.3 Pathogenesis of SSc vasculopathy. Endothelial injury and dysfunction is initiated by the actions of free radicals and environmental, chemical, or microbial agents that injure the endothelium either directly or indirectly by the induction of immune activation and the generation of autoantibodies and activated cellular immunity. The vascular injury leads to the activation of platelet and coagulation pathways that result in vascular microthrombosis. The resulting vasculopathy is associated with intimal hyperplasia in the small arterioles, and the ensuing luminal narrowing results in tissue hypoxia and the generation of the state of chronic ischemia. Released vascular products, in association with hypoxia and ischemia, collectively contribute to the activation of resident fibroblasts that transdifferentiate into profibrotic myofibroblasts and, in turn, perpetuate the vasculopathy by triggering vascular wall fibrosis

Microbial Triggers

Infectious agents may be part of the etiology of SSc, but the evidence is indirect. In one study, patients with RP were treated with triple antibiotics to eliminate *Helicobacter pylori* infection, a gastric bacterium associated with other vascular diseases [50]. The treatment regimen resulted in the disappearance of RP in 17 % of the patients and reduced symptoms in 72 % [51]. Other studies evaluated the incidence of *Helicobacter pylori* infection in SSc patients [52]; one study showed a higher correlation, while others showed none [53, 54].

Cytomegalovirus (CMV) infection may play a role in the pathogenesis of SSc vasculopathy. CMV infects ECs and monocytes/macrophages leading to dysregulation of the immune system and upregulation of fibrogenic cytokines [14, 55], events that are also characteristic of SSc. Indirect evidence supporting a role for CMV includes the presence of CMV antibodies in serum from SSc patients that could potentially interact with autoantigens [55, 56]. Rat and mouse models show that CMV infection leads to formation of intimal lesions [57, 58]. An immune-suppressed mouse model of CMV-induced neointima development has many characteristics of SSc including EC apoptosis, myofibroblast differentiation, and increased expression of transforming growth factor-β (TGF-β) and platelet-derived growth factor (PDGF). However, a significant difference between this model and human SSc is that the vascular lesions develop in the main abdominal vessels, while in SSc, the lesions occur in the microvasculature [59].

Parvovirus B19 has also been implicated in the pathogenesis of SSc. Parvovirus B19 is much more commonly found as an active infection in SSc patients (4 %) than the general population (0.6 %) [60]. Parvovirus B19 was detected in bone marrow biopsies from a high percentage of SSc patients (57 %), who did not have an active B19 infection [61]. Further studies found a correlation between B19 expression levels and the severity of endothelial dysfunction in SSc [62]. This suggests a potential role for this virus in SSc pathogenesis.

Endothelial Cell Cytotoxicity, Apoptosis, and Activation

The evidence of EC injury in SSc patients prompted studies to investigate the presence of potential cytotoxic factors in their serum. Some studies suggest that the cytotoxic effect of SSc plasma on ECs is antibody dependent [63–65]. Sgonc et al. showed that activated natural killer (NK) cells are required for antiendothelial cell antibody (AECA)-dependent apoptosis in human dermal microvascular ECs (MVECs) [66]. Two different cytotoxic mechanisms can be stimulated by NK cells: a granzyme/perforin synergistic mechanism and Fas/FasL interaction [67].

Kahaleh et al. reported a circulating proteolytic EC cytotoxic factor in plasma of SSc patients [68]. In a later study, they identified a granular enzyme, thought to be granzyme A that significantly inhibited EC growth [69].

Granzyme B (GrB), a serine protease found in cytoplasmic granules of NK cells and T lymphocytes, is protective against various pathogens [70, 71]. Some studies demonstrate that GrB cleaves vitronectin, fibronectin, and laminin, three proteins that have a primary role in ECM function, and consequently inhibits cell migration, spreading, and invasion [72]. Other studies have shown that the proteolytic activity of GrB and other proteases contained in T-cell granules cleaves plasminogen and plasmin into angiostatin fragments [73], which have multiple consequences in the ECM; plasminogen cleavage in the kringle domains produces antiangiogenic angiostatin, the pool of plasminogen that can be converted to plasmin is reduced, and subsequently, plasmin activity and its effects on regulating ECM composition become limited. Evidence indicates that this mechanism may be enhanced in SSc plasma contributing to increased levels of angiostatin [73].

A number of ECM cleavage products are inhibitors of angiogenesis; they all induce EC apoptosis. These antiangiogenic fragments include the collagen XV and XVIII breakdown product endostatin [74], collagen IV breakdown product tumstatin [75] and canstatin [76], plasminogen breakdown product angiostatin [73, 77], and 18-kDa prolactin fragment [78], among others [79]. Under normal conditions, antiangiogenic factors are tightly regulated to maintain a balance with proangiogenic factors. In addition to elevated plasma angiostatin levels [73], in SSc, there is evidence of elevated levels of endostatin [80, 81] which suggests an imbalance that favors angiogenesis inhibitors with proapoptotic activity.

Antibody-Dependent Cellular Cytotoxicity

Autoimmunity is a major component of SSc. Interestingly, all autoantigens are redistributed and clustered in blebs or apoptotic bodies on the cell surface of apoptotic cells despite their varied functions, structures, and cellular localization [82]. This led Casciola-Rosen et al. to propose that reactive oxygen species (ROS) in the blebs and apoptotic bodies may produce fragments of autoantigens which expose cryptic epitopes recognized by T cells [82]. This hypothesis has been supported by others showing that posttranslational protein alterations expose cryptic cleavage sites with significance in selection of autoantigens [83, 84]. The role of GrB cleavage of autoantigens is suggested by the presence of autoantibodies that recognize GrB-generated autoantigen fragments particularly in limited SSc (lSSc) patients with ischemic digital loss [85–87].

Antiendothelial Cell Antibodies (AECAs)

Circulating autoantibodies to ECs (AECAs) are found in 44–84 % of SSc patients in clinical trials [88, 89]. A greater incidence of AECAs is found in patients with digital ischemia or PAH [90, 91]. Interestingly, AECAs bind distinctly different micro- and macrovascular EC antigens in SSc patients with associated PAH and in patients with idiopathic PAH as compared to SSc patients without PAH [92]. The variant affinities could potentially be used as a predictor of more advanced vascular disease in SSc patients.

The role of AECAs in the induction of EC apoptosis is suggested by findings in the avian model of SSc (UCD 200/2006 chickens) [4]. EC apoptosis was noted following the transfer of AECAs into normal chick embryos [93]; however, apoptosis was also noted in other cell types making it difficult to determine if apoptosis results directly from AECAs binding or if it is part of normal embryogenesis.

SSc sera containing autoantibodies were shown to induce EC apoptosis [94]. A caspase inhibitor could only partially inhibit the apoptosis, suggesting that additional factors are involved in the induction of apoptosis. One such factor may be the ECM microfibrillar protein fibrillin-1. Autoantibodies to fibrillin-1 are found in a large proportion of SSc patients [95]. Fibrillin-1 expression was detected in apoptotic ECs (identified in the blebs and apoptotic bodies) exposed to SSc serum containing AECAs. These data suggest that AECAs found in SSc serum may induce fibrillin-1 expression and EC apoptosis, but the evidence is indirect.

Besides apoptosis, more recently, it has been reported that AECAs may play an important role in activating ECs [96]. Arends et al. demonstrated that immunoglobulins G (IgG) from AECA-positive SSc patients, patients with idiopathic PAH, and patients with systemic lupus erythematosus activate MVECs with increased expression of intercellular adhesion molecule-1 (ICAM-1) [96]. However, disease specificity for this observation is not established. Moreover, Wolf et al. reported significant elevation of anti-ICAM-1 IgM antibodies in the sera of both lSSc and diffuse SSc (dSSc) patients, while elevated anti-ICAM-1 IgG antibodies were found only in lSSc patients [97]. Moreover, anti-ICAM-1 IgG antibodies bind to ECs leading to a significant increase in ROS production [97].

Shear Stress and SSc Vascular Disease

Intimal hypertrophy and vascular remodeling are major contributors to vascular complications and mortality in SSc [98–100]. Key factors that contribute to vascular wall remodeling are shear stress, chronic hypoxia, and inflammation.

Increased shear stress impacts many aspects of the vascular wall. It can enhance EC and VSMC proliferation, increase levels of inflammatory molecules such as interleukin-8 (IL-8), promote ROS and collagen production, and inhibit eNOS levels and EC repair.

Increased cyclic stretch, which accompanies shear stress, plays an important role in regulating EC phenotype and gene expression by inducing ROS production. This leads to increased permeability, production of vascular endothelial growth factor (VEGF) and fibroblast growth factor (FGF), apoptosis and cytoskeletal remodeling and increased production of ECM, matrix-degrading enzymes, and inflammation [101, 102]. In this manner, increased cyclic stretch could partially explain the increased formation of ECM in disorders such as SSc. Cyclic stretch causes a much greater loss of endothelial barrier function in response to VEGF stimulation compared to no stretch controls; this effect is partially ameliorated by adding a ROS scavenger to the cells [101].

Reperfusion and Oxidative Injury

The concept that ischemia/reperfusion generates ROS was reported by McCord in 1985 [103]. Ischemia/reperfusion associated with RP leads to ROS generation that may contribute to vascular endothelial damage. Reactive oxygen and nitrogen species can contribute to vascular damage through peroxidation of lipids, oxidation of proteins, or a flawed antioxidant defense system such as that described for NO. Thus, significant decrease in total plasma antioxidant capacity was noted in SSc patients [104]. Moreover, antioxidant levels inversely correlated with the severity of RP and with capillary loss, suggesting that oxidative stress worsens in advanced microvasculature disease. In addition, increased levels of oxidative stress markers were reported and correlated with the overall severity of the disease [105]. A role for autoantibodies in deficient oxidative stress defense was suggested by the presence of autoantibodies that inhibit the oxidative stress repair enzyme methionine sulfoxide reductase A and B (MSRA and MSRB [106–108]) in SSc patients [109]. The antibody titer correlated with renal vascular damage and inversely correlated with pulmonary function [109].

Agonistic Antibodies to the Platelet-Derived Growth Factor Receptor and Generation of ROS

Baroni et al. identified autoantibodies in the sera of SSc patients that interact with and activate the receptor for platelet-derived growth factor (PDGFR), resulting in ROS accumulation in target cells that can potentially account for tissue injury [110]. Furthermore, these antibodies are capable of upregulating the expression of α-smooth muscle actin (α-SMA) and type I collagen in fibroblasts. Of note, these genes are characteristically overexpressed in SSc fibroblasts. It is interesting to note that PDGFR plays an important role in angiogenesis related to ischemic tissue and tumor growth [111]; nevertheless, the possible vascular consequences of the receptor activation in SSc are not known. Moreover, subsequent reports were unable to confirm the presence of stimulatory anti-PDGFR antibodies in SSc sera. Differences in the methodologies of these studies might account for the discrepant results, and further investigations are needed to further dissect the role of stimulatory anti-PDGFR antibodies in SSc [112].

Epigenetics and SSc Vasculopathy

The basis for EC dysfunction and altered cellular phenotype in SSc has not been determined, but primary metabolic abnormalities, responses to abnormal environmental signals, and clonal selection have all been hypothesized to play a role [113]. Nonetheless, SSc cellular abnormalities persist in multiple generations in vitro. The persistence of dysfunctional phenotype outside the disease environment suggests the possibility of an in vivo imprinting of disease phenotype that is inherited and is transmitted from one generation to the next. The term epigenetics describes all inherited changes in gene expression that are not coded in the DNA sequence itself. The two major mechanisms that are known to mediate epigenetic changes are DNA methylation and histone modification. More recently, microRNAs (miRNAs) have been identified as a major contributor to gene expression through posttranscriptional mechanisms [114] and thus were added to the epigenetic machinery.

Methylation of the CpG dinucleotides has long been recognized as a major epigenetic modification of the mammalian genome and is implicated in imprinting, X chromosome inactivation, embryonic development, defense against retroviral sequences, transcriptional repression of certain genes, and carcinogenesis [115, 116]. CpG islands are stretches of DNA located within the promoter regions of about 40 % of mammalian genes. The methylation of CpG islands leads to a stable, heritable repression of transcription of the affected gene. DNA methylation is the most widely studied epigenetic mechanism in autoimmune diseases and is considered the core epigenetic control mechanism. DNA methylation is accomplished by the de novo DNA methyltransferases (DNMTs) DNMT3a and DNMT3b, while an existing methylation pattern is maintained during cell division and thus inherited in proliferating cells by DNMT1 [117].

There is emerging evidence suggesting that alteration of DNA methylation profiles at global or gene-specific levels may contribute to SSc pathogenesis. Endothelial nitric oxide synthase gene (NOS3) expression is reduced in SSc skin and cultured ECs [118]. Data suggest that heavy methylation of the CpG sites in the promoter region of NOS3 gene leads to gene repression and that the addition of DNMT1 inhibitor 5-azacytidine leads to normalization of NOS3 expression. The significance of underexpression of NOS3 is illustrated by the fact that NOS3-null mice are characterized by systemic and pulmonary hypertension, impaired wound healing and angiogenesis, and impaired mobilization of stem and endothelial precursors, leading to failure of neovascularization [119, 120]. Another endothelial gene that appears to be regulated by epigenetic control is bone morphogenic protein receptor II (BMPRII). BMPs are members of the TGF-β superfamily of proteins that coordinate cell proliferation, differentiation, and survival. The latter is particularly true for ECs, since BMP signaling through BMPRII favors EC survival and apoptosis resistance. An inactivating mutation in the BMPRII gene has been linked to primary pulmonary hypertension suggesting a crucial role in the development of PAH-related vasculopathy [121]. In SSc, significant decrease in the expression levels of BMPRII in ECs and skin was described [122]. This was shown to be associated with enhanced responses of SSc ECs to apoptotic signals, including serum starvation and oxidation injury. Sequencing the BMPRII promoter region after bisulfite conversion demonstrated heavy methylation of CpG sites in BMPRII promoter in SSc ECs. BMPRII expression levels and the enhanced EC apoptotic responses were normalized by the addition of 5-azacytidine. These data suggest that epigenetic repression of BMPRII gene may play a central role in EC vulnerability to apoptosis and that impaired BMPRII signaling in SSc ECs may contribute to the pathogenesis of SSc vasculopathy [122].

The exact nature of epigenetic triggers in SSc is not known, but both hypoxia and oxidation injury are suggested triggers, as well as nutrients and other environmental factors [123].

Defective Vascular Regeneration in SSc

Vasculopathy in SSc is systemic, progressive, and often irreversible. This suggests that structural changes culminating in the obliteration and loss of the microvasculature are not normally repaired by either a compensatory growth of new vessels from existing vessels (angiogenesis) or de novo formation of new vessels (vasculogenesis). Both defective angiogenic pathways, as well as abnormalities in the release of bone marrow-derived progenitor cells, which have the potential to initiate vascular repair, have been identified in SSc patients.

Defective Angiogenesis: The Proangiogenic to Antiangiogenic Switch

Tissue ischemia and hypoxia are usually the main triggers for angiogenesis through the upregulation of proangiogenic factors, which then initiate angiogenic sprouting from preexisting microvessels by inducing vasodilation, proliferation, and migration of ECs, invasion of the surrounding extracellular matrix, and formation and stabilization of the vascular lumen of newly formed capillary vessels [124]. However, despite chronic tissue ischemia and progressive loss of microvessels in multiple vascular beds, compensatory angiogenesis is dysregulated and insufficient, and it does not allow vascular recovery in the course of SSc [125, 126].

Increasing evidence indicates that a dysregulated expression of a large array of proangiogenic and antiangiogenic factors may be largely responsible for the impaired angiogenic response found in patients with SSc [125, 126]. The nailfold capillaroscopic changes observed in the course of SSc may be explained by the action of different factors on angiogenesis. In the early stages of the disease, a proinflammatory state and an increased production of proangiogenic factors may stimulate angiogenesis. As a result, capillaroscopic analysis of the nailfold bed demonstrates the presence of microhemorrhages and tortuous, giant capillary loops, which are immature and instable microvessels presumably formed during an uncontrolled angiogenic response. This short proangiogenic response is followed by a dramatic impairment of the angiogenic process which might in part be explained by the action of several antiangiogenic factors, ultimately resulting in reduced capillary density and extensive avascular areas. Thus, the dramatic switch from proangiogenic to antiangiogenic characteristics suggests that the angiogenic process becomes impaired.

However, the functional role of angiogenic mediators in the disease pathogenesis is still poorly understood. Interestingly, while both several proangiogenic and antiangiogenic factors are overexpressed in SSc [125, 126], there appears to be an imbalance in the ratio of these mediators, favoring inhibition of angiogenesis and progressive vascular disease (Table 16.1).

Among the proangiogenic factors, VEGF is considered one of the most potent regulators of physiologic and pathologic angiogenesis and is overexpressed in most angiogenic conditions. Surprisingly, several studies have demonstrated enhanced expression of VEGF in both the skin and the circu-

Table 16.1 Dysregulated proangiogenic and antiangiogenic mediators in SSc

Proangiogenic	Antiangiogenic
VEGF	Endostatin
FGF-2	Angiostatin
Platelet-derived growth factor	Pentraxin 3
Interleukin-8/CXCL8	$VEGF_{165}b$
Stromal cell-derived factor 1/CXCL12	IP-10/CXCL10
Interleukin-6	MIG/CXCL9
CXCL16	Angiopoietin 2
EGFL7	Interleukin-4
Tissue kallikrein	Platelet factor 4
Kallikrein 9, 11, and 12	Soluble endoglin
Fractalkine/CX3CL1	Thrombospondin 1
Placental growth factor (PlGF)	Kallikrein 3

lation of SSc patients throughout different disease stages [125, 127–131]. The paradox is that VEGF levels, rather than being associated with evidence of angiogenesis, actually correlate with progressive microvascular loss and disease progression. In fact, a positive correlation was found between VEGF levels and the severity of nailfold capillary loss as well as with the extent of skin fibrosis measured by Rodnan skin thickness score [130]. Moreover, VEGFR-1 and VEGFR-2 are also upregulated on dermal ECs in SSc-affected skin [129, 131]. Nevertheless, there is also evidence suggesting that VEGF receptor signaling may be impaired in SSc based on the observation that dermal MVECs isolated from SSc patients show impaired response to VEGF in vitro [132].

As an explanation for the "VEGF paradox," it has been shown that VEGF-A primary transcript can be alternatively spliced in its terminal exon, producing two distinct mRNA splice variants that are translated to the proangiogenic $VEGF_{165}$ and antiangiogenic $VEGF_{165}b$ isoforms. Of interest, Manetti et al. reported that the increase in VEGF in SSc skin was the result of a significant increase in the antiangiogenic $VEGF_{165}b$ isoform instead of $VEGF_{165}$ [133]. Moreover, they provided evidence that circulating levels of $VEGF_{165}b$ were raised in SSc and that these increased levels were both early and persistent features of the disease. In addition, MVECs isolated from SSc skin constitutively expressed and released higher levels of $VEGF_{165}b$ than did MVECs from healthy individuals [133]. Interestingly, $VEGF_{165}$ and $VEGF_{165}b$ isoforms bind to the tyrosine kinase receptor VEGFR-2 with the same affinity, but binding of $VEGF_{165}b$ results in an insufficient tyrosine phosphorylation/activation of VEGFR-2 and incomplete or transient downstream signaling, which leads to an impaired angiogenic response [127]. Accordingly, SSc MVECs expressed higher levels of VEGFR-2 but also showed impaired phosphorylation/activation of this receptor, reduced activation of extracellular signal-regulated kinase (ERK)1/2, and impaired capillary morphogenesis in vitro [133]. Of note, treatment with recombinant $VEGF_{165}b$, as well as with conditioned media from SSc MVECs, inhibited $VEGF_{165}$-mediated VEGFR-2 phosphorylation, ERK1/2 signaling, and capillary morphogenesis in healthy MVECs, and these antiangiogenic effects could be abrogated by the administration of anti-$VEGF_{165}b$ neutralizing antibodies. The angiogenic potential of SSc MVECs is significantly impaired, but can be restored by the addition of combination of high-dose recombinant $VEGF_{165}$ and anti-$VEGF_{165}b$-blocking antibodies [133]. Finally, it is interesting to note that the switch from proangiogenic to antiangiogenic VEGF isoforms may be driven by TGF-β and the SRp55 splicing factor [133]. In another recent study, Manetti et al. [134] have reported that plasma levels of the antiangiogenic $VEGF_{165}b$ isoform correlated with the severity of capillary architectural loss and derangement, further suggesting that $VEGF_{165}b$ may participate in the loss of microvessels in SSc (Fig. 16.4).

A dysregulated expression of different chemokines and their receptors has also been linked to disturbed angiogenesis in SSc. In particular, antiangiogenic chemokines lacking the enzyme-linked receptor (ELR) motif, such as monokine induced by interferon-γ (IFN-γ) (MIG/CXCL9) and IFN-inducible protein 10 (IP-10/CXCL10), are elevated in SSc serum, whereas the expression of their receptor CXCR3 is downregulated on SSc dermal ECs [135]. In contrast, proangiogenic CXCL16 and its receptor CXCR6 are elevated in SSc serum and on SSc dermal ECs, respectively [135]. Thus, these findings may suggest that angiogenic chemokine receptor expression is likely regulated in an effort to promote angiogenesis.

Elevated levels of antiangiogenic pentraxin 3 (PTX3), a multifunctional pattern recognition protein that can suppress fibroblast growth factor 2 (FGF-2) proangiogenic function, have been associated with vascular manifestations of SSc [136]. Circulating PTX3 and FGF-2 levels were significantly higher in SSc patients than in healthy subjects. Moreover, circulating levels of PTX3 are elevated in SSc patients with digital ulcers or PAH, while FGF-2 is reduced in SSc patients with PAH. Multivariate analysis identified elevated PTX3 as an independent parameter associated with the presence of digital ulcers and PAH, and PTX3 levels were a useful predictor of future occurrences of digital ulcers. Reduced FGF-2 was independently associated with the presence of PAH [136].

In another recent study, Manetti et al. investigated the possible involvement of epidermal growth factor-like domain 7 (EGFL7), a unique proangiogenic molecule which is predominantly expressed and secreted by ECs and their progenitors and controls vascular development and integrity [137]. Circulating levels and dermal expression of EGFL7 were significantly decreased in SSc patients. Remarkably, the decrease of serum EGFL7 levels in SSc patients correlated with the severity of nailfold capillary abnormalities and

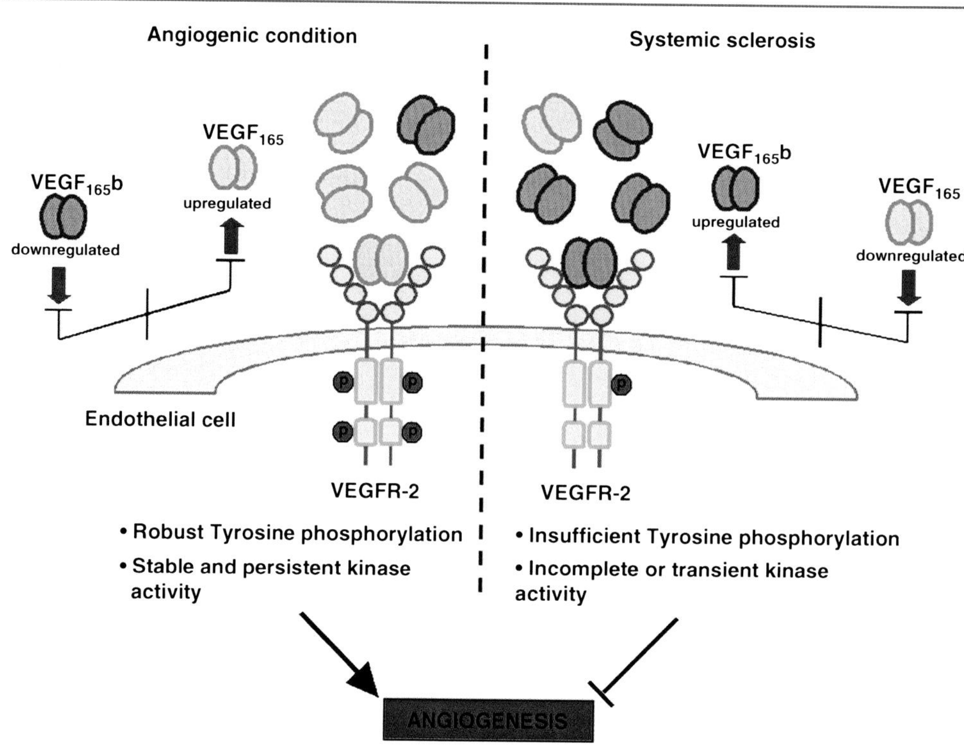

Fig. 16.4 In most angiogenic conditions, such as cancers, proangiogenic $VEGF_{165}$ predominates, whereas in deficient angiogenic conditions, such as SSc, the balance shifts to favor the expression of the $VEGF_{165}b$ antiangiogenic isoform. The two isoforms bind to VEGFR-2 with the same affinity, but binding of $VEGF_{165}b$ results in an insufficient tyrosine phosphorylation/activation of VEGFR-2 and incomplete or transient downstream signaling, which lead to impaired angiogenic response

presence of digital ulcers. In contrast to constitutive endothelial expression of EGFL7 in healthy skin, EGFL7 was found to be strongly reduced or even undetectable in SSc dermal microvessels. Furthermore, EGFL7 protein was found to be significantly downregulated in vitro in dermal MVECs obtained from SSc patients compared with control cells. Thus, it has been suggested that the loss of EGFL7 expression might contribute to the development and progression of peripheral microvascular damage and defective vascular repair process in SSc patients [137].

Defective Vasculogenesis

In the past, it had been thought that impaired angiogenesis and increased apoptosis of mature ECs were exclusively responsible for the microvascular abnormalities in SSc. However, several studies published over the last few years suggest that impairment of vasculogenesis (i.e., the generation of new blood vessels by stem or progenitor cells) and vascular repair may be also involved in SSc capillary loss, as shown by altered numbers and functional defects of circulating EPCs [125]. In fact, new blood vessels can be formed in the adult not only by the sprouting of fully differentiated ECs but also by recruitment of circulating progenitor cells, independently of the preexisting vasculature [138]. In particular, a subset of bone marrow-derived $CD34^+$ progenitor cells can acquire the characteristics of mature ECs, express EC markers, and incorporate into new capillary vessels at sites of ischemia [138]. Postnatal vasculogenesis contributes to vascular healing in response to vascular injury through the processes of rapid re-endothelialization of denuded vessels and collateral vessel formation in ischemic tissues. In this process, EPCs (identified as $CD34^+/CD133^+/VEGFR\text{-}2^+$ cells) are mobilized from their bone marrow niches into the circulation in response to stress- and/or damage-related signals and migrate through the bloodstream and home to the sites of vascular injury, where they extravasate through the endothelium and contribute to the formation of neovessels and the repair of damaged vasculature working in concert with preexisting mature ECs.

Several studies have analyzed the levels of circulating EPCs in the peripheral blood of SSc patients in comparison with healthy controls and/or other rheumatic conditions [125, 139, 140]. Although conflicting results have been reported, a possible correlation between reduction in the number of EPCs and severity of peripheral vascular manifestations has been demonstrated [141]. Moreover, it has been shown that SSc serum may induce EPC apoptosis and that this might account, at least in part, for the decreased numbers of circulating EPCs in SSc patients [142]. AECAs may also be directly responsible for apoptosis of EPCs in SSc [143]. In another study, EPC (defined as $CD34^+/CD133^+/CD309^+$) counts were significantly lower in SSc patients with digital ulcers or PAH and correlated negatively with circulating levels of antiangiogenic PTX3 [136]. Interestingly, PTX3 inhibited differentiation of EPCs in vitro [136]. Moreover, EPCs from SSc patients exhibited an impaired in vivo neovascularization capacity in a model of cotransplantation of immunomagnetically sorted circulating EPCs and murine colon carcinoma CT-26 cells beneath the skin of severe combined immunodeficiency (SCID) mice [144].

In addition to CD34+ EPCs, it has been proposed that bone marrow-derived CD14+ monocytes can serve as a subset of EPCs because of their expression of endothelial markers and ability to promote neovascularization in vitro and in vivo [145]. However, the current consensus is that monocytic cells do not give rise to ECs in vivo, but rather function as support cells, by promoting vascular formation and repair through their recruitment to the site of vascular injury, secretion of proangiogenic factors, and differentiation into mural cells (VSMCs and pericytes). These CD14+ monocytes that function in a supporting role in vascular repair are now termed monocytic proangiogenic hematopoietic cells (PHCs) [145]. Yamaguchi et al. recently showed that in patients with SSc, circulating monocytic PHCs increase dramatically in association with enhanced angiogenic potency, suggesting that these compensatory effects may be induced in response to defective vascular repair machinery [145].

Cipriani et al. examined the in vitro capacity of bone marrow-derived mesenchymal stem cells (MSCs) to differentiate toward the EC lineage [146]. In SSc patients, the percentage of VEGFR-2+ and CXCR4+ MSCs and endothelial-like MSCs was significantly lower than in controls. Accordingly, both SSc MSCs and endothelial-like MSCs displayed impaired responses to VEGF- and stromal cell-derived factor-1 (SDF-1)-induced migration, invasion and capillary-like structure formation on Matrigel, as well as an early senescence [146]. These data collectively suggest that endothelial repair may be affected in SSc starting from bone marrow stem niches. However, despite an impaired commitment toward the endothelial phenotype, Guiducci et al. [147] demonstrated that SSc bone marrow-derived MSCs exhibit an intact, or even potentiated, proangiogenic paracrine machinery that is suitable for autologous therapeutic approaches. Indeed, SSc MSCs overexpress different proangiogenic growth factors and are able to promote dermal EC sprouting angiogenesis in vitro [147]. In agreement with these findings, the same authors reported that intravenous infusion of culture-expanded autologous bone marrow-derived MSCs could regenerate the peripheral vascular network in a case of SSc complicated by acute gangrene of the extremities [148]. Other observations have provided support for the efficacy of MSCs in treating intractable digital ulcers, where autologous injection of MSCs led to a reduction in the size of the ulcers, an increase in blood flow, and the formation of new capillaries [149].

The Plasminogen Activator Pathway

The plasminogen activator (PA) pathway plays key roles in angiogenesis. Plasminogen is a precursor of proangiogenic plasmin [150] and a precursor of antiangiogenic angiostatin [77]; therefore, it plays a complicated role in the regulation of vascular homeostasis. Plasminogen can be cleaved at the carboxy terminus by PA to produce plasmin, a proteolytic and fibrinolytic protease. Its proteolytic activity activates many key proangiogenic factors including VEGF [151], TGF-β [152] and matrix metalloproteinases (MMPs) [153]. Plasminogen can also be cleaved within its amino terminus kringle domains by a number of proteases [154, 155]. The cleaved kringle domain fragments are angiostatin of various sizes with different antiangiogenic activity. Thus, alterations in plasminogen processing can have a profound effect on angiogenic homeostasis.

Plasmin activity is reduced in SSc while the amount of circulating angiostatin is increased [73]. This proangiogenic/antiangiogenic imbalance was manifested by reduced migration and proliferation of normal human dermal MVECs when exposed to SSc patients' plasma. Interestingly, exposure of normal dermal MVECs to angiostatin in amounts similar to those detected in SSc plasma resulted in a significant impairment of cell migration and ability to form vascular structures in collagen gels [73].

The PA pathway is further implicated in SSc by studies that examined the importance of urokinase plasminogen activator receptor (uPAR) in ECs isolated from SSc patients' skin biopsies. uPAR plays an important role in cell motility, adhesion, and matrix invasion through its binding interactions with urokinase plasminogen activator (uPA) [156], vitronectin [157], and intracellular signaling mediators, such as the integrin receptors [158]. D'Alessio et al. have shown that in dermal MVECs isolated from SSc skin, uPAR undergoes truncation between domains 1 and 2, a cleavage that is known to impair uPAR functions [132]. The uPAR cleavage in SSc MVECs was associated with the overexpression of MMP-12 [132]. Indeed, overproduction of MMP-12 by SSc dermal MVECs and fibroblasts accounts for endothelial uPAR cleavage leading to impaired uPA-induced MVECs migration, invasion, proliferation, and capillary morphogenesis on Matrigel [132]. Strikingly, treatment with an anti-MMP-12 monoclonal antibody was able to restore the angiogenic activity of normal MVECs treated with conditioned media from SSc MVECs [132, 159]. Furthermore, uPAR cleavage in SSc MVECs results in loss of integrin-mediated uPAR connection with the actin cytoskeleton [159]. The uncoupling of cleaved uPAR from β2 integrins impairs the activation of the small Rho GTPases Rac and Cdc42 and thus inhibits uPAR-dependent cytoskeletal rearrangement and cell motility, and ultimately resulting in impaired angiogenesis [159]. In a subsequent study, the same authors reported that MMP-12 gene silencing could in part restore the ability of SSc MVECs to produce capillary structures in vitro [160]. Moreover, elevated levels of MMP-12 in the circulation of SSc patients were associated with the severity of nailfold capillary abnormalities and the presence of digital ulcers [161]. Interestingly, elevated MMP-12 may suppress angiogenesis not only through the cleavage and subsequent inactivation of uPAR [132] but also through the proteolysis of plasminogen and generation of angiostatin [162].

Microarray Studies Revealing Altered Balance of Proangiogenic and Antiangiogenic Factors in SSc

Gene expression levels of proangiogenic and antiangiogenic factors have been analyzed in microarray studies which compared the transcriptome profiling of dermal MVECs isolated from skin biopsies from normal individuals and SSc patients [163, 164]. One microarray gene expression study detected important differences between normal and SSc MVECs in the kallikrein gene family [163]. Proangiogenic kallikreins 9, 11, and 12 were downregulated in SSc MVECs, whereas antiangiogenic kallikrein 3 was upregulated. The microarray data were further validated in experiments using normal MVECs treated with antibodies against kallikreins 9, 11, and 12 and subsequently analyzed in migration, proliferation, and capillary morphogenesis functional assays. All three antibodies were able to block angiogenesis in healthy MVECs [163]. Among the multiple kallikrein family members, tissue kallikrein (also known as kallikrein 1 or "true" tissue kallikrein) is a serine protease that cleaves kininogen and thereby regulates the kininogen–kinin pathway. Tissue kallikrein synthetized at the blood vessels acts through kinins which modulate a broad spectrum of vascular functions, playing an important role in the regulation of vascular homeostasis and angiogenesis [165–167]. Del Rosso et al. found that tissue kallikrein circulating levels are increased in SSc, particularly in patients with signs of early and active vascular disease, suggesting a role in the development of SSc microvascular abnormalities [168].

A second microarray gene expression study examined the expression of 14,000 genes in MVECs from skin biopsies obtained from normal subjects and dSSc patients [164]. Genes were categorized into functional groups based on gene ontology. Of those 14,000 genes, SSc MVECs overexpressed a number of proangiogenic transcripts but also a variety of genes that have a negative effect on angiogenesis [164]. Conversely, several genes that promote cell migration and adhesion to the ECM were downregulated in SSc MVECs, suggesting an anti-invasive phenotype of these cells [164]. In particular, the angiogenesis inhibitor PTX3, which is known to inhibit the proangiogenic effects of FGF-2, was strongly upregulated in SSc MVECs compared with normal MVECs [164]. Interestingly, in a subsequent study, Margheri et al. reported that silencing of PTX3 in SSc MVECs significantly increased their invasion in Matrigel and could in part restore their ability to produce capillary tubes in vitro [160]. Moreover, the 14,000 gene microarray study reported a reduced expression of desmoglein-2 (DSG2) in SSc MVECs [164]. Thus, to identify the role of DSG2 downregulation in the defective angiogenesis characteristic of SSc, Giusti et al. [169] studied the effect of silencing DSG2 in normal MVECs using DSG2-siRNA. The authors reported impaired actin stress fiber formation and diminished capillary morphogenesis in vitro. Of note, transfection of DSG2 into SSc MVECs restored their angiogenic properties in vitro to normal levels [169].

Avouac et al. investigated the gene expression profile of circulating EPC-derived ECs in normal and hypoxic conditions [170]. Their data revealed important gene expression changes in EPC-derived ECs from SSc patients, characterized by a proadhesive, proinflammatory, and activated phenotype [170].

Finally, the gene array study of Tinazzi et al. showed that circulating ECs from SSc patients display an altered expression of genes involved in the control of apoptosis and angiogenesis which may be modified by iloprost infusion [171].

Role of Perivascular Cells

Pericytes are located on the abluminal side of ECs in capillaries, precapillary arterioles, and postcapillary venules [172–174]. They are in close spatial proximity to and provide partial coverage for ECs [172]. Pericyte cell bodies and ECs are contained within the same basement membrane [175]. Vascular stabilization or maturation requires maintenance of established vessels and EC coverage by pericytes or VSMCs around the endothelial layer during angiogenesis [176].

Pericytes are contractile cells [177] which enable them to participate in hemodynamic regulation of microvascular blood flow and permeability by modifying (increase or decrease) inflammatory leakage at EC junctions. Additionally, pericytes contract in response to vasoactive mediators; ET-1, norepinephrine, angiotensin II, and bradykinin stimulate pericyte contraction, while NO, adenosine, adrenergic antagonists, and lipopolysaccharide induce pericyte relaxation [178–181].

Vascular permeability can be regulated by the extent of EC coverage by pericytes or by the extent of pericyte contraction that modifies EC intercellular junctions [182–185]. Pericyte coverage of EC junctions prevents leakage of proteins and cells from the vessel wall [174].

Pericytes are considered to be progenitor cells with the potential to differentiate into different cell types such as fibroblasts and myofibroblasts [186–189]; thus, they may link vascular injury to tissue fibrosis. Microvascular pericytes express PDGF receptors in wound healing and dermal scarring tissue [190, 191], as well as in early stages of SSc [192–194]. In another study [195], myofibroblasts were found in SSc skin biopsies, but not in normal skin. Two markers of myofibroblast differentiation were expressed in both pericytes and myofibroblasts in SSc but not in control biopsies [195], suggesting that pericytes may represent a source of myofibroblasts during dermal fibrosis. Asano et al. reported a decreased pericyte coverage of dermal capillaries in SSc [196].

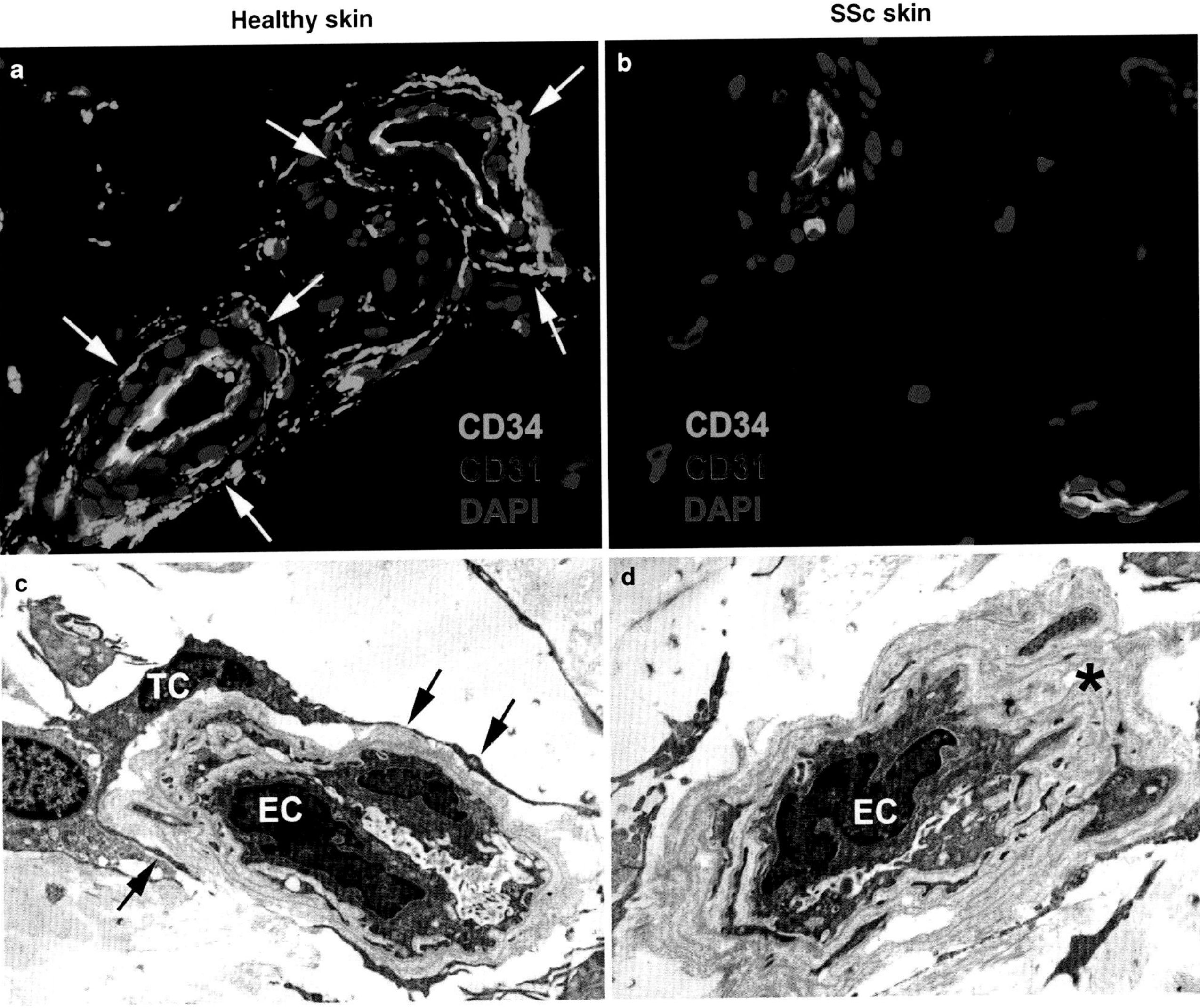

Fig. 16.5 (**a**, **b**) Representative photomicrographs of skin sections from healthy controls and SSc patients double immunostained for CD34 (*green*) and CD31 (*red*) and counterstained with DAPI (*blue*) to identify the nuclei. Telocytes are identified as CD34-positive/CD31-negative stromal cells, while endothelial cells are CD34/CD31 double positive. (**a**) Telocytes are numerous in healthy dermis, where they surround the microvessels (*arrows*). (**b**) No telocytes can be observed in SSc affected dermis. Original magnification: ×40. (**c**, **d**) Representative transmission electron microscopy (TEM) photomicrographs of healthy and SSc skin. (**c**) Healthy skin. The thin and long varicose processes of a perivascular telocyte (TC) encircle the basal lamina of a blood microvessel (*arrows*). (**d**) SSc skin. Telocytes are not identifiable around an occluded microvessel. Only a few cell debris are observed. The vessel basal lamina is thickened (*asterisk*). *EC* endothelial cell. TEM; Original magnification: ×6000

Besides fibroblasts, myofibroblasts, and pericytes, recent evidence indicates that other stromal cell types may be implicated in the pathophysiology of SSc. Telocytes, formerly called interstitial Cajal-like cells, are a distinct population of stromal cells that are characterized by very long cytoplasmic processes [197]. Telocytes act as supporting cells by forming a scaffold that defines the correct three-dimensional organization of tissues/organs during prenatal life and during tissue repair/renewal in postnatal life. It has been suggested that telocytes are involved in intercellular signaling that could influence the transcriptional activity of neighboring cells, either directly, by cell-to-cell contacts, or indirectly, by shedding microvesicles and exosomes or by secreting paracrine signaling molecules, including miRNAs [197]. Recently, Manetti et al. reported that telocytes display severe ultrastructural damage suggestive of ischemia-induced cell degeneration and are progressively lost from clinically affected SSc skin [198]. The authors proposed that, in SSc skin, the progressive loss of telocytes contributes to the altered three-dimensional organization of the ECM and may reduce the control of fibroblast and myofibroblast activity, thus favoring the fibrotic process [198]. Since telocytes are abundant in perivascular location, where they intimately surround the vessel basement membrane, and produce proangiogenic factors and participate to vascular stability [197], presumably their loss may even be linked to microvascular abnormalities in SSc. Immunofluorescence and transmission electron microscopy photomicrographs of telocytes and microvessels in healthy and SSc skin are shown in Fig. 16.5.

Vascular Wall Remodeling in SSc

Vascular remodeling follows microvascular injury and damage. Intimal and medial thickening and adventitial fibrosis are the common forms of remodeling found in SSc [149]. Intimal lesions change the vessel function and alter the composition and organization of the ECM. VSMCs are likely responsible for generating the fibrotic intimal lesions [149]. Under normal conditions, they assume a contractile or differentiated phenotype and regulate vessel diameter and blood flow. In pathological conditions, VSMCs become synthetic or dedifferentiated and generate intimal lesions through their secretion of ECM proteins in the absence of their contractile function [199–201]. Dysfunctional ECs, infiltrating leukocytes, and altered ECM in SSc provide the cues for intimal VSMCs to proliferate and form a fibrotic vascular lesion. In a recent study, Arts et al. demonstrated that a unique SSc IgG may induce growth and profibrotic state in VSMCs through the activation of the epidermal growth factor receptor signaling cascade [202].

Another theory is that transdifferentiation of ECs via the process of TGF-β-induced EndoMT may preferentially lead to subendothelial accumulation of myofibroblasts and fibrotic tissue with subsequent neointimal thickening, leading to a fibroproliferative vasculopathy [12, 203].

The ECM and basement membrane provide a support scaffold that is essential for blood vessel stability. Adhesion of ECs to the ECM enables them to undergo migration, proliferation, and morphogenesis, which are all necessary for neovascularization [204]. Degradation of the ECM/basement membrane leads to vessel collapse/regression [205–208]. Proteases that degrade the ECM/basement membrane play a key role in matrix remodeling during normal wound healing as well as in vascular diseases such as SSc.

The proteolytic activity of plasmin modifies many aspects of the ECM. It is the primary protease that degrades fibrin [207, 208], an ECM protein that forms a supportive scaffold for angiogenic vessels [209–211]. Fibrin, the major constituent of provisional matrix, enables ECs to adhere, spread, and proliferate [212, 213]. Fibrin or accumulated fibrinogen can be broken down by plasmin to negatively regulate angiogenesis [214, 215]. Reduced plasmin in SSc patients has been reported [73].

In addition to its own proteolytic activity, plasmin contributes to matrix remodeling by activating numerous MMPs [216, 217]. Of those, MMP-1, -3, -9, -10, and -13 promote capillary network regression followed by EC apoptosis [218, 219]. Several laboratories have examined plasma from SSc patients for the presence of various MMPs. One study reported that MMP-9 was downregulated in SSc patients, particularly those with PAH [220]. In another study, MMP-9 concentrations were greater in SSc plasma than controls [221].

Vascular Hypoxia in the Pathogenesis of SSc

Capillary rarefaction and disturbed blood flow, as well as excessive ECM accumulation, cause chronic tissue hypoxia in SSc. It was postulated that the avascular antiangiogenic areas visible in nailfold beds may result from tissue hypoxia and that the enlargement of capillaries may be a localized compensatory proangiogenic response to tissue hypoxia [125, 129]. In fact, intradermal skin oxygenation measurements verified hypoxic conditions in SSc patients with more advanced disease as compared to those with early disease and controls. Interestingly, expression of HIF-1α, a hypoxia-inducible transcriptional factor that upregulates VEGF, in the skin of SSc patients was lower than in controls. Additionally, HIF-1α expression did not correlate with VEGF expression pattern. Thus, it is concluded that increased VEGF expression in SSc patients is not stimulated by hypoxia, but could be the basis of megacapillaries [129]. However, subsequent studies demonstrated that the increase in VEGF expression in SSc skin was mainly the result of a significant increase in the antiangiogenic $VEGF_{165}b$ isoform instead of proangiogenic $VEGF_{165}$ [133].

The expression levels of VEGF, VEGFR-1, and VEGFR-2 have been examined also in late-outgrowth EPCs isolated from SSc patients and normal controls [222]. This study showed reduced mRNA and protein expression of VEGFR-1 in SSc EPCs under hypoxic conditions. Serum levels of soluble VEGFR-1 were significantly lower in SSc patients compared to controls, while soluble VEGF levels were elevated in SSc patients. Thickened skin in SSc may lead to hypoxia, as suggested by oxygen measurement in SSc skin [129, 223]. In both studies, the lowest oxygen levels were found in the thickened fibrotic skin. DNA microarray studies in human pulmonary arterial ECs exposed to normoxic or hypoxic conditions and in ECs infected with a constitutively active HIF-1α or β-galactosidase and exposed to nonhypoxic conditions [224] showed that genes upregulated by HIF-1α regulate collagen biosynthesis. The list includes COL1A2, COL4A1, COL4A2, COL5A1, COL9A1, COL18A1, procollagen prolyl hydroxylases, lysyl oxidase, and lysyl hydroxylases [224]. Thus, hypoxia could actively contribute to the fibroproliferative vasculopathy with intimal thickening characteristic of SSc.

In a recent study, Makarenko et al. [225] demonstrated that exposing human MVECs to intermittent hypoxia induces cell dysfunction associated with an increase in ROS formation and ERK phosphorylation. Of note, inhibition of the ERK signaling pathway and the use of antioxidants prevented the effect of intermittent hypoxia on MVECs [225]. This observation argues for a possible role for antioxidants in prevention of MVEC dysfunction mediated by intermittent hypoxia in vascular disorders such as SSc.

Relationship of Vasculopathy to Fibrosis

SSc is a connective tissue disease with markedly increased levels of collagen deposition that causes tissue fibrosis. Fibroblasts acquire abnormal characteristics that include increased proliferation, a switch to the activated state (myofibroblasts), and synthesis of abnormally high levels of collagen and other ECM components [226]. Excessive ECM deposition and accumulation in the heart, lung, vessels, skin, and kidney result in uncontrolled organ fibrosis and organ dysfunction, which are a major part of the SSc pathology. Despite the abnormal fibroblast activities that lead to the fibrotic state in SSc patients, the defective vasculature response to injury is considered to occur before fibrosis [149]. There are various hypotheses as to the mechanism by which the vascular system may contribute to fibrosis. One theory proposes that cytokines secreted by activated ECs form a gradient that attracts fibroblasts to the blood vessels which, in turn, stimulate fibroblast proliferation, activation, as well as synthesis and secretion of collagen. In support to this hypothesis, the deposition of ECM appears mostly clustered in perivascular regions in early fibrotic lesions. Another proposed mechanism is that ECs become permeable, which results in interstitial secretion of factors that stimulate fibroblast proliferation, activation, and production of collagen [226].

Two factors that have been implicated in the link between SSc vasculopathy and fibrosis are TGF-β and connective tissue growth factor (CTGF/CCN2). The TGF-β-dependent mechanism is linked to EC apoptosis and myofibroblast differentiation. Apoptotic ECs recruit phagocytes, particularly macrophages that engulf the apoptotic cells. This event stimulates upregulation of TGF-β, which promotes profibrotic myofibroblast differentiation and apoptosis resistance [227].

Another proposed mechanism is centered on CTGF and is independent of TGF-β pathway [228]. CTGF is a fibrinogenic protein that is constitutively expressed in dermal fibroblasts isolated from dSSc patients [229, 230]. Furthermore, CTGF injected subcutaneously into neonatal NIH Swiss mice stimulates tissue fibrosis without TGF-β upregulation. Further delineation of this mechanism was performed in C3H mice injected subcutaneously with serum-free medium conditioned by apoptotic murine aortic ECs. The mice that received the apoptotic ECs developed thickening of the skin with elevated expression of α-SMA, vimentin, and collagen and myofibroblast differentiation. Myofibroblast differentiation was reversed when caspase-3 expression was inhibited in ECs. CTGF was identified as the sole fibrinogenic protein whose expression was upregulated in mice treated with apoptotic ECs [228].

The notion that MVECs may play a central role in the pathogenesis of SSc, including activation of the fibrotic program, was reemphasized recently by a report from Serratì et al. [231], who demonstrated that conditioned media obtained from cultured SSc MVECs, but not control MVECs, evoked fibroblast activation as suggested by the overexpression of α-SMA, vimentin, and type I collagen. Moreover, the activated fibroblasts exhibited an aggressive mesenchymal cell behavior by upregulating MMP-2 and MMP-9 expression and acquiring the ability to invade Matrigel. The effect of SSc MVEC conditioned media on fibroblasts was mediated by elevated CTGF/CCN2, which in turn activates TGF-β. Interestingly, the use of CTGF/CCN2 inhibitor and TGF-β inhibitor peptides reversed fibroblast activation induced by SSc MVEC conditioned media [231].

Vascular injury can activate platelets to release serotonin and other profibrotic mediators, which ensures efficient and self-limited wound healing under physiologic conditions. By contrast, chronic vasculopathy may cause persistent increase in serotonin levels and perpetuate profibrotic tissue repair processes, thus linking vascular disease and fibrosis in SSc [232]. Indeed, serotonin stimulates fibroblasts to release excessive amounts of ECM proteins. The profibrotic effects of serotonin are exclusively mediated via $5HT_{2B}$ receptors which are overexpressed in SSc, suggesting an increased sensitivity of SSc fibroblasts to the profibrotic effects of serotonin [232].

Finally, an important link between vasculopathy and fibrosis in SSc pathogenesis may be represented by chronic overexpression of VEGF. In fact, Maurer et al. reported that double (+/+) VEGF transgenic mice spontaneously develop significant skin fibrosis, indicating profibrotic effect of VEGF in a gene-dosing manner [233]. Moreover, in vitro analysis revealed that VEGF is able to directly induce collagen synthesis in dermal fibroblasts [233].

Animal Models of SSc Vasculopathy

Animal models provided invaluable tools for unraveling the cellular and molecular events that drive the development of tissue fibrosis. All SSc models were discovered because of their fibrotic phenotype [234, 235]. However, only few animal models of SSc replicate the full spectrum of the human disease, including the fibrotic, vascular, inflammatory, and autoimmune features. Endothelial dysfunction occurs in various models [236]; however, it is not clear if EC dysfunction is a primary or secondary event in animals with chronic hypoxia and intense tissue fibrosis.

UCD 200/206 Chickens This chicken model manifests the entire spectrum of the clinical, histopathological, and serological features of SSc. EC apoptosis, induced by AECA-dependent cellular cytotoxicity, is considered to be a primary event in this model. Other immunologic features include the presence of antinuclear antibodies, anticardiolipin antibodies, and rheumatoid factors [237]. However, it has been difficult to use this model because of the high variability of disease course, the long generation time of chicken, the challenges in housing chicken, and the lack of easy availability of chicken reagents.

Chronic Graft-Versus-Host Disease (GVHD) This model is produced by the transplantation of immunologically incompatible spleen and bone marrow cells in a susceptible host. Tissue fibrosis is noted after host tissue infiltration by donor T cells and monocytes/macrophages. A very interesting chronic GVHD model, avoiding the need for irradiation, has been produced using the Rag-2 mouse, an immune-deficient mouse secondary to the loss of ability to rearrange immunoglobulin and T-cell receptor genes. In this model, not only fibrosis is noted but also vasoconstriction and intimal hyperplasia in both skin and kidney. In addition, there is an increase in ET-1 and adhesion molecule expression with circulating antinuclear antibodies and anti-Scl-70 antibodies in more than 90 % of these mice [238].

Endothelial Fli1-Deficient Mouse Friend leukemia integration-1 (Fli1) is a member of the Ets family of transcription factors that represses the transcription of collagen genes via Sp1-dependent pathway. Embryonic fibroblasts from Fli1-deficient mice exhibit significantly increased type I collagen expression levels in association with increased CTGF and decreased MMP-1 expression. Interestingly, a mouse model with a conditional deletion of Fli1 in ECs (Fli1 ECKO) develops disorganized dermal vascular network with greatly compromised vessel integrity and markedly increased vessel permeability. Downregulation of VE-cadherin and platelet-endothelial cell adhesion molecule 1, impaired development of basement membrane, and decreased pericyte coverage in dermal microvessels were also noted [196]. This phenotype is consistent with a role of Fli1 as a regulator of vessel maturation and stabilization. Importantly, a reduced expression level of Fli1 in SSc ECs was noted suggesting that Fli1 may play a critical role in the development of SSc vasculopathy [196].

Fra-2 Transgenic Mouse The fos-related antigen (Fra-2) belongs to the activator protein 1 (AP1) family of transcription factors. Fra-2 is overexpressed in SSc tissues and is shown to act as a novel downstream mediator of the profibrotic effects of TGF-β and PDGF. Mice with ectopic expression of Fra-2 in various organs develop generalized fibrosis and inflammation that is most pronounced in the lungs. Moreover, Fra-2 transgenic mice develop severe loss of small blood vessels in the skin that is paralleled by progressive skin fibrosis. Fra-2 transgenic mice display various features of SSc vasculopathy with decreased dermal capillary density and early EC apoptosis [239]. Interestingly, dermal EC apoptosis appears to occur before the onset of tissue fibrosis. The suppression of Fra-2 by small interfering RNA prevents EC apoptosis and improves parameters of EC angiogenic potential. However, no proliferative vasculopathy was detectable in the skin [239]. Conversely, Fra-2 transgenic mice have been reported to develop proliferative vasculopathy in the lungs closely resembling SSc-related PAH [240]. Thus, Fra-2 transgenic mice may be a potentially useful model for the investigation of the link between vasculopathy and fibrosis and for the exploration of the mechanisms of vasculopathy in different organs.

uPAR-Deficient Mouse The cleavage/inactivation of uPAR is a crucial step in fibroblast-to-myofibroblast transition and has been implicated in SSc peripheral microvasculopathy [132, 159, 241]. Therefore, Manetti et al. investigated whether uPAR gene knockout in mice could result in fibrosis and peripheral microvasculopathy resembling human SSc [242]. The skin of uPAR-deficient mice displays most of the typical pathological features of SSc. Dermal thickness, collagen content, and myofibroblast counts were significantly greater in uPAR-deficient mice than in wild-type mice. Similar to SSc, the skin of uPAR-deficient mice was characterized by the presence of thickened, closely packed and irregularly distributed collagen bundles, abundant perivascular fibrosis, and partial replacement of subcutaneous fat with connective tissue. Moreover, in the dermis of uPAR-deficient mice, there was a marked overexpression of the SSc-related profibrotic factors TGF-β, CTGF/CCN2, and ET-1. Of note, in uPAR-deficient mice, dermal fibrosis was paralleled by EC apoptosis and severe loss of microvessels similar to what is seen in SSc peripheral microvasculopathy [242]. In addition, uPAR-deficient mice also develop progressive lung fibrosis resembling the nonspecific interstitial pneumonia pattern of SSc. However, no evidence of vessel intima-media proliferation was reported either in the skin or the lungs [242]. Further studies are required to ascertain whether uPAR-deficient mice may develop SSc-like features in other internal organs. In this regard, it was reported that uPAR deficiency accelerates renal fibrosis in obstructive nephropathy [243].

Conclusions

The pathogenesis of the vascular disease in SSc appears to involve many cell types and signaling pathways. A complex interaction between ECs, immune cells, VSMCs, fibroblasts, pericytes, and the ECM is likely to contribute to the vascular reactivity, remodeling, and occlusive disease of SSc. EC activation/injury is an early and probably initiating event in disease pathogenesis. The exact mechanism for the widespread vascular disease in SSc is still unknown, but EC injury induced by an infectious agent, immune-mediated cytotoxicity, AECAs, and/or ischemia–reperfusion have all been suggested. Moreover, substantial evidence indicates that angiogenic and vasculogenic repair machineries are impaired and do not allow vascular recovery. The downstream effects of vascular dysfunction adversely affect organ function and determine clinical outcomes. Understanding the mechanisms underlying these processes provides the rationale for novel therapeutic strategies and specific targeted therapy. The definition of prefibrotic vascular lesions may have future therapeutic and preventive implications for SSc. Development of means to quantify endothelial injury and the activity of the vascular lesions are essential for the monitoring of therapies designed to block further vascular injury.

References

1. Fleischmajer R, Perlish JS, Shaw KV, Pirozzi DJ. Skin capillary changes in early systemic scleroderma. Electron microscopy and "in vitro" autoradiography with tritiated thymidine. Arch Dermatol. 1976;112(11):1553–7.
2. Grassi W, Core P, Carlino G, Blasetti P, Cervini M. Labial capillary microscopy in systemic sclerosis. Ann Rheum Dis. 1993;52(8):564–9.
3. Fleischmajer R, Perlish JS. Capillary alterations in scleroderma. J Am Acad Dermatol. 1980;2(2):161–70.
4. Sgonc R, Gruschwitz MS, Dietrich H, Recheis H, Gershwin ME, Wick G. Endothelial cell apoptosis is a primary pathogenetic event underlying skin lesions in avian and human scleroderma. J Clin Invest. 1996;98(3):785–92.
5. Chen F, Eriksson P, Kimura T, Herzfeld I, Valen G. Apoptosis and angiogenesis are induced in the unstable coronary atherosclerotic plaque. Coron Artery Dis. 2005;16(3):191–7.
6. Laurence J, Mitra D, Steiner M, Staiano-Coico L, Jaffe E. Plasma from patients with idiopathic and human immunodeficiency virus-associated thrombotic thrombocytopenic purpura induces apoptosis in microvascular endothelial cells. Blood. 1996;87(8):3245–54.
7. Albert ML, Pearce SF, Francisco LM, Sauter B, Roy P, Silverstein RL, Bhardwaj N. Immature dendritic cells phagocytose apoptotic cells via alphavbeta5 and CD36, and cross-present antigens to cytotoxic T lymphocytes. J Exp Med. 1998;188(7):1359–68.
8. Greeno EW, Bach RR, Moldow CF. Apoptosis is associated with increased cell surface tissue factor procoagulant activity. Lab Invest. 1996;75(2):281–9.
9. Tsuji S, Kaji K, Nagasawa S. Activation of the alternative pathway of human complement by apoptotic human umbilical vein endothelial cells. J Biochem. 1994;116(4):794–800.
10. Fleischmajer R, Perlish JS. [3H]Thymidine labeling of dermal endothelial cells in scleroderma. J Invest Dermatol. 1977;69(4):379–82.
11. Rodnan GP, Myerowitz RL, Justh GO. Morphologic changes in the digital arteries of patients with progressive systemic sclerosis (scleroderma) and Raynaud phenomenon. Medicine (Baltimore). 1980;59(6):393–408.
12. Manetti M, Guiducci S, Matucci-Cerinic M. The origin of the myofibroblast in fibroproliferative vasculopathy: does the endothelial cell steer the pathophysiology of systemic sclerosis? Arthritis Rheum. 2011;63(8):2164–7.
13. Youssef P, Englert H, Bertouch J. Large vessel occlusive disease associated with CREST syndrome and scleroderma. Ann Rheum Dis. 1993;52(6):464–6.
14. Pandey JP, LeRoy EC. Human cytomegalovirus and the vasculopathies of autoimmune diseases (especially scleroderma), allograft rejection, and coronary restenosis. Arthritis Rheum. 1998;41(1):10–5.
15. Cannon PJ, Hassar M, Case DB, Casarella WJ, Sommers SC, LeRoy EC. The relationship of hypertension and renal failure in scleroderma (progressive systemic sclerosis) to structural and functional abnormalities of the renal cortical circulation. Medicine (Baltimore). 1974;53(1):1–46.
16. Brown GE, O'Leary PA. Skin capillaries in scleroderma. Arch Intern Med. 1925;36:73–88.
17. Anderson ME, Allen PD, Moore T, Hillier V, Taylor CJ, Herrick AL. Computerized nailfold video capillaroscopy – a new tool for assessment of Raynaud's phenomenon. J Rheumatol. 2005;32(5):841–8.
18. Maricq HR, LeRoy EC. Patterns of finger capillary abnormalities in connective tissue disease by "wide-field" microscopy. Arthritis Rheum. 1973;16(5):619–28.
19. Blann AD, Illingworth K, Jayson MI. Mechanisms of endothelial cell damage in systemic sclerosis and Raynaud's phenomenon. J Rheumatol. 1993;20(8):1325–30.
20. Carpentier PH, Maricq HR. Microvasculature in systemic sclerosis. Rheum Dis Clin North Am. 1990;16(1):75–91.
21. Bukhari M, Herrick AL, Moore T, Manning J, Jayson MI. Increased nailfold capillary dimensions in primary Raynaud's phenomenon and systemic sclerosis. Br J Rheumatol. 1996;35(11):1127–31.
22. Cutolo M, Sulli A, Secchi ME, Paolino S, Pizzorni C. Nailfold capillaroscopy is useful for the diagnosis and follow-up of autoimmune rheumatic diseases. A future tool for the analysis of microvascular heart involvement? Rheumatology (Oxford). 2006;45 Suppl 4:iv43–6.
23. Meli M, Gitzelmann G, Koppensteiner R, Amann-Vesti BR. Predictive value of nailfold capillaroscopy in patients with Raynaud's phenomenon. Clin Rheumatol. 2006;25(2):153–8.
24. Miniati I, Guiducci S, Conforti ML, Rogai V, Fiori G, Cinelli M, Saccardi R, Guidi S, Bosi A, Tyndall A, Matucci-Cerinic M. Autologous stem cell transplantation improves microcirculation in systemic sclerosis. Ann Rheum Dis. 2009;68(1):94–8.
25. Albrecht HP, Hiller D, Hornstein OP, Bühler-Singer S, Mück M, Gruschwitz M. Microcirculatory functions in systemic sclerosis: additional parameters for therapeutic concepts? J Invest Dermatol. 1993;101(2):211–5.
26. Prescott RJ, Freemont AJ, Jones CJ, Hoyland J, Fielding P. Sequential dermal microvascular and perivascular changes in the development of scleroderma. J Pathol. 1992;166(3):255–63.
27. Lippton HL, Hauth TA, Summer WR, Hyman AL. Endothelin produces pulmonary vasoconstriction and systemic vasodilation. J Appl Physiol (1985). 1989;66(2):1008–12.
28. Vancheeswaran R, Azam A, Black C, Dashwood MR. Localization of endothelin-1 and its binding sites in scleroderma skin. J Rheumatol. 1994;21(7):1268–76.
29. Vancheeswaran R, Magoulas T, Efrat G, Wheeler-Jones C, Olsen I, Penny R, Black CM. Circulating endothelin-1 levels in systemic sclerosis subsets; a marker of fibrosis or vascular dysfunction? J Rheumatol. 1994;21(10):1838–44.
30. Cambrey AD, Harrison NK, Dawes KE, Southcott AM, Black CM, du Bois RM, Laurent GJ, McAnulty RJ. Increased levels of endothelin-1 in bronchoalveolar lavage fluid from patients with systemic sclerosis contribute to fibroblast mitogenic activity in vitro. Am J Respir Cell Mol Biol. 1994;11(4):439–45.
31. Kawaguchi Y, Suzuki K, Hara M, Hidaka T, Ishizuka T, Kawagoe M, Nakamura H. Increased endothelin-1 production in fibroblasts derived from patients with systemic sclerosis. Ann Rheum Dis. 1994;53(8):506–10.
32. Morelli S, Ferri C, Di Francesco L, Baldoncini R, Carlesimo M, Bottoni U, Properzi G, Santucci A. Plasma endothelin-1 levels in

patients with systemic sclerosis: influence of pulmonary or systemic arterial hypertension. Ann Rheum Dis. 1995;54(9):730–4.
33. Morelli S, Ferri C, Polettini E, Bellini C, Gualdi GF, Pittoni V, Valesini G, Santucci A. Plasma endothelin-1 levels, pulmonary hypertension, and lung fibrosis in patients with systemic sclerosis. Am J Med. 1995;99(3):255–60.
34. Abraham D, Distler O. How does endothelial cell injury start? The role of endothelin in systemic sclerosis. Arthritis Res Ther. 2007;9 Suppl 2:S2.
35. Frommer KW, Müller-Ladner U. Expression and function of ETA and ETB receptors in SSc. Rheumatology (Oxford). 2008;47 Suppl 5:v27–8.
36. Kasturi KN, Shibata S, Muryoi T, Bona CA. Tight-skin mouse an experimental model for scleroderma. Int Rev Immunol. 1994; 11(3):253–71.
37. Richard V, Solans V, Favre J, Henry JP, Lallemand F, Thuillez C, Marie I. Role of endogenous endothelin in endothelial dysfunction in murine model of systemic sclerosis: tight skin mice 1. Fundam Clin Pharmacol. 2008;22(6):649–55.
38. Cozzi F, Pigatto E, Rizzo M, Favaro M, Zanatta E, Cardarelli S, Riato L, Punzi L. Low occurrence of digital ulcers in scleroderma patients treated with bosentan for pulmonary arterial hypertension: a retrospective case-control study. Clin Rheumatol. 2013; 32(5):679–83.
39. Matucci-Cerinic M, Denton CP, Furst DE, Mayes MD, Hsu VM, Carpentier P, Wigley FM, Black CM, Fessler BJ, Merkel PA, Pope JE, Sweiss NJ, Doyle MK, Hellmich B, Medsger Jr TA, Morganti A, Kramer F, Korn JH, Seibold JR. Bosentan treatment of digital ulcers related to systemic sclerosis: results from the RAPIDS-2 randomised, double-blind, placebo-controlled trial. Ann Rheum Dis. 2011;70(1):32–8.
40. Guiducci S, Bellando Randone S, Bruni C, Carnesecchi G, Maresta A, Iannone F, Lapadula G, Matucci Cerinic M. Bosentan fosters microvascular de-remodelling in systemic sclerosis. Clin Rheumatol. 2012;31(12):1723–5.
41. Cutolo M, Zampogna G, Vremis L, Smith V, Pizzorni C, Sulli A. Long-term effects of endothelin receptor antagonism on microvascular damage evaluated by nailfold capillaroscopic analysis in systemic sclerosis. J Rheumatol. 2013;40(1):40–5.
42. Ignarro LJ. Biosynthesis and metabolism of endothelium-derived nitric oxide. Annu Rev Pharmacol Toxicol. 1990;30:535–60.
43. Ignarro LJ. Endothelium-derived nitric oxide: actions and properties. FASEB J. 1989;3(1):31–6.
44. Agostoni A, Marasini B, Biondi ML, Bassani C, Cazzaniga A, Bottasso B, Cugno M. L-arginine therapy in Raynaud's phenomenon? Int J Clin Lab Res. 1991;21(2):202–3.
45. Cailes J, Winter S, du Bois RM, Evans TW. Defective endothelially mediated pulmonary vasodilation in systemic sclerosis. Chest. 1998;114(1):178–84.
46. Livi R, Teghini L, Generini S, Matucci-Cerinic M. The loss of endothelium-dependent vascular tone control in systemic sclerosis. Chest. 2001;119(2):672–3.
47. Matucci-Cerinic M, Pietrini U, Marabini S. Local venomotor response to intravenous infusion of substance P and glyceryl trinitrate in systemic sclerosis. Clin Exp Rheumatol. 1990;8(6):561–5.
48. Cotton SA, Herrick AL, Jayson MI, Freemont AJ. Endothelial expression of nitric oxide synthases and nitrotyrosine in systemic sclerosis skin. J Pathol. 1999;189(2):273–8.
49. Dooley A, Gao B, Bradley N, Abraham DJ, Black CM, Jacobs M, Bruckdorfer KR. Abnormal nitric oxide metabolism in systemic sclerosis: increased levels of nitrated proteins and asymmetric dimethylarginine. Rheumatology (Oxford). 2006;45(6):676–84.
50. Mendall MA, Goggin PM, Molineaux N, Levy J, Toosy T, Strachan D, Camm AJ, Northfield TC. Relation of Helicobacter pylori infection and coronary heart disease. Br Heart J. 1994; 71(5):437–9.
51. Gasbarrini A, Massari I, Serricchio M, Tondi P, De Luca A, Franceschi F, Ojetti V, Dal Lago A, Flore R, Santoliquido A, Gasbarrini G, Pola P. Helicobacter pylori eradication ameliorates primary Raynaud's phenomenon. Dig Dis Sci. 1998;43(8):1641–5.
52. Aragona P, Magazzù G, Macchia G, Bartolone S, Di Pasquale G, Vitali C, Ferreri G. Presence of antibodies against Helicobacter pylori and its heat-shock protein 60 in the serum of patients with Sjögren's syndrome. J Rheumatol. 1999;26(6):1306–11.
53. Savarino V, Sulli A, Zentilin P, Raffaella Mele M, Cutolo M. No evidence of an association between Helicobacter pylori infection and Raynaud phenomenon. Scand J Gastroenterol. 2000;35(12): 1251–4.
54. Sulli A, Seriolo B, Savarino V, Cutolo M. Lack of correlation between gastric Helicobacter pylori infection and primary or secondary Raynaud's phenomenon in patients with systemic sclerosis. J Rheumatol. 2000;27(7):1820–1.
55. Vaughan JH, Shaw PX, Nguyen MD, Medsger Jr TA, Wright TM, Metcalf JS, Leroy EC. Evidence of activation of 2 herpesviruses, Epstein-Barr virus and cytomegalovirus, in systemic sclerosis and normal skins. J Rheumatol. 2000;27(3):821–3.
56. Neidhart M, Kuchen S, Distler O, Brühlmann P, Michel BA, Gay RE, Gay S. Increased serum levels of antibodies against human cytomegalovirus and prevalence of autoantibodies in systemic sclerosis. Arthritis Rheum. 1999;42(2):389–92.
57. Presti RM, Pollock JL, Dal Canto AJ, O'Guin AK, Virgin 4th HW. Interferon gamma regulates acute and latent murine cytomegalovirus infection and chronic disease of the great vessels. J Exp Med. 1998;188(3):577–88.
58. Zhou YF, Shou M, Harrell RF, Yu ZX, Unger EF, Epstein SE. Chronic non-vascular cytomegalovirus infection: effects on the neointimal response to experimental vascular injury. Cardiovasc Res. 2000;45(4):1019–25.
59. Hamamdzic D, Harley RA, Hazen-Martin D, LeRoy EC. MCMV induces neointima in IFN-gammaR/mice: intimal cell apoptosis and persistent proliferation of myofibroblasts. BMC Musculoskelet Disord. 2001;2:3.
60. Ferri C, Longombardo G, Azzi A, Zakrzewska K. Parvovirus B19 and systemic sclerosis. Clin Exp Rheumatol. 1999;17(2):267–8.
61. Magro CM, Nuovo G, Ferri C, Crowson AN, Giuggioli D, Sebastiani M. Parvoviral infection of endothelial cells and stromal fibroblasts: a possible pathogenetic role in scleroderma. J Cutan Pathol. 2004;31(1):43–50.
62. Zakrzewska K, Corcioli F, Carlsen KM, Giuggioli D, Fanci R, Rinieri A, Ferri C, Azzi A. Human parvovirus B19 (B19V) infection in systemic sclerosis patients. Intervirology. 2009;52(5): 279–82.
63. Drenk F, Deicher HR. Pathophysiological effects of endothelial cytotoxic activity derived from sera of patients with progressive systemic sclerosis. J Rheumatol. 1988;15(3):468–74.
64. Holt CM, Lindsey N, Moult J, Malia RG, Greaves M, Hume A, Rowell NR, Hughes P. Antibody-dependent cellular cytotoxicity of vascular endothelium: characterization and pathogenic associations in systemic sclerosis. Clin Exp Immunol. 1989;78(3): 359–65.
65. Penning CA, Cunningham J, French MA, Harrison G, Rowell NR, Hughes P. Antibody-dependent cellular cytotoxicity of human vascular endothelium in systemic sclerosis. Clin Exp Immunol. 1984;57(3):548–56.
66. Sgonc R, Gruschwitz MS, Boeck G, Sepp N, Gruber J, Wick G. Endothelial cell apoptosis in systemic sclerosis is induced by antibody-dependent cell-mediated cytotoxicity via CD95. Arthritis Rheum. 2000;43(11):2550–62.
67. Trapani JA. Dual mechanisms of apoptosis induction by cytotoxic lymphocytes. Int Rev Cytol. 1998;182:111–92.
68. Kahaleh MB, Leroy EC. Endothelial injury in scleroderma. A protease mechanism. J Lab Clin Med. 1983;101(4):553–60.

69. Kahaleh MB, Fan PS. Mechanism of serum-mediated endothelial injury in scleroderma: identification of a granular enzyme in scleroderma skin and sera. Clin Immunol Immunopathol. 1997; 83(1):32–40.
70. Müllbacher A, Waring P, Tha Hla R, Tran T, Chin S, Stehle T, Museteanu C, Simon MM. Granzymes are the essential downstream effector molecules for the control of primary virus infections by cytolytic leukocytes. Proc Natl Acad Sci U S A. 1999;96(24):13950–5.
71. Müller U, Sobek V, Balkow S, Hölscher C, Müllbacher A, Museteanu C, Mossmann H, Simon MM. Concerted action of perforin and granzymes is critical for the elimination of Trypanosoma cruzi from mouse tissues, but prevention of early host death is in addition dependent on the FasL/Fas pathway. Eur J Immunol. 2003;33(1):70–8.
72. Buzza MS, Zamurs L, Sun J, Bird CH, Smith AI, Trapani JA, Froelich CJ, Nice EC, Bird PI. Extracellular matrix remodeling by human granzyme B via cleavage of vitronectin, fibronectin, and laminin. J Biol Chem. 2005;280(25):23549–58.
73. Mulligan-Kehoe MJ, Drinane MC, Mollmark J, Casciola-Rosen L, Hummers LK, Hall A, Rosen A, Wigley FM, Simons M. Antiangiogenic plasma activity in patients with systemic sclerosis. Arthritis Rheum. 2007;56(10):3448–58.
74. Sasaki T, Larsson H, Tisi D, Claesson-Welsh L, Hohenester E, Timpl R. Endostatins derived from collagens XV and XVIII differ in structural and binding properties, tissue distribution and anti-angiogenic activity. J Mol Biol. 2000;301(5):1179–90.
75. Maeshima Y, Sudhakar A, Lively JC, Ueki K, Kharbanda S, Kahn CR, Sonenberg N, Hynes RO, Kalluri R. Tumstatin, an endothelial cell-specific inhibitor of protein synthesis. Science. 2002; 295(5552):140–3.
76. Kamphaus GD, Colorado PC, Panka DJ, Hopfer H, Ramchandran R, Torre A, Maeshima Y, Mier JW, Sukhatme VP, Kalluri R. Canstatin, a novel matrix-derived inhibitor of angiogenesis and tumor growth. J Biol Chem. 2000;275(2):1209–15.
77. Cao Y, Ji RW, Davidson D, Schaller J, Marti D, Söhndel S, McCance SG, O'Reilly MS, Llinás M, Folkman J. Kringle domains of human angiostatin. Characterization of the anti-proliferative activity on endothelial cells. J Biol Chem. 1996; 271(46):29461–7.
78. Ferrara N, Clapp C, Weiner R. The 16K fragment of prolactin specifically inhibits basal or fibroblast growth factor stimulated growth of capillary endothelial cells. Endocrinology. 1991;129(2):896–900.
79. Staton CA, Lewis CE. Angiogenesis inhibitors found within the haemostasis pathway. J Cell Mol Med. 2005;9(2):286–302.
80. Hebbar M, Peyrat JP, Hornez L, Hatron PY, Hachulla E, Devulder B. Increased concentrations of the circulating angiogenesis inhibitor endostatin in patients with systemic sclerosis. Arthritis Rheum. 2000;43(4):889–93.
81. Hummers LK, Hall A, Wigley FM, Simons M. Abnormalities in the regulators of angiogenesis in patients with scleroderma. J Rheumatol. 2009;36(3):576–82.
82. Casciola-Rosen LA, Anhalt G, Rosen A. Autoantigens targeted in systemic lupus erythematosus are clustered in two populations of surface structures on apoptotic keratinocytes. J Exp Med. 1994; 179(4):1317–30.
83. Sercarz EE, Lehmann PV, Ametani A, Benichou G, Miller A, Moudgil K. Dominance and crypticity of T cell antigenic determinants. Annu Rev Immunol. 1993;11:729–66.
84. Zhou Z, Ménard HA. Autoantigenic posttranslational modifications of proteins: does it apply to rheumatoid arthritis? Curr Opin Rheumatol. 2002;14(3):250–3.
85. Andrade F, Roy S, Nicholson D, Thornberry N, Rosen A, Casciola-Rosen L. Granzyme B directly and efficiently cleaves several downstream caspase substrates: implications for CTL-induced apoptosis. Immunity. 1998;8(4):451–60.
86. Casciola-Rosen L, Andrade F, Ulanet D, Wong WB, Rosen A. Cleavage by granzyme B is strongly predictive of autoantigen status: implications for initiation of autoimmunity. J Exp Med. 1999;190(6):815–26.
87. Schachna L, Wigley FM, Morris S, Gelber AC, Rosen A, Casciola-Rosen L. Recognition of Granzyme B-generated autoantigen fragments in scleroderma patients with ischemic digital loss. Arthritis Rheum. 2002;46(7):1873–84.
88. Youinou P, Revelen R, Bordron A. Is antiendothelial cell antibody the murder weapon in systemic sclerosis? Clin Exp Rheumatol. 1999;17(1):35–6.
89. Hill MB, Phipps JL, Cartwright RJ, Milford Ward A, Greaves M, Hughes P. Antibodies to membranes of endothelial cells and fibroblasts in scleroderma. Clin Exp Immunol. 1996;106(3):491–7.
90. Negi VS, Tripathy NK, Misra R, Nityanand S. Antiendothelial cell antibodies in scleroderma correlate with severe digital ischemia and pulmonary arterial hypertension. J Rheumatol. 1998; 25(3):462–6.
91. García de la Peña-Lefebvre P, Chanseaud Y, Tamby MC, Reinbolt J, Batteux F, Allanore Y, Kahan A, Meyer O, Benveniste O, Boyer O, Guillevin L, Boissier MC, Mouthon L. IgG reactivity with a 100-kDa tissue and endothelial cell antigen identified as topoisomerase 1 distinguishes between limited and diffuse systemic sclerosis patients. Clin Immunol. 2004;111(3):241–51.
92. Tamby MC, Chanseaud Y, Humbert M, Fermanian J, Guilpain P, Garcia-de-la-Peña-Lefebvre P, Brunet S, Servettaz A, Weill B, Simonneau G, Guillevin L, Boissier MC, Mouthon L. Anti-endothelial cell antibodies in idiopathic and systemic sclerosis associated pulmonary arterial hypertension. Thorax. 2005;60(9): 765–72.
93. Worda M, Sgonc R, Dietrich H, Niederegger H, Sundick RS, Gershwin ME, Wick G. In vivo analysis of the apoptosis-inducing effect of anti-endothelial cell antibodies in systemic sclerosis by the chorioallantoic membrane assay. Arthritis Rheum. 2003; 48(9):2605–14.
94. Bordron A, Dueymes M, Levy Y, Jamin C, Leroy JP, Piette JC, Shoenfeld Y, Youinou PY. The binding of some human antiendothelial cell antibodies induces endothelial cell apoptosis. J Clin Invest. 1998;101(10):2029–35.
95. Tan FK, Arnett FC, Reveille JD, Ahn C, Antohi S, Sasaki T, Nishioka K, Bona CA. Autoantibodies to fibrillin 1 in systemic sclerosis: ethnic differences in antigen recognition and lack of correlation with specific clinical features or HLA alleles. Arthritis Rheum. 2000;43(11):2464–71.
96. Arends SJ, Damoiseaux JG, Duijvestijn AM, Debrus-Palmans L, Boomars KA, Brunner-La Rocca HP, Cohen Tervaert JW, van Paassen P. Functional implications of IgG anti-endothelial cell antibodies in pulmonary arterial hypertension. Autoimmunity. 2013;46(7):463–70.
97. Wolf SI, Howat S, Abraham DJ, Pearson JD, Lawson C. Agonistic anti-ICAM-1 antibodies in scleroderma: activation of endothelial pro-inflammatory cascades. Vascul Pharmacol. 2013;59(1–2): 19–26.
98. Al-Dhaher FF, Pope JE, Ouimet JM. Determinants of morbidity and mortality of systemic sclerosis in Canada. Semin Arthritis Rheum. 2010;39(4):269–77.
99. Steen VD, Medsger TA. Changes in causes of death in systemic sclerosis, 1972–2002. Ann Rheum Dis. 2007;66(7):940–4.
100. Mathai SC, Hummers LK, Champion HC, Wigley FM, Zaiman A, Hassoun PM, Girgis RE. Survival in pulmonary hypertension associated with the scleroderma spectrum of diseases: impact of interstitial lung disease. Arthritis Rheum. 2009;60(2):569–77.
101. Birukov KG. Cyclic stretch, reactive oxygen species, and vascular remodeling. Antioxid Redox Signal. 2009;11(7):1651–67.
102. Grote K, Flach I, Luchtefeld M, Akin E, Holland SM, Drexler H, Schieffer B. Mechanical stretch enhances mRNA expression and

proenzyme release of matrix metalloproteinase-2 (MMP-2) via NAD(P)H oxidase-derived reactive oxygen species. Circ Res. 2003;92(11):e80–6.

103. McCord JM. Oxygen-derived free radicals in postischemic tissue injury. N Engl J Med. 1985;312(3):159–63.

104. Riccieri V, Spadaro A, Fuksa L, Firuzi O, Saso L, Valesini G. Specific oxidative stress parameters differently correlate with nailfold capillaroscopy changes and organ involvement in systemic sclerosis. Clin Rheumatol. 2008;27(2):225–30.

105. Valko M, Leibfritz D, Moncol J, Cronin MT, Mazur M, Telser J. Free radicals and antioxidants in normal physiological functions and human disease. Int J Biochem Cell Biol. 2007;39(1):44–84.

106. Kuschel L, Hansel A, Schönherr R, Weissbach H, Brot N, Hoshi T, Heinemann SH. Molecular cloning and functional expression of a human peptide methionine sulfoxide reductase (hMsrA). FEBS Lett. 1999;456(1):17–21.

107. Ogawa F, Sander CS, Hansel A, Oehrl W, Kasperczyk H, Elsner P, Shimizu K, Heinemann SH, Thiele JJ. The repair enzyme peptide methionine-S-sulfoxide reductase is expressed in human epidermis and upregulated by UVA radiation. J Invest Dermatol. 2006;126(5):1128–34.

108. Prentice HM, Moench IA, Rickaway ZT, Dougherty CJ, Webster KA, Weissbach H. MsrA protects cardiomyocytes against hypoxia/reoxygenation induced cell death. Biochem Biophys Res Commun. 2008;366(3):775–8.

109. Ogawa F, Shimizu K, Hara T, Muroi E, Komura K, Takenaka M, Hasegawa M, Fujimoto M, Takehara K, Sato S. Autoantibody against one of the antioxidant repair enzymes, methionine sulfoxide reductase A, in systemic sclerosis: association with pulmonary fibrosis and vascular damage. Arch Dermatol Res. 2010;302(1): 27–35.

110. Baroni SS, Santillo M, Bevilacqua F, Luchetti M, Spadoni T, Mancini M, Fraticelli P, Sambo P, Funaro A, Kazlauskas A, Avvedimento EV, Gabrielli A. Stimulatory autoantibodies to the PDGF receptor in systemic sclerosis. N Engl J Med. 2006; 354(25):2667–76.

111. Edelberg JM, Lee SH, Kaur M, Tang L, Feirt NM, McCabe S, Bramwell O, Wong SC, Hong MK. Platelet-derived growth factor-AB limits the extent of myocardial infarction in a rat model: feasibility of restoring impaired angiogenic capacity in the aging heart. Circulation. 2002;105(5):608–13.

112. Classen JF, Henrohn D, Rorsman F, Lennartsson J, Lauwerys BR, Wikström G, Rorsman C, Lenglez S, Franck-Larsson K, Tomasi JP, Kämpe O, Vanthuyne M, Houssiau FA, Demoulin JB. Lack of evidence of stimulatory autoantibodies to platelet-derived growth factor receptor in patients with systemic sclerosis. Arthritis Rheum. 2009;60(4):1137–44.

113. Derk CT, Jimenez SA. Systemic sclerosis: current views of its pathogenesis. Autoimmun Rev. 2003;2(4):181–91.

114. Reinhart BJ, Slack FJ, Basson M, Pasquinelli AE, Bettinger JC, Rougvie AE, Horvitz HR, Ruvkun G. The 21-nucleotide let-7 RNA regulates developmental timing in Caenorhabditis elegans. Nature. 2000;403(6772):901–6.

115. Razin A, Cedar H. DNA methylation and gene expression. Microbiol Rev. 1991;55(3):451–8.

116. Herman JG, Baylin SB. Gene silencing in cancer in association with promoter hypermethylation. N Engl J Med. 2003; 349(21):2042–54.

117. Richardson B. Primer: epigenetics of autoimmunity. Nat Clin Pract Rheumatol. 2007;3(9):521–7.

118. Romero LI, Zhang DN, Cooke JP, Ho HK, Avalos E, Herrera R, Herron GS. Differential expression of nitric oxide by dermal microvascular endothelial cells from patients with scleroderma. Vasc Med. 2000;5(3):147–58.

119. Huang PL, Huang Z, Mashimo H, Bloch KD, Moskowitz MA, Bevan JA, Fishman MC. Hypertension in mice lacking the gene for endothelial nitric oxide synthase. Nature. 1995;377(6546): 239–42.

120. Lee PC, Salyapongse AN, Bragdon GA, Shears 2nd LL, Watkins SC, Edington HD, Billiar TR. Impaired wound healing and angiogenesis in eNOS-deficient mice. Am J Physiol. 1999;277(4 Pt 2):H1600–8.

121. Rabinovitch M. Molecular pathogenesis of pulmonary arterial hypertension. J Clin Invest. 2012;122(12):4306–13.

122. Wang Y, Kahaleh B. Epigenetic repression of bone morphogenetic protein receptor II expression in scleroderma. J Cell Mol Med. 2013;17(10):1291–9.

123. Altorok N, Almeshal N, Wang Y, Kahaleh B. Epigenetics, the holy grail in the pathogenesis of systemic sclerosis. Rheumatology (Oxford). 2015;54(10):1759–70.

124. Carmeliet P. Mechanisms of angiogenesis and arteriogenesis. Nat Med. 2000;6(4):389–95.

125. Manetti M, Guiducci S, Ibba-Manneschi L, Matucci-Cerinic M. Mechanisms in the loss of capillaries in systemic sclerosis: angiogenesis versus vasculogenesis. J Cell Mol Med. 2010;14(6A): 1241–54.

126. Rabquer BJ, Koch AE. Angiogenesis and vasculopathy in systemic sclerosis: evolving concepts. Curr Rheumatol Rep. 2012; 14(1):56–63.

127. Manetti M, Guiducci S, Ibba-Manneschi L, Matucci-Cerinic M. Impaired angiogenesis in systemic sclerosis: the emerging role of the antiangiogenic VEGF(165)b splice variant. Trends Cardiovasc Med. 2011;21(7):204–10.

128. Distler O, Del Rosso A, Giacomelli R, Cipriani P, Conforti ML, Guiducci S, Gay RE, Michel BA, Brühlmann P, Müller-Ladner U, Gay S, Matucci-Cerinic M. Angiogenic and angiostatic factors in systemic sclerosis: increased levels of vascular endothelial growth factor are a feature of the earliest disease stages and are associated with the absence of fingertip ulcers. Arthritis Res. 2002;4(6):R11.

129. Distler O, Distler JH, Scheid A, Acker T, Hirth A, Rethage J, Michel BA, Gay RE, Müller-Ladner U, Matucci-Cerinic M, Plate KH, Gassmann M, Gay S. Uncontrolled expression of vascular endothelial growth factor and its receptors leads to insufficient skin angiogenesis in patients with systemic sclerosis. Circ Res. 2004;95(1):109–16.

130. Choi JJ, Min DJ, Cho ML, Min SY, Kim SJ, Lee SS, Park KS, Seo YI, Kim WU, Park SH, Cho CS. Elevated vascular endothelial growth factor in systemic sclerosis. J Rheumatol. 2003;30(7): 1529–33.

131. Mackiewicz Z, Sukura A, Povilenaité D, Ceponis A, Virtanen I, Hukkanen M, Konttinen YT. Increased but imbalanced expression of VEGF and its receptors has no positive effect on angiogenesis in systemic sclerosis skin. Clin Exp Rheumatol. 2002;20(5): 641–6.

132. D'Alessio S, Fibbi G, Cinelli M, Guiducci S, Del Rosso A, Margheri F, Serratì S, Pucci M, Kahaleh B, Fan P, Annunziato F, Cosmi L, Liotta F, Matucci-Cerinic M, Del Rosso M. Matrix metalloproteinase 12-dependent cleavage of urokinase receptor in systemic sclerosis microvascular endothelial cells results in impaired angiogenesis. Arthritis Rheum. 2004;50(10):3275–85.

133. Manetti M, Guiducci S, Romano E, Ceccarelli C, Bellando-Randone S, Conforti ML, Ibba-Manneschi L, Matucci-Cerinic M. Overexpression of VEGF165b, an inhibitory splice variant of vascular endothelial growth factor, leads to insufficient angiogenesis in patients with systemic sclerosis. Circ Res. 2011;109(3):e14–26.

134. Manetti M, Guiducci S, Romano E, Bellando-Randone S, Lepri G, Bruni C, Conforti ML, Ibba-Manneschi L, Matucci-Cerinic M. Increased plasma levels of the VEGF165b splice variant are associated with the severity of nailfold capillary loss in systemic sclerosis. Ann Rheum Dis. 2013;72(8):1425–7.

135. Rabquer BJ, Tsou PS, Hou Y, Thirunavukkarasu E, Haines 3rd GK, Impens AJ, Phillips K, Kahaleh B, Seibold JR, Koch

AE. Dysregulated expression of MIG/CXCL9, IP-10/CXCL10 and CXCL16 and their receptors in systemic sclerosis. Arthritis Res Ther. 2011;13(1):R18.

136. Shirai Y, Okazaki Y, Inoue Y, Tamura Y, Yasuoka H, Takeuchi T, Kuwana M. Elevated levels of pentraxin 3 in systemic sclerosis: associations with vascular manifestations and defective vasculogenesis. Arthritis Rheumatol. 2015;67(2):498–507.
137. Manetti M, Guiducci S, Romano E, Avouac J, Rosa I, Ruiz B, Lepri G, Bellando-Randone S, Ibba-Manneschi L, Allanore Y, Matucci-Cerinic M. Decreased expression of the endothelial cell-derived factor EGFL7 in systemic sclerosis: potential contribution to impaired angiogenesis and vasculogenesis. Arthritis Res Ther. 2013;15(5):R165.
138. Asahara T, Murohara T, Sullivan A, Silver M, van der Zee R, Li T, Witzenbichler B, Schatteman G, Isner JM. Isolation of putative progenitor endothelial cells for angiogenesis. Science. 1997; 275(5302):964–7.
139. Kuwana M, Okazaki Y, Yasuoka H, Kawakami Y, Ikeda Y. Defective vasculogenesis in systemic sclerosis. Lancet. 2004; 364(9434):603–10.
140. Allanore Y, Batteux F, Avouac J, Assous N, Weill B, Kahan A. Levels of circulating endothelial progenitor cells in systemic sclerosis. Clin Exp Rheumatol. 2007;25(1):60–6.
141. Avouac J, Juin F, Wipff J, Couraud PO, Chiocchia G, Kahan A, Boileau C, Uzan G, Allanore Y. Circulating endothelial progenitor cells in systemic sclerosis: association with disease severity. Ann Rheum Dis. 2008;67(10):1455–60.
142. Zhu S, Evans S, Yan B, Povsic TJ, Tapson V, Goldschmidt-Clermont PJ, Dong C. Transcriptional regulation of Bim by FOXO3a and Akt mediates scleroderma serum-induced apoptosis in endothelial progenitor cells. Circulation. 2008;118(21):2156–65.
143. Del Papa N, Quirici N, Scavullo C, Gianelli U, Corti L, Vitali C, Ferri C, Giuggioli D, Manfredi A, Maglione W, Onida F, Colaci M, Bosari S, Lambertenghi Deliliers G. Antiendothelial cell antibodies induce apoptosis of bone marrow endothelial progenitors in systemic sclerosis. J Rheumatol. 2010;37(10):2053–63.
144. Kuwana M, Okazaki Y. Brief report: impaired in vivo neovascularization capacity of endothelial progenitor cells in patients with systemic sclerosis. Arthritis Rheumatol. 2014;66(5):1300–5.
145. Yamaguchi Y, Kuwana M. Proangiogenic hematopoietic cells of monocytic origin: roles in vascular regeneration and pathogenic processes of systemic sclerosis. Histol Histopathol. 2013;28(2):175–83.
146. Cipriani P, Guiducci S, Miniati I, Cinelli M, Urbani S, Marrelli A, Dolo V, Pavan A, Saccardi R, Tyndall A, Giacomelli R, Cerinic MM. Impairment of endothelial cell differentiation from bone marrow-derived mesenchymal stem cells: new insight into the pathogenesis of systemic sclerosis. Arthritis Rheum. 2007;56(6): 1994–2004.
147. Guiducci S, Manetti M, Romano E, Mazzanti B, Ceccarelli C, Dal Pozzo S, Milia AF, Bellando-Randone S, Fiori G, Conforti ML, Saccardi R, Ibba-Manneschi L, Matucci-Cerinic M. Bone marrow-derived mesenchymal stem cells from early diffuse systemic sclerosis exhibit a paracrine machinery and stimulate angiogenesis in vitro. Ann Rheum Dis. 2011;70(11):2011–21.
148. Guiducci S, Porta F, Saccardi R, Guidi S, Ibba-Manneschi L, Manetti M, Mazzanti B, Dal Pozzo S, Milia AF, Bellando-Randone S, Miniati I, Fiori G, Fontana R, Amanzi L, Braschi F, Bosi A, Matucci-Cerinic M. Autologous mesenchymal stem cells foster revascularization of ischemic limbs in systemic sclerosis: a case report. Ann Intern Med. 2010;153(10):650–4.
149. Matucci-Cerinic M, Kahaleh B, Wigley FM. Review: evidence that systemic sclerosis is a vascular disease. Arthritis Rheum. 2013;65(8):1953–62.
150. Pepper MS. Role of the matrix metalloproteinase and plasminogen activator-plasmin systems in angiogenesis. Arterioscler Thromb Vasc Biol. 2001;21(7):1104–17.
151. Keck RG, Berleau L, Harris R, Keyt BA. Disulfide structure of the heparin binding domain in vascular endothelial growth factor: characterization of posttranslational modifications in VEGF. Arch Biochem Biophys. 1997;344(1):103–13.
152. Ihn H. The role of TGF-beta signaling in the pathogenesis of fibrosis in scleroderma. Arch Immunol Ther Exp (Warsz). 2002; 50(5):325–31.
153. Jinnin M, Ihn H, Mimura Y, Asano Y, Yamane K, Tamaki K. Effects of hepatocyte growth factor on the expression of type I collagen and matrix metalloproteinase-1 in normal and scleroderma dermal fibroblasts. J Invest Dermatol. 2005;124(2): 324–30.
154. Lijnen HR, Ugwu F, Bini A, Collen D. Generation of an angiostatin-like fragment from plasminogen by stromelysin-1 (MMP-3). Biochemistry. 1998;37(14):4699–702.
155. O'Reilly MS, Wiederschain D, Stetler-Stevenson WG, Folkman J, Moses MA. Regulation of angiostatin production by matrix metalloproteinase-2 in a model of concomitant resistance. J Biol Chem. 1999;274(41):29568–71.
156. Vassalli JD, Baccino D, Belin D. A cellular binding site for the Mr 55,000 form of the human plasminogen activator, urokinase. J Cell Biol. 1985;100(1):86–92.
157. Wei Y, Waltz DA, Rao N, Drummond RJ, Rosenberg S, Chapman HA. Identification of the urokinase receptor as an adhesion receptor for vitronectin. J Biol Chem. 1994;269(51):32380–8.
158. Ragno P. The urokinase receptor: a ligand or a receptor? Story of a sociable molecule. Cell Mol Life Sci. 2006;63(9):1028–37.
159. Margheri F, Manetti M, Serratì S, Nosi D, Pucci M, Matucci-Cerinic M, Kahaleh B, Bazzichi L, Fibbi G, Ibba-Manneschi L, Del Rosso M. Domain 1 of the urokinase-type plasminogen activator receptor is required for its morphologic and functional, beta2 integrin-mediated connection with actin cytoskeleton in human microvascular endothelial cells: failure of association in systemic sclerosis endothelial cells. Arthritis Rheum. 2006;54(12): 3926–38.
160. Margheri F, Serratì S, Lapucci A, Chillà A, Bazzichi L, Bombardieri S, Kahaleh B, Calorini L, Bianchini F, Fibbi G, Del Rosso M. Modulation of the angiogenic phenotype of normal and systemic sclerosis endothelial cells by gain-loss of function of pentraxin 3 and matrix metalloproteinase 12. Arthritis Rheum. 2010;62(8):2488–98.
161. Manetti M, Guiducci S, Romano E, Bellando-Randone S, Conforti ML, Ibba-Manneschi L, Matucci-Cerinic M. Increased serum levels and tissue expression of matrix metalloproteinase-12 in patients with systemic sclerosis: correlation with severity of skin and pulmonary fibrosis and vascular damage. Ann Rheum Dis. 2012;71(6):1064–72.
162. Xu Z, Shi H, Li Q, Mei Q, Bao J, Shen Y, Xu J. Mouse macrophage metalloelastase generates angiostatin from plasminogen and suppresses tumor angiogenesis in murine colon cancer. Oncol Rep. 2008;20(1):81–8.
163. Giusti B, Serratì S, Margheri F, Papucci L, Rossi L, Poggi F, Magi A, Del Rosso A, Cinelli M, Guiducci S, Kahaleh B, Matucci-Cerinic M, Abbate R, Fibbi G, Del Rosso M. The antiangiogenic tissue kallikrein pattern of endothelial cells in systemic sclerosis. Arthritis Rheum. 2005;52(11):3618–28.
164. Giusti B, Fibbi G, Margheri F, Serratì S, Rossi L, Poggi F, Lapini I, Magi A, Del Rosso A, Cinelli M, Guiducci S, Kahaleh B, Bazzichi L, Bombardieri S, Matucci-Cerinic M, Gensini GF, Del Rosso M, Abbate R. A model of anti-angiogenesis: differential transcriptosome profiling of microvascular endothelial cells from diffuse systemic sclerosis patients. Arthritis Res Ther. 2006; 8(4):R115.
165. Bhoola KD, Figueroa CD, Worthy K. Bioregulation of kinins: kallikreins, kininogens, and kininases. Pharmacol Rev. 1992;44(1): 1–80.

166. Plendl J, Snyman C, Naidoo S, Sawant S, Mahabeer R, Bhoola KD. Expression of tissue kallikrein and kinin receptors in angiogenic microvascular endothelial cells. Biol Chem. 2000;381(11): 1103–15.
167. Emanueli C, Madeddu P. Targeting kinin receptors for the treatment of tissue ischaemia. Trends Pharmacol Sci. 2001;22(9): 478–84.
168. Del Rosso A, Distler O, Milia AF, Emanueli C, Ibba-Manneschi L, Guiducci S, Conforti ML, Generini S, Pignone A, Gay S, Madeddu P, Matucci-Cerinic M. Increased circulating levels of tissue kallikrein in systemic sclerosis correlate with microvascular involvement. Ann Rheum Dis. 2005;64(3):382–7.
169. Giusti B, Margheri F, Rossi L, Lapini I, Magi A, Serratì S, Chillà A, Laurenzana A, Magnelli L, Calorini L, Bianchini F, Fibbi G, Abbate R, Del Rosso M. Desmoglein-2-integrin Beta-8 interaction regulates actin assembly in endothelial cells: deregulation in systemic sclerosis. PLoS One. 2013;8(7):e68117.
170. Avouac J, Cagnard N, Distler JH, Schoindre Y, Ruiz B, Couraud PO, Uzan G, Boileau C, Chiocchia G, Allanore Y. Insights into the pathogenesis of systemic sclerosis based on the gene expression profile of progenitor-derived endothelial cells. Arthritis Rheum. 2011;63(11):3552–62.
171. Tinazzi E, Dolcino M, Puccetti A, Rigo A, Beri R, Valenti MT, Corrocher R, Lunardi C. Gene expression profiling in circulating endothelial cells from systemic sclerosis patients shows an altered control of apoptosis and angiogenesis that is modified by iloprost infusion. Arthritis Res Ther. 2010;12(4):R131.
172. Allt G, Lawrenson JG. Pericytes: cell biology and pathology. Cells Tissues Organs. 2001;169(1):1–11.
173. Sima AA, Chakrabarti S, Garcia-Salinas R, Basu PK. The BB-rat; an authentic model of human diabetic retinopathy. Curr Eye Res. 1985;4(10):1087–92.
174. Sims DE. Recent advances in pericyte biology – implications for health and disease. Can J Cardiol. 1991;7(10):431–43.
175. Mandarino LJ, Sundarraj N, Finlayson J, Hassell HR. Regulation of fibronectin and laminin synthesis by retinal capillary endothelial cells and pericytes in vitro. Exp Eye Res. 1993;57(5):609–21.
176. Hirschi KK, D'Amore PA. Control of angiogenesis by the pericyte: molecular mechanisms and significance. EXS. 1997;79:419–28.
177. Herman IM, D'Amore PA. Microvascular pericytes contain muscle and nonmuscle actins. J Cell Biol. 1985;101(1):43–52.
178. Edelman DA, Jiang Y, Tyburski J, Wilson RF, Steffes C. Pericytes and their role in microvasculature homeostasis. J Surg Res. 2006;135(2):305–11.
179. Hirschi KK, Rohovsky SA, D'Amore PA. PDGF, TGF-beta, and heterotypic cell-cell interactions mediate endothelial cell-induced recruitment of 10T1/2 cells and their differentiation to a smooth muscle fate. J Cell Biol. 1998;141(3):805–14.
180. Kelley C, D'Amore P, Hechtman HB, Shepro D. Microvascular pericyte contractility in vitro: comparison with other cells of the vascular wall. J Cell Biol. 1987;104(3):483–90.
181. Tilton RG, Kilo C, Williamson JR. Pericyte-endothelial relationships in cardiac and skeletal muscle capillaries. Microvasc Res. 1979;18(3):325–35.
182. Cuevas P, Gutierrez-Diaz JA, Reimers D, Dujovny M, Diaz FG, Ausman JI. Pericyte endothelial gap junctions in human cerebral capillaries. Anat Embryol (Berl). 1984;170(2):155–9.
183. Miller FN, Sims DE. Contractile elements in the regulation of macromolecular permeability. Fed Proc. 1986;45(2):84–8.
184. Murphy DD, Wagner RC. Differential contractile response of cultured microvascular pericytes to vasoactive agents. Microcirculation. 1994;1(2):121–8.
185. Shepro D, Morel NM. Pericyte physiology. FASEB J. 1993;7(11): 1031–8.
186. Carmeliet P. Blood vessels and nerves: common signals, pathways and diseases. Nat Rev Genet. 2003;4(9):710–20.
187. Louissaint Jr A, Rao S, Leventhal C, Goldman SA. Coordinated interaction of neurogenesis and angiogenesis in the adult songbird brain. Neuron. 2002;34(6):945–60.
188. Palmer TD, Willhoite AR, Gage FH. Vascular niche for adult hippocampal neurogenesis. J Comp Neurol. 2000;425(4):479–94.
189. Rønnov-Jessen L, Petersen OW, Koteliansky VE, Bissell MJ. The origin of the myofibroblasts in breast cancer. Recapitulation of tumor environment in culture unravels diversity and implicates converted fibroblasts and recruited smooth muscle cells. J Clin Invest. 1995;95(2):859–73.
190. Sundberg C, Ivarsson M, Gerdin B, Rubin K. Pericytes as collagen-producing cells in excessive dermal scarring. Lab Invest. 1996;74(2):452–66.
191. Sundberg C, Ljungström M, Lindmark G, Gerdin B, Rubin K. Microvascular pericytes express platelet-derived growth factor-beta receptors in human healing wounds and colorectal adenocarcinoma. Am J Pathol. 1993;143(5):1377–88.
192. Rajkumar VS, Sundberg C, Abraham DJ, Rubin K, Black CM. Activation of microvascular pericytes in autoimmune Raynaud's phenomenon and systemic sclerosis. Arthritis Rheum. 1999; 42(5):930–41.
193. Jelaska A, Korn JH. Role of apoptosis and transforming growth factor beta1 in fibroblast selection and activation in systemic sclerosis. Arthritis Rheum. 2000;43(10):2230–9.
194. Sappino AP, Masouyé I, Saurat JH, Gabbiani G. Smooth muscle differentiation in scleroderma fibroblastic cells. Am J Pathol. 1990;137(3):585–91.
195. Rajkumar VS, Howell K, Csiszar K, Denton CP, Black CM, Abraham DJ. Shared expression of phenotypic markers in systemic sclerosis indicates a convergence of pericytes and fibroblasts to a myofibroblast lineage in fibrosis. Arthritis Res Ther. 2005;7(5):R1113–23.
196. Asano Y, Stawski L, Hant F, Highland K, Silver R, Szalai G, Watson DK, Trojanowska M. Endothelial Fli1 deficiency impairs vascular homeostasis: a role in scleroderma vasculopathy. Am J Pathol. 2010;176(4):1983–98.
197. Cretoiu SM, Popescu LM. Telocytes revisited. Biomol Concepts. 2014;5(5):353–69.
198. Manetti M, Guiducci S, Ruffo M, Rosa I, Faussone-Pellegrini MS, Matucci-Cerinic M, Ibba-Manneschi L. Evidence for progressive reduction and loss of telocytes in the dermal cellular network of systemic sclerosis. J Cell Mol Med. 2013;17(4):482–96.
199. Frid MG, Dempsey EC, Durmowicz AG, Stenmark KR. Smooth muscle cell heterogeneity in pulmonary and systemic vessels. Importance in vascular disease. Arterioscler Thromb Vasc Biol. 1997;17(7):1203–9.
200. Gittenberger-de Groot AC, DeRuiter MC, Bergwerff M, Poelmann RE. Smooth muscle cell origin and its relation to heterogeneity in development and disease. Arterioscler Thromb Vasc Biol. 1999; 19(7):1589–94.
201. Owens GK. Molecular control of vascular smooth muscle cell differentiation. Acta Physiol Scand. 1998;164(4):623–35.
202. Arts MR, Baron M, Chokr N, Fritzler MJ, Canadian Scleroderma Research Group (CSRG), Servant MJ. Systemic sclerosis immunoglobulin induces growth and a pro-fibrotic state in vascular smooth muscle cells through the epidermal growth factor receptor. PLoS One. 2014;9(6):e100035.
203. Jimenez SA. Role of endothelial to mesenchymal transition in the pathogenesis of the vascular alterations in systemic sclerosis. ISRN Rheumatol. 2013;2013:835948.
204. Rhodes JM, Simons M. The extracellular matrix and blood vessel formation: not just a scaffold. J Cell Mol Med. 2007;11(2):176–205.
205. Davis GE, Saunders WB. Molecular balance of capillary tube formation versus regression in wound repair: role of matrix metalloproteinases and their inhibitors. J Investig Dermatol Symp Proc. 2006;11(1):44–56.

206. Davis GE, Senger DR. Endothelial extracellular matrix: biosynthesis, remodeling, and functions during vascular morphogenesis and neovessel stabilization. Circ Res. 2005;97(11):1093–107.
207. Senger DR. Molecular framework for angiogenesis: a complex web of interactions between extravasated plasma proteins and endothelial cell proteins induced by angiogenic cytokines. Am J Pathol. 1996;149(1):1–7.
208. Vernon RB, Sage EH. Between molecules and morphology. Extracellular matrix and creation of vascular form. Am J Pathol. 1995;147(4):873–83.
209. Dvorak HF, Nagy JA, Berse B, Brown LF, Yeo KT, Yeo TK, Dvorak AM, van de Water L, Sioussat TM, Senger DR. Vascular permeability factor, fibrin, and the pathogenesis of tumor stroma formation. Ann N Y Acad Sci. 1992;667:101–11.
210. Dvorak HF, Senger DR, Dvorak AM. Fibrin as a component of the tumor stroma: origins and biological significance. Cancer Metastasis Rev. 1983;2(1):41–73.
211. Nagy JA, Brown LF, Senger DR, Lanir N, Van de Water L, Dvorak AM, Dvorak HF. Pathogenesis of tumor stroma generation: a critical role for leaky blood vessels and fibrin deposition. Biochim Biophys Acta. 1989;948(3):305–26.
212. Cheresh DA, Berliner SA, Vicente V, Ruggeri ZM. Recognition of distinct adhesive sites on fibrinogen by related integrins on platelets and endothelial cells. Cell. 1989;58(5):945–53.
213. Suehiro K, Gailit J, Plow EF. Fibrinogen is a ligand for integrin alpha-5beta1 on endothelial cells. J Biol Chem. 1997;272(8):5360–6.
214. Sahni A, Altland OD, Francis CW. FGF-2 but not FGF-1 binds fibrin and supports prolonged endothelial cell growth. J Thromb Haemost. 2003;1(6):1304–10.
215. Sahni A, Francis CW. Plasmic degradation modulates activity of fibrinogen-bound fibroblast growth factor-2. J Thromb Haemost. 2003;1(6):1271–7.
216. Bobik A, Tkachuk V. Metalloproteinases and plasminogen activators in vessel remodeling. Curr Hypertens Rep. 2003;5(6):466–72.
217. Garcia-Touchard A, Henry TD, Sangiorgi G, Spagnoli LG, Mauriello A, Conover C, Schwartz RS. Extracellular proteases in atherosclerosis and restenosis. Arterioscler Thromb Vasc Biol. 2005;25(6):1119–27.
218. Davis GE, Pintar Allen KA, Salazar R, Maxwell SA. Matrix metalloproteinase-1 and -9 activation by plasmin regulates a novel endothelial cell-mediated mechanism of collagen gel contraction and capillary tube regression in three-dimensional collagen matrices. J Cell Sci. 2001;114(Pt 5):917–30.
219. Saunders WB, Bayless KJ, Davis GE. MMP-1 activation by serine proteases and MMP-10 induces human capillary tubular network collapse and regression in 3D collagen matrices. J Cell Sci. 2005;118(Pt 10):2325–40.
220. Giannelli G, Iannone F, Marinosci F, Lapadula G, Antonaci S. The effect of bosentan on matrix metalloproteinase-9 levels in patients with systemic sclerosis-induced pulmonary hypertension. Curr Med Res Opin. 2005;21(3):327–32.
221. Kim WU, Min SY, Cho ML, Hong KH, Shin YJ, Park SH, Cho CS. Elevated matrix metalloproteinase-9 in patients with systemic sclerosis. Arthritis Res Ther. 2005;7(1):R71–9.
222. Avouac J, Wipff J, Goldman O, Ruiz B, Couraud PO, Chiocchia G, Kahan A, Boileau C, Uzan G, Allanore Y. Angiogenesis in systemic sclerosis: impaired expression of vascular endothelial growth factor receptor 1 in endothelial progenitor-derived cells under hypoxic conditions. Arthritis Rheum. 2008;58(11):3550–61.
223. Silverstein JL, Steen VD, Medsger Jr TA, Falanga V. Cutaneous hypoxia in patients with systemic sclerosis (scleroderma). Arch Dermatol. 1988;124(9):1379–82.
224. Manalo DJ, Rowan A, Lavoie T, Natarajan L, Kelly BD, Ye SQ, Garcia JG, Semenza GL. Transcriptional regulation of vascular endothelial cell responses to hypoxia by HIF-1. Blood. 2005;105(2):659–69.
225. Makarenko VV, Usatyuk PV, Yuan G, Lee MM, Nanduri J, Natarajan V, Kumar GK, Prabhakar NR. Intermittent hypoxia-induced endothelial barrier dysfunction requires ROS-dependent MAP kinase activation. Am J Physiol Cell Physiol. 2014;306(8):C745–52.
226. Kahaleh MB. The role of vascular endothelium in fibroblast activation and tissue fibrosis, particularly in scleroderma (systemic sclerosis) and pachydermoperiostosis (primary hypertrophic osteoarthropathy). Clin Exp Rheumatol. 1992;10 Suppl 7:51–6.
227. Tomasek JJ, Gabbiani G, Hinz B, Chaponnier C, Brown RA. Myofibroblasts and mechano-regulation of connective tissue remodelling. Nat Rev Mol Cell Biol. 2002;3(5):349–63.
228. Lauber K, Bohn E, Kröber SM, Xiao YJ, Blumenthal SG, Lindemann RK, Marini P, Wiedig C, Zobywalski A, Baksh S, Xu Y, Autenrieth IB, Schulze-Osthoff K, Belka C, Stuhler G, Wesselborg S. Apoptotic cells induce migration of phagocytes via caspase-3-mediated release of a lipid attraction signal. Cell. 2003;113(6):717–30.
229. Holmes A, Abraham DJ, Chen Y, Denton C, Shi-wen X, Black CM, Leask A. Constitutive connective tissue growth factor expression in scleroderma fibroblasts is dependent on Sp1. J Biol Chem. 2003;278(43):41728–33.
230. Shi-Wen X, Leask A, Abraham D. Regulation and function of connective tissue growth factor/CCN2 in tissue repair, scarring and fibrosis. Cytokine Growth Factor Rev. 2008;19(2):133–44.
231. Serratì S, Chillà A, Laurenzana A, Margheri F, Giannoni E, Magnelli L, Chiarugi P, Dotor J, Feijoo E, Bazzichi L, Bombardieri S, Kahaleh B, Fibbi G, Del Rosso M. Systemic sclerosis endothelial cells recruit and activate dermal fibroblasts by induction of a connective tissue growth factor (CCN2)/transforming growth factor β-dependent mesenchymal-to-mesenchymal transition. Arthritis Rheum. 2013;65(1):258–69.
232. Dees C, Akhmetshina A, Zerr P, Reich N, Palumbo K, Horn A, Jüngel A, Beyer C, Krönke G, Zwerina J, Reiter R, Alenina N, Maroteaux L, Gay S, Schett G, Distler O, Distler JH. Platelet-derived serotonin links vascular disease and tissue fibrosis. J Exp Med. 2011;208(5):961–72.
233. Maurer B, Distler A, Suliman YA, Gay RE, Michel BA, Gay S, Distler JH, Distler O. Vascular endothelial growth factor aggravates fibrosis and vasculopathy in experimental models of systemic sclerosis. Ann Rheum Dis. 2014;73(10):1880–7.
234. Christner PJ, Jimenez SA. Animal models of systemic sclerosis: insights into systemic sclerosis pathogenesis and potential therapeutic approaches. Curr Opin Rheumatol. 2004;16(6):746–52.
235. Smith GP, Chan ES. Molecular pathogenesis of skin fibrosis: insight from animal models. Curr Rheumatol Rep. 2010;12(1):26–33.
236. Marie I, Bény JL. Endothelial dysfunction in murine model of systemic sclerosis: tight-skin mice 1. J Invest Dermatol. 2002;119(6):1379–87.
237. Sgonc R. The vascular perspective of systemic sclerosis: of chickens, mice and men. Int Arch Allergy Immunol. 1999;120(3):169–76.
238. Ruzek MC, Jha S, Ledbetter S, Richards SM, Garman RD. A modified model of graft-versus-host-induced systemic sclerosis (scleroderma) exhibits all major aspects of the human disease. Arthritis Rheum. 2004;50(4):1319–31.
239. Maurer B, Busch N, Jüngel A, Pileckyte M, Gay RE, Michel BA, Schett G, Gay S, Distler J, Distler O. Transcription factor fos-related antigen-2 induces progressive peripheral vasculopathy in mice closely resembling human systemic sclerosis. Circulation. 2009;120(23):2367–76.
240. Maurer B, Reich N, Juengel A, Kriegsmann J, Gay RE, Schett G, Michel BA, Gay S, Distler JH, Distler O. Fra-2 transgenic mice as

a novel model of pulmonary hypertension associated with systemic sclerosis. Ann Rheum Dis. 2012;71(8):1382–7.
241. Bernstein AM, Twining SS, Warejcka DJ, Tall E, Masur SK. Urokinase receptor cleavage: a crucial step in fibroblast-to-myofibroblast differentiation. Mol Biol Cell. 2007;18(7):2716–27.
242. Manetti M, Rosa I, Milia AF, Guiducci S, Carmeliet P, Ibba-Manneschi L, Matucci-Cerinic M. Inactivation of urokinase-type plasminogen activator receptor (uPAR) gene induces dermal and pulmonary fibrosis and peripheral microvasculopathy in mice: a new model of experimental scleroderma? Ann Rheum Dis. 2014;73(9):1700–9.
243. Zhang G, Kim H, Cai X, López-Guisa JM, Alpers CE, Liu Y, Carmeliet P, Eddy AA. Urokinase receptor deficiency accelerates renal fibrosis in obstructive nephropathy. J Am Soc Nephrol. 2003;14(5):1254–71.

Biomarkers in Systemic Sclerosis

17

Robert Lafyatis and Sergio A. Jimenez

Introduction

Over the past 10 years, biomarkers have gone from a rarely considered subject of scientific inquiry to center stage in both clinical and translational science. The impetus for this is clear. They provide valuable information for more efficient performance of clinical trials while simultaneously creating a bridge to understanding disease pathogenesis. Strong correlations between biomarkers and disease activity suggest direct roles in pathogenesis for the biomarker; the stronger the correlation, the more likely a biomarker is implicated in pathogenesis. Thus, biomarkers provide unique opportunities to understand disease mechanisms. Biomarkers are also particularly valuable in clinical setting where the disease is hard to measure using clinical outcomes, as is the case for virtually all of SSc manifestations. However, the most exciting aspect of biomarkers is at the interface between clinical and translational medicine. The effect of drug treatment on biomarkers can lead to exciting insights into the roles of drug-targeted pathways in pathogenesis.

Biomarkers already permeate clinical care as commonly used laboratory tests. In the clinical setting, biomarkers are useful in several different contexts. In their most basic application, biomarkers are used in diagnosis of diseases or disease complications. Such laboratory tests are used in countless ways in diagnostics from TSH levels for thyroid disease to CK levels to assess the occurrence of muscle injury and myocardial infarction. However biomarkers have several other utilities that have been increasingly explored, which are particularly important in clinical trials. They can be used to track the progression or regression of disease, to select patients more likely to show progressive disease, and to predict which patients are most likely to respond to a given treatment. Utilizing biomarkers in such settings is also increasingly entering routine clinical care, paving the way for personalized medicine, in which care and drug therapy can be based on molecular characters of individual patients.

R. Lafyatis, MD (✉)
University of Pittsburgh School of Medicine, Pittsburgh, USA
e-mail: rlafyatis@gmail.com

S.A. Jimenez, MD
Department of Dermatology and Cutaneous Biology, Jefferson Institute of Molecular Medicine, Thomas Jefferson University, Philadelphia, PA, USA

Types of Biomarkers

The FDA has laid out categories of biomarkers, and the nomenclature they have established will be used here in referring to different types of biomarkers, see [1] and Figs. 17.1, 17.2, and 17.3.

Diagnostic Biomarkers

Diagnostic biomarkers are designed to indicate the presence of disease or its complications. Anti-nuclear and other autoantibodies have a long history of diagnostic utility in SSc. Other diagnostic biomarkers will be considered below, although the main utility of these may be in subtyping patients or predicting likely patient SSc complications.

Outcome Measures and Pharmacodynamic Biomarkers

Pharmacodynamic biomarkers are designed to change as the disease status changes. We will use the terms "status" or "severity" in our consideration of pharmacodynamic biomarkers rather than disease activity, as the latter might be confused with the disease trajectory, considered below in regard to prognostic biomarkers. These biomarkers are thus most usefully considered in the context of repeated measurement at different times and as such are comparable to clinical outcome measures.

J. Varga et al. (eds.), *Scleroderma*, DOI 10.1007/978-3-319-31407-5_17

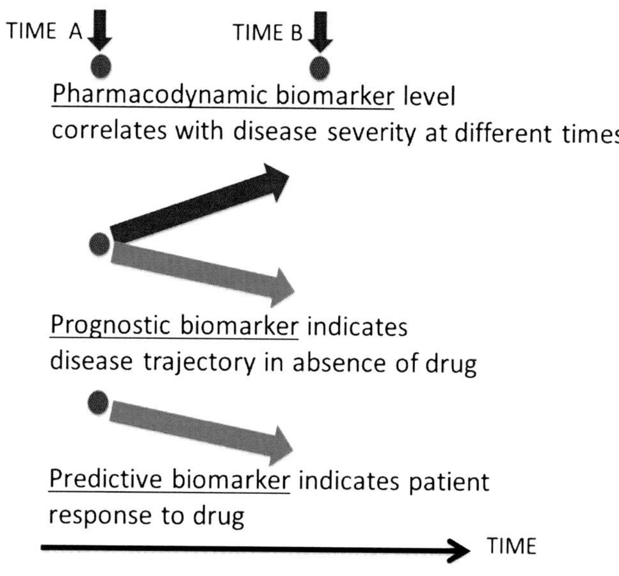

Fig. 17.1 Pharmacodynamic, prognostic, and predictive biomarkers. Pharmacodynamic biomarkers change with disease activity. Prognostic biomarkers indicate the disease trajectory in an untreated state. Predictive biomarkers indicate which patients will respond to a given drug treatment

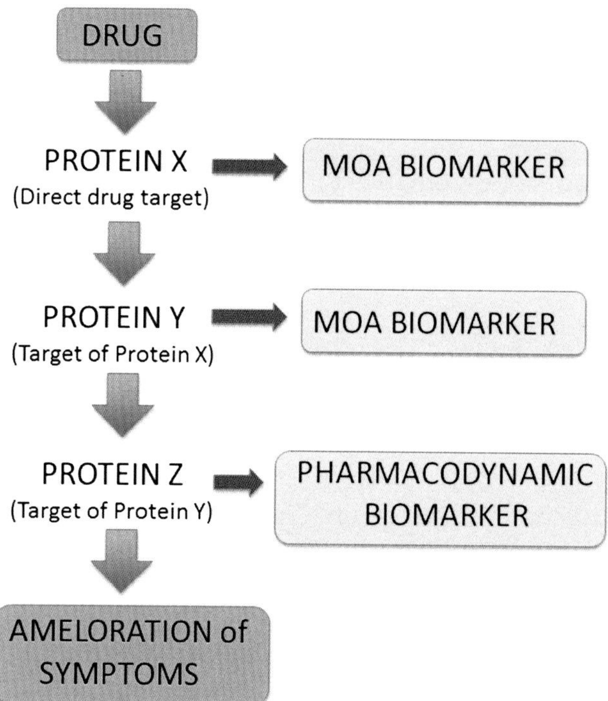

Fig. 17.2 Pharmacodynamic biomarkers. Pharmacodynamic biomarkers can serve to detect a drug's mechanisms of action (*MOA*). Typically these MOA biomarkers are identified on the basis of known targets of the drug. Pharmacodynamic biomarkers that serve as surrogate outcome measures are typically defined by a high association with the clinical outcome and are tightly associated with the pathogenic biochemical events leading to that outcome

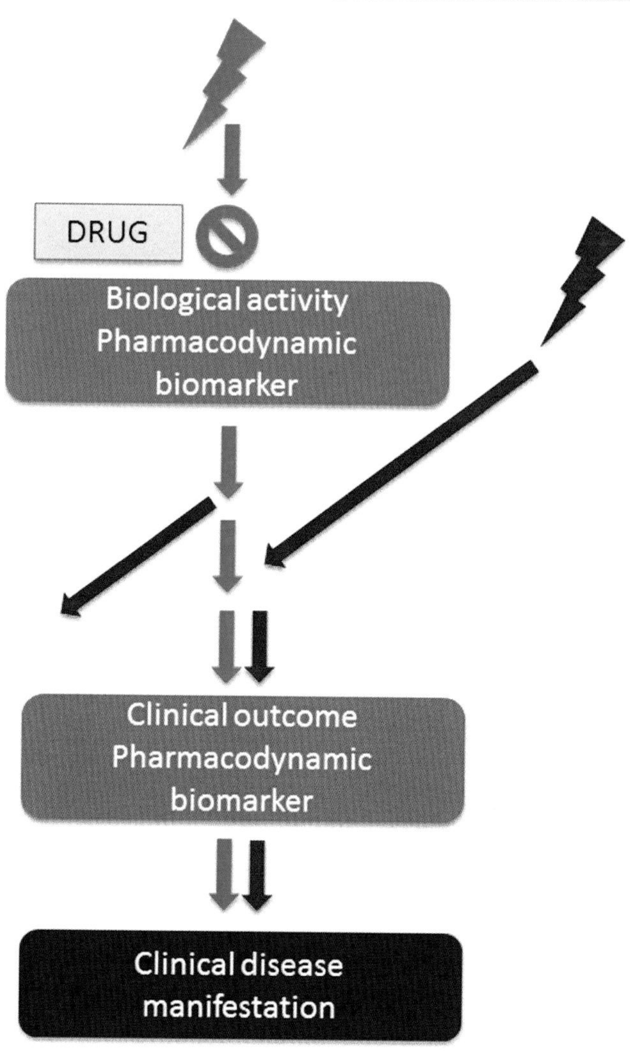

Fig. 17.3 Drug biological activity and clinical outcome pharmacodynamic biomarkers. The *green* lightning bolt and *arrows* indicate a drug that is successfully targeting a key pathogenic pathway. An effect of the drug on the biological activity biomarker indicates that the drug has successfully engaged a known biological target of the drug. The clinical response biomarker indicates that the drug is having an effect on the clinical outcome. The *red* lightning bolt and *arrows* indicate a pathogenic pathway in which the drug is unsuccessful. The drug may still succeed at blocking biological activity, but since this pathway is not involved in the pathogenic process, the clinical outcome biomarker is not affected. Note that it is important that the clinical outcome biomarker reflects biological processes directly in the route of pathogenesis and that it is proximal to the clinical outcome. If not, then a clinical outcome biomarker might respond like a drug biological activity biomarker, i.e., it might improve toward normal with drug treatment, but not reflect an improvement in clinical disease

A clinical outcome is typically used to anchor a pharmacodynamic biomarker. For SSc the most obvious anchors would be the MRSS or, in patients with interstitial lung disease (ILD), the forced vital capacity (FVC). The biomarker should thus change as the clinical outcome changes. If skin disease gets worse, then the biomarker should change proportionately. Pharmacodynamic biomarkers are particularly useful for clinical trials, where they can supplement a clinical outcome. However, pharmacodynamic biomarkers could also be useful for clinicians as a way of following disease severity. Pharmacodynamic biomarkers that meet certain criteria can graduate to become surrogate outcome measures.

Pharmacodynamic biomarkers can also serve to detect the expected mechanism of action of the therapeutic, if known. This is particularly important in early drug development when the proper dose of drug may not be known. These "mechanism of action (MOA)" biomarkers are easiest to identify for drugs with known discrete targets, for example, IL-6 or CRP levels in patients after treatment with anti-IL-6 or B cell levels in patients treated with anti-CD20. Although these biomarkers seem trivial for approved therapeutics, they are key for assessing target engagement for early drug development. Such MOA should be used in combination with a pharmacodynamic biomarker that is more closely associated with a clinical outcome measure to detect the likely drug effect on the disease (Fig. 17.2).

Biomarkers as Surrogate Outcome Measures

Surrogate outcome measures are pharmacodynamic biomarkers or other nonclinical outcomes that have achieved a status such that they can be used for drug approval, a feature generally given only to clinical outcomes. Clinical outcome measures are defined as a finding that reflects how a patient feels, functions, or survives. Several biomarkers have been found suitable for drug approval, such as LDL cholesterol and HbA1C. Neither of these directly measures patient symptoms, but both are tied to survival. Thus approval of biomarkers as surrogate outcomes must meet several criteria. They must be strongly associated with a relevant clinical outcome, but in addition they must be directly implicated in the pathogenic pathway of the disease.

The FDA has provided a mechanism for approval (referred to as qualification) of biomarkers meeting stringent criteria as surrogate outcome measures, making them approvable outcomes for a disease. However, the FDA expects that pharmacodynamic biomarkers will be most often used to guide drug development rather than as a basis for regulatory approval ([1] appendix 2 drug development tools). This conservative approach to qualification of biomarkers as surrogate outcomes is due to failures of past biomarkers to accurately reflect clinical outcomes. For example, biomarkers that reflect a drug's mechanism of action may not reflect a clinical response (Fig. 17.3).

Mechanism of Action (MOA) Biomarkers

Although increasingly drugs are designed to block or activate a specific molecular target, this may be far removed from the anticipated effect on the disease. This latter effect is better assessed with a pharmacodynamic biomarker and/or clinical outcome. All intervening steps in drug activation might be assessed by MOA biomarkers. In cases where the action of the drug is proximal to the effect on clinical markers, then pharmacodynamic and MOA biomarkers may be the same.

Prognostic Biomarkers

In contrast to pharmacodynamic biomarkers, which measure disease severity at a point in time, prognostic biomarkers measure where the disease is going. As such, they measure future disease trajectory. Will the skin get worse or better? Will ILD progress or stabilize? A particular challenge in identifying prognostic biomarkers is that they must be evaluated on an untreated patient population or be adjusted for treatment effects. As SSc patients are often treated with medications of unknown efficacy, prognostic biomarkers are particularly difficult to identify in SSc. Prognostic biomarkers in SSc include autoantibodies and genetic studies.

The highly variable clinical course of SSc makes prognostic biomarkers particularly important. In addition, they can be used effectively in clinical trial settings to help stratify patients for entry who are likely to show progressive disease.

Predictive Biomarkers

Predictive biomarkers tell whether a patient will respond to a given drug or other therapy. A prominent example of these is molecular markers used for patients with breast cancer [2]. These biomarkers have been widely embraced by both the FDA and the pharmaceutical industry. They are often identified during early phases of clinical development, where they can subsequently be used in Phase 3 trials to identify patients likely to respond to a given treatment. The identification of serum periostin in asthma as a predictive biomarker for response to anti-IL13 is a notable recent example of this approach [3]. These biomarkers are one of the major hopes of the concept of personalized medicine. These might consist of genetic markers or gene expression classifiers. The latter has been applied to SSc skin disease. A biomarker "classifier" that stratifies a disease phenotype by a molecular signature of genes has the potential to serve as both a prognostic and predictive biomarker.

Toxicity Biomarkers

Biomarkers of drug toxicity are of considerable importance for drug development, but will not be discussed further here.

Developing Biomarkers for Clinical Applications

Sources of Biomarker Information

Biomarkers can be assessed in many ways, including various measures of physiology such as EKG changes, blood pressure or hemodynamic monitoring, radiographic studies, as well as biochemical measures: protein and lipid mediator levels, mRNA expression, and DNA allelisms. The best biomarker for a given application depends on the biology of the disease or disease complication. However, high-throughput technologies, particularly microarray analyses of gene expression and emerging proteomics, appear to be favoring mRNA and proteins.

The relationship between a biomarker and disease pathogenesis is important in defining the best biomarker. If a disease is primarily genetic, then genetic markers would be expected to prove most useful. If driven by immune mediators or lipids, then interleukins or lipid mediators might, respectively, be more informative. Thus, one's bias about SSc pathogenesis might lead one investigator to focus more on genetic biomarkers, while another investigator focuses more on autoantibodies. In many cases the best biomarker measure will not be known and must be discovered empirically. Practical and innovative approaches based on clinical observations may prove particularly fruitful, such as assessing nailfold vascular changes. However, reproducibility and ease of applying a biomarker in a clinical setting may ultimately decide biomarker utility.

Generally speaking, getting as close as possible to the diseased tissue is likely to be most rewarding. When the diseased tissue is accessible, such as is often the case for tumor biomarkers and skin in SSc, that will typically be most informative. Skin is particularly attractive for analysis because of the ability to biopsy and re-biopsy. Major organs involved in SSc such as lungs and kidneys are much less accessible and so require other approaches.

Diseased Tissues

The advantage of analyzing diseased tissue is self-evident. Repeated sampling is currently only practical for skin. Because lung biopsy is not generally needed for diagnosis, tissue is rarely now available from patients with ILD. This may represent a significant loss for patients, as the biomarker information that could be obtained now from biopsies might have provided biomarkers that could guide therapy. However, studies discussed below have not yet identified a biomarker that provides a strong enough motive for obtaining biopsies to guide clinical care. Thus, most lung tissues have and will be obtained from patients at the time of transplant – of very limited value in terms of identifying clinically useful biomarkers.

Blood Biomarkers

Serum and plasma have been mainstays of biomarker studies. The obvious advantages are that blood circulates through all organs, so it samples disease at multiple sites. The ease of procurement and the ability to repetitively sample are also clear advantages of blood and blood element biomarkers. The main disadvantage of blood biomarkers is that they rely on what is discharged into the blood, which may or may not accurately represent what is happening in the diseased tissue. Although historically assessed mainly for proteins, blood also contains immune cells, microparticles, and other apparent "debris" possibly originating from cell turnover. Thus, recent novel approaches to biomarker discovery include measurements of mRNA, miRNA, and DNA.

Circulating miRNAs

Following the recent demonstration of the presence of nucleic acids in plasma and serum, and the highly productive NIH initiative providing strong support to study the role of extracellular RNA, there have been numerous publications describing the functional effects of extracellular RNA [4]. Most of these publications have focused on microRNAs (miRNAs) and in their potential utility as biomarkers of various disease processes [5]. MicroRNAs are small (~22 nucleotides), evolutionarily conserved noncoding RNA, which play important roles in the regulation of expression of a large number of protein-coding genes at the post-transcriptional level [6,7]. Although the role of miRNA in malignant disorders has been extensively studied [8,9], recent interest has been devoted to elucidating their participation in tissue fibrosis and fibrotic diseases [10–14]. Several miRNA have been shown to be involved in SSc tissue fibrosis, displaying either profibrotic or antifibrotic effects [15–21]. Furthermore, relevant targets of these miRNA are translated mRNAs involved in the pathogenesis of SSc-associated tissue fibrosis including collagens, matrix metalloproteinases, Smad signaling proteins, and even TGF-β [10,12,14]. One of the most extensively studied miRNA involved in SSc is miRNA29, which was found to be markedly decreased in SSc dermal fibroblasts and skin [15,16]. Overexpression of miR-29 in SSc fibroblasts decreased the levels of type I and type III collagens demonstrating a potent antifibrotic effect *in vitro*. Similar reduction of miR-29 was observed in fibrotic processes affecting other organs, including the heart, kidney, and lung. It was also shown that profibrotic stimuli including TGF-β, PDGF-B, and IL-4 reduced the levels of miR-29 in normal fibroblasts to levels similar to those observed in SSc fibroblasts, and a marked reduction in its levels was observed in the bleomycin model of skin fibrosis [15].

Besides the strong recent interest in the study of the functional role of miRNA in the regulation of important molecular pathways, the potential of circulating miRNAs as biomarkers has been extensively investigated in recent years [4,5,22]. MicroRNA were first detected in the blood plasma and serum in 2008 and have subsequently been shown to be present in other body fluids including urine, saliva, tears, and breast milk and thus, rendering them quite accessible for initial and serial determinations. Other reasons that render miRNAs excellent biomarker candidates include their remarkable stability in body fluids, and the fact that they can be easily measured with high sensitivity since they are amplifiable employing widely available PCR methods. The changes in circulating miRNA levels have been extensively used as diagnostic biomarkers for various types of cancer and numerous other clinical conditions [4,5,22]. However, their use as biomarkers for SSc is just becoming recognized.

Radiographic Studies

Radiographic tests provide a particularly rich opportunity for biomarker and biomarker development. CT scan, MRI, ultrasound, and PET scanning have each been applied to SSc with varying success. Newer technologies, particularly in quantitative CT and PET scanning, might yield much more informative biomarkers than those currently available.

Genetic Studies

Genetic associations with disease complications might be prognostic or predictive biomarkers. These biomarkers will be discussed in Chap. 3 on SSc genetics.

Autoantibodies

Autoantibodies have emerged as very useful markers for subsets of SSc patients. These disease subsets are associated with different disease complications and prognosis. Titers of anti-RNA pol3 have been reported to correlate with the extent of skin disease. Generally, autoantibody titers are relatively stable, so that their main value as biomarkers are as prognostic biomarkers of the risk of disease complications and perhaps in some cases of disease severity. These are discussed more fully in Chap. 15 on autoantibodies.

Other Biomarker Sources

Nailfold capillaroscopy, urine biomarkers, and digital plethysmography are examples of other modalities that might be utilized as biomarkers. This chapter will largely focus on biochemical biomarkers.

Biomarkers and High-Throughput Technologies

High-throughput technologies are increasingly driving biomarker studies as they permit non-hypothesis-driven identification of biomolecules. High-throughput mRNA technologies are well established. Microarrays can economically assess expression of all mRNAs in a single sample. However, RNA-sequencing is rapidly supplanting microarrays. This technology is able to look at noncoding RNAs and alternatively spliced mRNA that are not typically targeted on microarrays. Depending on the number of transcripts sequenced, RNA-seq can also be more sensitive than microarrays.

High-throughput proteomics have been more challenging particularly when applied to serum or plasma samples. Mass spectrometry is the most robust method for agnostically examining proteins in a biological sample. However, the utility of direct mass spectrometry measurements is restricted by the large dynamic range of serum proteins from abundant proteins such as albumins and immunoglobulins in blood (5–100 g/L) to rare cytokines (<1 fg/L) [23]. These proteins make it very difficult to see rarer (but potentially more informative) protein biomarkers in blood. Technologies aimed at depleting serum proteins before analysis have only partially mitigated this problem. New technologies, such as top-down proteomics [24] and SISCAPA [25], are beginning to show promise in translational research as well. Other technologies, such as Luminex and Somascan, use capture antibodies or aptamers to quantify proteins. These technologies can now permit identification or 200–1,000 proteins in a single sample, providing rich high-throughput methodologies for quantification of potential new protein biomarkers in serum and plasma.

Metabolomics provide another source of biomarker identification, though the value of this in biomarker identification is less proven.

Biomarker Performance: Correlations, Models, and ROC Curves

Biomarker utility is closely tied to how robustly they associate with the outcome they are modeling. Weak associations may tie the gene or protein marker to disease pathogenesis, but are unlikely to have much clinical utility. In some cases biomarkers weakly associated with a clinical outcome might be combined to provide more robust biomarkers. Developing biomarker models and evaluating biomarker performance depends on the type of biomarkers and, in particular, whether it is modeling a discrete or continuous variable.

Continuous variables are typically assessed using correlations or linear regression. Does the biomarker correlate with the MRSS or the FVC or other clinical measure? Multiple linear regression can be used to assess the value of using several analytes in a model. Methodologies for selecting analytes for models that include multiple analytes, such as forward selection and backward elimination and stepwise regression, have grown more complex [26]. More sophisticated statistical approaches are required to examine longitudinal changes in biomarkers and how these relate to longitudinal changes in clinical outcomes. General estimating equation or mixed models permit such analyses and also allow multiple analytes to be included in models.

Discrete variables include the presence or absence of disease or complication: i.e., diagnostic biomarkers. Does the patient have diffuse or limited SSc? Does the patient have ILD or PAH? Prognostic and predictive biomarkers can also be modeled as discrete variables. Is the patient going to show progressive or stable/regressive lung disease? Is the patient going to respond (or not respond) to a medication? Models of discreet variables can be developed using logistic regression and multiple logistic regression. Sensitivity and specificity of discrete variables can be assessed using receiver-operator characteristic (ROC) curves, plotting the sensitivity on the y-axis and 1-specificity on the x-axis. The area under the curve (AUC) of a ROC provides a global measure of performance and can be used for comparing biomarker performance, with AUC of 0.90–1 considered excellent, 0.80–0.90 considered good, 0.7–0.8 considered fair, 0.6–0.7 considered poor, and 0.5–0.06 considered without value. Various methods can be applied to choose the best threshold level of the biomarker to maximize sensitivity and specificity [27].

Other statistical methodologies can be applied to prognostic or predictive biomarkers, Patients can be divided into various trajectories and biomarkers used to predict which trajectory is most likely. Regardless of the model developed, validation using an independent dataset is critical. Models developed using a "discovery" dataset will almost always be less robust in a "validation" dataset. The more variables added to models and the less strong the independent associations, the more likely the model will not be robust.

Biomarkers of Disease Target Organs in SSc

Skin

Because of its easy accessibility and uniform involvement in patients with dcSSc, several groups have studied skin biomarkers. As the only tissue that can be easily biopsied and re-biopsied, skin biomarkers are particularly valuable for monitoring therapy as pharmacodynamic biomarkers. Generally biomarkers of skin disease have been examined in patients with dcSSc. Skin can also be used for assessing whether a drug is effectively engaging its target by examining expression of known drug targets. mRNA expression in skin has also been examined for biomarkers predictive of clinical responses and has been used to develop a classifier of skin disease. A gene classifier based on broad changes in gene expression has been developed that permits the division of patients into subsets of disease. This methodology and approach is discussed more completely in the Chap. YY on Precision Medicine.

Pharmacodynamic Biomarkers of Skin

mRNA Biomarkers Skin gene expression has provided the most robust pharmacodynamic biomarker of skin disease. Although skin shows many changes in gene expression, only a subset of these genes correlates with the MRSS. Several years ago a pharmacodynamic biomarker of skin disease was described [28]. This biomarker was composed of a combination of genes: two genes known to be regulated by TGF-β (THBS1 and COMP) and two other genes known to be regulated by interferons (SIGLEC1 and IFI44). These genes were combined into a "four-gene biomarker" using multiple linear regression. This biomarker correlated highly with the MRSS in a cross-sectional study. However, utility of a pharmacodynamic biomarker requires movement of the biomarker over time with disease severity, in this case assessed by MRSS. Only five patients were examined longitudinally using the four-gene biomarker.

More recently, Rice et al. systematically examined the best genes to use as pharmacodynamic biomarkers by examining microarray data [29]. The key step in identifying a more robust pharmacodynamic biomarker was focusing on the correlation between the longitudinal change in gene expression with the longitudinal change in MRSS. Using a general estimating equation, two genes (THBS1 and

MS4A4A) were found in combination to most closely change with change in MRSS. This "2GSSc skin biomarker" has been applied to samples from two open-label clinical trials. The biomarker changed dramatically in patients treated with anti-TGF-β, fresolimumab, whereas it did not change in patients treated with the c-abl inhibitor, nilotinib, providing valuable objective data for clinical efficacy of fresolimumab [30]. These studies show the promise of robust pharmacodynamic biomarkers, as they can provide an objective signal in early phase clinical trials.

Serum and Plasma Biomarkers Many serum and plasma biomarkers have been identified of dSSc skin disease. Some of these proteins appear to be markers of fibrosis and/or are regulated by TGF-β. Serum cartilage oligomeric protein 1 (COMP) is increased in sera from SSc patients and correlates moderately well with the MRSS ($r=0.57$) [31]. In one report, serum COMP levels changed longitudinally with change in the MRSS, indicating possible utility of COMP as a pharmacodynamic biomarker. Most other studies of dSSc skin biomarkers are cross-sectional. Plasma levels of osteopontin correlate, but only weakly, with the MRSS ($r=0.3$; $P=0.05$) [32]. Two other TGF-β-regulated proteins, thrombospondin-1 (TSP-1) and matrix metalloproteinase 9 (MMP9), are increased in SSc sera [33]. Serum MMP-9 concentrations correlate relatively well with the MRSS ($r=0.425$) [34]. Carboxy-terminal telopeptide of type I collagen (PICP) is elevated in patients with dSSc [35], and one study correlated highly with the skin score, $r=0.646$ [36]. In contrast, amino-terminal procollagen I (P1NP) did not correlate with the skin score in this study [36]. Amino-terminal III procollagen (PIIINP) levels are also higher in dcSSc patients and in one study were prognostic of poor survival [32,37]. However, in the CAT-192 study, where collagen propeptides were used as biomarkers, although both PINP and PIIINP levels were elevated in dSSc patients, only PINP levels showed statistically significant changes that correlated with the MRSS ($r=0.37$) [38]. Tissue inhibitor of metalloproteinases-1 (TIMP-1) is also higher in dSSc than lSSc [39]. Lysyl oxidase (LOX) levels were shown to trend toward a weak correlation with the MRSS in a small dSSc group of patients ($r=0.374$). Periostin levels were found in one study to correlate highly with the MRSS in SSc patients; however, most of the patients had lSSc ($r=0.79$) [40].

The relationship between inflammation and fibrosis is strongly supported by the co-upregulation of profibrotic and pro-inflammatory biomarkers. Sato showed that IL-6 and IL-10 correlate highly with the MRSS in SSc ($r=0.625$, and $r=0.663$, respectively) [41]. SSc patients express higher levels of IL-1RA and IL-13 CCL2, CCL3, CCL4, and CXCL8, but no clear associations were seen with the MRSS or other clinical parameters [42]. CCL2 was shown to correlate with MRSS in one study but most of the patients in this study had lSSc [43]. Pentraxin 3, a protein closely related to C-reactive protein, correlates weakly with the MRSS ($r=0.34$) [44]. sCD30, a member of the TNF receptor family (TNFR8), is an inflammatory marker elevated in many diseases. sCD30 levels have been shown to correlate moderately with the MRSS (rs=0.53) [45]. Elevated sCD30 and IL-6, particularly in patients with dSSc, were confirmed by Scala [46]. Markers of both B cell activation and B cell activating factor (BAFF), and T cell activation and soluble cytotoxic lymphocyte antigen 4 (CTLA-4) also correlate with the MRSS ($r=0.41$ and $r=0.37$, respectively) [47,48].

Several biomarkers that may reflect vascular injury are elevated in SSc patients. A vascular marker, L-selectin, correlates negatively with the MRSS [49]. Endostatin is elevated in SSc compared to controls and was higher in patients with more diffuse skin disease [50,51], though not shown to correlate directly with the MRSS longitudinally. Endothelin-1 and von Willebrand factor are also elevated in patients with SSc [52]. Adiponectin, an adipokine released by fat, correlates inversely with the MRSS [53].

The large number of serum biomarkers for skin disease in dSSc patients suggests that combining measures, particularly measures that are capturing different aspects of pathogenesis, might provide a successful approach for finding a serum biomarker of skin disease robust enough for utilization as a surrogate outcome measure in clinical trials.

Circulating miRNA Biomarkers Several recent studies have already demonstrated that the levels of selected miRNAs were altered in the serum of SSc patients [54–57]. One of the most extensive studies examined 95 miRNA that were predicted by *in silico* analyses to target SSc-related genes including IL-4, TGF-β, CTGF, PDGF-B, PDGF receptor (PDGFR) α/β, and COL1A2. The expression of these miRNA was measured by quantitative PCR in sera of SSc patients and healthy controls [56]. The results showed that 19 miRNAs were significantly downregulated in the serum of SSc patients as compared with healthy controls. Among them, miR-30b and the let-7 and miR-302 families of miRNAs were uniformly reduced in SSc patients. Other miRNA that were also significantly decreased in SSc patients included miR-19a, miR-26a, miR-106b, miR-181a, miR-181b, miR-191, miR-203, miR-376a, miR-409-3p, miR-410, miR-484, and miR-549. Consistent with previous reports, the levels of miR29a and miR142-3p tended to be higher in SSc patients. Of substantial interest were the results of comparison of miRNA levels in the serum of patients with limited (lcSSc) and diffuse (dcSSc) subsets of SSc patients. These showed that among the 19 miRNAs that were significantly lower in the serum of SSc patients, miR-30b was decreased more profoundly in dcSSc than in lcSSc and its levels were inversely correlated with the modified

Rodnan skin score. However, although the levels of miR-30b in lcSSc patients are less decreased than in the sera of dcSSc patients, they were still significantly lower than in healthy controls.

Other miRNA that have been studied as potential SSc biomarkers include miR-142-3p that was shown to be elevated in serum from SSc patients compared to patients with systemic lupus erythematosus and were also significantly different compared to the levels in serum from normal individuals and from patients with SSc-spectrum disorder [54]. The levels of miR-150 were found to be decreased in the serum of SSc patients compared to healthy controls and lower levels correlated with more severe clinical manifestations. Furthermore, patients with lower miR-150 levels had a higher ratio of dcSSc to lcSSc, a higher modified Rodnan skin score, and higher incidence of Scl-70 antibodies when compared with patients with normal serum miR-150 levels [19]. A similar correlation was observed for miR-196a, showing that patients with lower serum miR-196a levels had significantly higher ratio of dcSSc to lcSSc and higher extent and severity of skin involvement and showed higher prevalence of pitting scars [18]. Other studies demonstrated that the serum levels of miR-30b [56] and let-7a [21] were markedly decreased in SSc patients compared with healthy controls and levels of both miRNAs were more profoundly decreased in patients with dcSSc than in patients with lcSSc, and both were inversely correlated with the modified Rodnan skin score [54,56]. In contrast, other studies showed that serum levels of miR-92a [55] and miR-142-3p [54] were markedly higher in SSc patients when compared to healthy controls or to systemic lupus erythematosus, dermatomyositis, and SSc-spectrum disorder patients.

Another recent study analyzed differences in extracellular miRNA in the plasma of a Swedish cohort of 95 SSc patients and identified four miRNA (miRNA-223, miR-181b, miRNA-342-3p, and miRNA-184) that differed between the lcSSc and dcSSc subsets [57]. Also, these authors found that the levels of 10 miRNA displayed statistically significant differences between different autoantibody subgroups and that miRNA-233 correlated with the presence of anti-centromere antibodies. Thus, the authors suggested that miRNA played a role in SSc pathogenesis and clinical manifestations because specific miRNAs were found in significant association with distinct SSc autoantibody profiles and clinical SSc subsets.

Although the studies that examined circulating miRNA in SSc are relatively few and despite problems with the specificity and reproducibility [22], the studies published clearly indicate that the assessment of microRNA in the serum of SSc patients may provide valuable and reliable biomarkers for SSc diagnosis, and for assessment of its clinical subsets, extent of organ involvement and clinical course and potential outcomes.

Prognostic and Predictive Biomarkers of SSc Skin Disease

Prognostic mRNA biomarkers of SSc skin disease have generally been harder to identify. This may be biological, related to the variable and changing progression of the disease, or it may represent difficulty in assembling datasets from untreated patients. However, levels of one prognostic biomarker, skin CD14 mRNA levels, are prognostic for progressive disease in SSc patients [58]. As more skin RNA datasets become available from controlled trials we might anticipate that other prognostic biomarkers will be identified.

Several predictive biomarkers have been identified for SSc skin disease. However, none of these have been identified for proven therapeutics, which arguably have not been found for SSc skin disease. In a study of anti-TGFβ, THBS1 was shown to predict patients more likely to respond to the study medication [30] (Table 17.1)

Interstitial Lung Disease

mRNA Biomarkers of SSc-Associated ILD Christmann et al. compared gene expression in SSc lungs with the change in Fibmax score and FVC over time after lung biopsy in a small group of SSc patients. A series of collagen, interferon-regulated, and macrophage-associated genes were found to correlate most highly with progressive lung disease. These prognostic biomarkers provide important insights into the likely pathogenic drivers of the disease, but as lung biopsies are rarely performed, they are unlikely to play important roles in future clinical settings.

Autoantibodies Anti-Scl70 is associated with SSc-ILD and RNA-polymerase 3 negatively associated with ILD. These associations are discussed in the autoantibody chapter.

Serum/Plasma Biomarkers of ILD have generally been compared to pulmonary function tests (PFTs), typically the forced vital capacity (FVC) or total lung capacity (TLC). Several studies have shown that surfactant protein D (SP-D) and Krebs von den Lungen-6 (KL-6) are increased in patients with SSc-ILD. However, the degree of correlation with PFTs has been variable with SP-D correlations with the FVC ranging from $r=-0.61$ [48], −0.278 [60], to $r=-0.15$ [61]. SP-D does not act as a prognostic biomarker [62]. KL-6 levels have generally been shown to correlate less strongly with FVC ($r=-0.33$ to −0.17)) [61,63]. KL-6 levels also do not appear prognostic for decline in FVC [64].

A variety of matrix metalloproteinases (MMPs) have been examined in IPF. MMP7 levels are weakly prognostic for survival [65]. MMP7 levels are also associated with advanced SSc-ILD [66], and MMP-12 levels correlate

Table 17.1 Biomarkers of skin disease in systemic sclerosis

Biomarker group	Biomarkers of skin disease-MRSS	Correlation with MRSS (r)	Reference
Fibrotic	COMP	0.57	[31]
	Osteopontin	0.3	[32]
	Thrombospondin-1	?	[33]
	MMP-9	0.425	[34]
	TIMP-1	?	[39]
	Lysyl oxidase	0.374	[59]
	Periostin	0.79	[40]
Collagen	PICP	0.646	[36]
	P1NP	0.37	[38]
	P3NP	?	[32,37]
Immune	IL-6	0.625	[41]
	IL-10	0.663	[41]
	CCL2/MCP-1	0.56	[43]
	Pentraxin-3	0.34	[44]
	sCD30	0.53	[45]
	BAFF	0.41	[47]
	sCTLA-4	0.37	[48]
Vascular	L-selectin	−0.77	[49]
	Adiponectin	−0.28	[53]

Fibrotic markers refer to proteins known to be regulated by TGFβ. Collagen markers are amino-terminal (P1NP, P3NP) and carboxy-terminal (P1CP) propeptides of type I (P1CP, P1CP) or type III collagen (P3NP) collagen. Immune and vascular markers are known products from leukocytes and endothelial cells, respectively

both with the MRSS (r-0.62) and negatively with the FVC in SSc-ILD (r=−0.82) [67]. Neoepitopes of MMP-degraded extracellular matrix proteins were examined in a large IPF cohort. This group found that the rate of change in six of these neoepitopes correlated with progressive lung disease and mortality [68]. The rate of change at 3 months of a neoepitope of CRP, generated by MMP1/9 digestion, was most highly associated with mortality. In patients with rheumatoid arthritis, a combination biomarker that includes matrix metalloproteinase 7, pulmonary and activation-regulated chemokine, and surfactant protein D is highly sensitive and specific for the presence of ILD [69]. As mentioned in SSc skin disease, TIMP-1 levels have been shown to correlate weakly and negatively with the DLCO (r=−0.28) [39].

Several chemokines and cytokine markers have also been examined as biomarkers of SSc-ILD (reviewed in [70]. Serum pulmonary and activated chemokine (PARC/CCL18) levels correlate negatively with the TLC in SSc-ILD, r=−0.66 [71], or weakly, negatively with the FVC, r=−0.244 and DLCO, r=−0.326 [72]. CCL-18 has weak short-term prognostic value [62]. IL-6 appears to be a prognostic biomarker early in SSc-ILD, but only in patients with early disease, i.e., FVC >70% predicted [73]. Levels of IL-15, a cytokine in the IL2 family, also correlate negatively with the FVC r=−0.040 [74]. GDF-15, a member of the TGF-β superfamily, correlates with severity of lung disease (assessed by DLCO% predicted) and also with the change in lung disease longitudinally (prognostic) [75].

YKL-40, the human homolog of murine chitinase 3-like-1, is induced by and mediates downstream effects of IL-13, particularly induction of alternatively activated macrophages and tissue fibrosis [76]. YKL-40 is increased in SSc-ILD patients [77]. Chitinase-1 activity in serum is also elevated in SSc-ILD and levels correlate negatively with PFTs [78]. Also as seen for skin, serum levels of pentraxin 3 correlate negatively with FVC, r=−0.44 [44].

Soluble ICAM1 levels were shown to correlate with FVC longitudinally, and baseline sICAM1 is prognostic of declining FVC at 4 years in SSc patients [79]. Several markers for oxidative stress are increased in SSc-ILD. 8-isoprostane is increased in the sera of SSc-ILD, also correlating negatively (r=−0.42) [80]. Another biomarker of oxidative stress measured in the urine, 8-isoprostaglandin-F2a, correlates negatively with the DLCO (r=−0.044) [81]. Other studies in IPF patients have shown that leukocyte telomere length is prognostic for survival [82] (Table 17.2).

Bronchoalveolar Lavage Biomarkers of ILD

Bronchoalveolar lavage (BAL) fluid provides a source for biomarkers more closely in contact with lung tissues. A recent study examining a broad array of interleukins showed that IL-4, IL-8, and CCL2 levels correlated negatively with the FVC, r=−0.503, r=−0.394, and r=−0.441, respectively [83]. These correlations are higher than seen for most serum markers of ILD; however, BAL is difficult as a source for

Table 17.2 Biomarkers of lung disease in systemic sclerosis (or IPF)

Biomarker group	Biomarker	SSc-ILD	Tissue	FVC correlation (r)	References	Prognostic
Epithelium	Surfactant protein D (SP-D)	SSc-ILD	Blood	−0.61, −0.278, −0.15	[48,60,61]	No [62]
	Krebs von den Lungen-6 (KL-6)	SSc-ILD	Blood	−0.33, −0.17	[61,63]	No [64]
	MMP7	SSc-ILD; SSc-PAH	Blood	DLCO: −0.31		Weak [65]
	MMP12	IPF	Blood	−0.082	[67]	
	MMP neoepitopes	IPF	Blood	See reference	[68]	
	TIMP-1	SSc-ILD	Blood	$r=-0.28$	[39]	
	GDF-15	SSc-ILD	Blood	−0.316	[75]	
Immune	CCL18 (PARC)	SSc-ILD	Blood	−0.66, −0.244	[71,72]	
	IL-6	SSc-ILD	Blood			Yes [73]
	IL-15	SSc-ILD	Blood	−0.4	[74]	
	YKL-40	SSc-ILD	Blood	?	[77]	
	Chitinase-1	SSc-ILD	Blood	−0.62, −0.43	[78]	
	Pentraxin-3	SSc-ILD	Blood	−0.44	[44]	
Oxidative stress	8-isoprostane	SSc-ILD	Blood	−0.42	[80]	
	8-isoprostaglandin-F2a	SSc-ILD	Urine	−0.44	[81]	
Immune	IL-4	SSc-ILD	BAL	−0.503	[83]	
	IL-8	SSc-ILD	BAL	−0.394	[83]	
	CCL2	SSc-ILD	BAL	−0.441	[83]	

Epithelial cell markers refer to proteins known to be secreted by type II pneumocytes. Immune markers are known products from leukocytes, and oxidative stress proteins known are increased in cells undergoing oxidative stress. BAL refers to biomarkers found in bronchoalveolar lavage. A column showing several different correlations refer to different studies described in the text

repeated measure and may not be required in order to develop a robust marker for ILD.

Despite these many described biomarkers, there remains no widely validated and accepted biomarker for progressive SSc-ILD. In addition, a biochemical surrogate outcome for SSc-ILD might considerably enhance SSc-ILD clinical trials, as the currently most used outcome, the FVC, shows such great variability. The major block for identifying these biomarkers is assembling the proper clinical sample repository with associated clinical information. Such endeavors require national and international cooperation between SSc investigators.

Radiographic Studies of SSc-ILD

Radiographic methods provide a direct assessment of lung disease. Quantitative CT scanning, particularly quantitative lung fibrosis, appears a sensitive marker for treatment-related improvement in lung function [84]. Hyperpolarized gas has also been investigated in small numbers of patients with ILD [85]. FDG PET appears to have some utility in IPF, although its role is still being defined [86]. It seemed to predict aggressive ILD in one patient with DM, but was disappointing in another recent study of PM/DM showing positive in only 7/18 patients with ILD [87,88]. Newer radiolabeled compounds may prove increasingly useful as better targets for radioligands are discovered. However, sensitivity remains an issue with radiographic PET biomarkers.

Clinical and Biochemical Biomarkers of Pulmonary Arterial Hypertension

Many studies have examined clinical and serum/plasma biomarkers of idiopathic and SSc-associated pulmonary arterial hypertension (iPAH and SSc-PAH) (reviewed in [89]. Pulmonary arterial hypertension is defined by hemodynamic pressures measured on right heart catheterization (RHC): a mean pulmonary arterial pressure (PAP) of ≥25 mmHg, a pulmonary vascular resistance of >3, and Wood units and pulmonary capillary wedge pressure of ≤15 [90]. Early diagnosis in SSc-PAH may lead to better outcomes [91], so diagnostic biomarkers indicating the need for right heart catheterization (RHC) might improve survival.

Echocardiographic assessment of systolic PAP (sPAP) by assessing tricuspid velocity has been the most robust clinical biomarker to date, showing a good correlation with PAH on RHC (90% sensitivity and specificity of 75%) [92]. Numerous studies have shown the value, but also the limitations, of echocardiography (see [93]). Subsequent studies have shown enhanced detection of PAH using echocardiographic sPAP in combination with other measures. Echocardiographic sPAP in combination with the DLCO and proNT-BNP more accurately predicts the development of SSc-PAH [94]. Echocardiographic sPAP is a prominent component of recent algorithms for PAH diagnosis [95,96]. The latter of these, the DETECT study, devises a complex, two-step algorithm based on a large prospective study designed to determine the best clinical and biochemical biomarkers for SSc-PAH [96]. DLCO %predicted/FVC %predicted, current/past telangiectasia, anti-centromere antibody, NTpro-BNP, serum urate, and right axis deviation on electrocardiogram define patients needing echocardiography, and right atrial area and tricuspid velocity echocardiographic features define which patients should have RHC. Another echocardiographic measure, tricuspid annular plane systolic excursion (TAPSE), a measure that reflects right ventricular function, is prognostic for survival in SSc-PAH in one study [97].

Many biochemical measures have been shown to be diagnostic of PAH or prognostic of survival in patients with PAH. However, often studies of biochemical biomarkers of PAH do not include SSc-PAH patients or group SSc with other connective tissue disease (CTD) patients. SSc-PAH compared to iPAH is associated with increased mortality and show higher BNP levels and lower DLCO %predicted [98]. Thus, it is important that biomarkers of iPAH are evaluated discretely also in SSc-PAH patients. PAH biomarkers in SSc patients are also potentially confounded by co-morbid disease complications, including ILD and cardiac fibrosis. In SSc-ILD patients, PAH might also be secondary to hypoxia from ILD. However, this distinction has been rarely assessed in SSc-PAH biomarkers. Even biomarkers of pure SSc PAH might reflect different pathogenic processes. Biomarkers might reflect the effect of PAH on vascular remodeling, affecting endothelial or vascular smooth muscle cells, or they might measure inflammation, right heart failure, or hypoxia.

By far the most studied and only clinically available PAH biomarkers are markers of heart strain/failure: brain natriuretic peptide (BNP) and N-terminal fragment of pro-brain natriuretic peptide (NT-proBNP). These appear to have similar diagnostic accuracy [99]. In one study NT-proBNP had a diagnostic specificity for SSc-PAH of 95.1 % and a sensitivity of 55.9 % [100]. This is consistent with other PAH studies, indicating that BNP and NT-proBNP are generally specific for PH but lack sensitivity. NT-proBNP also correlates with mPAP, PVR, and survival. In patients with iPAH, BNP, and NT-proBNP are also both predictive of survival.

Inflammatory biomarkers have also shown some utility in PAH. Elevated CRP is associated with mortality, and in thromboembolic disease decreases with treatment, suggesting it may act as both a prognostic and PD biomarker [101]. More recently, human pentraxin 3 was shown to be another inflammatory biomarker for PAH and CTD-PAH [102]. Pentraxin 3 was much more robust than CRP for distinguishing CTD-PAH from CTD patients ($ROC_{AUC}=0.866$ compared to CRP $ROC_{AUC}=0.516$ and BNP $ROC_{AUC}=0.670$). However, only 59 % of the patients in the CTD and control groups had SSc. Using a proteomic approach, another study confirmed and extended inflammatory markers, showing that CRP, IL1, IL8, and TNFa are all increased in SSc-PAH compared to SSc-PAH [103]. This study included only patients with lSSc and most patients did not have ILD, thus it appears these markers are truly associated with SSc-PAH and not other disease manifestations. Urinary $15\text{-}F_{2t}$-isoprostane, a marker of lipid peroxidation and oxidative stress, is also highly prognostic of survival in PAH. In this study $15\text{-}F_{2t}$-isoprostane was more highly prognostic of survival than NT-proBNP, or big ET-1 [104].

Several markers of vascular disease are elevated in SSc-PAH. In an early study, endothelin1 (ET-1) levels were elevated in SSc-PAH but did not correlate with survival or PAP [105]. However, subsequent studies have shown that ET-1 levels correlate with PAP in PAH patients [106,107] and big ET-1 levels are shown to correlate with survival in PAH [108]. Endoglin levels are elevated in PAH and correlate with survival [109]. A proteomic approach showed that intercellular adhesion molecule-1 (ICAM-1), vascular cell adhesion molecular-1 VCAM, von Willebrand factor (vWF), and vascular endothelial cell growth factor (VEGF) are all elevated in lSSc-PAH patients compared to lSSc patients [103].

Several other biomarkers have been described for PAH. Osteopontin levels correlate with NT-BNP and survival in patients with iPAH [110]; osteopontin levels are also elevated in patients with SSc-ILD or SSc-PAH [111]. Provirus integration site for Moloney murine leukemia virus (Pim-1) has also been shown to be associated with iPAH, CTD-PAH, and SSc-PAH [112]. Pim-1 is also highly prognostic of survival. The SSc patients in this, as most PAH biomarker studies, were not phenotyped as to the presence of ILD, and for the main analysis were grouped with other CTD patients. In contrast to what is seen in the skin, adiponectin levels are elevated in patients with PAH [113] (Table 17.3)

Digital Ischemia, Digital Ulcers

Several vascular biomarkers correlate with digital ulcers (DU) in SSc [114]. sICAM-1 is elevated in SSc patients with DUs, but did not correlate with the MRSS [115]. Increased endoglin is associated with DUs and decreased DLCO [116]. Elevated endothelin-1 is associated with DUs as well as PAH [117,118]. sCD36 correlates with PAH on echocardiogram and with DLCO and is elevated in lSSc [119], but not in dSSc patients. PDGF-BB and PECAM1 were both found to be elevated in SSc patients with DU [120]. More recently,

Table 17.3 Biomarkers in patients with pulmonary arterial hypertension

Biomarker	Sensitivity	Specificity	ROC_{AUC}	Prognostic	Other	References
BNP	55.90 %	95.10 %	0.67	Yes		[100,102]
NT-BNP	Similar to BNP			Yes		[99,102]
CRP	62 %	63 %	0.516			
Pentraxin-3			0.866			[102]
Endoglin				Yes		[109]
Endothelin 1				Yes	$r=-0.4$ with TAPSE	[108]
Osteopontin				Yes		[110,111]
15-F_{2t}-isoprostane				Yes		[104]
Pim-1	75 %	77 %	0.82	Yes		[112]

PIGF and sVCAM have been shown to be elevated in patients with DUs, and PIGF levels strongly prognostic of future DUs [121].

In other studies IL-33 levels were found to correlate with DU [122] and microangiopathic changes [123]. IL-33 induces fibrosis dependent on the type 2 cytokines, IL-13 [124], suggesting a potential important role in SSc pathogenesis.

Biomarkers of Overall Disease in SSc

Although everyone agrees that the most exciting therapeutic advance would be discovery of a drug that treats overall disease of SSc patients, biomarker discovery in this area has been limited. The only widely accepted current methodology for assessing overall clinical disease activity is the European Scleroderma Study Group activity index (ESSGAI) [125,126]. The anchor for this index was expert assessment of disease activity. An ongoing study based on validation of longitudinal data, the combined response index for systemic sclerosis (CRISS), may prove a more robust measure of overall disease [127]. Microhemorrhages and giant capillaries on capillaroscopy correlate with the ESSGAI [128].

Angiopoietin-2 levels correlate with ESSGAI ($r=0.403$) [129], as do levels of GDF-15 [75] ($r=0.338$). GDF-15 levels were also shown to be associated with the change in ESSGAI over time [75]. Borrowing from biomarkers discovered for liver fibrosis, the enhanced liver fibrosis score was shown to correlate with the ESSGAI [130] as well as the MRSS. Although highly statistically significant, these correlations are relatively low ($r=0.28$–0.23, respectively). Leptin levels were found in a small study to be lower in active patients [131]. Elevated CRP is associated with ESSGAI, skin disease, and decreased FVC, though these correlations are all quite low [132]. CRP was also found to be weakly prognostic for long-term survival. Elevated COMP levels are associated with increased mortality [133].

Both clinical and biomarker approaches are under way to better classify SSc patients into subsets. Limited compared to diffuse skin disease has provided very useful information about prognosis of many disease complications. Using skin gene expression, Dr. Whitfield's group has developed methodologies for distinguishing patients with different patterns of skin gene expression that appear to reflect activation of different pathogenic pathways. This is described more completely elsewhere in this text.

Conclusion

Many biomarkers of SSc and its complications have already been identified. However, very few of these have been validated in multiple datasets and/or applied in a clinical setting. The burgeoning number of new therapeutics that might be tried for SSc patients makes the application of biomarkers to clinical trials increasingly important. Biomarkers help bridge our understanding of animal models to human disease. Pathways leading to fibrosis in mice may not be similar to those leading to fibrosis in human SSc. Biomarkers can indicate the vascular, fibrotic, and immunologic pathways most likely to be contributing to SSc pathogenesis and thus help in selecting drugs most likely to show efficacy. Biomarkers can also help in testing the effect of targeted therapeutics, as well as in patient selection. They will serve increasing roles in all aspects of medicine as we reach for a future of targeted therapeutics and precision medicine.

References

1. Qualification Process for Drug Development Tools. www.fdagov/downloads/Drugs//Guidances/UCM230597pdf. Food and drug administration-draft document. 2010.
2. Stopeck AT, Brown-Glaberman U, Wong HY, Park BH, Barnato SE, Gradishar WJ, et al. The role of targeted therapy and biomarkers in breast cancer treatment. Clin Exp Metastasis. 2012;29(7):807–19.
3. Corren J, Lemanske RF, Hanania NA, Korenblat PE, Parsey MV, Arron JR, et al. Lebrikizumab treatment in adults with asthma. N Engl J Med. 2011;365(12):1088–98.
4. Etheridge A, Gomes CP, Pereira RW, Galas D, Wang K. The complexity, function and applications of RNA in circulation. Front Genet. 2013;4:115. Pubmed Central PMCID: 3684799.
5. Etheridge A, Lee I, Hood L, Galas D, Wang K. Extracellular microRNA: a new source of biomarkers. Mutat Res. 2011;717(1–2):85–90. Pubmed Central PMCID: 3199035.

6. Bartel DP. MicroRNAs: genomics, biogenesis, mechanism, and function. Cell. 2004;116(2):281–97.
7. Eulalio A, Huntzinger E, Izaurralde E. Getting to the root of miRNA-mediated gene silencing. Cell. 2008;132(1):9–14.
8. Iorio MV, Croce CM. MicroRNA dysregulation in cancer: diagnostics, monitoring and therapeutics. A comprehensive review. EMBO Mol Med. 2012;4(3):143–59. Pubmed Central PMCID: 3376845.
9. Lages E, Ipas H, Guttin A, Nesr H, Berger F, Issartel JP. MicroRNAs: molecular features and role in cancer. Front Biosci. 2012;17:2508–40. Pubmed Central PMCID: 3815439.
10. Babalola O, Mamalis A, Lev-Tov H, Jagdeo J. The role of microRNAs in skin fibrosis. Arch Dermatol Res. 2013;305(9):763–76. Pubmed Central PMCID: 3979452.
11. Bowen T, Jenkins RH, Fraser DJ. MicroRNAs, transforming growth factor beta-1, and tissue fibrosis. J Pathol. 2013;229(2):274–85.
12. Jiang X, Tsitsiou E, Herrick SE, Lindsay MA. MicroRNAs and the regulation of fibrosis. FEBS J. 2010;277(9):2015–21. Pubmed Central PMCID: 2963651.
13. Patel V, Noureddine L. MicroRNAs and fibrosis. Curr Opin Nephrol Hypertens. 2012;21(4):410–6. Pubmed Central PMCID: 3399722.
14. Vettori S, Gay S, Distler O. Role of MicroRNAs in fibrosis. Open Rheumatol J. 2012;6:130–9. Pubmed Central PMCID: 3396185.
15. Maurer B, Stanczyk J, Jungel A, Akhmetshina A, Trenkmann M, Brock M, et al. MicroRNA-29, a key regulator of collagen expression in systemic sclerosis. Arthritis Rheum. 2010;62(6):1733–43.
16. Peng WJ, Tao JH, Mei B, Chen B, Li BZ, Yang GJ, et al. MicroRNA-29: a potential therapeutic target for systemic sclerosis. Expert Opin Ther Targets. 2012;16(9):875–9.
17. Zhu H, Li Y, Qu S, Luo H, Zhou Y, Wang Y, et al. MicroRNA expression abnormalities in limited cutaneous scleroderma and diffuse cutaneous scleroderma. J Clin Immunol. 2012;32(3):514–22.
18. Honda N, Jinnin M, Kajihara I, Makino T, Makino K, Masuguchi S, et al. TGF-beta-mediated downregulation of microRNA-196a contributes to the constitutive upregulated type I collagen expression in scleroderma dermal fibroblasts. J Immunol. 2012;188(7):3323–31.
19. Honda N, Jinnin M, Kira-Etoh T, Makino K, Kajihara I, Makino T, et al. miR-150 down-regulation contributes to the constitutive type I collagen overexpression in scleroderma dermal fibroblasts via the induction of integrin beta3. Am J Pathol. 2013;182(1):206–16.
20. Li H, Yang R, Fan X, Gu T, Zhao Z, Chang D, et al. MicroRNA array analysis of microRNAs related to systemic scleroderma. Rheumatol Int. 2012;32(2):307–13.
21. Makino K, Jinnin M, Hirano A, Yamane K, Eto M, Kusano T, et al. The downregulation of microRNA let-7a contributes to the excessive expression of type I collagen in systemic and localized scleroderma. J Immunol. 2013;190(8):3905–15.
22. Witwer KW. Circulating microRNA biomarker studies: pitfalls and potential solutions. Clin Chem. 2015;61(1):56–63.
23. Mitchell P. Proteomics retrenches. Nat Biotechnol. 2010;28(7):665–70.
24. Kelleher NL, Thomas PM, Ntai I, Compton PD, LeDuc RD. Deep and quantitative top-down proteomics in clinical and translational research. Expert Rev Proteomics. 2014;11(6):649–51. Pubmed Central PMCID: 4295490.
25. Weiss F, van den Berg BH, Planatscher H, Pynn CJ, Joos TO, Poetz O. Catch and measure-mass spectrometry-based immunoassays in biomarker research. Biochim Biophys Acta. 2014;1844(5):927–32.
26. Slinker BK, Glantz SA. Multiple linear regression: accounting for multiple simultaneous determinants of a continuous dependent variable. Circulation. 2008;117(13):1732–7.
27. Froud R, Abel G. Using ROC curves to choose minimally important change thresholds when sensitivity and specificity are valued equally: the forgotten lesson of pythagoras. Theoretical considerations and an example application of change in health status. PLoS One. 2014;9(12):e114468. Pubmed Central PMCID: 4256421.
28. Farina G, Lafyatis D, Lemaire R, Lafyatis R. A four-gene biomarker predicts skin disease in patients with diffuse cutaneous systemic sclerosis. Arthritis Rheum. 2010;62(2):580–8. Pubmed Central PMCID: 3018285.
29. Rice LM, Ziemek J, Stratton EA, McLaughlin S, Padilla CM, Mathes AL, et al. A Longitudinal biomarker for the extent of skin disease in patients with diffuse cutaneous systemic sclerosis. Arthritis Rheumatol. 2015 (In press).
30. Rice LM, Padilla CM, McLaughlin SR, Mathes A, Ziemek J, Goummih S, et al. Fresolimumab treatment decreases biomarkers and improves clinical symptoms in systemic sclerosis patients. J Clin Invest. 2015;125(7):2795–807.
31. Hesselstrand R, Kassner A, Heinegard D, Saxne T. COMP: a candidate molecule in the pathogenesis of systemic sclerosis with a potential as a disease marker. Ann Rheum Dis. 2008;67(9):1242–8. eng.
32. Horslev-Petersen K, Ammitzboll T, Engstrom-Laurent A, Bentsen K, Junker P, Asboe-Hansen G, et al. Serum and urinary aminoterminal type III procollagen peptide in progressive systemic sclerosis: relationship to sclerodermal involvement, serum hyaluronan and urinary collagen metabolites. J Rheumatol. 1988;15(3):460–7. eng.
33. Macko RF, Gelber AC, Young BA, Lowitt MH, White B, Wigley FM, et al. Increased circulating concentrations of the counter adhesive proteins SPARC and thrombospondin-1 in systemic sclerosis (scleroderma). Relationship to platelet and endothelial cell activation. J Rheumatol. 2002;29(12):2565–70. eng.
34. Kim WU, Min SY, Cho ML, Hong KH, Shin YJ, Park SH, et al. Elevated matrix metalloproteinase-9 in patients with systemic sclerosis. Arthritis Res Ther. 2005;7(1):R71–9. eng.
35. Kikuchi K, Ihn H, Sato S, Igarashi A, Soma Y, Ishibashi Y, et al. Serum concentration of procollagen type I carboxyterminal propeptide in systemic sclerosis. Arch Dermatol Res. 1994;286(2):77–80. eng.
36. Hunzelmann N, Risteli J, Risteli L, Sacher C, Vancheeswaran R, Black C, et al. Circulating type I collagen degradation products: a new serum marker for clinical severity in patients with scleroderma? Br J Dermatol. 1998;139(6):1020–5. eng.
37. Nagy Z, Czirjak L. Increased levels of amino terminal propeptide of type III procollagen are an unfavourable predictor of survival in systemic sclerosis. Clin Exp Rheumatol. 2005;23(2):165–72. eng.
38. Denton CP, Merkel PA, Furst DE, Khanna D, Emery P, Hsu VM, et al. Recombinant human anti-transforming growth factor beta1 antibody therapy in systemic sclerosis: a multicenter, randomized, placebo-controlled phase I/II trial of CAT-192. Arthritis Rheum. 2007;56(1):323–33. eng.
39. Kikuchi K, Kubo M, Sato S, Fujimoto M, Tamaki K. Serum tissue inhibitor of metalloproteinases in patients with systemic sclerosis. J Am Acad Dermatol. 1995;33(6):973–8. eng.
40. Yamaguchi Y, Ono J, Masuoka M, Ohta S, Izuhara K, Ikezawa Z, et al. Serum periostin levels are correlated with progressive skin sclerosis in patients with systemic sclerosis. Br J Dermatol. 2013;168(4):717–25.
41. Sato S, Hasegawa M, Takehara K. Serum levels of interleukin-6 and interleukin-10 correlate with total skin thickness score in patients with systemic sclerosis. J Dermatol Sci. 2001;27(2):140–6. eng.
42. Codullo V, Baldwin HM, Singh MD, Fraser AR, Wilson C, Gilmour A, et al. An investigation of the inflammatory cytokine and chemokine network in systemic sclerosis. Ann Rheum Dis. 2011;70(6):1115–21. eng.
43. Bandinelli F, Del Rosso A, Gabrielli A, Giacomelli R, Bartoli F, Guiducci S, et al. CCL2, CCL3 and CCL5 chemokines in systemic

sclerosis: the correlation with SSc clinical features and the effect of prostaglandin E1 treatment. Clin Exp Rheumatol. 2012;30(2 Suppl 71):S44–9.

44. Iwata Y, Yoshizaki A, Ogawa F, Komura K, Hara T, Muroi E, et al. Increased serum pentraxin 3 in patients with systemic sclerosis. J Rheumatol. 2009;36(5):976–83. eng.
45. Giacomelli R, Cipriani P, Lattanzio R, Di Franco M, Locanto M, Parzanese I, et al. Circulating levels of soluble CD30 are increased in patients with systemic sclerosis (SSc) and correlate with serological and clinical features of the disease. Clin Exp Immunol. 1997;108(1):42–6. eng.
46. Scala E, Pallotta S, Frezzolini A, Abeni D, Barbieri C, Sampogna F, et al. Cytokine and chemokine levels in systemic sclerosis: relationship with cutaneous and internal organ involvement. Clin Exp Immunol. 2004;138(3):540–6. eng.
47. Matsushita T, Hasegawa M, Yanaba K, Kodera M, Takehara K, Sato S. Elevated serum BAFF levels in patients with systemic sclerosis: enhanced BAFF signaling in systemic sclerosis B lymphocytes. Arthritis Rheum. 2006;54(1):192–201. eng.
48. Sato S, Fujimoto M, Hasegawa M, Komura K, Yanaba K, Hayakawa I, et al. Serum soluble CTLA-4 levels are increased in diffuse cutaneous systemic sclerosis. Rheumatology (Oxford). 2004;43(10):1261–6. eng.
49. Dunne JV, van Eeden SF, Keen KJ. L-selectin and skin damage in systemic sclerosis. PLoS One. 2012;7(9):e44814. Pubmed Central PMCID: 3441480.
50. Hebbar M, Peyrat JP, Hornez L, Hatron PY, Hachulla E, Devulder B. Increased concentrations of the circulating angiogenesis inhibitor endostatin in patients with systemic sclerosis. Arthritis Rheum. 2000;43(4):889–93.
51. Farouk HM, Hamza SH, El Bakry SA, Youssef SS, Aly IM, Moustafa AA, et al. Dysregulation of angiogenic homeostasis in systemic sclerosis. Int J Rheum Dis. 2013;16(4):448–54.
52. Vancheeswaran R, Magoulas T, Efrat G, Wheeler-Jones C, Olsen I, Penny R, et al. Circulating endothelin-1 levels in systemic sclerosis subsets – a marker of fibrosis or vascular dysfunction? J Rheumatol. 1994;21(10):1838–44. eng.
53. Lakota K, Wei J, Carns M, Hinchcliff M, Lee J, Whitfield ML, et al. Levels of adiponectin, a marker for PPAR-gamma activity, correlate with skin fibrosis in systemic sclerosis: potential utility as biomarker? Arthritis Res Ther. 2012;14(3):R102. Pubmed Central PMCID: 3446479.
54. Makino K, Jinnin M, Kajihara I, Honda N, Sakai K, Masuguchi S, et al. Circulating miR-142-3p levels in patients with systemic sclerosis. Clin Exp Dermatol. 2012;37(1):34–9.
55. Sing T, Jinnin M, Yamane K, Honda N, Makino K, Kajihara I, et al. microRNA-92a expression in the sera and dermal fibroblasts increases in patients with scleroderma. Rheumatology. 2012;51(9):1550–6.
56. Tanaka S, Suto A, Ikeda K, Sanayama Y, Nakagomi D, Iwamoto T, et al. Alteration of circulating miRNAs in SSc: miR-30b regulates the expression of PDGF receptor beta. Rheumatology. 2013;52(11):1963–72.
57. Wuttge DM, Carlsen AL, Teku G, Steen SO, Wildt M, Vihinen M, et al. Specific autoantibody profiles and disease subgroups correlate with circulating micro-RNA in systemic sclerosis. Rheumatology. 2015;54(11):2100–7.
58. Stifano G, Affandi AJ, Mathes AL, Rice LM, Nakerakanti S, Nazari B, et al. Chronic toll-like receptor 4 stimulation in skin induces inflammation, macrophage activation, transforming growth factor beta signature gene expression, and fibrosis. Arthritis Res Ther. 2014;16(4):R136. Pubmed Central PMCID: 4227089.
59. Rimar D, Rosner I, Nov Y, Slobodin G, Rozenbaum M, Halasz K, et al. Brief report: lysyl oxidase is a potential biomarker of fibrosis in systemic sclerosis. Arthritis Rheumatol. 2014;66(3):726–30.
60. Asano Y, Ihn H, Yamane K, Yazawa N, Kubo M, Fujimoto M, et al. Clinical significance of surfactant protein D as a serum marker for evaluating pulmonary fibrosis in patients with systemic sclerosis. Arthritis Rheum. 2001;44(6):1363–9. eng.
61. Hant FN, Ludwicka-Bradley A, Wang HJ, Li N, Elashoff R, Tashkin DP, et al. Surfactant protein D and KL-6 as serum biomarkers of interstitial lung disease in patients with scleroderma. J Rheumatol. 2009;36(4):773–80. eng.
62. Elhaj M, Charles J, Pedroza C, Liu X, Zhou X, Estrada YMRM, et al. Can serum surfactant protein D or CC-chemokine ligand 18 predict outcome of interstitial lung disease in patients with early systemic sclerosis? J Rheumatol. 2013;40(7):1114–20. Pubmed Central PMCID: 3728890.
63. Yanaba K, Hasegawa M, Takehara K, Sato S. Comparative study of serum surfactant protein-D and KL-6 concentrations in patients with systemic sclerosis as markers for monitoring the activity of pulmonary fibrosis. J Rheumatol. 2004;31(6):1112–20. eng.
64. Kumanovics G, Gorbe E, Minier T, Simon D, Berki T, Czirjak L. Follow-up of serum KL-6 lung fibrosis biomarker levels in 173 patients with systemic sclerosis. Clin Exp Rheumatol. 2014;32(6 Suppl 86):S-138–44.
65. Song JW, Do KH, Jang SJ, Colby TV, Han S, Kim DS. Blood biomarkers MMP-7 and SP-A: predictors of outcome in idiopathic pulmonary fibrosis. Chest. 2013;143(5):1422–9.
66. Moinzadeh P, Krieg T, Hellmich M, Brinckmann J, Neumann E, Muller-Ladner U, et al. Elevated MMP-7 levels in patients with systemic sclerosis: correlation with pulmonary involvement. Exp Dermatol. 2011;20(9):770–3.
67. Manetti M, Guiducci S, Romano E, Bellando-Randone S, Conforti ML, Ibba-Manneschi L, et al. Increased serum levels and tissue expression of matrix metalloproteinase-12 in patients with systemic sclerosis: correlation with severity of skin and pulmonary fibrosis and vascular damage. Ann Rheum Dis. 2012;71(6):1064–72.
68. Jenkins RG, Simpson JK, Saini G, Bentley JH, Russell AM, Braybrooke R, et al. Longitudinal change in collagen degradation biomarkers in idiopathic pulmonary fibrosis: an analysis from the prospective, multicentre PROFILE study. Lancet Respir Med. 2015;3(6):462–72.
69. Doyle TJ, Patel AS, Hatabu H, Nishino M, Wu G, Osorio JC, et al. Detection of rheumatoid arthritis-interstitial lung disease is enhanced by serum biomarkers. Am J Respir Crit Care Med. 2015;191(12):1403–12. Pubmed Central PMCID: 4476561.
70. Lota HK, Renzoni EA. Circulating biomarkers of interstitial lung disease in systemic sclerosis. Int J Rheumatol. 2012;2012:121439. Pubmed Central PMCID: 3439977.
71. Prasse A, Pechkovsky DV, Toews GB, Schafer M, Eggeling S, Ludwig C, et al. CCL18 as an indicator of pulmonary fibrotic activity in idiopathic interstitial pneumonias and systemic sclerosis. Arthritis Rheum. 2007;56(5):1685–93. eng.
72. Kodera M, Hasegawa M, Komura K, Yanaba K, Takehara K, Sato S. Serum pulmonary and activation-regulated chemokine/CCL18 levels in patients with systemic sclerosis: a sensitive indicator of active pulmonary fibrosis. Arthritis Rheum. 2005;52(9):2889–96. eng.
73. De Lauretis A, Sestini P, Pantelidis P, Hoyles R, Hansell DM, Goh NS, et al. Serum interleukin 6 is predictive of early functional decline and mortality in interstitial lung disease associated with systemic sclerosis. J Rheumatol. 2013;40(4):435–46.
74. Wuttge DM, Wildt M, Geborek P, Wollheim FA, Scheja A, Akesson A. Serum IL-15 in patients with early systemic sclerosis: a potential novel marker of lung disease. Arthritis Res Ther. 2007;9(5):R85. eng.
75. Lambrecht S, Smith V, De Wilde K, Coudenys J, Decuman S, Deforce D, et al. Growth differentiation factor 15, a marker of lung involvement in systemic sclerosis, is involved in fibrosis development but is not indispensable for fibrosis development. Arthritis Rheumatol. 2014;66(2):418–27.

76. Lee CG, Hartl D, Lee GR, Koller B, Matsuura H, Da Silva CA, et al. Role of breast regression protein 39 (BRP-39)/chitinase 3-like-1 in Th2 and IL-13-induced tissue responses and apoptosis. J Exp Med. 2009;206(5):1149–66. eng.
77. Nordenbaek C, Johansen JS, Halberg P, Wiik A, Garbarsch C, Ullman S, et al. High serum levels of YKL-40 in patients with systemic sclerosis are associated with pulmonary involvement. Scand J Rheumatol. 2005;34(4):293–7. eng.
78. Lee CG, Herzog EL, Ahangari F, Zhou Y, Gulati M, Lee CM, et al. Chitinase 1 is a biomarker for and therapeutic target in scleroderma-associated interstitial lung disease that augments TGF-beta1 signaling. J Immunol. 2012;189(5):2635–44. Pubmed Central PMCID: 4336775.
79. Hasegawa M, Asano Y, Endo H, Fujimoto M, Goto D, Ihn H, et al. Serum adhesion molecule levels as prognostic markers in patients with early systemic sclerosis: a multicentre, prospective, observational study. PLoS One. 2014;9(2):e88150. Pubmed Central PMCID: 3916412.
80. Ogawa F, Shimizu K, Muroi E, Hara T, Hasegawa M, Takehara K, et al. Serum levels of 8-isoprostane, a marker of oxidative stress, are elevated in patients with systemic sclerosis. Rheumatology (Oxford). 2006;45(7):815–8. eng.
81. Volpe A, Biasi D, Caramaschi P, Mantovani W, Bambara LM, Canestrini S, et al. Levels of F2-isoprostanes in systemic sclerosis: correlation with clinical features. Rheumatology (Oxford). 2006;45(3):314–20. eng.
82. Stuart BD, Lee JS, Kozlitina J, Noth I, Devine MS, Glazer CS, et al. Effect of telomere length on survival in patients with idiopathic pulmonary fibrosis: an observational cohort study with independent validation. Lancet Respir Med. 2014;2(7):557–65. Pubmed Central PMCID: 4136521.
83. Schmidt K, Martinez-Gamboa L, Meier S, Witt C, Meisel C, Hanitsch LG, et al. Bronchoalveoloar lavage fluid cytokines and chemokines as markers and predictors for the outcome of interstitial lung disease in systemic sclerosis patients. Arthritis Res Ther. 2009;11(4):R111. eng.
84. Kim HJ, Brown MS, Elashoff R, Li G, Gjertson DW, Lynch DA, et al. Quantitative texture-based assessment of one-year changes in fibrotic reticular patterns on HRCT in scleroderma lung disease treated with oral cyclophosphamide. Eur Radiol. 2011;21(12):2455–65.
85. Stewart NJ, Leung G, Norquay G, Marshall H, Parra-Robles J, Murphy PS, et al. Experimental validation of the hyperpolarized Xe chemical shift saturation recovery technique in healthy volunteers and subjects with interstitial lung disease. Magn Reson Med Off J Soc Magn Reson Med/Soc Magn Reson Med. 2014.
86. Hashefi M, Curiel R. Future and upcoming non-neoplastic applications of PET/CT imaging. Ann N Y Acad Sci. 2011;1228:167–74.
87. Morita Y, Kuwagata S, Kato N, Tsujimura Y, Mizutani H, Suehiro M, et al. 18F-FDG PET/CT useful for the early detection of rapidly progressive fatal interstitial lung disease in dermatomyositis. Intern Med. 2012;51(12):1613–8.
88. Owada T, Maezawa R, Kurasawa K, Okada H, Arai S, Fukuda T. Detection of inflammatory lesions by f-18 fluorodeoxyglucose positron emission tomography in patients with polymyositis and dermatomyositis. J Rheumatol. 2012;39(8):1659–65.
89. Foris V, Kovacs G, Tscherner M, Olschewski A, Olschewski H. Biomarkers in pulmonary hypertension: what do we know? Chest. 2013;144(1):274–83.
90. Hoeper MM, Bogaard HJ, Condliffe R, Frantz R, Khanna D, Kurzyna M, et al. Definitions and diagnosis of pulmonary hypertension. J Am Coll Cardiol. 2013;62(25 Suppl):D42–50.
91. Humbert M, Yaici A, de Groote P, Montani D, Sitbon O, Launay D, et al. Screening for pulmonary arterial hypertension in patients with systemic sclerosis: clinical characteristics at diagnosis and long-term survival. Arthritis Rheum. 2011;63(11):3522–30.
92. Denton CP, Cailes JB, Phillips GD, Wells AU, Black CM, Bois RM. Comparison of Doppler echocardiography and right heart catheterization to assess pulmonary hypertension in systemic sclerosis. Br J Rheumatol. 1997;36(2):239–43.
93. McGoon M, Gutterman D, Steen V, Barst R, McCrory DC, Fortin TA, et al. Screening, early detection, and diagnosis of pulmonary arterial hypertension: ACCP evidence-based clinical practice guidelines. Chest. 2004;126(1 Suppl):14S–34.
94. Allanore Y, Borderie D, Avouac J, Zerkak D, Meune C, Hachulla E, et al. High N-terminal pro-brain natriuretic peptide levels and low diffusing capacity for carbon monoxide as independent predictors of the occurrence of precapillary pulmonary arterial hypertension in patients with systemic sclerosis. Arthritis Rheum. 2008;58(1):284–91.
95. Galie N, Hoeper MM, Humbert M, Torbicki A, Vachiery JL, Barbera JA, et al. Guidelines for the diagnosis and treatment of pulmonary hypertension: the Task Force for the Diagnosis and Treatment of Pulmonary Hypertension of the European Society of Cardiology (ESC) and the European Respiratory Society (ERS), endorsed by the International Society of Heart and Lung Transplantation (ISHLT). Eur Heart J. 2009;30(20):2493–537.
96. Coghlan JG, Denton CP, Grunig E, Bonderman D, Distler O, Khanna D, et al. Evidence-based detection of pulmonary arterial hypertension in systemic sclerosis: the DETECT study. Ann Rheum Dis. 2014;73(7):1340–9. Pubmed Central PMCID: 4078756.
97. Mathai SC, Sibley CT, Forfia PR, Mudd JO, Fisher MR, Tedford RJ, et al. Tricuspid annular plane systolic excursion is a robust outcome measure in systemic sclerosis-associated pulmonary arterial hypertension. J Rheumatol. 2011;38(11):2410–8.
98. Chung L, Liu J, Parsons L, Hassoun PM, McGoon M, Badesch DB, et al. Characterization of connective tissue disease-associated pulmonary arterial hypertension from REVEAL: identifying systemic sclerosis as a unique phenotype. Chest. 2010;138(6):1383–94. Pubmed Central PMCID: 3621419.
99. Cavagna L, Caporali R, Klersy C, Ghio S, Albertini R, Scelsi L, et al. Comparison of brain natriuretic peptide (BNP) and NT-proBNP in screening for pulmonary arterial hypertension in patients with systemic sclerosis. J Rheumatol. 2010;37(10):2064–70.
100. Williams MH, Handler CE, Akram R, Smith CJ, Das C, Smee J, et al. Role of N-terminal brain natriuretic peptide (N-TproBNP) in scleroderma-associated pulmonary arterial hypertension. Eur Heart J. 2006;27(12):1485–94.
101. Quarck R, Nawrot T, Meyns B, Delcroix M. C-reactive protein: a new predictor of adverse outcome in pulmonary arterial hypertension. J Am Coll Cardiol. 2009;53(14):1211–8.
102. Tamura Y, Ono T, Kuwana M, Inoue K, Takei M, Yamamoto T, et al. Human pentraxin 3 (PTX3) as a novel biomarker for the diagnosis of pulmonary arterial hypertension. PLoS One. 2012;7(9):e45834. Pubmed Central PMCID: 3448700.
103. Pendergrass SA, Hayes E, Farina G, Lemaire R, Farber HW, Whitfield ML, et al. Limited systemic sclerosis patients with pulmonary arterial hypertension show biomarkers of inflammation and vascular injury. PLoS One. 2010;5(8):e12106. Pubmed Central PMCID: 2923145.
104. Dromparis P, Michelakis ED. F2-isoprostanes: an emerging pulmonary arterial hypertension biomarker and potential link to the metabolic theory of pulmonary arterial hypertension? Chest. 2012;142(4):816–20.
105. Morelli S, Ferri C, Polettini E, Bellini C, Gualdi GF, Pittoni V, et al. Plasma endothelin-1 levels, pulmonary hypertension, and lung fibrosis in patients with systemic sclerosis. Am J Med. 1995;99(3):255–60. eng.
106. Ciurzynski M, Bienias P, Irzyk K, Kostrubiec M, Bartoszewicz Z, Siwicka M, et al. Serum endothelin-1 and NT-proBNP, but not ADMA, endoglin and TIMP-1 levels, reflect impaired right ven-

tricular function in patients with systemic sclerosis. Clin Rheumatol. 2014;33(1):83–9. Pubmed Central PMCID: 3890053.

107. Rubens C, Ewert R, Halank M, Wensel R, Orzechowski HD, Schultheiss HP, et al. Big endothelin-1 and endothelin-1 plasma levels are correlated with the severity of primary pulmonary hypertension. Chest. 2001;120(5):1562–9.

108. Cracowski JL, Degano B, Chabot F, Labarere J, Schwedhelm E, Monneret D, et al. Independent association of urinary F2-isoprostanes with survival in pulmonary arterial hypertension. Chest. 2012;142(4):869–76.

109. Malhotra R, Paskin-Flerlage S, Zamanian RT, Zimmerman P, Schmidt JW, Deng DY, et al. Circulating angiogenic modulatory factors predict survival and functional class in pulmonary arterial hypertension. Pulm Circ. 2013;3(2):369–80. Pubmed Central PMCID: 3757832.

110. Lorenzen JM, Nickel N, Kramer R, Golpon H, Westerkamp V, Olsson KM, et al. Osteopontin in patients with idiopathic pulmonary hypertension. Chest. 2011;139(5):1010–7.

111. Lorenzen JM, Kramer R, Meier M, Werfel T, Wichmann K, Hoeper MM, et al. Osteopontin in the development of systemic sclerosis – relation to disease activity and organ manifestation. Rheumatology (Oxford). 2010;49(10):1989–91. eng.

112. Renard S, Paulin R, Breuils-Bonnet S, Simard S, Pibarot P, Bonnet S, et al. Pim-1: a new biomarker in pulmonary arterial hypertension. Pulm Circ. 2013;3(1):74–81. Pubmed Central PMCID: 3641743.

113. Santos M, Reis A, Goncalves F, Ferreira-Pinto MJ, Cabral S, Torres S, et al. Adiponectin levels are elevated in patients with pulmonary arterial hypertension. Clin Cardiol. 2013.

114. Chora I, Guiducci S, Manetti M, Romano E, Mazzotta C, Bellando-Randone S, et al. Vascular biomarkers and correlation with peripheral vasculopathy in systemic sclerosis. Autoimmun Rev. 2015;14(4):314–22.

115. Sfikakis PP, Tesar J, Baraf H, Lipnick R, Klipple G, Tsokos GC. Circulating intercellular adhesion molecule-1 in patients with systemic sclerosis. Clin Immunol Immunopathol. 1993;68(1):88–92. eng.

116. Wipff J, Avouac J, Borderie D, Zerkak D, Lemarechal H, Kahan A, et al. Disturbed angiogenesis in systemic sclerosis: high levels of soluble endoglin. Rheumatology (Oxford). 2008;47(7):972–5.

117. Sulli A, Soldano S, Pizzorni C, Montagna P, Secchi ME, Villaggio B, et al. Raynaud's phenomenon and plasma endothelin: correlations with capillaroscopic patterns in systemic sclerosis. J Rheumatol. 2009;36(6):1235–9.

118. Kim HS, Park MK, Kim HY, Park SH. Capillary dimension measured by computer-based digitalized image correlated with plasma endothelin-1 levels in patients with systemic sclerosis. Clin Rheumatol. 2010;29(3):247–54.

119. Bassyouni IH, Gheita TA, Talaat RM. Clinical significance of serum levels of sCD36 in patients with systemic sclerosis: preliminary data. Rheumatology (Oxford). 2011;50(11):2108–12.

120. Riccieri V, Stefanantoni K, Vasile M, Macri V, Sciarra I, Iannace N, et al. Abnormal plasma levels of different angiogenic molecules are associated with different clinical manifestations in patients with systemic sclerosis. Clin Exp Rheumatol. 2011;29(2 Suppl 65):S46–52.

121. Avouac J, Meune C, Ruiz B, Couraud PO, Uzan G, Boileau C, et al. Angiogenic biomarkers predict the occurrence of digital ulcers in systemic sclerosis. Ann Rheum Dis. 2012;71(3):394–9.

122. Terras S, Opitz E, Moritz RK, Hoxtermann S, Gambichler T, Kreuter A. Increased serum IL-33 levels may indicate vascular involvement in systemic sclerosis. Ann Rheum Dis. 2013;72(1):144–5.

123. Manetti M, Guiducci S, Ceccarelli C, Romano E, Bellando-Randone S, Conforti ML, et al. Increased circulating levels of interleukin 33 in systemic sclerosis correlate with early disease stage and microvascular involvement. Ann Rheum Dis. 2011;70(10):1876–8.

124. Rankin AL, Mumm JB, Murphy E, Turner S, Yu N, McClanahan TK, et al. IL-33 induces IL-13-dependent cutaneous fibrosis. J Immunol. 2010;184(3):1526–35.

125. Valentini G, Bencivelli W, Bombardieri S, D'Angelo S, Della Rossa A, Silman AJ, et al. European Scleroderma Study Group to define disease activity criteria for systemic sclerosis. III. Assessment of the construct validity of the preliminary activity criteria. Ann Rheum Dis. 2003;62(9):901–3. Pubmed Central PMCID: 1754649.

126. Valentini G, Della Rossa A, Bombardieri S, Bencivelli W, Silman AJ, D'Angelo S, et al. European multicentre study to define disease activity criteria for systemic sclerosis. II. Identification of disease activity variables and development of preliminary activity indexes. Ann Rheum Dis. 2001;60(6):592–8. Pubmed Central PMCID: 1753669.

127. Khanna D, Distler O, Avouac J, Behrens F, Clements PJ, Denton C, et al. Measures of response in clinical trials of systemic sclerosis: the Combined Response Index for Systemic Sclerosis (CRISS) and Outcome Measures in Pulmonary Arterial Hypertension related to Systemic Sclerosis (EPOSS). J Rheumatol. 2009;36(10):2356–61.

128. Sambataro D, Sambataro G, Zaccara E, Maglione W, Polosa R, Afeltra AM, et al. Nailfold videocapillaroscopy micro-haemorrhage and giant capillary counting as an accurate approach for a steady state definition of disease activity in systemic sclerosis. Arthritis Res Ther. 2014;16(5):462. Pubmed Central PMCID: 4212098.

129. Michalska-Jakubus M, Kowal-Bielecka O, Chodorowska G, Bielecki M, Krasowska D. Angiopoietins-1 and -2 are differentially expressed in the sera of patients with systemic sclerosis: high angiopoietin-2 levels are associated with greater severity and higher activity of the disease. Rheumatology (Oxford). 2011;50(4):746–55. eng.

130. Abignano G, Cuomo G, Buch MH, Rosenberg WM, Valentini G, Emery P, et al. The enhanced liver fibrosis test: a clinical grade, validated serum test, biomarker of overall fibrosis in systemic sclerosis. Ann Rheum Dis. 2014;73(2):420–7.

131. Budulgan M, Dilek B, Dag SB, Batmaz I, Yildiz I, Sariyildiz MA, et al. Relationship between serum leptin level and disease activity in patients with systemic sclerosis. Clin Rheumatol. 2014;33(3):335–9.

132. Muangchan C, Harding S, Khimdas S, Bonner A, Canadian Scleroderma Research g, Baron M, et al. Association of C-reactive protein with high disease activity in systemic sclerosis: results from the Canadian Scleroderma Research Group. Arthritis Care Res. 2012;64(9):1405–14.

133. Hesselstrand R, Andreasson K, Wuttge DM, Bozovic G, Scheja A, Saxne T. Increased serum COMP predicts mortality in SSc: results from a longitudinal study of interstitial lung disease. Rheumatology (Oxford). 2012;51(5):915–20.

Pathophysiology of Fibrosis in Systemic Sclerosis

18

Maria Trojanowska and John Varga

Fibrosis is characterized by excessive accumulation of connective tissue in the extracellular matrix of parenchymal organs and replacement of normal tissue architecture with stiff collagen-rich connective tissue, resulting in failure of the affected organs. Fibrosis in the skin and multiple visceral organs is the hallmark of scleroderma, in common with a diverse group of chronic human diseases (Fig. 18.1). While in the latter fibrosis is confined to a single target organ such as the lung or kidney, in scleroderma fibrosis can occur in most internal organs as well as the skin and musculoskeletal structures.

In fibrotic conditions, fibrosis is the end result of a complex cascade of vascular and immune-mediated responses to environmental injury in a genetically predisposed individual [1]. As illustrated in Fig. 18.2, injured or activated vascular, epithelial, and immune cells produce paracrine mediators, autoantibodies, and reactive oxygen species (ROS) such as hydrogen peroxide (H_2O_2) or superoxide anion (O_2^-) that trigger the activation, differentiation, and persistent survival of stromal mesenchymal cells, leading to excessive matrix deposition and increasing stiffness and, ultimately, tissue remodeling and fibrosis.

The Extracellular Matrix

The extracellular matrix (ECM) is composed of collagens and other large structural proteins such as proteoglycans, fibrillins, fibronectin, and adhesion molecules. In addition to its passive role as a structural scaffold, the ECM also plays a dynamic role in instructing the behavior (differentiation, proliferation, migration, adhesion, biosynthetic capacity, and survival) of stromal cells and serves as a major reservoir for sequestering growth factors and matricellular proteins. In scleroderma, excessive connective tissue accumulation results from its overproduction by fibroblasts activated in response to soluble factors, hypoxia and ROS, or biochemical and mechanical signals from the surrounding ECM or via cell-cell interactions [2]. Impaired matrix degradation and turnover and expansion of the pool of ECM-producing mesenchymal cells are also important.

Collagen Synthesis and Its Regulation

The collagen family comprises over two dozen structural proteins with critical roles in organ development, growth, and differentiation. The ECM of the skin, bones, and tendons is composed largely of type I collagen, with smaller amounts of associated type III collagen. In contrast, type II collagen is found mainly in articular cartilage. Type VI collagen, made primarily by macrophages and adipocytes, is a widely distributed heterotrimer. Enzymatic cleavage of its α3 chain gives rise to endotrophin, which has profibrotic activity. The characteristic triple-helix structure of the fibrillar collagens is made possible by the presence of a glycine at every third residue of a repeating Gly-X-Y sequence, where X is a proline and Y is a hydroxyproline. During their biosynthesis, fibrillar collagens undergo extensive enzymatic modifications both inside the cell and additional processing following their secretion. Covalent cross-linking catalyzed by enzymes such as lysyl oxidase-like 2 (LOXL2) stabilizes the collagen fiber network in the extracellular space and impedes matrix turnover.

Type I collagen synthesis is regulated by a number of cues including cytokines and other soluble extracellular factors, ROS, and cell-cell and cell-matrix contact (Table 18.1). Environmental cues allow fibroblasts to respond to dynamic tissue requirements during development and tissue repair [3].

M. Trojanowska, PhD (✉)
Department of Medicine, Boston University Medical Center, Boston, MA, USA
e-mail: trojanme@bu.edu

J. Varga, MD
John and Nancy Hughes Professor, Feinberg School of Medicine, Northwestern University, Chicago, IL, USA

J. Varga et al. (eds.), *Scleroderma*, DOI 10.1007/978-3-319-31407-5_18

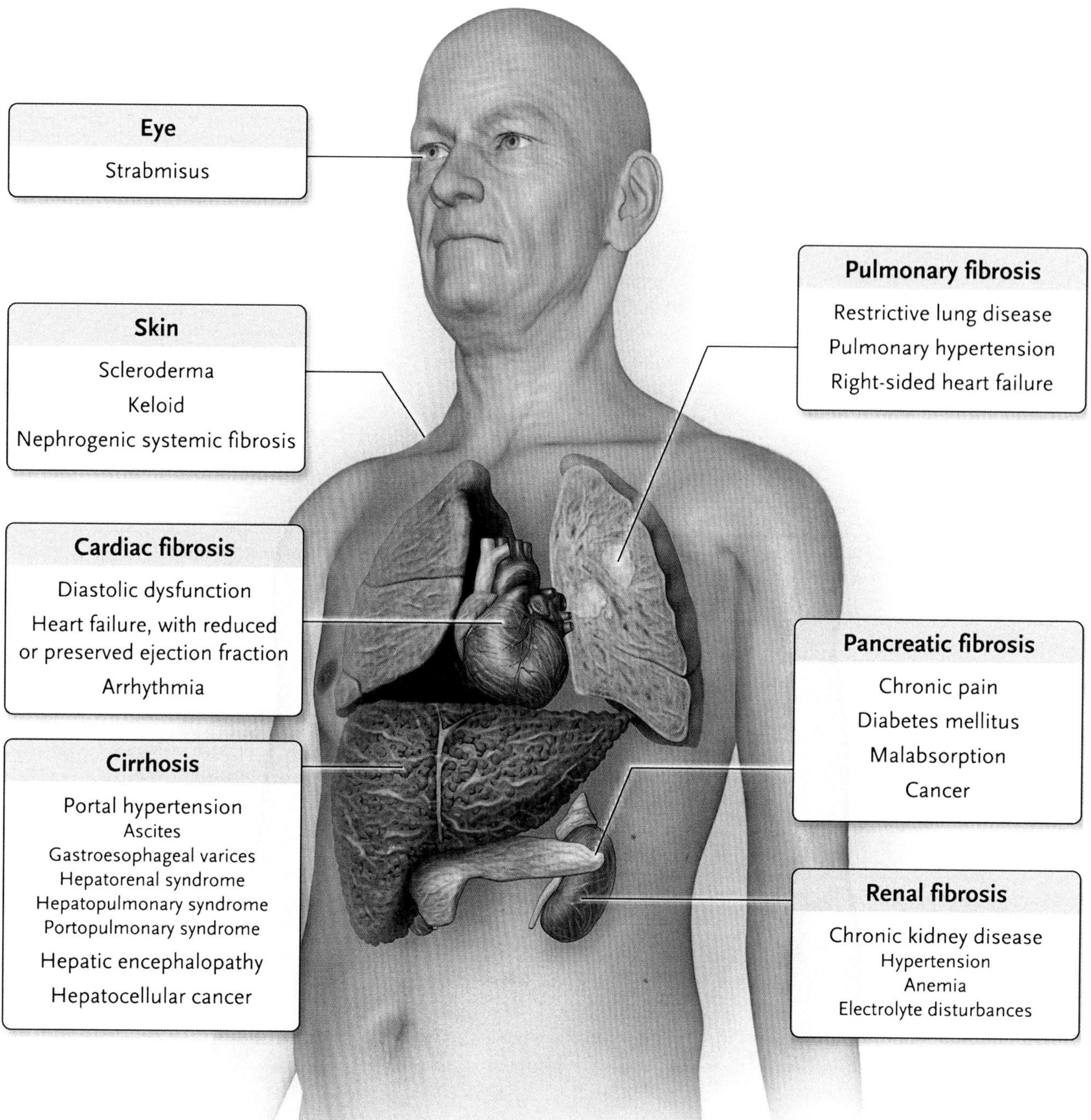

Fig. 18.1 Fibrosis in multiple organs. Pathological scarring of fibrosis occurs in multiple organs, leading to loss of function. Fibrosis in the bone marrow, heart, intestinal tract, kidney, liver, and lungs together contributes to more than one-third of all deaths worldwide. The stroma of solid tumors also represents a fibrotic lesion. Effective therapies to prevent, or halt the progression, or promote regression, of fibrosis are not yet available (With permission, Rockey et al. [138])

The genes encoding the various collagens harbor cis-acting conserved regulatory elements that are recognized by DNA-binding transcription factors. Among these, Sp1, Ets1, Smad2/3, Egr-1, and CCAAT-binding factor (CBF) stimulate, and C/EBP, YB1, c-Krox, and Fli-1 suppress transcription [4]. These transcription factors interact with one another as well as with non-DNA-binding cofactors, scaffold proteins, and chromatin-modifying enzymes such as p300/CBP, PCAF, sirtuins, and histone deacetylases (HDACs). The activities and interactions of transcription factors and cofactors are controlled by extracellular cues. Chromatin-modifying enzymes such as acetyltransferases and HDACs facilitate the access of DNA-binding factors to cognate cis-acting regulatory DNA sequences and enhance transcription [5]. Alterations in the levels, intracellular compartmentalization, activities or interactions among the various transcription factors, cofactors, and chromatin-modifying enzymes contribute to persistent fibroblast activation in scleroderma.

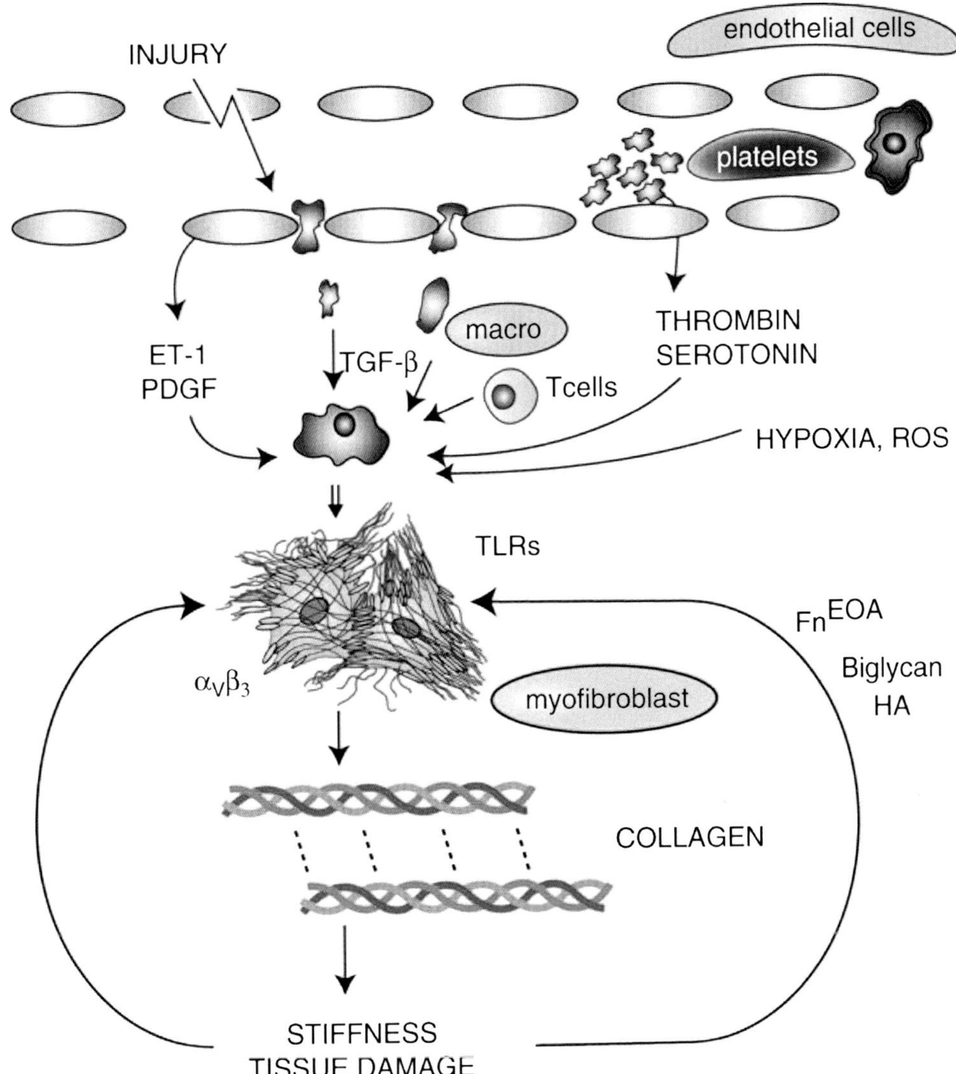

Fig. 18.2 Pathogenesis of fibrosis in scleroderma. Vascular injury triggers endothelial cell activation and perivascular inflammation, intravascular platelet activation, altered fibrinolysis, and reduced blood flow. Consequent tissue hypoxia and oxidative stress lead to generation of reactive oxygen species (*ROS*), which directly activates fibroblasts. Activated endothelial cells and platelets secrete endothelin-1, platelet-derived growth factors, thrombin, and serotonin, each of which can further activate fibroblasts. Inflammation is associated with secretion of TGF-β, IL-6, IL-13, and chemokines that drive further activation of fibroblasts and their differentiation into contractile myofibroblasts. Myofibroblasts produce collagen and other matrix components, and via surface integrins activate matrix-bound latent TGF-β, resulting in self-amplifying stimulatory loops. The matrix undergoes remodeling resulting in increased mechanical stiffness and accumulation of damage-associated matricellular proteins such as the alternately spliced EDA-fibronectin, tenascin C, and hyaluronic acid (*HA*) that are not normally present in adult tissue. Damage-associated molecular patterns are sensed by fibroblasts via Toll-like receptors (*TLRs*) and elicit activation. Self-sustaining and cell-autonomous persistent fibroblast activation results in the progression of fibrosis and formation of an intractable scar. Studies with animal models of fibrosis indicate that organ fibrosis is potentially reversible

Effector Cells of Fibrosis: Fibroblasts

Fibroblasts are versatile stromal cells that are capable of both synthesis and degradation of ECM. While some markers are in common use as research tools to identify all fibroblasts (e.g., α-smooth muscle actin, vimentin, FSP1, desmin, and prolyl hydroxylase), no unique markers that specifically identify fibroblasts have been described, and the developmental origins of these specialized cells remain unsettled. While unstimulated fibroblasts are biosynthetically quiescent, under the influence of appropriate extracellular cues, fibroblasts become activated and secrete ECM macromolecules, growth factors, and cytokines. Additionally, activated fibroblasts migrate, adhere to, contract, and remodel connective tissue and transdifferentiate into contractile myofibroblasts. Together, these biosynthetic, proinflammatory, contractile, and adhesive functions enable fibroblasts to execute their primary function, which is rapid and effective wound healing

Table 18.1 Selected extracellular signals that contribute to fibrosis in scleroderma

Signal	Cellular source	Elevated in scleroderma
TGF-β family	Inflammatory cells, platelets, fibroblasts, macrophages Release from latent form sequestered within ECM	+
PDGF	Platelets, macrophages, fibroblasts, endothelial cells	+
Thrombin	Circulation	+
CTGF/CCN2	Fibroblasts, endothelial cells	+
Insulin-like growth factor-1	Fibroblasts	+
IL-1ß	Monocytes via inflammasome	+
IL-1 alpha	Keratinocytes	
IL-4, IL-13	Th2 lymphocytes, mast cells	+
IL-6	Macrophages, B cells, T cells, fibroblasts	+
Chemokines (MCP-1, MCP-3, CXCL12, CXCR4)	Neutrophils, epithelial cells, endothelial cells, fibroblasts	+
Angiotensin II	Liver/circulation	+
Endothelin-1	Endothelial cells	+
Adenosine	Multiple cells	
Wnt ligands	Developmental pathway aberrantly reactivated	+
Notch/jagged	Developmental pathway aberrantly reactivated	+
Hedgehog	Developmental pathway aberrantly reactivated	+
Endogenous ligands for TLR4 (alternately spliced forms of fibronectin, tenascin)	Generated during tissue injury	
Agonistic functional autoantibodies (against ET1 receptor, PDGF receptor, Ang II receptor)	B cells	+
Lysophosphatidic acid	Generated during tissue injury	+
Hypoxia	Underperfused tissue	+
Reactive oxygen species (H_2O_2, $O2^-$)	Generated spontaneously from scleroderma fibroblasts and during ischemia reperfusion	+

[6]. Whereas under physiologic conditions the fibroblast repair program is tightly regulated and self-limited, pathological fibrosis is characterized by uncontrolled fibroblast activation that results in exaggerated ECM accumulation and remodeling, culminating in scarring in the skin, lungs, kidneys, heart, and other organs [1].

Genome-wide DNA microarray studies reveal that skin fibroblasts explanted from different anatomic locations differ markedly in their pattern of gene expression, suggesting that fibroblasts at different positions in the body axis could be considered distinct differentiated cell types [7, 8]. The apparent "positional memory" of fibroblasts is governed by epigenetic mechanisms via imprinting by the homeobox (HOX) family transcription factors that are for the "hox code." Lineage tracing studies in transgenic mice are providing a nuanced and increasingly complex picture of the developmental origins, lineage specificities, and diversity of dermal fibroblasts. These studies reveal that fibroblasts residing within the derma arise from at least two distinct lineages. One lineage gives rise to the cells of the papillary (upper) dermis, including dermal papilla, whereas the other lineage gives rise to cells in the lower dermis, including reticular fibroblasts, preadipocytes, and adipocytes [9]. A remarkable series of recent studies further illuminate the lineage specificity of cells responsible for fibrosis in the dermis [10]. A fibroblast lineage defined by the embryonic expression of *Engrailed-1* (En1) within the dermis appears to be almost exclusively responsible for the synthesis of connective tissue during skin fibrogenesis. The fibrogenic En1 dermal fibroblasts express the CD26/dipeptidyl peptidase-4 (DPP4) cell surface marker. Ablation of CD26-positive fibroblasts in mice results in diminished experimental skin fibrosis, identifying CD26 as a potential target for anti-fibrotic therapy.

Additional Effector Cells of Fibrosis: Myofibroblasts, Pericytes, Endothelial Cells, and Cellular Plasticity

In fibrotic tissues, the pool of biosynthetically activated mesenchymal cells is expanded not only by proliferation of resident fibroblasts, which is not robust, but also by transdifferentiation from other cell lineages, as well as the influx of bone marrow-derived myeloid cells and mesenchymal progenitor cells. Recent advances in cell fate mapping approaches in mice facilitate increasingly accurate characterization of the origin of activated fibroblasts in fibrotic lesions. Several recent studies point to perivascular mesenchymal stem cells called pericytes as the main precursors of collagen-producing cells in fibrosis [10]. Pericytes are mesenchymal cells in the walls of small blood vessels that are normally in intimate contact with the underlying endothelium. Their primary physiologic function is to regulate vascular homeostasis [11]. Such profibrotic precursors were further characterized as a progeny of perivascular PDGFRα[+]/ADAM12[+] cells during acute skin and muscle injury [12]. In scleroderma patients, a marked increase in microvascular pericyte compartment and an increased expression of PDGF receptors have been reported. It has been demonstrated that activated pericytes can give rise to collagen-producing myofibroblasts, thus linking microvascular injury and fibrosis [13].

Interestingly, analyses of lung and kidney fibrosis implicated a heterogenous origin of activated fibroblasts/myofibroblasts. For example, in a mouse model of kidney fibrosis, ~50 % of myofibroblasts originated from resident fibroblasts through proliferation, while the rest were derived through differentiation from bone marrow progenitors, with a small proportion originating from endothelial or epithelial cells through endothelial/epithelial to mesenchymal transition [14]. Expansion of PDGFRα-positive, collagen-producing local fibroblasts was also observed in bleomycin-induced lung fibrosis [15]. Another major population of collagen-producing myofibroblasts in this model derived from the FoxD1+ PDGFRα + NG2+ pericytes [15]. Expansion of PDGFRα-positive cells during organ fibrosis is consistent with the phenotype of transgenic mice expressing activated PDGFRα, which develop fibrosis in multiple organs [16]. Lineage tracing studies of dermal fibrosis support the existence of multiple profibrotic precursor cells. One study showed that Sox2-positive progenitor cells residing within dermal papillae give rise to myofibroblasts accumulating in the fibrotic dermis in response to bleomycin injury [17]. Furthermore, endogenous CTGF was required for the expansion of these progenitor cells. A more recent study using murine lineage tracing indicated that the majority of myofibroblasts in the fibrotic dermis arise from intradermal adipocyte progenitors [18]. These studies need to be interpreted with caution as the precise markers to identify specific cell populations are still lacking. Furthermore, the relevance of the findings from models of experimental injury using lineage tracing transgenic mice to the respective human disease conditions remains to be established and will continue to be a significant challenge.

Myofibroblasts, characterized by expression of cytoskeletal protein alpha-smooth muscle actin, synthesize collagens, tissue inhibitors of metalloproteinases (TIMPs), and most other ECM components and are a major source of TGF-β secretion and activation during the fibrotic response [19]. Myofibroblasts can originate from resident fibroblasts upon stimulation by TGF-ß, a process that also requires the presence of alternately spliced fibronectin (EDA), as well as mechanical tension. In normal wound healing, myofibroblasts are detected transiently in the early granulation tissue and then progressively disappear via apoptosis. Timely elimination of myofibroblasts is a crucial step in successful wound resolution [20]. In pathological fibrogenesis, myofibroblasts persist in lesional tissue, resulting in excessively contracted and mechanically stressed matrix characteristic of chronic scar [21].

Under certain conditions, epithelial cells can undergo transformation to fibroblasts. This process, referred to as epithelial-mesenchymal transition (EMT), plays a vital role during vertebrate embryonic development. Upon stimulation, epithelial cells lose characteristic markers of cell-cell adhesion such as E-cadherin; acquire fibroblast markers such as alpha-smooth muscle actin, desmin, and podoplanin; and display fibroblast features such as collagen synthesis and contractility. Pathological EMT occurs prominently in cancer and is potentially implicated in renal fibrosis, cirrhosis, and idiopathic pulmonary fibrosis [22]. Recent studies suggest that chronic epithelial cell injury is associated with endoplasmic reticulum stress, which may contribute to their apoptosis or transdifferentiation in fibrosis [23]. Similar to epithelial cells, vascular endothelial cells can, upon injury, undergo a transition to fibroblasts. This process, called EndMT, has been demonstrated in the liver and other organs in various forms of experimentally induced fibrosis. Both EMT and EndMT processes are triggered by TGF-β and Notch, via Snail, and both appear to be implicated in the generation of tissue fibrosis in scleroderma [24].

Bone Marrow-Derived Fibrocytes and Monocyte-Derived Macrophages

Fibrocytes are bone marrow-derived CD34+ mesenchymal progenitor cells that are normally detected in small numbers in the peripheral blood. Fibrocytes can present antigen, secrete proinflammatory and profibrotic mediators, and also synthesize collagen [25]. These bone marrow-derived cells express CD14+ (a monocyte marker), as well as chemokine receptors (CCR3, CCR5, and CXCR4), which allows them to home to and accumulate within target tissues. The role for circulating fibrocytes and their tissue trafficking in the pathogenesis of fibrosis was established in animal models using neutralizing antibodies and in CXCR4-deficient mice. Mice with accelerated senescence have an increased number of circulating fibrocytes and exhibit increased sensitivity to bleomycin-induced fibrosis. It is thought that within lesional tissue, fibrocytes undergo differentiation into activated myofibroblasts, losing the CD14+ and CD34+ markers in the process, and contribute to the progression of fibrosis.

Accumulation of fibrocytes in mouse models of lung, liver, kidney, and skin fibrosis is well established; however, how these cells contribute to fibrosis remains a matter of debate [26]. Although, fibrocytes are able to produce some collagen type I and differentiate into myofibroblasts, a recent study has found that the main source of intracellular collagen in fibrocytes is through the uptake from the neighboring collagen-producing cells [27]. Fibrocytes may contribute to the process of fibrosis through secretion of profibrotic and proinflammatory mediators, including TGF-ß, TNFα, IL-1ß, and selected chemokines [26].

Other studies have identified multipotent monocyte-derived progenitor cells in peripheral blood. Certain monocyte populations might undergo differentiation within injured tissue to generate M2a-like macrophages that produce TGF-ß along with other fibrogenic growth factors and cytokines, including PDGF, IGFBP-5, and galectin, along with metalloproteinases such as MMP7. However, the significance of fibrocytes and other bone marrow-derived progenitor cells in the pathogenesis of scleroderma-associated fibrosis remains speculative [28].

Stiff Extracellular Matrix Provides Signaling That Amplifies Fibrosis Through Mechanotransduction and YAP/TAZ

Although soluble paracrine mediators as pivotal signals for fibroblast activation have been extensively characterized (see below), recent studies indicate that the mechanical properties of the matrix microenvironment also have profound effects on fibroblast morphology, migration, proliferation, differentiation, and biosynthetic properties [29]. These findings have led to the emergence of a novel paradigm stating that matrix rigidity and tension as not solely consequences of fibrosis, but are also themselves responsible for promoting, amplifying, and sustaining the fibrotic process [30]. It has been shown that stiffness in an injured organ can increase rapidly and may even precede morphologic or biochemical evidence of fibrosis [31]. Indeed, fibrosis in the skin, lungs, and other organs is associated with sometimes striking increases in matrix stiffness. Explanted fibroblasts show activation when plated on substrates of increasing stiffness. Stiffness-dependent fibroblast activation has been variously attributed to activation of matrix-bound latent TGF-β in biomechanically stressed fibroblasts mediated via cell surface integrins [32] or suppression of Cox-2 with reduced endogenous PGE2, an autocrine inhibitor of fibroblast activation [30].

The precise mechanisms whereby changes in matrix stiffness are sensed by the resident fibroblast and converted into durable alterations in cell function are not well understood. It has been proposed that signaling cascades involving cell surface integrins, focal adhesion kinase (FAK) or ROCK, and changes in focal adhesion assembly and cytoskeletal tension may be responsible. The implication of these findings is that progressive increase in matrix rigidity and mechanical tension drives increased fibroblast activation, matrix deposition, and remodeling, promoting a self-reinforcing vicious cycle of fibrosis.

Significant progress has been made in characterizing signaling pathways and transcription factors that underlie the fibrotic responses elicited by mechanical and adhesive signals. The Hippo-TAZ/YAP and myocardin/MRTF pathways have emerged as key mediators of cellular responses to mechanical inputs. Furthermore, the Hippo-YAP/TAZ pathway by interacting with several other signaling pathways such as TGF-β Smad and Wnt/β-catenin may play a central role in coordinating inputs from the intracellular signaling network with the cues from the cell's environment [33, 34]. Transcriptional cofactors TAZ and YAP, which are regulated by the integrity of the actomyosin cytoskeleton, are the key sensors, as well as mediators of mechanical signals [35]. Disruption of F-actin or inhibition of the small GTPase RhoA results in TAZ/YAP inactivation [35, 36]. GPRC signaling can also activate the YAP/TAZ signaling in a Rho GTPase-dependent manner depending on the coupled G protein [37] (Fig. 18.3). Studies in lung fibroblasts confirmed the role of TAZ and YAP as sensors of matrix stiffness [38]. Functional studies revealed that YAP/TAZ regulate profibrotic gene expression, including PAI-1 and collagen in a TGF-β-independent manner. YAP and, especially, TAZ are prominently expressed in fibrotic, but not in healthy lung tissues [38]. Myocardin (MAL) and the related factors MRTF-A and MRTF-B represent another group of mechanosensitive transcription activators regulated by matrix stiffness; however, the mode of their activation appears to be distinct from that of YAP/TAZ [39]. MRTF-A is sequestered in the cytoplasm by monomeric G-actin and is released upon Rho-induced actin polymerization [39]. MRTF-A promotes a myofibroblast phenotype by inducing α-SMA and collagen expression [40]. Understanding the mechanotransductive pathways that couple alterations in matrix stiffness to fibroblast activation might identify novel strategies to control fibrosis.

Molecular Determinants of Repair and Fibrosis

The expression of ECM genes is normally tightly regulated to meet the dynamic needs of tissue remodeling upon injury. Expression of key genes is regulated by TGF-ß and other paracrine/autocrine mediators, cell-cell contact, hypoxia,

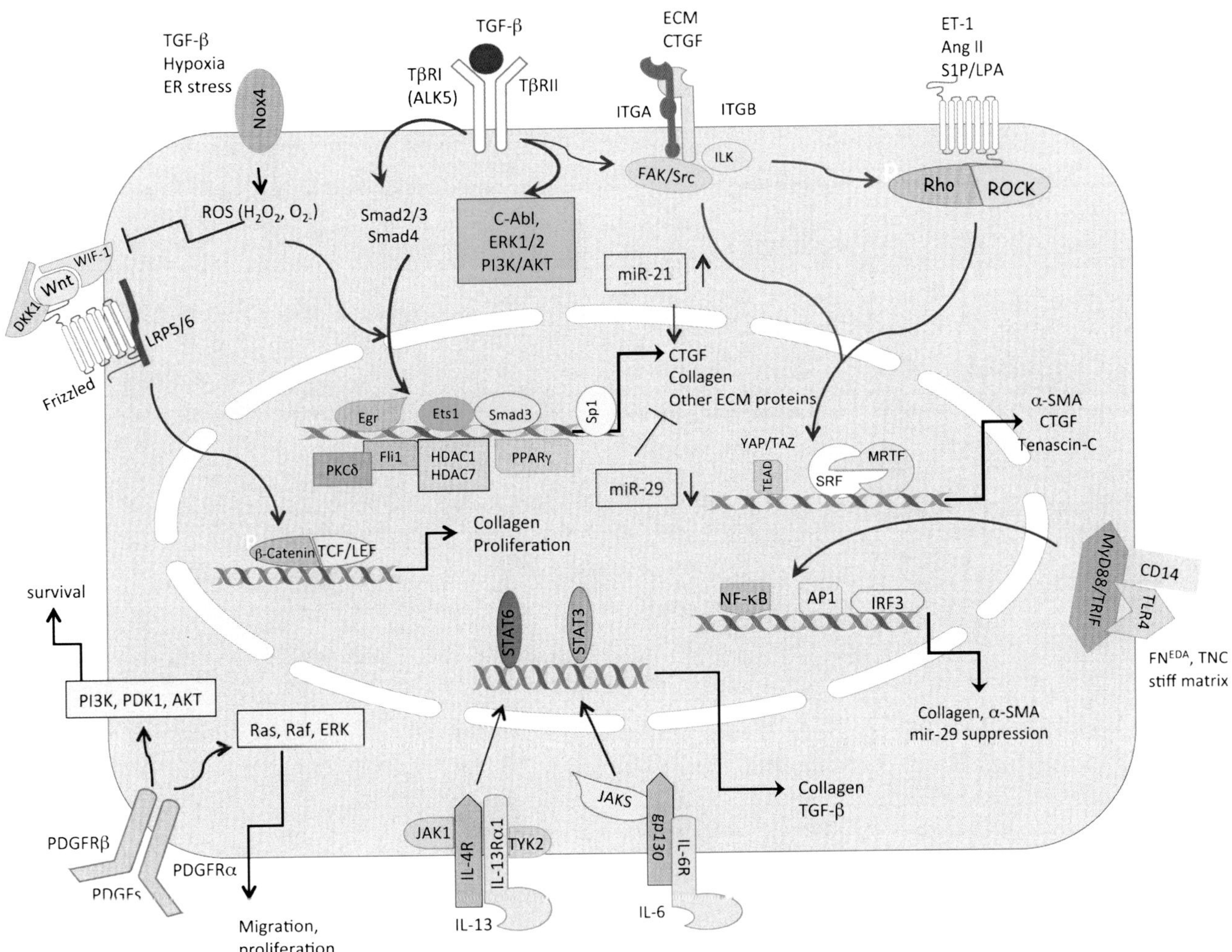

Fig. 18.3 Fibroblast regulation. TGF-β has a central role in SSc fibroblast activation and myofibroblast differentiation. Upon engagement of the cell surface TGF-β receptors, TGF-β induces profibrotic gene expression through activation of canonical (Smad2/3 dependent) and noncanonical pathways and through cross talk with other intracellular signaling pathways. Smad2/Smad3 cooperates with other transcriptional activators (e.g., Ets1 on the promoters of CTGF, COL1A2, and other profibrotic genes) [43–45]. Transcription activators recruit co-activators, such as p300 and CBP that relax chromatin structure by catalyzing histone acetylation, with recruitment of the basal transcription machinery and increasing activator-dependent transcription. Levels of p300 are constitutively elevated in SSc fibroblasts [46]. Profibrotic TGF-β responses also involve inactivation of transcriptional repressors, including Fli1 and PPAR-γ [47–49]. Sp1 is important for regulating basal expression of extracellular matrix genes and a target of the anti-fibrotic effects of bortezomib [50, 51]. Noncanonical TGF-β signaling pathways with relevance to fibrosis include Erk-MAPK, FAK/c-Abl/PI3 kinase/Akt, TAK1/JNK/p38, and Endoglin-Smad1 pathways [52]. Transcription factor Egr-1 is induced by TGF-ß and is a direct downstream target of c-Abl. Notably, hypoxia and TGF-β converge on Egr-1 to stimulate NOX4 expression, leading to enhanced ROS generation [53]. Canonical Wnt signaling, shown to be hyperactivated in SSc tissues with lesions, is a potent inducer of fibrosis in vivo. Wnt3a induces fibrogenic response in dermal fibroblasts [54]. The endogenous Wnt inhibitor, WIF1, is a ROS target, and its expression is constitutively downregulated in SSc fibroblasts [55]. TGF-β requires a stiff matrix and activation of FAK with focal adhesion assembly for myofibroblast transdifferentiation [56]. Integrins are heterodimeric glycoproteins composed of α (*ITGA*) and β (*ITGB*) subunits that mediate cell attachment to the ECM and serve as mechanosensors of the cell. Mechanotransduction mediated by surface integrins triggers the formation of an intracellular multiprotein signaling complex composed of FAK/Src/MEK and integrin-linked kinase (*ILK*)/RhoA/F-actin. Profibrotic effects of CTGF are also mediated through the αvβ5 integrin and Src in dermal fibroblasts [57]. In addition to TGF-β and CTGF, ET1, S1P/LPA, and Ang II also converge onto Rho/F-actin signaling. Two known transcriptional regulatory pathways mediate cell responses to mechanical signals: myocardin-related transcription factors, MRTF-A and MRTF-B/SRF, and the components of the Hippo pathway, YAP, and TAZ [39]. Connective tissue molecules, such as alternately spliced variant of FnEDA and tenascin C, are induced by TGF-β and constitutively upregulated in SSc, representing "damage-associated molecular patterns" (DAMPs) that serve as endogenous TLR4 ligands to elicit profibrotic responses [58]. The TLR4-mediated profibrotic pathways might involve suppression of anti-fibrotic mir-29. IL-6 and IL-13 are pleiotropic cytokines, which directly, or indirectly through TGF-β, drive collagen production and promote fibrotic matrix deposition [59, 60]. PDGFs stimulate fibroblast migration, proliferation, and matrix gene expression [61]. Abbreviations: *ECM* extracellular matrix, *PDGF* platelet-derived growth factor, *ROS* reactive oxygen species

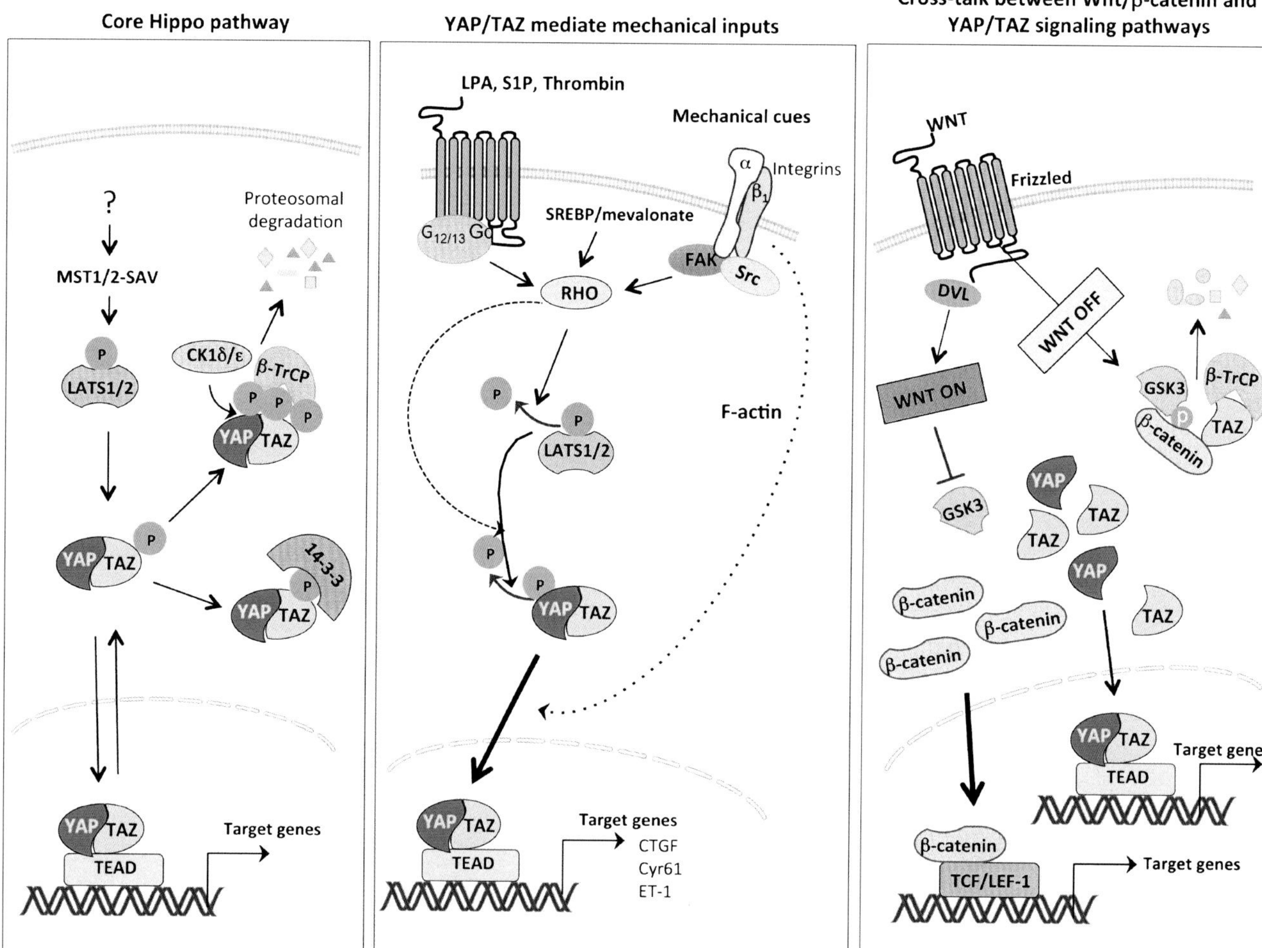

Fig. 18.4 YAP/TAZ function as intracellular mediators of cytoskeletal and mechanical inputs and the Wnt signaling pathway. (*Left panel*) The core Hippo signaling pathway consists of serine/threonine protein kinases MST1/2 and their cofactor Salvador (also known as WW45) and LATS1/2, which upon activation phosphorylate transcription co-activators YAP and TAZ. Phosphorylated TAZ and YAP are sequestered by a scaffolding protein 14-3-3 and retained in the cytoplasm. Further phosphorylation of YAP or TAZ by caseine kinase 1δ/ε triggers the recruitment of β-TrCP/SCF ubiquitin ligase, which facilitates TAZ/YAP ubiquitylation and degradation. Phosphorylated YAP/TAZ are excluded from the nucleus and accumulate in the cytoplasm, where they become degraded by the proteasome. (*Middle panel*) Selected GPRC agonists activate TAZ/YAP by inhibiting LATS1/2 phosphorylation in a Rho GTPase-dependent manner [37]. In contrast, the SREBP/mevalonate pathway activates YAP/TAZ through Rho GTPase independently of LATS1/2 [41]. (*Right panel*) YAP/TAZ are closely integrated with the Wnt/β-catenin pathway [42]. TAZ through association with Axin is required for recruitment of β-TrCP to the β-catenin destruction complex leading to β-catenin degradation. Activation of Wnt signaling leads to simultaneous induction of β-catenin and TAZ/YAP-mediated gene expression

and ROS, as well as through the biomechanical properties of the surrounding ECM (Fig. 18.4).

Transforming Growth Factor-ß

Multiple cytokines implicated in scleroderma have potent effects on the maintenance of ECM homeostasis (Table 18.1). Of these, TGF-β is undoubtedly most fundamental and is widely considered to be the master regulator of both physiologic fibrogenesis (wound healing and tissue repair) and pathological fibrosis in all organs.

The TGF-ß Superfamily and Mechanisms for Activation

Transforming growth factor-ß is a member of a large superfamily of signaling proteins that also includes activin, inhibins, growth differentiation factors, bone morphogenetic proteins (BMPs), and myostatin. There are three TGF-ß isoforms encoded by three different genes (TGF-β1, TGF-β2, and TGF-β3). TGF-βs are secreted by platelets, monocytes/macrophages, T cells, and dendritic cells and fibroblasts, and most cell types express surface receptors for TGF-β. Importantly, a large pool of inactive TGF-β is sequestered within connective tissue in a latent form bound to fibronectin and fibrillin through latent TGF-ß binding proteins (LTBPs).

The type of cellular response elicited by TGF-β is specific for the target cell lineage and is exquisitely context dependent. While TGF-ß suppresses the proliferation of epithelial cells, it stimulates the proliferation of fibroblasts. In mesenchymal cells, TGF-β acts as a potent inducer of fibrillar collagen synthesis and stimulates migration, adhesion, and transdifferentiation into myofibroblasts. Moreover, TGF-ß also induces ROS generation from the cytosol as well as mitochondria and suppresses the production of most matrix-degrading metalloproteinases (Table 18.2). In endothelial and epithelial cells, TGF-β elicits cell fate changes called epithelial-mesenchymal transition (EMT) and endothelial-mesenchymal transition (EndMT), resulting in fibroblast transdifferentiation [62]. A recent study suggests that adipocytic progenitor cells also undergo a similar myofibroblast transition in response to TGF-ß. In contrast to TGF-ß, BMP7, a member of the TGF-ß superfamily, has largely anti-fibrotic effects, reverses EMT, and antagonizes most TGF-ß responses.

TGF-β is exceedingly pleiotropic in its function and plays essential roles in normal tissue repair, angiogenesis, and immune regulation. Aberrant TGF-β function is implicated in cancer, fibrosis, and autoimmunity, along with a large and diverse group of inherited disorders [63]. A single nucleotide polymorphism (SNP) at the TGF-ß locus (rs1982073) has been implicated as a risk allele for organ fibrosis, but appears to have only a modest effect. Virtually all cells secrete TGF-β as a latent complex that is sequestered within the ECM. Under appropriate conditions, tissue-bound latent TGF-β is converted to its biologically active form that is capable of binding to surface receptors and eliciting cellular responses. The activation of latent TGF-β is a complex process controlled in part by fibrillin-1 and is mediated by surface integrins including αvß6 (on epithelial cells), αvß8 (on dendritic cells), αvß5 (on fibroblasts), and potentially additional integrins expressed in cell type-specific manner, thrombospondins, and proteolytic enzymes such as MMP14, thrombin, and plasmin. These findings highlight the fact that TGF-ß bioavailability and activity are regulated primarily through its spatially and temporally restricted activation from the latent form, and deregulation of this complex process is implicated in diseases such as Marfan syndrome. Because of its central role in orchestrating fibrotic responses, TGF-β is considered as a potential therapeutic target in scleroderma. Blocking TGF-β activity using neutralizing antibodies or receptor antagonists and selectively blocking intracellular TGF-β signaling using small molecular kinase inhibitors are promising therapeutic strategies for a variety of conditions and are undergoing evaluation in preclinical and clinical studies.

Intracellular Signaling by TGF-β: Canonical Smad Pathways

Activated TGF-β binds to its type II cell membrane receptor (ALK5), triggering an intracellular signal transduction cascade that leads to the induction of target genes. The evolutionarily conserved canonical TGF-β signal transduction pathway involves phosphorylation of the type I TGF-β receptor, a serine/threonine kinase that in turn phosphorylates downstream cytosolic signal transducers called Smads [64]. Ligand-induced phosphorylation of Smad2/3 allows them to form heterocomplexes with Smad4 and translocate into the nucleus where they bind to a consensus Smad-binding element (SBE) and recruit transcriptional cofactors such as the histone acetylase p300/CBP. Conserved SBE sequences are found in many TGF-β-inducible genes, including type I collagens, PAI-1, alpha-smooth muscle actin, and connective tissue growth factor (CTGF). Ligand-induced signal transduction through the Smad pathway is tightly controlled by endogenous inhibitors such as Smad7 and BAMBI, which are themselves regulated by TGF-β [65].

Table 18.2 Fibrogenic activities of transforming growth factor-β that are potentially relevant to the pathogenesis of systemic sclerosis

Recruits monocytes
Stimulates synthesis of collagens, fibronectin, proteoglycans, elastin, PAI-1, and TIMPs; inhibits matrix metalloproteinases
Stimulates fibroblast proliferation, chemotaxis
Induces fibrogenic cytokine/chemokine production: CTGF; autoinduction
Blocks type II interferon (IFN-γ) synthesis and activity
Stimulates production of endothelin-1
Stimulates generation of Nox4-dependent and mitochondrial reactive oxygen species (ROS)
Promotes telomere shortening via hTERT
Stimulates expression of surface receptors for TGF-β, PDGF
Induces fibroblast mitogenic responses to PDGF-AA
Promotes fibroblast-myofibroblast differentiation, monocyte-fibrocyte differentiation
Promotes epithelial-mesenchymal transition (EMT), endothelial-mesenchymal transition (EndMT)
Inhibits myofibroblast apoptosis

Noncanonical TGF-β Signaling

Although the Smad pathway appears to be the central mediator of profibrotic signals from the TGF-β receptors, there are alternative non-Smad pathways. Non-Smad signaling molecules activated by TGF-β include non-receptor protein tyrosine kinases (c-Abl, p38 and JNK, integrin-associated focal adhesion kinase FAK, and TGF-β-activated kinase TAK1), lipid kinases such as PI3 kinase and its downstream target Akt, and the calcium-dependent phosphatase calcineurin. Signaling via c-Abl is particularly relevant to scleroderma. This non-receptor tyrosine kinase implicated in chronic myelogenous leukemia (CML) mediates profibrotic signals induced by TGF-β as well as PDGF [66]. Moreover, c-Abl is constitutively activated in scleroderma fibroblasts [67]. In explanted scleroderma skin fibroblasts, multiple small molecule tyrosine kinase inhibitors reversed the abnormal ECM gene expression, and treatment prevented the development of skin fibrosis in mouse models of scleroderma and prevented the development of skin fibrosis [68].

Cytokines, Growth Factors, Chemokines, Peptides, and Lipid Mediators

Paracrine mediators important in scleroderma include cytokines, growth factors, chemokines, and eicosanoids. These mediators regulate ECM accumulation and mesenchymal cell function and show aberrant expression or activity in scleroderma (Table 18.2). Soluble mediators such as CTGF, PDGF, IL-4, IL-6, IL-13, adenosine, prostaglandin $F2_a$, and lysophosphatidic acid (LPA1) contribute to the pathogenesis of fibrosis and therefore potentially represent both biomarkers and druggable therapeutic targets.

Connective Tissue Growth Factor (CCN2)

Connective tissue growth factor (CCN2) is a 40 kDa cysteine-rich member of the CCN early-response gene family increasingly implicated, along with TGF-ß, in all forms of pathological fibrosis. This matricellular growth factor is involved in normal angiogenesis, wound healing, and development, and mice lacking CCN2 die at birth. Normal tissues have undetectable levels of CTGF, but its expression is markedly elevated in fibrotic conditions. Serum levels of CTGF correlate with the extent of skin and pulmonary fibrosis in scleroderma patients. The expression of CTGF is readily induced in normal fibroblasts by TGF-β, IL-4, and VEGF, whereas tumor necrosis factor-α and iloprost block stimulation. Transgenic mice overexpressing CTGF develop scleroderma-like skin fibrosis and microvascular pathology [69]. Further support for the pathogenic role of CTGF in fibrosis was provided by a study that showed that ablation of CCN2 in the fibroblast precursor cells attenuated the development of bleomycin-induced in mice [17]. In vitro, CTGF exerts multiple profibrotic effects in normal fibroblasts. Because many of these CTGF effects parallel those induced by TGF-β, it has been suggested that TGF-β responses are mediated through endogenous CTGF. However, the nature of the cellular CTGF receptors and the mechanism underlying CTGF profibrotic responses remain incompletely characterized.

Platelet-Derived Growth Factors

Platelet-derived growth factors are disulfide-bonded heterodimeric proteins that act mainly on stromal cells and regulate the wound healing process. Originally isolated from platelets, PDGF isoforms are also secreted from macrophages, endothelial cells, and fibroblasts. PDGF, signaling via the alpha and beta receptors, acts as a potent mitogen and chemoattractant for fibroblasts. Moreover, in fibroblasts PDGF induces ROS generation and stimulates the synthesis of collagen, fibronectin, and proteoglycans and the secretion of TGF-β1, MCP-1, and IL-6 [70]. Transgenic mice expressing a constitutively active mutant PDGF alpha receptor (PDGFRα) develop progressive fibrosis in the skin and multiple organs [16]. Lesional skin fibroblasts explanted from scleroderma patients show elevated expression of both PDGF and PDGF beta receptor [71, 72], and PDGF levels are increased in the bronchoalveolar lavage fluid. In some scleroderma patients, functional circulating antibodies targeting the PDGF receptor have been described [73]. These serum autoantibodies induce fibroblast activation and ROS generation in vitro; however, they are not specific for scleroderma and have also been detected in patients with graft-versus-host disease.

Developmental Pathways: Wnt, Hippo, Jagged/Notch, and Hedgehog

Wnt and Notch developmental pathways play fundamental roles in normal embryogenesis, and their deregulation is implicated in various disorders. These pathways appear to be deregulated in fibrosis and scleroderma. The Wnts comprise a family of poorly soluble glycoproteins with dual roles in cell-cell adhesion and transcriptional regulation. While Wnts have essential roles in morphogenesis, stem cell homeostasis, and cell fate determination, abnormal Wnt signaling is implicated in cancer, as well as rheumatoid arthritis, osteoporosis, PAH, and even aging [74]. Intracellular Wnt signaling is mediated via canonical (β-catenin), YAP/TAZ, and noncanonical pathways. Additionally, there is extensive cross talk with intracellular TGF-β signaling. Transcription of a large number of genes with diverse biological functions, many of which are associated with tissue remodeling and pathological fibrosis, is induced by Wnts through β-catenin. Transgenic mice overexpressing Wnt10b, or a constitutively active mutant β-catenin, develop exuberant wound healing, scleroderma-like dermal fibrosis, and increased collagen accumulation in the skin [54, 75, 76]. Lungs from patients with idiopathic and scleroderma-associated pulmonary fibrosis show increased nuclear β-catenin accumulation at fibrotic foci [77, 78]. Transcriptome profiling of scleroderma skin biopsies shows elevated expression of multiple Wnt ligands, Wnt receptors, and Wnt targets.

The Hippo pathway is an evolutionarily conserved intracellular cascade involved in regulation of cell proliferation, apoptosis, and differentiation [79–81]. The core Hippo signaling pathway consists of serine/threonine protein kinases MST1/2 (the sterile 20-like kinases) and LATS1/2 (large tumor suppressor like kinases 1 and 2) regulating phosphorylation of transcriptional co-activators YAP (Yes-associated protein) and TAZ (transcriptional co-activator with PDZ binding motif, WWTR1) (Fig. 18.4). In the nucleus TAZ/YAP function as transcriptional co-activators by interacting with their primary partner TEAD, as well as a number of other transcription factors, including Smads, Egr1, and Runx, to regulate specific subsets of genes [33]. TAZ and YAP are closely integrated with the Wnt/β-catenin pathway as components of the β-catenin destruction complex [42]. Consequently, activation of Wnt signaling leads to concurrent induction of β-catenin and TAZ/YAP-mediated responses (Fig. 18.4). On the other hand, TAZ/YAP can also dampen Wnt responses by sequestering β-catenin in the cytoplasm. The functional outcomes of the interplay between these two signaling pathways depend on the activation status of each pathway and the cellular context [34].

Notch is a transmembrane receptor that is activated by its ligand Jagged. The Jagged/Notch axis has fundamental roles in embryonic development, wound healing, and tissue repair. Notch signaling via Snail regulates endothelial cell and fibroblast responses including myofibroblast differentiation. A mouse model of scleroderma exhibited activated Notch signaling in the skin and lungs, and ADAM17, a proteinase induced by TGF-β and ROS that initiates Notch signal transduction, was elevated in scleroderma skin biopsies [82].

The Hedgehog (Hh) signaling pathway is a key developmental pathway also involved in tissue repair and regeneration in adults [83]. Sonic hedgehog (Shh), the most widely expressed and best characterized Hh ligand in mammalian tissues, binds to its transmembrane receptor Patched 1 (Ptch1), relieves repression of the transmembrane protein Smoothened (Smo), and triggers intracellular signaling cascades downstream from Smo. The transcription factors Gli-1, Gli-2, and Gli-3 mediate hedgehog target gene expression. Accumulating evidence links aberrant hedgehog signaling to fibrosis in the liver, kidney, and lungs [84]. Activation of the Hh signaling pathway has also been implicated in scleroderma. Several of the components of the Hh signaling pathway, including SHH, Gli-1, and Gli-2, are overexpressed in scleroderma skin [85]. Both TGF-ß and canonical Wnt signaling stimulated SHH expression in dermal fibroblasts. In fibroblasts treatment with SHH stimulated collagen gene expression and myofibroblast transdifferentiation. In vivo studies confirmed the profibrotic role of the Hh pathway in dermal fibrosis [85]. Although Wnt, Hippo, Notch, and Hedgehog developmental pathways are attractive targets for anti-fibrotic therapies, due to their important role in stem cell function, long-term blockade may be associated with substantial toxicity, especially in tissues with high cell turnover. However, therapeutic effect with minimal toxicity was achieved by low doses of combined Hedgehog/Wnt or Hedgehog/Notch inhibitors. Combination therapies demonstrated additive anti-fibrotic effects in preventive and therapeutic regimes and were well tolerated [86].

T Cells and Interleukins: IL-1, IL-4, IL-6, and IL-13

Interleukin-1ß is an inflammatory cytokine produced by multiple cell types, and its intracellular maturation and secretion are controlled by the inflammasome. Epidermal keratinocytes from scleroderma skin biopsies constitutively secreted IL-1α [87]. Coculture of scleroderma keratinocytes with normal skin fibroblasts resulted in fibroblast activation and myofibroblast differentiation that was mediated by IL-1α secreted by keratinocytes. Mice with deleted T-bet, a transcription factor that is required for Th1 differentiation, exhibit exaggerated fibrosis upon bleomycin challenge [88]. Indeed, a type II immune response, associated with a predominance of Th2 cytokines, promotes fibrogenesis and is a consistent observation in multiple fibrotic conditions [89]. The Th2 cytokine IL-4 stimulates fibroblast proliferation, chemotaxis and collagen synthesis, and production of TGF-β, CTGF, and TIMP. Serum levels of IL-4 are elevated in scleroderma, and the number of IL-4-producing T lymphocytes is increased in peripheral blood and skin.

Interleukin-6 is a multifunctional cytokine belonging to a family that also includes oncostatin M, IL-11, and leukemia inhibitory factor. IL-6 is produced by monocytes, activated B cells, fibroblasts, fibrocytes, and endothelial cells. The biological activities of IL-6 are mediated through the gp130 receptors (also known as CD130), which forms a heterodimer with IL-6Ra to induce Jak-Stat intracellular signaling pathway shared with other cytokines. Intracellular IL-6 signaling is tightly regulated by PIAS and SOCS, which block STAT and JAK signaling, respectively, and the tyrosine phosphatase SHP-2, which dephosphorylates activated JAK and STAT proteins. Transgenic mice carrying a mutated gp130 receptor exhibited worse lung fibrosis when challenged with bleomycin, whereas knockdown of IL-6 ameliorated bleomycin-induced fibrosis [90, 91]. In cultured fibroblasts, IL-6 stimulates proliferation and collagen synthesis and prevents Fas-induced apoptosis. Serum levels of IL-6 are elevated in patients with pulmonary fibrosis and scleroderma, and correlated with the severity and progression of skin and lung involvement. An ongoing phase III clinical trial is examining the efficacy of tocilizumab, which binds to the IL-6 receptor and blocks IL-6 signaling, in patients with scleroderma.

The Th2 cytokine IL-13 is implicated in asthma and fibrotic conditions. The profibrotic effects of IL-13 involve both indirect mechanisms via stimulation of TGF-β production by macrophages, as well as direct effects on fibroblast proliferation and collagen synthesis. Circulating monocytes, as well as CD8+ T cells, from patients with scleroderma produce increased IL-13, and serum levels of IL-13 are elevated [92, 93]. IL-13 represents a potential target for therapy in scleroderma.

Chemokines

Chemokines were originally identified based on their chemotactic effects on leukocytes, but are now recognized to have a broad range of cellular targets and biological activities. The CC chemokine MCP-1 stimulates collagen production directly, as well as through induction of endogenous TGF-β production. Serum levels of MCP-1, along with those of MIP-1 alpha, IL-8, CXCL8, and CCL18, are elevated in scleroderma and correlate with the severity of skin fibrosis. Mononuclear cells and dermal fibroblasts from scleroderma patients spontaneously produce these chemokines, and lesional scleroderma fibroblasts show constitutive upregulation of CCR2, the MCP-1 receptor. The MCP-1-CCR2 axis is thought to play a major role in the pathogenesis of scleroderma by amplifying collagen stimulation and promoting Th2 cytokine production. Significantly, MCP-1 null mice are resistant to the development of fibrosis induced by subcutaneous injections of bleomycin [94]. Enhanced MCP-1 and MCP-3 expression was noted in lesional skin in scleroderma, particularly in early-stage disease. The levels of MIP-1 alpha, CXCL8, and CCL18 are also elevated in scleroderma bronchoalveolar lavage (BAL) fluid. In one study, elevated CCL18 levels in the BAL fluid identified scleroderma patients who had pulmonary fibrosis, and changes in CCL18 serum levels showed a strong negative correlation with changes in lung function in this cohort. Additional chemokines overexpressed in lesional tissue or serum in patients with scleroderma or in animal models of scleroderma include RANTES and PARC (CC chemokines) and IL-8, MIP-2, and fractalkine (CXC chemokines).

The insulin-like growth factor binding protein-1 (IGFBP-1) stimulates collagen synthesis and fibroblast proliferation and induces TGF-β. Patients with scleroderma have elevated levels of IGF-1 in BAL fluids. Expression of IGFBP-3 is markedly elevated in scleroderma fibroblasts. Adenoviral delivery of IGFBP-5 resulted in the induction of chronic scleroderma-like fibrosis in mice [95].

Fibrogenic and Vasoactive Peptides Implicated in Scleroderma: Angiotensin II and Endothelin-1

Angiotensin II (Ang II), a key component of the renin-angiotensin system (RAS), is a vasoactive peptide that regulates vascular constriction, salt, and water retention and increases vascular blood pressure [96]. Recent studies have demonstrated that Ang II is also a potent profibrotic molecule that induces kidney, liver, heart, and skin fibrosis in animal models [97]. Ang II signals through two receptors, angiotensin receptor 1 (AT_1R) and angiotensin receptor 2 (AT_2R). Locally, AT_1R activation stimulates many of the signaling pathways including tyrosine kinases, c-Src, FAK, and PI3K, as well as RhoA/Rho kinase and MAP kinase families [96]. The fibrogenic effects of Ang II are also mediated through activation of TGF-ß signaling, as well as through the upregulation of NOX4 and subsequent generation of ROS. The role of AT_2R in pathogenesis is less known, and some studies suggest that it may have a protective and anti-fibrotic function by counteracting many AT_1R-mediated effects. Other components of the "protective arm" of RAS include the newly described Ang-derived small peptides Ang (1–7), which signal through the G-protein-coupled receptor Mas, as well as angiotensin-converting enzyme 2 (ACE2) that selectively degrades Ang II and generates Ang(1–7). Studies in rodent models of pulmonary and dermal fibrosis demonstrated that blockade of the Ang II/ AT_1R axis has beneficial therapeutic effects [98, 99]. A different strategy of upregulating the ACE2/Ang-(1–7)/Mas axis similarly prevented lung fibrosis and pulmonary hypertension [100, 101].

The endothelin 1 (ET1) signaling network consists of a family of three vasoactive peptides, ET1, ET2, and ET3 that signal through two distinct G-protein-coupled receptors, ET_AR and ET_BR. ET1, the best characterized isoform, is known for its pleiotropic biological effects, including a well-documented role in tissue fibrosis [102]. ET1 is induced by TGF-β in dermal fibroblasts and mediates some of its profibrotic effects. Potent profibrotic effects of ET1 were confirmed in vivo either by overexpressing ET1 in murine skin or lungs or by blocking ET1 signaling in bleomycin-induced pulmonary or dermal fibrosis [103, 104]. Expression of ET1 and its receptors is elevated in SSc skin [105]. Moreover, functional, pathogenic antibodies directed against AT_1R and ET_AR were identified in patients with SSc and linked to increased prevalence of SSc-related vascular and fibrotic complications and higher risk for SSc-induced mortality [106, 107].

Bioactive Lipids

Bioactive lipids are potent modulators of fibroblast function. While several prostanoids inhibit fibrotic responses through a variety of direct and indirect mechanisms, prostaglandin F (PGF_{2a}) was shown to be elevated in patients with pulmonary fibrosis and to stimulate collagen production and fibroblast proliferation [108]. Mice with targeted deletion of the PGF receptor are protected from bleomycin-induced pulmonary fibrosis.

Lysophosphatidic acid (LPA), generated locally via the hydrolysis of membrane phospholipids, exerts multiple biological activities via G-protein-coupled transmembrane receptors. LPA was shown to induce fibroblast chemotaxis and CTGF production [109, 110]. Significantly, levels of LPA are elevated in the lungs of patients with pulmonary fibrosis [111, 112]. Moreover, LPA1 knockout mice are protected from bleomycin-induced skin and lung fibrosis. A recent study indicates that LPA induces avβ6 integrin-mediated activation of latent TGF-β in epithelial cells, contributing to sustained autocrine and paracrine TGF-β signaling [110]. Recent clinical trials have examined the effects of LPA antagonism in patients with scleroderma.

Regulation of Fibroblast Function and Fibrosis via Innate Immune Signaling and the Inflammasome

The IFN signature observed in inflammatory myeloid cells from patients with scleroderma, coupled with the strong and consistent genetic association of scleroderma with molecules mediating innate immunity and IFN signaling, provides strong support for the involvement of innate immunity in the pathogenesis of scleroderma [113]. Toll-like receptors (TLRs) are key components of the innate immune system that serve as the first line of defense against pathogens. As primary pattern recognition receptors, TLRs sense and react rapidly to proteins, lipids, and nucleic acids from infectious pathogens or from the damaged host. TLRs are located at the cell surface (TLR2 and TLR4) or on endosomal membranes (TLR3, TLR7, and TLR9). Activation of TLR4 by lipopolysaccharide (LPS) plays a causal role in liver fibrosis, with sensitization of hepatic stellate cells to TGF-β as the underlying mechanism [114]. In addition, TLR4 also induced the expression of the profibrotic transcription factors Egr-1 and Egr-2. In scleroderma, activation of fibroblast TLRs during sterile inflammation might be triggered by endogenous TLR ligands. These so-called damage-associated molecular patterns (DAMPs) are generated at sites of tissue injury in response to mechanical damage, inflammation, autoimmunity, and oxidative stress. Three general classes of endogenous TLR ligands are recognized: matricellular molecules such as hyaluronan, alternatively spliced form of fibronectin (extra domain A [EDA]) and tenascin C, and biglycan; intracellular stress proteins (alarmins) such as HMGB1 and Hsp60; and nucleic acids and immune complexes released from damaged or necrotic cells.

The expression of both TLR3 and TLR4 is elevated in scleroderma skin and lung biopsies, and levels correlate with disease severity and progression. Elevated TLR4 expression is accompanied by substantial tissue accumulation of putative endogenous TLR ligands including alternately spliced isoforms of fibronectin and tenascin C. Mice lacking either TLR4 or endogenous TLR4 ligands fibronectin-EDA or tenascin C exhibit reduced skin, lung, and cardiac fibrosis when challenged with bleomycin or angiotensin II. These observations suggest that fibroblasts exposed to endogenous TLR4 ligands generated during tissue injury switch to an activated phenotype. In this way, fibroblast signaling initiated by damage-associated endogenous TLR ligands in scleroderma might be responsible for transformation of self-limited regenerative tissue repair into aberrant and intractable fibrotic scar formation. TLR9, expressed on endosomes, recognizes nucleic acids, primarily unmethylated CpG-containing bacterial and viral DNA. By also recognizing endogenous damage-associated DNA as well as mitochondrial DNA released during cell injury and death, TLR9 plays a major pathogenic role in autoimmune diseases such as systemic lupus erythematosus. While TLR9 stimulation on fibroblasts elicits fibrotic responses in vitro, the precise role of TLR9 in fibrosis and scleroderma remains to be clarified. The TLR3 ligand poly(I:C) causes dramatic induction of type I IFN, as well as IL-6 and other inflammatory cytokines in normal fibroblasts, and blocks TGF-ß-induced fibrotic responses [115].

In addition to the TLRs, both immune and nonimmune cells have a variety of cytosolic innate immune sensors including NOD-like receptors (NLR), RIG-I, and Nalp3 that recognize and respond to nucleic acids, damage-associated endogenous molecules, as well as environmental signals such as silica, bleomycin, and gadolinium. Once activated, these pattern recognition receptors facilitate inflammasome assembly with activation of caspase-1 and secretion of proIL-1β and IL-18. Nlrp1, a key scaffolding protein for inflammasome assembly, is a susceptibility gene for scleroderma and associated pulmonary fibrosis. Moreover, expression of the NLRP3 inflammasome is elevated in scleroderma skin biopsies. A20, a critical intracellular negative regulator of both TLR signaling and inflammasome activation, is a genetic risk allele in scleroderma, and its impaired activity might contribute to unchecked innate immunity, fibroblast activation, and consequent tissue fibrosis in scleroderma patients. Inflammasome activation and IL-1β secretion play pathogenic roles in experimental lung fibrosis in the mouse and are increasingly recognized as important factors and potential therapeutic targets in scleroderma and other fibrosing conditions [116, 117].

Negative Regulation of ECM Accumulation

To avoid excessive matrix accumulation and scarring in response to injury, redundant control mechanisms have evolved. Fibroblasts are equipped with a plethora of cell-intrinsic mechanisms for negatively regulating ECM gene expression, myofibroblast accumulation, and TGF-β stimulation. For example, Smad7 blocks TGF-β signaling by accelerating TGF-β receptor degradation. Functional impairment of Smad7 was demonstrated in scleroderma fibroblasts. Other cell-intrinsic endogenous repressors of collagen synthesis include the transcription factors Sp3, Fli-1, p53, Ras, Nrf2, cofactors such as Nab2 and HDACs, microRNAs, and nuclear receptors such as peroxisome proliferator-activated receptor (PPAR)-γ. Impaired expression, regulation, or function of these endogenous inhibitors may contribute to failure to limit fibroblast activation in scleroderma.

Interferon-γ

The inflammatory cytokine interferon-γ, produced primarily by Th1 lymphocytes, is a major negative regulator of fibroblast activation. Interferon-γ represses collagen gene expression and abrogates stimulation induced by TGF-β [118]. Interferon-γ is also a potent inhibitor of fibroblast proliferation and migration, fibroblast-mediated matrix contraction, and myofibroblast transdifferentiation. However, IFN-γ may have an indirect profibrotic effect by stimulating TGF-β and ET1 synthesis in microvascular endothelial cells and inducing endothelial-to-mesenchymal transition [119]. Significantly, some studies have shown that fibroblasts explanted from scleroderma patients are relatively resistant to the inhibitory effects of IFN-γ. Clinical trials of IFN-γ in scleroderma have demonstrated modest and inconsistent improvement in skin fibrosis, but a large randomized trial in idiopathic pulmonary fibrosis showed no benefit [120, 121].

Adiponectin and Peroxisome Proliferator-Activated Receptor-γ

Peroxisome proliferator-activated receptor-γ (PPAR-γ) is a type II orphan nuclear receptor present on adipocytes, macrophages, and other cell types. PPAR-γ modulates TGF-β signaling and mesenchymal cell plasticity and is implicated in fibrosis. Originally identified as a key regulator of adipogenesis and lipid metabolism, PPAR-γ is a dual function molecule acting as both a nuclear receptor and ligand-inducible transcription factor in diverse tissues. Various lipid moieties and electrophilic prostanoids such 15d-prostaglandin J_2 (15d-PGJ_2) serve as endogenous ligands for PPAR-γ. Insulin-sensitizing drugs such as rosiglitazone or pioglitazone were found to be potent pharmacological PPAR-γ agonists. Many target genes positively regulated by PPAR-γ play key roles in adipogenesis, including adiponectin. PPAR-γ also controls a plethora of vascular and immune processes, and abnormal PPAR-γ function is implicated in lipodystrophy, atherosclerosis, PAH, and inflammatory diseases. In skin and lung fibroblasts, 15d-PGJ_2 or pharmacological PPAR-γ ligands caused virtual abrogation of TGF-β-induced collagen production, myofibroblast transdifferentiation, EMT, and other Smad3-dependent profibrotic responses [49]. These anti-fibrotic effects include both direct transrepression, as well as negative regulation mediated through adiponectin, which activates AMP kinase and disrupts focal adhesion assembly and FAK activation. The expression and activity of PPAR-γ in the skin are impaired in patients with scleroderma and scarring alopecia. Both candidate gene and GWA studies have identified SNPs in *PPARG* associated with scleroderma, but the functional consequences of these genetic polymorphisms and their contribution to disease manifestations such as fibrosis and PAH remain to be elucidated. Recent studies have indicated that expression of adipogenic genes, and peroxisomal biogenesis, is compromised in patients with pulmonary fibrosis. Additionally, circulating levels of adiponectin, a direct transcriptional target of PPAR-γ and a marker for its activity, are reduced in scleroderma patients and correlate with disease severity [122]. Furthermore, PPAR-γ expression in lesional tissue shows an inverse relationship with TGF-β signaling. Of note, many factors implicated in fibrosis including TGF-β, Wnt ligands, IL-13, hypoxia, LPA, and CTGF potently inhibit PPAR-γ expression or function [123]. Compromised PPAR-γ expression and function in scleroderma and other fibrotic conditions of the skin and lungs may be an important pathogenic factor that contributes to the persistence and progression of fibrosis as well as vascular damage [124].

The Scleroderma Fibroblast

Fibroblasts explanted from lesional skin or fibrotic lungs of patients with scleroderma represent a heterogeneous and poorly defined cell population. In mass culture, these fibroblasts display relatively stable phenotypic alterations that persist during their serial passage in vitro. Hallmarks of the so-called "scleroderma phenotype" of fibroblasts are characterized by the following: constitutively enhanced ECM synthesis, secretion of profibrotic cytokines and chemokines, resistance to apoptosis, insensitivity to IFN-α, and other inhibitory signals. Additionally scleroderma fibroblasts spontaneously generate both mitochondrial and Nox4-dependent ROS (Fig. 18.5).

Moreover, scleroderma fibroblasts show spontaneous myofibroblast transdifferentiation and mature focal adhesions, due in part to constitutive activation of the FAK focal adhesion kinase. Several of the scleroderma fibroblast hallmarks are shared with aged fibroblasts. These include altered balance of oxidants and antioxidant defenses such as Nox4/Nrf2, impaired expression or compromised function of antiaging histone deacetylase mechanisms such as sirtuins (SIRT1 and SIRT3), and deregulated autophagic flux [125]. It remains unsettled whether the scleroderma fibroblast phenotype represents a fixed cell-intrinsic abnormality, likely due to acquired epigenetic modifications, or activation in response to exogenous stimuli in the fibrotic microenvironment.

Numerous intracellular signaling molecules have been reported to be abnormally expressed or constitutively activated in scleroderma fibroblasts in culture. The list includes protein kinase C, Smad3, Smad7, Egr-1, p300, sirtuins, and NOX4, as well as several microRNA species [126]. Elevated expression of the pro-survival factors Bcl-2 and Akt in scleroderma fibroblasts may play a role in their relative resistance to apoptosis [127, 128]. Because most of the scleroderma fibroblast characteristics can be induced in normal fibroblasts by treatment with TGF-β, it has been suggested that the scleroderma phenotype could be due to autocrine TGF-β signaling. Of note, cell surface TGF-β receptor expression is elevated on scleroderma fibroblasts, which could sensitize these cells to endogenously produced TGF-β or to low levels of TGF-β within the cellular milieu. Notably, scleroderma fibroblasts have elevated levels of thrombospondin and αvß3 integrins, both of which catalyze latent TGF-β activation at the cell surface. Consistent with the autocrine TGF-β hypothesis, scleroderma fibroblasts show constitutive Smad3 activation and interaction with the histone acetyltransferase p300/CBP. Additional studies demonstrate defective expression or function of endogenous

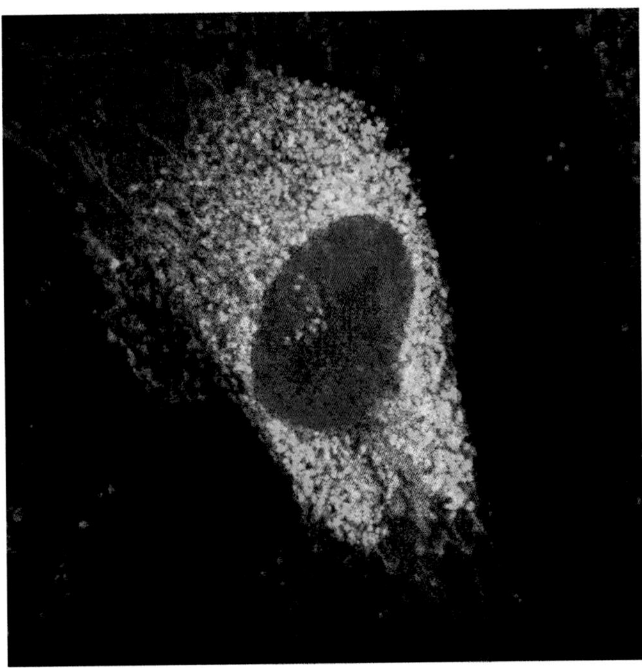

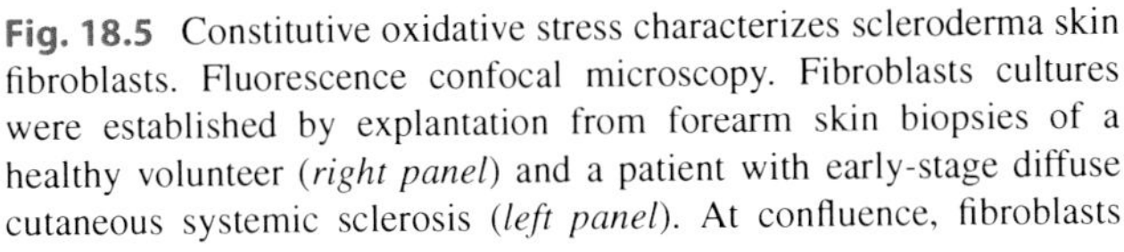

Fig. 18.5 Constitutive oxidative stress characterizes scleroderma skin fibroblasts. Fluorescence confocal microscopy. Fibroblasts cultures were established by explantation from forearm skin biopsies of a healthy volunteer (*right panel*) and a patient with early-stage diffuse cutaneous systemic sclerosis (*left panel*). At confluence, fibroblasts were incubated with MitoSOX Red to identify mitochondrial ROS (*red color*) and H_2CFDA probe to identify intracellular ROS (*green color*). Note marked increase in both mitochondrial and cytosolic ROS is scleroderma fibroblasts (Courtesy of Jun Wei and John Varga)

suppressors of TGF-β signaling, suggesting that failure to terminate fibroblast activation may represent a fundamental defect in scleroderma. Autocrine TGF-β signaling cannot fully account for all of the phenotypic hallmarks of scleroderma fibroblasts such as constitutive CTGF production, indicating that both Smad-independent TGF-β signaling mechanisms, as well as non-TGF-β-mediated activation events, are involved in the induction or maintenance of the scleroderma phenotype. The cell-autonomous scleroderma phenotype could also result from integrin-mediated mechanotransduction from the surrounding ECM, particularly as the stiffness of the fibrotic pericellular matrix is elevated in tissue fibrosis.

Epigenetic Reprogramming, Noncoding RNA, and the Scleroderma Fibroblast Phenotype

Epigenetic alterations in scleroderma fibroblasts are associated with persistent and heritable acquired changes in fibroblast function. Silencing endogenous negative regulators of collagen gene expression by DNA methylation or chromatin histone deacetylation or through microRNAs could suppress their expression with resultant derepression of collagen synthesis [129]. Indeed, a genome-wide DNA methylation analysis revealed a large number of differentially methylated CpG sites in scleroderma fibroblasts [130]. The majority of the differentially methylated genes were hypomethylated in both lcSSc and dcSSc fibroblasts. Although lcSSc and dcSSc show largely distinct methylation patterns, a subgroup of genes, including genes with known profibrotic roles, such as ADAM12, and transcription factors RUNX1, RUNX2, and RUNX3 were present in both scleroderma subsets. Moreover, components of the Wnt/γ-catenin pathway were among the hypomethylated genes in both scleroderma subsets. Additional studies demonstrated that two transcription factors shown to inhibit fibrotic gene expression, KLF5 and FLI1, were simultaneously repressed at the epigenetic level owing to promoter methylation and silencing [131]. The pathogenic significance of altered regulation of these two genes was highlighted by the observation that transgenic mice with deletions of a single copy of *Klf5* and *Fli1* spontaneously developed a phenotype that recapitulated all three key features of systemic sclerosis; skin fibrosis, vasculopathy, and B-cell activation with autoantibody production [131]. Moreover, fibroblasts isolated from SSc patients showed elevated levels of methylation-regulating genes and global DNA hypermethylation coupled with transcriptional silencing of Wnt signaling pathway inhibitor 1 (DKK1), Wnt inhibitory factor 1 (WIF1), and secreted frizzled-related protein 1 (SFRP1), genes that control Wnt signaling [55, 132]. Posttranslational histone modifications, including acetylation/deacetylation and methylation, are also implicated in SSc. Although levels of histone deacetylases (HDACs) have been reported to be either elevated or reduced in SSc, pharmacological HDAC inhibition in healthy subject fibroblasts resulted in suppression of fibrotic responses [133, 134]. The levels of p300, a histone acetyltransferase, are elevated in SSc fibroblasts, and p300 promotes fibrotic responses by enhancing stimulation of collagen gene transcription [46].

MicroRNAs represent a large family of 18–23 nucleotide noncoding RNAs that function as intracellular regulators of gene expression. Of particular interest are miR-21 and miR-29. Both microRNAs show aberrant expression in patients with SSc and may contribute to pathogenesis. On one hand, miR-21, the level of which is elevated in SSc fibroblasts, suppresses the expression of anti-fibrotic Smad7, thereby promoting expression of profibrotic genes [135]. On the other hand, miR-29, the level of which is reduced in SSc fibroblasts and which is suppressed by fibrotic stimuli, has inhibitory effects on fibrotic gene expression [136, 137]. Remarkably, microRNAs can be detected in the circulation and exert biological activities when incorporated into microvesicles. Although much remains to be learned about the full spectrum, regulation, and mechanism of action of aberrant miRNAs in SSc, these noncoding RNAs may serve as both biomarkers and therapeutic targets in the future.

References

1. Bhattacharyya S, Wei J, Varga J. Understanding fibrosis in systemic sclerosis: shifting paradigms, emerging opportunities. Nat Rev Rheumatol. 2012;8:42–54.
2. Ho YY, Lagares D, Tager AM, Kapoor M. Fibrosis – a lethal component of systemic sclerosis. Nat Rev Rheumatol. 2014;10:390–402.
3. Rosenbloom J, Mendoza FA, Jimenez SA. Strategies for anti-fibrotic therapies. Biochim Biophys Acta. 1832;2013:1088–103.
4. Ramirez F, Tanaka S, Bou-Gharios G. Transcriptional regulation of the human alpha2(I) collagen gene (COL1A2), an informative model system to study fibrotic diseases. Matrix Biol: J Int Soc Matrix Biol. 2006;25:365–72.
5. Ghosh AK, Wei J, Wu M, Varga J. Constitutive Smad signaling and Smad-dependent collagen gene expression in mouse embryonic fibroblasts lacking peroxisome proliferator-activated receptor-gamma. Biochem Biophys Res Commun. 2008;374:231–6.
6. Watsky MA, Weber KT, Sun Y, Postlethwaite A. New insights into the mechanism of fibroblast to myofibroblast transformation and associated pathologies. Int Rev Cell Mol Biol. 2010;282: 165–92.
7. Chang HY, Chi JT, Dudoit S, Bondre C, van de Rijn M, Botstein D, Brown PO. Diversity, topographic differentiation, and positional memory in human fibroblasts. Proc Natl Acad Sci U S A. 2002;99:12877–82.
8. Rinn JL, Bondre C, Gladstone HB, Brown PO, Chang HY. Anatomic demarcation by positional variation in fibroblast gene expression programs. PLoS Genet. 2006;2:e119.
9. Driskell RR, Lichtenberger BM, Hoste E, Kretzschmar K, Simons BD, Charalambous M, Ferron SR, Herault Y, Pavlovic G, Ferguson-Smith AC, Watt FM. Distinct fibroblast lineages determine dermal architecture in skin development and repair. Nature. 2013;504:277–81.

10. Rinkevich Y, Walmsley GG, Hu MS, Maan ZN, Newman AM, Drukker M, Januszyk M, Krampitz GW, Gurtner GC, Lorenz HP, Weissman IL, Longaker MT. Skin fibrosis. Identification and isolation of a dermal lineage with intrinsic fibrogenic potential. Science. 2015;348(6232):aaa2151. doi:10.1126/science.aaa2151. PMID: 25883361.
11. Schrimpf C, Duffield JS. Mechanisms of fibrosis: the role of the pericyte. Curr Opin Nephrol Hypertens. 2011;20:297–305.
12. Dulauroy S, Di Carlo SE, Langa F, Eberl G, Peduto L. Lineage tracing and genetic ablation of ADAM12(+) perivascular cells identify a major source of profibrotic cells during acute tissue injury. Nat Med. 2012;18:1262–70.
13. Rajkumar VS, Howell K, Csiszar K, Denton CP, Black CM, Abraham DJ. Shared expression of phenotypic markers in systemic sclerosis indicates a convergence of pericytes and fibroblasts to a myofibroblast lineage in fibrosis. Arthritis Res Ther. 2005;7:R1113–23.
14. LeBleu VS, Taduri G, O'Connell J, Teng Y, Cooke VG, Woda C, Sugimoto H, Kalluri R. Origin and function of myofibroblasts in kidney fibrosis. Nat Med. 2013;19:1047–53.
15. Hung C, Linn G, Chow YH, Kobayashi A, Mittelsteadt K, Altemeier WA, Gharib SA, Schnapp LM, Duffield JS. Role of lung pericytes and resident fibroblasts in the pathogenesis of pulmonary fibrosis. Am J Respir Crit Care Med. 2013;188:820–30.
16. Olson LE, Soriano P. Increased PDGFRalpha activation disrupts connective tissue development and drives systemic fibrosis. Dev Cell. 2009;16:303–13.
17. Liu S, Shi-wen X, Abraham DJ, Leask A. CCN2 is required for bleomycin-induced skin fibrosis in mice. Arthritis Rheum. 2011;63:239–46.
18. Marangoni RG, Korman B, Wei J, Wood TA, Graham L, Whitfield ML, Scherer PE, Tourtellotte WG, Varga J. Myofibroblasts in cutaneous fibrosis originate from adiponectin-positive intradermal progenitors. Arthritis Rheum. 2015;67:1062–1073.
19. Hinz B. The myofibroblast: paradigm for a mechanically active cell. J Biomech. 2010;43:146–55.
20. Jun JI, Lau LF. The matricellular protein CCN1 induces fibroblast senescence and restricts fibrosis in cutaneous wound healing. Nat Cell Biol. 2010;12:676–85.
21. Chan MW, Hinz B, McCulloch CA. Mechanical induction of gene expression in connective tissue cells. Methods Cell Biol. 2010;98:178–205.
22. Kalluri R, Neilson EG. Epithelial-mesenchymal transition and its implications for fibrosis. J Clin Invest. 2003;112:1776–84.
23. Korfei M, Ruppert C, Mahavadi P, Henneke I, Markart P, Koch M, Lang G, Fink L, Bohle RM, Seeger W, Weaver TE, Guenther A. Epithelial endoplasmic reticulum stress and apoptosis in sporadic idiopathic pulmonary fibrosis. Am J Respir Crit Care Med. 2008;178:838–46.
24. Li Z, Jimenez SA. Protein kinase Cdelta and c-Abl kinase are required for transforming growth factor beta induction of endothelial-mesenchymal transition in vitro. Arthritis Rheum. 2011;63:2473–83.
25. Abe R, Donnelly SC, Peng T, Bucala R, Metz CN. Peripheral blood fibrocytes: differentiation pathway and migration to wound sites. J Immunol. 2001;166:7556–62.
26. Xu J, Cong M, Park TJ, Scholten D, Brenner DA, Kisseleva T. Contribution of bone marrow-derived fibrocytes to liver fibrosis. Hepatobiliary Surg Nutr. 2015;4:34–47.
27. Kleaveland KR, Velikoff M, Yang J, Agarwal M, Rippe RA, Moore BB, Kim KK. Fibrocytes are not an essential source of type I collagen during lung fibrosis. J Immunol. 2014;193:5229–39.
28. Herzog EL, Bucala R. Fibrocytes in health and disease. Exp Hematol. 2010;38:548–56.
29. Hinz B. Formation and function of the myofibroblast during tissue repair. J Invest Dermatol. 2007;127:526–37.
30. Liu F, Mih JD, Shea BS, Kho AT, Sharif AS, Tager AM, Tschumperlin DJ. Feedback amplification of fibrosis through matrix stiffening and COX-2 suppression. J Cell Biol. 2010;190:693–706.
31. Georges PC, Hui JJ, Gombos Z, McCormick ME, Wang AY, Uemura M, Mick R, Janmey PA, Furth EE, Wells RG. Increased stiffness of the rat liver precedes matrix deposition: implications for fibrosis. Am J Physiol Gastrointest Liver Physiol. 2007;293: G1147–54.
32. Wipff PJ, Rifkin DB, Meister JJ, Hinz B. Myofibroblast contraction activates latent TGF-beta1 from the extracellular matrix. J Cell Biol. 2007;179:1311–23.
33. Mauviel A, Nallet-Staub F, Varelas X. Integrating developmental signals: a Hippo in the (path)way. Oncogene. 2012;31:1743–56.
34. Piccolo S, Dupont S, Cordenonsi M. The biology of YAP/TAZ: hippo signaling and beyond. Physiol Rev. 2014;94:1287–312.
35. Aragona M, Panciera T, Manfrin A, Giulitti S, Michielin F, Elvassore N, Dupont S, Piccolo S. A mechanical checkpoint controls multicellular growth through YAP/TAZ regulation by actin-processing factors. Cell. 2013;154:1047–59.
36. Dupont S, Morsut L, Aragona M, Enzo E, Giulitti S, Cordenonsi M, Zanconato F, Le Digabel J, Forcato M, Bicciato S, Elvassore N, Piccolo S. Role of YAP/TAZ in mechanotransduction. Nature. 2011;474:179–83.
37. Yu FX, Zhao B, Panupinthu N, Jewell JL, Lian I, Wang LH, Zhao J, Yuan H, Tumaneng K, Li H, Fu XD, Mills GB, Guan KL. Regulation of the Hippo-YAP pathway by G-protein-coupled receptor signaling. Cell. 2012;150:780–91.
38. Liu F, Lagares D, Choi KM, Stopfer L, Marinkovic A, Vrbanac V, Probst CK, Hiemer SE, Sisson TH, Horowitz JC, Rosas IO, Fredenburgh LE, Feghali-Bostwick C, Varelas X, Tager AM, Tschumperlin DJ. Mechanosignaling through YAP and TAZ drives fibroblast activation and fibrosis. Am J Physiol Lung Cell Mol Physiol. 2015;308:L344–57.
39. Janmey PA, Wells RG, Assoian RK, McCulloch CA. From tissue mechanics to transcription factors. Differ; Res Biol Divers. 2013;86:112–20.
40. Luchsinger LL, Patenaude CA, Smith BD, Layne MD. Myocardin-related transcription factor-A complexes activate type I collagen expression in lung fibroblasts. J Biol Chem. 2011;286:44116–25.
41. Sorrentino G, Ruggeri N, Specchia V, Cordenonsi M, Mano M, Dupont S, Manfrin A, Ingallina E, Sommaggio R, Piazza S, Rosato A, Piccolo S, Del Sal G. Metabolic control of YAP and TAZ by the mevalonate pathway. Nat Cell Biol. 2014;16:357–66.
42. Azzolin L, Zanconato F, Bresolin S, Forcato M, Basso G, Bicciato S, Cordenonsi M, Piccolo S. Role of TAZ as mediator of Wnt signaling. Cell. 2012;151:1443–56.
43. Asano Y, Trojanowska M. Fli1 represses transcription of the human alpha2(I) collagen gene by recruitment of the HDAC1/p300 complex. PLoS One. 2013;8:e74930.
44. Koinuma D, Tsutsumi S, Kamimura N, Taniguchi H, Miyazawa K, Sunamura M, Imamura T, Miyazono K, Aburatani H. Chromatin immunoprecipitation on microarray analysis of Smad2/3 binding sites reveals roles of ETS1 and TFAP2A in transforming growth factor beta signaling. Mol Cell Biol. 2009;29:172–86.
45. Van Beek JP, Kennedy L, Rockel JS, Bernier SM, Leask A. The induction of CCN2 by TGFbeta1 involves Ets-1. Arthritis Res Ther. 2006;8:R36.
46. Ghosh AK, Bhattacharyya S, Lafyatis R, Farina G, Yu J, Thimmapaya B, Wei J, Varga J. p300 is elevated in systemic sclerosis and its expression is positively regulated by TGF-beta: epigenetic feed-forward amplification of fibrosis. J Invest Dermatol. 2013;133:1302–10.
47. Asano Y, Trojanowska M. Phosphorylation of Fli1 at threonine 312 by protein kinase C delta promotes its interaction with p300/CREB-binding protein-associated factor and subsequent acetyla-

tion in response to transforming growth factor beta. Mol Cell Biol. 2009;29:1882–94.

48. Ghosh AK, Bhattacharyya S, Lakos G, Chen SJ, Mori Y, Varga J. Disruption of transforming growth factor beta signaling and profibrotic responses in normal skin fibroblasts by peroxisome proliferator-activated receptor gamma. Arthritis Rheum. 2004;50:1305–18.
49. Ghosh AK, Bhattacharyya S, Wei J, Kim S, Barak Y, Mori Y, Varga J. Peroxisome proliferator-activated receptor-gamma abrogates Smad-dependent collagen stimulation by targeting the p300 transcriptional coactivator. FASEB J: Off Publ Fed Am Soc Exp Biol. 2009;23:2968–77.
50. Goffin L, Seguin-Estevez Q, Alvarez M, Reith W, Chizzolini C. Transcriptional regulation of matrix metalloproteinase-1 and collagen 1A2 explains the anti-fibrotic effect exerted by proteasome inhibition in human dermal fibroblasts. Arthritis Res Ther. 2010;12:R73.
51. Verrecchia F, Rossert J, Mauviel A. Blocking sp1 transcription factor broadly inhibits extracellular matrix gene expression in vitro and in vivo: implications for the treatment of tissue fibrosis. J Invest Dermatol. 2001;116:755–63.
52. Nakerakanti S, Trojanowska M. The role of TGF-beta receptors in fibrosis. Open Rheumatol J. 2012;6:156–62.
53. Bhattacharyya S, Fang F, Tourtellotte W, Varga J. Egr-1: new conductor for the tissue repair orchestra directs harmony (regeneration) or cacophony (fibrosis). J Pathol. 2013;229:286–97.
54. Wei J, Melichian D, Komura K, Hinchcliff M, Lam AP, Lafyatis R, Gottardi CJ, MacDougald OA, Varga J. Canonical Wnt signaling induces skin fibrosis and subcutaneous lipoatrophy: a novel mouse model for scleroderma? Arthritis Rheum. 2011;63:1707–17.
55. Svegliati S, Marrone G, Pezone A, Spadoni T, Grieco A, Moroncini G, Grieco D, Vinciguerra M, Agnese S, Jungel A, Distler O, Musti AM, Gabrielli A, Avvedimento EV. Oxidative DNA damage induces the ATM-mediated transcriptional suppression of the Wnt inhibitor WIF-1 in systemic sclerosis and fibrosis. Sci Signal. 2014;7:ra84.
56. Leask A. Integrin 1: a mechanosignaling sensor essential for connective tissue deposition by fibroblasts. Adv Wound Care. 2013;2:160–6.
57. Nakerakanti SS, Bujor AM, Trojanowska M. CCN2 is required for the TGF-beta induced activation of Smad1-Erk1/2 signaling network. PLoS One. 2011;6:e21911.
58. Bhattacharyya S, Tamaki Z, Wang W, Hinchcliff M, Hoover P, Getsios S, White ES, Varga J. FibronectinEDA promotes chronic cutaneous fibrosis through Toll-like receptor signaling. Sci Transl Med. 2014;6:232ra50.
59. Duncan MR, Berman B. Stimulation of collagen and glycosaminoglycan production in cultured human adult dermal fibroblasts by recombinant human interleukin 6. J Invest Dermatol. 1991;97:686–92.
60. Jinnin M, Ihn H, Yamane K, Tamaki K. Interleukin-13 stimulates the transcription of the human alpha2(I) collagen gene in human dermal fibroblasts. J Biol Chem. 2004;279:41783–91.
61. Trojanowska M. Role of PDGF in fibrotic diseases and systemic sclerosis. Rheumatology. 2008;47 Suppl 5:v2–4.
62. Iwano M. EMT and TGF-beta in renal fibrosis. Front Biosci. 2010;2:229–38.
63. Varga J, Pasche B. Transforming growth factor beta as a therapeutic target in systemic sclerosis. Nat Rev Rheumatol. 2009;5:200–6.
64. Feng XH, Derynck R. Specificity and versatility in tgf-beta signaling through Smads. Annu Rev Cell Dev Biol. 2005;21:659–93.
65. Briones-Orta MA, Tecalco-Cruz AC, Sosa-Garrocho M, Caligaris C, Macias-Silva M. Inhibitory Smad7: emerging roles in health and disease. Curr Mol Pharmacol. 2011;4:141–53.
66. Daniels CE, Wilkes MC, Edens M, Kottom TJ, Murphy SJ, Limper AH, Leof EB. Imatinib mesylate inhibits the profibrogenic activity of TGF-beta and prevents bleomycin-mediated lung fibrosis. J Clin Invest. 2004;114:1308–16.
67. Bhattacharyya S, Ishida W, Wu M, Wilkes M, Mori Y, Hinchcliff M, Leof E, Varga J. A non-Smad mechanism of fibroblast activation by transforming growth factor-beta via c-Abl and Egr-1: selective modulation by imatinib mesylate. Oncogene. 2009;28:1285–97.
68. Distler JH, Jungel A, Huber LC, Schulze-Horsel U, Zwerina J, Gay RE, Michel BA, Hauser T, Schett G, Gay S, Distler O. Imatinib mesylate reduces production of extracellular matrix and prevents development of experimental dermal fibrosis. Arthritis Rheum. 2007;56:311–22.
69. Sonnylal S, Shi-Wen X, Leoni P, Naff K, Van Pelt CS, Nakamura H, Leask A, Abraham D, Bou-Gharios G, de Crombrugghe B. Selective expression of connective tissue growth factor in fibroblasts in vivo promotes systemic tissue fibrosis. Arthritis Rheum. 2010;62:1523–32.
70. Svegliati S, Cancello R, Sambo P, Luchetti M, Paroncini P, Orlandini G, Discepoli G, Paterno R, Santillo M, Cuozzo C, Cassano S, Avvedimento EV, Gabrielli A. Platelet-derived growth factor and reactive oxygen species (ROS) regulate Ras protein levels in primary human fibroblasts via ERK1/2. Amplification of ROS and Ras in systemic sclerosis fibroblasts. J Biol Chem. 2005;280:36474–82.
71. Klareskog L, Gustafsson R, Scheynius A, Hallgren R. Increased expression of platelet-derived growth factor type B receptors in the skin of patients with systemic sclerosis. Arthritis Rheum. 1990;33:1534–41.
72. Yamakage A, Kikuchi K, Smith EA, LeRoy EC, Trojanowska M. Selective upregulation of platelet-derived growth factor alpha receptors by transforming growth factor beta in scleroderma fibroblasts. J Exp Med. 1992;175:1227–34.
73. Baroni SS, Santillo M, Bevilacqua F, Luchetti M, Spadoni T, Mancini M, Fraticelli P, Sambo P, Funaro A, Kazlauskas A, Avvedimento EV, Gabrielli A. Stimulatory autoantibodies to the PDGF receptor in systemic sclerosis. N Engl J Med. 2006;354:2667–76.
74. Rao TP, Kuhl M. An updated overview on Wnt signaling pathways: a prelude for more. Circ Res. 2010;106:1798–806.
75. Atit R, Sgaier SK, Mohamed OA, Taketo MM, Dufort D, Joyner AL, Niswander L, Conlon RA. Beta-catenin activation is necessary and sufficient to specify the dorsal dermal fate in the mouse. Dev Biol. 2006;296:164–76.
76. Cheon S, Poon R, Yu C, Khoury M, Shenker R, Fish J, Alman BA. Prolonged beta-catenin stabilization and tcf-dependent transcriptional activation in hyperplastic cutaneous wounds. Lab Invest; J Techn Methods Pathol. 2005;85:416–25.
77. Konigshoff M, Eickelberg O. WNT signaling in lung disease: a failure or a regeneration signal? Am J Respir Cell Mol Biol. 2010;42:21–31.
78. Lam AP, Flozak AS, Russell S, Wei J, Jain M, Mutlu GM, Budinger GR, Feghali-Bostwick CA, Varga J, Gottardi CJ. Nuclear beta-catenin is increased in systemic sclerosis pulmonary fibrosis and promotes lung fibroblast migration and proliferation. Am J Respir Cell Mol Biol. 2011;45:915–22.
79. Halder G, Dupont S, Piccolo S. Transduction of mechanical and cytoskeletal cues by YAP and TAZ. Nat Rev Mol Cell Biol. 2012;13:591–600.
80. Moroishi T, Hansen CG, Guan KL. The emerging roles of YAP and TAZ in cancer. Nat Rev Cancer. 2015;15:73–9.
81. Varelas X. The Hippo pathway effectors TAZ and YAP in development, homeostasis and disease. Development. 2014;141:1614–26.
82. Kavian N, Servettaz A, Mongaret C, Wang A, Nicco C, Chereau C, Grange P, Vuiblet V, Birembaut P, Diebold MD, Weill B, Dupin N, Batteux F. Targeting ADAM-17/notch signaling abrogates the development of systemic sclerosis in a murine model. Arthritis Rheum. 2010;62:3477–87.

83. Yao E, Chuang PT. Hedgehog signaling: from basic research to clinical applications. J Formos Med Assoc = Taiwan yi zhi. 2015;114:569–76.
84. Hu L, Lin X, Lu H, Chen B, Bai Y. An overview of hedgehog signaling in fibrosis. Mol Pharmacol. 2015;87:174–82.
85. Horn A, Palumbo K, Cordazzo C, Dees C, Akhmetshina A, Tomcik M, Zerr P, Avouac J, Gusinde J, Zwerina J, Roudaut H, Traiffort E, Ruat M, Distler O, Schett G, Distler JH. Hedgehog signaling controls fibroblast activation and tissue fibrosis in systemic sclerosis. Arthritis Rheum. 2012;64:2724–33.
86. Distler A, Lang V, Del Vecchio T, Huang J, Zhang Y, Beyer C, Lin NY, Palumbo-Zerr K, Distler O, Schett G, Distler JH. Combined inhibition of morphogen pathways demonstrates additive antifibrotic effects and improved tolerability. Ann Rheum Dis. 2014;73:1264–8.
87. Aden N, Nuttall A, Shiwen X, de Winter P, Leask A, Black CM, Denton CP, Abraham DJ, Stratton RJ. Epithelial cells promote fibroblast activation via IL-1alpha in systemic sclerosis. J Invest Dermatol. 2010;130:2191–200.
88. Lakos G, Melichian D, Wu M, Varga J. Increased bleomycin-induced skin fibrosis in mice lacking the Th1-specific transcription factor T-bet. Pathobiology: J Immunopathol Mol Cell Biol. 2006;73:224–37.
89. Wynn TA. Fibrotic disease and the T(H)1/T(H)2 paradigm. Nat Rev Immunol. 2004;4:583–94.
90. Khan K, Xu S, Nihtyanova S, Derrett-Smith E, Abraham D, Denton CP, Ong VH. Clinical and pathological significance of interleukin 6 overexpression in systemic sclerosis. Ann Rheum Dis. 2012;71:1235–42.
91. Kitaba S, Murota H, Terao M, Azukizawa H, Terabe F, Shima Y, Fujimoto M, Tanaka T, Naka T, Kishimoto T, Katayama I. Blockade of interleukin-6 receptor alleviates disease in mouse model of scleroderma. Am J Pathol. 2012;180:165–76.
92. Fuschiotti P, Medsger Jr TA, Morel PA. Effector CD8+ T cells in systemic sclerosis patients produce abnormally high levels of interleukin-13 associated with increased skin fibrosis. Arthritis Rheum. 2009;60:1119–28.
93. O'Reilly S. Role of interleukin-13 in fibrosis, particularly systemic sclerosis. Biofactors. 2013;39:593–6.
94. Ferreira AM, Takagawa S, Fresco R, Zhu X, Varga J, DiPietro LA. Diminished induction of skin fibrosis in mice with MCP-1 deficiency. J Invest Dermatol. 2006;126:1900–8.
95. Yasuoka H, Hsu E, Ruiz XD, Steinman RA, Choi AM, Feghali-Bostwick CA. The fibrotic phenotype induced by IGFBP-5 is regulated by MAPK activation and egr-1-dependent and -independent mechanisms. Am J Pathol. 2009;175:605–15.
96. Montezano AC, Nguyen Dinh Cat A, Rios FJ, Touyz RM. Angiotensin II and vascular injury. Curr Hypertens Rep. 2014;16:431.
97. Stawski L, Haines P, Fine A, Rudnicka L, Trojanowska M. MMP-12 deficiency attenuates angiotensin II-induced vascular injury, M2 macrophage accumulation, and skin and heart fibrosis. PLoS One. 2014;9:e109763.
98. Marut W, Kavian N, Servettaz A, Hua-Huy T, Nicco C, Chereau C, Weill B, Dinh-Xuan AT, Batteux F. Amelioration of systemic fibrosis in mice by angiotensin II receptor blockade. Arthritis Rheum. 2013;65:1367–77.
99. Tanaka J, Tajima S, Asakawa K, Sakagami T, Moriyama H, Takada T, Suzuki E, Narita I. Preventive effect of irbesartan on bleomycin-induced lung injury in mice. Respir Invest. 2013;51:76–83.
100. Meng Y, Yu CH, Li W, Li T, Luo W, Huang S, Wu PS, Cai SX, Li X. Angiotensin-converting enzyme 2/angiotensin-(1-7)/Mas axis protects against lung fibrosis by inhibiting the MAPK/NF-kappaB pathway. Am J Respir Cell Mol Biol. 2014;50:723–36.
101. Shenoy V, Ferreira AJ, Qi Y, Fraga-Silva RA, Diez-Freire C, Dooies A, Jun JY, Sriramula S, Mariappan N, Pourang D, Venugopal CS, Francis J, Reudelhuber T, Santos RA, Patel JM, Raizada MK, Katovich MJ. The angiotensin-converting enzyme 2/angiogenesis-(1–7)/Mas axis confers cardiopulmonary protection against lung fibrosis and pulmonary hypertension. Am J Respir Crit Care Med. 2010;182:1065–72.
102. Rodriguez-Pascual F, Busnadiego O, Gonzalez-Santamaria J. The profibrotic role of endothelin-1: is the door still open for the treatment of fibrotic diseases? Life Sci. 2014;118:156–64.
103. Lagares D, Garcia-Fernandez RA, Jimenez CL, Magan-Marchal N, Busnadiego O, Lamas S, Rodriguez-Pascual F. Endothelin 1 contributes to the effect of transforming growth factor beta1 on wound repair and skin fibrosis. Arthritis Rheum. 2010;62:878–89.
104. Makino K, Jinnin M, Aoi J, Kajihara I, Makino T, Fukushima S, Sakai K, Nakayama K, Emoto N, Yanagisawa M, Ihn H. Knockout of endothelial cell-derived endothelin-1 attenuates skin fibrosis but accelerates cutaneous wound healing. PLoS One. 2014;9:e97972.
105. Abraham DJ, Vancheeswaran R, Dashwood MR, Rajkumar VS, Pantelides P, Xu SW, du Bois RM, Black CM. Increased levels of endothelin-1 and differential endothelin type A and B receptor expression in scleroderma-associated fibrotic lung disease. Am J Pathol. 1997;151:831–41.
106. Kill A, Tabeling C, Undeutsch R, Kuhl AA, Gunther J, Radic M, Becker MO, Heidecke H, Worm M, Witzenrath M, Burmester GR, Dragun D, Riemekasten G. Autoantibodies to angiotensin and endothelin receptors in systemic sclerosis induce cellular and systemic events associated with disease pathogenesis. Arthritis Res Ther. 2014;16:R29.
107. Riemekasten G, Philippe A, Nather M, Slowinski T, Muller DN, Heidecke H, Matucci-Cerinic M, Czirjak L, Lukitsch I, Becker M, Kill A, van Laar JM, Catar R, Luft FC, Burmester GR, Hegner B, Dragun D. Involvement of functional autoantibodies against vascular receptors in systemic sclerosis. Ann Rheum Dis. 2011;70:530–6.
108. Oga T, Matsuoka T, Yao C, Nonomura K, Kitaoka S, Sakata D, Kita Y, Tanizawa K, Taguchi Y, Chin K, Mishima M, Shimizu T, Narumiya S. Prostaglandin F(2alpha) receptor signaling facilitates bleomycin-induced pulmonary fibrosis independently of transforming growth factor-beta. Nat Med. 2009;15:1426–30.
109. Rancoule C, Pradere JP, Gonzalez J, Klein J, Valet P, Bascands JL, Schanstra JP, Saulnier Blache JS. Lysophosphatidic acid-1-receptor targeting agents for fibrosis. Expert Opin Investig Drugs. 2011;20:657–67.
110. Xu MY, Porte J, Knox AJ, Weinreb PH, Maher TM, Violette SM, McAnulty RJ, Sheppard D, Jenkins G. Lysophosphatidic acid induces alphavbeta6 integrin-mediated TGF-beta activation via the LPA2 receptor and the small G protein G alpha(q). Am J Pathol. 2009;174:1264–79.
111. Castelino FV, Seiders J, Bain G, Brooks SF, King CD, Swaney JS, Lorrain DS, Chun J, Luster AD, Tager AM. Amelioration of dermal fibrosis by genetic deletion or pharmacologic antagonism of lysophosphatidic acid receptor 1 in a mouse model of scleroderma. Arthritis Rheum. 2011;63:1405–15.
112. Tager AM, LaCamera P, Shea BS, Campanella GS, Selman M, Zhao Z, Polosukhin V, Wain J, Karimi-Shah BA, Kim ND, Hart WK, Pardo A, Blackwell TS, Xu Y, Chun J, Luster AD. The lysophosphatidic acid receptor LPA1 links pulmonary fibrosis to lung injury by mediating fibroblast recruitment and vascular leak. Nat Med. 2008;14:45–54.
113. Kim D, Peck A, Santer D, Patole P, Schwartz SM, Molitor JA, Arnett FC, Elkon KB. Induction of interferon-alpha by scleroderma sera containing autoantibodies to topoisomerase I: association of higher interferon-alpha activity with lung fibrosis. Arthritis Rheum. 2008;58:2163–73.
114. Seki E, De Minicis S, Osterreicher CH, Kluwe J, Osawa Y, Brenner DA, Schwabe RF. TLR4 enhances TGF-beta signaling and hepatic fibrosis. Nat Med. 2007;13:1324–32.

115. Fang F, Ooka K, Sun X, Shah R, Bhattacharyya S, Wei J, Varga J. A synthetic TLR3 ligand mitigates profibrotic fibroblast responses by inducing autocrine IFN signaling. J Immunol. 2013;191:2956–66.
116. Gasse P, Mary C, Guenon I, Noulin N, Charron S, Schnyder-Candrian S, Schnyder B, Akira S, Quesniaux VF, Lagente V, Ryffel B, Couillin I. IL-1R1/MyD88 signaling and the inflammasome are essential in pulmonary inflammation and fibrosis in mice. J Clin Invest. 2007;117:3786–99.
117. Kawaguchi M, Takahashi M, Hata T, Kashima Y, Usui F, Morimoto H, Izawa A, Takahashi Y, Masumoto J, Koyama J, Hongo M, Noda T, Nakayama J, Sagara J, Taniguchi S, Ikeda U. Inflammasome activation of cardiac fibroblasts is essential for myocardial ischemia/reperfusion injury. Circulation. 2011;123:594–604.
118. Varga J, Olsen A, Herhal J, Constantine G, Rosenbloom J, Jimenez SA. Interferon-gamma reverses the stimulation of collagen but not fibronectin gene expression by transforming growth factor-beta in normal human fibroblasts. Eur J Clin Invest. 1990;20:487–93.
119. Chrobak I, Lenna S, Stawski L, Trojanowska M. Interferon-gamma promotes vascular remodeling in human microvascular endothelial cells by upregulating endothelin (ET)-1 and transforming growth factor (TGF) beta2. J Cell Physiol. 2013;228:1774–83.
120. King Jr TE, Albera C, Bradford WZ, Costabel U, Hormel P, Lancaster L, Noble PW, Sahn SA, Szwarcberg J, Thomeer M, Valeyre D, du Bois RM, Group IS. Effect of interferon gamma-1b on survival in patients with idiopathic pulmonary fibrosis (INSPIRE): a multicentre, randomised, placebo-controlled trial. Lancet. 2009;374:222–8.
121. Varga J. Recombinant cytokine treatment for scleroderma. Can the antifibrotic potential of interferon-gamma be realized clinically? Arch Dermatol. 1997;133:637–42.
122. Wei J, Ghosh AK, Sargent JL, Komura K, Wu M, Huang QQ, Jain M, Whitfield ML, Feghali-Bostwick C, Varga J. PPARgamma downregulation by TGFss in fibroblast and impaired expression and function in systemic sclerosis: a novel mechanism for progressive fibrogenesis. PLoS One. 2010;5:e13778.
123. Wei J, Bhattacharyya S, Varga J. Peroxisome proliferator-activated receptor gamma: innate protection from excessive fibrogenesis and potential therapeutic target in systemic sclerosis. Curr Opin Rheumatol. 2010;22:671–6.
124. Oruqaj G, Karnati S, Vijayan V, Kotarkonda LK, Boateng E, Zhang W, Ruppert C, Gunther A, Shi W, Baumgart-Vogt E. Compromised peroxisomes in idiopathic pulmonary fibrosis, a vicious cycle inducing a higher fibrotic response via TGF-beta signaling. Proceedings of the National Academy of Sciences of the United States of America. 2015.
125. Piera-Velazquez S, Jimenez SA. Role of cellular senescence and NOX4-mediated oxidative stress in systemic sclerosis pathogenesis. Curr Rheumatol Rep. 2015;17:473.
126. Trojanowska M, Varga J. Molecular pathways as novel therapeutic targets in systemic sclerosis. Curr Opin Rheumatol. 2007;19:568–73.
127. Samuel GH, Lenna S, Bujor AM, Lafyatis R, Trojanowska M. Acid sphingomyelinase deficiency contributes to resistance of scleroderma fibroblasts to Fas-mediated apoptosis. J Dermatol Sci. 2012;67:166–72.
128. Santiago B, Galindo M, Rivero M, Pablos JL. Decreased susceptibility to Fas-induced apoptosis of systemic sclerosis dermal fibroblasts. Arthritis Rheum. 2001;44:1667–76.
129. Wang Y, Fan PS, Kahaleh B. Association between enhanced type I collagen expression and epigenetic repression of the FLI1 gene in scleroderma fibroblasts. Arthritis Rheum. 2006;54:2271–9.
130. Altorok N, Tsou PS, Coit P, Khanna D, Sawalha AH. Genome-wide DNA methylation analysis in dermal fibroblasts from patients with diffuse and limited systemic sclerosis reveals common and subset-specific DNA methylation aberrancies. Ann Rheum Dis. 2014;74:1612–20.
131. Noda S, Asano Y, Nishimura S, Taniguchi T, Fujiu K, Manabe I, Nakamura K, Yamashita T, Saigusa R, Akamata K, Takahashi T, Ichimura Y, Toyama T, Tsuruta D, Trojanowska M, Nagai R, Sato S. Simultaneous downregulation of KLF5 and Fli1 is a key feature underlying systemic sclerosis. Nat Commun. 2014;5:5797.
132. Dees C, Schlottmann I, Funke R, Distler A, Palumbo-Zerr K, Zerr P, Lin NY, Beyer C, Distler O, Schett G, Distler JH. The Wnt antagonists DKK1 and SFRP1 are downregulated by promoter hypermethylation in systemic sclerosis. Ann Rheum Dis. 2014;73:1232–9.
133. Ghosh AK, Mori Y, Dowling E, Varga J. Trichostatin A blocks TGF-beta-induced collagen gene expression in skin fibroblasts: involvement of Sp1. Biochem Biophys Res Commun. 2007;354:420–6.
134. Huber LC, Distler JH, Moritz F, Hemmatazad H, Hauser T, Michel BA, Gay RE, Matucci-Cerinic M, Gay S, Distler O, Jungel A. Trichostatin A prevents the accumulation of extracellular matrix in a mouse model of bleomycin-induced skin fibrosis. Arthritis Rheum. 2007;56:2755–64.
135. Zhu H, Luo H, Li Y, Zhou Y, Jiang Y, Chai J, Xiao X, You Y, Zuo X. MicroRNA-21 in scleroderma fibrosis and its function in TGF-beta-regulated fibrosis-related genes expression. J Clin Immunol. 2013;33:1100–9.
136. Bhattacharyya S, Kelley K, Melichian DS, Tamaki Z, Fang F, Su Y, Feng G, Pope RM, Budinger GR, Mutlu GM, Lafyatis R, Radstake T, Feghali-Bostwick C, Varga J. Toll-like receptor 4 signaling augments transforming growth factor-beta responses: a novel mechanism for maintaining and amplifying fibrosis in scleroderma. Am J Pathol. 2013;182:192–205.
137. Maurer B, Stanczyk J, Jungel A, Akhmetshina A, Trenkmann M, Brock M, Kowal-Bielecka O, Gay RE, Michel BA, Distler JH, Gay S, Distler O. MicroRNA-29, a key regulator of collagen expression in systemic sclerosis. Arthritis Rheum. 2010;62:1733–43.
138. Rockey DC, Darwin Bell P, Hill JA. Fibrosis – a common pathway to organ injury and failure. N Engl J Med. 2015;372:1138–49.

Overview of Animal Models

19

Yoshihide Asano and Jörg H.W. Distler

Introduction

The ability to sample fibrotic tissue in SSc by performing skin biopsy has been a major strength in trying to understand the pathobiology of this disease in comparison to other forms of organ-based fibrosis. It has permitted the identification of cardinal histological features of scleroderma and has defined key phases of the pathology in a temporal sequence so that there is now a clear understanding that as the disease develops, the first changes occur at the level of the dermal microcirculation followed by the development of inflammation that first involves cells of the innate immune and later adaptive immune system. Finally, there is the fibrotic stage of the disease that results in the replacement of specialized structures with rather vascular fibrotic connective tissue. The final component is the most important in determining the morbidity and mortality of SSc as it occurs in all target tissues. It is noteworthy that the activated pathways are largely overlapping with the biological responses during normal wound healing, but in contrast to physiological tissue responses to injury, they are not effectively terminated, but become chronically activated. In addition to defining these components of the SSc disease process, skin biopsy material has also proven valuable as a starting point to identify deregulated signaling cascades and to generate novel hypotheses. To test the importance of a candidate pathway, process, or mediator, it is necessary to explore the relevance experimentally. While experiments on cellular components isolated from affected tissues such as primary fibroblasts are essential to provide first proof of concept, there is a pressing need to further validate the results in vivo. Animal models of SSc are crucially required to close the gap between in vitro studies and clinical trials.

However, this translation from bench to bedside has long been hindered by a paucity of suitable animal models, as well as insufficient characterization of the existing models; however, this has changed over the last years. Several promising animal models of SSc have recently been described. Moreover, intensive characterization of the existing models greatly improved our understanding of the strengths and limitations of preexisting models.

Traditionally, murine models of SSc have been considered primarily in the context of skin fibrosis. As skin fibrosis is seen in the vast majority of patients, this is a reasonable starting point. However, as our understanding of the disease process has evolved, the breadth of animal models addressing these pathogenic mechanisms has also evolved. In particular, models of immunity and inflammation and vascular injury, as well as pathogenic processes in other organ systems, particularly the lungs, need to be considered as models of SSc. Unfortunately, no current animal model manifests the whole range of pathological features seen in patients. Instead, in most models, only a fraction of disease manifestations are modeled, reflecting the limitations of our understanding of underlying pathogenesis. Thus, a comprehensive description of mouse models of SSc requires consideration of a vast array of animal models of fibrosis, inflammation, autoimmunity, and vascular injury. This chapter describes traditional models of SSc in more detail but also provides a more comprehensive review of models, including emerging disease models. We will outline strengths and weaknesses of each model. Models will be somewhat arbitrarily divided into models with fibrosis as predominant clinical feature; models with immune and inflammatory deregulation and subsequent, inflammation-dependent fibrosis; and models with SSc-like vascular disease. We will demonstrate that there is not one perfect model of SSc that resembles all features of human SSc [1]. However, we aim to highlight that a wise combination of complimentary models can boost our understanding of the molecular pathogenesis of SSc and

Y. Asano, MD, PhD (✉)
Department of Dermatology, University of Tokyo Graduate School of Medicine, Tokyo, Japan
e-mail: yasano-tky@umin.ac.jp

J.H.W. Distler, MD
Department of Internal Medicine, University of Erlangen-Nuremberg, Erlangen-Nuremberg, Germany

J. Varga et al. (eds.), *Scleroderma*, DOI 10.1007/978-3-319-31407-5_19

Table 19.1 Key features of common animal models of SSc

	Fibrosis: skin/internal organs	SSc-like vasculopathy	Inflammation	Autoimmunity
Bleomycin-induced skin fibrosis	+++/(+)	Ø	+++	+
HOCl-induced fibrosis	+++/+	Ø	+++	+
cGvHD models	+++/+	Ø	++	+
Tsk-1 mice	+++/Ø	Ø	(+)	++
Tsk-2 mice	+++/Ø	Ø	(+)	++
Fra2 tg mice	+++/+++	+++	++	Ø
uPAR$^{-/-}$ mice	+++/+++	++	++	?
Caveolin-1$^{-/-}$ mice	+++/++	(+)	++	Ø
TβRI^{CA} mice	+++ / Ø or (+)*	Ø	Ø	Ø
TβRIIΔk × Col1a2; CreER mice	+++/++	++	Ø	Ø
CTGF × Col1a2; CreER mice	+++/++	?	Ø	?
Wnt10 tg mice	+++ / Ø	?	Ø	Ø
β-catenin$^{\Delta Exon3}$ × Col1a2; CreER mice	+++/(+)**	Ø	Ø	Ø
Klf5$^{+/-}$;*Fli1*$^{+/-}$ mice	+++/+++	+++	+++	+
UCD200/206 chicken	++/++	+++	+	+

Among these animal models, Fra2 tg mice, uPAR–/– mice, and *Klf5*$^{+/-}$;*Fli1*$^{+/-}$ mice mimic the histology of nonspecific interstitial pneumonia and pulmonary vascular changes characteristic of SSc

* means no in the case of adeno-associated viral vector-induced overexpression and modestly in the case of Col1a2CreER-mediated overexpression of TGF-betaRCA (CA is upper case).

** means that there are different stains with different Cre lines that vary in phenotype.

might support the development of novel targeted therapies. Key features of common animal models of SSc are outlined in Table 19.1.

Models of SSc with Fibrosis as Predominant Clinical Feature

Although fibrosis is a feature of several organs in SSc, the predominantly affected sites are the skin, seen in most patients, and lung, seen in many patients and one of the major causes of morbidity and mortality.

The Tight-Skin-1 Mouse (Tsk-1)

One of the best-characterized and most widely used genetic mouse models for SSc is the tight-skin-1 mouse (Tsk-1). This strain, originally identified as a spontaneous mutant, shows diffusely tethered skin that can be detected shortly after birth but is more easily appreciated as tightening over the intercapsular skin as the mice age [2]. A stable mouse strain was derived and through backcross linked to the pallid locus for skin color. A series of elegant genetic mapping studies identified fibrillin 1 as the responsible gene, and sequencing of this gene showed that an in-frame tandem partial reduplication was the mutation responsible for the phenotype [3] (Fig. 19.1). Heterozygous mice manifest the phenotype, while homozygous mutant mice die in utero at ~day 8. Skin pathology causing skin tethering is due to thickening of the fascial layers of the skin rather than the dermis. Histologically, this manifests as thickening of the so-called hypodermis without major collagen accumulation in the dermis. However, this process may be relevant to the subcutaneous fascia hyperplasia seen in SSc skin. Of interest, fibroblasts isolated from Tsk-1 display an activated phenotype in vitro with increased release of collagen, thus resembling the endogenous activation of SSc fibroblasts in culture. In addition to skin fibrosis, Tsk-1 mice show more widespread effects linked to the central structural role fibrillin plays in microfibrils and elastic fibers, including muscle fascia and tendon hyperplasia, skeletal overgrowth and pulmonary emphysema, and other microfibril or elastic fiber-rich tissues, including emphysema. The mutant fibrillin-1 protein leads to altered microfibril structure, stability and turnover, and altered depositions of other fibrillin-associated microfibril proteins [4, 5]. The molecular pathways activated by mutant fibrillin in Tsk-1 mice resemble those in SSc with activation of central pro-fibrotic pathways including transforming growth factor beta (TGF-β), canonical Wnt, and activator protein 1 (AP-1) signaling [6–8].

Inflammatory infiltrates are absent in Tsk-1 mice. However, several publications demonstrate that B cells are activated in Tsk-1 mice and that inhibition of B-cell function ameliorates the Tsk-1 phenotype [9, 10]. Indeed, Tsk-1 mice display autoantibodies [11, 12], and passive transfer of Tsk-1

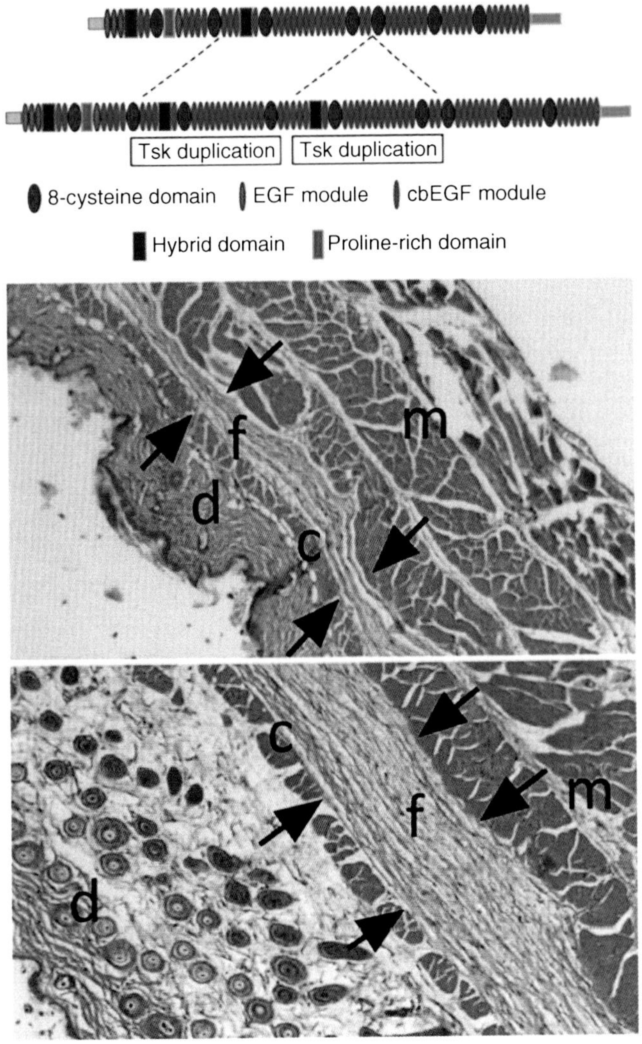

Fig. 19.1 Mutant fibrillin in Tsk-1 mice leads to fascia hyperplasia. *Upper panel*: Protein structure resulting from the in-frame duplication seen in Tsk-1 mice. *Middle and lower panels*: Cross section of skin to body wall from control (*middle panel*) and Tsk-1 (*lower panel*) mice showing increased fascia thickness (*f*, marked with *arrows*), dermis (*d*), panniculus carnosus (*c*), and skeletal muscle (*m*), hematoxylin and eosin stain. Proper measurement of fascia thickness requires full-thickness biopsy including subcutaneous muscle in this model. The increased subcutaneous fat seen here in Tsk-1 skin is not a feature of this mouse but an irregular feature of mouse skin depending on the location of the skin and weight/age of the mouse

immune cells partially reproduces the Tsk-1 phenotype [13, 14]. On the contrary, the Tsk-1 phenotype has been reported to be largely preserved in recombination activating gene (RAG)-deficient mice [15, 16].

The Tight-Skin 2 Mouse (Tsk-2)

The Tsk-2 mouse strain was a product of chemical mutagenesis using ethylnitrosourea that led to a similar phenotype in the skin as Tsk-1 [17]. Tsk-2/+ mouse fibrotic phenotype has recently been shown to be due to a gain-of-function mutation in the N-terminal propeptide of type III collagen (PIIINP) segment of the Col3a1 gene [18]. It is reported that some histological differences in this phenotype compared to Tsk-1 suggest a more generalized fibrotic phenotype associated with inflammatory change in the skin and autoantibodies. In an intriguing experiment, Tsk-1 and Tsk-2 strains were intercrossed, and a mouse with more marked skin tightness was produced. The Tsk-2 strain has not been extensively validated, and so the validity or utility of this strain cannot be concluded.

TGF-ß-Mediated Models of Fibrosis

The overwhelming evidence supporting a role of enhanced TGF-β signaling in human SSc led to the development of mouse strains in which there is a more defined abnormality of TGF-β activity.

Inducible Expression of Activated TGF-βRI

Expression of a mutated, constitutively active form of the type I TGF-β receptor (TGF-βRI^{CA}) offers the possibility for sustained ligand-independent activation of TGF-β signaling. Two different strategies are currently employed to overexpress TGF-βRI^{CA}: an elegant compound genetic strategy with fibroblast-specific overexpression of TGF-βRI^{CA} and overexpression with adeno-associated viral vectors. In the genetic approach, TGF-βRI^{CA} was conditionally expressed by insertion after a floxed STOP cassette. When these mice were bred to estrogen-inducible Cre recombinase mice and challenged with tamoxifen, the stop codon is excised, and TGF-βRI^{CA} expression is selectively activated in fibroblasts. This proved very effective, and mice demonstrated severe skin fibrosis and abnormalities in multiple organs [19]. Replication-deficient type V adeno-associated viral vectors encoding for TGF-βRI^{CA} offer a technically less-complex approach to locally overexpress TGF-βRI^{CA} in tissues of interest. Both approaches have been extensively used to study TGF-β signaling in vivo [20–23].

Fibroblast-Specific Deletion of the TGF-βRII-Kinase Domain-TβRIIΔk

Another mouse model with aberrant TGF-β signaling was developed by fibroblast-specific overexpression of a non-signaling mutant type II TGF-β receptor using the same promoter construct as in TGF-βRI^{CA} mice [24] lacking in the intracellular kinase domain. Although this construct had been shown to operate as a dominant negative inhibitor of TGF-β signaling in tissue culture, in vivo paradoxical upregulation of

TGF-β signaling was observed, and mice developed fibrosis [24]. Lungs of TGF-βRII-kinase domain-TβRIIΔk-fib mice treated with intratracheal saline, a treatment not resulting in any pathology in normal mice, or bleomycin showed epithelial injury or increased epithelial injury and fibrosis, respectively. The strain provided the first evidence that upregulated fibroblast TGF-β activity leads to perivascular fibrosis [25]. Moreover, this strain is more sensitive to SU5416-induced pulmonary arterial hypertension (PAH) (inhibitor of the fetal liver kinase 1 (Flk-1), kinase domain receptor (KDR), vascular endothelial growth factor (VEGF) receptor tyrosine kinase, a common model of PAH) with pulmonary arteriolar luminal obliteration caused by proliferating endothelial cells [26]. One potential limitation of this strain is the relatively mild nature of baseline fibrosis, and its future probably lies in studies aiming to better understand the interplay between TGF-β and other candidate pathways and in understanding second events in the pathogenesis of organ-based disease in SSc.

Fibroblast-Specific Transgenic Overexpression of Connective Tissue Growth Factor (CTGF)

The matricellular protein connective tissue growth factor (CTGF), a member of the CCN family or proteins (CCN2), is a common target gene of TGF-β and mediates in part the pro-fibrotic effects of TGF-β. Although its pro-fibrotic effects on cultured fibroblasts are modest, CTGF is expressed at sustained high levels in SSc tissues and by explanted SSc fibroblasts. A similar approach to the experiments examining TGF-β signaling has been employed to overexpress CTGF in fibroblasts. Fibroblast-specific CTGF-overexpressing mice develop fibrosis in the skin and internal organs [27]. This model may be an elegant tool to study CTGF signaling in vivo.

Models of Fibrosis Induced by Activation of Canonical Wnt Signaling

Wnt10b Transgenic Mice

A new model of fibrosis has recently been described that results from transgenic overexpression of Wnt10b under control of the adipocyte promoter FABP4 [28]. These mice show massive skin fibrosis with up to fivefold increase in dermal thickness and up to tenfold increase in hydroxyproline content and prominent hypodermal atrophy with replacement of subcutaneous fat by collagen as in SSc. Consistent with these in vivo effects, Wnt overexpression in vitro in fibroblasts and pre-adipocytes shows blockade of adipogenesis and upregulated pro-fibrotic gene expression. These effects are similar to changes seen in SSc skin and suggest that Wnt's might contribute to fibrosis in SSc by activating resident fibroblasts and through altered developmental programming of pre-adipocytes [20, 29].

Fibroblast-Specific Overexpression of a Constitutively Active β-Catenin

Another model with selective activation of canonical Wnt signaling is the β-catenin^{CA} fib model. In this model, an exon-3-deficient mutant of β-catenin that is resistant to phosphorylation and subsequent degradation of β-catenin is overexpressed in an inducible manner selectively in fibroblasts using the same Col1a2 CreER line as described for TGF-βRI^{CA} mice [30]. These mice rapidly develop skin fibrosis within 2–4 weeks. However, other features of SSc such as vasculopathy have not been studied in those mice.

Caveolin-1-Deficient Mice

Caveolin-1 deficiency in mice leads to a complex phenotype partially resembling SSc with both vascular and fibrotic features, including lung fibrosis, cardiomyopathy, and pulmonary hypertension [31–37]. While data on the effects of caveolin-1 vascular permeability are conflicting, several lines of evidence suggest that caveolin-1 regulates vasoreaction. Aortic rings of caveolin-1-deficient mice show enhanced relaxation to acetylcholine challenge. Aortic endothelial cells isolated from caveolin-deleted mice produce increased levels of NO, possibly due to disruption of the normal inhibitory interaction of caveolin with endothelial nitric oxide synthase (eNOS). In addition, small arteries in caveolin-deficient mice show decreased vascular smooth muscle cell-dependent endothelin-1 or angiotensin-II-elicited vasoconstriction. Notably, these mice also show marked changes in lung morphology with large areas of the lungs displaying markedly thickened septa; increased immunostaining for Flk-1-positive cells, a marker of endothelial and hematopoietic progenitors; increased extracellular matrix; and hypertrophy of type II pneumocytes. Increased matrix is also seen in the dermis of these fibrotic mice, possibly related to enhanced TGF-β activity as caveolin-1 overexpression inhibits TGF-β signaling [36, 38].

Xenograft Model of SSc Skin in SCID Mice

In other areas of experimental medicine, the use of models in which disease tissue is grafted onto immunodeficient mice has been fruitful in understanding aspects of the human disease. This approach has been applied in a limited way to SSc by transplanting skin onto severe combined immunodeficiency (SCID) mice that lack most components of a competent immune system [39, 40]. The skin survives and 30 days after transplant shows increased intranuclear phospho-smad 2 and phospho-smad 3 and decreased smad 7 staining, compared to control skin, and a similar pattern of expression was seen in untransplanted skin. The extent to which this adds to studies of tissue samples or from cultured cells or tissue-equivalent models derived from these skin biopsies is unclear. Moreover, standardization of this model is challenging. However, this is a promising area for future evaluation and deserves further exploration.

Models of SSc with Immune and Inflammatory Deregulation and Subsequent Fibrosis

Mice have provided a powerful experimental system for immunology research. It is not surprising that this has led to the development of immunologically based mouse models for SSc. In some cases, this has been through genetic modification of other strains, but the best-characterized immune models are those based upon transplantation of splenocyte with or without bone marrow cells with minor human leukocyte antigen (HLA) mismatches and subsequent chronic graft-versus-host disease (cGvHD). Like some of the models described above, these models not only provide mimics of the disease and a platform to explore potential targeted therapies but also shed important light upon possible key immunopathology relevant to human SSc.

Murine Sclerodermatous Chronic Graft-Versus-Host Disease (cGvHD)

Many forms of cGvHD have been described in mice with the common theme of transfer of immune cells, typically splenocytes and/or bone marrow cells from a donor animal to a recipient with minor histocompatibility mismatch (Fig. 19.2). cGvHD models of SSc have several appeals: the similarity to human chronic graft-versus-host disease, which sometimes manifests sclerodermatous skin changes in addition to other autoimmune features. Moreover, cGvHD is clearly immune driven and further thought to require adaptive immunity, representing the only available models requiring the adaptive immune system.

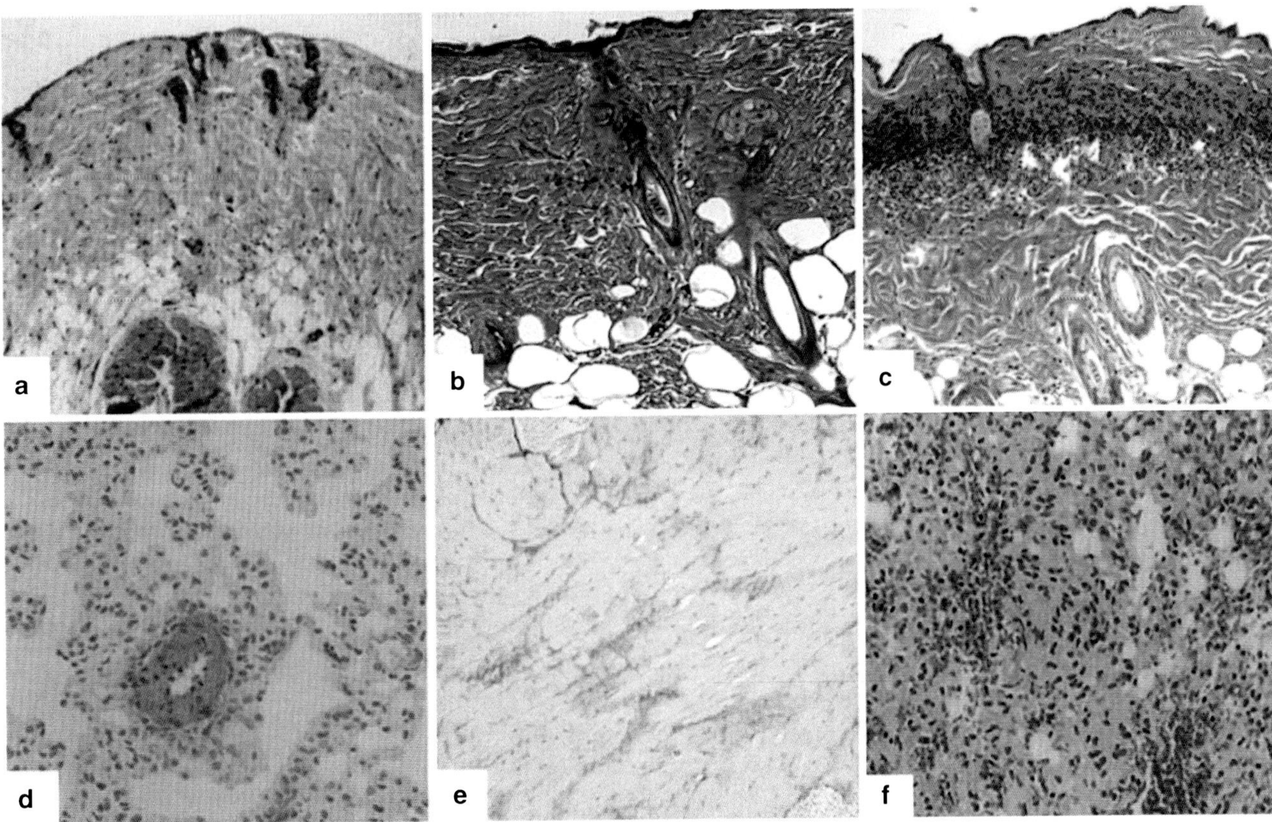

Fig. 19.2 Genetic models of SSc with directed activation of TGF-β signaling. Two complementary mouse models with fibroblast-specific activation of TGF-β signaling are shown. Both express mutated TGF-β receptors. Panels (**a–c**) show skin fibrosis. The strain TβRIIΔk-fib has a mutant form of TβRII and develops mild skin fibrosis (**a**). The strain TβRI-CA-fib expresses a constitutively active TβRI receptor and has high-level activation of TGF-β signaling. There is marked fibrosis in the skin shown by H&E stain (**b**) and Masson's trichrome (**c**). The TβRIIΔk-fib strain also shows susceptibility to relevant organ-based features of scleroderma including pulmonary vasculopathy (**d**), cardiac fibrosis (**e**), and in a minority of cases, lung fibrosis (**f**)

Several cGvHD models, a subset of the large number of graft-versus-host disease (GVHD) models, have been described (reviewed in [41]). Model strains mismatched for minor histocompatibility differences more typically drive a chronic immunological activation reminiscent of SSc, while models utilizing mismatched major histocompatibility complex (MHC) donors and recipients more typically lead to systemic lupus erythematosus (SLE)-like disease. The most common strain combination for SSc-GVHD utilizes splenocytes and bone marrow cells from B10.D2 (H-2^d) into irradiated BALB/c (H-2^d) hosts (B10.D2 (H-2^d) ½ BALB/c (H-2^d) model) [42–46]. The phenotype is observed in the skin and some viscera, including the lungs, persists for some time, and then usually undergoes some degree of spontaneous resolution after very long follow-up. The histological characteristics show a mononuclear cell infiltrate with T cells and monocyte-macrophage cells that resemble some of the features of human GVHD and SSc. In general, there is activation of dermal connective tissue synthesis and thickened fibrosis of affected tissues, although the degree of persistent cellular infiltrate is rather more than is typical of human SSc.

A further modification of this model was the use of a genetically immunodeficient mouse that lacks any adaptive immune system due to the genomic deletion of both copies of the critical recombination activation gene-2 (RAG2) that encodes for an enzyme which is essential for T- and B-lymphocyte maturation by combining constituent genes to assemble T-cell receptor and immunoglobulin. RAG2-deleted mice develop several features of SSc including autoantibodies, vascular disease, and skin and intestinal fibrosis. These mice lack lung fibrosis described in the irradiated model. They apparently develop more robust skin disease due to a radio-resistant host CD4+CD25+cell population possibly representing regulatory T cells (Fig. 19.3). Development of disease in this model requires either donor or host antigen-presenting cells (APCs), CD4+ T cells, and CD80/86-dependent costimulation [47, 48].

Another common model for sclerodermatous cGvHD is the LP/J (H-2^b) ½ C57Bl/6 (H-2^b) model. In this model, cGvHD is induced by transplantation of splenocytes from LP/J (H-2^b) donor mice into C57Bl/6 (H-2^b) mice after sublethal irradiation. Allogeneically transplanted mice develop systemic inflammation and subsequent fibrosis as described for the B10.D2 (H-2^d) ½ BALB/c (H-2^d) model. The onset of inflammation is more acute and severe as in the B10.D2 (H-2^d) ½ BALB/c (H-2^d) model. However, the major advantage is that C57Bl/6 mice serve as recipients. As most genetically modified strains are available on a C57Bl/6 background, those strains are accessible to evaluation in this model.

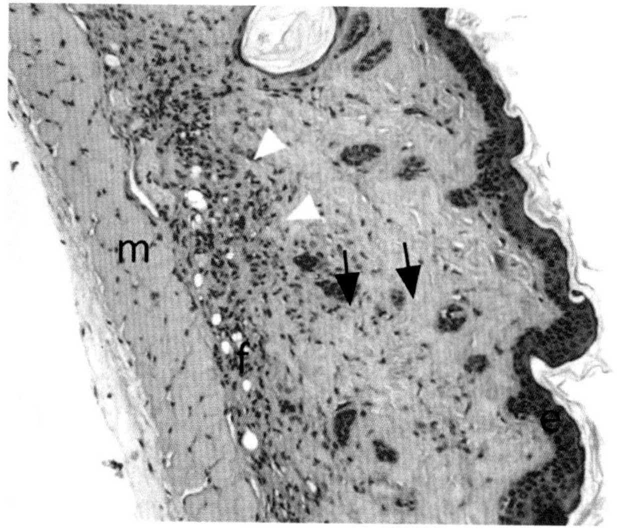

Fig. 19.3 Graft-versus-host disease induced skin fibrosis. Skin pathology, hematoxylin, and eosin stain, 4 weeks after B10. D2 splenocyte injection into BALB/c RAG2-/- mice, showing intact hypodermal muscle (*m*, panniculus carnosus), fat largely replaced by inflammatory cell infiltrate (*f*) epidermal hyperplasia (*e*), collagen deposition (*black arrows*), and dermal inflammation (*white arrowheads*)

Bleomycin-Induced Inflammation and Fibrosis

Bleomycin is a cancer chemotherapeutic that has established itself as a potent initiator of tissue injury and fibrosis. It has become associated with two models that have become a cornerstone of experimental biology that is highly relevant to studies of SSc. Bleomycin can be given through intravenous, intraperitoneal (i.p.), subcutaneous, or intratracheal routes to initiate lung fibrosis. This only occurs in certain susceptible mouse strains, the basis of this susceptibility defined genetically by the expression levels of the inactivating enzyme. The mechanisms for bleomycin-induced tissue injury and fibrosis are complex, including pro-fibrotic mediators such as TGF-β, Wnt, Notch, hedgehog, and its activator avb6 integrin; innate immune and inflammasome mediators such as interleukin-1 (IL-1), interleukin- 6 (IL-6), High Mobility Group Box 1 (HMGB1); as well as the lipid mediator lysophosphatidic acid [20, 49–57]. This may represent one of the strengths of this model, as it is likely to replicate some of the complexity of fibrotic initiation in human disease. As a consequence of tissue damage, there is inflammation and subsequent activation of myofibroblasts.

In wild-type mice challenged intratracheally with bleomycin, fibrosis can be lethal, but if mice survive, there is generally slow resolution of the fibrotic pathology. This is in contrast to most human lung pathology but is an important reminder that fibrosis may be reversible under some circumstances. As well as being a well-established model for lung fibrosis, there has been considerable use of bleomycin as an inducer of skin changes that reflect SSc (Fig. 19.4). The model of bleomycin-induced skin fibrosis has become one of the most widely used models for pathogenetic studies of SSc and has been very widely used to explore candidate therapies for SSc that may address the inflammatory as well as the fibrotic phase of the disease. However, one has to be

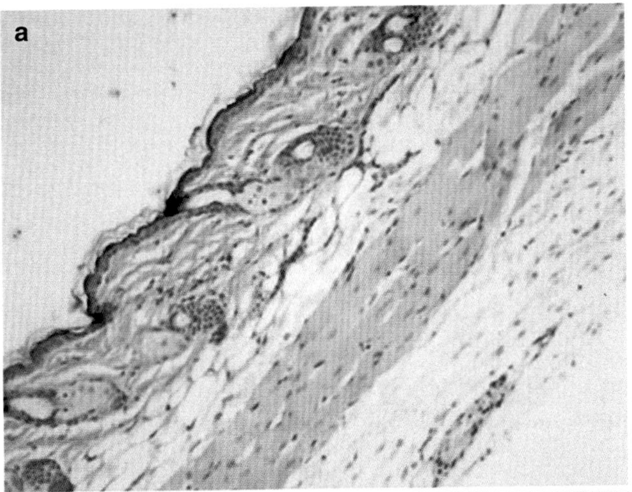

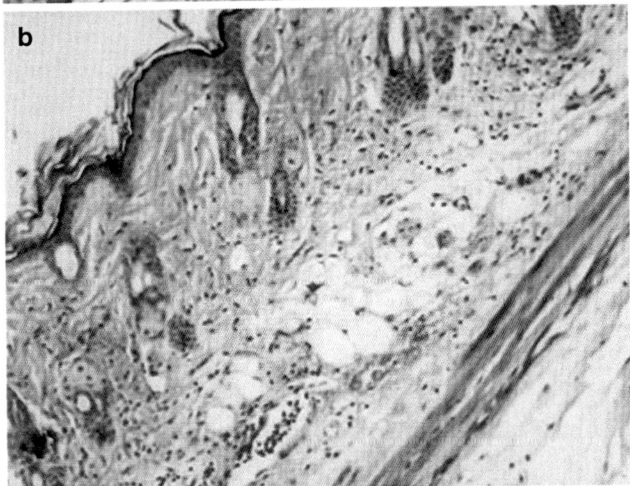

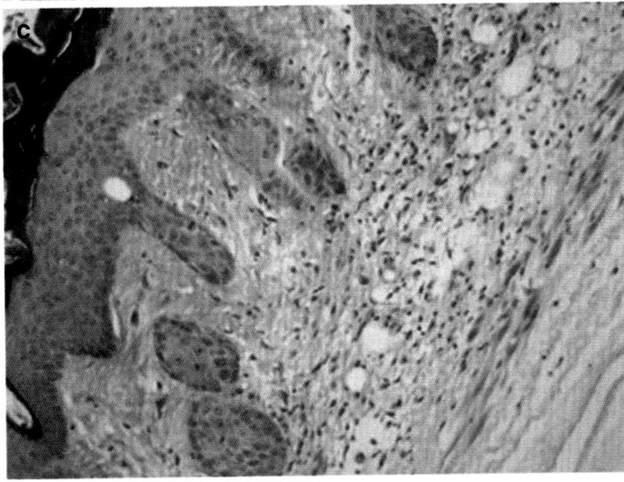

Fig. 19.4 Bleomycin-induced skin fibrosis. Intradermal bleomycin injected daily for 21 days induces inflammation and fibrosis (panels **b** and **c**) and epidermal hyperplasia (panel **c**) compared to control skin (panel **a**), hematoxylin and eosin stain

aware of the limitations of this approach: Bleomycin-induced fibrosis is dependent on an initial phase of inflammation. In preventive setups, treatments that interfere with this early inflammatory phase will also prevent the development of fibrosis. Bleomycin-induced fibrosis is thus hyper-responsive to anti-inflammatory treatment, in particular with preventive-dosing schedules. Models of bleomycin-induced fibrosis are thus suited for therapeutic evaluation of the anti-fibrotic effects of drugs with anti-inflammatory mode of action. Nevertheless, the bleomycin skin model tests facets of the pathogenic process that may not be included in genetically determined models and has a number of practical advantages in terms of ease of use. Another advantage of this model is that it can be used in various genetically manipulated mice to explore the relationship between inflammatory and fibrotic pathways.

Models of Reactive Oxygen Species in SSc

Another intriguing recently described model utilizes subcutaneous injection of oxidating agents to induce many SSc-like features. Peroxynitrites induced skin fibrosis and serum anti-centromere protein B (CENP-B), while hypochlorite or hydroxyl radicals induced skin and lung fibrosis and anti-DNA topoisomerase 1 autoantibodies. This model promises to provide a more clear definition of the importance of reactive oxygen species in SSc pathogenesis [58, 59].

Models with SSc-Like Vascular Disease

Although several promising models have been described in the last years, murine models with SSc-like vascular disease are still very limited and often not generally available. However, given the prominent vascular features of SSc and the high risk of serious vascular complications in SSc patients, effective model systems are crucially required to improve our understanding of the vascular pathogenesis of SSc.

Models of Pulmonary Arterial Hypertension (PAH)

Several methods are used for detecting features of PAH, including endothelial injury, perivascular muscular hyperplasia, perivascular inflammation, and right heart hypertrophy. However, most of those models resemble idiopathic PAH rather than SSc/CTD-PAH. Those models have been extensively reviewed elsewhere and will not be discussed here.

Vascular Hyperplasia and Fibrosis in Fra2 Transgenic Mice

Fra2 is a member of the AP-1 family of transcription factors. AP-1 signaling has been shown to be activated by pro-fibrotic mediators such as TGF-β and hedgehog signaling in SSc, resulting in a prominent overexpression of Fra2 in SSc patients. Mice with transgenic, non-conditional overexpression of Fra2 (Fra2 tg) recapitulate the major vascular and fibrotic manifestations of SSc [60–62]. Fra2 tg mice demonstrate a major pulmonary phenotype that includes fibrosis and vasculopathy with a marked proliferative pattern. Neointimal hyperplasia induced by proliferation of vascular smooth muscle cells and obliteration of pulmonary arteries accompanied by perivascular inflammation appears first [60]. This is followed by interstitial inflammation and progressive collagen deposition. In addition to lung disease, these mice develop a similar process in the skin, also showing endothelial cell apoptosis followed by loss of capillaries and fibrosis, thus replicating the pathological cascade of human SSc (Fig. 19.5). Moreover, other organ manifestations of SSc such as cardiac and intestinal involvement also occur in Fra2 tg mice. First studies indicate that Fra2 tg mice may provide a novel platform for interventional studies for vasomodulatory as well as for anti-fibrotic therapies.

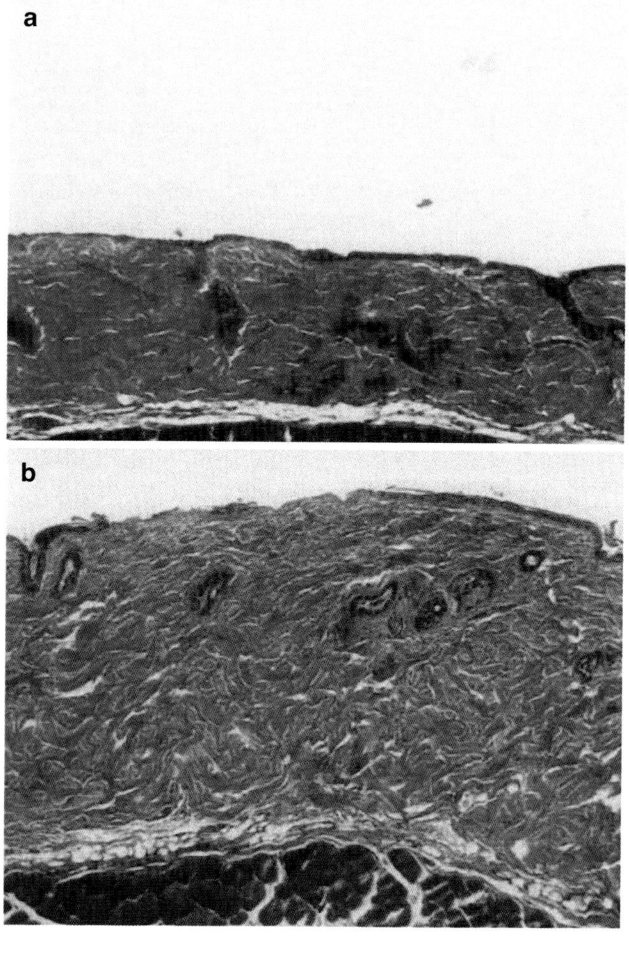

a

b

Fig. 19.5 Skin pathology in Fra-2 transgenic mice. Fra-2 transgenic mice show increased dermal thickness (panel **b**) compared to control skin (panel **a**), trichrome stain and collagen stains *blue*

Urokinase-Type Plasminogen Activator Receptor (uPAR)-Deficient Mice

Another exciting new model with vascular and fibrotic features of SSc are urokinase-type plasminogen activator receptor (uPAR)-deficient mice. uPAR is a key component of the fibrinolytic system and is also involved in extracellular matrix remodeling and in angiogenesis. Full-length uPAR is downregulated in fibrotic skin of SSc patients, and this downregulation may contribute to fibroblast activation. uPAR-deficient mice present with endothelial cell apoptosis, loss of microvessels, and collagen accumulation in the skin [63]. This strain also displays pulmonary disease with nonspecific interstitial pneumonia-like features, inflammation, and thickening of the alveolar septa. Further studies to investigate other organs and to determine the chronology of the pathologic findings are ongoing. However, uPAR-deficient mice may also be an exciting model to study the interplay between vascular manifestations and fibrosis in SSc.

Allograft Arteriopathy

Vascular occlusion is frequently the main pathogenic process limiting allograft survival in late allograft failure. These vascular lesions are similar to SSc vascular changes with smooth muscle cell hyperplasia and associated perivascular extracellular matrix accumulation and inflammation [64, 65]. Heterotopic cardiac or intra-aortic transplants are most widely used and several different host and donor strains, more severe mismatches requiring immunosuppression for survival. Though cellular immunity mediated by CD4+ T cell is mainly responsible for initiating alloreactivity, macrophages and releasing a variety of mediators, including interferon-gamma (IFNγ), are thought to mediate vascular injury [66]. Notably, in addition to inflammatory cells, a portion of neointimal cells in murine aortic arteriopathy are host derived. In rats, allogeneic aorta transplants revealed increased TGF-β-signaling protein, phospho-smad 2 [67]. Thus, this model provides further evidence that TGF-β is an important mediator of vascular damage. A major challenge of these models is the surgical skill required for successful transplants.

UCD200 Chicken

The best characterized of the non-mouse models of SSc is the UCD200 chicken model [68]. There is evidence of endothelial cell apoptosis and microvascular damage, and this is associated with some areas of localized skin fibrosis i.p. at the crown [69, 70]. Those manifestations seem to be triggered by skin traumata. Some very elegant studies using this chicken strain have been undertaken, and the model has value in testing interventions that may influence early vascular changes in SSc. However, the practical challenge of working with chickens and the limited genetic and functional biological data to apply to these studies hinder widespread use of this model.

New Murine SSc Models with Fli1 Deficiency

SSc is believed to be a multifactorial disease caused by the complex interplay between hereditary and environmental factors [71]. Various combinations of predisposing factors may explain the disease heterogeneity and a variety of organ involvement of this disease. Transcription factor Friend leukemia virus integration 1 (Fli1), a member of the Ets transcription factor family, may represent such a predisposing factor for the development of SSc. Fli1 expression is constitutively suppressed in dermal fibroblasts, dermal microvascular endothelial cells and perivascular inflammatory cells in the lesional and non-lesional skin of SSc patients, which is likely to be mediated at least partially by an epigenetic mechanism [72]. Epigenetic suppression of *Fli1* gene is clearly proved by the increased methylation of CpG island and the decreased acetylation of histone H3 and H4 in the *Fli1* promoter using genomic DNA isolated from bulk skin and/or cultivated dermal fibroblasts of SSc patients [73]. Although Fli1 deficiency induces SSc-like phenotypes in dermal fibroblasts and dermal microvascular endothelial cells at molecular levels [72, 74], *Fli1*$^{+/-}$ mice do not spontaneously develop apparent clinical symptoms characteristic of SSc [75]. Therefore, *Fli1* haploinsufficiency is not enough to induce clinical features of SSc in vivo, suggesting that additional factors are required to generate genetic animal models of SSc. Based on this idea, two genetic animal models were generated: endothelial cell-specific *Fli1* knockout (*Fli1* ECKO) mice and double heterozygous mice for *Fli1* and *Klf5* genes. The former mice reproduce vascular changes, and the latter mice recapitulate immune abnormalities, vasculopathy, and tissue fibrosis of SSc [74, 76].

Endothelial Cell-Specific Fli1 Knockout Mice

Endothelial cell-specific *Fli1* knockout (*Fli1* ECKO) mice generated by crossing *Fli1*$^{flox/flox}$ mice with *Tie2*-Cre transgenic mice mimic the structural and functional abnormalities of SSc vasculopathy, such as stenosis of arterioles, dilation of capillaries, and increased vascular permeability of small vessels. This vascular phenotype is largely attributable to the altered expression of several molecules regulating vascular integrity, such as the decreased expression of VE-cadherin, PECAM1, PDGF-B, and $S1P_1$ receptor and the increased expression of MMP-9. The reduction of VE-cadherin and PECAM1 expression results in a weak endothelial cell-cell interaction. Increased expression of MMP-9 leads to altered remodeling of vascular basement membrane, such as loss of type IV collagen and compensatory increase of proteoglycans. Furthermore, downregulation of VE-cadherin, PDGF-B, and $S1P_1$ receptor causes the loss of endothelial cell-mural cell interaction. Importantly, the expression profile of these molecules is identical to that seen in dermal small vasculature of SSc lesional skin [74]. Thus, *Fli1* ECKO mice recapitulate the vascular phenotype of SSc, suggesting the involvement of endothelial Fli1 deficiency in the pathogenesis of SSc vasculopathy.

Klf5$^{+/-}$; *Fli1*$^{+/-}$ Mice

Krüppel-like factor 5 (KLF5) is a member of the SP/KLF transcription factor family [77]. *KLF5* gene expression is downregulated in SSc skin [78], and *Klf5* haploinsufficiency alters the fibrotic response following experimental tissue damage in the heart and kidney [79, 80]. In addition, the increased methylation of CpG island and the decreased acetylation of histones H3 and H4 are noted in the *KLF5* promoter of SSc dermal fibroblasts [59]. Therefore, the downregulated expression of *KLF5* gene is likely to be a potential predisposing factor of SSc as well as the suppression of *FLI1* gene expression. Consistent with this notion, double heterozygous mice for *Klf5* and *Fli1* genes spontaneously develop three cardinal features of SSc such as immune abnormalities, vasculopathy, and extensive tissue fibrosis of the skin and lung. *Klf5*$^{+/-}$; *Fli1*$^{+/-}$ mice develop inflammation and vascular changes such as stenosis of arterioles and dilation of capillaries in the skin around 4 weeks of age and autoantibody production and the decrease of vascular beds around 8 weeks of age. Dermal and pulmonary fibrosis becomes apparent around 3 months and 4 months of age, respectively. Abnormal collagen fibril assembly similar to SSc is also induced after 2 months of age, and tissue hypoxia and decreased blood flow velocity are noted around 4 months of age in the skin. In the lung, diffuse uniform expansion of alveolar septa with patchy septal lymphocytic infiltration is present, reminiscent of human nonspecific interstitial pneumonia, while the pathological findings indicating usual interstitial pneumonia, honeycombing or fibroblastic foci, are rarely seen. Pulmonary vascular changes characteristic of pulmonary arterial hypertension and pulmonary veno-occlusive disease become remarkable around 8 months of age. *Klf5*$^{+/-}$;*Fli1*$^{+/-}$ mice also exhibit CD19 upregulation in B cells, which has been shown to largely contribute to the pathogenesis of SSc [81]. A series of studies with

Klf5$^{+/-}$;*Fli1*$^{+/-}$ mice suggests a novel concept that the downregulation of these two transcription factors may be the primary event triggering the three major manifestations in SSc [76]. These findings support the idea that environmental factors determine the clinical phenotype of SSc, while genetic factors contribute to the susceptibility and the severity of this disease [82, 83].

Myocardial Disease in Mouse Models

Myocardial involvement is a major cause of death in SSc and may account for up to one third of deaths in SSc patients [84–87]. Cardiac involvement is believed to occur in the majority, if not all, SSc patients, although it is often clinically occult [88, 89]. Abnormal vasoreactivity and structural defects of small arterioles and of capillaries in the myocardium lead to repeated local hypoperfusion, which subsequently could trigger myocardial fibrosis, which is often patchy and affects both ventricles [90, 91].

Despite its clinical relevance, only few studies analyzed myocardial alterations in murine models of SSc so far. A recent study compared myocardial changes in Tsk-1, B10.D2 (H-2d) ½ BALB/c (H-2d) cGvHD model and Fra2 tg mice to those of SSc patients [92]. Tsk-1 mice and mice with cGvHD mimicked only few features of SSc-associated cardiomyopathy and were not considered as suitable models of SSc-related cardiomyopathy. However, heart involvement of Fra2 tg mice resembled all major histopathological features of SSc-associated myocardial disease with apoptosis of endothelial cells and decreased capillary counts, perivascular inflammatory infiltrates, and activation of fibroblasts with subsequent accumulation of collagen. Fra2 tg mice may indeed share a similar molecular pathophysiology, as Fra2 is also overexpressed in the heart of SSc patients, and the expression pattern of Fra2 in SSc patients resembled the one in Fra2 tg mice with predominant expression in capillaries. Caveolin-1 knockout mice have been shown to suffer from severe biventricular hypertrophy with systolic and diastolic severe heart failure [93]. Although caveolin-1 is not expressed in cardiomyocytes, caveolin-1 knockout mice are characterized by a severe eNOS hyperactivation yielding increased systemic NO levels, which are thought to mediate the cardiac phenotype of caveolin-1 knockout mice [94]. However, no microvascular alterations have been reported in caveolin-1-deficient mice. A fibrotic cardiomyopathy has also been described in TβRIIΔk-fib mice, whereas other histopathologic findings of myocardial disease in humans were not noted [24]. Conclusive data on other mouse models of SSc are not yet available. However, it would be of major interest to study the myocardial involvement in particular of other systemic models of SSc.

What Have We Learned from Analyzing Animal Models?

It can clearly be observed that there is no lack of interesting animal models for SSc, and there has been a major increase in the number and type of models used in recent studies. It has become commonplace to use gene-targeted mice to help to understand facet of the disease, and inducible models for SSc such as the bleomycin skin or lung models are central to this. There must however be caution. No single model reflects the entire pathology of human SSc in its complexity and chronicity, and so each model needs to be considered carefully on its merits and the strengths and weaknesses that it can bring to any study. It is of critical importance to test any hypothesis in several complementary models before drawing firm conclusions.

The use of conditional genetic strategies has substantially increased the power and relevance of many experiments that use mouse models of SSc. The advantages of some of these approaches are that genes can be turned on or off in selected cell lineages at particulate timer points. This allows molecular triggering events to be replicated, and the impact of gene expression changes at defined time points in experimental pathology to be explored (e.g., treatment or reversal rather than prevention). Also genes that are lethal in germ line manipulation or even conventional lineage-specific disruption can be investigated. This has been a fruitful area and one that is set to continue to be productive and informative in the immediate future.

References

1. Beyer C, Schett G, Distler O, Distler JH. Animal models of systemic sclerosis: prospects and limitations. Arthritis Rheum. 2010;62(10):2831–44.
2. Green MC, Sweet HO, Bunker LE. Tight-skin, a new mutation of the mouse causing excessive growth of connective tissue and skeleton. Am J Pathol. 1976;82(3):493–512.
3. Siracusa LD, McGrath R, Ma Q, Moskow JJ, Manne J, Christner PJ, et al. A tandem duplication within the fibrillin 1 gene is associated with the mouse tight skin mutation. Genome Res. 1996;6(4):300–13.
4. Kielty CM, Raghunath M, Siracusa LD, Sherratt MJ, Peters R, Shuttleworth CA, et al. The Tight skin mouse: demonstration of mutant fibrillin-1 production and assembly into abnormal microfibrils. J Cell Biol. 1998;140(5):1159–66.
5. Lemaire R, Farina G, Kissin E, Shipley JM, Bona C, Korn JH, et al. Mutant fibrillin 1 from tight skin mice increases extracellular matrix incorporation of microfibril-associated glycoprotein 2 and type I collagen. Arthritis Rheum. 2004;50(3):915–26.
6. Bayle J, Fitch J, Jacobsen K, Kumar R, Lafyatis R, Lemaire R. Increased expression of Wnt2 and SFRP4 in Tsk mouse skin: role of Wnt signaling in altered dermal fibrillin deposition and systemic sclerosis. J Invest Dermatol. 2008;128(4):871–81.
7. Dees C, Akhmetshina A, Zerr P, Reich N, Palumbo K, Horn A, et al. Platelet-derived serotonin links vascular disease and tissue fibrosis. J Exp Med. 2011;208(5):961–72.

8. Avouac J, Palumbo K, Tomcik M, Zerr P, Dees C, Horn A, et al. Inhibition of activator protein 1 signaling abrogates transforming growth factor beta-mediated activation of fibroblasts and prevents experimental fibrosis. Arthritis Rheum. 2012;64(5):1642–52.
9. Komura K, Fujimoto M, Yanaba K, Matsushita T, Matsushita Y, Horikawa M, et al. Blockade of CD40/CD40 ligand interactions attenuates skin fibrosis and autoimmunity in the tight-skin mouse. Ann Rheum Dis. 2008;67(6):867–72.
10. Saito E, Fujimoto M, Hasegawa M, Komura K, Hamaguchi Y, Kaburagi Y, et al. CD19-dependent B lymphocyte signaling thresholds influence skin fibrosis and autoimmunity in the tight-skin mouse. J Clin Invest. 2002;109(11):1453–62.
11. Murai C, Saito S, Kasturi KN, Bona CA. Spontaneous occurrence of anti-fibrillin-1 autoantibodies in tight-skin mice. Autoimmunity. 1998;28(3):151–5.
12. Shibata S, Muryoi T, Saitoh Y, Brumeanu TD, Bona CA, Kasturi KN. Immunochemical and molecular characterization of anti-RNA polymerase I autoantibodies produced by tight skin mouse. J Clin Invest. 1993;92(2):984–92.
13. Walker MA, Harley RA, DeLustro FA, LeRoy EC. Adoptive transfer of tsk skin fibrosis to +/+ recipients by tsk bone marrow and spleen cells. Proc Soc Exp Biol Med Soc Exp Biol Med (New York, NY). 1989;192(2):196–200.
14. Phelps RG, Daian C, Shibata S, Fleischmajer R, Bona CA. Induction of skin fibrosis and autoantibodies by infusion of immunocompetent cells from tight skin mice into C57BL/6 Pa/Pa mice. J Autoimmun. 1993;6(6):701–18.
15. Siracusa LD, McGrath R, Fisher JK, Jimenez SA. The mouse tight skin (Tsk) phenotype is not dependent on the presence of mature T and B lymphocytes. Mamm Genome: Off J Int Mamm Genome Soc. 1998;9(11):907–9.
16. Kasturi KN, Hatakeyama A, Murai C, Gordon R, Phelps RG, Bona CA. B-cell deficiency does not abrogate development of cutaneous hyperplasia in mice inheriting the defective fibrillin-1 gene. J Autoimmun. 1997;10(6):505–17.
17. Christner PJ, Peters J, Hawkins D, Siracusa LD, Jimenez SA. The tight skin 2 mouse. An animal model of scleroderma displaying cutaneous fibrosis and mononuclear cell infiltration. Arthritis Rheum. 1995;38(12):1791–8.
18. Long KB, Li Z, Burgwin CM, Choe SG, Martyanov V, Sassi-Gaha S, et al. The Tsk2/+ mouse fibrotic phenotype is due to a gain-of-function mutation in the PIIINP segment of the Col3a1 gene. J Invest Dermatol. 2015;135(3):718–27.
19. Sonnylal S, Denton CP, Zheng B, Keene DR, He R, Adams HP, et al. Postnatal induction of transforming growth factor beta signaling in fibroblasts of mice recapitulates clinical, histologic, and biochemical features of scleroderma. Arthritis Rheum. 2007;56(1):334–44.
20. Akhmetshina A, Palumbo K, Dees C, Bergmann C, Venalis P, Zerr P, et al. Activation of canonical Wnt signalling is required for TGF-beta-mediated fibrosis. Nat Commun. 2012;3:735.
21. Beyer C, Zenzmaier C, Palumbo-Zerr K, Mancuso R, Distler A, Dees C, et al. Stimulation of the soluble guanylate cyclase (sGC) inhibits fibrosis by blocking non-canonical TGFbeta signalling. Ann Rheum Dis. 2015;74(7):1408–16.
22. Tomcik M, Zerr P, Pitkowski J, Palumbo-Zerr K, Avouac J, Distler O, et al. Heat shock protein 90 (Hsp90) inhibition targets canonical TGF-beta signalling to prevent fibrosis. Ann Rheum Dis. 2014;73(6):1215–22.
23. Zerr P, Vollath S, Palumbo-Zerr K, Tomcik M, Huang J, Distler A, et al. Vitamin D receptor regulates TGF-beta signalling in systemic sclerosis. Ann Rheum Dis. 2015;74(3):e20.
24. Denton CP, Zheng B, Evans LA, Shi-wen X, Ong VH, Fisher I, et al. Fibroblast-specific expression of a kinase-deficient type II transforming growth factor beta (TGFbeta) receptor leads to paradoxical activation of TGFbeta signaling pathways with fibrosis in transgenic mice. J Biol Chem. 2003;278(27):25109–19.
25. Derrett-Smith EC, Dooley A, Khan K, Shi-wen X, Abraham D, Denton CP. Systemic vasculopathy with altered vasoreactivity in a transgenic mouse model of scleroderma. Arthritis Res Ther. 2010;12(2):R69.
26. Derrett-Smith EC, Dooley A, Gilbane AJ, Trinder SL, Khan K, Baliga R, et al. Endothelial injury in a transforming growth factor beta-dependent mouse model of scleroderma induces pulmonary arterial hypertension. Arthritis Rheum. 2013;65(11):2928–39.
27. Sonnylal S, Shi-Wen X, Leoni P, Naff K, Van Pelt CS, Nakamura H, et al. Selective expression of connective tissue growth factor in fibroblasts in vivo promotes systemic tissue fibrosis. Arthritis Rheum. 2010;62(5):1523–32.
28. Longo KA, Wright WS, Kang S, Gerin I, Chiang SH, Lucas PC, et al. Wnt10b inhibits development of white and brown adipose tissues. J Biol Chem. 2004;279(34):35503–9.
29. Wei J, Melichian D, Komura K, Hinchcliff M, Lam AP, Lafyatis R, et al. Canonical Wnt signaling induces skin fibrosis and subcutaneous lipoatrophy: a novel mouse model for scleroderma? Arthritis Rheum. 2011;63(6):1707–17.
30. Beyer C, Schramm A, Akhmetshina A, Dees C, Kireva T, Gelse K, et al. beta-catenin is a central mediator of pro-fibrotic Wnt signaling in systemic sclerosis. Ann Rheum Dis. 2012;71(5):761–7.
31. Castello-Cros R, Whitaker-Menezes D, Molchansky A, Purkins G, Soslowsky LJ, Beason DP, et al. Scleroderma-like properties of skin from caveolin-1-deficient mice: implications for new treatment strategies in patients with fibrosis and systemic sclerosis. Cell Cycle (Georgetown, Tex). 2011;10(13):2140–50.
32. Del Galdo F, Sotgia F, de Almeida CJ, Jasmin JF, Musick M, Lisanti MP, et al. Decreased expression of caveolin 1 in patients with systemic sclerosis: crucial role in the pathogenesis of tissue fibrosis. Arthritis Rheum. 2008;58(9):2854–65.
33. Le Saux O, Teeters K, Miyasato S, Choi J, Nakamatsu G, Richardson JA, et al. The role of caveolin-1 in pulmonary matrix remodeling and mechanical properties. Am J Physiol Lung Cell Mol Physiol. 2008;295(6):L1007–17.
34. Tourkina E, Richard M, Gooz P, Bonner M, Pannu J, Harley R, et al. Antifibrotic properties of caveolin-1 scaffolding domain in vitro and in vivo. Am J Physiol Lung Cell Mol Physiol. 2008;294(5):L843–61.
35. Tourkina E, Richard M, Oates J, Hofbauer A, Bonner M, Gooz P, et al. Caveolin-1 regulates leucocyte behaviour in fibrotic lung disease. Ann Rheum Dis. 2010;69(6):1220–6.
36. Wang XM, Zhang Y, Kim HP, Zhou Z, Feghali-Bostwick CA, Liu F, et al. Caveolin-1: a critical regulator of lung fibrosis in idiopathic pulmonary fibrosis. J Exp Med. 2006;203(13):2895–906.
37. Yamaguchi Y, Yasuoka H, Stolz DB, Feghali-Bostwick CA. Decreased caveolin-1 levels contribute to fibrosis and deposition of extracellular IGFBP-5. J Cell Mol Med. 2011;15(4):957–69.
38. Del Galdo F, Lisanti MP, Jimenez SA. Caveolin-1, transforming growth factor-beta receptor internalization, and the pathogenesis of systemic sclerosis. Curr Opin Rheumatol. 2008;20(6):713–9.
39. Dong C, Zhu S, Wang T, Yoon W, Li Z, Alvarez RJ, et al. Deficient Smad7 expression: a putative molecular defect in scleroderma. Proc Natl Acad Sci U S A. 2002;99(6):3908–13.
40. Distler JH, Jungel A, Kowal-Bielecka O, Michel BA, Gay RE, Sprott H, et al. Expression of interleukin-21 receptor in epidermis from patients with systemic sclerosis. Arthritis Rheum. 2005;52(3):856–64.
41. Chu YW, Gress RE. Murine models of chronic graft-versus-host disease: insights and unresolved issues. Biol Blood Marrow Transplant: J Am Soc Blood Marrow Transplant. 2008;14(4):365–78.
42. Huu DL, Matsushita T, Jin G, Hamaguchi Y, Hasegawa M, Takehara K, et al. FTY720 ameliorates murine sclerodermatous chronic graft-versus-host disease by promoting expansion of

splenic regulatory cells and inhibiting immune cell infiltration into skin. Arthritis Rheum. 2013;65(6):1624–35.
43. McCormick LL, Zhang Y, Tootell E, Gilliam AC. Anti-TGF-beta treatment prevents skin and lung fibrosis in murine sclerodermatous graft-versus-host disease: a model for human scleroderma. J Immunol. 1999;163(10):5693–9.
44. Zhang Y, McCormick LL, Desai SR, Wu C, Gilliam AC. Murine sclerodermatous graft-versus-host disease, a model for human scleroderma: cutaneous cytokines, chemokines, and immune cell activation. J Immunol. 2002;168(6):3088–98.
45. Zerr P, Distler A, Palumbo-Zerr K, Tomcik M, Vollath S, Dees C, et al. Combined inhibition of c-Abl and PDGF receptors for prevention and treatment of murine sclerodermatous chronic graft-versus-host disease. Am J Pathol. 2012;181(5):1672–80.
46. Zerr P, Palumbo-Zerr K, Distler A, Tomcik M, Vollath S, Munoz LE, et al. Inhibition of hedgehog signaling for the treatment of murine sclerodermatous chronic graft-versus-host disease. Blood. 2012;120(14):2909–17.
47. Anderson BE, McNiff JM, Matte C, Athanasiadis I, Shlomchik WD, Shlomchik MJ. Recipient CD4+ T cells that survive irradiation regulate chronic graft-versus-host disease. Blood. 2004;104(5):1565–73.
48. Anderson BE, McNiff JM, Jain D, Blazar BR, Shlomchik WD, Shlomchik MJ. Distinct roles for donor- and host-derived antigen-presenting cells and costimulatory molecules in murine chronic graft-versus-host disease: requirements depend on target organ. Blood. 2005;105(5):2227–34.
49. Akhmetshina A, Venalis P, Dees C, Busch N, Zwerina J, Schett G, et al. Treatment with imatinib prevents fibrosis in different preclinical models of systemic sclerosis and induces regression of established fibrosis. Arthritis Rheum. 2009;60(1):219–24.
50. Beyer C, Huang J, Beer J, Zhang Y, Palumbo-Zerr K, Zerr P, et al. Activation of liver X receptors inhibits experimental fibrosis by interfering with interleukin-6 release from macrophages. Ann Rheum Dis. 2015;74(6):1317–24.
51. Beyer C, Reichert H, Akan H, Mallano T, Schramm A, Dees C, et al. Blockade of canonical Wnt signalling ameliorates experimental dermal fibrosis. Ann Rheum Dis. 2013;72(7):1255–8.
52. Dees C, Zerr P, Tomcik M, Beyer C, Horn A, Akhmetshina A, et al. Inhibition of Notch signaling prevents experimental fibrosis and induces regression of established fibrosis. Arthritis Rheum. 2011;63(5):1396–404.
53. Palumbo K, Zerr P, Tomcik M, Vollath S, Dees C, Akhmetshina A, et al. The transcription factor JunD mediates transforming growth factor {beta}-induced fibroblast activation and fibrosis in systemic sclerosis. Ann Rheum Dis. 2011;70(7):1320–6.
54. Gasse P, Mary C, Guenon I, Noulin N, Charron S, Schnyder-Candrian S, et al. IL-1R1/MyD88 signaling and the inflammasome are essential in pulmonary inflammation and fibrosis in mice. J Clin Invest. 2007;117(12):3786–99.
55. Horan GS, Wood S, Ona V, Li DJ, Lukashev ME, Weinreb PH, et al. Partial inhibition of integrin alpha(v)beta6 prevents pulmonary fibrosis without exacerbating inflammation. Am J Respir Crit Care Med. 2008;177(1):56–65.
56. Tager AM, LaCamera P, Shea BS, Campanella GS, Selman M, Zhao Z, et al. The lysophosphatidic acid receptor LPA1 links pulmonary fibrosis to lung injury by mediating fibroblast recruitment and vascular leak. Nat Med. 2008;14(1):45–54.
57. Avouac J, Elhai M, Tomcik M, Ruiz B, Friese M, Piedavent M, et al. Critical role of the adhesion receptor DNAX accessory molecule-1 (DNAM-1) in the development of inflammation-driven dermal fibrosis in a mouse model of systemic sclerosis. Ann Rheum Dis. 2013;72(6):1089–98.
58. Servettaz A, Goulvestre C, Kavian N, Nicco C, Guilpain P, Chereau C, et al. Selective oxidation of DNA topoisomerase 1 induces systemic sclerosis in the mouse. J Immunol. 2009;182(9):5855–64.
59. Kavian N, Servettaz A, Mongaret C, Wang A, Nicco C, Chereau C, et al. Targeting ADAM-17/notch signaling abrogates the development of systemic sclerosis in a murine model. Arthritis Rheum. 2010;62(11):3477–87.
60. Maurer B, Busch N, Jungel A, Pileckyte M, Gay RE, Michel BA, et al. Transcription factor fos-related antigen-2 induces progressive peripheral vasculopathy in mice closely resembling human systemic sclerosis. Circulation. 2009;120(23):2367–76.
61. Maurer B, Distler JH, Distler O. The Fra-2 transgenic mouse model of systemic sclerosis. Vascul Pharmacol. 2013;58(3):194–201.
62. Reich N, Maurer B, Akhmetshina A, Venalis P, Dees C, Zerr P, et al. The transcription factor Fra-2 regulates the production of extracellular matrix in systemic sclerosis. Arthritis Rheum. 2010;62(1):280–90.
63. Manetti M, Rosa I, Milia AF, Guiducci S, Carmeliet P, Ibba-Manneschi L, et al. Inactivation of urokinase-type plasminogen activator receptor (uPAR) gene induces dermal and pulmonary fibrosis and peripheral microvasculopathy in mice: a new model of experimental scleroderma? Ann Rheum Dis. 2014;73(9):1700–9.
64. Mitchell RN. Graft vascular disease: immune response meets the vessel wall. Annu Rev Pathol. 2009;4:19–47.
65. Mitchell RN, Libby P. Vascular remodeling in transplant vasculopathy. Circ Res. 2007;100(7):967–78.
66. Nagano H, Mitchell RN, Taylor MK, Hasegawa S, Tilney NL, Libby P. Interferon-gamma deficiency prevents coronary arteriosclerosis but not myocardial rejection in transplanted mouse hearts. J Clin Invest. 1997;100(3):550–7.
67. Dong C, Zhu S, Wang T, Yoon W, Goldschmidt-Clermont PJ. Upregulation of PAI-1 is mediated through TGF-beta/Smad pathway in transplant arteriopathy. J Heart Lung Transplant: Off Publ Int Soc Heart Transplant. 2002;21(9):999–1008.
68. Wick G, Andersson L, Hala K, Gershwin ME, Selmi C, Erf GF, et al. Avian models with spontaneous autoimmune diseases. Adv Immunol. 2006;92:71–117.
69. Gruschwitz MS, Moormann S, Kromer G, Sgonc R, Dietrich H, Boeck G, et al. Phenotypic analysis of skin infiltrates in comparison with peripheral blood lymphocytes, spleen cells and thymocytes in early avian scleroderma. J Autoimmun. 1991;4(4):577–93.
70. Sgonc R, Gruschwitz MS, Dietrich H, Recheis H, Gershwin ME, Wick G. Endothelial cell apoptosis is a primary pathogenetic event underlying skin lesions in avian and human scleroderma. J Clin Invest. 1996;98(3):785–92.
71. Asano Y, Sato S. Animal models of scleroderma: current state and recent development. Curr Rheumatol Rep. 2013;15(12):382.
72. Kubo M, Czuwara-Ladykowska J, Moussa O, Markiewicz M, Smith E, Silver RM, et al. Persistent down-regulation of Fli1, a suppressor of collagen transcription, in fibrotic scleroderma skin. Am J Pathol. 2003;163(2):571–81.
73. Wang Y, Fan PS, Kahaleh B. Association between enhanced type I collagen expression and epigenetic repression of the FLI1 gene in scleroderma fibroblasts. Arthritis Rheum. 2006;54(7):2271–9.
74. Asano Y, Stawski L, Hant F, Highland K, Silver R, Szalai G, et al. Endothelial Fli1 deficiency impairs vascular homeostasis: a role in scleroderma vasculopathy. Am J Pathol. 2010;176(4):1983–98.
75. Taniguchi T, Asano Y, Akamata K, Noda S, Takahashi T, Ichimura Y, et al. Fibrosis, vascular activation, and immune abnormalities resembling systemic sclerosis in bleomycin-treated Fli-1-haploinsufficient mice. Arthritis Rheumatol (Hoboken, NJ). 2015;67(2):517–26.
76. Noda S, Asano Y, Nishimura S, Taniguchi T, Fujiu K, Manabe I, et al. Simultaneous downregulation of KLF5 and Fli1 is a key feature underlying systemic sclerosis. Nat Commun. 2014;5:5797.
77. Dong JT, Chen C. Essential role of KLF5 transcription factor in cell proliferation and differentiation and its implications for human diseases. Cellul Mol Life Sci: CMLS. 2009;66(16):2691–706.
78. Whitfield ML, Finlay DR, Murray JI, Troyanskaya OG, Chi JT, Pergamenschikov A, et al. Systemic and cell type-specific gene

expression patterns in scleroderma skin. Proc Natl Acad Sci U S A. 2003;100(21):12319–24.
79. Takeda N, Manabe I, Uchino Y, Eguchi K, Matsumoto S, Nishimura S, et al. Cardiac fibroblasts are essential for the adaptive response of the murine heart to pressure overload. J Clin Invest. 2010;120(1):254–65.
80. Fujiu K, Manabe I, Nagai R. Renal collecting duct epithelial cells regulate inflammation in tubulointerstitial damage in mice. J Clin Invest. 2011;121(9):3425–41.
81. Sato S, Fujimoto M, Hasegawa M, Takehara K, Tedder TF. Altered B lymphocyte function induces systemic autoimmunity in systemic sclerosis. Mol Immunol. 2004;41(12):1123–33.
82. Feghali-Bostwick C, Medsger Jr TA, Wright TM. Analysis of systemic sclerosis in twins reveals low concordance for disease and high concordance for the presence of antinuclear antibodies. Arthritis Rheum. 2003;48(7):1956–63.
83. Sharif R, Mayes MD, Tan FK, Gorlova OY, Hummers LK, Shah AA, et al. IRF5 polymorphism predicts prognosis in patients with systemic sclerosis. Ann Rheum Dis. 2012;71(7):1197–202.
84. Ferri C, Valentini G, Cozzi F, Sebastiani M, Michelassi C, La Montagna G, et al. Systemic sclerosis: demographic, clinical, and serologic features and survival in 1,012 Italian patients. Medicine. 2002;81(2):139–53.
85. Ioannidis JP, Vlachoyiannopoulos PG, Haidich AB, Medsger Jr TA, Lucas M, Michet CJ, et al. Mortality in systemic sclerosis: an international meta-analysis of individual patient data. Am J Med. 2005;118(1):2–10.
86. Steen VD, Medsger Jr TA. Severe organ involvement in systemic sclerosis with diffuse scleroderma. Arthritis Rheum. 2000;43(11): 2437–44.
87. Ferri C, Valentini G, Cozzi F, Sebastiani M, Michelassi C, La Montagna G, et al. Systemic sclerosis: demographic, clinical, and serologic features and survival in 1,012 Italian patients. Medicine (Baltimore). 2002;81(2):139–53.
88. Allanore Y, Meune C. Primary myocardial involvement in systemic sclerosis: evidence for a microvascular origin. Clin Exp Rheumatol. 2010;28(5 Suppl 62):S48–53.
89. Hachulla AL, Launay D, Gaxotte V, de Groote P, Lamblin N, Devos P, et al. Cardiac magnetic resonance imaging in systemic sclerosis: a cross-sectional observational study of 52 patients. Ann Rheum Dis. 2009;68(12):1878–84.
90. Bulkley BH, Ridolfi RL, Salyer WR, Hutchins GM. Myocardial lesions of progressive systemic sclerosis. A cause of cardiac dysfunction. Circulation. 1976;53(3):483–90.
91. Tzelepis GE, Kelekis NL, Plastiras SC, Mitseas P, Economopoulos N, Kampolis C, et al. Pattern and distribution of myocardial fibrosis in systemic sclerosis: a delayed enhanced magnetic resonance imaging study. Arthritis Rheum. 2007;56(11):3827–36.
92. Venalis P, Kumanovics G, Schulze-Koops H, Distler A, Dees C, Zerr P, et al. Cardiomyopathy in murine models of systemic sclerosis. Arthritis Rheumatol (Hoboken, NJ). 2015;67(2):508–16.
93. Zhao YY, Liu Y, Stan RV, Fan L, Gu Y, Dalton N, et al. Defects in caveolin-1 cause dilated cardiomyopathy and pulmonary hypertension in knockout mice. Proc Natl Acad Sci U S A. 2002;99(17):11375–80.
94. Wunderlich C, Schober K, Lange SA, Drab M, Braun-Dullaeus RC, Kasper M, et al. Disruption of caveolin-1 leads to enhanced nitrosative stress and severe systolic and diastolic heart failure. Biochem Biophys Res Commun. 2006;340(2):702–8.

Part IV

Cardiovascular Manifestations and Management

Raynaud's Phenomenon, Digital Ulcers and Nailfold Capillaroscopy

20

Ariane L. Herrick, Fredrick M. Wigley, and Marco Matucci-Cerinic

Raynaud's phenomenon (RP) is characterised by a tri- or biphasic colour change (pallor, cyanosis and hyperaemia) due to an exaggeration or perturbation of normal responses to low temperature or emotional stress. It affects mainly the fingers, with relative sparing of the thumbs, but may also occur in the toes, tongue, ears and nose. Typically, RP attacks are symmetrical, involving both hands with patients noting that there is often a dominant or more sensitive finger(s), usually the index and middle fingers. After the first phase of blanching, RP will continue with signs and symptoms of ischaemia (blue) and rewarming (red). This review of the pathogenesis of RP will address the normal physiology of the thermoregulatory vessel and then focus on potential physiological and pathological mechanisms that can alter vasoreactivity.

Historical Review

Maurice Raynaud in 1862 stated that 'local asphyxia of the extremities' was a result of 'increased irritability of the central parts of the cord presiding over the vascular innervation'. Sir Jonathan Hutchinson realised that the symptoms described by Raynaud could be associated with a number of disorders and were not due to one disease. In 1896, he proposed the term 'Raynaud's phenomenon' to describe these vasospastic attacks. In 1930, Sir Thomas Lewis observed that even when reflex vasodilation is produced by warming the body, vasospasm could still be induced by putting the hands in cold water; conversely, vasospasm could not be produced by body cooling if the hands were kept warm. He concluded that RP was due to a 'local fault' in the blood vessels rather than a defect in the central nervous system as Maurice Raynaud had proposed. Currently, a local defect(s) is still hypothesised to be responsible for RP. In 1992, LeRoy and Medsger proposed new criteria for primary RP which included serology and nailfold capillary findings [1]. They recognised that RP was the manifestation of a widespread systemic vascular disease in SSc patients. In the modern era, new understanding of the complex regulation of the cutaneous circulation and its role in the regulation of body temperature (and how this becomes dysfunctional in patients with RP) has emerged [2, 3]. Clinical scientists now are working with the help of industry to discover and develop new therapies for patients with RP.

Thermoregulation

The perception of temperature is a critical function of the somatosensory system that protects us from extreme environmental temperatures [4]. Afferent nerve fibres of the somatosensory system detect environmental stimuli and, in cold temperatures, activate both Aδ and unmyelinated C fibres. Temperature-sensitive ion channels on specialised dorsal root ganglion neurons allow cutaneous nerves to respond to both heat and cold temperature. A cold receptor, transient receptor potential ion channel (TRPM8), is responsible for detection of various degrees of cold temperature [5]. These primary afferent neurons convert thermal stimuli into action potentials that relay sensory information to the spinal cord and brain [6]. While TRPM8 neurons are a molecularly diverse population, a direct association with a defect or unique subtype of these receptors causing RP has not been shown. The preoptical/anterior hypothalamus in the brain is now known to act as a 'thermostat' receiving information from peripheral signals and coordinating

A.L. Herrick, MD, FRCP (✉)
Centre for Musculoskeletal Research, The University of Manchester, Salford Royal NHS Foundation Trust, Manchester Academic Health Science Centre, Manchester, UK
e-mail: ariane.herrick@manchester.ac.uk

F.M. Wigley, MD
Department of Medicine/Rheumatology, The Johns Hopkins University School of Medicine, Baltimore, MD, USA

M. Matucci-Cerinic, MD, PhD
Department of Experimental and Clinical Medicine, University of Florence, Florence, Italy

J. Varga et al. (eds.), *Scleroderma*, DOI 10.1007/978-3-319-31407-5_20

efferent responses [7]. Sympathetic-mediated vasoconstrictor and vasodilator nerves innervate arterioles and regulate regional blood flow in the skin. Sympathetic noradrenergic nerves via the release of norepinephrine maintain increased tone to cutaneous thermoregulatory vessels during normal environmental temperatures.

The vascular endothelium, smooth muscle cells and nerve terminals form an integrated unit in which specific interactions and soluble mediators released in the microenvironment contribute together to determine the final balance between vasodilatation and vasoconstriction. These interactions are influenced by a variety of factors including the level of physical activity, the ambient temperature, the individual's emotional state and direct traumatic or inflammatory insults to the vessels. The skin circulation is unique in that it plays a role in both bringing nutrition to the skin and in regulating central body temperature. There are two components of blood flow to the skin of the digits, thermoregulatory and nutritional [8]. Approximately 80–90 % of blood flow through the digits is controlled by thermoregulatory mechanisms. The cutaneous blood flow can shift from very low to high flow via a complex mechanism that involves both centrally controlled and locally mediated reflexes [7]. Environmental temperatures influence skin blood flow by triggering a rapid decrease in skin blood flow in the cold, thus shifting blood to deeper plexus and preserving body heat. In warm ambient temperatures, there is an increase in cutaneous blood flow seen as a skin blush. This occurs rapidly during small increases in body temperature such as during vigorous exercise. The increase in skin blood flow coupled with sweating cools the blood and allows heat loss at the surface of the skin by convection. This critical thermoregulation by skin circulation is altered by exercise, reproductive hormones, ageing, diseases that affect vascular function and normal reflex mechanisms [7]. In addition, there is acclimation to ambient conditions by physical conditioning.

The sympathetic nervous system regulates the thermoregulatory process by controlling the supply of blood through arteriovenous (A-V) shunts present in the microcirculation of the skin. Numerous arteriovenous (A-V) shunts in peripheral sites of the skin provide low-resistance conduits that allow shunting of blood from arterioles to venules at high flow rates. During heat exposure, these shunts open allowing a large increase in blood flow into the skin surface with heat dissipation. Skin blood flow can increase to as much as 6–8 L/min or 60 % of cardiac output [7]. In response to body cooling, the shunts close under increased sympathetic tone and redirect blood centrally to maintain core temperature. Nutritional flow is constitutive and provided through a network of capillary vessels [9]. Normal vascular smooth muscle also has inherent contractile activity (phasic and tonic) that can be dramatically increased following activation of the vascular smooth muscle cell. For example, the degree of vasoreactivity can be affected by a vasoconstrictor agonist or by an increase in transmural pressure. Thus, repeated episodes of vasoconstriction may enhance smooth muscle responses. The degree of vasoconstriction also depends on local activation of adrenergic nerves and an increase in number and affinity of the postsynaptic a-2 receptors on cutaneous vessels.

Systemic Sclerosis and Raynaud's Phenomenon

Patients with RP can demonstrate dramatic colour changes (usually a blue discoloration of cyanosis) on the surface of the skin, due to shunting of blood in the thermoregulatory vessels, yet maintain reasonable nutritional flow. Predominately, vasoconstriction of thermoregulatory vessels alone during cold exposure with maintenance of nutritional flow accounts for the absence of ischaemic lesions among patients with uncomplicated RP. Constriction of thermoregulatory vessels is manifested by a cyanotic skin typically of blue discoloration (Fig. 20.1a) during an RP attack. This cyanotic appearance is caused by reduced blood flow and venous pooling, which allows blood to deoxygenate. Coffman demonstrated that when measuring total digital blood flow, there is a difference between primary RP patients and those with SSc [8]. Critical ischaemic events occur when digital artery closure affects both thermoregulatory and nutritional blood flow; total flow ceases long enough for tissue hypoxia to reach a critical stage. When total digital blood flow is compromised, the skin will appear white or pale (Fig. 20.1b). Episodes of cold temperature-induced vasospasm are typically self-limited, but when the vasospasm is sustained, then progressive tissue ischaemia occurs and tissue necrosis or ulceration can develop. For example, prolonged cold exposure in a normal individual may lead to frostbite.

Primary RP appears to be primarily functional in nature. The vessels appear normal in structure, and there is little evidence for progression of the process with time. In fact, studies suggest that RP improves [10] and the intensity is influenced by gender, environment, stress and physiological hormonal changes. The defect in primary RP is unknown but is clearly genetically derived in that family clustering with primary RP exists. Studies suggest that about 30 % of first-degree relatives of a proband have RP [11].

In contrast, in SSc and other secondary forms of RP, it is thought that the underlying vascular disease disrupts the normal mechanisms responsible for control of vessel reactivity. It should be emphasised that almost all patients with SSc experience RP – over 95 % [12]. Structural vascular abnormalities of both the microvasculature and digital artery are well recognised in SSc [13]. A widespread obliterative vasculopathy of the peripheral arteries and microcirculation is seen. Although a popular model to explain the pathogenesis of the underlying SSc vascular disease is not yet fully proven,

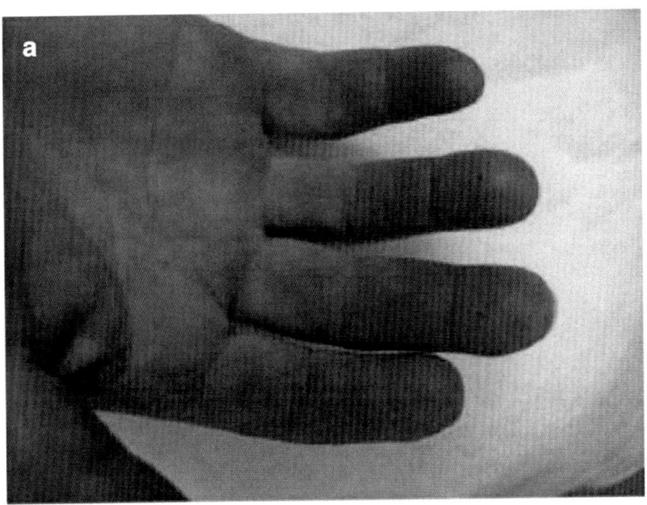

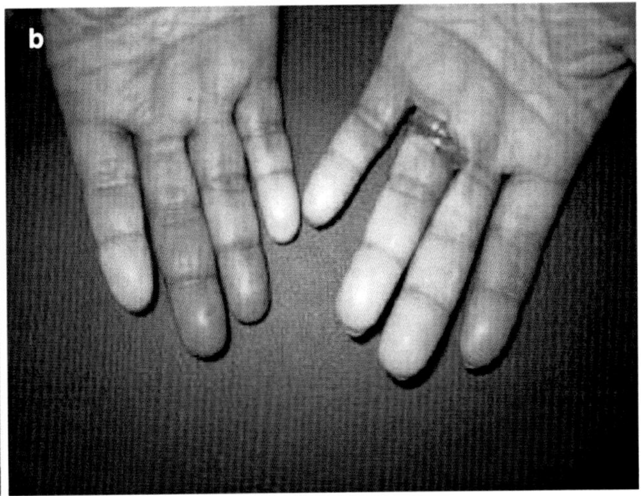

Fig. 20.1 Active Raynaud's phenomenon. (**a**) Cyanotic phase with blue discoloration of the distal fingers. (**b**) Pallor phase with white discoloration of the distal fingers

it suggests that the endothelial cell layer of the microvascular is activated/injured early in the disease process leading to endothelial cell dysfunction, over-expression of adhesion molecules, enhanced leukocyte migration, proliferation of pericytes, adhesion and activation of platelets and influx of a perivascular infiltrate. Cellular growth factors, oxidative stress and immune mediators stimulate the appearance of myofibroblasts in the vessel wall that synthesise a thickened intima layer, compromising regional blood flow by narrowing the vascular lumen. Unlike patients with primary RP who have mild episodes that rarely interfere with daily activities, patients with SSc experience intense and frequent ischaemic events associated with recurrent digital ulcers in 25–39 % of cases [14]. Structural disease of muscular peripheral arteries is known to occur in SSc, and, thus, diseased vessels have altered flow, aggravating normal responses to cold and sympathetic stimulation of cutaneous vessels. Although larger vessels (e.g. digital artery) are involved, the vascular disease of SSc involves predominantly the microcirculation and arterioles. The peripheral microvascular damage in SSc is mainly characterised by increasing structural alterations of the capillaries of the skin with a progressive decrease in their density and a decrease in cutaneous blood flow [15]. Thus, RP associated with SSc has structural disease of the involved vessels. The process causing the structural disease leads to functional abnormalities that manifest at the skin as RP. These functional abnormalities are thought to disrupt normal neural control of vascular reactivity.

Neural Mechanism of Raynaud's Phenomenon

The thermoregulatory vessels are potentially influenced by an array of mediators, but there is compelling evidence that the increased sensitivity to cold temperatures is mediated in part by α-adrenergic responses [16]. During decline in core body temperature, there is increased sympathetic tone in the A-V shunts, forcing blood flow into deeper venous plexus and thus reducing heat loss. Decreased sympathetic tone leads to vasodilatation and increased skin blood flow. Cold also activates vasoconstriction by selectively amplifying vascular smooth muscle reactivity to the sympathetic neurotransmitter. Norepinephrine initiates cutaneous vasoconstriction by activating two distinct families of receptors on vascular smooth muscle, α_1 and α_2-adrenoreceptor. Although α_1-receptors are ubiquitous, the functional activity of α_2-receptors is prominent on the vascular smooth muscle of cutaneous vessels [16]. The administration of 'selective' α_1- and α_2-adrenergic agonists to human volunteers causes a marked reduction in skin or finger blood flow [17], while inhibition of the α_2-receptor inhibited cold-induced vasoconstriction in patients with RP [18]. Experiments using isolated murine tail artery revealed that the α_{2C}-subtype is responsible for the thermoregulatory function of the α_2-receptors [16]. Chotani et al. [19] demonstrated in ex vivo studies that α_{2C}-adrenoreceptor plays a prominent role in vasoconstriction of cutaneous arteries after moderate cooling. Under normal conditions (37 °C), α_{2C}-adrenoceptors are silently stored within the Golgi apparatus and translocate to the cell surface after cold exposure, contributing to the adrenergic constrictive response. This suggests that an altered pattern of expression of these α 2 subtypes could modify α_2-receptor sensitivity during cold exposure, but not at normal temperatures. Cold-induced cutaneous vasoconstriction is also restrained by simultaneous cold-induced vasodilation from sympathetic nerves; thus a defect in the regulation of sympathetic-induced vasodilation could lead to excessive vasoconstriction.

Bailey et al. [20] showed that cooling induces activation of Rho/Rho kinase signalling pathway, and this prompts translocation of α_{2C}-adrenoreceptor from Golgi complex to the plasma membrane, together with augmented sensitivity to Ca^{++} of contractile proteins. This study suggests that the Rho-kinase pathway is important in trafficking molecules through microtubule depolymerisation inside cells like vascular smooth muscle. This implies that surface cooling of the skin can increase the sensitivity of the thermoregulatory vessel to local cooling by enhancing the expression of α_{2C}-adrenoreceptor and thus exaggerating the vessel's response to sympathetic signalling by the neurotransmitter norepinephrine. However, experts suggest that α_{2C}-receptors do not appear to respond directly to cold and therefore should be considered 'thermoeffectors' rather than 'thermosensors' [16].

In patients with primary RP, the pathogenic importance of α_2-receptors is suggested by experiments with selective receptor antagonists. In one report of 23 patients, for example, the number of fingers with cold-induced vasospastic attacks was markedly reduced with yohimbine (an α_2-receptor blocker) compared with prazosin (an α_1-receptor blocker) [21]. In SSc, an increased activity of α_2-receptors is demonstrated ex vivo in cutaneous vessels from patients [22]. This suggests that part of the disease process in SSc activates increased expression of α_2-receptors and thus enhances the vascular response to norepinephrine.

Increased contractile responses to α_2-adrenergic agonists and cooling observed in patients with RP compared to healthy controls are associated with increased protein tyrosine kinase (PTK) activity and tyrosine phosphorylation. These abnormalities are described in arteries from both primary and secondary RP subjects, providing a theoretical unifying explanation for the cold-induced vascular reactivity. Studies by Furspan et al. [23, 24] provide evidence that the increased contractile response to α_2-adrenergic agonists and cooling observed in patients with RP compared with healthy controls is associated with increased protein tyrosine kinase (PTK) activity and tyrosine phosphorylation. The identity of the ultimate target protein for tyrosine phosphorylation is still unknown, and it is possible that PTK activity may increase secondary to abnormal levels of other mediators (i.e. platelet-derived growth factor, transforming growth factor-b, other cytokines or reactive oxygen species), but while confirmation of this work is needed, the potential use of PTK inhibitor to treat RP is intriguing.

Neuropeptides and Raynaud's Phenomenon

Sympathetic nerves also release neuropeptides that act as co-transmitters that can either enhance vasoconstriction (neuropeptide Y) or mediate vasodilatation (vasoactive intestinal peptide (VIP), substance P). Local increases in skin temperature cause vasodilatation by stimulating local neuropeptide release from cutaneous sensory nerves (including calcitonin gene-related peptide [CGRP], substance P [SP] and neurokinin A [NKA]). Abnormality of the vasodilatory neuropeptides substance P and CGRP is postulated to occur in both primary RP and in secondary Raynaud's associated with SSc [25]. Substance P and nitric oxide (NO) are also released from endothelial cells. Bunker et al. found a reduced number of CGRP immunoreactive neurons in the skin and improved RP after intravenous delivery of CGRP in patients with RP or SSc [26, 27]. While these data support the concept that there is a deficiency of CGRP release or other vasodilating neuropeptides, there is no clear evidence that this pathway is a dominant problem in RP. Stephens et al. [28] confirmed that the sympathetic co-transmitter neuropeptide Y can induce a reflex cutaneous vasoconstrictor response after mild cooling (31.7 °C), and this effect is independent of norepinephrine. These studies were performed on human participants after total body cooling and measured skin blood flow by laser Doppler flowmetry following locally injected antagonist of neuropeptide Y-Y_1 receptors. It is of interest that peripheral neuropathy is associated with disrupted cutaneous blood flow. For example, there is an association of cold hands and RP in patients with carpal tunnel syndrome [29].

Endothelial Cell Function and Raynaud's Phenomenon

Although vascular smooth muscle can respond directly to the neurotransmitter norepinephrine, neuropeptides, physical or environmental stimuli, important physiologic control of smooth muscle activity is also indirectly mediated by factors released by endothelial cells. The endothelium is a metabolically active tissue that, under normal circumstances, regulates regional blood flow, transportation of nutrients, coagulation and fibrinolysis and migration of blood cells while maintaining an antithrombotic lining in the vasculature. These important biologic functions are achieved through production of a complex array of molecules including vasodilators (e.g. NO and prostacyclin), vasoconstrictors (e.g. endothelin-1 and platelet-activating factor) and cell adhesion molecules (e.g. selectins and integrins). Perturbation of endothelial cell homeostasis driven by a disturbed state (inflammation, cytokine activation, trauma/vibration) can lead to a significant imbalance in the profile of mediators secreted by the endothelium. Vasoconstriction may thus result when there is imbalance towards release of active vasoconstrictive mediators even without underlying permanent structural vascular damage. These include increased production of endothelin-1 [30], decreased sensory nerve innervation (CGRP-containing nerve fibres) [26] and impaired release of vasodilators from the endothelium such as NO or prostacyclin [31]. In SSc, there is evidence that endothelial cell dysfunction is abnormal perhaps due to immune-mediated injury. This process then can disturb the natural balance of vasoactive mediators leading to a tendency for exaggerated vasoconstriction. Clinically, this can be manifest by cold sensitivity and RP. Repeated episodes of RP may lead to ischaemia-reperfusion injury that creates a cycle of repeated vascular injury and propagation of the disease process. Physical trauma to blood vessels can also disturb normal endothelial cell function. The hand-arm vibration syndrome is caused by chronic trauma from the use of vibration tools and devices. RP is part of the clinical manifestations of this syndrome.

Endothelin-1 (ET-1) is a 21-amino-acid peptide with potent vasoconstrictor properties that can mediate vascular injury and abnormal vascular reactivity in SSc [32]. ET-1 is released from the endothelial cells, macrophages, epithelial cells and mesenchymal cells and can act directly on vascular smooth muscle cells. ET-1 is elevated in the plasma of SSc patients compared to controls, and it increases during cold exposure in selected SSc patients [33]. There is no clear evidence that altered activity of ET-1 plays a role in primary RP. The localisation of ET-1 on specimens obtained by skin biopsies, with ET-1 deposits in the endothelial cells and dermal fibroblasts, has a positive correlation with the serum levels of ET-1 [30]. Increased ET-1 production can cause oxidant stress and endothelial dysfunction and likely contributes to SSc-related vascular dysfunction including RP and ischaemia-reperfusion tissue injury. Therefore, inhibiting ET-1 activity is considered an attractive target in treating SSc vascular disease.

Circumstantial evidence for a defect in vascular NO production comes from laboratory studies that demonstrate a decreased response to endothelium-dependent challenges but not to endothelium-independent pathways [31]. In addition, intra-arterial infusion of nitroprusside or L-arginine, the physiologic substrate for NO, decreased cold-induced vasospasm in SSc [34]. Endothelial dysfunction can also be assessed by quantifying plasma asymmetric dimethylarginine (ADMA), an endogenous inhibitor of endothelial NO synthase (NOS). ADMA levels are reported high in the plasma of SSc patients suggesting abnormal NO production by inhibition of NOS [35, 36]. An impaired availability of NO, related to polymorphisms in the endothelial NOS (eNOS) gene, is also postulated [37]. Paradoxically, under circumstances of ischaemia/hypoxia-reperfusion (i.e. RP associated with SSc), NO can mediate free radical tissue injury by interacting with superoxide anion to produce peroxynitrate, a powerful oxidising agent [38]. Clearly, the pathological role of NO in SSc is complex, but endothelial injury and defective NO production remains a viable target for therapeutic intervention.

Endothelial cells also release prostaglandins that are vasodilatory. Epoprostenol (prostacyclin) is a potent vasodilator that acts to activate membrane-bound adenylate cyclase to increase cyclic adenosine monophosphate (AMP). Defects in release of prostacyclin are thought to occur in RP, particularly in secondary forms with endothelial dysfunction such as seen in SSc.

Other Intravascular Factors

Vascular reactivity is also affected by shear stress, vasoactive substances released during platelet activation (thromboxane, serotonin), a change in blood viscosity and potentially changes in rheological properties of blood such as altered red blood cell deformability. Several studies give evidence for activation of platelets in SSc including elevated levels of circulating platelet aggregates, increased plasma levels of β-thromboglobulin, enhanced adhesion of SSc-derived platelets, increased circulating microparticles containing platelet fragments, increased circulating platelet-leukocyte complexes and increased urinary levels of thromboxane likely derived from activated platelets [39–41]. Thus, it is in theory possible that both serotonin and thromboxane release from platelets mediate vasoconstriction in SSc.

Circulating hormones such as oestrogen may have a role as a mediator of changes in vascular tone [25]. Epidemiological studies suggest that oestrogen use is associated with RP, but the biologic evidence demonstrates that oestrogens may actually act as a vasodilator. Arterial vessel relaxation is linked to the ability of 17-b estradiol to increase NO synthase expression and to induce calcium-dependent NO production. Endothelial function and vasomotor changes in patients with RP suggest that acute and chronic oestrogen administration has some positive effect on flow-mediated dilation of the brachial artery [42]. Oestrogen is known to increase the expression of α_{2C}-adrenoreceptor on the smooth muscle of cutaneous vessels and increases the α_2-receptor-mediated response to cold exposure [43]. However, information about effects of oestrogen on the distal circulation or about variation of clinical manifestations such as the symptoms, number and duration of RP attacks is not defined.

Ischaemia is a potent stimulus for free radical formation, and thus, hypoxia from SSc vascular disease likely creates free radial formation. Oxidative stress is thought to be an important causative factor in tissue and cellular injury in SSc. Free radicals can be released in a vascular wall from macrophages, endothelial cells and vascular smooth muscle cells. Studies have demonstrated increased levels of oxidised lipoproteins and an increased susceptibility of low-density lipoproteins to oxidation in SSc patients [44], giving further support for oxygen-free radicals playing a role in SSc vascular disease. Probucol, an antioxidant, may reduce lipoprotein

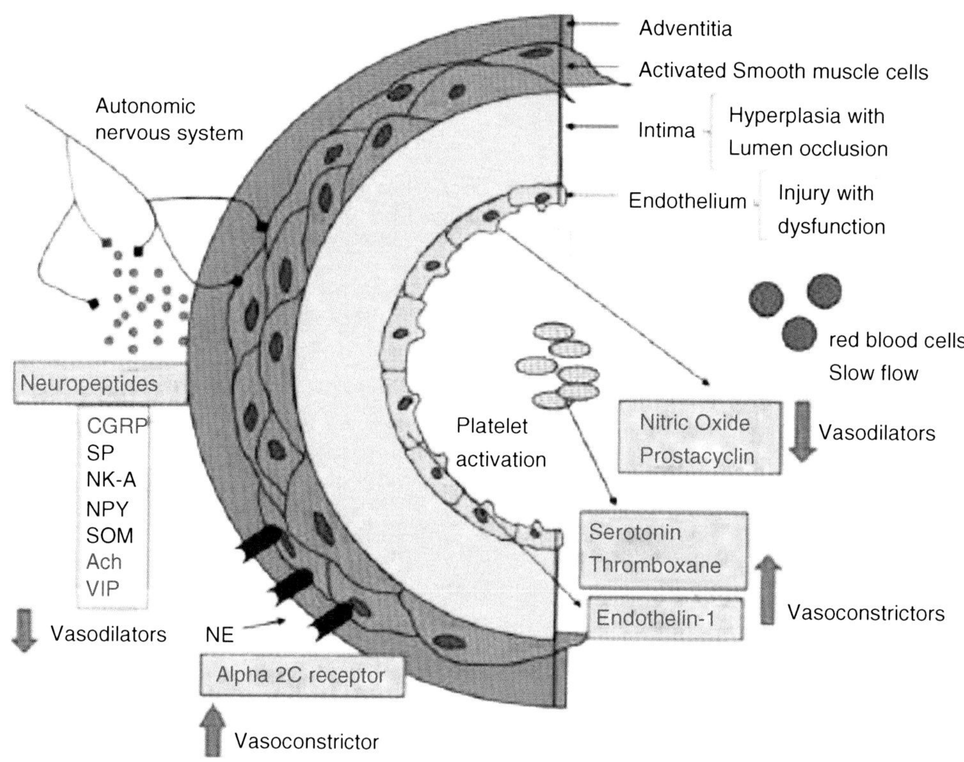

Fig. 20.2 Raynaud's phenomenon in scleroderma. *CGRP* calcitonin gene-related peptide, *SP* substance P, *NKA* neurokinin A, *SOM* somatostatin, *Ach* acetylcholine, *VIP* vasoactive intestinal polypeptide, *NE norepinephrine*. Scleroderma vascular disease leads to intimal hyperplasia and lumen narrowing and slow flow which enhances vasoconstriction. Injury to the endothelium causes decreased production of the vasodilators nitric oxide and prostacyclin and increased production of the potent vasoconstrictor endothelin-1. An activated smooth muscle layer has increased expression of α_{2C}-receptors and thus an increased vasoconstriction to the neurotransmitter norepinephrine. Cutaneous nerve injury decreases the production of vasodilating neuropeptides including CGRP. The scleroderma vascular disease causes an imbalance of vasodilators and vasoconstrictors leading to the vasospasm of Raynaud's phenomenon

oxidation in patients with Raynaud's phenomenon [45]. It is interesting to speculate that vasoconstriction and reduction in tissue perfusion can result in tissue hypoxia that further alters cell function and could aggravate RP. There is evidence that endothelial cell response to hypoxia can affect the cell physiology in many ways including the induction of genes encoding vasoconstrictors and smooth muscle mitogens [46].

Summary of Pathogenesis

The pathogenesis of Raynaud's phenomenon (RP) is currently not fully explained, but an imbalance between the normal regulation of vasoconstriction and vasodilation of cutaneous vessels is postulated (Fig. 20.2). Vascular reactivity is regulated by both intrinsic vascular mediators and extrinsic factors including the neural control of vascular tone and the influence of circulating mediators that affect thermoregulatory vessels. A complex interaction of these regulators creates a delicate balance that provides important physiological responses including regulating regional blood flow and maintaining normal core body temperature. RP is an exaggeration of the normal responses to our environmental temperatures. In SSc, abnormal vasoreactivity and RP are caused by the disease process disrupting digital and thermoregulatory vessels and usual neurovascular control.

Ischaemic Complications: Digital Ulcers and Critical Ischaemia

RP in patients with SSc can be very severe and may progress to irreversible tissue injury. The main ischaemic complications are digital ulceration and critical ischaemia: these can coexist [47, 48]. Both can result in the loss of the affected digit and are therefore medical emergencies. Early intervention is essential, and patients should be advised to seek early medical advice in the event of a digit becoming permanently discoloured or if an ulcer develops. Both digital ulcers and critical ischaemia are usually extremely painful and may result in tissue loss and major disability (including work disability [49, 50]), with loss of hand function and a major negative impact on quality of life [51–54].

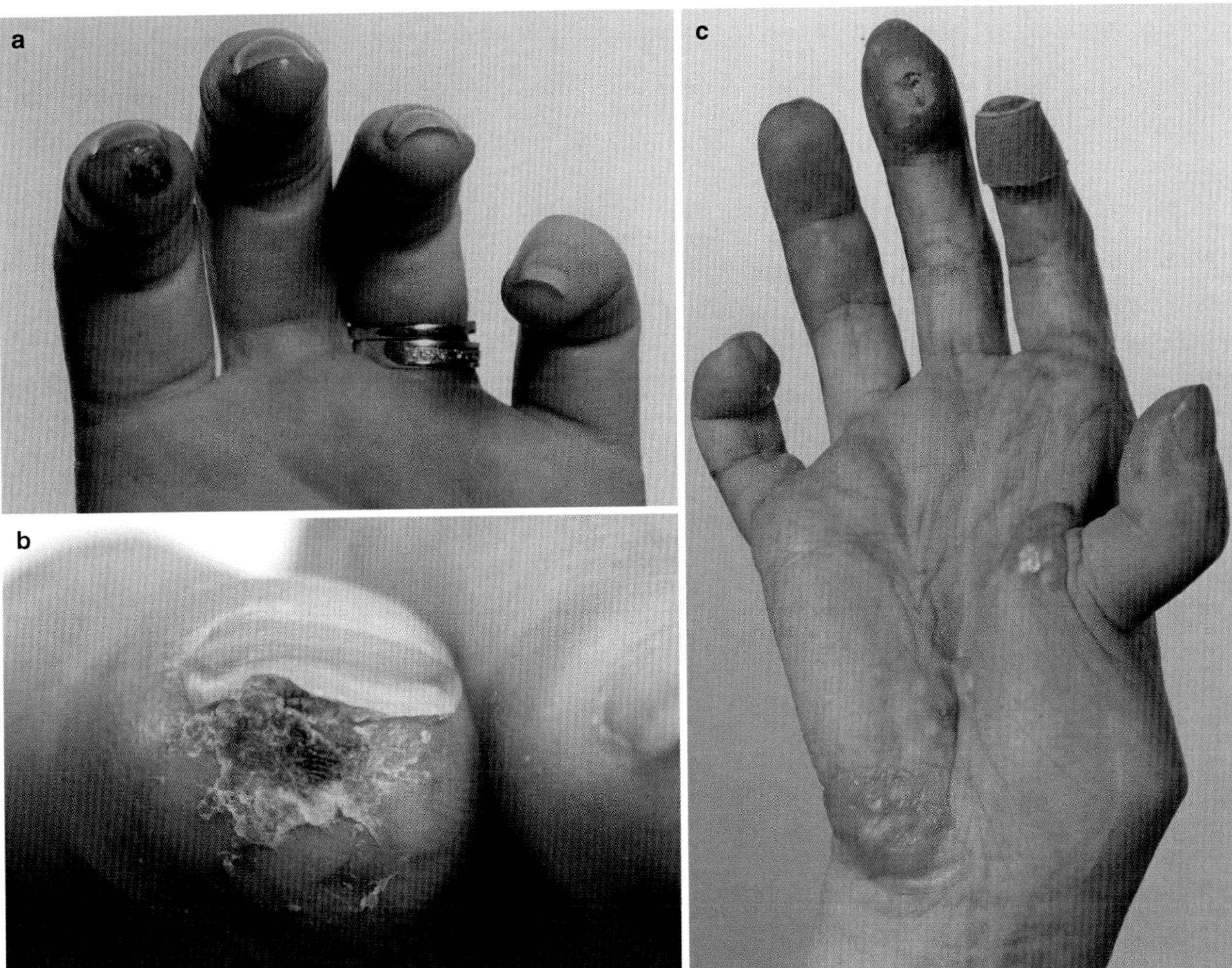

Fig. 20.3 Digital ulcers in patients with SSc: (a, b) show examples of fingertip ulcers and (c) an ulcer overlying calcinosis (distal phalanx of middle finger)

Digital Ulcers

Digital ulcers are common [55, 56], occurring in up to 50% of patients with SSc, and often early on in the disease course [57]. They tend to occur over the fingertips in patients with limited cutaneous SSc and over the extensor surfaces in patients with diffuse cutaneous SSc, who often have marked contractures and are at risk of micro-trauma (Figs. 20.3 and 20.4). Due to the poor digital blood supply, digital ulcers can be very difficult to heal and can become infected, sometimes with bone involvement, which can be detected early using magnetic resonance (MR) imaging, before changes on plain radiography [58] (Fig. 20.4). Ulcers overlying areas of calcinosis (Fig. 20.3c) are especially difficult to heal.

As well as being painful and disabling, a further significance of digital ulcers is that they may be a 'sentinel sign' for early internal organ involvement and predict a worse disease course in the patient with SSc [59, 60].

Critical Ischaemia

Although this is usually due to progression of the noninflammatory angiopathy of SSc, which affects both microvessels and digital arteries, three questions must always be asked, in order not to miss a potentially treatable problem:

1. Is there concomitant large vessel (proximal) disease? If so, then an urgent vascular opinion should be sought. It has been suggested that patients with SSc have an increased prevalence of large vessel disease [61–63]. Whether or not this is the case, the combination of small and large vessel disease is potentially very serious and must not be overlooked.
2. Is there concomitant vasculitis? This is rare in SSc but has been reported and should be considered especially in patients with overlap syndromes, for example, with systemic lupus erythematosus.

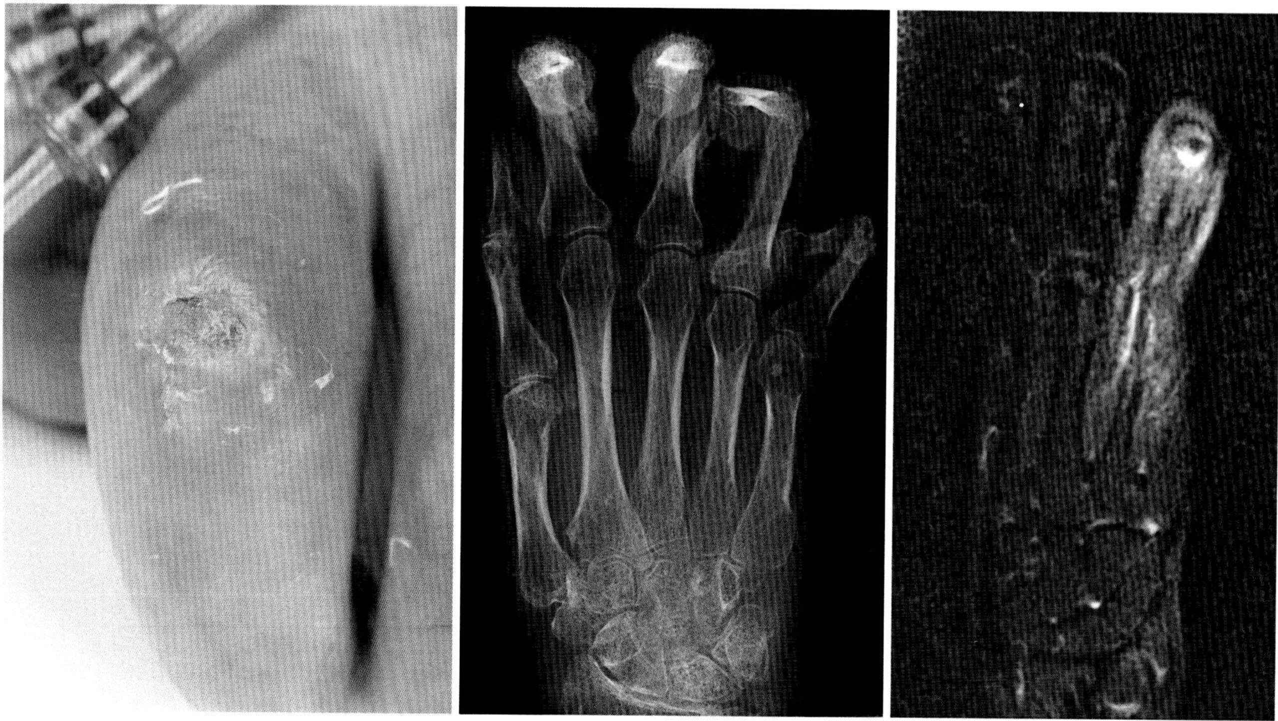

Fig. 20.4 Extensor surface ulcer (overlying proximal interphalangeal joint) in a patient with diffuse cutaneous SSc. Plain radiograph (*middle panel*) shows the marked flexion contractures. MR scan (*right*) shows underlying bone marrow oedema, suggestive of osteomyelitis

3. Is there a concomitant coagulopathy? This is also rare, but the possibility of, for example, an antiphospholipid syndrome should always be considered.

Imaging of Raynaud's Phenomenon

There are three main indications for imaging in patients with RP who have either a suspected or known diagnosis of SSc:

1. To help differentiate between primary and SSc-related RP.
2. To identify problems which require specific intervention. This is usually in the context of the patient with SSc and critical ischaemia and/or digital ulceration. The key points are to diagnose coexisting large vessel disease, underlying bone infection and calcinosis.
3. To study pathogenesis and assess disease severity/treatment response in the research setting.

Differentiating Between Primary and SSc-Related Raynaud's Phenomenon

Different methods have been used to differentiate between primary and SSc-related Raynaud's phenomenon, including nailfold capillaroscopy [64, 65], thermography [66–70], laser Doppler imaging [71] and finger systolic pressure measurement [72]. Of these, only nailfold capillaroscopy and (to a much lesser extent) thermography are applied in the clinical setting.

Nailfold Capillaroscopy

Abnormal nailfold capillaries are an early feature of SSc. At the nailfold, capillaries run parallel to, as opposed to perpendicular to, the skin surface, and this allows them to be visualised non-invasively. The main rationale for nailfold capillaroscopy is that it facilitates early diagnosis of a SSc-spectrum disorder [73, 74] because abnormal nailfold capillaries are a predictor of development of SSc in the patient presenting with RP [75, 76]. Nailfold capillaroscopy can help in identifying patients with *very early* systemic sclerosis [77]. Moreover, abnormal nailfold capillaries are one of the new 2013 American College of Rheumatology (ACR)/European league Against Rheumatism (EULAR) criteria for SSc [78, 79] reinforcing the need for rheumatologists to be familiar with the technique. Normal capillaries are reassuring, whereas a 'SSc pattern' (including capillary dilation, haemorrhages and often areas of avascularity) suggests an underlying SSc-spectrum disorder [65, 80]. However, it is important to recognise that there is a spectrum of normality and abnormality, with the result that appearances can be equivocal when some loops appear borderline dilated. In this situation, the pragmatic approach is to repeat the capillaroscopy in 1–2 years' time if there remains clinical concern.

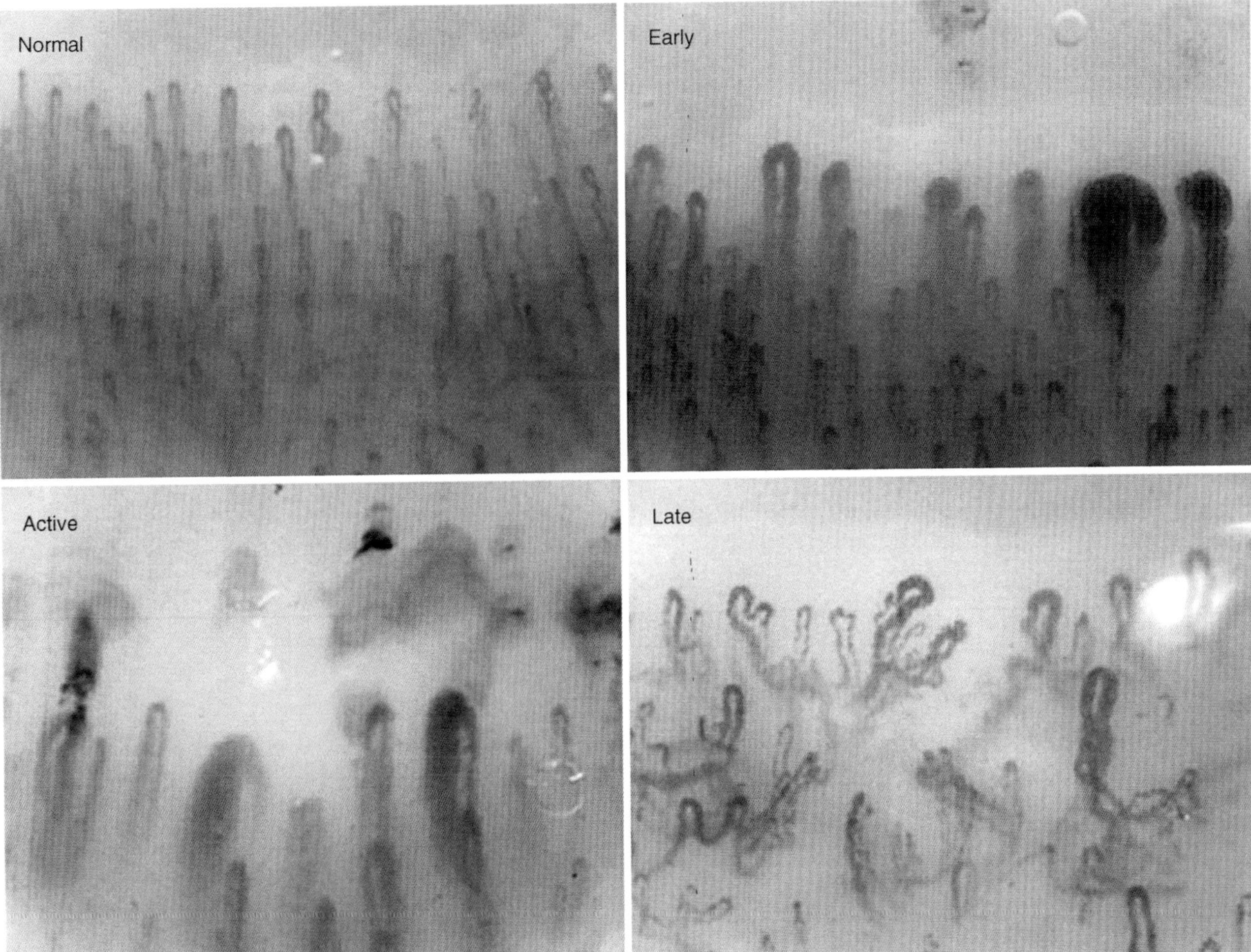

Fig. 20.5 Classification of the scleroderma pattern. NVC qualitative patterns that include an 'early' pattern (few giant capillaries, few capillary microhaemorrhages, no evident loss of capillaries and relatively well-preserved capillary distribution), an 'active' pattern (frequent giant capillaries, frequent capillary microhaemorrhages, moderate loss of capillaries, absent or mild ramified capillaries with mild disorganisation of the capillary architecture) and a 'late' pattern (almost absent giant capillaries and microhaemorrhages, severe loss of capillaries with extensive avascular areas, neovascularisation with ramified/bushy capillaries and intense disorganisation of the normal capillary array). (Of note, the *left upper* panel contains a normal capillaroscopic image). Image is adapted from Cutolo M and Smith V and used with permission

Cutolo and colleagues have described three patterns of the 'SSc pattern' of nailfold capillaroscopic change: 'early', 'active' and 'late', on the basis of numbers of giant capillaries and of microhaemorrhages, the extent of capillary loss and of disorganisation of the capillary architecture and the presence of neoangiogenesis [81] (Fig. 20.5).

While the main use of nailfold capillaroscopy in the clinical setting is early detection of SSc, there is increasing interest in the concept of using capillaroscopy to predict risk of different clinical features of SSc, especially digital ulcers, because the degree of capillaroscopic abnormality has been shown to be predictive of risk of digital ulceration [82–84].

Different Capillaroscopy Techniques There are a number of different techniques for visualising the nailfold capillaries (Fig. 20.6). For all of these, applying a drop of oil to the nailbed will improve visualisation of the capillaries. The original widefield technique (magnification 12–14×) described by Maricq and colleagues [64, 80] is still used, although nailfold videomicroscopy, which allows much higher magnification (200–600×), is gaining popularity. For clinicians without access to either of these techniques, an ophthalmoscope [85], handheld dermatoscope [86] or (more recently) USB microscope can be used. The dermatoscope magnifies capillaries in the order of 10×. So far dermoscopy has been relatively little researched in patients with Raynaud's, but early reliability studies are promising [87, 88], and capillary abnormalities detected on dermoscopy improve the sensitivity of diagnosis of limited cutaneous SSc [89]. A recent study (involving 48 rheumatologists) which compared dermoscopy and high-magnification videocapillaroscopy suggested that the techniques are comparable and that most nailfolds can be assessed by either technique [90].

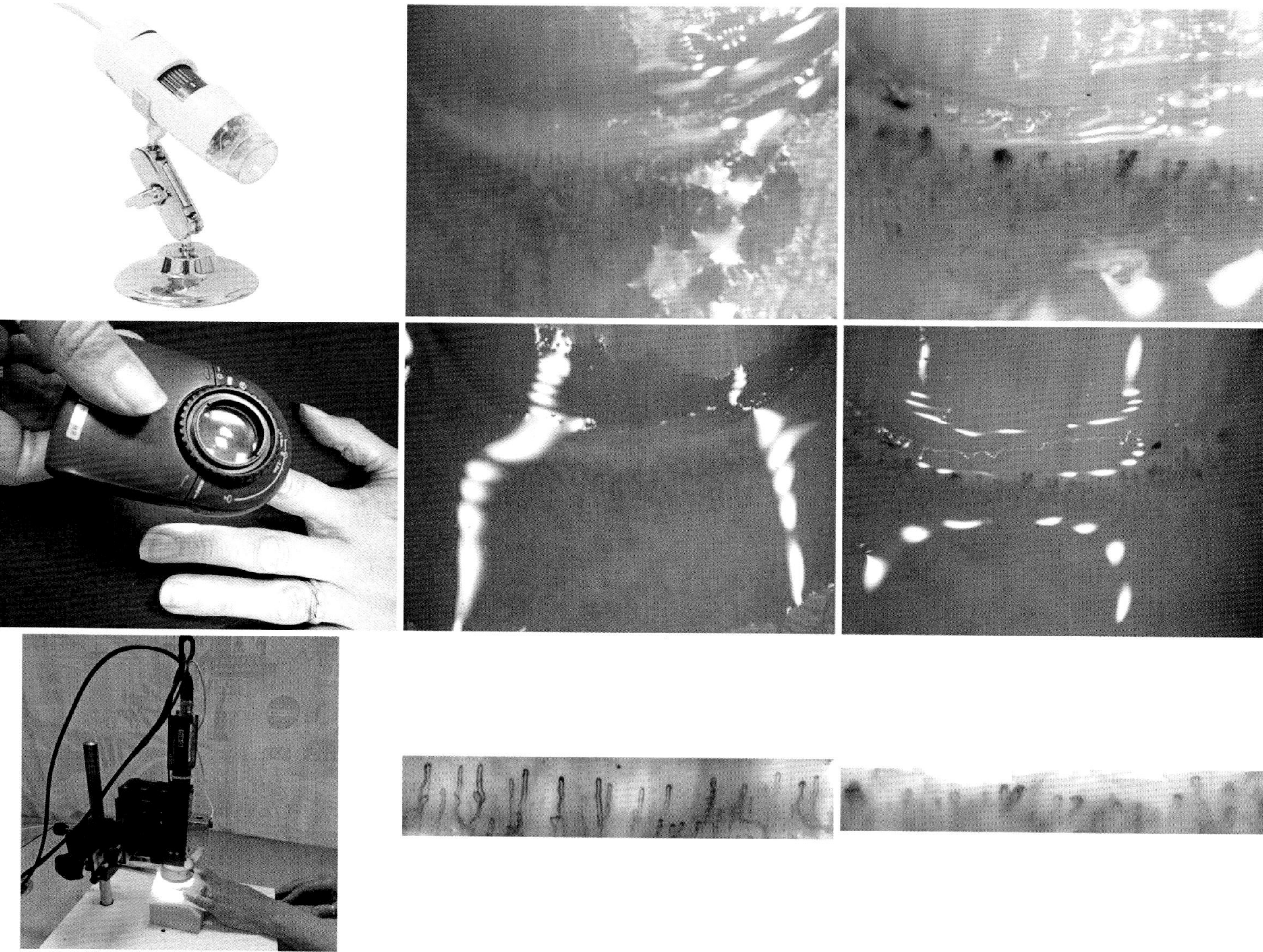

Fig. 20.6 Different capillaroscopic techniques. The different techniques are shown on the left side column: USB microscope (*top*), dermatoscope (*middle*), videomicroscope (*bottom*). The *middle* and *right* side columns show the images acquired using each technique from a healthy control subject (*middle column*: same digit imaged using each technique) and a patient with SSc (*right column*: same digit imaged using each technique). The images from the patient with SSc show some dilated capillaries and areas of avascularity

However, more images (i.e. nailfolds) could be graded by nailfold videocapillaroscopy than by dermoscopy, and images were graded more 'severely' by videocapillaroscopy than by dermoscopy [90]. An advantage of low magnification techniques (widefield microscopy, dermoscopy, USB microscopy) is that they image the whole of the nailfold 'at a glance', allowing any abnormalities to be easily detected. However, low magnification inevitably limits accurate measurement of capillary density and dimensions which may be useful in clinical research studies.

Thermography

Infrared thermography images surface temperature (Fig. 20.7) and is therefore an indirect measure of blood flow. Dynamic imaging, examining response to a cold challenge, helps to differentiate between patients with primary RP and SSc [66, 67], as does the finding of a temperature gradient along a finger of greater than 1 °C (cold fingertips) at a room temperature of 30 °C [68, 69]. However, a recent study suggested that 'baseline' images are more discriminatory between primary and secondary RP than imaging after cold challenge testing [70].

However, thermography requires expensive equipment, and ideally a temperature-controlled laboratory, and its use is therefore restricted to specialist centres. Standardisation of imaging protocols across centres is needed to encourage increased use of this technique.

Identifying Problems Which Require Specific Intervention

Imaging plays a role in the assessment of ischaemic complications (critical digital ischaemia and refractory digital ulceration) described below. The key investigations used in everyday clinical practice are as follows:

(a) Assessment of arterial pulses by Doppler ultrasound [91] and imaging of large vessels (by X-ray, MR or computed tomography (CT) angiography) if large (proximal) vessel disease is suspected. Doppler ultrasound can be performed in the outpatient clinic and is indicated if the peripheral pulses cannot readily be felt. The peripheral pulses and arterial Dopplers should be normal in patients with primary Raynaud's and SSc. If not, then the patient should be referred for a vascular surgical opinion which will most likely include large vessel imaging [92]. Advances in MR angiography are now allowing detailed visualisation of the digital arteries in patients with SSc [93–95].

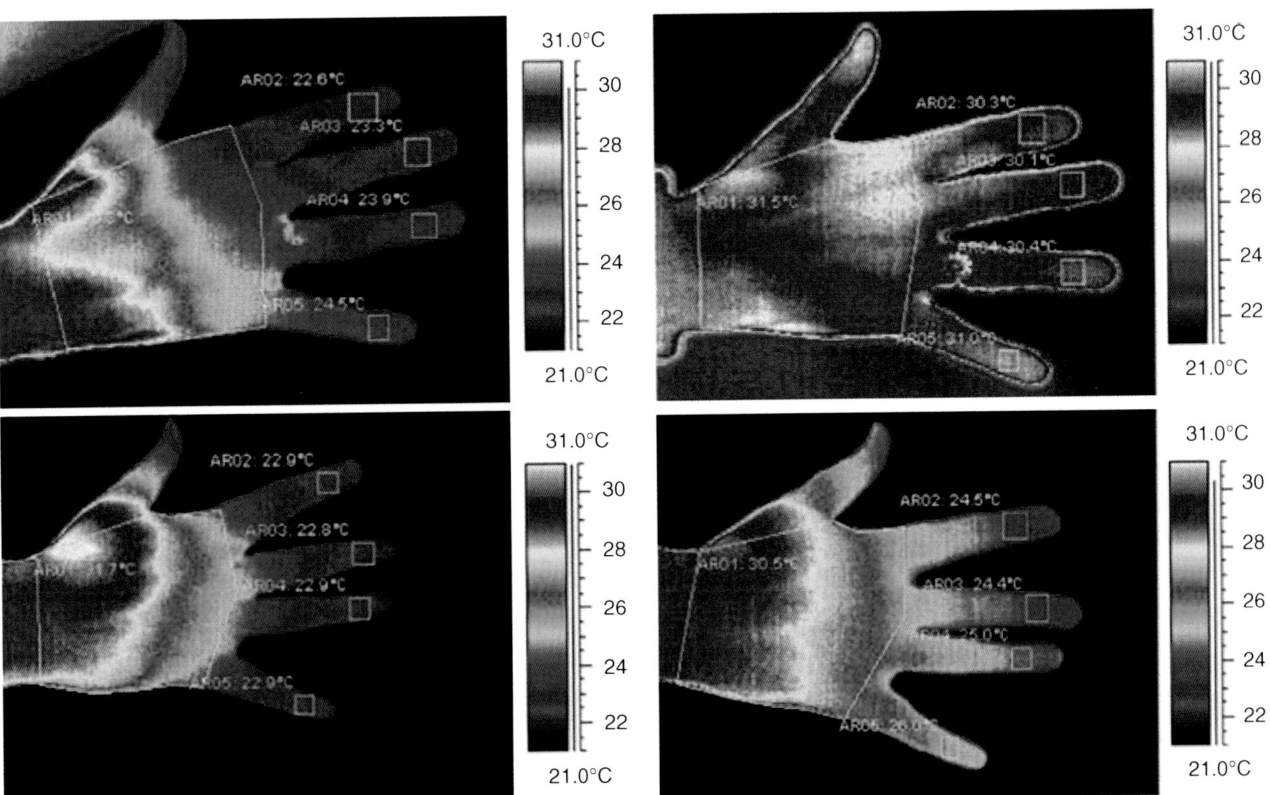

Fig. 20.7 Upper panels show a patient with PRP, lower panels a patient with SSc. Left hand panels at a room temperature of 23°C (the fingers rewarm), right hand panels at a room temperature of 30°C (the fingers do not rewarm)

(b) Plain radiographs. These may demonstrate calcinosis, acro-osteolysis and (usually in the context of an infected digital ulcer) bone infection.
(c) MR imaging is useful in the early diagnosis of bone infection (Fig. 20.4).

Research Applications: To Study Pathogenesis and Assess Disease Severity/Treatment Response

This is an exciting time for researchers interested in imaging the digital vasculature in patients with SSc, because several imaging modalities are in the process of being developed or refined [96]. The main challenge is to develop reliable outcome measures of digital vascular disease, which are sensitive to change. Robust endpoints of SSc-related digital vascular disease would allow clinical trials in smaller numbers of patients than currently considered necessary, to be adequately powered. A detailed discussion of these is out with the scope of this chapter, but they include advances in:

(a) MR angiography, which may in the future allow measurement of change in digital artery disease [93–95].
(b) Nailfold videocapillaroscopy, with the potential to quantify change over time or in response to drug treatment [97]. Increasingly investigators are including capillaroscopy in studies of treatment response [98–100]. This is an exciting but challenging area of research. Challenges include how best to quantify abnormality and to ensure that the same part of the nailbed is examined on each occasion over time (for this reason ideally the whole nailbed should be included) [101].
(c) Laser Doppler, which measures microvascular perfusion. There are a number of different laser Doppler methods [96, 102]. Early studies in RP used single-probe laser Doppler flowmetry, which had the problem of large site-to-site variation leading to poor reproducibility. Laser Doppler imaging ('scanning' laser Doppler) measures blood flow over an area and is non-contact [103]. The technique continues to evolve, with faster scanning times, the use of different wavelengths (allowing different levels of the microcirculation to be examined) and laser speckle contrast imaging [102, 104, 105], which allows measurement of microvascular perfusion over an area without the need for sequential scans, thus reducing imaging time.

Management of Raynaud's Phenomenon

This section will outline the general approach to management but focus on key recent developments, highlighting how advances in our understanding of pathogenesis are driving advances in therapeutics. Possible future treatment approaches will be discussed.

General (Nondrug Measures)

Avoiding cold exposure, reduction of emotional stress and stopping smoking are key aspects of patient education. Patients with SSc who smoke have an increased severity of RP compared to those who do not [106, 107].

Drug Treatment

Because of the complex pathogenesis of SSc-related RP, a large number of different drugs are of either proven or potential benefit. All will have one or more of the following properties: (1) enhance vasodilation, (2) inhibit vasoconstriction, (3) reduce vascular injury and (4) inhibit platelet aggregation/procoagulant tendency (Table 20.1). In general, the evidence base for drug treatment in SSc-related RP is weak: a meta-analysis of calcium channel blockers, considered first-line treatment, included only 109 patients from eight clinical trials [108]. However, the situation is changing, with an increasing number of multinational studies in recent years.

Figure 20.8 summarises our approach to treatment of SSc-related Raynaud's phenomenon. All patients should be on a calcium channel blocker (unless intolerant). If calcium channel blockade is ineffective, or only partially effective, another vasodilator should be substituted or added in, possibly (if Raynaud's phenomenon is severe) in combination with an antiplatelet agent.

Drugs Which Enhance Vasodilation

Calcium Channel Blockers

Sustained release nifedipine and amlodipine are most commonly used, but other dihydropyridines are also prescribed [109]. Starting with a low dose and gradually increasing and using a sustained release preparation are likely to increase tolerability. As well as being vasodilators, calcium channel blockers have antiplatelet [110] and possibly antioxidant effects [111].

Prostanoids

Similarly, to calcium channel blockers, prostanoids are thought to have multiple modes of action, including vasodilation, inhibition of platelet aggregation and vascular remodelling [112]. They are effective in reducing frequency and severity of Raynaud's attacks and in healing digital ulcers [113, 114]. Intravenous (IV) prostanoids are the first-line treatment for SSc-related critical digital ischaemia and refractory digital ulceration. Many clinicians also give IV prostanoids to patients with severe RP at the onset of

Table 20.1 Drug treatment of Raynaud's phenomenon – current and future treatment approaches

Drug or group of drugs	Action (s)	Comments on present or future use
Vasodilators		
Calcium channel blockers	Act on smooth muscle cells to produce vasodilation. Also have antiplatelet effects and possibly antioxidant effects	First line drug treatment. Commence in low dose and gradually increase
Prostanoids	Vasodilate, inhibit platelet aggregation and may have vascular remodelling properties	Intravenous prostanoids used in the treatment of acute digital ischaemia/ulceration
Supplementation of L-arginine/NO pathway, including with phosphodiesterase inhibitors	L-arginine is a substrate for NO in endothelial cells. NO acts on smooth muscle cells to produce vasodilation via cGMP Phosphodiesterase type V inhibitors inhibit degradation of cGMP	Topical NO donation (including with GTN) to produce local rather than systemic vasodilation is currently being researched. Phosphodiesterase inhibitors are also being researched and are being used increasingly in patients with severe Raynaud's phenomenon
Drugs which reduce vasoconstriction		
ACE inhibitors	Prevent conversion of angiotensin I to angiotensin II. May have effects on endothelial function and on vascular remodelling	Reasonable choice if calcium channel blockers are ineffective or not tolerated, although no good evidence base
Angiotensin II receptor blockers	Block action of angiotensin II on vascular smooth muscle	Reasonable choice if calcium channel blockers are ineffective or not tolerated, although no good evidence base
α-adrenergic blockers	Block vasoconstriction	Reasonable choice if calcium channel blockers are ineffective or not tolerated. Research on-going into selective α_{2C}-adrenergic blockers
Endothelin-1 receptor antagonists	Block vasoconstriction via action of endothelin-1 on smooth muscle cells	Indicated for prevention of digital ulceration in patients with SSc-spectrum disorders and a history of digital ulcers
Serotonin reuptake inhibitors	Block uptake of serotonin, a vasoconstrictor	May be effective in some patients, although there is a need for further research
Drugs with 'intravascular' effects		
Antioxidants	Reduce oxidative stress (e.g. from hypoxic/reperfusion injury)	Good therapeutic rationale in SSc-spectrum disorders but require further study before these can be recommended
Antithrombotics		
Antiplatelet agents	Inhibit platelet aggregation	Good therapeutic rationale in SSc-spectrum disorders but require further study before these can be recommended. However, reasonable to give low-dose aspirin in patients with SSc and severe digital ischaemia, although it has to be recognised there is no good evidence base for this

winter, with the aim of reducing severity of Raynaud's attacks and preventing digital ulceration. However, IV prostanoids require hospitalisation and what are required are safe, effective oral prostanoids. So far experience with oral prostanoids has been disappointing [115, 116]. A recent study of oral treprostinil in the treatment of SSc-related digital ulcers did not meet its primary endpoint but did show a trend towards reduction in net ulcer burden compared to placebo [117].

Supplementation of the L-Arginine/NO Pathway, Including Phosphodiesterase Inhibitors

This is an area of 'moving' therapeutics. NO is a potent vasodilator, and there has been recent interest in topical (transdermal) NO donation. Applying glyceryl trinitrate, an NO donor, produces both local [118] and systemic [119] vasodilation. The ideal would be to have an easy to use, topical NO donor which is effective but free from adverse effects, in other words a preparation which maximises local but minimises systemic effects. A randomised placebo-controlled trial of topical nitrate therapy [120] in 219 patients, administered as a novel formulation of nitroglycerin, MQX-503, demonstrated benefit in terms of improvement in Raynaud's Condition Score (RCS). The improvement in RCS after 4 weeks' treatment was less in patients with SSc-related RP than in those with primary RP, although there was a placebo response in patients with primary Raynaud's. There were no differences in side effects (including headaches and dizziness) between groups. Topical nitrate therapy deserves further research.

Phosphodiesterase type 5 (PDE5) inhibitors enhance the effect of NO by inhibiting degradation of cyclic guanosine monophosphate. Although earlier controlled clinical trials of phosphodiesterase inhibitors in RP including patients with SSc gave somewhat conflicting results [121–123], recent studies suggest that phosphodiesterase inhibitors confer benefit

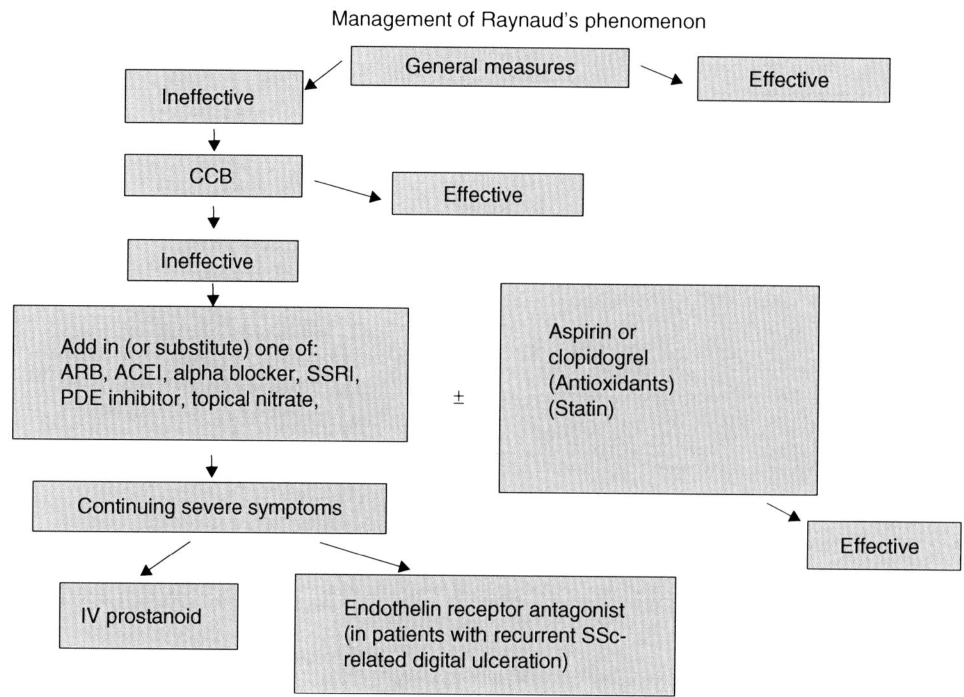

Fig. 20.8 Management of Raynaud's phenomenon. Drugs in parentheses indicate possible future approaches. General measures: avoid stress, cold exposure, trauma and smoking. *CCB* calcium channel blocker, *ARB* angiotensin II receptor blocker, *ACEI* angiotensin-converting enzyme inhibitor, *SSRI* serotonin reuptake inhibitor, *PDE* phosphodiesterase inhibitor

[123–125] and a very recent study [126] showed comparable efficacy with udenafil 100 mg/day and amlodipine 10 mg/day in terms of improving RP attacks. A meta-analysis suggested that phosphodiesterase inhibitors conferred benefit in patients with secondary RP in terms of Raynaud's Condition Score and frequency and duration of RP attacks [127]. Phosphodiesterase inhibitors are now being used increasingly in SSc-related RP, especially in severe Raynaud's which does not respond to calcium channel blockers. It is important to highlight that to date, controlled trials have been of short duration (6 weeks or less on active treatment). Further clinical trials of longer duration are required to establish the place of phosphodiesterase inhibition in SSc-related digital ischaemia.

Drugs Which Inhibit Vasoconstriction

Angiotensin-Converting Enzyme (ACE) Inhibitors and Angiotensin II Receptor Blockers

Angiotensin II is not only vasoconstrictive but also profibrotic, and so there is a strong rationale for angiotensin-converting enzyme (ACE) and angiotensin II receptor blockers in SSc-related RP. However, the evidence base for their use is weak. A multicentre, double-blind, placebo-controlled trial of quinapril in 210 patients with either limited cutaneous SSc (186 patients) or antibody positive RP reported no benefit in peripheral vascular manifestations after 2–3 years' treatment [128]. Although losartan has been reported to be more effective than nifedipine, this was in a small open study and the dose of nifedipine was low (20 mg) [129]. Further studies are required especially of angiotensin II receptor blockers.

α-Adrenergic Blockers

There is a limited evidence base for non-selective α-receptor blockade in SSc-related Raynaud's phenomenon [130]. If an α-receptor blocker is used in combination with a calcium channel blocker, then a low initial dose must be used because of concerns about the combination leading to hypotension. Increased understanding of the role of the cold-sensitive α_{2C}-adrenoreceptor in the pathogenesis of RP may lead to further research into selective blockade of α_{2C}-adrenoreceptor [18, 131].

Endothelin-1 Receptor Antagonists

The considerable interest in the role of ET-1 in the pathogenesis of SSc has been matched by the investigation of the therapeutic effects of ET-1 receptor antagonism including in the treatment of SSc-related digital vascular disease. Two large multicentre studies [132, 133] both found that bosentan, which antagonises both ET_A and ET_B ET-1 receptors, reduced the number of new digital ulcers but had no effect on the healing of existing ulcers. In the first study (RAPIDS-1) of 122 patients with SSc [132], the number of new ulcers during the 16-week study period was 1.4 in the bosentan versus 2.7 in the placebo-treated group. In addition, there were beneficial effects on hand function. Therefore, ET-1 receptor antagonism should be considered in patients with recurrent digital ulcers refractory to other treatments.

Serotonin Reuptake Inhibitors

Serotonin is a vasoconstrictor; therefore, drugs antagonising its effects or limiting its availability may prevent vasoconstriction. An open-label study in 53 patients [134] suggested that fluoxetine, a selective serotonin reuptake inhibitor, was beneficial in both primary and secondary RP. An advantage of this class of drugs is that they are less likely to cause vasodilatory side effects than some of the other drugs discussed above. However, further research is required to establish their place in SSc-related RP.

Drugs Which Prevent or Reduce SSc-Related Vasculopathy

There is no drug currently known to prevent SSc-related digital vasculopathy. Yet this is the ideal and, as a next step, to remodel the distorted vasculature. This will be an area of active research over the next 10 years. Although current treatment recommendations are confined to vasodilation (with some clinicians favouring addition of an antiplatelet agent as discussed below), the aim in the future is to be in a position to recommend additional therapies, some of which are given in parentheses in Fig. 20.8.

Antithrombotics

Platelet activation is well recognised in SSc, and amputated digits from patients with SSc often show thrombotic occlusion. Thus, there is a strong therapeutic rationale for antithrombotics, although there is no good evidence base for this and it seems unlikely that a well-designed clinical trial of antiplatelet therapy will ever be performed. The pragmatic approach is to give low-dose aspirin to patients with severe digital ischaemia, bearing in mind that many patients have upper gastrointestinal disease and another antiplatelet agent such as clopidogrel may therefore be preferable. As discussed above, several drugs whose predominant benefit in RP is likely to be vasodilation may also have antiplatelet effects, including prostanoids and calcium channel blockers. Low molecular weight heparin [135], tissue plasminogen activator followed by warfarin [136] and *FXIII* [137] have been reported to confer benefit in small open studies, but further studies are required before these can be recommended even for severe digital ischaemia.

Antioxidants

On the assumption that oxidant stress is an important contributor to pathogenesis, antioxidants should be beneficial [138]. Yet despite there having been a number of trials of different antioxidants, none of these trials has shown definite benefit, reasons including small numbers of patients studied, short durations of treatment and patients often having late disease and possibly irreversible vascular injury. Although N-acetylcysteine was recently reported to confer benefit in SSc-related digital ulceration [139], this was in an open study and so results need to be confirmed in a controlled trial.

Future Approaches

Several other drugs might have beneficial effect on SSc-related digital vascular problems.

Statins could be effective via a number of different mechanisms: Abou-Raya et al. reported improvements in both clinical and laboratory measurements in patients with SSc treated with atorvastatin, indicating that statins deserve further research [140, 141]. RhoA/Rho-kinase inhibitors [16] have mechanisms of action which could prevent SSc-related vasculopathy (see Pathogenesis). A laboratory-based cold challenge study showed no benefit from fasudil, a Rho-kinase inhibitor, in terms of skin temperature recovery and digital blood flow after acute dosing [142]. A number of different drugs currently prescribed predominantly for their vasodilatory actions – prostanoids, ACE inhibitors and ET-1 receptor antagonists – have effects on vascular remodelling [112, 143, 144]: although it is premature to recommend prescribing these, singly or in combination, with the aim of preventing progression of SSc-related vasculopathy, what are required are clinical trials of these drugs in early disease.

Surgery

Surgery will be discussed under below under treatment of 'Ischaemic complications': it has no role in SSc-related RP unless this progresses to near critical ischaemia and/or digital ulceration.

Treatment Approach to Digital Ulceration and Critical Ischaemia

Critical ischaemia and digital ulceration often coexist, and the principles of management are the same with the emphasis on early intervention (Fig. 20.9). Ideally, there should be an open-door policy to allow early assessment and treatment. The use of iloprost infusions and endothelin-1 receptor antagonists in patients with digital ulceration has already been referred to above. The EULAR treatment recommendations for treatment of SSc [145] include recommendations for digital ulcers. A recent meta-analysis of clinical trials of SSc-related digital ulcers highlights the need for larger studies and for standardised outcome measures [146].

Critical ischaemia is always a medical emergency: after checking that there is no concomitant problem requiring

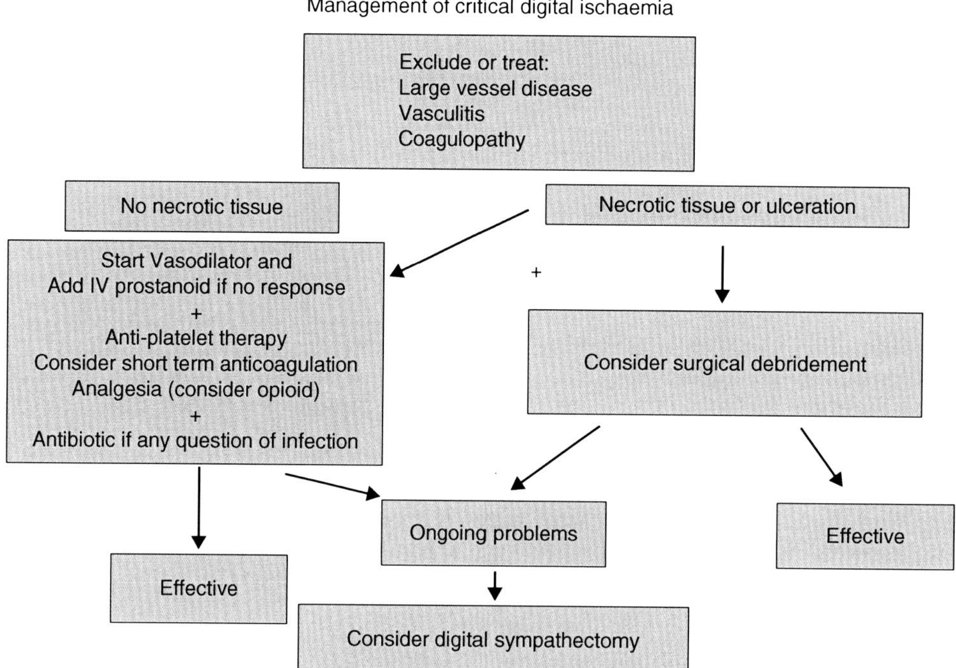

Fig. 20.9 Management of critical digital ischaemia. Intravenous prostaglandins can be used if no rapid response to oral vasodilators. Anticoagulation can be used for 48–72 h. Antiplatelet therapy with aspirin is recommended

specific treatment (proximal vessel disease, vasculitis or a coagulopathy), the key points are:

1. Adequate analgesia. These lesions can be excruciatingly painful, and opiates are often required.
2. Intravenous prostanoids, to maximise perfusion.
3. Antibiotics if there is any possibility of infection.
4. Skilled nursing care, with tissue viability input.
5. Surgical invention if indicated. The commonest procedure is debridement of necrotic tissue and release of any pus. This is likely to be indicated when the affected area, for example, the fingertip, is acutely tender. It is best to involve the surgical team early, before bone infection becomes established. In recent years, there has been increasing interest in digital (palmar) sympathectomy [147–149], sometimes in combination with decompression arteriolysis of the radial and ulnar arteries proximal to the wrist, and vascular reconstruction [150]. Some of the benefit of digital sympathectomy is likely to be from the decompression resulting from the adventitial strip [151]. Digital sympathectomy is a highly specialised procedure, performed only in specialist centres. When an ulcer overlies an area of calcinosis, surgical debulking of the calcinosis may facilitate ulcer healing. It is important to highlight that there are no controlled trials of any form of surgical intervention for RP [152].
6. Botulinum toxin. Injections of botulinum toxin are being increasingly used in patients with severe RP and digital ulceration or critical ischaemia [153–155]. However, controlled clinical trials are required.
7. Possible future new treatment approaches These may include injectable cell-based therapy, the rationale being that bone marrow cells might stimulate angiogenesis. However, such approaches need to be put to the test in clinical trials.

References

1. LeRoy EC, Medsger Jr TA. Raynaud's phenomenon: a proposal for classification. Clin Exp Rheumatol. 1992;10:485–8.
2. Flavahan NA. A vascular mechanistic approach to understanding Raynaud phenomenon. Nat Rev Rheumatol. 2015;11:146–58.
3. Flavahan NA. Pathophysiological regulation of the cutaneous vascular system. In: Wigley FM, Herrick AL, Flavahan NA, editors. Raynaud's phenomenon: a guide to pathogenesis and treatment. New York: Springer Science+Business Media; 2015. doi:10.1007/978-1-4939-1526-2.
4. McKemy DD. How cold is it? TRPM8 and TRPA1 in the molecular logic of cold sensation. Mol Pain. 2005;1:16.
5. Schepers RJ, Ringkamp M. Thermoreceptors and thermosensitive afferents. Neurosci Biobehav Rev. 2010;34:177–84.
6. McKemy DD, Neuhausser WM, Julius D. Identification of a cold receptor reveals a general role for TRP channels in thermosensation. Nature. 2002;416:52–8.
7. Charkoudian N. Mechanisms and modifiers of reflex induced cutaneous vasodilation and vasoconstriction in humans. J Appl Physiol. 2010;109:1221–8.
8. Coffman JD, Cohen AS. Total and capillary fingertip blood flow in Raynaud's phenomenon. N Engl J Med. 1971;285:259–63.
9. Hummers LK, Wigley FM. Management of Raynaud's phenomenon and digital ischemic lesions in scleroderma. Rheum Dis Clin N Am. 2003;29:293–313.
10. Suter LG, Murabito JM, Felson DT, et al. The incidence and natural history of Raynaud's phenomenon in the community. Arthritis Rheum. 2005;52:1259–63.

11. Freedman RR, Mayes MD. Familial aggregation of primary Raynaud's disease. Arthritis Rheum. 1996;39:1189–91.
12. Meier FM, Frommer KW, Dinser R, et al. Update on the profile of the EUSTAR cohort: an analysis of the EULAR Scleroderma Trials and Research group database. Ann Rheum Dis. 2012;71: 1355–60.
13. Matucci-Cerinic M, Kahaleh B, Wigley FM. Evidence that systemic sclerosis is a vascular disease. Arthritis Rheum. 2013;65: 1953–62.
14. Steen V, Denton CP, Pope JE, et al. Digital ulcers: overt vascular disease in systemic sclerosis. Rheumatology (Oxford). 2009;48 Suppl 3:iii19–24.
15. Maricq HR, Downey JA, LeRoy EC. Standstill of nailfold capillary blood flow during cooling in scleroderma and Raynaud's syndrome. Blood Vessels. 1976;13:338–49.
16. Flavahan NA. Regulation of vascular reactivity in scleroderma: new insights into Raynaud's phenomenon. Rheum Dis Clin N Am. 2008;34:81–7.
17. Freedman RR, Moten M, Migály P, et al. Cold-induced potentiation of alpha 2-adrenergic vasoconstriction in primary Raynaud's disease. Arthritis Rheum. 1993;36:685–90.
18. Wise RA, Wigley FM, White B, et al. Efficacy and tolerability of a selective alpha(2 C)-adrenergic receptor blocker in recovery from cold-induced vasospasm in scleroderma patients: a single-center, double-blind, placebo-controlled, randomized crossover study. Arthritis Rheum. 2004;50:3994–4001.
19. Chotani MA, Flavahan S, Mitra S, et al. Silent alpha(2 C)-adrenergic receptors enable cold-induced vasoconstriction in cutaneous arteries. Am J Physiol Heart Circ Physiol. 2000;27: H1075–83.
20. Bailey SR, Mitra S, Flavahan S, et al. Reactive oxygen species from smooth muscle mitochondria initiate cold-induced constriction of cutaneous arteries. Am J Physiol Heart Circ Physiol. 2005;289:H243–50.
21. Freedman RR, Baer RP, Mayes MD. Blockade of vasospastic attacks by α_2-adrenergic but not alpha 1-adrenergic antagonists in idiopathic Raynaud's disease. Circulation. 1995;92:1448–51.
22. Flavahan NA, Flavahan S, Liu Q, et al. Increased alpha2-adrenergic constriction of isolated arterioles in diffuse scleroderma. Arthritis Rheum. 2000;43:1886–90.
23. Furspan PB, Chatterjee S, Mayes MD, et al. Cooling-induced contraction and protein tyrosine kinase activity of isolated arterioles in secondary Raynaud's phenomenon. Rheumatology (Oxford). 2005;44:488–94.
24. Furspan PB, Chatterjee S, Freedman RR. Increased tyrosine phosphorylation mediates the cooling-induced contraction and increased vascular reactivity of Raynaud's disease. Arthritis Rheum. 2004;50:1578–85.
25. Generini S, Seibold JR, Matucci-Cerinic M. Estrogens and neuropeptides in Raynaud's phenomenon. Rheum Dis Clin N Am. 2005;31:177–86.
26. Bunker CB, Terenghi G, Springall DR, et al. Deficiency of calcitonin gene-related peptide in Raynaud's phenomenon. Lancet. 1990;336:1530–3.
27. Bunker CB, Reavley C, O'Shaughnessy DJ, et al. Calcitonin gene-related peptide in treatment of severe peripheral vascular insufficiency in Raynaud's phenomenon. Lancet. 1993;342:80–3.
28. Stephens DP, Saad AR, Bennett LA, et al. Neuropeptide Y antagonism reduces reflex cutaneous vasoconstriction in humans. Am J Physiol Heart Circ Physiol. 2004;287:H1404–9.
29. Chung MS, Gong HS, Baek GH. Prevalence of Raynaud's phenomenon in patients with idiopathic carpal tunnel syndrome. J Bone Joint Surg Br. 1999;81:1017–9.
30. Tabata H, Yamakage A, Yamazaki S. Cutaneous localization of endothelin-1 in patients with systemic sclerosis: immunoelectron microscopic study. Int J Dermatol. 1997;36:272–5.
31. Freedman RR, Girgis R, Mayes MD. Endothelial and adrenergic dysfunction in Raynaud's phenomenon and scleroderma. J Rheumatol. 1999;26:2386–8.
32. Abraham DJ, Krieg T, Distler J, et al. Overview of pathogenesis of systemic sclerosis. Rheumatology (Oxford). 2009;48 Suppl 3:iii3–7.
33. Kahaleh MB. Endothelin, an endothelial-dependent vasoconstrictor in scleroderma. Enhanced production and profibrotic action. Arthritis Rheum. 1991;34:978–83.
34. Freedman RR, Girgis R, Mayes MD. Acute effect of nitric oxide on Raynaud's phenomenon in scleroderma. Lancet. 1999;354:739.
35. Blaise S, Maas R, Trocme C, et al. Correlation of biomarkers of endothelium dysfunction and matrix remodelling in patients with systemic sclerosis. J Rheumatol. 2009;36:984–8.
36. Sinici I, Kalyoncu U, Karahan S, et al. Endothelial nitric oxide gene polymorphism and risk of systemic sclerosis: predisposition effect of T-786 C promoter and protective effect of 27 bp repeats in Intron 4. Clin Exp Rheumatol. 2010;28:169–75.
37. Matucci Cerinic M, Kahaleh MB. Beauty and the beast. The nitric oxide paradox in systemic sclerosis. Rheumatology (Oxford). 2002;41:843–7.
38. Reilly IA, Roy L, Fitzgerald GA. Biosynthesis of thromboxane in patients with systemic sclerosis and Raynaud's phenomenon. Br Med J (Clin Res Ed). 1986;292:1037–9.
39. Pamuk GE, Turgut B, Pamuk ON, et al. Increased circulating platelet-leucocyte complexes in patients with primary Raynaud's phenomenon and Raynaud's phenomenon secondary to systemic sclerosis: a comparative study. Blood Coagul Fibrinolysis. 2007;18:297–302.
40. Wigley FM. Raynaud's phenomenon is linked to unopposed estrogen replacement therapy in postmenopausal women. Clin Exp Rheumatol. 2001;19:10–1.
41. Eid AH, Maiti K, Mitra S, et al. Estrogen increases smooth muscle expression of α_{2C}-adrenoceptors and cold-induced constriction of cutaneous arteries. Am J Physiol Heart Circ Physiol. 2007;293: H1955–61.
42. Bruckdorfer KR, Hillary JB, Bunce T, et al. Increased susceptibility to oxidation of low-density lipoproteins isolated from patients with systemic sclerosis. Arthritis Rheum. 1995;38:1060–7.
43. Denton CP, Bunce TD, Dorado MB, et al. Probucol improves symptoms and reduces lipoprotein oxidation susceptibility in patients with Raynaud's phenomenon. Rheumatology (Oxford). 1999;38:309–15.
44. Faller DV. Endothelial cell responses to hypoxic stress. Clin Exp Pharmacol Physiol. 1999;26:74–84.
45. Amanzi L, Braschi F, Fiori G, Galluccio F, Miniati I, Guiducci S, et al. Digital ulcers in scleroderma: staging, characteristics and sub-setting through observation of 1614 digital lesions. Rheumatology. 2010;49:1374–82.
46. Nihtyanova SI, Brough GM, Black CM, Denton CP. Clinical burden of digital vasculopathy in limited and diffuse systemic sclerosis. Ann Rheum Dis. 2008;67:120–3.
47. Berezne A, Seror R, Morell-Dubois S, et al. Impact of systemic sclerosis on occupational and professional activity with attention to patients with digital ulcers. Arthritis Care Res. 2011;63:277–85.
48. Guillevin L, Hunsche E, Denton CP, Kreig T, Schwierin B, Rosenberg D, et al. Functional impairment of systemic scleroderma patients with digital ulcerations: results from the DUO registry. Clin Exp Rheumatol. 2013;31(2 Suppl 76):71–80.
49. Rannou F, Poiraudeau S, Berezne A, et al. Assessing disability and quality of life in systemic sclerosis: construct validities of the Cochin Hand Function Scale, Health Assessment Questionnaire (HAQ), systemic sclerosis HAQ, and Medical Outcomes Study 36-Item Short Form health survey. Arthritis Rheum. 2007;57:94–102.
50. Mouthon L, Mestre-Stanilas C, Berezne A, et al. Impact of digital ulcers on disability and health related quality of life in systemic sclerosis. Ann Rheum Dis. 2010;69:214–7.

51. Ennis H, Vail A, Wragg E, Taylor A, Moore T, Murray A, et al. A prospective study of systemic sclerosis-related digital ulcers: prevalence, location, and functional impact. Scand J Rheumatol. 2013;42:483–6.
52. Mouthon L, Carpentier P, Lok C, Clerson P, Gressin V, Hachulla E, et al. Ischemic digital ulcers affect hand disability and pain in systemic sclerosis. J Rheumatol. 2014;41:1317–23.
53. Khimdas S, Harding S, Bonner A, et al. Associations with digital ulcers in a large cohort of systemic sclerosis: results from the Canadian Scleroderma Research Group Registry. Arthritis Care Res (Hoboken). 2011;63:142–9.
54. Denton CP, Krieg T, Guillevin L, et al. Demographic, clinical and antibody characteristics of patients with digital ulcers in systemic sclerosis: data from the DUO Registry. Ann Rheum Dis. 2012;71:718–21.
55. Hachulla E, Clerson P, Launay D, et al. Natural history of ischemic digital ulcers in systemic sclerosis: single-center retrospective longitudinal study. J Rheumatol. 2007;34:2423–30.
56. Zhou A, Muir L, Harris J, Herrick A. The impact of magnetic resonance (MR) imaging in early diagnosis of hand osteomyelitis in patients with systemic sclerosis. Clin Exp Rheumatol. 2014;32(6 Suppl 86):S-232.
57. Bruni C, Guiducci S, Bellando-Randone S, et al. Digital ulcers as a sentinel sign for early internal organ involvement in very early systemic sclerosis. Rheumatology. 2015;54:72–6.
58. Mihai C, Landewé R, van der Heijde D, et al. Digital ulcers predict a worse disease course in patients with systemic sclerosis. Ann Rheum Dis. 2015. doi:10.1136/annrheumdis-2014-205897.
59. Veale DJ, Collidge TA, Belch JJF. Increased prevalence of symptomatic macrovascular disease in systemic sclerosis. Ann Rheum Dis. 1995;54:853–5.
60. Ho M, Veale D, Eastmond C, et al. Macrovascular disease and systemic sclerosis. Ann Rheum Dis. 2000;59:39–43.
61. Youseff P, Brama T, Englert H, et al. Limited scleroderma is associated with increased prevalence of macrovascular disease. J Rheumatol. 1995;22:469–72.
62. Maricq HR, LeRoy EC. Patterns of finger capillary abnormalities in connective tissue disease by 'widefield' microscopy. Arthritis Rheum. 1973;16:619–28.
63. Herrick AL, Cutolo M. Clinical implications from capillaroscopic analysis in patients with Raynaud's phenomenon and systemic sclerosis. Arthritis Rheum. 2010;62:2595–604.
64. Darton K, Black CM. Pyroelectric vidicon thermography and cold challenge quantify the severity of Raynaud's phenomenon. Br J Rheumatol. 1991;30:190–5.
65. O'Reilly D, Taylor L, El-Hadidy K, et al. Measurement of cold challenge responses in primary Raynaud's phenomenon and Raynaud's phenomenon associated with systemic sclerosis. Ann Rheum Dis. 1992;51:1193–6.
66. Clark S, Hollis S, Campbell F, et al. The 'distal-dorsal difference' as a possible predictor of secondary Raynaud's phenomenon. J Rheumatol. 1999;26:1125–8.
67. Anderson ME, Moore TL, Lunt M, et al. The 'distal-dorsal difference': a thermographic parameter by which to differentiate between primary and secondary Raynaud's phenomenon. Rheumatology. 2007;46:533–8.
68. Pauling JD, Flower V, Shipley JA, Harris ND, McHugh NJ. Influence of the cold challenge on the discriminatory capacity of the digital distal-dorsal difference in the thermographic assessment of Raynaud's phenomenon. Microvasc Res. 2011;82:364–8.
69. Clark S, Campbell F, Moore T, et al. Laser Doppler imaging - a new technique for quantifying microcirculatory flow in patients with primary Raynaud's phenomenon and systemic sclerosis. Microvasc Res. 1999;57:284–91.
70. Maricq HR, Weinrich MC, Valter I, et al. Digital vascular responses to cooling in subjects with cold sensitivity, primary Raynaud's phenomenon, or scleroderma-spectrum disorders. J Rheumatol. 1996;23:2068–78.
71. LeRoy EC, Medsger TA. Criteria for the classification of early systemic sclerosis. J Rheumatol. 2001;28:1573–6.
72. Matucci-Cerinic M, Allanore Y, Czirják L, et al. The challenge of early systemic sclerosis for the EULAR Scleroderma Trial and Research Group (EUSTAR) community: it is time to cut the Gordian knot and develop a prevention or rescue strategy. Ann Rheum Dis. 2009;68:1377–80.
73. Koenig M, Joyal F, Fritzler MJ, et al. Autoantibodies and microvascular damage are independent predictive factors for the progression of Raynaud's phenomenon to systemic sclerosis: a twenty-year prospective study of 586 patients, with validation of proposed criteria for early systemic sclerosis. Arthritis Rheum. 2008;58:3902–12.
74. Ingegnoli F, Boracchi P, Gualtierotti R, et al. Improving outcome prediction of systemic sclerosis from isolated Raynaud's phenomenon: role of autoantibodies and nail-fold capillaroscopy. Rheumatology. 2010;49:797–805.
75. Avouac J, Fransen J, Walker UA, et al. Preliminary criteria for the very early diagnosis of systemic sclerosis: results of a Delphi Consensus Study from EULAR Scleroderma Trials and Research Group. Ann Rheum Dis. 2011;70:476–81.
76. Van den Hoogen F, Khanna D, Fransen J, Johnson SR, Baron M, Tyndall A, et al. 2013 classification criteria for systemic sclerosis. Arthritis Rheum. 2013;65:2737–47.
77. Van den Hoogen F, Khanna D, Fransen J, Johnson SR, Baron M, Tyndall A, et al. 2013 classification criteria for systemic sclerosis. Ann Rheum Dis. 2013;72:1747–55.
78. Maricq HR. Widefield capillary microscopy. Technique and rating scale for abnormalities seen in scleroderma and related disorders. Arthritis Rheum. 1981;24:1159–65.
79. Cutolo M, Sulli A, Smith V. How to perform and interpret capillaroscopy. Best Pract Res Clin Rheumatol. 2013;27:237–48.
80. Sebastiani M, Manfredi A, Colaci M, et al. Capillaroscopic skin ulcer risk index: a new prognostic tool for digital skin ulcer development in systemic sclerosis patients. Arthritis Rheum. 2009;61:688–94.
81. Smith V, De Keyser F, Pizzorni C, et al. Nailfold capillaroscopy for day-to-day clinical use: construction of a simple scoring modality as a clinical prognostic index for digital trophic lesions. Ann Rheum Dis. 2011;70:180–3.
82. Cutolo M, Herrick AL, Distler O, et al. Nailfold videocapillaroscopic and other clinical risk factors for digital ulcers in systemic sclerosis: a multicenter, prospective cohort study. Arthritis Rheumatol 2016 (Epub ahead of print).
83. Anders HJ, Sigl T, Schattenkirchner M. Differentiation between primary and secondary Raynaud's phenomenon: a prospective study comparing nailfold capillaroscopy using an ophthalmoscope or stereomicroscope. Ann Rheum Dis. 2001;60:407–9.
84. Bergman R, Sharony L, Shapira D, et al. The handheld dermatoscope as a nail-fold capillaroscopic instrument. Arch Dermatol. 2003;139:1027–30.
85. Baron M, Bell M, Bookman A, et al. Office capillaroscopy in systemic sclerosis. Clin Rheumatol. 2007;26:1268–74.
86. Moore TL, Murray AK, Roberts C, et al. Reliability of dermoscopy in the assessment of patients with Raynaud's phenomenon. Rheumatology. 2010;49:542–7.
87. Hudson M, Taileerfer S, Steele R, et al. Improving the sensitivity of the American College of Rheumatology classification criteria for systemic sclerosis. Clin Exp Rheumatol. 2007;25:754–7.
88. Hughes M, Moore T, O'Leary N, Tracey A, Ennis H, Dinsdale G, et al. A study comparing videocapillaroscopy and dermoscopy in the assessment of nailfold capillaries in patients with systemic sclerosis-spectrum disorders. Rheumatology 2015;154:251–9.

89. White C. Intermittent claudication. N Engl J Med. 2007;356:1241–50.
90. Hasegawa M, Nagai Y, Tamura A, et al. Arteriographic evaluation of vascular changes of the extremities in patients with systemic sclerosis. Br J Dermatol. 2006;155:1159–64.
91. Allanore Y, Seror R, Chevrot A, et al. Hand vascular involvement assessed by magnetic resonance angiography in systemic sclerosis. Arthritis Rheum. 2007;56:2747–54.
92. Sheehan JJ, Fan Z, Davarpanah AH, et al. Nonenhanced MR angiography of the hand with flow-sensitive dephasing-prepared balanced SSFP sequence: initial experience with systemic sclerosis. Radiology. 2011;259:248–56.
93. Zhang W, Xu JR, Lu Q, Ye S, Liu XS. High-resolution magnetic resonance angiography or digital arteries in SSc patients on 3 Tesla: preliminary study. Rheumatology. 2011;50:1712–9.
94. Murray A, Pauling JD, Flavahan. Non-invasive methods of assessing Raynaud's phenomenon. In: Wigley FM, Herrick AL, Flavahan NA, editors. Raynaud's phenomenon: a guide to pathogenesis and treatment. New York: Springer Science+Business Media; 2015. doi:10.1007/978-1-4939-1526-2_4.
95. Anderson ME, Allen PD, Moore T, et al. Computerised nailfold video capillaroscopy – a new tool for the assessment of Raynaud's phenomenon. J Rheumatol. 2005;32:841–8.
96. Moore TL, Vail A, Herrick AL. Assessment of digital vascular structure and function in response to bosentan in patients with systemic sclerosis-related Raynaud's phenomenon. Rheumatology. 2007;46:363–4.
97. Guiducci S, Bellando Randone S, Bruni C, Carnesecchi G, Maresta A, Iannone F, et al. Bosentan fosters de-remodelling in systemic sclerosis. Clin Rheumatol. 2012;31:1723–5.
98. Cutolo M, Zampogna G, Vremis L, Smith V, Pizzorna C, Sulli A. Longterm effects of endothelin receptor antagonism on microvascular damage evaluated by nailfold capillaroscopic analysis in systemic sclerosis. J Rheumatol. 2013;40:40–5.
99. Murray AK, Vail A, Moore TL, Manning JB, Taylor CJ, Herrick AL. The influence of measurement location on reliability of quantitative nailfold videocapillaroscopy in patients with SSc. Rheumatology. 2012;51:1323–30.
100. Allen J, Howell K. Microvascular imaging: techniques and opportunities for clinical physiological measurements. Physiol Meas. 2014;35:R91–141.
101. Murray A, Herrick AL, King TA. Laser Doppler imaging: a developing technique for application in the rheumatic diseases. Rheumatology. 2004;43:1210–8.
102. Murray AK, Moore TL, Manning JB, et al. Noninvasive imaging techniques in the assessment of scleroderma spectrum disorders. Arthritis Care Res. 2009;61:1103–11.
103. Ruaro B, Sulli A, Alessandri E, Pizzorni C, Ferrari G, Cutolo M. Laser speckle contrast analysis: a new method to evaluate peripheral blood perfusion in systemic sclerosis patients. Ann Rheum Dis. 2014;73:1181–5.
104. Harrison BJ, Silman AJ, Hider SL, Herrick AL. Cigarette smoking: a significant risk factor for digital vascular diseases in patients with systemic sclerosis. Arthritis Rheum. 2002;46:3312–6.
105. Hudson M, Lo E, Lu Y, Canadian Scleroderma Research Group, et al. Cigarette smoking in patients with systemic sclerosis. Arthritis Rheum. 2011;63(1):230–8.
106. Thompson AE, Shea B, Welch V, et al. Calcium-channel blockers for Raynaud's phenomenon in systemic sclerosis. Arthritis Rheum. 2001;44:1841–7.
107. Sturgill MG, Seibold JR. Rational use of calcium-channel antagonists in Raynaud's phenomenon. Curr Opin Rheumatol. 1998;10:584–8.
108. Malamet R, Wise RA, Ettinger WH, et al. Nifedipine in the treatment of Raynaud's phenomenon. Evidence for inhibition of platelet activation. Am J Med. 1985;78:602–8.
109. Allanore Y, Borderie D, Lemarechal H, et al. Acute and sustained effects of dihydropyridine-type calcium channel antagonists on oxidative stress in systemic sclerosis. Am J Med. 2004;116:595–600.
110. Fishman AP. Pulmonary hypertension – beyond vasodilator therapy. N Engl J Med. 1998;338:321–2.
111. Wigley FM, Wise RA, Seibold JR, et al. Intravenous iloprost infusion in patients with Raynaud phenomenon secondary to systemic sclerosis. A multicenter, placebo-controlled, double-blind study. Ann Intern Med. 1994;120:199–206.
112. Pope J, Fenlon D, Thompson A, et al. Iloprost and cisaprost for Raynaud's phenomenon in progressive systemic sclerosis. Cochrane Database Syst Rev. 2000;2:CD000953.
113. Wigley FM, Korn JH, Csuka ME, et al. Oral iloprost treatment in patients with Raynaud's phenomenon secondary to systemic sclerosis: a multi-center, placebo-controlled, double-blind study. Arthritis Rheum. 1998;41:670–7.
114. Vayssairat M. Preventative effect of an oral prostacyclin analog, beraprost sodium, on digital necrosis in systemic sclerosis. French Microcirculation Society Multicentre Group for the Study of Vascular Acrosyndromes. J Rheumatol. 1999;26:2173–88.
115. Seibold JR, Wigley FM, Schiopu E, et al. Digital ischemic ulcers in systemic sclerosis treated with oral treprostinil diethanolamine: a randomized, double-blind, placebo-controlled, multicenter study. Arthritis Rheum. 2011;63(10 Suppl S):S968–9 (abstract).
116. Anderson ME, Moore TL, Hollis S, et al. Digital vascular response to topical glyceryl trinitrate, as measured by laser Doppler imaging, in primary Raynaud's phenomenon and systemic sclerosis. Rheumatology. 2002;41:324–8.
117. Teh LS, Manning J, Moore T, et al. Sustained-release transdermal glyceryl trinitrate patches as a treatment for primary and secondary Raynaud's phenomenon. Br J Rheumatol. 1995;34:636–41.
118. Chung L, Shapiro L, Fiorentino D, et al. MQX-503, a novel formulation of nitroglycerin, improves the severity of Raynaud's phenomenon. Arthritis Rheum. 2009;60:870–7.
119. Fries R, Shariat K, von Wilmowsky H, et al. Sildenafil in the treatment of Raynaud's phenomenon resistant to vasodilatory therapy. Circulation. 2005;112:2980–5.
120. Schiopu E, Hsu VM, Impens AJ, et al. Randomized placebo-controlled crossover trial of tadalafil in Raynaud's phenomenon secondary to systemic sclerosis. J Rheumatol. 2009;36:2264–8.
121. Herrick AL, van den Hoogen F, Gabrielli A, et al. Modified-release sildenafil reduces Raynaud's attack frequency in limited cutaneous systemic sclerosis. Arthritis Rheum. 2011;63:775–82.
122. Shenoy PD, Kumar S, Jha LK, Choudhary SK, Singh U, Misra R, et al. Efficacy of tadalafil in secondary Raynaud's phenomenon resistant to vasodilator therapy: a double-blind randomized crossover trial. Rheumatology. 2010;49:2420–8.
123. Caglayan E, Axmann S, Hellmich M, Moinzadeh P, Rosenkranz S. Vardenafil for the treatment of Raynaud phenomenon: a randomized, double-blind, placebo-controlled crossover study. Arch Intern Med. 2012;172:1182–4.
124. Lee EY, Park JK, Lee W, Kim YK, Park CS, Giles JT, et al. Head-to-head comparison of udenafil vs amlodipine in the treatment of secondary Raynaud's phenomenon: a double-blind, randomized, cross-over study. Rheumatology. 2014;53(4):658–64.
125. Roustit M, Blaise S, Allanore Y, et al. Phosphodiesterase-5 inhibitors for the treatment of secondary Raynaud's phenomenon: systematic review and meta-analysis of randomised trials. Ann Rheum Dis. 2013;72:1696–9.
126. Gliddon AE, Doré CJ, Black CM, et al. Prevention of vascular damage in scleroderma and autoimmune Raynaud's phenomenon: a randomised controlled trial of the ACE-inhibitor quinapril. Arthritis Rheum. 2007;56:3837–46.
127. Dziadzio M, Denton CP, Smith R, et al. Losartan therapy for Raynaud's phenomenon and scleroderma: clinical and biochemical

findings in a fifteen-week, randomized, parallel-group, controlled trial. Arthritis Rheum. 1999;42:2646–55.
128. Pope J, Fenlon D, Thompson A, Shea B, Furst D, Wells G, et al. Prazosin for Raynaud's phenomenon in progressive systemic sclerosis. Cochrane Database Syst Rev. 2000;2:CD000956.
129. Herrick AL, Murray AK, Ruck A, Rouru J, Moore TL, Whiteside J, Hakulinen P, Wigley F, Snapir A. A double-blind randomised placebo-controlled crossover trial of the alpha2 C-adrenoceptor antagonist ORM-12741 for prevention of cold-induced vasospasm in patients with systemic sclerosis. Rheumatology. 2014;53(5): 948–52.
130. Korn JH, Mayes M, Matucci-Cerinic M, et al. For the RAPIDS-1 study group. Digital ulcers in systemic sclerosis. Prevention by treatment with bosentan, an oral endothelin receptor antagonist. Arthritis Rheum. 2004;50:3985–93.
131. Matucci-Cerinic M, Denton CP, Furst DE, et al. Bosentan treatment of digital ulcers related to systemic sclerosis: results from the RAPIDS-2 randomised, double-blind, placebo-controlled trial. Ann Rheum Dis. 2011;70:32–8.
132. Coleiro B, Marshall SE, Denton CP, et al. Treatment of Raynaud's phenomenon with the selective serotonin reuptake inhibitor fluoxetine. Rheumatology. 2001;40:1038–43.
133. Denton CP, Howell K, Stratton RJ, et al. Long-term low molecular weight heparin therapy for severe Raynaud's phenomenon: a pilot study. Clin Exp Rheumatol. 2000;18:499–502.
134. Lakshminarayanan S, Maestrello SJ, Vazquez-Abad D, et al. Treatment of severe Raynaud's phenomenon and ischemic ulcerations with tissue plasminogen activator. Clin Exp Rheumatol. 1999;17:260.
135. Dickneite G, Herwald H, Korte W, Allanore Y, Denton CP, Matucci Cerinic M. Coagulation factor XIII: a multifunctional transglutaminase with clinical potential in a range of conditions. Thromb Haemost. 2015;113:686–97.
136. Herrick AL, Matucci CM. The emerging problem of oxidative stress and the role of antioxidants in systemic sclerosis. Clin Exp Rheumatol. 2001;19:4–8.
137. Rosato E, Borghese F, Pisarri S, et al. The treatment with N-acetylcysteine of Raynaud's phenomenon and ischemic ulcers therapy in sclerodermic patients: a prospective observational trial of 50 patients. Clin Exp Rheumatol. 2009;28: 1379–84.
138. Abou-Raya A, Abou-Raya S, Helmii M. Statins as immunomodulators in systemic sclerosis. Ann N Y Acad Sci. 2007;1110:670–80.
139. Abou-Raya A, Abou-Raya S, Helmii M. Statins: potentially useful in therapy of systemic sclerosis-related Raynaud's phenomenon and digital ulcers. J Rheumatol. 2008;35:1801–8.
140. Fava A, Wung PK, Wigley FM, Hummers LK, Daya NR, Ghazarian SR, Boin F. Efficacy of Rho kinase inhibitor fasudil in secondary Raynaud's phenomenon. Arthritis Care Res (Hoboken). 2012;64(6):925–9.
141. Chrysant SG. Vascular remodeling: the role of angiotensin-converting enzyme inhibitors. Am Heart J. 1998;135:S21–30.
142. Kirchengast M, Munter K. Endothelin-1 and endothelin receptor antagonists in cardiovascular remodeling. PSEBM. 1999;221: 312–25.
143. Kowal-Bielecka O, Landewe R, Avouac J, Chwiesko S, Miniati I, Czirjak L, et al. EULAR recommendations for the treatment of systemic sclerosis: a report from the EULAR Scleroderma Trials and Research group (EUSTAR). Ann Rheum Dis. 2009;68: 620–8.
144. Tingey T, Shu J, Smuczek J, Pope J. Meta-analysis of healing and prevention of digital ulcers in systemic sclerosis. Arthritis Care Res (Hoboken). 2013;65:1460–71.
145. Hartzell TL, Makhni EC, Sampson C. Long-term results of periarterial sympathectomy. J Hand Surg Am. 2009;34:1454–60.
146. Kotsis SV, Chung KC. A systematic review of the outcomes of digital sympathectomy for treatment of chronic digital ischemia. J Rheumatol. 2003;30:1788–92.
147. Bogoch ER, Gross DK. Surgery of the hand in patients with systemic sclerosis: outcomes and considerations. J Rheumatol. 2005;32:642–8.
148. Tomaino MM, Goitz RJ, Medsger TA. Surgery for ischemic pain and Raynaud's phenomenon in scleroderma: a description of treatment protocol and evaluation of results. Microsurgery. 2001;21:75–9.
149. Yee AMF, Hotchkiss RN, Paget SA. Adventitial stripping: a digit saving procedure in refractory Raynaud's phenomenon. J Rheumatol. 1998;25:269–76.
150. Herrick A, Muir L. Raynaud's phenomenon (secondary). Clinical evidence. BMJ Publishing Group Ltd. London. 2015.
151. Neumeister MW. Botulinum toxin type A in the treatment of Raynaud's phenomenon. J Hand Surg Am. 2010;35A:2085–92.
152. Iorio ML, Masden DL, Higgins JP. Botulinum toxin A treatment of Raynaud's phenomenon: a review. Semin Arthritis Rheum. 2012;41:599–603.
153. Rajendram R, Hayward A. Ultrasound-guided digital sympathectomy using botulinum toxin. Anaesthesia. 2013;68(10):1077.
154. Guiducci S, Porta F, Saccardi R, et al. Autologous mesenchymal stem cells foster revascularization of ischemic limbs in systemic sclerosis: a case report. Ann Intern Med. 2010;153:650–4.
155. Takagi G, Miyamoto M, Tara S, Kirinoki-Ichikawa S, Kubota Y, Hada T, Takagi I, Mizuno K. Therapeutic vascular angiogenesis for intractable macroangiopathy-related digital ulcer in patients with systemic sclerosis: a pilot study. Rheumatology (Oxford). 2014;53(5):854–9.

Renal Crisis and Other Renal Manifestations of Scleroderma

21

Christopher P. Denton and Marie Hudson

Introduction

Renal complications are an important clinical manifestation of systemic sclerosis. In particular, scleroderma renal crisis (SRC) is a hallmark internal organ complication and historically was the predominant mechanism of scleroderma-related death. Outcomes of SRC have improved, but it remains a critical manifestation of the disease that must be diagnosed early and managed appropriately in collaboration with renal specialists. It is also now appreciated that other renal complications occur in SSc [1]. In many cases there is co-occurrence of these different manifestations, and this may account for the particular severity of SSc. Other causes of renal pathology should however always be considered in SSc and with better treatment for SRC are becoming more relevant to management of the disease [2].

There have certainly been improvements in survival after SRC in current practice compared with historical data [3]. Several factors are probably relevant, but undoubtedly the routine use of angiotensin-converting enzyme (ACE) inhibitor agents to treat SRC, together with other advances in renal replacement therapy, has transformed outcome, thereby representing one of the most significant advances in scleroderma therapeutics [4]. There is clear improvement in early mortality from renal crisis, but this better outcome has highlighted the poor long-term outcome for scleroderma patients through complications of long-term dialysis or from other scleroderma complications.

C.P. Denton, PhD, FRCP (✉)
Division of Medicine, Department of Inflammation, Centre for Rheumatology and Connective Tissue Diseases, UCL Division of Medicine, Royal Free Hospital, London, UK
e-mail: c.denton@ucl.ac.uk

M. Hudson, MD, MPH
Division of Rheumatology and Lady Davis Institute for Medical Research, Jewish General Hospital, Montréal, QC, Canada

Faculty of Medicine, McGill University, Montréal, QC, Canada

Renal Disease in SSc: The Spectrum of Involvement

Although SRC is the most important renal complication, manifested as accelerated phase hypertension accompanied by acute kidney injury (AKI), other processes that need to be considered in scleroderma include interstitial nephritis, glomerulonephritis and renal vasculitis [5]. In addition there is chronic renal vasculopathy and renal parenchymal fibrosis [6]. There is a high frequency of microscopic glomerular or tubular proteinuria for which the long-term significance is uncertain. These different complications will be discussed below.

Historical Aspects of SSc Renal Disease

Renal failure was first described in scleroderma in 1863 [7]. There was initial controversy concerning the specificity of this complication to scleroderma, but the link was established over the next 80 years, and numerous case reports linked scleroderma with renal disease and increased mortality [8]. Microvascular changes showing the classic vascular changes were described even in patients who died of nonrenal causes [9]. It was not until 1952, however, that Moore and Sheehan [10] identified a specific renal lesion as a major syndrome. They reported three scleroderma patients who developed acute hypertension and renal failure and died 6–8 weeks later. Concentric thickening of the intralobular arteries was found in all three cases and led to the term scleroderma renal crisis. Although bearing similarities to other forms of thrombotic microangiopathy associated AKI, there appear to be specific features of SRC that reflect the background autoimmune rheumatic disease and which impact on severity and outcome [11].

J. Varga et al. (eds.), *Scleroderma*, DOI 10.1007/978-3-319-31407-5_21

Scleroderma Renal Crisis

Definition

Scleroderma renal crisis (SRC) is defined as the new onset of accelerated arterial hypertension and/or rapidly progressive oliguric renal failure during the course of SSc. One should not assume that non-malignant hypertension alone without uraemia or other renal abnormalities is renal crisis. Likewise, urine abnormalities and/or mild uraemia in a scleroderma patient are likely to have other explanations and should not be considered SRC [1]. There are some differences between the criteria used to define SRC in different studies, and this may in part account for some of the different outcomes that are reported. Although a hallmark of SSc, SRC was not retained in the ACR/EULAR 2013 classification criteria for SSc because it did not add to sensitivity and specificity of the final set of items retained [12]. On the other hand, anti-RNA polymerase III, which are strongly associated with SRC (see below), were included [13]. There is no accepted gold standard to diagnose SRC. Two sets of criteria have been proposed (Table 21.1), with one including 'renal biopsy findings consistent with SRC (microangiopathy)' as an additional diagnostic feature for normotensive SRC [13, 14] and the other including 'hypertensive encephalopathy' as a diagnostic feature of either hypertensive or normotensive SRC [15]. The recently reported International Scleroderma Renal Crisis Survey included 75 incident SRC cases using physician-diagnosed SRC. Seventy (70) subjects were identified as hypertensive and 5 as normotensive, although none of the latter underwent kidney biopsy. In the absence of a renal biopsy, diagnosis of normotensive SRC is challenging. Indeed, all of the subjects diagnosed with hypertensive SRC met both sets of criteria presented in Table 21.1, whereas only two out of five subjects diagnosed with normotensive SRC by a physician met either of the criteria. Thus, although the current definitions of hypertensive SRC appear highly sensitive, additional work will be required to improve the definition of normotensive SRC and in particular to determine the value of kidney biopsy and/or other serological and genetic biomarkers in this subset of disease. The issue of specificity is also important, as other forms of thrombotic microangiopathy may have striking similarity to SRC and so the presence of SSc becomes a critical aspect to diagnosis (Box 21.1).

Table 21.1 Factors that occur prior to SRC that may be predictive for future SRC

Predictive of SRC	Not predictive of SRC
Disease symptoms <4 years	Previous blood pressure elevations
Diffuse skin involvement	Abnormal urinalysis
Rapid progression of skin thickening	Stable, mildly elevated serum creatinine
Anti-RNA polymerase III antibody	Anti-topoisomerase or anti-centromere antibodies
New anaemia	Pathologic abnormalities in renal blood vessels
New cardiac events	
Pericardial effusion	
Congestive heart failure	
Antecedent high-dose corticosteroid	

Box 21.1 Clinical Criteria for Definition of Scleroderma Renal Crisis (SRC)

Scleroderma renal crisis is defined as follows, requiring both of:

1. A new onset of blood pressure >150/85 obtained at least twice over a consecutive 24-h period. This blood pressure is chosen because it is that defined by the New York Heart Association as significant hypertension.
2. Decrease in the renal function as defined by a decrement of at least 10 % in the calculated glomerular filtration rate (eGFR) or measured GFR of below 90. When possible, a repeat serum creatinine and recalculation of the GFR should be obtained to corroborate the initial results.

In order to corroborate further the occurrence of acute renal crisis, it would be desirable to have any of the following, if available:

- Microangiopathic haemolytic anaemia on blood smear
- Retinopathy typical of acute hypertensive crisis
- New onset of urinary RBCs (excluding other causes)
- Flash pulmonary oedema
- Oliguria or anuria
- Renal biopsy with typical features including onion skin proliferation within the walls of intra-renal arteries and arterioles, fibrinoid necrosis and glomerular shrinkage.

Notes

1. Cases of typical SRC histological appearance have been associated with systemic sclerosis in the absence of hypertension; these cases of normotensive SRC are reported to have a particularly poor outcome, and their precise relationship to the more typical hypertensive SRC is not known.
2. Up to one fifth of cases of SRC with hypertension have been identified as the presenting feature of SSc, and so, in these cases, pre-existing diagnosis of SSc will not be present. These cases represent an important diagnostic and management challenge.

Epidemiology

SRC was previously reported to affect up to 25 % of SSc patients with early diffuse disease, but contemporary series seem to suggest that this may have fallen to as low as 5 % [2, 3]. A limitation is that previous data were generated in largely prevalent cohorts. There are now several prospective cohorts of SSc cases, although the frequency of SRC may vary in different populations. For diffuse SSc, the current estimate of the frequency of SRC is approximately 10 %. This comes from the US Prospective Registry in Systemic Sclerosis (PRESS) cohort which, to date, has recruited 97 early diffuse SSc subjects and 12 have developed SRC (D. Khanna and T. Frech, personal communication). The frequency in limited SSc is much lower and some populations, such as Japanese, appear to have a much lower frequency of SRC. A recent UK cohort suggests overall frequency in diffuse SSc of 14 % compared with 3 % in limited SSc [16]. Interestingly, the incidence of renal crisis appears to have decreased since ACE inhibitors (ACEi) have been available, although there is no evidence that ACEi prevent renal crisis. Indeed, prior use of ACEi has been associated with worse long-term outcome and a higher frequency of long-term dialysis after SRC, as suggested by two independent cohort studies [17, 18] and most persuasively by the recent International Scleroderma Renal Crisis Survey [19]. The mechanism for this is unknown, but it is possible that the low dose used in non-hypertensive patients is inadequate to handle the surge of renin when SRC is triggered but masks the acute manifestations which normally bring the patient to the attention of physicians early in the episode, turning the event into a less reversible, more chronic process.

Renal crisis is most often encountered early in the course of the disease, with 75 % of SRC cases occurring less than 4 years after the first symptom attributable to scleroderma and males are proportionately more frequently affected than females [15]. However, late occurrences, even 20 years after disease onset, also occur, and the impact of other treatment for SSc skin- or organ-based disease might further change the timing and frequency of SRC. Early studies suggested that African-American patients are three times as likely as Caucasians to develop SRC [16]. In one series, it was reported that 22 % of SRC may have this as the presenting feature of the disease or at least not have a pre-existing diagnosis of SSc even if attributable clinical features are present.

Factors Predicting SRC

The characteristics of a typical patient are well recognised from several cohort studies. Many of these features or laboratory characteristics can be identified before the development of a renal crisis, and therefore careful baseline assessment of all scleroderma cases for risk of crisis is essential. Patients with a greatly increased risk to develop this complication must be followed extremely closely for any hints of renal crisis. Patients with diffuse cutaneous scleroderma with skin thickening on the proximal extremities and/or the trunk are at greatest risk for SRC, with 20–25 % of this patient subgroup getting SRC [21, 22]. Far fewer patients with limited cutaneous scleroderma (previously termed the CREST syndrome) who have long-standing skin changes restricted to distal extremities ever develop renal crisis. There are even fewer cases of renal crisis documented in limited scleroderma patients with anti-centromere antibody [23, 24]. Thus, the vast majority of SRC cases (75–80 %) occur in patients with diffuse skin involvement, and rapid progression of skin thickening has been shown to be associated with development of SRC [24].

Some SRC cases occur in patients with less severe skin involvement but who are destined to develop typical diffuse scleroderma, although they only have minimal or even no skin changes at the time of the diagnosis of renal crisis. It is not infrequent for this type of patient with such minimal cutaneous and systemic findings to have the diagnosis of renal crisis made only at the time of kidney biopsy [25, 26]. There are several distinguishing features that are helpful to identify those patients who are likely to evolve to diffuse cutaneous disease. These patients almost always have a short duration of symptoms, often less than 1 year. Polyarthritis/arthralgias, puffy or swollen hands and legs and carpal tunnel syndrome are a common complex of symptoms in patients with early diffuse scleroderma [13]. Although Raynaud's phenomenon eventually is almost universally found in scleroderma, its absence in early diffuse scleroderma is not uncommon. The presence of palpable tendon friction rubs, which occur in 65 % of diffuse scleroderma patients, is an extremely helpful and predictive sign of diffuse scleroderma even prior to the development of diffuse cutaneous skin involvement [27]. Less than 5 % of limited scleroderma patients ever have tendon rubs. Tendon friction rubs have recently been confirmed to be independent predictors of SRC (HR 2.33, 95 % CI 1.03, 6.19) in a prospective EUSTAR cohort study that included 1,301 SSc patients with disease duration ≤3 years and follow-up of at least 2 years [41].

Patients without known scleroderma who present with new isolated malignant hypertension should be carefully questioned for the presence of the aforementioned set of symptoms.

Autoantibodies may be helpful in predicting SRC. Antinuclear antibodies are seen in 95 % of scleroderma so their presence may be helpful in determining whether a malignant hypertension patient could possibly have scleroderma. Anti-RNA polymerase III is a scleroderma specific antibody that is seen almost exclusively in diffuse scleroderma, and 24–33 % of patients with this antibody develop SRC [28–30]. In contrast, renal crisis occurs in only 10 % of patients with anti-topoisomerase antibodies, which are also associated with diffuse skin disease [22]. The anti-centromere antibody, the antibody seen in classic limited scleroderma (or CREST syndrome), is rarely associated with renal crisis [24]. It is recommended that patients with early diffuse scleroderma should monitor their own blood pressure regularly and notify their physicians immediately when their blood pressure is persistently increased.

Anti-RNA polymerase III antibodies have now been established as a robust risk factor for SRC, being present in more than 50 % of SSc patients who develop SRC in some series [31] and associated with a significant increase in the odds of SRC (odds ratio [OR] 6.4, 95 % confidence interval [CI] 3.4–12.2, $p<0.001$) [31]. Interestingly, a recent report from The Royal Free cohort compared outcomes of SRC in anti-RNA polymerase III antibody positive and negative subjects [32]. Of the 150 cases with confirmed SRC, 61 (41 %) were positive for anti-RNA polymerase III antibodies. The anti-RNA polymerase III antibody positive cases were more likely to require dialysis compared to the negative patients (51 % vs 29 %, $p=0.07$), but they were also more likely to discontinue dialysis (53 % vs 26 %, $p=0.01$) and had better survival (log rank $p=0.003$). Whether this reflects differences in presentation and diagnosis or in the underlying pathology remains unclear.

Most SSc sera that react with anti-RNA polymerases recognise more than one class of RNA polymerases. Anti-RNA polymerases I and III almost always coexist, and among those, some sera also contain anti-RNA polymerase II [29, 33]. A group of Japanese investigators recently published a study of 583 SSc subjects, among whom 37 (6 %) were positive for anti-RNA polymerase III by a commercially available ELISA and 17 (2.9 %) developed SRC. There was a significantly higher frequency of SRC in anti-RNA polymerase III-positive compared to anti-RNA polymerase III-negative SSc patients (9 of 37 [24 %] positive vs 8 of 546 [1 %] negative, OR 21.6, 95 % CI 7.8–60.3, $p<0.00001$) [34]. The investigators further characterized the profiles of the 37 anti-RNA polymerase III antibody positive subjects by immunoprecipitation and defined two groups, according to the presence or absence of anti-RNA polymerase II: 17 had anti-RNA polymerase I/II/III and 20 had anti-RNA polymerase I/III or III alone. In multivariate Cox proportional analysis, both anti-RNA polymerase I/II/III positivity (OR 11.0, 95 % CI 1.6–222.8, $p=0.0118$) and an ELISA index for anti-RNA polymerase III of ≥157 (OR 2.4×109, 95 % CI 2.1-uncalculated, $p=0.0093$) were independent factors associated with the development of SRC. These results were validated in an independent cohort [35] and pooled analysis of both cohorts [36]. Although the clinical usefulness of anti-RNA polymerase II may be limited by the fact that detection requires complex immunoprecipitation assays that are conducted in a limited number of laboratories, the higher ELISA index for anti-RNA polymerase III has better potential utility as a biomarker for SRC.

Antecedent hypertension is not usually present prior to SRC. Most often there is a very acute onset of markedly elevated blood pressure. Normal blood pressures have been documented within 24 h prior to the onset of SRC hypertension [21]. In isolation, an abnormal urinalysis or increased serum creatinine do not predict SRC.

Several non-renal abnormalities may precede SRC, including asymptomatic pericardial effusion, congestive heart failure and/or arrhythmias [24, 37]. New anaemia, an uncommon manifestation of scleroderma, can be an early clue to renal crisis [20], particularly when microangiopathic haemolysis and thrombocytopenia are present.

Prior use of high-dose glucocorticoid frequently precedes the development of SRC [38–40]. A case control study matched 106 patients with renal crisis to other scleroderma patients based on features that would be associated with increased risks for renal crisis or the use of steroids [1, 15]. Sex, disease subset, disease duration, extent of skin thickening, the presence of tendon friction rubs and inflammatory myopathy were similar in both groups. Patients who received high-dose prednisone (>15 mg/day) were three times more likely to develop renal crisis in the next 6 months. High-dose steroids should be used with great caution and very close monitoring in patients with early diffuse scleroderma. In a recent cohort study from France, Guillevin et al. [3] found that the majority of SRC cases had been exposed to glucocorticoids prior to SRC and that this was significantly greater than control cases of SSc without SRC. However, this study has all of the well-appreciated limitations of a retrospective cohort design in a multicentre heterogeneous population of SSc.

Some of the most robust data regarding glucocorticoid exposure that are available come from the recent International Scleroderma Renal Crisis Survey, which recruited 75 incident SRC cases [19]. Among these, median disease duration from onset of the first non-Raynaud's symptom to the diagnosis of SRC was 1.5 years and 75 % had diffuse cutaneous systemic sclerosis (dcSSc). In addition, of the 19 subjects who were identified as having limited cutaneous systemic sclerosis (lcSSc) ($n=16$) or systemic sclerosis sine scleroderma ($n=3$) at baseline, almost half had antibodies associated with diffuse skin involvement (ATA $n=6$ and anti-RNA polymerase III $n=2$). Thus, progression to dcSSc in some of these patients is likely, suggesting an even stronger association between SRC and dcSSc. In addition, exposure to glucocorticoids was associated with SRC, with a strong association between prednisone dose and mortality in the International Scleroderma Renal Crisis Survey: for every milligram of prednisone, the risk of death increased by 4 % (hazard ratio [HR] 1.04, 95 % CI 1.02, 1.07, $p<0.01$).

Clinical Presentation

Patients may complain of severe headache, blurred vision or other encephalopathic symptoms with the onset of accelerated hypertension. Seizures may occur, although earlier diagnosis and better management of SRC should reduce the frequency of these events. Otherwise, the symptoms of renal crisis are non-specific: increased fatigue, headache, dyspnea or malaise. High-risk patients must be taught to take these symptoms seriously and should check their own blood pressure if these symptoms occur.

Most patients have striking elevations of blood pressure at the onset of SRC. Ninety percent have blood pressure levels greater than 150/90 mmHg, and 30 % have diastolic recordings greater than 120 mmHg. Up to 10 % of cases have been reported to have a normal blood pressure, although 'normal' has to be interpreted case by case. Indeed, an increase of 20 mmHg in blood pressure in a patient with usually low normal pressures (e.g. increase from 95/60 to 140/85) can represent renal crisis. Thus, any change in blood pressure should lead to further testing and close monitoring. Normotensive renal crisis requires the presence of other features, primarily rapidly progressive unexplained azotemia and/or microangiopathic haemolytic anaemia with thrombocytopenia. Pulmonary haemorrhage is a rare life-threatening problem, which has occurred in several of these patients [38, 42]. It complicates the diagnosis and is a poor prognostic sign. Paradoxically, it appears that higher systolic or diastolic blood pressure at presentation may be associated with better long-term outcome in hypertensive SRC [17].

Patients with SRC often present with congestive heart failure (dyspnea, paroxysmal nocturnal dyspnea or even pulmonary oedema), serious ventricular arrhythmias (even cardiac arrest) and/or large pericardial effusions [49, 50]. This is primarily from the stress of the hypertension on the heart, from effects of hyperreninemia and from fluid overload secondary to oliguric renal failure, although some patients with very severe disease also have primary scleroderma myocardial involvement contributing to these problems. Severe pulmonary hypertension secondary to the malignant systemic hypertension has also been seen but has a different course than the more frequent chronic pulmonary hypertension seen in limited scleroderma patients. Prompt control of the blood pressure usually improves these cardiac problems.

In some situations, SRC may be confused with other illnesses. Several cases of thrombotic thrombocytopenic purpura (TTP) have been reported in scleroderma patients, but it is unclear whether it was an isolated coexistent disease or just a different interpretation of SRC [43]. A review of the eight cases of TTP and scleroderma in the literature found that there were few differences between the patient subsets. Although a few 'responded' to plasmapheresis, most were also treated with ACE inhibitors [44]. Fever and haemorrhagic manifestations were the only findings that distinguished the two conditions. New research in the pathophysiology of TTP has led to the observation that vWF-cleaving protease activity is decreased or deficient in TTP [45]. A pilot study did not find abnormalities of the vWF-cleaving protease activity in ten SRC patients [46]. If a diagnosis of TTP is made in a scleroderma patient, an ACE inhibitor should be used in conjunction with TTP treatment [47].

Laboratory Findings

Laboratory investigation of AKI in SRC is the main focus of initial investigations. There is usually both proteinuria and microscopic haematuria on dipstick urinalysis. Proteinuria is mild or moderate (generally <2 g per day), and microscopy can show microscopic haematuria (5–100 rbc/hpf) and granular casts [48]. Serum creatinine is typically at least 150 % of baseline value at presentation. This represents Stage 1 AKI in the most recent international consensus guidelines for AKI care [49]. Again, 'normal' renal function needs to be interpreted cautiously since the creatinine value can reach this relative increase without rising above the normal absolute range in scleroderma patients with low muscle mass.

Creatinine can rise rapidly in the first few days following onset of renal crisis and will usually continue to rise even once blood pressure has been adequately controlled. Although a slower increase of serum creatinine can occur over days to weeks, it is much more likely to increase by 0.5–1.0 mg/dl creatinine per day. It is important to recognise that even after antihypertensive therapy has effectively controlled blood pressure, the serum creatinine may continue to rise. The issue of whether the ACE inhibitor itself contributes to such increases is often raised, but in that setting, we have not had any patient who has had significant improvement in serum creatinine after stopping the ACE inhibitor. Unfortunately, there are still situations where the serum creatinine continues to rise and the patient develops renal failure in spite of adequate control of the blood pressure with ACE inhibitors. In these circumstances, the addition of glucocorticoids, immunosuppressive therapy or plasmapheresis is never helpful.

Microangiopathic haemolytic anaemia, which is characterized by normochromic, fragmented red blood cells, reticulocytosis and thrombocytopenia, occurs in almost half of patients with SRC. The platelet count is rarely lower than 20,000/mm^3, and its improvement is often the first sign of adequate response to therapy even though the serum creatinine is continuing to increase. Patients are not usually symptomatic from this process although anaemia may contribute to congestive heart failure. One series found a reduced platelet count in 50 % of SRC patients and red cell fragments in 52 % [17]. Other evidence of haemolysis, including a reduced

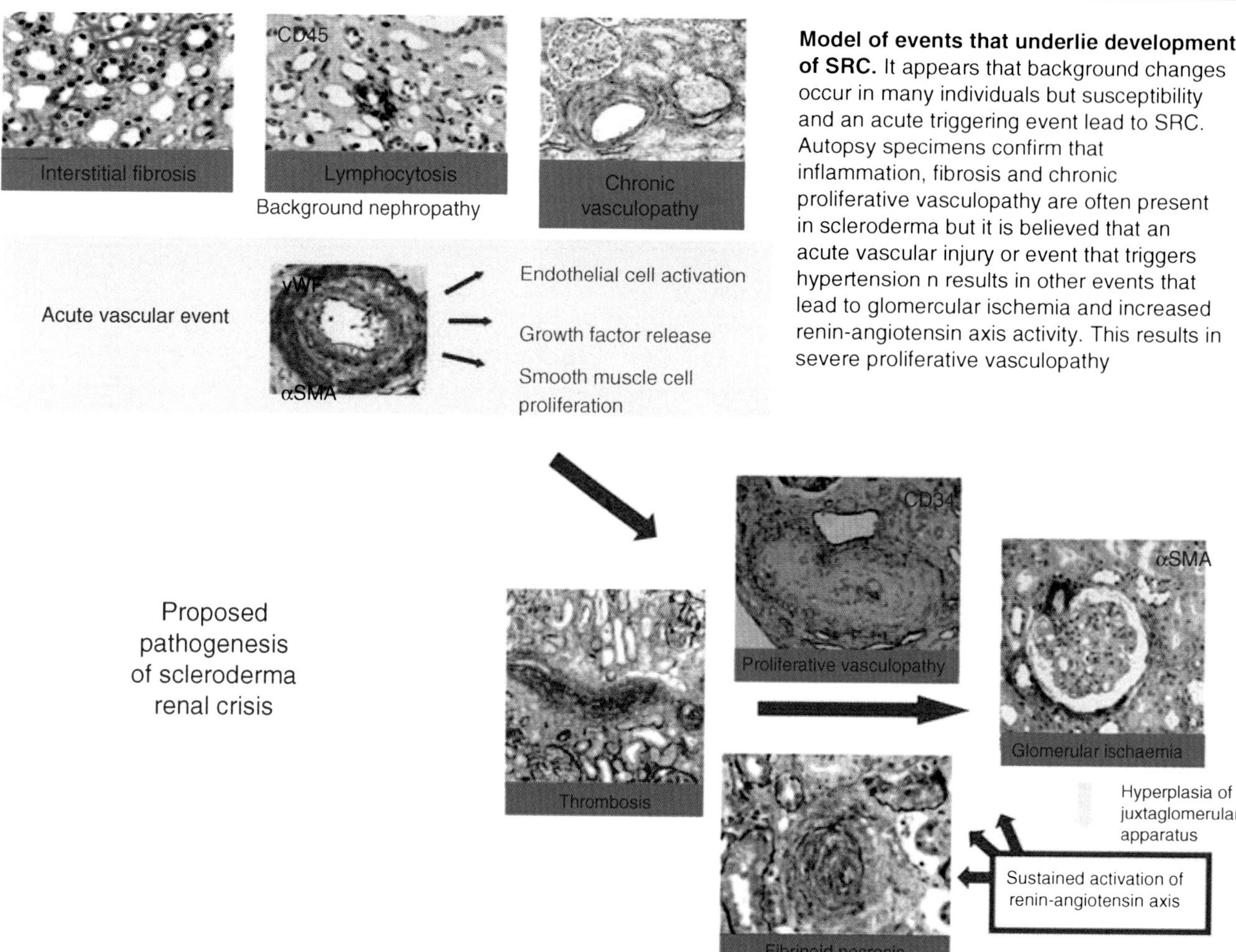
Interstitial fibrosis
CD45
Lymphocytosis
Chronic vasculopathy
Background nephropathy
Model of events that underlie development of SRC. It appears that background changes occur in many individuals but susceptibility and an acute triggering event lead to SRC. Autopsy specimens confirm that inflammation, fibrosis and chronic proliferative vasculopathy are often present in scleroderma but it is believed that an acute vascular injury or event that triggers hypertension n results in other events that lead to glomerular ischemia and increased renin-angiotensin axis activity. This results in severe proliferative vasculopathy
Acute vascular event
vWF
αSMA
Endothelial cell activation
Growth factor release
Smooth muscle cell proliferation
Proposed pathogenesis of scleroderma renal crisis
CD34
Proliferative vasculopathy
αSMA
Glomerular ischaemia
Thrombosis
Fibrinoid necrosis
Hyperplasia of juxtaglomerular apparatus
Sustained activation of renin-angiotensin axis

Fig. 21.1 Model of events that underlie development of SRC. It appears that background changes occur in many individuals, but susceptibility and an acute triggering event lead to SRC. Autopsy specimens confirm that inflammation, fibrosis and chronic proliferative vasculopathy are often present in scleroderma, but it is believed that an acute vascular injury or event that triggers hypertension results in other events that lead to glomerular ischemia and increased renin-angiotensin axis activity. This results in severe proliferative vasculopathy

serum haptoglobin level and/or a raised lactate dehydrogenase, should be sought. Given the remaining diagnostic uncertainty in this field, if a diagnosis of TTP or HUS is suspected in a scleroderma patient, we recommend that an ACE inhibitor should be used in conjunction with plasmapheresis.

Pathogenesis

Although the pathology of SSc focuses on interplay between the innate and adaptive immune system, connective tissue and extracellular matrix metabolism and vasculopathy in the microcirculation and microvasculature, SRC is principally an impairment of arterial blood flow in the kidney. First suggested by Steen et al. [24], a plausible model that explains clinical heterogeneity and the time course of the disease is that specific organ-based injury or damage occurs in susceptible individuals within the context of a unifying background of vasculopathy, fibrosis and autoimmunity [1]. It is noteworthy that there is evidence of all of these different processes in the kidney in SSc [51]. It is particularly important to observe that these abnormalities are present even in the absence of SRC. Thus, they may reflect a background pathological state upon which SRC is superimposed. The triggering event or events may include vascular injury. The end result is the initiation of a positive feedback loop that is driven by increased activity of the renin-angiotensin axis. The pathogenic mechanisms that lead to SRC have been defined though a number of studies examining biopsy material and circulating molecular markers. The clinical efficacy of ACEi confirms the central role of the renin-angiotensin axis in driving the process. Elevated levels of rennin are a hallmark of the condition. However, it is clear that background fibrosis, vasculopathy and inflammatory lesions occur frequently in SSc and that these do not inevitably lead to established scleroderma renal crisis (SRC). The likely pathogenic process is summarised in Fig. 21.1. An acute event, probably vascular, appears to initiate a self-perpetuating cascade that leads to glomerular hypoperfusion and increased renin release. These events lead to release or activation of cytokines and growth factors that result in the typical proliferative vascular lesion of SRC. Hypertensive changes add to this constellation of events. Consistent with this model is the link between histopathological features and outcome that has been established in several recent studies. Thus, acute vascular injury is associated with worse outcome based upon studies that have linked biopsy appearance to long-term outcome, such as the need for permanent dialysis [17, 52]. Although anti-RNA polymerase III antibodies are strongly associated with SRC occurrence, there is no evidence for direct pathogenicity [53].

In the acute setting, the main diagnostic benefit of renal biopsy is to exclude other pathologies. In the longer term, it may help to inform renal prognosis (see below). Biopsy needs to be delayed until the patient is clinically stable with good blood pressure control and the platelet count has recovered. The renal pathological findings in SRC are broadly the same as those seen in other causes of accelerated hypertension [10]. Fibrinoid necrosis is seen either in arterial walls or in the subintima in small arteries and arterioles (characteristically the interlobular and arcuate arteries). The resulting intimal thickening leads to narrowing or total obliteration of the lumen and a typical 'onion skin' appearance (Fig. 21.1). Adventitial and periadventitial fibrosis, an indication of chronic vasculopathy seen in patients with SRC, is rarely seen in accelerated hypertension without scleroderma. Glomeruli are collapsed with wrinkling of the basement membrane. Interestingly, unlike in other renal diseases, the extent of interstitial scarring does not have prognostic value, whereas markers of acute vascular injury (including fibrinoid necrosis and thrombosed vessels) do predict poor renal outcome [17, 52].

The dramatic response to therapeutic inhibition of the renin-angiotensin system in SRC in SRC (and previous apparent improvement after nephrectomy) implicates renin overproduction as a central part of the pathogenesis of SRC. However, hyperreninemia is uncommon before the acute onset of SRC and if present does not predict future events. Thus, the initial trigger of SRC remains largely unknown.

Markers of renal injury have been reported to be increased prior to SRC. Studies examining serum levels of sVCAM-1 or vWF have shown that these may be increased at the onset or preceding SRC [54, 55]. Studies of other markers of damage such as adipokines and SSc are emerging. Lipocalin-2 is an adipokine that has been reported elevated in acute kidney injury and immunity. Its role in SSc was therefore explored in 50 SSc subjects with relatively early disease (mean duration of 3 years) who had not been previously treated with glucocorticoids or immunosuppressants [56, 57]. Although the investigators reported that the prevalence of SRC was significantly higher in those with elevated serum lipocalin-2 levels compared to those with normal levels, the actual numbers were very small, with only two cases of SRC in the cohort. In addition, serum lipocalin-2 levels were inversely correlated with eGFR in SSc patients with eGFR <60 ml/min/1,73 m2 ($r=-0.68$, $p=0.035$) but not in those with eGFR >60 ml/min/1,73 m2 ($r=0.04$, $p=0.79$). Along with these preliminary finding, the investigators also reported interesting associations between serum lipocalin-2 and skin scores (positive correlation) and right ventricular systolic pressures in subjects with normal eGFR (negative correlation), between lipocalin-2 expression in dermal fibroblasts and endothelial cells of lesional skin, and in dermal fibroblasts, but not endothelial cells, of bleomycin-treated mice. Finally, deficiency of transcription factor Fli1, which is implicated in SSc vasculopathy, induced lipocalin-2 expression in cultured endothelial cells. Further studies to confirm these results, in particular the role of lipocalin-1 as a biomarker for SRC, and to determine whether lipocalin-1 has a causal role in the pathogenesis SSc are required.

Although challenging in a rare disease with specific clinical and serological associations, there have been initial attempts to try to define genetic susceptibility for SRC. A first study reported an association between SRC and distinct MHC class I haplotypes, namely, HLA-DRB1*0407 and *1304 [58]. In addition association between anti-RNA polymerase antibody reactivity and endothelin receptor polymorphism has been suggested in one cohort study, but not yet confirmed independently [59]. More recently, a study focused on patients with anti-RNA polymerase positive disease and attempted to define differences between those cases with SRC and a cohort of ARA positive cases followed for at least 5 years without developing SRC. This latter group may reasonably be assumed to have protection from this complication. Patients with these extreme phenotypes of anti-RNA polymerase III antibody positive disease were genotyped: 50 with SRC (all within 18 months of disease onset) and 50 without SRC (all with >5 years of disease). Reported data suggest a number of SRC associated single nucleotide polymorphisms (SNPs) within genes and gene regions. The top associations were found in the complement region ($p = 1.66 \times 10–5$) and in other genes including EPHA5, GRIA3, HECW2 and CTNND2 [55]. These findings are of clear biological relevance. On the one hand, renal pathological changes in SRC resemble those of the thrombotic microangiopathy (TMA) syndromes, in which dysregulation of the complement system is increasingly recognised [60] and peritubular capillary complement 4d deposits have been associated with an increased risk of prolonged renal failure [52]. On the other hand, catenin (cadherin-associated protein) delta 2 (CTNND2) is known to regulate adhesion molecules relevant to fibrosis. Further validation of these findings is ongoing.

To date, there are no robust animal models that replicate the features of SRC. Attempts to induce hypertensive renal injury in transgenic strains that manifest features of SSc have been undertaken. So far these studies support the concept that reduced renal inflammatory lesions may be important in the uncontrolled proliferative vascular changes of SSc but have not provided fundamental insight into specific mechanisms of SRC [61].

Treatment

The most important aspect of management of renal crisis is early detection and diagnosis. It is essential that high-risk patients are identified and that there is clear patient education and blood pressure monitoring. There should also be regular assessment of urine and biochemical indices of renal function. In general, all SSc patients should receive education about the importance of having blood pressure monitoring, both regularly and at any time if symptoms like headache, breathlessness, dizziness or syncope develop. This is especially important in cases of dcSSc within 4 years of onset. We usually recommend home BP monitoring twice weekly with instructions about individualised levels that should prompt medical review. Specialist nurses and patient 'warning cards' can provide invaluable patient support in this context [62]. If new onset hypertension or other relevant symptoms develop or if there is incidental finding of hypertension, urinalysis abnormality or renal impairment, it is essential to obtain urgent specialist medical advice. In this way, appropriate tests can be performed and treatment initiated.

Once SRC is diagnosed, patients should be aggressively managed, preferably with hospitalisation and careful daily monitoring. Reflecting evidence-based recommendations [63], hypertension in SSc should prompt an ACEi being introduced or dose increased if already being taken. A short acting ACE inhibitor may be preferable in haemodynamically unstable cases. However, ACEi resistance is frequent, and our practice is to initiate a long-acting drug as soon as possible and escalate the dose daily to maximum. There is close monitoring with daily blood tests and aim for reduction of blood pressure to target as soon as possible, although in established SRC, this often takes some days. Renal function may continue to deteriorate during that time. It is important to increase the ACEi dose to maximum – our practice is to double this every 24 h. Often it takes several days for BP to fall to normal, and renal function may continue to deteriorate even after the initiation of ACEi. This is an important point as it may lead to inappropriate reduction or discontinuation of ACEi. We usually add an ARB to treatment once the ACEi is in the therapeutic range and to introduce other antihypertensives including calcium channel blockers, doxazosin and clonidine if blood pressure remains unacceptably high. The goal is to achieve normal pre-SRC blood pressure. There are reports suggesting that ARB alone is less effective than ACEi in treating SRC [64, 65]. Beta-blocking drugs are contraindicated due to effects on peripheral circulation, and parenteral antihypertensives are usually not needed, although nitrate infusion is sometimes beneficial when pulmonary oedema complicates SRC. There have been reports of using endothelin receptor antagonists in SRC [66], and this may be logical based upon the high circulating levels of ET-1 reported in patients at the time of SRC [67] and also studies demonstrating that endothelin ligand and receptor expression may be increased in SRC [68, 69]. In addition, polymorphism in the endothelin ligand receptor axis [59] but not the ACE axis [50] has been associated with scleroderma. There has been one open-label trial of bosentan added to standard treatment for SRC, but the place of endothelin axis blockade is unclear and requires additional investigation. The similarity of the pathology of SRC ad precapillary PAH in SSc makes it plausible that an ERA might be beneficial for vascular repair post-SRC.

In cases where renal replacement is required, this is generally by haemofiltration or haemodialysis, the choice of method being determined by haemodynamic stability and local facilities. Occasionally in more indolent cases, it may be possible to move to peritoneal dialysis as the first form of renal replacement. It is important to emphasise patient education and vigilance amongst patient and health professionals since it is critical to diagnose SRC as soon as possible. The unique challenges of managing renal crisis during pregnancy are discussed in elsewhere in this textbook.

Renal biopsy is particularly important in patients where there is any uncertainty about the diagnosis. If anything is atypical in the presentation, the patient or the course, it is important to confirm diagnosis and rule out other aetiologies of kidney pathology, particularly glomerulonephritis. Renal biopsy can provide valuable prognostic information and scores have been developed. Interestingly the chronic damage index that predicts long-term outcome in many renal pathologies does not appear to do so in SRC [50]. This emphasises that SRC is an acute event often superimposed upon background nephropathy. We perform renal biopsy as soon as clotting and blood pressure permit this to be safely undertaken and this often provides useful prognostic information (see Fig. 21.2).

The place for plasma exchange in SRC is uncertain as it has not been shown to be of benefit in SRC but is a central part of the management of some related conditions such as thrombotic thrombocytopenic purpura. It may be considered in cases that have severe MAHA and consumptive coagulopathy. However, there are no controlled clinical trial data available, and case reports provide a mixed message concerning the benefits of this approach [44]. ACEi must be

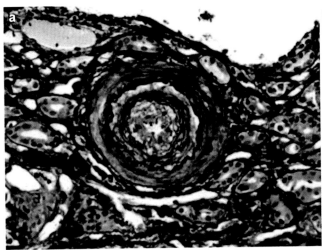

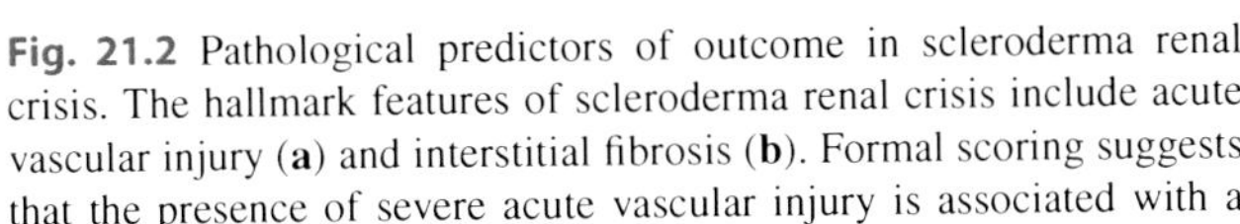

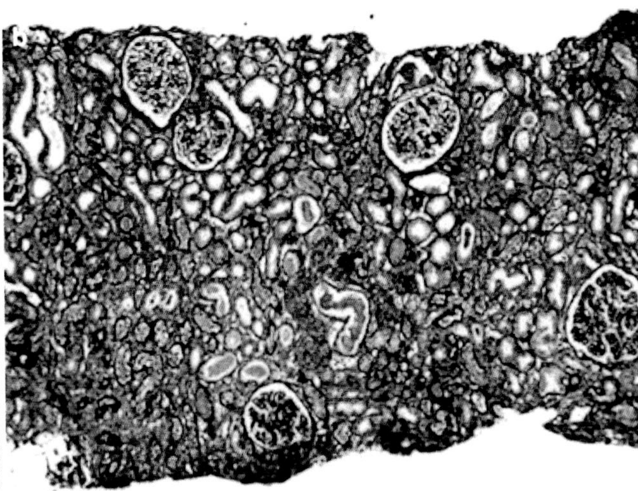

Fig. 21.2 Pathological predictors of outcome in scleroderma renal crisis. The hallmark features of scleroderma renal crisis include acute vascular injury (**a**) and interstitial fibrosis (**b**). Formal scoring suggests that the presence of severe acute vascular injury is associated with a poor prognosis and increased likelihood of permanent need for dialysis. Conversely, the extent of fibrotic scarring does not appear to reflect long-term renal outcome (discussed further in reference [17])

used in conjunction with plasma exchange in the setting of scleroderma.

Organ-based complications are managed supportively, and this may include management of pulmonary oedema or encephalopathy using standard approaches such as supplementary oxygen, ventilatory support, sedation and/or antiseizure medications according to clinical circumstances.

Prevention

Patient education is critical together with risk stratification and vigilant monitoring of BP, urine and renal function. There is no clear evidence that ACEi have prophylactic benefit. Recent data from UK and French cohorts both point to a worse long-term outcome in cases requiring dialysis in patients taking ACEi or ARB at the time of SRC diagnosis. The basis for this is unclear and may relate to delays in diagnosis and additional therapy. A large controlled study of an ACEi, quinapril, did not show any preventative effect on vascular complications of SSc [70]. Of note in that study, though, is that only subjects with either lcSSc or Raynaud's phenomenon were included, both groups at low risk of SRC. The International Scleroderma Renal Crisis Study was undertaken to investigate the *prophylactic role* of ACE inhibitors. We found that exposure to ACE inhibitors *prior to the onset* of SRC was associated with a greater than twofold increase in the risk of mortality (hazard ratio 2.42, 95 % CI 1.0–5.75, $p=0.046$). Of note, though, is that all of the 16 subjects on ACE inhibitors prior to the onset of their SRC had some indication for this, including systemic hypertension ($n=12$), Raynaud's phenomenon ($n=2$), prophylaxis because of concurrent corticosteroid exposure ($n=2$) and chronic renal insufficiency ($n=1$). None of the subjects exposed to ACE inhibitors prior to SRC were on it as simple prophylaxis from SRC. Thus, it is possible that confounding by indication may have contributed to the poor outcomes. Thus, at this time, the question of a prophylactic role of ACE inhibitors to prevent SRC remains largely unresolved.

Long-Term Outcome

Since ACE inhibitors have become available, survival in SRC has improved dramatically, from roughly a 1-year 10 % survival to a 5-year 60 % survival. In 1990, the long-term outcome of the initial 145 cases of SRC treated with ACE inhibitors at the University of Pittsburgh was reported: 61 % had a good outcome as defined by not requiring or only requiring temporary dialysis [59]. A prospective international cohort and three large recent retrospective cohort studies showed data very similar to those of Steen in the 1990s [3, 17–19]. Thirty-five to 45 % of patients with renal crisis do not require dialysis. After their creatinine peaks, it slowly improves and patients rarely go on to develop chronic renal failure after 'surviving' renal crisis, as long as their blood pressure continues to be controlled. The use of ACE inhibitors should be indefinite as recurrences years after the initial event have occurred when these drugs were discontinued. More than half of patients who initially require dialysis are able to discontinue it 3–18 months later. In the 20 % of SRC patients whose blood pressure is controlled soon enough and the kidney heals, the patients are able to come off dialysis and in most cases continue to slowly improve, similar to an acute tubular necrosis. Most patients that discontinue dialysis have adequate kidney function that does not further deteriorate as long as the blood pressure is controlled.

Unfortunately, up to 40% of SRC still have a poor outcome with premature death or long-term renal replacement therapy. Twenty percent require chronic dialysis and have similar types and frequency of vascular access and peritoneal clearance problems compared to other dialysis patients. Survival of scleroderma patients on dialysis is similar to other multisystem diseases such as diabetes. And there continues to be about 20% of patients who have an early death within 6 months. In general, the patients with a poor prognosis are older, male and have a lower blood pressure. Education of patients and physicians, early diagnosis and aggressive treatment with ACE inhibitors remain our best hopes for improving outcomes at this time.

An Australia and New Zealand series quoted above showed a median survival of 2.4 years for scleroderma patients on dialysis compared with 6.0 years for other patients [71]. In a US study of dialysis patients with scleroderma between 1992 and 1997, 2-year survival in the scleroderma group was 49% compared with 64% in all other patients [64]. Likewise, a review of scleroderma renal transplant cases from the United Network for Organ Sharing registry from 1987 to 1996 showed both lower graft and patient survival times than in renal transplant patients without systemic diseases [52].

Transplantation in SSc

It is well established that renal transplants are feasible after SRC in those cases that require permanent dialysis [72]. This may be considered in patients that have a suitable live related donor or match in an unrelated programme. The rate of recurrence is reported at up to 20%, although it can be difficult to distinguish SRC from transplant vasculopathy in chronic rejection [73]. Decisions about transplant should be delayed for 18–24 months because renal recovery can occur in this time frame. Registry data confirm the very poor survival of SRC cases on long-term dialysis, and suitable cases should be considered for transplant.

Interstitial Renal Disease

Postmortem studies have confirmed that expression of fibrillar collagens is increased in SSc even in the absence of any clinical evidence of renal abnormality. However, there are some cases in which interstitial renal disease occurs as a consequence of drugs or other stimuli [52]. It is unclear whether SSc cases are more susceptible to this but interstitial nephritis remains an important differential diagnosis in any case of SSc with renal insufficiency.

Glomerulonephritis

Glomerulonephritis occurs in the context of overlap connective tissue disease, and there are often clinical or serological clues. In our cohort all, cases of glomerulonephritis had some serological features of lupus or positive ANCA. This is consistent with other reported cases [74]. Glomerulonephritis may occur as an isolated pathology and clues are often present in the autoantibody profile of cases. On occasion there may have been a scleroderma renal crisis before development of glomerulonephritis. Representative biopsies from cases of GN in SSc are shown in Fig. 21.3.

Vasculitis

The significance of ANCA in SSc is important [75]. Series in the literature suggest that typical ANCA may be associated with glomerulonephritis [76] or small vessel vasculitis [77]. Typical and atypical ANCA are reported – the most frequent being MPO [78]. This provides strong justification for early renal biopsy as treatment for the vasculitis is paramount and will involve high-dose glucocorticoids (and immunosuppression) that would otherwise be contraindicated in SSc. The association of ANCA vasculitis with SSc has recently been reviewed. Interestingly, MHC associations have been identified that may fit with this association for both conditions, and also it is suggested that the distribution of vasculitic lesions is different for SSc-associated disease that could reflect concurrence of two distinct vasculopathic processes [78].

Other Causes of Renal Dysfunction in SSc

Other than SRC and the entities mentioned above, renal disease in SSc has been reported to be common (up to 20% of subjects) and to result from a variety of causes, including both scleroderma-related (concomitant heart, lung and gastrointestinal disease) and non-scleroderma-related (hypertension, diabetes, infection and drugs such as non-steroidal antiinflammatory drugs, penicillamine and angiotensin-converting enzyme (ACE) inhibitors) [6, 79, 80] However, in these situations, renal abnormalities tend to be mild, renal function does not appear to deteriorate meaningfully over time and prognosis of the renal disease tends to be generally favourable.

Future Perspectives

Despite the marked improvement in outcome for the majority of patients with scleroderma renal crisis since the introduction of ACE inhibitors, there is a significant subgroup for

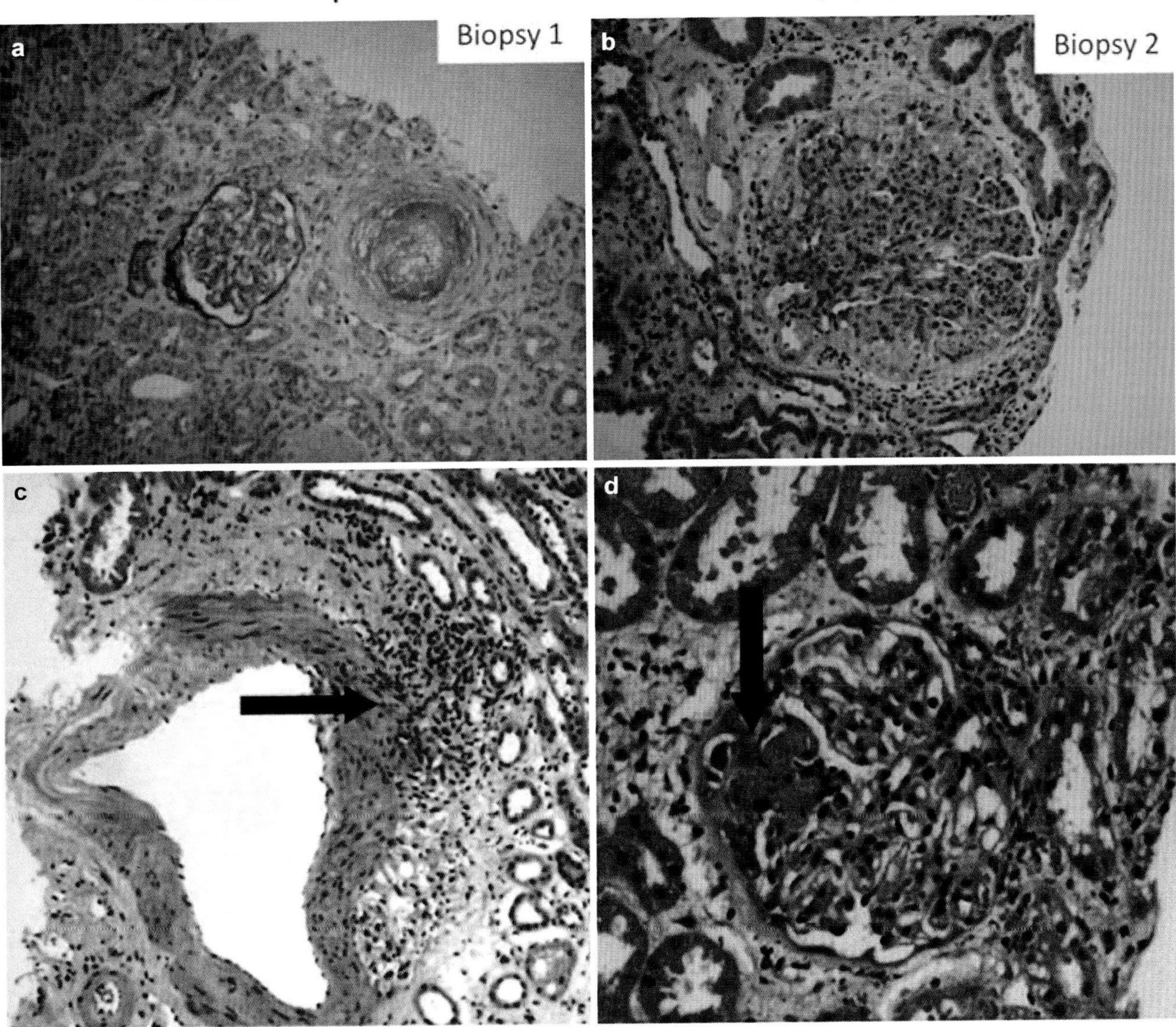

Fig. 21.3 Inflammatory renal pathology in scleroderma biopsy specimens. It is important to perform renal biopsy in cases of suspected glomerulonephritis. Clues for this include increased proteinuria, active urinary sediment and/or serology. (**a**) In the upper case, this patient had previously demonstrated typical SRC on biopsy (**a**) with good outcome. There was later deterioration in renal function, increased proteinuria and high-titre anti-dsDNA antibodies. Repeat renal biopsy showed membranoproliferative glomerulonephritis (**b**). The lower case had early dcSSc and high-titre ANCA and haematuria with normal renal function. The renal biopsy demonstrated vasculitis (**c**) and early crescentic glomerulonephritis (**d**)

whom mortality remains high. The poor long-term outcomes of SRC justify a continued search for novel treatment strategies. Some of the most exciting data emerging on the pathophysiology of SRC relates to endothelin-1, mostly because this is an actionable target. Endothelin-1 is known to contribute to other vascular manifestations of SSc including digital ulcers and pulmonary arterial hypertension. Elevated serum levels of endothelin-1 have now been reported in a small series of 27 SRC subjects [73] and increased endothelin-1 and both endothelin-A and endothelin-B receptor expression was increased in SRC biopsies [63, 64]. In 2013, the Bosentan in Renal Disease-1 (BIRD-1) study reported the safety of bosentan, a non-selective endothelin-1 receptor antagonist, in addition to ACE inhibition in an open-label study of six SRC patients [73]. Bosentan is currently being further investigated for SRC in the Effect of Bosentan in Scleroderma Renal Crisis (ScS-REINBO), an open-label safety and efficacy study of 16 incident SRC patients undertaken by French investigators in Paris (ClinicalTrials.gov identifier: NCT01241383). Data collection is expected to be completed in 2015. In addition, a phase II, single centre, randomised, placebo-controlled study of Zibotentan, a novel selective endothelin-A antagonists underway (ClinicalTrials.gov identifier: NCT02047708). Three study arms are included, that is, patients with mild or moderate chronic kidney disease associated with SSc, SRC patients who do not require dialysis and patients who have had SRC and are on dialysis. The primary outcome measure will be soluble vascular cell adhesion molecule 1 (sVCAM 1). A number of other actionable targets of SRC, including direct renin inhibition and inhibitors of the complement cascade, remain to be studied. The role of immunosuppression during the acute context of SRC or for the management of other renal manifestations of SSc needs to be delineated. In conclusion, outcomes and early mortality have improved dramatically but more needs to be achieved. Our ability to identify a subset of patients at high risk of developing the condition – those with early diffuse cutaneous systemic sclerosis and anti-RNA polymerase III antibodies in particular – offers hope that early diagnosis will improve this serious manifestation of SSc.

References

1. Denton CP, Lapadula G, Mouthon L, Muller-Ladner U. Renal complications and scleroderma renal crisis. Rheumatology (Oxford). 2009;48 Suppl 3:iii32–5.
2. Steen VD, Mayes MD, Merkel PA. Assessment of kidney involvement. Clin Exp Rheumatol. 2003;21(3 Suppl 29):S29–31.
3. Guillevin L, Bérezné A, Seror R, Teixeira L, Pourrat J, Mahr A, et al. Scleroderma renal crisis: a retrospective multicentre study on 91 patients and 427 controls. Rheumatology (Oxford). 2012;51(3): 460–7.
4. Steen VD, Costantino JP, Shapiro AP, Medsger Jr TA. Outcome of renal crisis in systemic sclerosis: relation to availability of angiotensin converting enzyme (ACE) inhibitors [see comments]. Ann Intern Med. 1990;113(5):352–7.
5. Arnaud L, Huart A, Plaisier E, Francois H, Mougenot B, Tiev K, et al. ANCA-related crescentic glomerulonephritis in systemic sclerosis: revisiting the "normotensive scleroderma renal crisis". Clin Nephrol. 2007;68(3):165–70.
6. Steen VD, Syzd A, Johnson JP, Greenberg A, Medsger Jr TA. Kidney disease other than renal crisis in patients with diffuse scleroderma. J Rheumatol. 2005;32(4):649–55.
7. Auspitz H. Ein beit zur lehre vom haute-sklerem der erwachsenen. Wrin Med Wschr. 1863;13:739–55.
8. Osler W. The principles and practice of medicine. New York: Appleton; 1892. p. 993–8.
9. Goetz RH. The pathology of progressive systemic sclerosis (generalized scleroderma) with special reference to changes in the viscera. Clin Proc Grad Med Assoc. 1945;4:337–92.
10. Moore HC, Sheehan HL. The kidney of scleroderma. Lancet. 1952;1:68.
11. Keeler E, Fioravanti G, Samuel B, Longo S. Scleroderma renal crisis or thrombotic thrombocytopenic purpura: seeing through the masquerade. Lab Med. 2015;46(2):e39–44. doi:10.1309/LM72AM5XFHZYOQCB.
12. Leroy EC, Black C, Fleischmajer R, Jablonska S, Krieg T, Medsger Jr TA, et al. Scleroderma (systemic sclerosis): classification, subsets and pathogenesis. J Rheumatol. 1988;15(2):202–5.
13. Phan TG, Cass A, Gillin A, Trew P, Fertig N, Sturgess A. Anti-RNA polymerase III antibodies in the diagnosis of scleroderma renal crisis sine scleroderma. J Rheumatol. 1999;26(11):2489–92.
14. van den Hoogen F, et al. 2013 classification criteria for systemic sclerosis: an American college of rheumatology/European league against rheumatism collaborative initiative. Ann Rheum Dis. 2013;72(11):1747–55.
15. Steen VD, Medsger Jr TA. Case-control study of glucocorticoids and other drugs that either precipitate or protect from the development of scleroderma renal crisis. Arthritis Rheum. 1998;41(9): 1613–9.
16. Nihtyanova SI, Schreiber BE, Ong VH, Rosenberg D, Moinzadeh P, Coghlan JG, Wells AU, Denton CP. Prediction of pulmonary complications and long-term survival in systemic sclerosis. Arthritis Rheumatol. 2014;66(6):1625–35.
17. Penn H, Howie AJ, Kingdon EJ, Bunn CC, Stratton RJ, Black CM, et al. Scleroderma renal crisis: patient characteristics and long-term outcomes. QJM. 2007;100(8):485–94.
18. Teixeira L, Mouthon L, Mahr A, Berezne A, Agard C, Mehrenberger M, et al. Mortality and risk factors of scleroderma renal crisis: a French retrospective study of 50 patients. Ann Rheum Dis. 2008;67(1):110–6.
19. Hudson M, et al. Exposure to ACE inhibitors prior to the onset of scleroderma renal crisis-results from the International Scleroderma Renal Crisis Survey. Semin Arthritis Rheum. 2014;43(5):666–72.
20. Steen VD, Lanz Jr JK, Conte C, Owens GR, Medsger Jr TA. Therapy for severe interstitial lung disease in systemic sclerosis. A retrospective study. Arthritis Rheum. 1994;37(9):1290–6.
21. Traub YM, Shapiro AP, Rodnan GP, Medsger TA, McDonald Jr RH, Steen VD, et al. Hypertension and renal failure (scleroderma renal crisis) in progressive systemic sclerosis. Review of a 25-year experience with 68 cases. Medicine (Baltimore). 1983;62(6): 335–52.
22. Steen VD, Medsger Jr TA. Epidemiology and natural history of systemic sclerosis. Rheum Dis Clin N Am. 1990;16(1):1–10.
23. Steen VD, Ziegler GL, Rodnan GP, Medsger Jr TA. Clinical and laboratory associations of anticentromere antibody in patients with progressive systemic sclerosis. Arthritis Rheum. 1984;27(2): 125–31.
24. Steen VD, Medsger Jr TA, Osial Jr TA, Ziegler GL, Shapiro AP, Rodnan GP. Factors predicting development of renal involvement in progressive systemic sclerosis. Am J Med. 1984;76(5):779–86.
25. Korzets Z, Schneider M, Savin H, Ben Chetrit S, Bernheim J, Shitrit P, et al. Intriguing presentation of scleroderma renal crisis (scleroderma renal crisis sine scleroderma sine hypertension). Nephrol Dial Transplant. 1998;13(11):2953–6.
26. Molina JF, Anaya JM, Cabrera GE, Hoffman E, Espinoza LR. Systemic sclerosis sine scleroderma: an unusual presentation in scleroderma renal crisis. J Rheumatol. 1995;22(3):557–60.
27. Steen VD, Medsger Jr TA. The palpable tendon friction rub: an important physical examination finding in patients with systemic sclerosis [see comments]. Arthritis Rheum. 1997;40(6):1146–51.
28. Bunn CC, Denton CP, Shi-wen X, Knight C, Black CM. Anti-RNA polymerases and other autoantibody specificities in systemic sclerosis. Br J Rheumatol. 1998;37(1):15–20.
29. Okano Y, Steen VD, Medsger Jr TA. Autoantibody reactive with RNA polymerase III in systemic sclerosis. Ann Intern Med. 1993;119(10):1005–13.
30. Rivolta R, Mascagni B, Berruti V, Quarto DP, Elli A, Scorza R, et al. Renal vascular damage in systemic sclerosis patients without clinical evidence of nephropathy. Arthritis Rheum. 1996;39(6): 1030–4.
31. Nguyen B, et al. Association of RNA polymerase III antibodies with scleroderma renal crisis. J Rheumatol. 2010;37(5):1068; author reply 1069.
32. Lynch B, et al. The prognosis of scleroderma renal crisis in RNA-polymerase III antibody-positive compared to RNA-polymerase III antibody-negative patients. Rheumatology. 2014;53 suppl 1:i179.
33. Kuwana M, et al. Autoantibody reactive with three classes of RNA polymerases in sera from patients with systemic sclerosis. J Clin Invest. 1993;91(4):1399–404.

34. Hamaguchi Y, et al. Clinical and immunologic predictors of scleroderma renal crisis in Japanese systemic sclerosis patients with anti-RNA polymerase III autoantibodies. Arthritis Rheumatol. 2015; 67(4):1045–52.
35. Patel V, et al. Anti-RNA polymerase II antibodies in a US cohort of systemic sclerosis patients: comment on the article by Hamaguchi et al. Arthritis Rheumatol. 2015;67:2547–8.
36. Steen VD. Scleroderma renal crisis. Rheum Dis Clin N Am. 2003;29(2):315–33.
37. McWhorter JE, Leroy EC. Pericardial disease in scleroderma (systemic sclerosis). Am J Med. 1974;57(4):566–75.
38. Helfrich DJ, Banner B, Steen VD, Medsger Jr TA. Normotensive renal failure in systemic sclerosis. Arthritis Rheum. 1989;32(9): 1128–34.
39. Kohno K, Katayama T, Majima K, Fujisawa M, Iida S, Fukami K, et al. A case of normotensive scleroderma renal crisis after high-dose methylprednisolone treatment. Clin Nephrol. 2000;53(6):479–82 [In Process Citation].
40. Yamanishi Y, Yamana S, Ishioka S, Yamakido M. Development of ischemic colitis and scleroderma renal crisis following methylprednisolone pulse therapy for progressive systemic sclerosis. Intern Med. 1996;35(7):583–6.
41. Avouac J, et al. Joint and tendon involvement predict disease progression in systemic sclerosis: a EUSTAR prospective study. Ann Rheum Dis 2016;75(1):103–9.
42. Bar J, Ehrenfeld M, Rozenman J, Perelman M, Sidi Y, Gur H. Pulmonary-renal syndrome in systemic sclerosis. Semin Arthritis Rheum. 2001;30(6):403–10.
43. Kapur A, Ballou SP, Renston JP, Luna E, Chung-Park M. Recurrent acute scleroderma renal crisis complicated by thrombotic thrombocytopenic purpura. J Rheumatol. 1997;24(12):2469–72.
44. Kfoury Baz EM, Mahfouz RA, Masri AF, Jamaleddine GW. Thrombotic thrombocytopenic purpura in a case of scleroderma renal crisis treated with twice-daily therapeutic plasma exchange. Ren Fail. 2001;23(5):737–42.
45. Manadan AM, Harris C, Block JA. Thrombotic thrombocytopenic purpura in the setting of systemic sclerosis. Semin Arthritis Rheum. 2005;34(4):683–8.
46. Torok KS, Cortese Hassett A, Kiss JE, Lucas M, Medsger TA. ACR presentation 2008. Scleroderma renal crisis and thrombotic thrombocytopenic purpura – are they related? ACR presentation 2008.
47. Lian EC. Pathogenesis of thrombotic thrombocytopenic purpura: ADAMTS13 deficiency and beyond. Semin Thromb Hemost. 2005;31(6):625–32.
48. Penn H, Denton CP. Diagnosis, management and prevention of scleroderma renal disease. Curr Opin Rheumatol. 2008;20(6): 692–6.
49. KDIGO. Clinical practice guideline for acute kidney injury (AKI). Kidney Int Suppl. 2012;2(1):4.
50. Wipff J, Gallier G, Dieude P, Avouac J, Tiev K, Hachulla E, et al. Angiotensin-converting enzyme gene does not contribute to genetic susceptibility to systemic sclerosis in European Caucasians. J Rheumatol. 2009;36(2):337–40.
51. Stratton RJ, Coghlan JG, Pearson JD, Burns A, Sweny P, Abraham DJ, et al. Different patterns of endothelial cell activation in renal and pulmonary vascular disease in scleroderma. QJM. 1998;91(8): 561–6.
52. Batal I, Domsic RT, Medsger TA, Bastacky S. Scleroderma renal crisis: a pathology perspective. Int J Rheumatol. 2010;54:3704.
53. Nihtyanova SI, Parker JC, Black CM, Bunn CC, Denton CP. A longitudinal study of anti-RNA polymerase III antibody levels in systemic sclerosis. Rheumatology (Oxford). 2009;48(10):1218–21.
54. Penn H, et al. Targeting the endothelin axis in scleroderma renal crisis: rationale and feasibility. QJM. 2013;106(9):839–48.
55. Denton CP, Bickerstaff MC, Shiwen X, Carulli MT, Haskard DO, Dubois RM, Black CM. Serial circulating adhesion molecule levels reflect disease severity in systemic sclerosis. Br J Rheumatol. 1995;34(11):1048–54.
56. Takahashi T, et al. A possible contribution of lipocalin-2 to the development of dermal fibrosis, pulmonary vascular involvement, and renal dysfunction in systemic sclerosis. Br J Dermatol. 2015;173:681–9.
57. Guerra S, et al. Defining genetic risk for scleroderma renal crisis: a genome-wide analysis of anti-RNA polymerase antibody-positive systemic sclerosis. Rheumatology. 2014;54 suppl 1:i159.
58. Nguyen B, et al. HLA-DRB1*0407 and *1304 are risk factors for scleroderma renal crisis. Arthritis Rheum. 2011;63:530–4.
59. Fonseca C, Renzoni E, Sestini P, Pantelidis P, Lagan A, Bunn C, McHugh N, Welsh KI, Du Bois RM, Denton CP, Black C, Abraham D. Endothelin axis polymorphisms in patients with scleroderma. Arthritis Rheum. 2006;54:3034–42.
60. George JN, Nester CM. Syndromes of thrombotic microangiopathy. N Engl J Med. 2014;371(7):654–66.
61. Derrett-Smith E, et al. Perturbed response to experimental renal injury in a mouse model of systemic sclerosis. Rheumatology. 2014;53 suppl 1:i176.
62. Shapiro L, et al. Development of a "Renal Crisis Prevention Card" as an educational tool aimed at improving outcomes in high-risk patients with systemic sclerosis. Arthritis Rheumatol. 2014; 66:abstract Suppl. 2716.
63. Kowal-Bielecka O, Landewe R, Avouac J, Chwiesko S, Miniati I, Czirjak L, et al. EULAR recommendations for the treatment of systemic sclerosis: a report from the EULAR Scleroderma Trials and Research group (EUSTAR). Ann Rheum Dis. 2009;68(5):620–8.
64. Steen VD, Medsger Jr TA. Long-term outcomes of scleroderma renal crisis. Ann Intern Med. 2000;133(8):600–3.
65. Cheung WY, Gibson IW, Rush D, Jeffery J, Karpinski M. Late recurrence of scleroderma renal crisis in a renal transplant recipient despite angiotensin II blockade. Am J Kidney Dis. 2005; 45(5):930–4.
66. Dhaun N, Macintyre IM, Bellamy CO, Kluth DC. Endothelin receptor antagonism and renin inhibition as treatment options for scleroderma kidney. Am J Kidney Dis. 2009;54(4):726–31.
67. Vancheeswaran R, Magoulas T, Efrat G, Wheeler-Jones C, Olsen I, Penny R, et al. Circulating endothelin-1 levels in systemic sclerosis subsets a marker of fibrosis or vascular dysfunction? [see comments]. J Rheumatol. 1994;21(10):1838–44.
68. Kobayashi H, Nishimaki T, Kaise S, Suzuki T, Watanabe K, Kasukawa R, et al. Immunohistological study endothelin-1 and endothelin-A and B receptors in two patients with scleroderma renal crisis. Clin Rheumatol. 1999;18(5):425–7.
69. Mouthon L, Mehrenberger M, Teixeira L, Fakhouri F, Berezne A, Guillevin L, et al. Endothelin-1 expression in scleroderma renal crisis. Hum Pathol. 2011;42(1):95–102.
70. Gliddon AE, Doré CJ, Black CM, McHugh N, Moots R, Denton CP, Herrick A, Barnes T, Camilleri J, Chakravarty K, Emery P, Griffiths B, Hopkinson ND, Hickling P, Lanyon P, Laversuch C, Lawson T, Mallya R, Nisar M, Rhys-Dillon C, Sheeran T, Maddison PJ. Prevention of vascular damage in scleroderma and autoimmune Raynaud's phenomenon: a multicenter, randomized, double-blind, placebo-controlled trial of the angiotensin-converting enzyme inhibitor quinapril. Arthritis Rheum. 2007;56:3837–46.
71. Siva B, McDonald SP, Hawley CM, Rosman JB, Brown FG, Wiggins KJ, et al. End-stage kidney disease due to scleroderma—outcomes in 127 consecutive ANZDATA registry cases. Nephrol Dial Transplant. 2011;26:3165–71.
72. Chang YJ, Spiera H. Renal transplantation in scleroderma. Medicine (Baltimore). 1999;78(6):382–5.
73. Gibney EM, Parikh CR, Jani A, Fischer MJ, Collier D, Wiseman AC. Kidney transplantation for systemic sclerosis improves survival and may modulate disease activity. Am J Transplant. 2004;4(12):2027–31.

74. Herrera-Esparza R, Aguilar JL, Saucedo A, Gonzalez I, Lopez-Robles E, Avalos-Diaz E. Scleroderma with type III glomerulonephritis and MPO-ANCA antibodies in the serum. J Eur Acad Dermatol Venereol. 2005;19(5):617–20.
75. Casari S, Haeney M, Farrand S, Herrick A. Antineutrophil cytoplasmic antibodies a "Red Flag" in patients with systemic sclerosis. J Rheumatol. 2002;29(12):2666–7.
76. Mimura I, Hori Y, Matsukawa T, Uozaki H, Tojo A, Fujita T. Noncrescentic ANCA-associated renal crisis in systemic sclerosis. Clin Nephrol. 2008;70(2):183–5.
77. Anders HJ, Wiebecke B, Haedecke C, Sanden S, Combe C, Schlondorff D. MPO-ANCA-positive crescentic glomerulonephritis: a distinct entity of scleroderma renal disease? Am J Kidney Dis. 1999;33:e3.
78. Derrett-Smith EC, Nihtyanova SI, Harvey J, Salama AD, Denton CP. Revisiting ANCA-associated vasculitis in systemic sclerosis: clinical, serological and immunogenetic factors. Rheumatology (Oxford). 2013;52(10):1824–31.
79. Shanmugam VK, Steen VD. Renal manifestations in scleroderma: evidence for subclinical renal disease as a marker of vasculopathy. Int J Rheumatol. 2010;2010. pii: 538589. doi: 10.1155/2010/538589. Epub 2010 Aug 17. PMID: 20827302.
80. Caron, Hudson, et al. Longitudinal study of renal function in systemic sclerosis. J Rheumatol. 2012;39(9):1829–34. doi:10.3899/jrheum.111417.

Cardiac Involvement: Evaluation and Management

22

Sanjiv J. Shah, Ahmad Mahmood, and J. Gerry Coghlan

Introduction

Cardiac involvement in systemic sclerosis (SSc) is common and can present with protean manifestations, and when symptomatic portends a poor prognosis [1–6]. SSc can affect virtually any cardiac structure, thereby causing myocardial abnormalities (including myocardial fibrosis, left ventricular [LV] systolic dysfunction, and LV diastolic dysfunction), coronary microvascular ischemia, pericardial disease, conduction abnormalities (including brady- and tachyarrhythmias), and less commonly valvular disease [1–5]. Furthermore, cardiac manifestations of SSc can be primary (i.e., direct cardiac involvement due to the SSc disease process) or secondary to pulmonary arterial hypertension, interstitial lung disease, or significant kidney disease, all of which are common in patients with SSc [1, 6]. The purpose of the present chapter is to focus on primary, direct cardiac involvement in SSc, with discussion of: (1) epidemiology of cardiac involvement in SSc; (2) screening for cardiac involvement in SSc; (3) characterization of the pathophysiology, diagnosis, and management of specific cardiac lesions in SSc; (4) noninvasive and invasive tools for the detection and monitoring of cardiac involvement; and (5) areas of uncertainty in the study of cardiac involvement in SSc.

The successful evaluation and management of cardiac involvement in patients with SSc requires careful screening, a high index of suspicion given the broad and nonspecific symptoms associated with cardiac manifestations, and a multidisciplinary approach involving rheumatologists, cardiologists, and imaging specialists [6]. With the advent of novel noninvasive tests such as new biomarkers, tissue Doppler imaging, speckle-tracking echocardiography, and diffuse fibrosis imaging using cardiac magnetic resonance imaging (MRI), the screening, diagnosis, and research of cardiac manifestations of SSc should expand rapidly in the near future.

Epidemiology of Cardiac Involvement in Systemic Sclerosis

Defining the epidemiology of cardiac involvement in SSc has proven to be difficult because of the wide variety of possible cardiac manifestations and variability in the types of diagnostic techniques used to diagnose SSc heart disease. Clinical symptoms can be considered as "late" events in a significant number of patients. Electrocardiography and chest radiography are insensitive techniques, whereas echocardiography (especially tissue Doppler imaging and speckle-tracking techniques), single-photon emission computerized tomography (SPECT), radionuclide ventriculography, and MRI allow the detection of structural and functional cardiac lesions at a much earlier stage. From published studies, it appears that cardiac manifestations are quite common in SSc, but the exact prevalence depends greatly on the patient population, definition of cardiac manifestations, and tests used to diagnose cardiac involvement. For example, rates of cardiac involvement in SSc for reduced LV ejection fraction [7], clinical cardiac involvement (defined as pericarditis, heart failure, severe arrhythmias, or conduction abnormalities) [8], abnormal tissue Doppler systolic or diastolic function [4, 9–11], and abnormal results on thallium scanning [12] have been found to be 5.4 %, 30–35 %, 40–60 %, and >60–70 %, respectively.

Besides difficulties in estimating prevalence of cardiac manifestations, there is some controversy regarding the frequency of cardiac involvement in limited cutaneous versus diffuse cutaneous forms of SSc. Whereas some studies have found that both types of SSc have similar rates of cardiac involvement, others have found increased prevalence

S.J. Shah, MD (✉)
Northwestern University Feinberg School of Medicine, Chicago, IL, USA
e-mail: sanjiv.shah@northwestern.edu

J.G. Coghlan, MD • Ahmad Mahmood, MD
Department of Pulmonary Hypertension, Royal Free Hospital, London, UK
e-mail: gerry.coghlan@nhs.net; mahmood.ahmad2@nhs.net

J. Varga et al. (eds.), *Scleroderma*, DOI 10.1007/978-3-319-31407-5_22

of cardiac manifestations in diffuse cutaneous SSc [1, 4, 8]. In a study of 1012 Italian patients with SSc, cardiac involvement was present in 32 % of diffuse cutaneous SSc versus 23 % in limited cutaneous SSc [8]. This finding was replicated in a large study of LV systolic dysfunction in SSc. Of 7073 patients with SSc, 383 had LV systolic dysfunction (defined as LV ejection fraction <55 %), whereas 6690 had normal LV systolic function. SSc patients with LV systolic dysfunction were more likely to have diffuse cutaneous SSc compared to patients with normal LV systolic function (48 % vs. 32 %, respectively; $P=0.001$) [7]. A recent study also found that patients with diffuse cutaneous SSc develop cardiac involvement sooner after diagnosis than limited cutaneous SSc patients [13]. Additional studies have found that the prevalence of cardiac involvement is especially high in the subset of patients with rapidly evolving skin involvement [14], anti-U3RNP antibodies [15], and/or skeletal myopathy [16]. From these studies, we can conclude that cardiac involvement occurs frequently in both limited and diffuse cutaneous forms of SSc but appears to be more common in the latter, and SSc patients at highest risk are those who have rapidly progressive skin disease, anti-U3RNP antibodies, and/or concomitant skeletal myopathy.

Several studies have examined the influence of cardiac involvement on death in SSc. In large series of SSc patients, when cardiac involvement appeared to be clinically evident, it was found to be a poor prognostic factor [17]. In a study of patients with the diffuse cutaneous form of SSc, cardiac symptoms were observed in 15 % of patients; at 10-year follow-up, cardiac involvement explained 20 % of disease–attributed deaths [18]. In a large cohort of Italian patients, 35 % had cardiac symptoms or arrhythmia, with cardiac involvement alone accounting for 36 % of deaths [8]. In French Canadian patients, 11.4 % of deaths involved the heart [19]. An international meta-analysis of pooled cohorts of 11,526 person-years of follow-up [20] found that clinical cardiac involvement was present in 10 % of patients. A multivariate analysis in this study demonstrated an increased hazard ratio for mortality of 2.8 (95 % confidence interval 2.1–3.8) if cardiac involvement was present, and presence of cardiac involvement was the strongest predictor of mortality in this study [20]. These findings have been affirmed by more recent studies, the largest of which was a European study involving 5860 patients [21–24]. In this study, 55 % of deaths were due to SSc while 45 % of deaths were thought to be unrelated to SSc. Of the SSc-related deaths, 26 % were cardiac (predominantly heart failure and arrhythmias), whereas 29 % of non-SSc-related deaths were due to cardiac causes. Thus, in patients with SSc, death due to cardiac disease is common and presence of cardiac involvement is an independent risk factor for death.

Screening and Diagnosis of Cardiac Involvement in Systemic Sclerosis

Given the poor prognosis associated with cardiac involvement in SSc, screening for the detection of subclinical cardiac disease (in addition to thorough evaluation of cardiac symptoms) is highly desirable. Often times, details from the clinical history and physical examination provide important clues for the presence of cardiac involvement. Exertional lightheadedness, dizziness, or syncope can be a sign of pulmonary arterial hypertension, RV dysfunction, or arrhythmias. Chronic pericardial disease (both constrictive pericarditis and chronic pericardial effusion) often presents with symptoms of right-sided heart failure (lethargy, abdominal fullness, early satiety, and leg swelling). Myocardial disease and microvascular ischemia often do not cause specific symptoms until severe, at which point chest pain, shortness of breath, and overt left heart failure can occur. The sudden worsening of Raynaud's phenomenon (e.g., digital necrosis) may be an ominous sign of severe cardiac microvascular dysfunction and/or myocardial dysfunction leading to reduced cardiac output and reflexive systemic vasoconstriction. In these cases, urgent evaluation is often necessary so that therapies can be instituted to improve cardiac function.

Unlike interstitial lung disease and pulmonary arterial hypertension, optimal screening for direct cardiac involvement in SSc is unknown. Patients with SSc undergo routine Doppler echocardiography for pulmonary hypertension screening, so evaluation of possible direct cardiac involvement can and should be performed simultaneously. Given the ability of tissue Doppler imaging to detect subclinical systolic and diastolic dysfunction, this widely available technique should be performed on all patients with SSc.

Along with Doppler and tissue Doppler echocardiography, cardiac biomarker testing (with natriuretic peptides) is the other cornerstone in screening for cardiac involvement in SSc. In patients with symptoms or signs of cardiac involvement, and in patients with abnormal results on screening tests, detailed evaluation of possible forms of cardiac involvement should be undertaken as outlined in Table 22.1.

Specific Cardiac Manifestations of Systemic Sclerosis

Given the diverse cardiac manifestations of SSc, understanding pathophysiology, clinical manifestations, diagnosis, and management of the various possibilities of cardiac involvement is essential. Figure 22.1 displays a schematic of the possible primary cardiac manifestations of SSc. In the following section, we review each of these specific forms of cardiac involvement in SSc in further detail. Primary cardiac

Table 22.1 Recommendations for evaluation of abnormal cardiac symptoms, signs, or screening studies in systemic sclerosis

Abnormal cardiac symptom, sign, or screening study	Recommendation for further evaluation specific to systemic sclerosis
Chest pain	Evaluate for myocardial microvascular ischemia with perfusion imaging (either nuclear or cardiac MRI); evaluate for pericarditis or pericardial effusion with ECG, echo, and cardiac MRI
Shortness of breath, exercise intolerance	If alternative causes (interstitial lung disease, pulmonary arterial hypertension) have been excluded, evaluate with natriuretic peptides (BNP or NT-proBNP); consider exercise testing to objectively document dyspnea and exercise intolerance (cardiopulmonary exercise testing can distinguish cardiac from pulmonary causes). If cardiac involvement suspected, evaluate further with echocardiography and cardiac MRI
Left heart failure (pulmonary edema or pulmonary vascular congestion)	Echocardiography, cardiac MRI with perfusion; consider constrictive pericarditis
Right heart failure (elevated jugular venous pressure, pleural effusion, hepatomegaly, ascites, and/or leg swelling)	Echocardiography, cardiac MRI to look for constrictive pericarditis; if strong suspicion for constrictive pericarditis, evaluate further with simultaneous right and left heart catheterization
Palpitations	48-h Holter monitor; if symptoms are infrequent, may need 30-day event monitor
Lightheadedness, dizziness, or syncope	48-h Holter monitor; if symptoms are infrequent, may need 30-day event monitor; echocardiography to evaluate for structural heart disease and to exclude pulmonary arterial hypertension which can cause exertional lightheadedness or syncope
RV systolic dysfunction TAPSE <1.6 cm [125] RV tissue Doppler S' <10 cm/s [125] RV fractional area change <0.35 [125] Septal flattening in systole or diastole ("D-shaped" LV in short axis)	Consider right heart catheterization to differentiate primary RV involvement (low or normal RV and PA systolic pressures) vs. secondary RV involvement due to pulmonary hypertension (high RV and PA systolic pressures)
LV systolic dysfunction LV ejection fraction <55 % [7, 171]	Perfusion study (nuclear or cardiac MRI) to evaluate for microvascular (or macrovascular) ischemia; check for signs and symptoms of heart failure; consider coronary angiography to exclude epicardial coronary disease, especially in patients with EF <40–45 % or if angina or atherosclerotic coronary artery disease risk factors are present
LV diastolic dysfunction Impaired relaxation and/or evidence of elevated LV filling pressures [121]	Evaluate for coronary artery disease, systemic hypertension, or microvascular ischemia; check for signs and symptoms of heart failure
Reduced LV tissue Doppler velocities Lateral s' <10 cm/s [122] Lateral e' <10 cm/s if age <54 years; lateral e' <9 if age 55–65 years; or lateral e' <8 cm/s if age >65 years [122, 172]	More data is needed to determine optimal evaluation of systemic sclerosis patients with subclinical reduction in tissue Doppler velocities
Elevated natriuretic peptide levels BNP >60 pg/ml [117] NT-proBNP >125 pg/ml [107]	If DLCO is decreased and/or RV dysfunction is present on echocardiography, proceed to right heart catheterization to evaluate for pulmonary hypertension; evaluate for LV systolic or diastolic dysfunction; check for signs and symptoms of heart failure

MRI magnetic resonance imaging, *RV* right ventricle, *LV* left ventricle, *S'* systolic longitudinal tissue Doppler velocity, *E'* early diastolic longitudinal tissue Doppler velocity, *BNP* B-type natriuretic peptide, *NT-proBNP* N-terminal pro-B-type natriuretic peptide, *DLCO* diffusing capacity of carbon monoxide

involvement in SSc must be differentiated from secondary involvement, which can occur in the setting of pulmonary arterial hypertension, interstitial lung disease, systemic hypertension, and significant renal disease.

Intrinsic Myocardial Disease: Myocardial Fibrosis and Microvascular Ischemia

Direct myocardial involvement in SSc often involves a combination of myocardial ischemia and fibrosis. As in other organs involved in SSc, there is a complex interplay between microvascular disease, possible low-grade inflammation, and the ultimate development of fibrosis, which is the hallmark of SSc-related myocardial disease.

Pathophysiology In patients with SSc, the primary problem that ultimately leads to cardiac fibrosis and ventricular dysfunction is an abnormality of the coronary microcirculation, including vasospasm and recurrent ischemia-reperfusion injury [1, 4, 9]. There are several lines of evidence which support the conclusion that the microcirculation, and not traditional atherosclerotic coronary disease, is the site of abnormal myocardial blood flow in SSc. Histological examinations have revealed

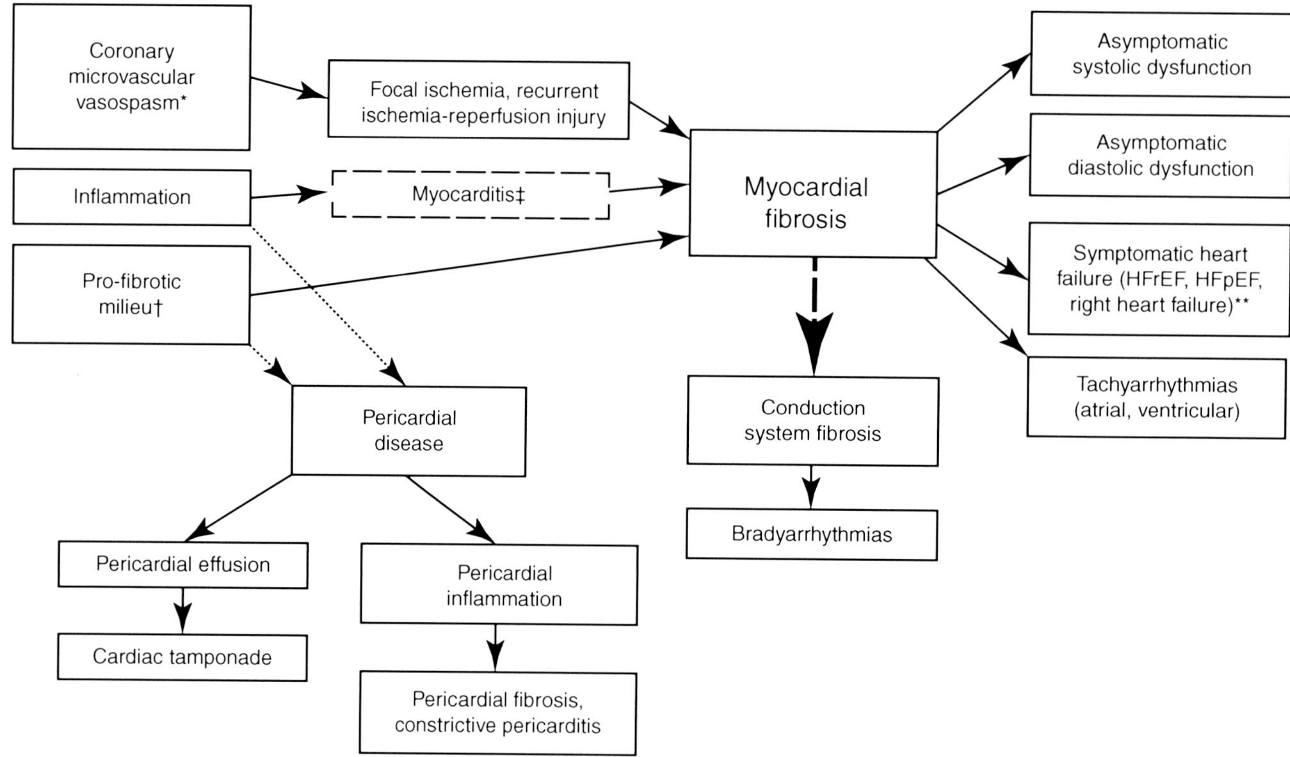

Fig. 22.1 Schematic diagram of primary cardiac manifestations of systemic sclerosis. *Coronary microvascular vasospasm may directly induce asymptomatic (or symptomatic) systolic and diastolic dysfunction and tachyarrhythmias. †Factors such as TGF-β1, reactive oxygen species [168, 169]; ‡Clinically active myocarditis can occur but is uncommon and typically associated with myositis; anecdotal reports of common "low-grade" cardiac inflammation have been reported [3], but there are no systematic studies which corroborate this observation; ***HFrEF* heart failure with reduced LV ejection fraction, *HFpEF* heart failure with preserved LV ejection fraction

diffuse patchy fibrosis, with contraction band necrosis unrelated to epicardial coronary artery stenosis [25, 26] and concentric intimal hypertrophy associated with fibrinoid necrosis of intramural coronary arteries [27]. SSc cardiac fibrosis can be distinguished from atherosclerotic coronary artery disease because SSc involves the immediate subendocardium, which is usually spared in atherosclerotic heart disease. In addition, hemosiderin deposits are not typically seen in SSc but are found in atherosclerosis [3]. Furthermore, angina pectoris and myocardial infarction have been observed in SSc patients whose epicardial coronary arteries were normal. These findings suggest that extensive microvascular disease can occur in patients with SSc via mechanisms that are independent from atherosclerosis.

Vasospasm of the small coronary arteries and arterioles play a major role in the early myocardial abnormalities in patients with SSc. These functional and reversible abnormalities were first demonstrated using thallium-201 SPECT; these studies, allowing the assessment of myocardial perfusion, provided evidence of early reversible ischemia. Myocardial perfusion defects in SSc patients were demonstrated either at rest, after exercise, or after cold stimulation [28–32]. Exercise-induced perfusion defects observed by scintigraphy were predictive of developing subsequent cardiac disease or death [33]. As these vasospastic lesions progress, they often lead to recurrent ischemia and reperfusion which leads to myocyte apoptosis and leads to replacement with fibroblasts and collagen deposits as fibrosis ensues.

Besides coronary vasospasm, there is also evidence to implicate impaired coronary vasodilator reserve in patients with SSc. Coronary vasodilator reserve at cardiac catheterization has been investigated in clinically symptomatic SSc patients with the diffuse cutaneous form of the disease [34]: at rest, the mean coronary sinus blood flow was not significantly different compared to control subjects; in contrast, after maximal coronary artery vasodilation with intravenous dipyridamole, the coronary vasodilator reserve was strikingly reduced. All the SSc patients had evidence of established myocardial involvement, confirmed using noninvasive procedures. Their coronary arteriograms were normal; endomyocardial biopsies showed fibrotic tissue and a typical SSc vascular lesion with concentric intimal hypertrophy. These results demonstrated that despite normal epicardial coronary arteries, structural abnormalities of small coronary arteries or arterioles explained the strikingly reduced coronary reserve. Subsequent studies using contrast enhanced transthoracic Doppler before and after adenosine infusion confirmed the impaired coronary flow reserve in SSc patients without clinical evidence of cardiac involvement [35, 36].

Finally, myocardial inflammation can also occur and may cause acute myocarditis with resultant myocardial fibrosis. Myocardial inflammation may be acute or subacute and can result in rapid decline in cardiac function; whether low-grade chronic inflammation is present in SSc and contributes to the generalized fibrotic process and the slow decline of cardiac function in SSc is unknown and has only been reported anecdotally [3]. When severe myocarditis is present, it is often associated with skeletal muscle myositis [3, 37, 38], a finding which may represent a specific subset of SSc patient with an overlap syndrome of SSc and polymyositis.

Clinical Manifestations and Diagnosis Recurrent vasospasm, poor vasodilator reserve, focal ischemia, and recurrent ischemia-reperfusion injury, and inflammation (when present) all culminate in the same end result: myocardial fibrosis. All of these pathologic insults can lead to the varied clinical manifestations of myocardial disease in SSc, which include asymptomatic LV systolic or diastolic dysfunction (which can occur several years prior to becoming clinically evident) and clinically overt heart failure (Fig. 22.2). Overt heart failure, in turn, can present as acute myocarditis or myopericarditis with a rapid decline in LV ejection fraction; chronic heart failure with reduced ejection fraction (systolic heart failure); or chronic heart failure with preserved ejection fraction (diastolic heart failure). In addition, patients with SSc occasionally develop acute vasospastic crisis, which manifests as severe peripheral and cardiac Raynaud's phenomenon. These patients develop a rapid decline in cardiac output due to ischemia and reduced LV systolic function. This in turn leads to poor perfusion of the extremities, which exacerbates the severe Raynaud's phenomenon and can rapidly lead to digital necrosis if left untreated.

LV Systolic and Diastolic Dysfunction Several studies, using radionuclide ventriculography, have demonstrated a decreased global LV ejection fraction (LVEF) in a minority of patients, although segmental dysfunction and exercise-induced LV dysfunction are more prevalent [39]. Studies of LV regional wall motion in SSc have shown that 29% of patients have one or more areas of hypokinesis [40]. In SSc patients with diffuse cutaneous disease, the group with thallium defect scores above the median had a significantly lower mean LVEF than the other group and all patients with abnormal resting LVEF had thallium scores above the median [12]. The link between myocardial perfusion abnormalities and dysfunction suggests a similar underlying mechanism for myocardial involvement in SSc.

Several studies have reported on the prevalence of diastolic dysfunction in SSc [41–45], and have shown that diastolic dysfunction is more common in SSc compared to controls [11]. Such abnormalities have been correlated with disease duration [46, 47], and have suggested that impaired diastolic relaxation of the LV together is associated with a defective cardiac functional reserve [41]. Whether LV diastolic dysfunction in SSc is primary or secondary to other cardiac abnormalities is a subject of debate [42, 43]. Importantly, when diastolic dysfunction is present in SSc, it is associated with worse survival [47, 48], underscoring its importance as a marker of cardiac involvement in SSc.

RV Dysfunction Several studies have demonstrated a primary abnormality of RV function in SSc, independent of pulmonary hypertension [49–57]. A study by Meune et al. focused on cardiac function in 42 SSc patients with normal pulmonary arterial pressure and less than 5 years of disease duration compared to matched controls; radionuclide ventriculography showed that 16 SSc patients had reduced RVEF, 3 had reduced LVEF, and 10 had reduced peak filling rate, highlighting early RV systolic and left diastolic dysfunction [57]. Moreover, RVEF was correlated with both LVEF and peak filling rate, whereas no correlation was found with either pulmonary function impairment or pulmonary arterial pressure, strongly suggesting intrinsic myocardial involvement in these patients [57]. Others have found abnormalities in RV diastolic function using tissue Doppler imaging [56, 58] and tricuspid annular plane systolic excursion (TAPSE) [55].

Approach to the Patient with Clinical Symptoms or Signs of Possible Myocardial Involvement In patients with shortness of breath, chest pain, heart failure symptoms, or frequent palpitations or arrhythmias, investigation of direct myocardial involvement is warranted. In these cases, echocardiography with tissue Doppler imaging and natriuretic peptides (BNP or NT-proBNP) can be very helpful as a first step. If microvascular ischemia is suspected, either SPECT or adenosine perfusion cardiac MRI can be performed. If available, we prefer cardiac MRI because of its increased sensitivity, higher spatial resolution, and ability to simultaneously evaluate the RV and pericardium along with LV structure and perfusion. In selected cases, coronary angiography, invasive hemodynamic testing, or endomyocardial biopsy can be performed to assist in diagnosis and therapeutic decision-making. Patients who are found to have reduced LV ejection fraction (even if mildly reduced) should be monitored very closely for the possibility of acute vasospastic crisis or acute myocarditis since these can be life-threatening conditions.

Management In SSc, treatment of myocardial involvement varies by clinical manifestation. It should be noted that there is a general lack of randomized controlled trials of therapies for cardiac involvement in SSc. Nevertheless, in single-arm, open label studies, several vasodilators have been suggested

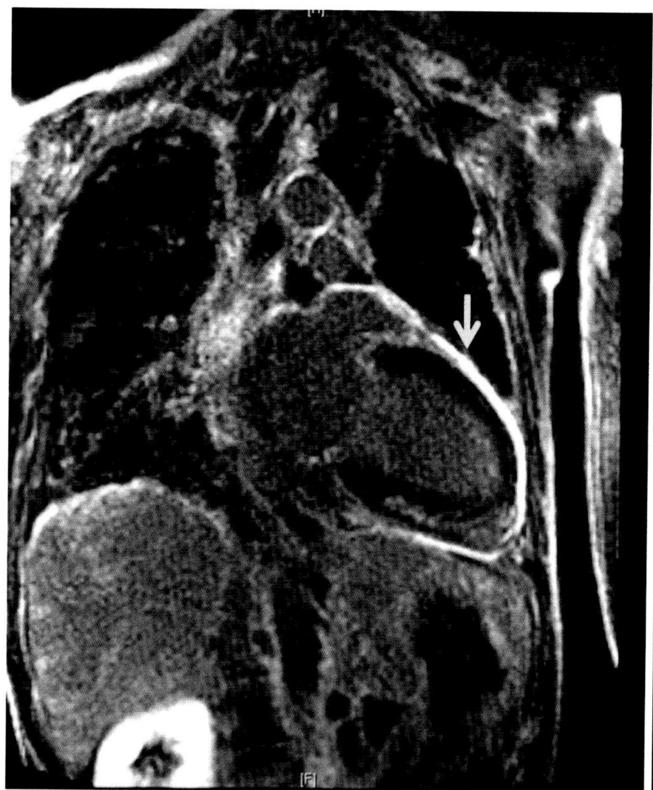

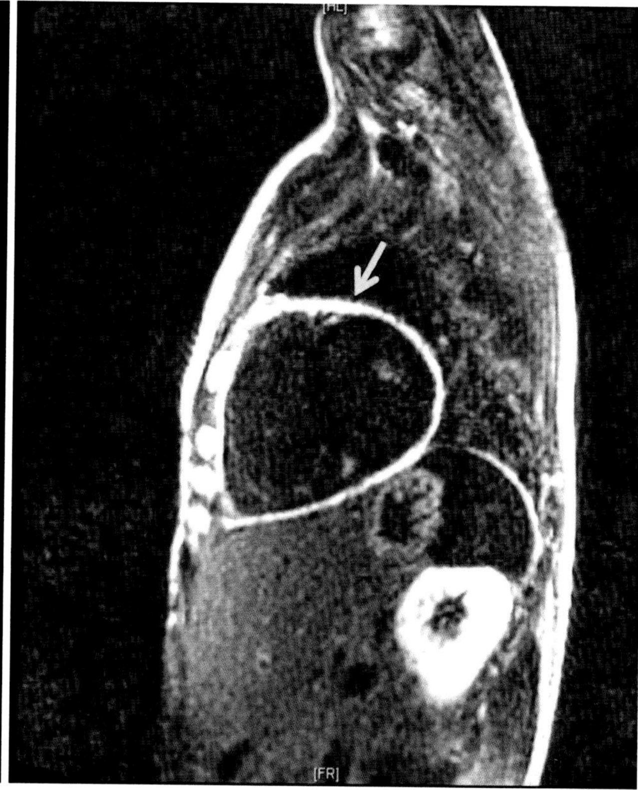

Fig. 22.2 Pericardial enhancement in a patient with diffuse cutaneous systemic sclerosis and constrictive pericarditis. Cardiac magnetic resonance imaging demonstrates intense signal uptake in the pericardium along with pericardial thickening in a 39-year-old man with severe, long-standing diffuse cutaneous systemic sclerosis and right heart failure due to constrictive pericarditis

to improve perfusion in SSc, further emphasizing the potential role of reversible vasospasm of the small coronary arteries. After intravenous administration of dipyridamole [59], as well as after treatment with nifedipine [60], nicardipine [61], or captopril [62], improved myocardial perfusion has been demonstrated in SSc patients using thallium-201 SPECT. Some myocardial perfusion defects were reversible, whereas others remained fixed, suggesting the co-existence of ischemic (functional) lesions accessible to reperfusion after relief of small coronary artery vasospasm and irreversible (fixed) lesions due to organic vessel disease or myocardial fibrosis [63]. The beneficial effect of nifedipine on myocardial perfusion and metabolism in SSc patients was also demonstrated using positron emission tomography [64], nifedipine caused a significant increase in 38 K myocardial uptake, a significant decrease in 18FDG myocardial uptake, and a significant increase in the myocardial 38 K/18FDG ratio, indicating improvement in both myocardial perfusion and myocardial metabolism. Nifedipine-induced improvement was also seen using cardiac MRI, with a mean 38 % increase of the global perfusion index and a significant decrease in the number of SSc patients with more than one segmental perfusion defect [65]. Similar results were observed using cardiac MRI for the assessment of the beneficial effect of bosentan, an oral dual endothelin receptor antagonist, on myocardial perfusion in SSc patients [66]. These findings suggest a role for vasodilators in treating and potentially preventing progression of microvascular disease in SSc.

Effects of vasodilators on ventricular dysfunction have also been demonstrated. Nicardipine was shown to acutely improve global LVEF and segmental abnormalities [67]. Improvements in both LVEF and RVEF after oral treatment with nicardipine and a correlation between improvement in LVEF and RVEF were demonstrated [57]. These results provide further evidence for the same pathogenic pathway, with reversible vasospastic small coronary artery disease inducing segmental and global cardiac dysfunction. Nifedipine significantly increased segmental (posterior wall) systolic and diastolic strain rates [65]. As peak systolic and early diastolic strain rates are respective markers of regional contractility and diastolic function, this study strongly suggested that nifedipine improved intrinsic myocardial properties; strain rate determined by tissue Doppler echocardiography is less load-dependant than other methods [68], and the afterload estimated by the systolic blood pressure heart rate product did not change significantly after nifedipine [65]. These results, together with the increased perfusion shown by MRI, suggested that an increase in myocardial perfusion might be the main determinant in the observed increased contractility, highlighting the global intrinsic beneficial effects of vasodilators such as nifedipine.

Thus, in open label studies vasodilators, such as calcium channel blockers mostly of dihydropyridine type, angiotensin converting enzyme inhibitors, and endothelin receptor antagonist, have been demonstrated in SSc patients, to induce improvement in the early vasospastic reversible component of the "primary" SSc myocardial disease. The possibility of long-term beneficial effects of calcium channel blockers was demonstrated in a large series of 7073 SSc patients: age, male gender, digital ulcerations, myositis, and lung involvement were independently associated with increased prevalence of LV dysfunction; in contrast, calcium channel blocker use appeared to be protective (odds ratio 0.41; 95 % confidence interval 0.22–0.74) [7]. Although these data are highly promising, it should be noted that the aforementioned study was observational and therefore cannot prove a cause-and-effect relationship between calcium channel blocker use and reduction in incidence of LV dysfunction. Currently, vasodilators such as calcium channel blockers remain the best studied for established myocardial disease in SSc, and given the aforementioned data may be considered for preventive therapy as well. It is unknown whether immunosuppressive therapy for myocardial disease is beneficial outside the realm of myocarditis (discussed below) or whether antifibrotic therapies will be beneficial based on available data. Dihydropyridine calcium channel blockers (e.g., amlodipine, nifedipine) have minimal negative inotropic effect and are generally well tolerated except for reflex tachycardia and lower extremity edema in some patients. All systemic vasodilators, including calcium channel blockers, should be used with caution in patients with severe pulmonary arterial hypertension as there is a potential for harm in nonvasoreactive forms of pulmonary hypertension such as SSc (see European Society of Cardiology [ESC] guidelines 2015) [69].

In SSc patients with overt LV systolic dysfunction (i.e., LVEF <40 %), we advocate treatment with neurohormonal blockade given the beneficial effects of this therapeutic strategy in all forms of LV systolic dysfunction. ACE-inhibitors or angiotensin receptor blockers are first-line treatments for SSc-associated LV systolic dysfunction given their utility in other manifestations of SSc (e.g., Raynaud's phenomenon, scleroderma renal disease). Beta-blockers can also be used, but we recommend the use of carvedilol given its combined beta- and alpha-blocking effects, which may help prevent exacerbation of Raynaud's phenomenon with other, more selective beta-blockers such as metoprolol. Mineralocorticoid receptor antagonists, such as spironolactone or eplerenone, can also be used in these patients. As with all patients with systolic dysfunction, the role of cardiac resynchronization therapy should be explored where the ejection fraction is reduced (<35 %) in association with left bundle branch block, and preventative ICD (implantable converter defibrillator) where regional scarring is associated with reduced ejection fraction (see ESC Guidelines published in 2013) [70].

In patients with acute myocarditis or myopericarditis, administration of immunosuppressive medications has been reported to improve LV ejection fraction and reduction in clinical symptoms [37, 71, 72]. Intravenous cyclophosphamide and corticosteroids have been used in this scenario, and a recent case series of myocarditis in SSc highlighted the importance of early diagnosis for successful treatment [72]. In patients with acute vasospastic crisis with myocardial involvement, urgent hospitalization (typically in an intensive care unit setting) and evaluation should be undertaken. These patients can have reduced LV ejection fraction and frequent arrhythmias along with worsening peripheral vasoconstriction. Unfortunately, there is little data on optimal treatment for this rare but life-threatening clinical scenario. Intravenous vasodilators, such as nitroprusside, may be useful to treat both LV systolic dysfunction and vasospasm; calcium channel blockers and ACE-inhibitors can also be helpful in this situation. Intravenous prostacyclin has been used for acute worsening of peripheral vasoconstriction to prevent digital necrosis [73]; however, prostacyclins should be used with caution in patients with symptomatic heart failure due to LV systolic dysfunction because of their association with increased mortality in this patient population [74].

Coronary Artery Disease

Although coronary microvascular disease, and not epicardial coronary artery disease, has been thought to be the primary coronary manifestation of SSc, a prior study found that coronary artery calcium scores were higher in SSc compared to controls [75]. Newer studies, including a national cross-sectional cohort study and a systematic review with meta-analysis, have found that coronary heart disease is more prevalent in SSc despite a lower number of cardiovascular risk factors in SSc compared to non-SSc controls [76, 77]. The relationship between epicardial coronary artery disease and coronary microvascular dysfunction in SSc, however, requires further investigation.

Pericardial Disease

Patients with SSc can develop a range of complications due to pericardial disease, including pericardial inflammation, fibrinous pericarditis, fibrous pericarditis, pericardial effusion, pericardial adhesions, cardiac tamponade, and constrictive pericarditis [3]. Although rarely symptomatic, when significant pericardial disease is present, it can cause considerable morbidity in patients with SSc. The pathophysiology of pericardial disease in SSc is not well known.

Pericardial effusion is common in SSc and often asymptomatic. At autopsy, the prevalence of pericardial involvement has been reported to be as high as 78%; however, clinically symptomatic pericardial disease is only present in 5–16% [3, 78, 79]. Although pericardial abnormalities can often be detected in SSc, the presence of pericardial effusion should not be ignored because it can be a clue to impending scleroderma renal crisis and it can be seen in patients with pulmonary arterial hypertension. In patients with idiopathic pulmonary arterial hypertension, the presence of a pericardial effusion has been associated with poor prognosis [80, 81], the mechanism thought to be one of impaired lymphatic drainage of pericardial fluid due to elevated right atrial pressure. In SSc patients with pulmonary arterial hypertension who have pericardial effusion, the etiology could be SSc, pulmonary arterial hypertension, or both. Regardless of the etiology, drainage of the pericardial effusion should be avoided in patients with pulmonary arterial hypertension [3]. In patients with SSc but no pulmonary arterial hypertension, the decision to drain the effusion should be made on a case-by-case basis, but is generally reserved for patients who have developed life-threatening cardiac tamponade [81]. If symptoms of heart failure are present and can be attributed to the pericardial effusion, gentle diuresis is warranted.

Constrictive pericarditis is a syndrome that often presents as right-side heart failure, shortness of breath, fatigue, anorexia, and wasting. It can be difficult to diagnose in patients with SSc who are susceptible to both constriction (due to pericardial involvement) and restriction (due to myocardial involvement with fibrosis) [84]. Thus, differentiation typically requires a multimodality approach, including echocardiography, simultaneous RV and LV invasive hemodynamics, and cardiac MRI or CT [85]. Factors which increase the likelihood of constrictive pericarditis in SSc include diastolic septal bounce with increased respiratory variation in mitral inflow and preserved (or increased) tissue Doppler e′ velocity on echocardiography [86], discordance of peak LV and RV pressures at peak inspiration on invasive hemodynamic testing [84], normal (or near-normal) BNP or NT-proBNP [87], and enhanced and/or thickened pericardium on cardiac MRI (see example, Fig. 22.2) or cardiac CT. Some patients with SSc will simultaneously have both constrictive and restrictive physiology, which can be very difficult to manage since pericardial stripping will not be beneficial and could result in severe morbidity or death in this situation. In these cases (and in patients in whom comorbidities preclude the possibility of pericardial stripping), intensive management with diuretics and sodium/fluid restriction will be essential in limiting symptoms and preserving quality of life.

Conduction Disease and Arrhythmias

Arrhythmias are frequent in SSc and have been reviewed in detail recently by Vacca et al. [88]. Fibrosis of the conduction system disease can occur in SSc, and its relationship to myocardial fibrosis is variable [89]. When conduction system fibrosis occurs, it most commonly involves the sinoatrial node [90], though conduction system abnormalities in SSc are rarely symptomatic [91]. However, patients with SSc can develop palpitations, syncope, and even sudden death. Thus, recognition and identification of brady- and tachyarrhythmias is essential. Several ECG abnormalities have been reported in SSc, including P-wave notching, nonspecific ST-T wave abnormalities, RV or LV hypertrophy, and low-voltage QRS, along with other abnormalities such as increased QT dispersion and decreased heart rate variability (a marker of autonomic dysfunction) summarized in detail by Lubitz et al. [91]. A recent study found that abnormal spatial QRS-T angle, a marker of ventricular repolarization, predicts life-threatening ventricular arrhythmias in SSc [92]. Electrocardiographic abnormalities are also predictive of survival, although it is unclear whether these changes reflect overall disease burden or contribute to morbidity and mortality.

As opposed to the relatively low incidence of symptomatic conduction system disease and bradyarrhythmias, ventricular and supraventricular arrhythmias are common [3, 91, 93]. Up to two-thirds of patients have documented premature ventricular contractions (PVCs) and the prevalence of nonsustained ventricular tachycardia ranges from 7 to 30% [94]. Advanced age and SSc disease burden, and possibly extent of lung involvement, have been associated with arrhythmic burden. Unfortunately, there is very limited data on the use of SSc-specific therapies, vasodilators, antiarrhythmics, or devices such as pacemakers or defibrillators in patients with SSc, which makes determining the best course of treatment difficult [91].

Based on available data for cardiac electrophysiologic abnormalities in SSc, we recommend screening for arrhythmias using ambulatory Holter or event monitoring in patients with symptoms of palpitations, lightheadedness, dizziness, or syncope. Exercise treadmill ECG testing can help identify arrhythmias that are exertional in nature. If arrhythmias are identified, they should be correlated to cardiac imaging (echocardiography) and given the lack of SSc-specific studies for treatment of arrhythmias, therapy should follow current treatment guidelines such as those available from the American Heart Association and ESC.

Cardiac Complications of Systemic Sclerosis Therapies

Some drugs used in the treatment of SSc have adverse cardiovascular effects which should be considered when treating patients with SSc. Of the drugs used to treat SSc, the ones with the best studied and most often reported adverse cardiac effects include cyclophosphamide [95] and hydroxychloroquine [96]. Cyclophosphamide-induced cardiac toxicity is uncommon when used at nonmyeloablative doses for the treatment of SSc. However, cyclophosphamide can be associated with LV or RV systolic dysfunction at high doses, which are used prior to stem cell transplantation (which has been used to treat patients with SSc [97, 98]). Older age and an abnormal LV or RV ejection fraction prior to high-dose cyclophosphamide are known risk factors for the development of ventricular dysfunction and subsequent symptomatic heart failure. In rare cases, cyclophosphamide has been associated with the development of hemorrhagic myopericarditis [99], which can be variably associated with pericardial effusion and cardiac tamponade, and typically occurs early on after administration of the drug.

Although there is little data to support the use of hydroxychloroquine in SSc, some patients with SSc are nonetheless prescribed hydroxychloroquine as a treatment for symptomatic control of joint pain. Despite a lack of studies for hydroxychloroquine's use in SSc, there has been a report in the literature of restrictive cardiomyopathy associated with hydroxychloroquine in a patient with SSc [100], a complication which has been well described in the literature in patients with other rheumatologic diseases such as rheumatoid arthritis and systemic lupus erythematosus who are often prescribed the drug. Hydroxychloroquine cardiotoxicity typically presents as symptomatic heart failure; however, it can also be associated with conduction system disease. If suspected, hydroxychloroquine toxicity can be diagnosed by endomyocardial biopsy, which shows vacuolization of myocytes on light microscopy and myelin figures and megamitochondria on electron microscopy [96, 100].

Aside from cyclophosphamide and hydroxychloroquine, imatinib mesylate and autologous stem cell transplantation are experimental therapies for SSc that can adversely affect the heart. Cardiotoxicity and severe heart failure have been reported in cancer patients treated with imatinib mesylate [101, 102]. Cardiotoxicity may be enhanced or more common in SSc patients treated with imatinib and related compounds given their antiangiogenic effects. Although stem cell transplantation itself most likely does not cause cardiotoxicity, myeloablative doses of cyclophosphamide used prior to stem cell transplantation can result in cardiac toxicity (as described above), and patients with pre-existing cardiac dysfunction are at increased risk for morbidity and mortality with stem cell transplantation [97, 103]. Thus, prior to stem cell transplantation, careful screening is mandatory (typically with echocardiography, cardiac MRI, and cardiac catheterization) to exclude LV or RV dysfunction, pulmonary arterial hypertension, or significant pericardial disease [97, 104].

Tools for the Assessment of Cardiac Dysfunction in Systemic Sclerosis

Serum Biomarkers

Several biomarkers have been studied in SSc to determine their utility in diagnosing cardiac involvement and assisting with the management of SSc patients. Of these, natriuretic peptide and troponin tests have been the most frequently studied in SSc and appear to provide the most diagnostic information.

There are several types of natriuretic peptides, but the two most widely studied types are atrial natriuretic peptide (ANP) and B-type natriuretic peptide (BNP). ANP is primarily secreted by the atria, whereas BNP is primarily secreted by both the left and right ventricle [RV] [105]. Both ANP and BNP act to enhance systemic vasodilation, natriuresis, and diuresis via membrane-bound natriuretic peptide receptors, which are coupled to a cyclic GMP-dependent signaling cascade. As opposed to ANP, which is stored in preformed granules and can be released with minimal stimuli, BNP is synthesized and requires BNP gene expression. Therefore, BNP is more likely to be elevated after sustained elevation in ventricular wall stress and therefore has become the preferred natriuretic peptide for diagnostic use in the clinical setting. BNP originates from a precursor protein, pre-proBNP, which is cleaved into $proBNP_{1-108}$ and then further cleaved into the biologically active BNP_{1-32} and the biologically inert amino-terminal (NT)-proBNP. Current commercial BNP assays measure both BNP_{1-108} and BNP_{1-32}, whereas NT-proBNP assays measure only NT-proBNP [104, 105].

BNP and NT-proBNP were initially studied as biomarkers for the identification of pulmonary hypertension in SSc patients. However, it is well known that BNP and NT-proBNP can increase not only in the setting of RV dysfunction (e.g., in pulmonary hypertension) but also in LV systolic dysfunction, LV diastolic dysfunction, and myocardial ischemia [106, 107]. Thus, natriuretic peptides may be better utilized as a screen for overall cardiac involvement in SSc as opposed to simply screening for pulmonary hypertension [108]. Indeed, in a study of 69 consecutive patients Allanore and colleagues found that NT-proBNP diagnosed overall cardiac involvement (either LV systolic dysfunction, RV systolic dysfunction, or elevated pulmonary artery pressure) with an excellent area under the curve of 0.94 (95% CI 0.87–0.99) on receiver operator characteristic (ROC) analysis [109]. These authors additionally found that an NT-proBNP cut-off of 125 pg/ml (well within the "normal" range in non-SSc patients [106]) was optimal for the detection of cardiac involvement in SSc.

BNP vs. NT-proBNP in SSc Most studies to date in SSc have examined NT-proBNP [108–118]. The main theoretical advantage to NT-proBNP is its longer half-life and increased stability [106]. However, since NT-proBNP is not cleared by the natriuretic peptide clearance receptor and is primarily excreted by the kidneys, renal dysfunction is more likely to cause higher NT-proBNP levels with less of an effect on BNP. In a single-center study, Cavagna and colleagues compared the utility of BNP and NT-proBNP for the diagnosis of pulmonary arterial hypertension in SSc and found that although pulmonary artery pressure correlated with both BNP and NT-proBNP, the former was slightly superior to the latter with higher area under the ROC curve (0.74 vs. 0.63, respectively) [119]. Furthermore, only BNP (and not NT-proBNP) was independently associated with pulmonary arterial hypertension diagnosis. Nonetheless, at the present time, there is insufficient data to determine whether one type of natriuretic peptide is superior to another in the diagnosis of cardiovascular disease in SSc. Given the importance of early identification of cardiovascular disease in SSc, either BNP or NT-proBNP should be used routinely in patients with SSc, as outlined below.

Practical Use of Natriuretic Peptides in Patients with SSc Based on available studies it appears that either BNP or NT-proBNP can be used in SSc for screening, diagnosis, and prognosis. As compared to the general population, it is also apparent that lower thresholds for BNP and NT-proBNP should be used to signify possible cardiovascular involvement in the patient with SSc. Levels of BNP >60 pg/ml or NT-proBNP >125 pg/ml should alert the clinician that there is potential for cardiovascular involvement in SSc. However, it should be noted that both cardiac and noncardiac conditions can influence natriuretic peptide levels (Table 22.2), and these should be taken into consideration when interpreting results of BNP (or NT-proBNP) testing in SSc. Finally, when screening or diagnosing pulmonary hypertension in SSc, natriuretic peptides will likely perform best when coupled with other noninvasive data such as pulmonary artery systolic pressure and RV function on echocardiography, and carbon monoxide diffusing capacity on pulmonary function testing.

Cardiac troponins have been studied extensively in the setting of coronary- and noncoronary causes of myocyte necrosis. An initial small study found that cardiac troponin T was not elevated in patients with SSc [120]. However, a larger study ($n = 161$ SSc patients, $n = 213$ controls) that measured high-sensitivity troponin T (hsTnT) found that hsTnT levels were higher in SSc compared to controls and was associated with diffuse cutaneous SSc and pulmonary arterial hypertension [121]. If troponin is elevated in a patient with SSc, other potential causes include myopericarditis or non-SSc cardiovascular disease such as acute coronary syndrome or pulmonary embolism.

Echocardiography

Echocardiography, including Doppler and tissue Doppler imaging, serves a critical role in the assessment of cardiac involvement in SSc by providing information on cardiac structure, systolic dysfunction, diastolic dysfunction, pericardial disease, valvular disease, RV function, and pulmonary hypertension. Many patients with SSc undergo routine annual screening with echocardiography. Routine echocardiographic measurements in SSc include LV dimensions and volumes (including ejection fraction) and wall thickness (for assessment of hypertrophy), Doppler echocardiography for the evaluation of stenotic and regurgitant valvular lesions, identification of pericardial effusion, and estimation of pulmonary artery systolic pressure. Although these routine assessments are important, several newer echocardiographic techniques such as tissue Doppler imaging and RV quantification are available and should be utilized in all patients with SSc.

Tissue Doppler Imaging The assessment of myocardial tissue velocities using the Doppler technique has provided immense insight into longitudinal function of the heart. Since the heart is composed of longitudinal, circumferential, and radial fibers, global indices (such as ejection fraction) do not capture the full extent of myocardial dysfunction, especially in patients who have subclinical cardiac involvement. Because subendocardial fibers, which are mostly longitudinal in orientation, are most susceptible to microvascular ischemia, longitudinal systolic and diastolic dysfunctions are often the earliest signs of cardiac impairment in SSc. By using a modified Doppler technique to identify low velocity, high amplitude signals found in myocardial tissue (as opposed to high velocity, low amplitude signals generated by red blood cells during traditional Doppler evaluation of blood flow) Doppler imaging is able to measure longitudinal tissue velocities. Typically, velocities are measured at the septal and lateral mitral annulus. Waves generated include isovolumic contraction, systolic longitudinal velocity (s'), isovolumic relaxation, early diastolic longitudinal velocity (e'), and late (atrial) diastolic longitudinal velocity (a') (Fig. 22.3) [122]. Of these, s' can be used to identify early, subclinical LV systolic dysfunction in patients with SSc, whereas e' is critically important as a marker of LV diastolic dysfunction, particularly impaired relaxation.

The advent of tissue Doppler imaging has revolutionized the assessment of diastolic dysfunction because of the difficulties encountered with traditional Doppler mitral inflow imaging. Virtually all traditional Doppler imaging indices, including transmitral E and A waves, E/A ratio, pulmonary venous flow, and early mitral deceleration time, suffer from a bimodal distribution during the progression from normal

Table 22.2 Factors which can influence natriuretic peptide levels

Factors associated with increased NP levels
LV systolic or diastolic dysfunction
RV systolic or diastolic dysfunction
Acute coronary syndrome
Valvular heart disease
Atrial arrhythmias (atrial fibrillation)
Pulmonary arterial hypertension, pulmonary venous hypertension
Interstitial lung disease if associated pulmonary hypertension
Pulmonary embolism
Older age
Female gender
Weight loss, cachexia
Renal insufficiency
Sepsis/critical illness
Anemia
High-output state (e.g., cirrhosis)
Glucocorticoids, excess cortisol levels
Hyperthyroidism
Malignancies
CNS injury (e.g., stroke, subarachnoid hemorrhage)
Factors associated with normal or decreased NP levels
Obesity
Constrictive pericarditis
Flash pulmonary edema
Cardiac medications (ACE-inhibitors, ARBs, beta-blockers, diuretics, spironolactone)

Data presented in table derived from literature on natriuretic peptides [103, 105, 173–175]
NP natriuretic peptides (i.e., BNP or NT-proBNP), *LV* left ventricle, *RV* right ventricle, *ACE* angiotensin converting enzyme, *ARB* angiotensin receptor blocker

to abnormal [123]. For example, in normals, E/A ratio is > 1. As diastolic dysfunction ensues, E/A ratio reversal occurs and decreases to below 0.8 due to impaired LV relaxation. However, as diastolic dysfunction worsens, left atrial pressure rises and E/A ratio normalizes. Thus, mitral inflow and pulmonary venous flow patterns in normal and moderate ("pseudonormal") diastolic dysfunction can appear similar. Tissue Doppler e′ has the advantage of decreasing linearly with worsening diastolic function and therefore can be used to differentiate normal diastolic function from moderate or severe diastolic dysfunction. Tissue Doppler e′ velocity does decrease with normal aging, so the age of the patient must be considered when interpreting e′ velocity and diastolic function in general. Fortunately, age-specific cut-offs for abnormal e′ velocity exist [123, 124]. Thus, by using age-appropriate cut-offs for tissue Doppler e', one can identify diastolic dysfunction early in the patient with SSc. Although a secondary effect of LV dysfunction (systolic or diastolic) left atrial enlargement is an extremely useful parameter and should be measured in all patients (left atrial volume index > 28 ml/m^2) in the absence of atrial fibrillation or mitral valve disease confirms that significant LV dysfunction is present [125].

Right Ventricular Quantification Although previously considered a passive conduit in the cardiopulmonary system, it is now well known that the RV is extremely important in a wide variety of disease states, including SSc. In SSc, RV dysfunction can be primary (due to direct myocardial involvement) or secondary (due to pulmonary hypertension from pulmonary vascular disease, LV dysfunction, or interstitial lung disease). Thus, careful evaluation of the RV can provide considerable insight into cardiovascular manifestations of SSc. Assessment of the RV by echocardiography has been challenging due to its nonuniform, pyramidal shape [126]. However, advances in echocardiographic RV imaging [127], along with published guidelines for the quantification of the RV [125], now allow for routine evaluation of the RV in SSc. Five parameters (RV fractional area change, TAPSE, tricuspid annular tissue Doppler S', pulmonary artery systolic pressure, and the ratio of tricuspid regurgitant velocity to pulmonary artery velocity time integral [a noninvasive marker of pulmonary vascular resistance]) form the cornerstone of echocardiographic RV assessment in SSc (Figs. 22.4, 22.5, and 22.6). Finally it should be remembered that as an independent predictor of pulmonary hypertension right atrial area should be assessed in all patients (normal <18 cm^2) (DETECT study) [128].

Nuclear Imaging, Cardiac MRI, and Cardiac Computed Tomography (CT)

Nuclear imaging techniques such as SPECT are currently the most commonly used method for the detection of abnormal myocardial perfusion. As described above, this technique, which relies on both a stressor (e.g., exercise, vasodilator, or cold stimuli in SSc) and an isotope (e.g., thallium-201), has been utilized to investigate myocardial ischemia in SSc [59]. Advances in nuclear imaging techniques, especially the use of positron emission tomography (PET) scanning allows for enhanced resolution of the heart and may increase sensitivity for detection of microvascular ischemia in SSc [129]. However, detection of subendocardial ischemia by nuclear imaging is limited and inferior to perfusion imaging with cardiac MRI, which is discussed in detail below. Combined cardiac SPECT or PET and cardiac CT overcomes some of these limitations and can offer comprehensive assessment of the heart [133], though it remains to be seen if this type of study will be useful in SSc.

Both cardiac MRI and cardiac CT can provide valuable information on cardiac involvement in SSc. Either tech-

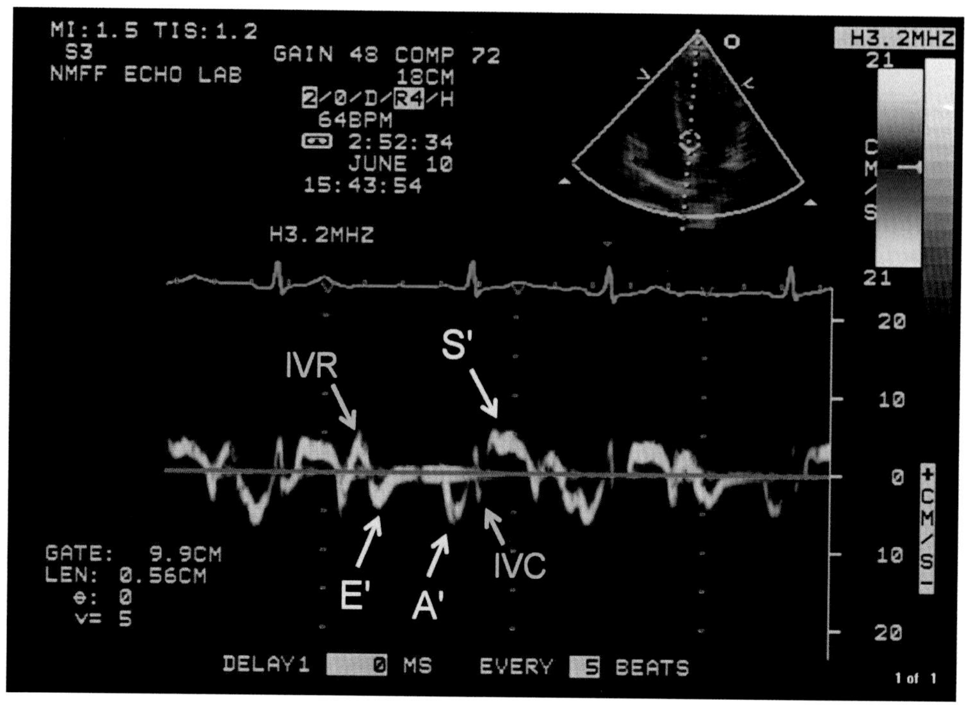

Fig. 22.3 Tissue Doppler imaging of the mitral annulus. *S'* systolic tissue velocity, *E'* early diastolic tissue velocity, *A'* late (atrial) diastolic tissue velocity, *IVC* isovolumic contraction, *IVR* isovolumic relaxation. Systolic and diastolic tissue velocities are decreased in this example of septal (medial) mitral annulus longitudinal tissue Doppler imaging from a 51-year-old woman with long-standing diffuse cutaneous systemic sclerosis

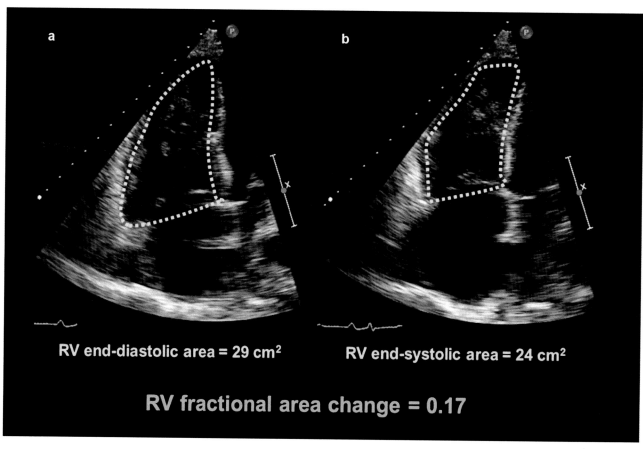

Fig. 22.4 Right ventricular fractional area change. *RV* right ventricle. Right ventricular fractional area change in a 63-year-old woman with limited cutaneous systemic sclerosis and pulmonary arterial hypertension. (**a**) RV end-diastolic area. (**b**) RV end-systolic area. RV fractional area change (= [RV end-diastolic area – RV end-systolic area]/RV end-diastolic area; normal [125] >0.35) is an echocardiographic marker of global RV systolic function

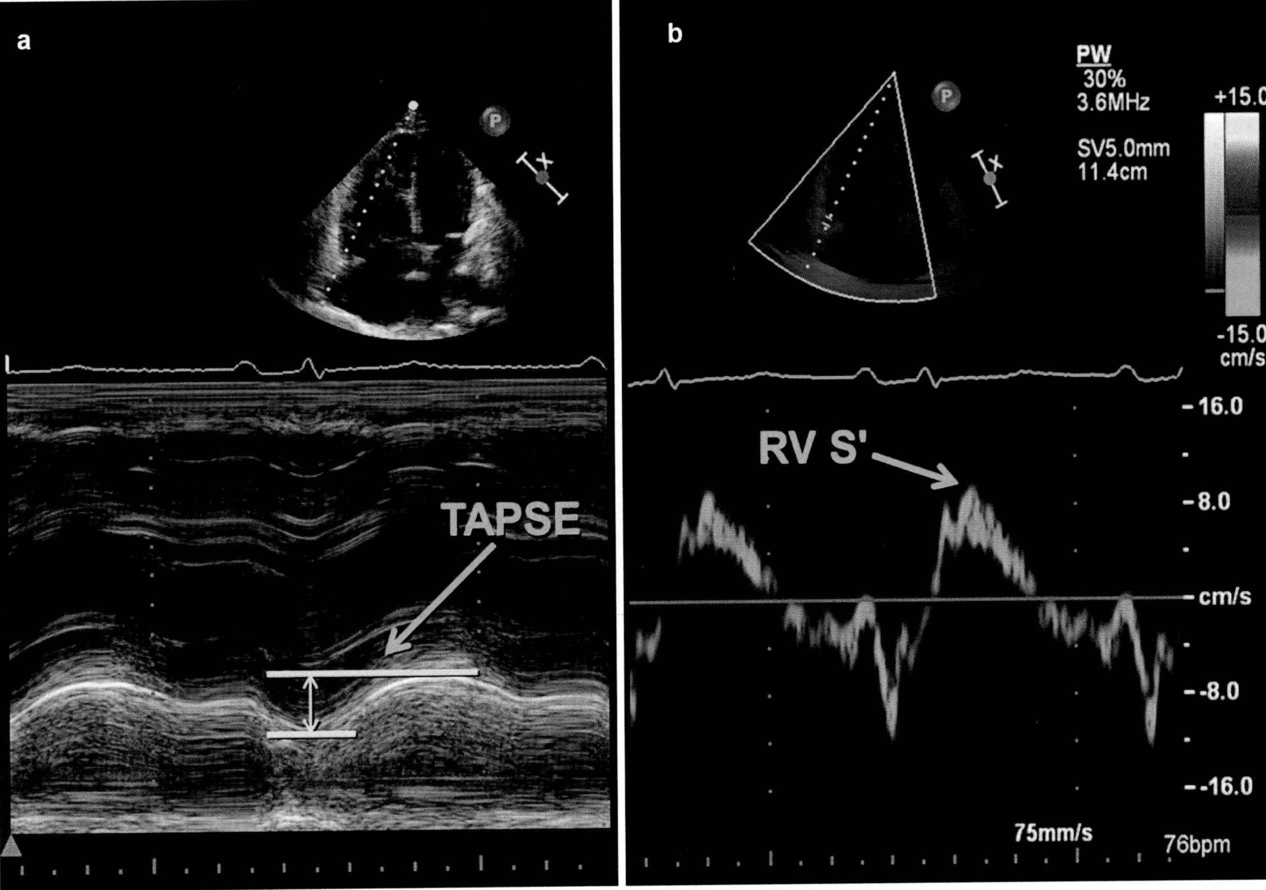

Fig. 22.5 Right ventricular longitudinal systolic function. (**a**) *TAPSE* tricuspid annular plane systolic excursion (normal [125] >1.6 cm); (**b**) *RV* S' right ventricular systolic longitudinal tissue Doppler velocity (normal [125] >10 cm/s). Images are from the same patient described in Fig. 22.2. Both TAPSE and RV S' are reduced, indicating a decrease in longitudinal RV systolic function. Both TAPSE and RV S' can be very useful if the RV is not well visualized or for the diagnosis of early RV dysfunction (prior to the reduction in global RV systolic function)

nique can be used to evaluation for pericardial disease and is invaluable for this purpose since echocardiography cannot reliably evaluate pericardial thickness and/or inflammation. However, given the frequent use of chest CT for evaluation of lung involvement in SSc, radiation exposure in these patients is not trivial. Therefore, cardiac MRI (which does not involve radiation exposure) may be preferable to cardiac CT.

Besides evaluation of pericardial disease, cardiac MRI is also the gold standard for assessment of cardiac structure given its high spatial resolution [2, 49, 76, 132]. Cardiac MRI has been investigated in SSc and found to detect cardiac abnormalities with high sensitivity [133–136]. In one study of 52 patients with SSc, 75 % had at least one detectable abnormality on cardiac MRI [76]. On gadolinium-enhanced cardiac MRI images in SSc, if diffuse enhancement is detected, the possibility of infiltrative disease is often entertained. Most often, however, severe diffuse fibrosis of the heart is the cause of the diffuse enhancement (thus, the "infiltrative process" is infiltration by fibroblasts and collagen). Traditional vasodilator perfusion cardiac MRI can also reliably detect subendocardial ischemia (Fig. 22.7) by displaying a circumferential loss of perfusion in the subendocardium, a finding that is thought to be due to microvascular disease in SSc [132]. Finally, since evaluation of the RV is difficult using routine echocardiography, cardiac MRI is emerging as a vital technique for evaluation of RV structure and function [49] and may be useful in SSc for the differentiation of primary RV involvement from secondary RV involvement due to pulmonary arterial hypertension. In a cardiac MRI study of 50 SSc patients, Bezante and colleagues found that RV ejection fraction was decreased in SSc compared to controls (47 ± 7 % vs. 58 ± 4 %; $P < 0.0001$) and lower in diffuse cutaneous SSc when compared to limited cutaneous SSc (44 ± 6 % vs. 48 ± 7 %; $P = 0.03$) [49].

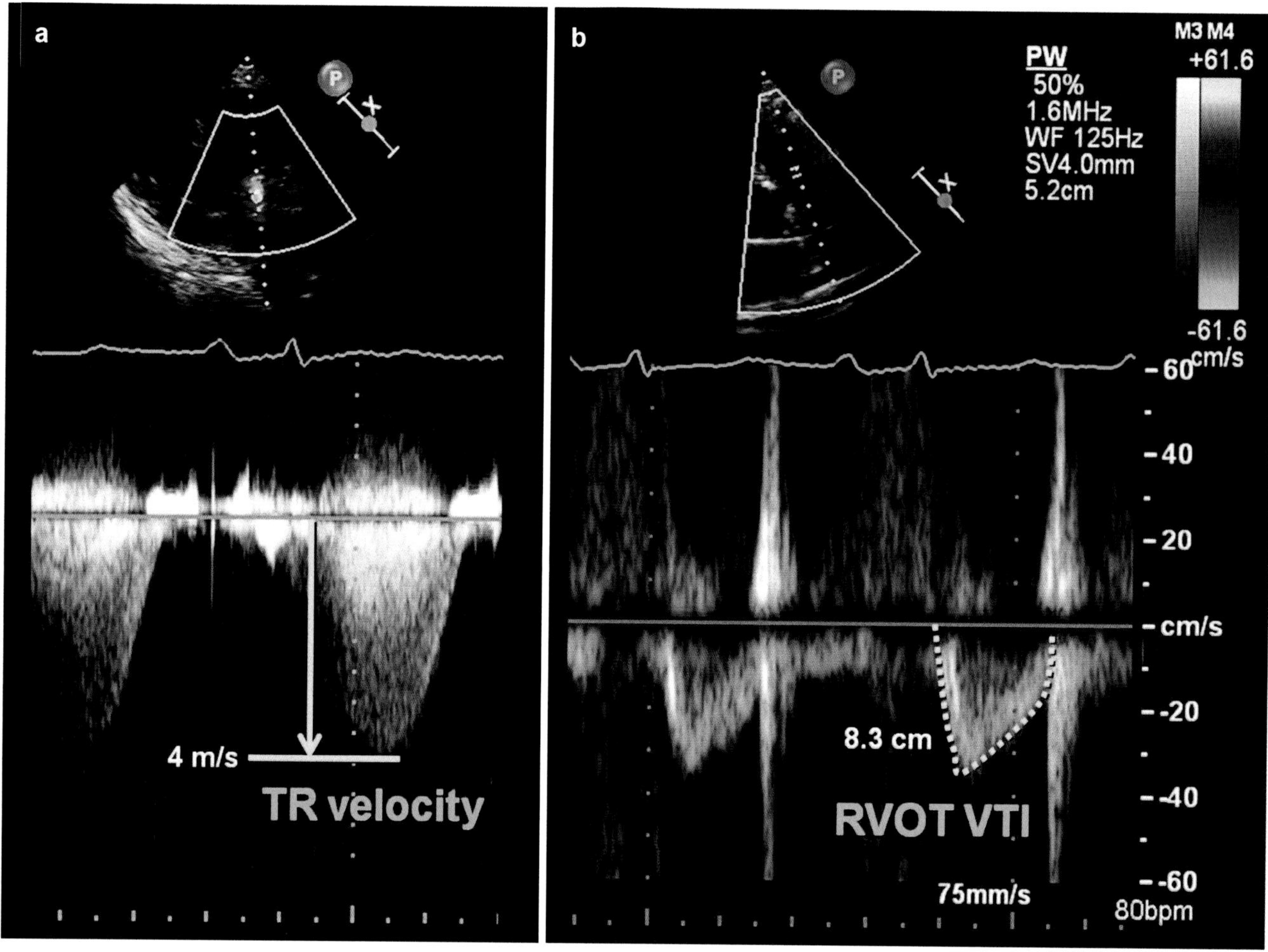

Fig. 22.6 Non-invasive estimation of pulmonary artery systolic pressure and pulmonary vascular resistance. *TR* tricuspid regurgitation, *RVOT VTI* right ventricular outflow tract velocity time integral (a measure of flow). Pulmonary vascular resistance can be estimated from the ratio of TR velocity (Panel **a**) to RVOT VTI (Panel **b**) which can help determine whether RV dysfunction is primary (due to intrinsic RV involvement) or secondary (due to pulmonary hypertension). If RV dysfunction is primary, TR velocity will be low and RVOT VTI will be low (with a normal or near-normal ratio [<0.18] [170]). If RV dysfunction is secondary to pulmonary hypertension, the ratio of TR velocity to RVOT VTI will be high (>0.18) [170]. In this example, from the patient described in Figs. 22.2 and 22.3, ratio of TR velocity to RVOT VTI = 0.48; thus, estimated PVR is elevated and indicative of secondary RV dysfunction due to pulmonary hypertension

Cardiac Catheterization

Cardiac catheterization, the gold standard tool for assessment of hemodynamics and epicardial coronary anatomy, is necessary in patients with SSc when the diagnoses of pulmonary arterial hypertension, constrictive pericarditis, cardiac tamponade, or epicardial coronary artery disease are entertained. Cardiac catheterization also offers the opportunity for endomyocardial biopsy which may be necessary in SSc if there is suspicion of infiltrative cardiac disease, side effects of medications (e.g., hydroxychloroquine cardiomyopathy [100]), or active myocarditis [137]. Recent studies have also highlighted the utility of exercise testing at the time of right heart catheterization to determine the cause of unexplained dyspnea in SSc [138, 139]. Using a systematic strategy of identifying SSc patients with exercise-induced elevation in PA systolic pressure on echocardiography, Hager et al. were able to demonstrate the ability of exercise invasive hemodynamic testing to differentiate exercise-induced precapillary pulmonary hypertension from the much more common exercise-induced pulmonary venous hypertension due to LV diastolic dysfunction [138].

Although cardiac catheterization is an invasive procedure, it is minimally invasive and can be performed with minimal risks by experienced operators. Therefore, although it should be used judiciously, cardiac catheterization should not be avoided since it can provide a definitive diagnosis.

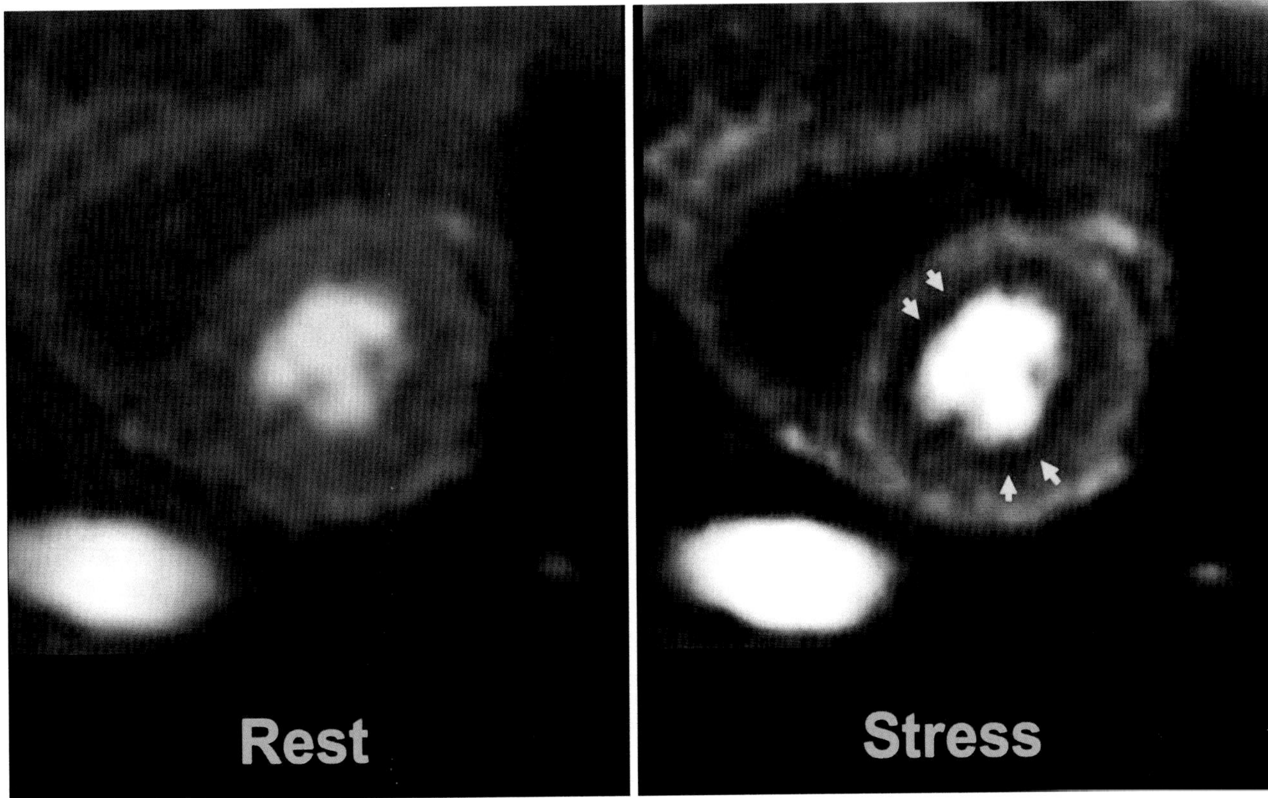

Fig. 22.7 Cardiac magnetic resonance imaging in systemic sclerosis: subendocardial ischemia. Short axis slice through the left ventricle showing subendocardial ischemia (*arrows*) due to microvascular disease. At rest there is homogeneous uptake of contrast in the myocardium. At peak stress, the subendocardium is dark circumferentially (*arrows*), indicating that there is decreased perfusion in this territory (indicative of microvascular ischemia) (MRI images courtesy of Daniel C. Lee, M.D., Northwestern University Feinberg School of Medicine)

Arrhythmia Monitoring

Arrhythmias are common in SSc and can cause significant morbidity [3, 24, 140–142]. Several options are available for monitoring of arrhythmias. In SSc patients with frequent palpitations, 24- or 48-h Holter monitoring is likely to detect the cause of symptoms. However, in patients with less frequent symptoms or in patients with symptoms such as syncope, longer-term (typically 30-day) event monitors are typically necessary. Newer devices for arrhythmia detection, such as the Zio patch (which collect electrocardiographic data for up to 14 days) and implantable loop recorders, which can detect arrhythmias indefinitely, are available and may extend the ability to detect arrhythmias in SSc.

Emerging Tools

Future tools likely to be important in SSc heart disease include speckle-tracking echocardiography for the evaluation of myocardial strain [143–146], MRI T1 mapping for the evaluation of diffuse cardiac fibrosis [147–149], and absolute perfusion cardiac MRI for the evaluation of microvascular coronary ischemia [150].

Speckle-Tracking Echocardiography for Measurement of Myocardial Strain Although tissue Doppler imaging is widely available, this technique is used primarily for the measurement of tissue velocities. However, because different parts of the myocardium move at different velocities, the heart changes shape during its movement across the cardiac cycle and deformation occurs. Thus, tissue velocities do not tell the entire story of cardiac motion and cardiac mechanics. Myocardial strain is the fractional change in length of a segment of myocardium compared to its original length [143]. Strain is therefore a measure of cardiac deformation that differs from velocity. The fundamentals of strain imaging have been described in detail elsewhere [139, 151, 152]. Based on the association between cardiac fibrosis, circulating markers of fibrosis, and reduced myocardial strains in prior non-SSc studies [153, 154], measurement of strain in SSc may be a valuable tool for the assessment of preclinical myocardial involvement in SSc.

Myocardial strain, which occurs in the radial, circumferential, and longitudinal directions in the heart, is difficult to measure using tissue Doppler techniques because this technique requires alignment of the Doppler ultrasound beam with the direction of myocardial motion [143, 144, 155]. Speckle-tracking echocardiography, which solves this problem by providing an angle-independent solution for measurement of myocardial deformation, uses a pattern-recognition type of software to follow naturally occurring acoustic markers (ultrasound speckles) throughout the cardiac cycle. Detection of spatial movement of this "fingerprint" (Fig. 22.8a) during the cardiac cycle allows direct calculation of strain (Fig. 22.8b, c). Speckle-tracking echocardiography is possible with commercially available echocardiography machines and thus can be applied to patients with SSc. Cardiac MRI also has the capability of measuring myocardial strain (e.g., MRI tagging technique [156]) and is considered the gold standard for noninvasive assessment of strain given the higher spatial resolution (albeit lower temporal resolution) of cardiac MRI compared with echocardiography. In the past 5 years, several speckle-tracking echocardiography studies in SSc have been published (Table 22.3) [157–164]. These studies demonstrate the power of speckle-tracking echocardiography in detecting subclinical myocardial dysfunction in patients with SSc.

Other advances in echocardiography that may have a role include three dimensional imaging, particularly important in assessing the RV. Single beat 3D echo has the advantage of being rhythm independent; however, the resolution available means that to date interobserver reproducibility remains inadequate [165]. By contrast, two-dimensional knowledge-based reconstruction, by using a standard echo probe and views coupled with a database of known RV shapes and sizes obtained from CMR studies, shows a high degree of interobserver reproducibility. In the future these techniques may provide access to volumetric RV data in situations where CMR is not accessible or acceptable [166] .

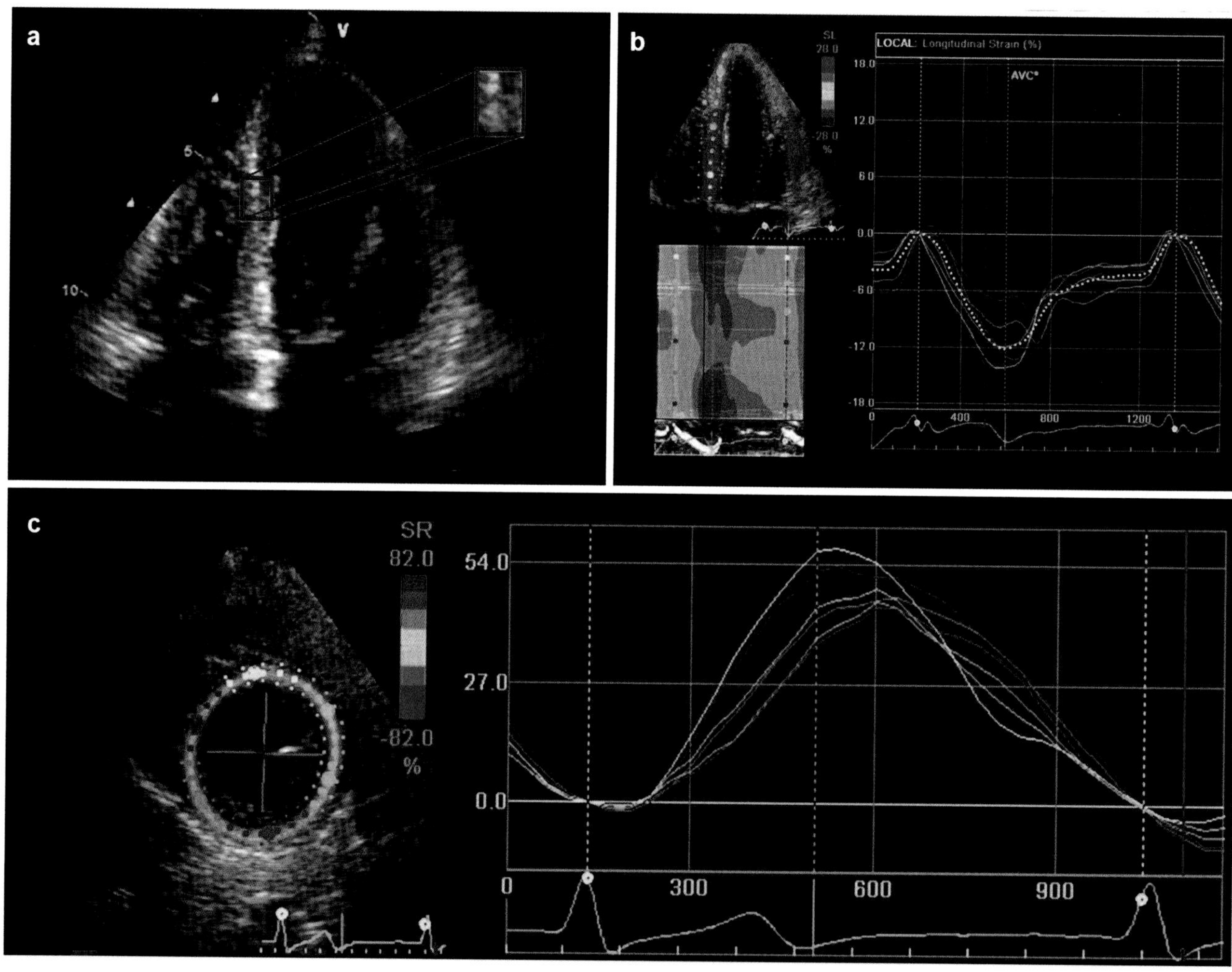

Fig. 22.8 Speckle-tracking echocardiography. (a) Speckle-tracking methodology showing "fingerprint" of ultrasound speckles which are tracked over the cardiac cycle. (b) Longitudinal and (c) radial strain curves from a patient with diffuse cutaneous systemic sclerosis. Note the reduction in peak global longitudinal strain (−12 %) with preserved radial strain (+49 %) suggestive of early subendocardial cardiac involvement

Table 22.3 Recent speckle-tracking echocardiography studies in systemic sclerosis

First author	Year	Sample size	Primary findings	Clinical implications
Agoston [153]	2014	42 SSc 42 controls	Despite similarly normal LVEF, pulmonary pressures, and left atrial (LA) volumes in SSc patients and controls, patients with SSc had significantly worse LA strain parameters.	Patients with SSc may have intrinsic left atrial dysfunction which can be an early sign of HFpEF
Atas [154]	2015	41 SSc 38 controls	Patients with SSc had had more frequent LV diastolic dysfunction, larger LA volumes, and worse LA strain parameters compared to controls.	
Cadeddu [155]	2015	45 SSc 20 controls	Compared to controls, SSc patients had higher E/e′ (a marker of LV filling pressures), larger LA volumes, and reduced LV contractile reserve, as assessed by exercise echocardiography with speckle-tracking (reduced global longitudinal strain at peak exercise).	Impaired LV contractile reserve may be reflective of underlying cardiac involvement in SSc and can be detected with speckle-tracking analysis of images obtained during exercise stress echocardiography
Cusma [156]	2013	29 SSc 30 controls	LV longitudinal and circumferential strains were lower (worse) in SSc compared to controls, and there was a significant correlation between anti-Scl-70 antibodies and longitudinal and circumferential strain parameters in SSc.	Patients with SSc have worse (more impaired) indices of cardiac mechanics compared to controls; these intrinsic abnormalities in myocardial function appear to be more prominent in patients with elevated anti-Scl-70 antibodies
Spethmann [157]	2012	22 SSc 22 controls	LV global longitudinal strain and strain rate were significantly worse in SSc compared to controls, particularly in the basal segments of the LV.	
Spethmann [158]	2014	19 SSc	In this pilot study, 19 SSc patients without pulmonary hypertension underwent speckle-tracking echocardiography at baseline and at 2 years of follow-up. LV ejection fraction and diastolic function remained unchanged, but LV global longitudinal strain decreased during follow-up.	LV global longitudinal strain, measured using speckle-tracking echocardiography, may be a sensitive marker of the longitudinal decline in LV function in SSc.
Tigen [159]	2014	53 SSc 26 controls	SSc patients had significantly lower longitudinal, circumferential, and radial LV strain compared to controls. Within the SSc group, 13/53 patients had a fragmented QRS on electrocardiography; SSc patients with a fragmented QRS had lower longitudinal strain values.	A fragmented QRS complex on routine 12-lead electrocardiography may be indicative of abnormal LV mechanics in SSc patients.
Yiu [160]	2011	104 SSc 37 controls	SSc patients had significantly worse LV longitudinal and circumferential strain compared to controls, despite similar LV ejection fraction between the 2 groups. Within the SSc groups, worse strain parameters correlated with (1) lower peak VO_2 on cardiopulmonary exercise testing and (2) more abnormal findings on 24-h electrocardiography (Holter monitoring).	Abnormal LV longitudinal and circumferential strain, detected by speckle-tracking echocardiography, is a marker of early LV systolic dysfunction in SSc and may underlie exercise intolerance and arrhythmias in these patients.

Cardiac MRI T1 Mapping (Diffuse Fibrosis Imaging) Cardiac MRI has emerged as the gold standard tool for the detection of myocardial scar (focal fibrosis), such as that found in patients who have suffered a myocardial infarction and in some types of cardiomyopathies. This technique, which uses late gadolinium enhancement, relies on differential uptake of gadolinium in scarred (fibrotic) and adjacent nonscarred (nonfibrotic) myocardial tissue [167]. In patients with SSc, fibrosis is relatively diffuse and therefore cannot be detected readily using traditional late gadolinium enhancement. Fortunately, recent advances in cardiac MRI now allow determination of diffuse myocardial fibrosis using a T1 mapping technique [147–151]. Preliminary studies have now shown that the T1 mapping technique can be useful in SSc to detect diffuse interstitial fibrosis [71–170]. In addition, T2 imaging, which detects myocardial edema, may be useful in the detection of early or overt myocarditis [172]. Table 22.4 summarizes recent studies published within the last 5 years that have investigated the utility of cardiac MRI in SSc.

Cardiac MRI Absolute Perfusion Like the detection of myocardial scar, traditional methods for detecting abnormalities in myocardial perfusion (i.e., ischemia) also rely on relative differences between adjacent myocardial territories. Thus, currently available perfusion techniques are most helpful for focal epicardial coronary disease and less helpful for diffuse microvascular ischemia such as that seen in SSc. However, a novel technique of "absolute perfusion" has been developed using cardiac MRI and may solve the problem of detection of diffuse myocardial ischemia [6, 150]. By evaluating differences between enhancement of the myocardium and blood pool using mathematical techniques of deconvolution, absolute perfusion imaging with cardiac MRI may be a new way to diagnose and quantify myocardial ischemia in SSc and may provide insight on the effects of different classes of vasodilator therapy in SSc.

Summary: Recommendations and Unanswered Questions

Early diagnosis and treatment of direct cardiac involvement in SSc is essential given the considerable morbidity and mortality associated with cardiac manifestations. Based on available data, we recommend yearly screening with comprehensive echocardiography (including tissue Doppler imaging) and natriuretic peptide testing (either BNP or NT-proBNP). If present, symptoms and signs of possible cardiac involvement should be thoroughly investigated, thereby ensuring timely intervention in the at-risk patient. For the most common type of cardiac involvement, intrinsic myocardial disease, treatment with vasodilators improves myocardial perfusion and may deter the development of overt LV systolic dysfunction by reducing progression to myocardial fibrosis. Nevertheless, despite considerable advances in our understanding of SSc cardiac involvement, several unanswered questions remain:

- Are there truly differences between diffuse and limited forms of SSc in terms of frequency of cardiac involvement? Although most studies have found that primary cardiac involvement is more common in diffuse cutaneous SSc, especially in patients with rapid progression of skin findings, gene expression data from skin biopsies in SSc patients [173] suggests that current skin-based classification of SSc is somewhat arbitrary. Therefore, it will be of interest to determine whether certain molecular subsets of patients will have more frequent cardiac involvement, while others do not.
- What are the best ways to screen for cardiac involvement? Current screening for cardiac involvement involves natriuretic peptides and echocardiography, including tissue Doppler imaging. However, the frequency of screening, and whether screening and early diagnosis of cardiac involvement changes clinical outcome, has yet to be determined. Furthermore, the utility of newer technologies such as speckle-tracking echocardiography, cardiac MRI diffuse fibrosis imaging, and absolute perfusion imaging is still unknown.
- Although vasodilator therapy with drugs such as calcium channel blockers and ACE-inhibitors forms the cornerstone of treatment for myocardial involvement in SSc, randomized controlled trials are lacking, and the effect of these drugs on long-term outcomes is unknown. Furthermore, there are several novel medications currently in development (e.g., neprilysin inhibitors [174], soluble guanylate stimulators [175]) that may be particular beneficial for cardiac involvement in SSc given their mechanisms of action. However, the large number of patients required for adequately powered randomized clinical trials, coupled with the widespread use of vasodilators for Raynaud's phenomenon in SSc, will likely make the conduct of clinical studies challenging. Nevertheless, such studies must be performed, and the formation of large collaborative SSc research groups for multicenter clinical trials will assist in these endeavors.
- Can immunosuppressive therapy prevent progressive heart disease? Is cardiac fibrosis reversible? Current and newer drugs on the horizon for SSc may be able to address these questions, with the caveat that any improvement in cardiac function will have to be balanced with the potential for toxicity with these drugs.
- Are device therapies under-used in scleroderma? Would more widespread use of ICDs and biventricular

Table 22.4 Recent cardiac magnetic resonance imaging studies in systemic sclerosis

First author	Year	Sample size	Primary findings	Clinical implications
Barison [162]	2015	30 SSc 10 controls	On MRI T1 mapping, patients with SSc had increased extracellular volume (ECV) fraction in both the heart and the skeletal muscle, reflecting increased diffuse interstitial fibrosis in these tissues.	MRI T1 mapping ECV values appear to be useful in SSc for the detection of interstitial fibrosis. In SSc, the diffuse fibrosis that occurs in the heart may also occur in the skeletal muscle in parallel.
Di Cesare [129]	2013	58 SSc (all female)	Myocardial fibrosis (late gadolinium enhancement) was present in 25/58 (43 %) of the SSc in a linear pattern (16 patients) and nodular pattern (9 patients).	In patients with SSc, cardiac MRI can detect focal scar (late gadolinium enhancement), diffuse interstitial fibrosis (T1 mapping), myocardial edema suggestive of myocarditis (T2 imaging), and subendocardial ischemia (perfusion imaging). These abnormalities have been correlated with biomarkers, NYHA functional class, and other imaging parameters indicative of cardiac dysfunction in SSc.
Mavrogeni [164]	2015	46 SSc (all dcSSc)	Of the 46 dcSSc patients, 2 had evidence of early myocarditis (myocardial edema on T2 imaging); the other 44 patients underwent a myocardial stress perfusion-fibrosis protocol and were found to have reduced myocardial perfusion reserve index (MPRI) compared to controls. Of the 11 SSc patients with 2-year follow-up MRI, all had deterioration in MPRI and 8/11 had diffuse subendocardial late gadolinium enhancement.	
Moroncini [130]	2014	26 SSc 13 controls	Of the 26 SSc patients, 54 % had perfusion defects and 25 % had late gadolinium enhancement.	
Rodriguez-Reyna [131]	2015	62 SSc	Of the 62 SSc patients, 79 % had subendocardial perfusion detects, and 45 % had late gadolinium enhancement, which was more common in dcSSc (59 %) compared to lcSSc (33 %) ($P=0.04$). Patients with perfusion defects had higher values of high-sensitivity C-reactive protein.	
Sano [132]	2012	40 SSc	Of the 40 SSc patients, 17.5 % had evidence of late gadolinium enhancement, the presence of which was associated with worse NYHA functional class.	
Thuny [163]	2014	33 SSc 16 controls	All 33 SSc patients studied had no significant echocardiographic abnormalities and no late gadolinium enhancement. SSc patients had higher ECV values on MRI T1 mapping compared to controls. ECV correlated with LA volume and grade of diastolic dysfunction.	

pacemakers improve prognosis and functional status in this population?

Despite these unanswered questions, much has been learned about the cardiac manifestations of SSc, and it is hoped that ongoing investigations in this area will shed new light on prevention and treatment of cardiac disease in SSc.

Conclusions

Direct cardiac involvement is a frequent and early finding in SSc patients, both in the diffuse and limited cutaneous forms of the disease. There are several cardiac manifestations of SSc, each of which can cause considerable morbidity. The pathogenesis of direct cardiac involvement typically involves a vasospastic mechanism that is thought to play a major role in SSc in general. Evidence suggests that vasospasm of the small coronary arteries or arterioles initially impairs perfusion and function, which is reversible early but over time is followed by structural coronary arteriolar lesions leading to irreversible abnormalities. Therefore, early detection through screening is critical to prevent irreversible cardiac damage, especially since the presence of clinically overt cardiac involvement due to SSc is associated with adverse outcomes. Natriuretic peptides (either BNP or NT-proBNP) and tissue Doppler imaging have emerged as the most useful screening tools for cardiac involvement and form the cornerstone of cardiac assessment in SSc. Delayed enhancement cardiac MRI has also emerged as an extremely useful tool to evaluate abnormal cardiac structure, pericardial disease, perfusion, and diffuse fibrosis. Although the optimal strategies for combating cardiac manifestations of SSc have not been completely defined, there is accumulating evidence to suggest a major role of vasodilators early in the course of disease for the prevention of long-term cardiac morbidity and mortality. In the future, drugs that might prevent or treat structural vascular lesions (and fibrosis) might be extremely important. Therefore, more understanding of the molecular pathophysiology and optimal treatment of cardiac involvement in SSc is necessary, with the hope that novel treatments for cardiac disease can limit the morbidity and mortality of SSc overall.

Acknowledgment The authors would like to thank and acknowledge André Kahan MD, PhD, for his important contributions as a co-author of the first edition of this chapter.

References

1. Kahan A, Coghlan G, McLaughlin V. Cardiac complications of systemic sclerosis. Rheumatology (Oxford). 2009;48 Suppl 3:iii45–8.
2. Allanore Y, Meune C, Kahan A. Systemic sclerosis and cardiac dysfunction: evolving concepts and diagnostic methodologies. Curr Opin Rheumatol. 2008;20:697–702.
3. Champion HC. The heart in scleroderma. Rheum Dis Clin North Am. 2008;34:181–90; viii.
4. Meune C, Vignaux O, Kahan A, Allanore Y. Heart involvement in systemic sclerosis: evolving concept and diagnostic methodologies. Arch Cardiovasc Dis. 2010;103:46–52.
5. Parks JL, Taylor MH, Parks LP, Silver RM. Systemic sclerosis and the heart. Rheum Dis Clin North Am. 2014;40:87–102.
6. Desai CS, Lee DC, Shah SJ. Systemic sclerosis and the heart: current diagnosis and management. Curr Opin Rheumatol. 2011;23:545–54.
7. Allanore Y, Meune C, Vonk MC, Airo P, Hachulla E, Caramaschi P, Riemekasten G, Cozzi F, Beretta L, Derk CT, Komocsi A, Farge D, Balbir A, Riccieri V, Distler O, Chiala A, Papa ND, Simic KP, Ghio M, Stamenkovic B, Rednic S, Host N, Pellerito R, Zegers E, Kahan A, Walker UA, Matucci-Cerinic M. Prevalence and factors associated with left ventricular dysfunction in the EULAR Scleroderma Trial and Research group (EUSTAR) database of patients with systemic sclerosis. Ann Rheum Dis. 2010;69: 218–21.
8. Ferri C, Valentini G, Cozzi F, Sebastiani M, Michelassi C, La Montagna G, Bullo A, Cazzato M, Tirri E, Storino F, Giuggioli D, Cuomo G, Rosada M, Bombardieri S, Todesco S, Tirri G. Systemic sclerosis: demographic, clinical, and serologic features and survival in 1,012 Italian patients. Medicine (Baltimore). 2002;81:139–53.
9. Kahan A, Allanore Y. Primary myocardial involvement in systemic sclerosis. Rheumatology (Oxford). 2006;45 Suppl 4: iv14–7.
10. Meune C, Avouac J, Wahbi K, Cabanes L, Wipff J, Mouthon L, Guillevin L, Kahan A, Allanore Y. Cardiac involvement in systemic sclerosis assessed by tissue-doppler echocardiography during routine care: a controlled study of 100 consecutive patients. Arthritis Rheum. 2008;58:1803–9.
11. Plazak W, Zabinska-Plazak E, Wojas-Pelc A, Podolec P, Olszowska M, Tracz W, Bogdaszewska-Czabanowska J. Heart structure and function in systemic sclerosis. Eur J Dermatol. 2002;12:257–62.
12. Follansbee WP, Curtiss EI, Medsger TA, Steen VD, Uretsky BF, Owens GR, Rodnan GP. Physiologic abnormalities of cardiac function in progressive systemic sclerosis with diffuse scleroderma. N Engl J Med. 1984;310:142–8.
13. Fernandez-Codina A, Simeon-Aznar CP, Pinal-Fernandez I, Rodriguez-Palomares J, Pizzi MN, Hidalgo CE, Del Castillo AG, Prado-Galbarro FJ, Sarria-Santamera A, Fonollosa-Pla V, Vilardell-Tarres M. Cardiac involvement in systemic sclerosis: differences between clinical subsets and influence on survival. Rheumatol Int. 2015; Epub ahead of print.
14. Perera A, Fertig N, Lucas M, Rodriguez-Reyna TS, Hu P, Steen VD, Medsger Jr TA. Clinical subsets, skin thickness progression rate, and serum antibody levels in systemic sclerosis patients with anti-topoisomerase I antibody. Arthritis Rheum. 2007;56:2740–6.
15. Steen VD. Autoantibodies in systemic sclerosis. Semin Arthritis Rheum. 2005;35:35–42.
16. Ranque B, Authier FJ, Berezne A, Guillevin L, Mouthon L. Systemic sclerosis-associated myopathy. Ann N Y Acad Sci. 2007;1108:268–82.
17. Clements PJ, Lachenbruch PA, Furst DE, Paulus HE, Sterz MG. Cardiac score. A semiquantitative measure of cardiac involvement that improves prediction of prognosis in systemic sclerosis. Arthritis Rheum. 1991;34:1371–80.
18. Steen VD, Medsger Jr TA. Severe organ involvement in systemic sclerosis with diffuse scleroderma. Arthritis Rheum. 2000;43: 2437–44.
19. Scussel-Lonzetti L, Joyal F, Raynauld J-P, Roussin A, Rich E, Goulet J-R, Raymond Y, Senecal J-L. Predicting mortality in systemic sclerosis: analysis of a cohort of 309 French Canadian patients with emphasis on features at diagnosis as predictive factors for survival. Medicine (Baltimore). 2002;81:154–67.
20. Ioannidis JP, Vlachoyiannopoulos PG, Haidich AB, Medsger Jr TA, Lucas M, Michet CJ, Kuwana M, Yasuoka H, van den Hoogen F, Te Boome L, van Laar JM, Verbeet NL, Matucci-Cerinic M, Georgountzos A, Moutsopoulos HM. Mortality in systemic sclerosis: an international meta-analysis of individual patient data. Am J Med. 2005;118:2–10.
21. Al-Dhaher FF, Pope JE, Ouimet JM. Determinants of morbidity and mortality of systemic sclerosis in Canada. Semin Arthritis Rheum. 2010;39:269–77.
22. Czirjak L, Kumanovics G, Varju C, Nagy Z, Pakozdi A, Szekanecz Z, Szucs G. Survival and causes of death in 366 Hungarian patients with systemic sclerosis. Ann Rheum Dis. 2008;67:59–63.

23. Joven BE, Almodovar R, Carmona L, Carreira PE. Survival, causes of death, and risk factors associated with mortality in Spanish systemic sclerosis patients: results from a single university hospital. Semin Arthritis Rheum. 2010;39:285–93.
24. Tyndall AJ, Bannert B, Vonk M, Airo P, Cozzi F, Carreira PE, Bancel DF, Allanore Y, Muller-Ladner U, Distler O, Iannone F, Pellerito R, Pileckyte M, Miniati I, Ananieva L, Gurman AB, Damjanov N, Mueller A, Valentini G, Riemekasten G, Tikly M, Hummers L, Henriques MJ, Caramaschi P, Scheja A, Rozman B, Ton E, Kumanovics G, Coleiro B, Feierl E, Szucs G, Von Muhlen CA, Riccieri V, Novak S, Chizzolini C, Kotulska A, Denton C, Coelho PC, Kotter I, Simsek I, de la Pena Lefebvre PG, Hachulla E, Seibold JR, Rednic S, Stork J, Morovic-Vergles J, Walker UA. Causes and risk factors for death in systemic sclerosis: a study from the EULAR Scleroderma Trials and Research (EUSTAR) database. Ann Rheum Dis. 2010;69:1809–15.
25. Follansbee WP, Miller TR, Curtiss EI, Orie JE, Bernstein RL, Kiernan JM, Medsger TA. A controlled clinicopathologic study of myocardial fibrosis in systemic sclerosis (scleroderma). J Rheumatol. 1990;17:656–62.
26. Bulkley BH, Ridolfi RL, Salyer WR, Hutchins GM. Myocardial lesions of progressive systemic sclerosis. A cause of cardiac dysfunction. Circulation. 1976;53:483–90.
27. James TN. De subitaneis mortibus. VIII. Coronary arteries and conduction system in scleroderma heart disease. Circulation. 1974;50:844–56.
28. Alexander EL, Firestein GS, Weiss JL, Heuser RR, Leitl G, Wagner HN, Brinker JA, Ciuffo AA, Becker LC. Reversible cold-induced abnormalities in myocardial perfusion and function in systemic sclerosis. Ann Intern Med. 1986;105:661–8.
29. Gustafsson R, Mannting F, Kazzam E, Waldenstrom A, Hallgren R. Cold-induced reversible myocardial ischaemia in systemic sclerosis. Lancet. 1989;2:475–9.
30. Lekakis J, Mavrikakis M, Emmanuel M, Prassopoulos V, Papazoglou S, Papamichael C, Moulopoulou D, Kostamis P, Stamatelopoulos S, Moulopoulos S. Cold-induced coronary Raynaud's phenomenon in patients with systemic sclerosis. Clin Exp Rheumatol. 1998;16:135–40.
31. Long A, Duffy G, Bresnihan B. Reversible myocardial perfusion defects during cold challenge in scleroderma. Br J Rheumatol. 1986;25:158–61.
32. Mizuno R, Fujimoto S, Saito Y, Nakamura S. Cardiac Raynaud's phenomenon induced by cold provocation as a predictor of long-term left ventricular dysfunction and remodelling in systemic sclerosis: 7-year follow-up study. Eur J Heart Fail. 2010;12: 268–75.
33. Steen VD, Follansbee WP, Conte CG, Medsger Jr TA. Thallium perfusion defects predict subsequent cardiac dysfunction in patients with systemic sclerosis. Arthritis Rheum. 1996;39: 677–81.
34. Kahan A, Nitenberg A, Foult JM, Amor B, Menkes CJ, Devaux JY, Blanchet F, Perennec J, Lutfalla G, Roucayrol JC. Decreased coronary reserve in primary scleroderma myocardial disease. Arthritis Rheum. 1985;28:637–46.
35. Montisci R, Vacca A, Garau P, Colonna P, Ruscazio M, Passiu G, Iliceto S, Mathieu A. Detection of early impairment of coronary flow reserve in patients with systemic sclerosis. Ann Rheum Dis. 2003;62:890–3.
36. Sulli A, Ghio M, Bezante GP, Deferrari L, Craviotto C, Sebastiani V, Setti M, Filaci G, Puppo F, Barsotti A, Cutolo M, Indiveri F. Blunted coronary flow reserve in systemic sclerosis: a sign of cardiac involvement in asymptomatic patients. Ann Rheum Dis. 2004;63:210–1.
37. Kerr LD, Spiera H. Myocarditis as a complication in scleroderma patients with myositis. Clin Cardiol. 1993;16:895–9.
38. West SG, Killian PJ, Lawless OJ. Association of myositis and myocarditis in progressive systemic sclerosis. Arthritis Rheum. 1981;24:662–8.
39. Follansbee WP, Zerbe TR, Medsger Jr TA. Cardiac and skeletal muscle disease in systemic sclerosis (scleroderma): a high risk association. Am Heart J. 1993;125:194–203.
40. Hegedus I, Czirjak L. Left ventricular wall motion abnormalities in 80 patients with systemic sclerosis. Clin Rheumatol. 1995;14:161–4.
41. Valentini G, Vitale DF, Giunta A, Maione S, Gerundo G, Arnese M, Tirri E, Pelaggi N, Giacummo A, Tirri G, Condorelli M. Diastolic abnormalities in systemic sclerosis: evidence for associated defective cardiac functional reserve. Ann Rheum Dis. 1996;55:455–60.
42. Aguglia G, Sgreccia A, Bernardo ML, Carmenini E, Giusti De Marle M, Reali A, Morelli S. Left ventricular diastolic function in systemic sclerosis. J Rheumatol. 2001;28:1563–7.
43. Nakajima K, Taki J, Kawano M, Higuchi T, Sato S, Nishijima C, Takehara K, Tonami N. Diastolic dysfunction in patients with systemic sclerosis detected by gated myocardial perfusion SPECT: an early sign of cardiac involvement. J Nucl Med. 2001;42:183–8.
44. Rosato E, Maione S, Vitarelli A, Giunta A, Fontanella L, de Horatio LT, Cacciatore F, Proietti M, Pisarri S, Salsano F. Regional diastolic function by tissue Doppler echocardiography in systemic sclerosis: correlation with clinical variables. Rheumatol Int. 2009;29:913–9.
45. Kazzam E, Waldenstrom A, Landelius J, Hallgren R, Arvidsson A, Caidahl K. Non-invasive assessment of left ventricular diastolic function in patients with systemic sclerosis. J Intern Med. 1990;228:183–92.
46. Armstrong GP, Whalley GA, Doughty RN, Gamble GD, Flett SM, Tan PL, Sharpe DN. Left ventricular function in scleroderma. Br J Rheumatol. 1996;35:983–8.
47. Hinchcliff M, Desai CS, Varga J, Shah SJ. Prevalence, prognosis, and factors associated with left ventricular diastolic dysfunction in systemic sclerosis. Clin Exp Rheumatol. 2012;30:S30–7.
48. Faludi R, Kolto G, Bartos B, Csima G, Czirjak L, Komocsi A. Five-year follow-up of left ventricular diastolic function in systemic sclerosis patients: determinants of mortality and disease progression. Semin Arthritis Rheum. 2014;44:220–7.
49. Bezante GP, Rollando D, Sessarego M, Panico N, Setti M, Filaci G, Molinari G, Balbi M, Cutolo M, Barsotti A, Indiveri F, Ghio M. Cardiac magnetic resonance imaging detects subclinical right ventricular impairment in systemic sclerosis. J Rheumatol. 2007;34:2431–7.
50. George BJ, Kwan MD, Morris MJ. Isolated right ventricular failure in scleroderma heart disease. Cardiol Rev. 2004;12:279–81.
51. Giunta A, Tirri E, Maione S, Cangianiello S, Mele A, De Luca A, Valentini G. Right ventricular diastolic abnormalities in systemic sclerosis. Relation to left ventricular involvement and pulmonary hypertension. Ann Rheum Dis. 2000;59:94–8.
52. Gonzalez A, Seres L, Ferrer E, Valle V. Isolated right ventricular systolic dysfunction in scleroderma. Rev Esp Cardiol. 2008;61: 990–1.
53. Hsiao SH, Lee CY, Chang SM, Lin SK, Liu CP. Right heart function in scleroderma: insights from myocardial Doppler tissue imaging. J Am Soc Echocardiogr. 2006;19:507–14.
54. Huez S, Roufosse F, Vachiery JL, Pavelescu A, Derumeaux G, Wautrecht JC, Cogan E, Naeije R. Isolated right ventricular dysfunction in systemic sclerosis: latent pulmonary hypertension? Eur Respir J. 2007;30:928–36.
55. Lee CY, Chang SM, Hsiao SH, Tseng JC, Lin SK, Liu CP. Right heart function and scleroderma: insights from tricuspid annular plane systolic excursion. Echocardiography. 2007;24:118–25.
56. Lindqvist P, Caidahl K, Neuman-Andersen G, Ozolins C, Rantapaa-Dahlqvist S, Waldenstrom A, Kazzam E. Disturbed

right ventricular diastolic function in patients with systemic sclerosis: a Doppler tissue imaging study. Chest. 2005;128:755–63.
57. Meune C, Allanore Y, Devaux JY, Dessault O, Duboc D, Weber S, Kahan A. High prevalence of right ventricular systolic dysfunction in early systemic sclerosis. J Rheumatol. 2004;31:1941–5.
58. Meune C, Khanna D, Aboulhosn J, Avouac J, Kahan A, Furst DE, Allanore Y. A right ventricular diastolic impairment is common in systemic sclerosis and is associated with other target-organ damage. Semin Arthritis Rheum. 2016;45(4):439–45.
59. Kahan A, Devaux JY, Amor B, Menkes CJ, Weber S, Foult JM, Venot A, Guerin F, Degeorges M, Roucayrol JC. Pharmacodynamic effect of dipyridamole on thallium-201 myocardial perfusion in progressive systemic sclerosis with diffuse scleroderma. Ann Rheum Dis. 1986;45:718–25.
60. Kahan A, Devaux JY, Amor B, Menkes CJ, Weber S, Nitenberg A, Venot A, Guerin F, Degeorges M, Roucayrol JC. Nifedipine and thallium-201 myocardial perfusion in progressive systemic sclerosis. N Engl J Med. 1986;314:1397–402.
61. Kahan A, Devaux JY, Amor B, Menkes CJ, Weber S, Venot A, Guerin F, Degeorges M, Roucayrol JC. Nicardipine improves myocardial perfusion in systemic sclerosis. J Rheumatol. 1988;15:1395–400.
62. Kahan A, Devaux JY, Amor B, Menkes CJ, Weber S, Venot A, Strauch G. The effect of captopril on thallium 201 myocardial perfusion in systemic sclerosis. Clin Pharmacol Ther. 1990;47:483–9.
63. Ishida R, Murata Y, Sawada Y, Nishioka K, Shibuya H. Thallium-201 myocardial SPET in patients with collagen disease. Nucl Med Commun. 2000;21:729–34.
64. Duboc D, Kahan A, Maziere B, Loc'h C, Crouzel C, Menkes CJ, Amor B, Strauch G, Guerin F, Syrota A. The effect of nifedipine on myocardial perfusion and metabolism in systemic sclerosis. A positron emission tomographic study. Arthritis Rheum. 1991;34:198–203.
65. Vignaux O, Allanore Y, Meune C, Pascal O, Duboc D, Weber S, Legmann P, Kahan A. Evaluation of the effect of nifedipine upon myocardial perfusion and contractility using cardiac magnetic resonance imaging and tissue Doppler echocardiography in systemic sclerosis. Ann Rheum Dis. 2005;64:1268–73.
66. Allanore Y, Meune C, Vignaux O, Weber S, Legmann P, Kahan A. Bosentan increases myocardial perfusion and function in systemic sclerosis: a magnetic resonance imaging and Tissue-Doppler echography study. J Rheumatol. 2006;33:2464–9.
67. Kahan A, Devaux JY, Amor B, Menkes CJ, Weber S, Guerin F, Venot A, Strauch G. Pharmacodynamic effect of nicardipine on left ventricular function in systemic sclerosis. J Cardiovasc Pharmacol. 1990;15:249–53.
68. Smiseth OA, Ihlen H. Strain rate imaging: why do we need it? J Am Coll Cardiol. 2003;42:1584–6.
69. Galiè N, Humbert M, Vachiery JL, Gibbs S, Lang I, Torbicki A, Simonneau G, Peacock A, Vonk Noordegraaf A, Beghetti M, Ghofrani A, Gomez Sanchez MA, Hansmann G, Klepetko W, Lancellotti P, Matucci M, McDonagh T, Pierard LA, Trindade PT, Zompatori M, Hoeper M. 2015 ESC/ERS Guidelines for the diagnosis and treatment of pulmonary hypertension: The Joint Task Force for the Diagnosis and Treatment of Pulmonary Hypertension of the European Society of Cardiology (ESC) and the European Respiratory Society (ERS): endorsed by: Association for European Paediatric and Congenital Cardiology (AEPC), International Society for Heart and Lung Transplantation (ISHLT). Eur Respir J. 2015;46(4):903–75.
70. European Society of Cardiology (ESC); European Heart Rhythm Association (EHRA), Brignole M, Auricchio A, Baron-Esquivias G, Bordachar P, Boriani G, Breithardt OA, Cleland J, Deharo JC, Delgado V, Elliott PM, Gorenek B, Israel CW, Leclercq C, Linde C, Mont L, Padeletti L, Sutton R, Vardas PE. 2013 ESC guidelines on cardiac pacing and cardiac resynchronization therapy: the task force on cardiac pacing and resynchronization therapy of the European Society of Cardiology (ESC). Developed in collaboration with the European Heart Rhythm Association (EHRA). Europace. 2013;15(8):1070–118.
71. Stack J, McLaughlin P, Sinnot C, Henry M, MacEneaney P, Eltahir A, Harney S. Successful control of scleroderma myocarditis using a combination of cyclophosphamide and methylprednisolone. Scand J Rheumatol. 2010;39:349–50.
72. Pieroni M, De Santis M, Zizzo G, Bosello S, Smaldone C, Campioni M, De Luca G, Laria A, Meduri A, Bellocci F, Bonomo L, Crea F, Ferraccioli G. Recognizing and treating myocarditis in recent-onset systemic sclerosis heart disease: potential utility of immunosuppressive therapy in cardiac damage progression. Semin Arthritis Rheum. 2014;43:526–35.
73. Chung L, Fiorentino D. Digital ulcers in patients with systemic sclerosis. Autoimmun Rev. 2006;5:125–8.
74. Califf RM, Adams KF, McKenna WJ, Gheorghiade M, Uretsky BF, McNulty SE, Darius H, Schulman K, Zannad F, Handberg-Thurmond E, Harrell Jr FE, Wheeler W, Soler-Soler J, Swedberg K. A randomized controlled trial of epoprostenol therapy for severe congestive heart failure: the Flolan International Randomized Survival Trial (FIRST). Am Heart J. 1997;134:44–54.
75. Mok MY, Lau CS, Chiu SS, Tso AW, Lo Y, Law LS, Mak KF, Wong WS, Khong PL, Lam KS. Systemic sclerosis is an independent risk factor for increased coronary artery calcium deposition. Arthritis Rheum. 2011;63:1387–95.
76. Ngian GS, Sahhar J, Proudman SM, Stevens W, Wicks IP, Van Doornum S. Prevalence of coronary heart disease and cardiovascular risk factors in a national cross-sectional cohort study of systemic sclerosis. Ann Rheum Dis. 2012;71:1980–3.
77. Ungprasert P, Charoenpong P, Ratanasrimetha P, Thongprayoon C, Cheungpasitporn W, Suksaranjit P. Risk of coronary artery disease in patients with systemic sclerosis: a systematic review and meta-analysis. Clin Rheumatol. 2014;33:1099–104.
78. Hachulla AL, Launay D, Gaxotte V, de Groote P, Lamblin N, Devos P, Hatron PY, Beregi JP, Hachulla E. Cardiac magnetic resonance imaging in systemic sclerosis: a cross-sectional observational study of 52 patients. Ann Rheum Dis. 2009;68:1878–84.
79. Byers RJ, Marshall DA, Freemont AJ. Pericardial involvement in systemic sclerosis. Ann Rheum Dis. 1997;56:393–4.
80. Hinderliter AL, Willis PW, Long W, Clarke WR, Ralph D, Caldwell EJ, Williams W, Ettinger NA, Hill NS, Summer WR, de Biosblanc B, Koch G, Li S, Clayton LM, Jobsis MM, Crow JW. Frequency and prognostic significance of pericardial effusion in primary pulmonary hypertension. PPH Study Group. Primary pulmonary hypertension. Am J Cardiol. 1999;84:481–4, A410.
81. Park B, Dittrich HC, Polikar R, Olson L, Nicod P. Echocardiographic evidence of pericardial effusion in severe chronic pulmonary hypertension. Am J Cardiol. 1989;63:143–5.
82. Habib G, Torbicki A. The role of echocardiography in the diagnosis and management of patients with pulmonary hypertension. Eur Respir Rev. 2010;19:288–99.
83. Wooten MD, Reddy GV, Johnson RD. Cardiac tamponade in systemic sclerosis: a case report and review of 18 reported cases. J Clin Rheumatol. 2000;6:35–40.
84. Nishimura RA. Constrictive pericarditis in the modern era: a diagnostic dilemma. Heart. 2001;86:619–23.
85. Hancock EW. Differential diagnosis of restrictive cardiomyopathy and constrictive pericarditis. Heart. 2001;86:343–9.
86. Dal-Bianco JP, Sengupta PP, Mookadam F, Chandrasekaran K, Tajik AJ, Khandheria BK. Role of echocardiography in the diagnosis of constrictive pericarditis. J Am Soc Echocardiogr. 2009;22:24–33; quiz 103–4.
87. Leya FS, Arab D, Joyal D, Shioura KM, Lewis BE, Steen LH, Cho L. The efficacy of brain natriuretic peptide levels in differentiating

constrictive pericarditis from restrictive cardiomyopathy. J Am Coll Cardiol. 2005;45:1900–2.

88. Vacca A, Meune C, Gordon J, Chung L, Proudman S, Assassi S, Nikpour M, Rodriguez-Reyna TS, Khanna D, Lafyatis R, Matucci-Cerinic M, Distler O, Allanore Y. Cardiac arrhythmias and conduction defects in systemic sclerosis. Rheumatology (Oxford). 2014;53:1172–7.
89. D'Angelo WA, Fries JF, Masi AT, Shulman LE. Pathologic observations in systemic sclerosis (scleroderma). A study of fifty-eight autopsy cases and fifty-eight matched controls. Am J Med. 1969;46:428–40.
90. Ridolfi RL, Bulkley BH, Hutchins GM. The cardiac conduction system in progressive systemic sclerosis. Clinical and pathologic features of 35 patients. Am J Med. 1976;61:361–6.
91. Lubitz SA, Goldbarg SH, Mehta D. Sudden cardiac death in infiltrative cardiomyopathies: sarcoidosis, scleroderma, amyloidosis, hemachromatosis. Prog Cardiovasc Dis. 2008;51:58–73.
92. Gialafos E, Konstantopoulou P, Voulgari C, Giavri I, Panopoulos S, Vaiopoulos G, Mavrikakis M, Moyssakis I, Sfikakis PP. Abnormal spatial QRS-T angle, a marker of ventricular repolarisation, predicts serious ventricular arrhythmia in systemic sclerosis. Clin Exp Rheumatol. 2012;30:327–31.
93. Wozniak J, Dabrowski R, Luczak D, Kwiatkowska M, Musiej-Nowakowska E, Kowalik I, Szwed H. Evaluation of heart rhythm variability and arrhythmia in children with systemic and localized scleroderma. J Rheumatol. 2009;36:191–6.
94. Kostis JB, Seibold JR, Turkevich D, Masi AT, Grau RG, Medsger Jr TA, Steen VD, Clements PJ, Szydlo L, D'Angelo WA. Prognostic importance of cardiac arrhythmias in systemic sclerosis. Am J Med. 1988;84:1007–15.
95. Fraiser LH, Kanekal S, Kehrer JP. Cyclophosphamide toxicity. Characterising and avoiding the problem. Drugs. 1991;42:781–95.
96. Cotroneo J, Sleik KM, Rene Rodriguez E, Klein AL. Hydroxychloroquine-induced restrictive cardiomyopathy. Eur J Echocardiogr. 2007;8:247–51.
97. Burt RK, Oliveira MC, Shah SJ, Moraes DA, Simoes B, Gheorghiade M, Schroeder J, Ruderman E, Farge D, Chai ZJ, Marjanovic Z, Jain S, Morgan A, Milanetti F, Han X, Jovanovic B, Helenowski IB, Voltarelli J. Cardiac involvement and treatment-related mortality after non-myeloablative haemopoietic stem-cell transplantation with unselected autologous peripheral blood for patients with systemic sclerosis: a retrospective analysis. Lancet. 2013;381:1116–24.
98. Burt RK, Shah SJ, Dill K, Grant T, Gheorghiade M, Schroeder J, Craig R, Hirano I, Marshall K, Ruderman E, Jovanovic B, Milanetti F, Jain S, Boyce K, Morgan A, Carr J, Barr W. Autologous non-myeloablative haemopoietic stem-cell transplantation compared with pulse cyclophosphamide once per month for systemic sclerosis (ASSIST): an open-label, randomised phase 2 trial. Lancet. 2011;378:498–506.
99. Yamamoto R, Kanda Y, Matsuyama T, Oshima K, Nannya Y, Suguro M, Chizuka A, Hamaki T, Takezako N, Miwa A, Kami M, Mori S, Kojima T, Saito K, Itaoka Y, Kashida M. Myopericarditis caused by cyclophosphamide used to mobilize peripheral blood stem cells in a myeloma patient with renal failure. Bone Marrow Transplant. 2000;26:685–8.
100. Soong TR, Barouch LA, Champion HC, Wigley FM, Halushka MK. New clinical and ultrastructural findings in hydroxychloroquine-induced cardiomyopathy--a report of 2 cases. Hum Pathol. 2007;38:1858–63.
101. Distler JH, Distler O. Cardiotoxicity of imatinib mesylate: an extremely rare phenomenon or a major side effect? Ann Rheum Dis. 2007;66:836.
102. Kerkela R, Grazette L, Yacobi R, Iliescu C, Patten R, Beahm C, Walters B, Shevtsov S, Pesant S, Clubb FJ, Rosenzweig A, Salomon RN, Van Etten RA, Alroy J, Durand JB, Force T. Cardiotoxicity of the cancer therapeutic agent imatinib mesylate. Nat Med. 2006;12:908–16.
103. Fujimaki K, Maruta A, Yoshida M, Sakai R, Tanabe J, Koharazawa H, Kodama F, Asahina S, Minamizawa M, Matsuzaki M, Fujisawa S, Kanamori H, Ishigatsubo Y. Severe cardiac toxicity in hematological stem cell transplantation: predictive value of reduced left ventricular ejection fraction. Bone Marrow Transplant. 2001;27:307–10.
104. Burt RK, Oliveira MC, Shah SJ. Cardiac assessment before stem cell transplantation for systemic sclerosis. JAMA. 2014;312:1803.
105. Daniels LB, Maisel AS. Natriuretic peptides. J Am Coll Cardiol. 2007;50:2357–68.
106. Maisel A, Mueller C, Adams Jr K, Anker SD, Aspromonte N, Cleland JG, Cohen-Solal A, Dahlstrom U, DeMaria A, Di Somma S, Filippatos GS, Fonarow GC, Jourdain P, Komajda M, Liu PP, McDonagh T, McDonald K, Mebazaa A, Nieminen MS, Peacock WF, Tubaro M, Valle R, Vanderhyden M, Yancy CW, Zannad F, Braunwald E. State of the art: using natriuretic peptide levels in clinical practice. Eur J Heart Fail. 2008;10:824–39.
107. Weber M, Hamm C. Role of B-type natriuretic peptide (BNP) and NT-proBNP in clinical routine. Heart. 2006;92:843–9.
108. Allanore Y, Meune C. N-terminal pro brain natriuretic peptide: the new cornerstone of cardiovascular assessment in systemic sclerosis. Clin Exp Rheumatol. 2009;27:59–63.
109. Allanore Y, Wahbi K, Borderie D, Weber S, Kahan A, Meune C. N-terminal pro-brain natriuretic peptide in systemic sclerosis: a new cornerstone of cardiovascular assessment? Ann Rheum Dis. 2009;68:1885–9.
110. Allanore Y, Borderie D, Meune C, Cabanes L, Weber S, Ekindjian OG, Kahan A. N-terminal pro-brain natriuretic peptide as a diagnostic marker of early pulmonary artery hypertension in patients with systemic sclerosis and effects of calcium-channel blockers. Arthritis Rheum. 2003;48:3503–8.
111. Mukerjee D, Yap LB, Holmes AM, Nair D, Ayrton P, Black CM, Coghlan JG. Significance of plasma N-terminal pro-brain natriuretic peptide in patients with systemic sclerosis-related pulmonary arterial hypertension. Respir Med. 2003;97:1230–6.
112. Williams MH, Handler CE, Akram R, Smith CJ, Das C, Smee J, Nair D, Denton CP, Black CM, Coghlan JG. Role of N-terminal brain natriuretic peptide (N-TproBNP) in scleroderma-associated pulmonary arterial hypertension. Eur Heart J. 2006;27:1485–94.
113. Mathai SC, Hassoun PM. N-terminal brain natriuretic peptide in scleroderma-associated pulmonary arterial hypertension. Eur Heart J. 2007;28:140–1; author reply 141.
114. Allanore Y, Borderie D, Avouac J, Zerkak D, Meune C, Hachulla E, Mouthon L, Guillevin L, Meyer O, Ekindjian OG, Weber S, Kahan A. High N-terminal pro-brain natriuretic peptide levels and low diffusing capacity for carbon monoxide as independent predictors of the occurrence of precapillary pulmonary arterial hypertension in patients with systemic sclerosis. Arthritis Rheum. 2008;58:284–91.
115. Choi HJ, Shin YK, Lee HJ, Kee JY, Shin DW, Lee EY, Lee YJ, Lee EB, Song YW. The clinical significance of serum N-terminal pro-brain natriuretic peptide in systemic sclerosis patients. Clin Rheumatol. 2008;27:437–42.
116. Dimitroulas T, Giannakoulas G, Karvounis H, Settas L. Limitations of the findings regarding the relationship between N-terminal pro-brain natriuretic peptide and systemic sclerosis-related pulmonary arterial hypertension: comment on the article by Allanore et al. Arthritis Rheum. 2008;58:2215–6; author reply 2216.
117. Carlo-Stella N, Belloli L, Biondi ML, Marasini B. Serum N-terminal pro-brain natriuretic peptide, a marker of skin thickness in systemic sclerosis? Clin Rheumatol. 2009;28:241–2.
118. Mathai SC, Bueso M, Hummers LK, Boyce D, Lechtzin N, Le Pavec J, Campo A, Champion HC, Housten T, Forfia PR, Zaiman AL, Wigley FM, Girgis RE, Hassoun PM. Disproportionate eleva-

tion of N-terminal pro-brain natriuretic peptide in scleroderma-related pulmonary hypertension. Eur Respir J. 2010;35:95–104.

119. Cavagna L, Caporali R, Klersy C, Ghio S, Albertini R, Scelsi L, Moratti R, Bonino C, Montecucco C. Comparison of brain natriuretic peptide (BNP) and NT-proBNP in screening for pulmonary arterial hypertension in patients with systemic sclerosis. J Rheumatol. 2010;37:2064–70.
120. Montagnana M, Lippi G, Volpe A, Salvagno GL, Biasi D, Caramaschi P, Cesare GG. Evaluation of cardiac laboratory markers in patients with systemic sclerosis. Clin Biochem. 2006;39: 913–7.
121. Avouac J, Meune C, Chenevier-Gobeaux C, Borderie D, Lefevre G, Kahan A, Allanore Y. Cardiac biomarkers in systemic sclerosis: contribution of high-sensitivity cardiac troponin in addition to N-terminal pro-brain natriuretic peptide. Arthritis Care Res (Hoboken). 2015;67:1022–30.
122. Ho CY, Solomon SD. A clinician's guide to tissue Doppler imaging. Circulation. 2006;113:e396–8.
123. Nagueh SF, Appleton CP, Gillebert TC, Marino PN, Oh JK, Smiseth OA, Waggoner AD, Flachskampf FA, Pellikka PA, Evangelista A. Recommendations for the evaluation of left ventricular diastolic function by echocardiography. J Am Soc Echocardiogr. 2009;22:107–33.
124. Rossi A, Temporelli PL, Quintana M, Dini FL, Ghio S, Hillis GS, Klein AL, Marsan NA, Prior DL, Yu CM, Poppe KK, Doughty RN, Whalley GA, MeRGE Heart Failure Collaborators. Independent relationship of left atrial size and mortality in patients with heart failure: an individual patient meta-analysis of longitudinal data (MeRGE Heart Failure). Eur J Heart Fail. 2009; 11(10):929–36.
125. Henein M, Lindqvist P, Francis D, Morner S, Waldenstrom A, Kazzam E. Tissue Doppler analysis of age-dependency in diastolic ventricular behaviour and filling: a cross-sectional study of healthy hearts (the Umea General Population Heart Study). Eur Heart J. 2002;23:162–71.
126. Ho SY, Nihoyannopoulos P. Anatomy, echocardiography, and normal right ventricular dimensions. Heart. 2006;92 Suppl 1:i2–13.
127. Coghlan JG, Denton CP, Grünig E, Bonderman D, Distler O, Khanna D, Müller-Ladner U, Pope JE, Vonk MC, Doelberg M, Chadha-Boreham H, Heinzl H, Rosenberg DM, McLaughlin VV, Seibold JR, DETECT Study Group. Evidence-based detection of pulmonary arterial hypertension in systemic sclerosis: the DETECT study. Ann Rheum Dis. 2014;73(7):1340–9.
128. Horton KD, Meece RW, Hill JC. Assessment of the right ventricle by echocardiography: a primer for cardiac sonographers. J Am Soc Echocardiogr. 2009;22:776–92; quiz 861–2.
129. Rudski LG, Lai WW, Afilalo J, Hua L, Handschumacher MD, Chandrasekaran K, Solomon SD, Louie EK, Schiller NB. Guidelines for the echocardiographic assessment of the right heart in adults: a report from the American Society of Echocardiography endorsed by the European Association of Echocardiography, a registered branch of the European Society of Cardiology, and the Canadian Society of Echocardiography. J Am Soc Echocardiogr. 2010;23:685–713; quiz 786–8.
130. Schindler TH, Schelbert HR, Quercioli A, Dilsizian V. Cardiac PET imaging for the detection and monitoring of coronary artery disease and microvascular health. JACC Cardiovasc Imaging. 2010;3:623–40.
131. Kaufmann PA, Di Carli MF. Hybrid SPECT/CT and PET/CT imaging: the next step in noninvasive cardiac imaging. Semin Nucl Med. 2009;39:341–7.
132. Kobayashi H, Yokoe I, Hirano M, Nakamura T, Nakajima Y, Fontaine KR, Giles JT, Kobayashi Y. Cardiac magnetic resonance imaging with pharmacological stress perfusion and delayed enhancement in asymptomatic patients with systemic sclerosis. J Rheumatol. 2009;36:106–12.
133. Di Cesare E, Battisti S, Di Sibio A, Cipriani P, Giacomelli R, Liakouli V, Ruscitti P, Masciocchi C. Early assessment of subclinical cardiac involvement in systemic sclerosis (SSc) using delayed enhancement cardiac magnetic resonance (CE-MRI). Eur J Radiol. 2013;82:e268–73.
134. Moroncini G, Schicchi N, Pomponio G, Dziadzio M, della Costanza OP, Pierfederici A, Ferretti L, Pupita G, Valeri G, Agliata G, Salvolini L, Giovagnoni A, Gabrielli A. Myocardial perfusion defects in scleroderma detected by contrast-enhanced cardiovascular magnetic resonance. Radiol Med. 2014;119: 885–94.
135. Rodriguez-Reyna TS, Morelos-Guzman M, Hernandez-Reyes P, Montero-Duarte K, Martinez-Reyes C, Reyes-Utrera C, Vazquez-La Madrid J, Morales-Blanhir J, Nunez-Alvarez C, Cabiedes-Contreras J. Assessment of myocardial fibrosis and microvascular damage in systemic sclerosis by magnetic resonance imaging and coronary angiotomography. Rheumatology (Oxford). 2015;54:647–54.
136. Sano M, Satoh H, Suwa K, Nobuhara M, Saitoh T, Saotome M, Urushida T, Katoh H, Shimoyama K, Suzuki D, Ogawa N, Takehara Y, Sakahara H, Hayashi H. Characteristics and clinical relevance of late gadolinium enhancement in cardiac magnetic resonance in patients with systemic sclerosis. Heart Vessels. 2015;30:779–88.
137. Cooper LT, Baughman KL, Feldman AM, Frustaci A, Jessup M, Kuhl U, Levine GN, Narula J, Starling RC, Towbin J, Virmani R. The role of endomyocardial biopsy in the management of cardiovascular disease: a scientific statement from the American Heart Association, the American College of Cardiology, and the European Society of Cardiology. Circulation. 2007;116:2216–33.
138. Hager WD, Collins I, Tate JP, Azrin M, Foley R, Lakshminarayanan S, Rothfield NF. Exercise during cardiac catheterization distinguishes between pulmonary and left ventricular causes of dyspnea in systemic sclerosis patients. Clin Respir J. 2013;7:227–36.
139. Ciurzynski M, Bienias P, Irzyk K, Kostrubiec M, Bartoszewicz Z, Siwicka M, Kurzyna M, Demkow U, Pruszczyk P. Exaggerated increase of exercise-induced pulmonary artery pressure in systemic sclerosis patients predominantly results from left ventricular diastolic dysfunction. Clin Res Cardiol. 2013;102:813–20.
140. Ciftci O, Onat AM, Yavuz B, Akdogan A, Aytemir K, Tokgozoglu L, Sahiner L, Deniz A, Ureten K, Kizilca G, Calguneri M, Oto A. Cardiac repolarization abnormalities and increased sympathetic activity in scleroderma. J Natl Med Assoc. 2007;99:232–7.
141. Can I, Onat AM, Aytemir K, Akdogan A, Ureten K, Kiraz S, Ertenli I, Ozer N, Tokgozoglu L, Oto A. Assessment of atrial conduction in patients with scleroderma by tissue Doppler echocardiography and P wave dispersion. Cardiology. 2007;108:317–21.
142. Sergiacomi G, De Nardo D, Capria A, Manenti G, Fabiano S, Borzi M, De Sanctis G, Konda D, Sperandio M, Schillaci O, Masala S, Simonetti G, Fontana L. Non-invasive diagnostic and functional evaluation of cardiac and pulmonary involvement in systemic sclerosis. In Vivo. 2004;18:229–35.
143. Geyer H, Caracciolo G, Abe H, Wilansky S, Carerj S, Gentile F, Nesser HJ, Khandheria B, Narula J, Sengupta PP. Assessment of myocardial mechanics using speckle tracking echocardiography: fundamentals and clinical applications. J Am Soc Echocardiogr. 2010;23:351–69; quiz 453–5.
144. Blessberger H, Binder T. NON-invasive imaging: two dimensional speckle tracking echocardiography: basic principles. Heart. 2010;96:716–22.
145. Pavlopoulos H, Nihoyannopoulos P. Strain and strain rate deformation parameters: from tissue Doppler to 2D speckle tracking. Int J Cardiovasc Imaging. 2008;24:479–91.
146. Teske AJ, De Boeck BW, Melman PG, Sieswerda GT, Doevendans PA, Cramer MJ. Echocardiographic quantification of myocardial function using tissue deformation imaging, a guide to image

acquisition and analysis using tissue Doppler and speckle tracking. Cardiovasc Ultrasound. 2007;5:27.
147. Iles L, Pfluger H, Phrommintikul A, Cherayath J, Aksit P, Gupta SN, Kaye DM, Taylor AJ. Evaluation of diffuse myocardial fibrosis in heart failure with cardiac magnetic resonance contrast-enhanced T1 mapping. J Am Coll Cardiol. 2008;52:1574–80.
148. Messroghli DR, Greiser A, Frohlich M, Dietz R, Schulz-Menger J. Optimization and validation of a fully-integrated pulse sequence for modified look-locker inversion-recovery (MOLLI) T1 mapping of the heart. J Magn Reson Imaging. 2007;26:1081–6.
149. Messroghli DR, Radjenovic A, Kozerke S, Higgins DM, Sivananthan MU, Ridgway JP. Modified Look-Locker inversion recovery (MOLLI) for high-resolution T1 mapping of the heart. Magn Reson Med. 2004;52:141–6.
150. Lee DC, Johnson NP. Quantification of absolute myocardial blood flow by magnetic resonance perfusion imaging. JACC Cardiovasc Imaging. 2009;2:761–70.
151. Abraham TP, Dimaano VL, Liang HY. Role of tissue Doppler and strain echocardiography in current clinical practice. Circulation. 2007;116:2597–609.
152. Marwick TH. Measurement of strain and strain rate by echocardiography: ready for prime time? J Am Coll Cardiol. 2006;47:1313–27.
153. Plaksej R, Kosmala W, Frantz S, Herrmann S, Niemann M, Stork S, Wachter R, Angermann CE, Ertl G, Bijnens B, Weidemann F. Relation of circulating markers of fibrosis and progression of left and right ventricular dysfunction in hypertensive patients with heart failure. J Hypertens. 2009;27:2483–91.
154. Popovic ZB, Kwon DH, Mishra M, Buakhamsri A, Greenberg NL, Thamilarasan M, Flamm SD, Thomas JD, Lever HM, Desai MY. Association between regional ventricular function and myocardial fibrosis in hypertrophic cardiomyopathy assessed by speckle tracking echocardiography and delayed hyperenhancement magnetic resonance imaging. J Am Soc Echocardiogr. 2008;21:1299–305.
155. Mondillo S, Galderisi M, Mele D, Cameli M, Lomoriello VS, Zaca V, Ballo P, D'Andrea A, Muraru D, Losi M, Agricola E, D'Errico A, Buralli S, Sciomer S, Nistri S, Badano L. Speckle-tracking echocardiography: a new technique for assessing myocardial function. J Ultrasound Med. 2011;30:71–83.
156. Shehata ML, Cheng S, Osman NF, Bluemke DA, Lima JA. Myocardial tissue tagging with cardiovascular magnetic resonance. J Cardiovasc Magn Reson. 2009;11:55.
157. Agoston G, Gargani L, Miglioranza MH, Caputo M, Badano LP, Moreo A, Muraru D, Mondillo S, Moggi Pignone A, Matucci Cerinic M, Sicari R, Picano E, Varga A. Left atrial dysfunction detected by speckle tracking in patients with systemic sclerosis. Cardiovasc Ultrasound. 2014;12:30.
158. Atas H, Kepez A, Tigen K, Samadov F, Ozen G, Cincin A, Sunbul M, Bozbay M, Direskeneli H, Basaran Y. Evaluation of left atrial volume and function in systemic sclerosis patients using speckle tracking and real-time three-dimensional echocardiography. Anatol J Cardiol. 2016;16(5):316–22.
159. Cadeddu C, Deidda M, Giau G, Lilliu M, Cadeddu F, Binaghi G, Mura MN, Farci M, Del Giacco S, Manconi PE, Mercuro G. Contractile reserve in systemic sclerosis patients as a major predictor of global cardiac impairment and exercise tolerance. Int J Cardiovasc Imaging. 2015;31:529–36.
160. Cusma Piccione M, Zito C, Bagnato G, Oreto G, Di Bella G, Carerj S. Role of 2D strain in the early identification of left ventricular dysfunction and in the risk stratification of systemic sclerosis patients. Cardiovasc Ultrasound. 2013;11:6.
161. Spethmann S, Dreger H, Schattke S, Riemekasten G, Borges AC, Baumann G, Knebel F. Two-dimensional speckle tracking of the left ventricle in patients with systemic sclerosis for an early detection of myocardial involvement. Eur Heart J Cardiovasc Imaging. 2012;13:863–70.
162. Spethmann S, Rieper K, Riemekasten G, Borges AC, Schattke S, Burmester GR, Hewing B, Baumann G, Dreger H, Knebel F. Echocardiographic follow-up of patients with systemic sclerosis by 2D speckle tracking echocardiography of the left ventricle. Cardiovasc Ultrasound. 2014;12:13.
163. Tigen K, Sunbul M, Ozen G, Durmus E, Kivrak T, Cincin A, Ozben B, Atas H, Direskeneli H, Basaran Y. Regional myocardial dysfunction assessed by two-dimensional speckle tracking echocardiography in systemic sclerosis patients with fragmented QRS complexes. J Electrocardiol. 2014;47:677–83.
164. Knight DS, Grasso AE, Quail MA, Muthurangu V, Taylor AM, Toumpanakis C, Caplin ME, Coghlan JG, Davar J. Accuracy and reproducibility of right ventricular quantification in patients with pressure and volume overload using single-beat three-dimensional echocardiography. J Am Soc Echocardiogr. 2015;28(3):363–74.
165. Knight DS, Schwaiger JP, Krupickova S, Davar J, Muthurangu V, Coghlan JG. Accuracy and test-retest reproducibility of two-dimensional knowledge-based volumetric reconstruction of the right ventricle in pulmonary hypertension. J Am Soc Echocardiogr. 2015;28(8):989–98.
166. Yiu KH, Schouffoer AA, Marsan NA, Ninaber MK, Stolk J, Vlieland TV, Scherptong RW, Delgado V, Holman ER, Tse HF, Huizinga TW, Bax JJ, Schuerwegh AJ. Left ventricular dysfunction assessed by speckle-tracking strain analysis in patients with systemic sclerosis: relationship to functional capacity and ventricular arrhythmias. Arthritis Rheum. 2011;63:3969–78.
167. Vohringer M, Mahrholdt H, Yilmaz A, Sechtem U. Significance of late gadolinium enhancement in cardiovascular magnetic resonance imaging (CMR). Herz. 2007;32:129–37.
168. Barison A, Gargani L, De Marchi D, Aquaro GD, Guiducci S, Picano E, Cerinic MM, Pingitore A. Early myocardial and skeletal muscle interstitial remodelling in systemic sclerosis: insights from extracellular volume quantification using cardiovascular magnetic resonance. Eur Heart J Cardiovasc Imaging. 2015;16: 74–80.
169. Thuny F, Lovric D, Schnell F, Bergerot C, Ernande L, Cottin V, Derumeaux G, Croisille P. Quantification of myocardial extracellular volume fraction with cardiac MR imaging for early detection of left ventricle involvement in systemic sclerosis. Radiology. 2014;271:373 80.
170. Mavrogeni S, Bratis K, Karabela G, Spiliotis G, van Wijk K, Hautemann D, Reiber JH, Koutsogeorgopoulou L, Markousis-Mavrogenis G, Kolovou G, Stavropoulos E. Cardiovascular Magnetic Resonance Imaging clarifies cardiac pathophysiology in early, asymptomatic diffuse systemic sclerosis. Inflamm Allergy Drug Targets. 2015;14(1):29–36.
171. Milano A, Pendergrass SA, Sargent JL, George LK, McCalmont TH, Connolly MK, Whitfield ML. Molecular subsets in the gene expression signatures of scleroderma skin. PLoS One. 2008;3: e2696.
172. Solomon SD, Zile M, Pieske B, Voors A, Shah A, Kraigher-Krainer E, Shi V, Bransford T, Takeuchi M, Gong J, Lefkowitz M, Packer M, McMurray JJ. The angiotensin receptor neprilysin inhibitor LCZ696 in heart failure with preserved ejection fraction: a phase 2 double-blind randomised controlled trial. Lancet. 2012;380:1387–95.
173. Pieske B, Butler J, Filippatos G, Lam C, Maggioni AP, Ponikowski P, Shah S, Solomon S, Kraigher-Krainer E, Samano ET, Scalise AV, Muller K, Roessig L, Gheorghiade M. Rationale and design of the SOluble guanylate Cyclase stimulatoR in heArT failurE Studies (SOCRATES). Eur J Heart Fail. 2014;16:1026–38.
174. Kapur NK. Transforming growth factor-{beta}: governing the transition from inflammation to fibrosis in heart failure with preserved left ventricular function. Circ Heart Fail. 2011;4:5–7.
175. Gabrielli A, Avvedimento EV, Krieg T. Scleroderma. N Engl J Med. 2009;360:1989–2003.

176. Abbas AE, Fortuin FD, Schiller NB, Appleton CP, Moreno CA, Lester SJ. A simple method for noninvasive estimation of pulmonary vascular resistance. J Am Coll Cardiol. 2003;41:1021–7.
177. Lang RM, Bierig M, Devereux RB, Flachskampf FA, Foster E, Pellikka PA, Picard MH, Roman MJ, Seward J, Shanewise JS, Solomon SD, Spencer KT, Sutton MS, Stewart WJ. Recommendations for chamber quantification: a report from the American Society of Echocardiography's Guidelines and Standards Committee and the Chamber Quantification Writing Group, developed in conjunction with the European Association of Echocardiography, a branch of the European Society of Cardiology. J Am Soc Echocardiogr. 2005;18:1440–63.
178. Solomon SD, Janardhanan R, Verma A, Bourgoun M, Daley WL, Purkayastha D, Lacourciere Y, Hippler SE, Fields H, Naqvi TZ, Mulvagh SL, Arnold JM, Thomas JD, Zile MR, Aurigemma GP. Effect of angiotensin receptor blockade and antihypertensive drugs on diastolic function in patients with hypertension and diastolic dysfunction: a randomised trial. Lancet. 2007;369:2079–87.
179. Baggish AL, van Kimmenade RR, Januzzi Jr JL. The differential diagnosis of an elevated amino-terminal pro-B-type natriuretic peptide level. Am J Cardiol. 2008;101:43–8.
180. Bettencourt PM. Clinical usefulness of B-type natriuretic peptide measurement: present and future perspectives. Heart. 2005;91:1489–94.
181. Rehman SU, Januzzi Jr JL. Natriuretic peptide testing in clinical medicine. Cardiol Rev. 2008;16:240–9.

Part V

Pulmonary Manifestations and Management

Overview of Lung Involvement: Diagnosis, Differential Diagnosis and Monitoring

23

Christopher P. Denton

Introduction

Lung complications have the highest mortality of any of the disease-related complications of systemic sclerosis following improvements in outcome of scleroderma renal crisis [1]. Currently these complications are spread between lung fibrosis and pulmonary arterial hypertension, with a particularly poor survival when both of these lung processes occur concurrently [2]. Since there is symptomatic overlap between the lung complications and other manifestations of SSc that lead to breathlessness and limited exercise capacity, the differential diagnosis of pulmonary complications is important. In addition therapeutic options for lung complications have increased as evidence supporting current treatment strategies grows; new options for the treatment of pulmonary arterial hypertension emerge and potential use of antifibrotic agents that are now licensed for the treatment of idiopathic pulmonary fibrosis for other forms of lung fibrosis such as systemic sclerosis. In addition there is a growing interest in the academic community and the commercial arena for testing potential agents for lung fibrosis in systemic sclerosis including agents targeting novel mechanism such as targeted immunosuppression or anti-integrin mechanisms. However, evaluation of new treatments in SSc lung fibrosis and pulmonary hypertension can be challenging as endpoints that are effective or validated in other disease starts may not be transferable to systemic sclerosis. These issues are considered elsewhere in other chapters, but a brief discussion below served as an introduction to key points relevant to investigation and treatment of systemic sclerosis. Finally, other lung complications can occur in systemic sclerosis. For example, in overlap polymyositis or SLE, the cardinal parenchymal lung complications of this disease may occur. Similarly vasculitis may be relevant. ANCA-associated vasculitis occurs in overlap with SSc and usually has anti-MPO specificity [3]. This form is especially associated with lung fibrosis.

C.P. Denton, PhD, FRCP
Division of Medicine, Department of Inflammation, Centre for Rheumatology and Connective Tissue Diseases, UCL Division of Medicine, Royal Free Hospital, London, UK
e-mail: c.denton@ucl.ac.uk

Differential Diagnosis

All patients diagnosed with systemic sclerosis should undergo assessment for pulmonary complications [4]. This is important so that a baseline is well established for future serial investigation. Thus all patients will routinely undergo chest radiography, which although insensitive for fibrosis may alert to the presence of other relevant pathology or comorbidity and also allow future radiographs to be compared and so more useful. Lung function tests are important to define restrictive lung disease, raise suspicion of pulmonary vascular disease and asses the presence of comorbidity such as concomitant airways disease such as emphysema. This is important to allow reliable interpretation of subsequent test performed during follow-up and also to help to stage the disease defined by more robust approaches such as high-resolution computed tomography (HRCT) scan. It is generally recommended that all patients with SSc should have an HRCT performed, and if this is looking for early parenchymal disease, it should be performed prone, although a limited number of slices may be as effective as a full scan to reduce radiation exposure [5]. In more advanced disease, this is not important, but for comparative purposes, it is sensible to use similar scanning protocols. The combination of lung function and HRCT can be used for simple staging of lung fibrosis that can be used as an early indicator of the need for treatment or likelihood of stability over time. This will be reinforced by protocoled serial investigation with repeat lung function tests every 3–6 months initially or if there is a sustained change in symptoms. The HRCT will generally indicate the type of parenchymal lung disease, NSIP is the most frequent pattern on CT, and this correlates well with

J. Varga et al. (eds.), *Scleroderma*, DOI 10.1007/978-3-319-31407-5_23

histological classification [6]. Usual interstitial pneumonia (UIP) is less common in SSc, and there is less clear evidence that it is associated with a worse outcome than NSIP, in contrast to data from idiopathic lung fibrosis [7]. Other forms of parenchymal disease may be present such as organising pneumonia that is typically seen in overlap myositis cases and LIP that may be associated with SLE. If features are atypical or there is concern about concurrent malignancy, then a VATS lung biopsy may be considered, but in most cases of SSc lung fibrosis, this is outside current practice. Similarly, infection or other concerns may require bronchoalveolar lavage (BAL) analysis, but this is not usually performed as part of routine investigation. The main reason for this is that it has not been shown to provide useful information about activity or risk of progression that is superior to other less invasive modalities such as HRCT. Other investigations to evaluate epithelial damage have been assessed in the research setting and may provide additional useful information but are not usually feasible in routine care. Serum KL-6 has been used in other forms of lung fibrosis as a marker of damage of severity and can be monitored to assess treatment response in idiopathic lung fibrosis, but this test is not yet fully validated in lung fibrosis in SSc [8]. Nevertheless there are some encouraging preliminary data and studies that suggest that this may become part of the routine baseline assessment of lung fibrosis in SSc and could even have some value in longitudinal follow-up. Interestingly serum IL-6 levels appear to predict worse outcome for SSc with mild but not in severe lung fibrosis, suggesting this may be relevant in earlier or less extensive lung disease [9].

As well as lung fibrosis, the other most common intrinsic lung complication of SSc is pulmonary arterial hypertension. This occurs in the context of other forms of pulmonary hypertension and so diagnosis and classification may be very challenging. Thus, patients appear to develop PH at approximately 1–2 % frequency per year under follow-up [10]. This generally occurs in more established disease and the risk of development persisted throughout follow-up. This probably explains the difference in apparent frequency that has been reported in different series and cohort studies, due to different durations of follow-up and inclusion of a mixture of incident and prevalent cases in most studies. The best cross-sectional data probably come from the recent DETECT study [11]. Nearly one third of cases with disease duration over 3 years and a moderately severe impairment of gas transfer (DLco) had elevated mean PAP, above 25 mmHg, at rest. These cases all had PH, and around two thirds had PAH (group I PH) based on normal PCWP and the absence of major lung fibrosis. The remaining cases of PH were equally split between those apparently associated with left heart disease (group II) and those with significant lung fibrosis (group III). The availability of licensed PAH therapies that can be used in SSc PAH together with the need for careful investigation and expert management of PH makes the appropriate routine screening of cases of SSc mandatory although the best screening approaches are still being defined. It is clear that systematic investigation of SSc patients with at least an annual lung function tests and echocardiogram together with pre-specified criteria for further investigation, especially for progress to RHC, has been associated with improved long-term survival [12].

Management of Parenchymal Lung Disease in SSc

Current approaches to the management of parenchymal lung disease in SSc focus on detection of lung fibrosis and assessment of severity. This is important as it suggests the need for treatment and also because the extent of fibrosis has been demonstrated in independent studies to be the best predictor of future worsening. Thus cases with significant lung fibrosis are bit in most need for treatments and more likely to worsen. The simple RSA-UKSSG staging system has been used to rapidly stage cases of SSc lung fibrosis [13]. It has been shown that HRCT examination to differentiate clearly extensive or mild disease combined with FVC measurement using a threshold of 70 % for indeterminate cases allows most cases with more or less than 20 % of the lung involved to be discriminated, compared with more rigorous formal assessment of the extent of fibrosis on CT. This is important since the 20 % threshold seems to associate with greater risk of decline ad significant impact on survival.

Once the extent of disease has been assessed, cases that need treatment can be identified. All patients should have background treatment including rigorous anti-reflux therapy. Other supportive measures such as antioxidants may be considered. Immunosuppression is usually considered and MMF or cyclophosphamide is currently the most frequent treatment [14]. Some centres stratify cases and treat the most severe with cyclophosphamide, usually by the intravenous route. This is considered standard treatment in many centres, but after a series of infusions, many consider switching to oral immunosuppression with MMF. This has been shown to be better tolerated than azathioprine that was included in previous regimens. Emerging results from the recently completed second Scleroderma Lung Study (SLS-II) suggest that MMF might be as good as oral cyclophosphamide and this may increase the use of oral MMF as primary treatments for SSc. The onset of benefit appeared more rapid compared with oral cyclophosphamide. In cases that continue to worsen despite this treatment, there are rare relatively few options. It may be possible to refer cases to specialist transplant centres although SSc comorbidity and especially gastro-oesophageal reflux make this problematic. However, a series of cases of SSc-PF transplanted suggest reasonable outcome, and anti-reflux surgery may be considered at the time of transplantation [15]. Other medical approaches include the use of rituximab and this is widely used in many European centres. The evidence base is largely from observational series and drawing analogy with other forms of CTD-associated lung fibrosis such as anti-synthetase syndrome where the benefit can be substantial and rapid [16]. Formal recommendation of this approach will require further high-quality evidence to be available. Clinical trials to compare cyclophosphamide with rituximab for primary treatment for SSc-associated lung fibrosis are ongoing. Another approach has been to consider adding treatments licensed for IPF such as pirfenidone or nintedanib to immune suppression in SSc-PF, but clinical trial data are lacking. Studies are ongoing as are clinical trials evaluating other potential treatment strategies specifically in SSc-PF.

Management of Pulmonary Vascular Disease in SSc

Inclusion of cases of CTD-associated group I PH (PAH) was a landmark in the recent history of SSc therapeutics since it allowed CTD-PAH to be included within the licensed indication of the emerging oral therapies. Thus bosentan and then sildenafil became available and rapidly established themselves as treatments for PAH in SSc and were used in combination for more severe or progressive cases with apparent benefit [17]. Although early studies suggested blunted response in CTD-PAH, the more recent and robust morbidity mortality trials have not shown this differentiation between PAH-SSc compared with patients that had idiopathic or familial forms. Other agents have emerged so that there are now licensed therapies targeting the prostacyclin, nitric oxide and endothelin pathways in PAH that can be used in SSc [18]. The specific use of these agents is considered in more detail in later chapters, but combination treatment is now well established, and there is ongoing discussion about timing of this and the best combination. Some form of stratification of cases is generally used so that these expensive drugs are used in those that need the best therapy and are likely to derive benefit.

Other aspects of PH are also important in SSc; first, there is a high frequency of cases with postcapillary PH [19]. This may confound diagnosis of PAH and also requires different treatments. In addition there are many patients with PH and lung fibrosis. Dissecting our group I and group III components remains a challenge. Operationally this is usually based upon the extent of the lung fibrosis and the haemodynamic characteristics of the RHC at diagnosis, but it remains a concern that AH components of the disease may be undertreated and at least in a small number of cases targeted PAH treatment may be detrimental. If there is significant lung fibrosis, then PAH therapies should be introduced with caution and careful follow-up looking for signs of desaturation that may reflect detrimental effects of ventilation perfusion mismatch. Another diagnostic and management challenge is the occurrence of pulmonary veno-occlusive disease (PVOD) in some cases of SSc [20]. It is not clear how common this is especially as the CT appearances of PVOD resemble common changes in SSc, but it is certainly an issue, and some cases of SSc show typical worsening of disease with pulmonary vasodilator therapy. For these reasons it is critical that specialist PH centres are involved in management of PH in SSc. A consequence of screening programmes is that cases of SSc with borderline elevation of PH are identified. These appear to be at substantial risk of progression or PAH and so may represent an opportunity for early intervention. This needs to be assessed in prospective studies, but around one third of borderline mPAP elevation cases progressed to PAH within 3 years, so this is an important and relevant problem. Some cases that do not progress may have milder group II PH or stable group III PH, so these have relevance to differential diagnosis and also mandate careful assessment of PH in SSc.

Concluding Remarks

Lung complications of SSc are very common and have a major impact on survival. They also require expert assessment and management. This is confounded by the very high frequency of other causes for breathlessness in SSc and the absence of high-quality evidence-based treatments for SSc lung fibrosis. This is an active area for clinical investigation and it is likely that cases will be detected better, stratified more appropriately and treated more effectively over coming years. Since more than half of SSc-associated deaths are due to cardiorespiratory complications, this is a priority area for clinical progress in SSc, but one that is likely to continue to benefit from clinical advances in related non-SSc lung disease [21].

References

1. Steen VD, Medsger TA. Changes in causes of death in systemic sclerosis, 1972–2002. Ann Rheum Dis. 2007;66(7):940–4.
2. Condliffe R, Kiely DG, Peacock AJ, Corris PA, Gibbs JS, Vrapi F, Das C, Elliot CA, Johnson M, DeSoyza J, Torpy C, Goldsmith K, Hodgkins D, Hughes RJ, Pepke-Zaba J, Coghlan JG. Connective tissue disease-associated pulmonary arterial hypertension in the modern treatment era. Am J Respir Crit Care Med. 2009;179(2):151–7.
3. Derrett-Smith EC, Nihtyanova SI, Harvey J, Salama AD, Denton CP. Revisiting ANCA-associated vasculitis in systemic sclerosis: clinical, serological and immunogenetic factors. Rheumatology (Oxford). 2013;52(10):1824–31.
4. Wells AU, Steen V, Valentini G. Pulmonary complications: one of the most challenging complications of systemic sclerosis. Rheumatology (Oxford). 2009;48 Suppl 3:iii40–4.

5. Frauenfelder T, Winklehner A, Nguyen TD, Dobrota R, Baumueller S, Maurer B, Distler O. Screening for interstitial lung disease in systemic sclerosis: performance of high-resolution CT with limited number of slices: a prospective study. Ann Rheum Dis. 2014;73(12):2069–73.
6. Desai SR, Veeraraghavan S, Hansell DM, Nikolakopolou A, Goh NS, Nicholson AG, Colby TV, Denton CP, Black CM, du Bois RM, Wells AU. CT features of lung disease in patients with systemic sclerosis: comparison with idiopathic pulmonary fibrosis and non-specific interstitial pneumonia. Radiology. 2004;232(2):560–7.
7. Bouros D, Wells AU, Nicholson AG, Colby TV, Polychronopoulos V, Pantelidis P, Haslam PL, Vassilakis DA, Black CM, du Bois RM. Histopathologic subsets of fibrosing alveolitis in patients with systemic sclerosis and their relationship to outcome. Am J Respir Crit Care Med. 2002;165(12):1581–6.
8. Goh NS, Desai SR, Anagnostopoulos C, Hansell DM, Hoyles RK, Sato H, Denton CP, Black CM, du Bois RM, Wells AU. Increased epithelial permeability in pulmonary fibrosis in relation to disease progression. Eur Respir J. 2011;38(1):184–90.
9. De Lauretis A, Sestini P, Pantelidis P, Hoyles R, Hansell DM, Goh NS, Zappala CJ, Visca D, Maher TM, Denton CP, Ong VH, Abraham DJ, Kelleher P, Hector L, Wells AU, Renzoni EA. Serum interleukin 6 is predictive of early functional decline and mortality in interstitial lung disease associated with systemic sclerosis. J Rheumatol. 2013;40(4):435–46.
10. Nihtyanova SI, Schreiber BE, Ong VH, Rosenberg D, Moinzadeh P, Coghlan JG, Wells AU, Denton CP. Prediction of pulmonary complications and long-term survival in systemic sclerosis. Arthritis Rheumatol. 2014;66(6):1625–35.
11. Coghlan JG, Denton CP, Grünig E, Bonderman D, Distler O, Khanna D, Müller-Ladner U, Pope JE, Vonk MC, Doelberg M, Chadha-Boreham H, Heinzl H, Rosenberg DM, McLaughlin VV, Seibold JR, DETECT study group. Evidence-based detection of pulmonary arterial hypertension in systemic sclerosis: the DETECT study. Ann Rheum Dis. 2014;73(7):1340–9.
12. Nihtyanova SI, Tang EC, Coghlan JG, Wells AU, Black CM, Denton CP. Improved survival in systemic sclerosis is associated with better ascertainment of internal organ disease: a retrospective cohort study. QJM. 2010;103(2):109–15.
13. Goh NS, Desai SR, Veeraraghavan S, Hansell DM, Copley SJ, Maher TM, Corte TJ, Sander CR, Ratoff J, Devaraj A, Bozovic G, Denton CP, Black CM, du Bois RM, Wells AU. Interstitial lung disease in systemic sclerosis: a simple staging system. Am J Respir Crit Care Med. 2008;177(11):1248–54.
14. Kowal-Bielecka O, Landewé R, Avouac J, Chwiesko S, Miniati I, Czirjak L, Clements P, Denton C, Farge D, Fligelstone K, Földvari I, Furst DE, Müller-Ladner U, Seibold J, Silver RM, Takehara K, Toth BG, Tyndall A, Valentini G, van den Hoogen F, Wigley F, Zulian F, Matucci-Cerinic M; EUSTAR Co-Authors. EULAR recommendations for the treatment of systemic sclerosis: a report from the EULAR Scleroderma Trials and Research group (EUSTAR). Ann Rheum Dis. 2009 May;68(5):620–8.
15. Volkmann ER, Saggar R, Khanna D, Torres B, Flora A, Yoder L, Clements PJ, Elashoff RM, Ross DJ, Agrawal H, Borazan N, Furst DE, Saggar R. Improved transplant-free survival in patients with systemic sclerosis-associated pulmonary hypertension and interstitial lung disease. Arthritis Rheumatol. 2014;66(7):1900–8.
16. Keir GJ, Maher TM, Hansell DM, Denton CP, Ong VH, Singh S, Wells AU, Renzoni EA. Severe interstitial lung disease in connective tissue disease: rituximab as rescue therapy. Eur Respir J. 2012;40(3):641–8.
17. Williams MH, Das C, Handler CE, Akram MR, Davar J, Denton CP, Smith CJ, Black CM, Coghlan JG. Systemic sclerosis associated pulmonary hypertension: improved survival in the current era. Heart. 2006;92(7):926–32.
18. Pulido T, Adzerikho I, Channick RN, Delcroix M, Galiè N, Ghofrani HA, Jansa P, Jing ZC, Le Brun FO, Mehta S, Mittelholzer CM, Perchenet L, Sastry BK, Sitbon O, Souza R, Torbicki A, Zeng X, Rubin LJ, Simonneau G, SERAPHIN Investigators. Macitentan and morbidity and mortality in pulmonary arterial hypertension. N Engl J Med. 2013;369(9):809–18.
19. Fox BD, Shimony A, Langleben D, Hirsch A, Rudski L, Schlesinger R, Eisenberg MJ, Joyal D, Hudson M, Boutet K, Serban A, Masetto A, Baron M. High prevalence of occult left heart disease in scleroderma-pulmonary hypertension. Eur Respir J. 2013;42(4):1083–91.
20. O'Callaghan DS, Dorfmuller P, Jaïs X, Mouthon L, Sitbon O, Simonneau G, Humbert M, Montani D. Pulmonary veno-occlusive disease: the bête noire of pulmonary hypertension in connective tissue diseases? Presse Med. 2011;40(1 Pt 2):e65–78.
21. Tyndall AJ, Bannert B, Vonk M, Airò P, Cozzi F, Carreira PE, Bancel DF, Allanore Y, Müller-Ladner U, Distler O, Iannone F, Pellerito R, Pileckyte M, Miniati I, Ananieva L, Gurman AB, Damjanov N, Mueller A, Valentini G, Riemekasten G, Tikly M, Hummers L, Henriques MJ, Caramaschi P, Scheja A, Rozman B, Ton E, Kumánovics G, Coleiro B, Feierl E, Szucs G, Von Mühlen CA, Riccieri V, Novak S, Chizzolini C, Kotulska A, Denton C, Coelho PC, Kötter I, Simsek I, de la Pena Lefebvre PG, Hachulla E, Seibold JR, Rednic S, Stork J, Morovic-Vergles J, Walker UA. Causes and risk factors for death in systemic sclerosis: a study from the EULAR Scleroderma Trials and Research (EUSTAR) database. Ann Rheum Dis. 2010;69(10):1809–15.

24 Clinical Assessment of Lung Disease

Gregory J. Keir, Richard M. Silver, and Athol U. Wells

Epidemiology of Systemic Sclerosis-Associated Interstitial Lung Disease

For a variety of reasons, the epidemiology of systemic sclerosis-associated interstitial lung disease (SSc-ILD) has been difficult to accurately define. SSc is not a common disease (with an estimated prevalence of 50–300 per 1 million) [1], and it may follow a clinically heterogeneous course, often with widely varying pulmonary manifestations. SSc-ILD may range from limited, nonprogressive lung involvement to major pulmonary inflammation and fibrosis progressing to respiratory failure and death. The accuracy of epidemiological data has been further hampered by methodological differences in case ascertainment and differences in the definition of pulmonary disease.

Many of these shortcomings are now being addressed. The development of international collaborative databases has facilitated the collection of clinical data on a large scale, and a major reclassification of the diffuse parenchymal lung diseases has standardized the diagnostic criteria and nomenclature in this sometimes confusing area of respiratory medicine [2]. In addition, the growing acceptance of the multidisciplinary clinical–radiological–pathologic correlation as the diagnostic gold standard in interstitial lung diseases has contributed to our understanding of these conditions enormously. In SSc, lung biopsy is now seldom performed, but the integration of clinical and radiological data provides a robust means of collecting standardized data.

G.J. Keir, MBBS, FRACP (✉)
Department of Respiratory Medicine, Princess Alexandra Hospital, Brisbane, QLD, Australia
e-mail: Gregory.Keir@health.qld.gov.au

R.M. Silver, MD, MACR
Division of Rheumatology and Immunology, Medical University of South Carolina, Charleston, SC, USA

A.U. Wells, MD, FRCP
Interstitial Lung Disease Unit, National Heart & Lung Institute, London, UK

J. Varga et al. (eds.), *Scleroderma*, DOI 10.1007/978-3-319-31407-5_24

The recently reported EUSTAR database has confirmed ILD as the leading cause of death in the SSc population. In this cohort of over 5,800 patients, 35 % of all SSc-related deaths were directly attributable to pulmonary fibrosis, with 26 % of deaths due to pulmonary arterial hypertension (PAH) and 4 % due to renal disease [3]. This major shift in mortality patterns over recent decades, with pulmonary disease now far surpassing renal disease as the major cause of mortality in SSc, reflects improvements in the diagnosis and management of SSc renal disease and gives further impetus to strive for similar improvement in our understanding and treatment of SSc-related lung disease.

Women are at considerably higher risk for developing scleroderma than men, with a variably reported ratio of 3:1 to 14:1 and a peak age of onset of 30–50 years [1]. In the USA, several large series have consistently identified African–American ethnicity as a risk factor for the development of SSc-ILD, with male gender and SSc cardiac involvement being additional features associated with the development of severe restrictive lung disease [4, 5]. African–American and Hispanic patients tend to have more severe disease than their Caucasian counterparts, with disease onset in African–Americans also tending to occur at an earlier age [6].

Early autopsy studies reported a degree of interstitial lung involvement in the majority of patients with SSc [7]. In the largest surgical biopsy series to date, Bouros and co-workers reported non-specific interstitial pneumonia (NSIP) as the most common histopathologic pattern seen in SSc-ILD [8]. In this series of 80 patients, NSIP was present in 78 % (predominantly of the fibrotic NSIP subtype). The variety of patterns present in the remainder of patients included usual interstitial pneumonia (UIP) in 8 %, changes of end-stage lung disease in 8 % and respiratory bronchiolitis-associated interstitial lung disease due to smoking in a handful of cases. As discussed in more detail below, mortality in this cohort was more strongly linked to physiological impairment at presentation and change during follow-up than to the histopathologic subtype of disease. This finding contrasts strikingly with idiopathic interstitial lung disease in which histologic patterns of UIP (denoting a clinical diagnosis of idiopathic pulmonary fibrosis) and NSIP are both well represented and overall have very different outcomes. For this reason, the performance of diagnostic surgical lung biopsy in selected cases remains a central part of the investigation algorithm in idiopathic disease but not in SSc-ILD.

The advent of high-resolution computed tomography (HRCT) has greatly enhanced the detection of SSc-ILD, with HRCT changes seen in 55–65 % of SSc patients and up to 96 % of those with abnormal pulmonary function tests [9, 10]. An HRCT appearance compatible with NSIP is the most frequently observed pattern [11], corresponding to the typical histopathologic lesion of SSc-ILD. However, the high diagnostic sensitivity of HRCT, allowing the confident identification of interstitial abnormalities at an earlier stage than ever before, has presented the conundrum of when, and in whom, to commence treatment for SSc-ILD. An understanding of the natural history of SSc-ILD, based on large historical cohorts [12–14] and further informed by the evaluation of HRCT data in recent major series [15, 16], has led to the more accurate identification of patient subgroups at high and low risk of disease progression. This, in turn, has helped substantially in clarifying decisions on whether to institute therapy, as discussed in more detail below.

Risk Factors for the Presence of Interstitial Lung Disease

Several factors have proved useful in predicting the presence and longitudinal behaviour of interstitial lung involvement in SSc. The autoantibody profile and the distinction between limited and diffuse cutaneous disease have both been linked to the presence of interstitial lung disease. Disease progression is linked to the duration of systemic disease, the severity of impairment of pulmonary function tests (PFTs), the extent of abnormal lung on HRCT, and the observed recent disease progression during short-term monitoring. Several groups have demonstrated genetic associations between various MHC alleles and non-MHC genes with pulmonary disease which may eventually add useful information to prognostic algorithms. As in the evaluation of any interstitial lung disease patient, a careful occupational exposure history should be obtained. A recent meta-analysis confirms the century-old observation that occupational silica exposure is associated with SSc, particularly in males, and also confirms the more recent observations that such patients are more likely to have diffuse cutaneous (dcSSc) disease with anti-topoisomerase I autoantibodies (ATAs, also known as anti-Scl-70 antibody) and ILD [17].

Diffuse Versus Limited Cutaneous SSc

Depending on the extent of skin involvement, SSc is classified as limited cutaneous (lcSSc) or diffuse cutaneous (dcSSc) disease subtypes. In patients with lcSSc, skin involvement does not extend proximal to the elbows or knees, although involvement of the face or neck may occur. In dcSSc, skin disease is more extensive often involving the trunk, shoulder and pelvic girdles, as well as the face and acral areas. The prevalence of SSc-ILD has been reported at 53 % in those with dcSSc compared with 35 % in those with lcSSc [18]. In an analysis of almost 400 patients with recently diagnosed SSc, 42 % of dcSSc patients and 22 % of lcSSc developed significant pulmonary fibrosis during follow-up over 15 years. In this series, 'significant' pulmonary fibrosis was defined as a forced vital capacity (FVC) or diffusing capacity for carbon monoxide (DLco) of ≤55 % predicted, or a decline in FVC or DLco of ≥15 % [19]. Five-, 10- and 15-year survival rates were 94 %, 81.7 % and 69.2 %, respectively, in lcSSc patients and 85.5 %, 71.6 % and 55.1 %, respectively, in dcSSc, without a significant gender mortality difference.

It has been suggested that these observations are accounted for by more powerful associations between the autoantibody profile and the presence and course of SSc-ILD. In a multivariate analysis from the EUSTAR database, autoantibody profile contributed to 15 of the organ complications, whereas division into clinical SSc subtype provided an explanatory effect in 11 of the organ complications. This implies that autoantibody status may be a more useful predictor of organ involvement than categorization into lcSSc or dcSSc disease [18].

Autoantibodies

Anti-nuclear antibodies (ANAs) are present in greater than 90 % of SSc patients, and specific ANA profiles provide useful predictive and prognostic information regarding different clinical phenotypes.

The topoisomerases are a family of enzymes involved in altering the tertiary structure of the DNA molecule, and of the six distinct topoisomerase enzymes identified in humans, only autoantibodies against topoisomerase I have been detected [20]. Anti-topoisomerase I autoantibodies (ATAs, also known as anti-Scl-70 antibody) are found in approximately 20 % of SSc patients, predominantly in association with dcSSc. They are strongly linked to the development ILD, with over 85 % of ATA-positive SSc patients developing pulmonary fibrosis [21]. In a group of 202 SSc patients with well-defined clinical phenotypes, 48 of 54 patients who were positive for ATA had evidence of pulmonary fibrosis. Despite this high degree of specificity, ATA lacked sensitivity with only 48 of 120 (40 %) of patients with ATA positivity having pulmonary fibrosis [22]. Several studies have reported a correlation between ATA titer and SSc disease severity and activity, including SSc-ILD [23–25]. In contrast to ATAs, the presence of anti-centromere antibody (ACA) appears to be associated with a much lower likelihood of the development of significant SSc-ILD. ACA occurs in 20–30 % of SSc patients and tends to be associated with lcSSc and an increased risk of pulmonary arterial hypertension [26].

The mechanism of production of these autoantibodies and how this relates to the development of the clinical phenotypes with which they are associated is poorly understood. However, it is believed that MHC class II HLA molecules play an important role, as will be discussed in the next section.

Genetic Associations

The genetic complexity of systemic sclerosis is well recognized, and it has been proposed that a variety of environmental factors influence differing genotypes to give rise to clinically heterogeneous phenotypes which are a defining characteristic of SSc. Although specific genetic associations related to SSc-ILD have emerged, consistency across differing populations and ethnicities is often lacking.

Several lines of evidence support a genetic predisposition in SSc, including familial cases (including twins) [27], the increased prevalence of autoantibodies and other rheumatic diseases in family members and the association of the major histocompatibility complex (MHC) with specific autoantibodies. However, given the low prevalence of disease, clinical heterogeneity and likelihood that multiple genetic loci contribute to disease susceptibility, unravelling the genetic basis of SSc has proven difficult.

Much of our knowledge regarding the genetic basis for SSc has come from the study of a unique population of Choctaw Indians in southeastern Oklahoma who were found to have tenfold increased disease prevalence and a relatively homogeneous phenotype. Affected Choctaw Indians tend to have diffuse cutaneous disease with pulmonary fibrosis and a high prevalence of ATA positivity (>80 %). A genome-wide screen in the members of this population has revealed multiple microsatellite markers in different chromosome regions associated with SSc. Candidate regions include the MHC, fibrillin 1 gene (15q), the topoisomerase 1 gene (chromosome 20q) and the SPARC gene (secreted protein, acid rich in cysteine, chromosome 5q) [28].

A number of MHC, or human leucocyte antigen-class II (HLA-class II), allelic associations with SSc and various SSc-related autoantibodies have been identified [29]. HLA-class II is an area of particular genetic interest in SSc given its potential role in autoantibody production and the association of certain autoantibody profiles with differing disease phenotypes. Although the mechanism of autoantibody production is not completely understood, current evidence suggests that the processed antigen is presented by HLA-class II molecules to helper T cells resulting in activation and proliferation of an antigen-specific autoantibody response. As discussed, ATA is strongly associated with the development of SSc-ILD. Gilchrist and co-workers have demonstrated ATA positivity to be strongly linked to the carriage of the HLA-DRB1*11 and HLA-DPB*1301 alleles [22].

Several other non-MHC-related genes have also been identified which may influence the development of ILD in SSc. In a study of 127 Japanese patients, Sumita and colleagues reported that single-nucleotide polymorphisms (SNPs) in the surfactant protein B (SP-B) gene (resulting in the T/T genotype at nt1580in) are associated with a lower risk of SSc-ILD [30]. Surfactant proteins are produced by alveolar-lining type II cells and act to maintain alveolar structural stability and contribute to host defence functions. Polymorphisms in the surfactant protein genes are associated with a variety of pulmonary diseases, in particular SP-C gene mutations and associations with familial IPF [31]. Recently, a single-nucleotide polymorphism of the MUC5B gene promoter region has been strongly associated with both familial interstitial pneumonia and sporadic idiopathic pulmonary fibrosis, although the same association has not been observed in SSc, suggesting a potential fundamental difference in the genetic susceptibility between these conditions [32]. Several other genetic polymorphisms have also been reported to predispose to interstitial lung involvement in SSc, including the IL-1α and IL-1β genes [33, 34].

Clinical Presentation of SSc-ILD

The multisystem involvement of SSc poses significant challenges to the clinician attempting to unravel symptomatology. Respiratory symptoms in particular are often non-specific and may be a manifestation of disease in one or more thoracic or extrathoracic 'domains'. Dyspnoea and exercise limitation occur frequently and may be the result of interstitial lung involvement, pulmonary vascular disease, extrathoracic restriction due to skin involvement or muscle and joint disease. General deconditioning with loss of fitness may also be a significant unrecognized contributor. Occam's razor teaches that 'plurality must not be posited without necessity', but in a multisystem disease such as SSc, a symptom such as dyspnoea usually can be ascribed to more than one cause.

History and Examination

The multiplicity of mechanisms contributing to dyspnoea and exercise limitation in SSc emphasizes the importance of an accurate history and physical examination. A significant loss of pulmonary reserve may occur before dyspnoea becomes overt, with breathlessness at rest being a symptom of advanced lung disease. SSc patients often limit the degree of exertion, often for non-pulmonary reasons, and therefore may not have complaints of dyspnoea even when there is an evidence of significant interstitial disease. History taking should aim to establish the duration of SSc symptoms, given that decline in FVC early in the disease course is associated with poorer pulmonary outcomes (as discussed earlier). If dyspnoea is present, subjective measures of limitation and impact on daily living and quality of life are important to quantify. If dyspnoea is progressive, establishing the rate of decline of symptoms is vital. Potential non-respiratory contributions to dyspnoea and exercise limitation should also be explored including muscle and joint involvement and potential cardiac disease.

Chest auscultation may reveal fine bi-basal crackles if pulmonary fibrosis has developed. Physical signs of pulmonary hypertension may not be recognizable until disease is advanced with a loud pulmonary component (P2) of the second heart sound, a right ventricular heave, an elevated JVP and signs of peripheral oedema. Widespread skin thickening, particularly over the thorax, may result in impaired expansion of the thoracic cage during respiration, further contributing to dyspnoea.

Change in examination findings may not be a sensitive indicator of progressive pulmonary disease, and there should be an emphasis on correlating examination findings with robust and reproducible investigations in order to detect change over time. Exercise tolerance may be reduced in SSc patients even in the absence of demonstrable ILD or pulmonary hypertension. In a cohort of 13 SSc patients with normal FVC and DLco, no evidence of pulmonary vascular disease on echocardiogram and no ILD on HRCT, this group had a significantly lower VO_2 peak during exercise compared with a matched control group [35]. Potential explanations for this reduced exercise capacity include the development of exercise-induced pulmonary hypertension and muscle hypoxia due to microvasculature abnormalities. A similar observation by Battle and co-workers demonstrated the frequency of respiratory symptoms to be similar in SSc patients with and without concurrent lung disease [36]. Elucidating the cause of these symptoms, and potential targets for therapeutic intervention, involves a thorough history and examination and the strategic use of investigations such as CT imaging, lung function testing, cardiopulmonary exercise testing and assessment of the pulmonary vasculature.

Imaging

High-resolution computed tomography (HRCT) has become the radiological investigation of choice in patients with suspected SSc-ILD. The chest radiograph is a valuable initial screening tool, particularly when interpreted with knowledge of physical examination findings and pulmonary function testing; however, it lacks diagnostic sensitivity and specificity particularly in early SSc interstitial lung involvement. The chest radiograph remains a useful imaging modality for the SSc patient who has acute dyspnoea, cough or chest pain.

Although initial reports suggested SSc-ILD was synonymous with the changes observed in idiopathic pulmonary fibrosis (a histologic pattern of usual interstitial pneumonia) [37], recent work has confirmed non-specific interstitial pneumonia (NSIP) to be the most frequently observed pattern of lung disease in SSc. Desai and co-workers compared HRCT changes in a group of 225 SSc patients against patients with biopsy-confirmed idiopathic UIP (a clinical diagnosis of IPF) or NSIP. The imaging features in the SSc patient group were most similar to the imaging changes in the NSIP biopsy group, with a greater proportion of ground-glass change and fine reticular opacity compared with the IPF group [11]. A more detailed discussion of imaging in SSc-ILD is undertaken in a subsequent chapter.

Pulmonary Function Tests

Pulmonary function tests (PFTs) form a crucial part in the staging of disease severity and the serial monitoring of SSc-ILD. Whilst SSc-ILD is most often associated with a restrictive ventilatory defect, the coexistence of pulmonary vascular disease, extra-pulmonary restriction or airflow obstruction may make PFT interpretation more complicated. Typical measurements made during pulmonary function testing include spirometric volumes, lung volumes performed with body plethysmography and diffusing capacity of the lung. A variety of other tests including lung compliance, airways resistance and ventilatory capacity may also be measured should the need arise.

Spirometric volumes are the most readily available measures of lung function and are highly reproducible when performed by trained personnel. Measurements consist of the forced expiratory volume in 1 s (FEV1) and the total exhaled volume (the vital capacity, VC) following a maximal inspiration. The VC is a clinically invaluable measure of lung volume and may be performed as a slow or forced manoeuvre (forced vital capacity, FVC). Reduction in FVC (<80 % predicted) and an increased FEV1/FVC ratio of >0.8 are hallmark features of a restrictive ventilatory defect.

Body plethysmography is a more complex measurement performed inside a sealed, airtight chamber (the 'body box') and is used to calculate the total lung capacity (TLC) and residual volume (RV) of the lung following expiration and a variety of airway resistance measures. Reduction in TLC and RV is a characteristic of ILD, although serial measurements offer little additional information over and above serial FVC manoeuvres.

Diffusing capacity of the lung (DLco) is a measure of the rate of diffusion of carbon monoxide (CO) across the blood–gas barrier into the pulmonary capillaries. Based on Fick's law of diffusion, DLco is proportional to the surface area of the blood–gas membrane, the difference in partial pressure of CO and a diffusing constant, and inversely proportional to the thickness of the blood–gas barrier. It is most often measured by the single-breath method, during which a single inhalation of dilute CO is made, and the rate of disappearance of CO from the alveolar gas is calculated. The diffusion coefficient (Kco) is calculated by dividing the DLco by the volume of ventilated lung (VA) and has been proposed as a more specific measure of diffusion given it incorporates the available lung surface for diffusion (represented by VA) into its derivation.

DLco may be affected by a variety of pulmonary pathologic processes, including diseases of the lung parenchyma (e.g. emphysema), the interstitium and the pulmonary vasculature, all leading to ventilation–perfusion mismatch. Of all lung function measures, DLco is most prone to measurement variation.

SSc-ILD is typically characterized by a restrictive ventilatory defect (FVC <70 % predicted and/or FEV1/FVC ratio of >0.8), reduced diffusing capacity and reduced lung compliance. Up to 40 % of SSc patients have evidence of moderate restriction (FVC 50–70 % predicted), and up to 15 % will have a severe restrictive pattern on spirometry (FVC <50 % predicted) [4]. An analysis of SSc-related mortality published by the EUSTAR database researchers has identified, in a multivariate Cox proportional hazard analysis, independent risk factors associated with increased mortality including a forced vital capacity (FVC) <80 % predicted, a reduced DLco and the presence of dyspnoea on exertion [3].

Prognostic Evaluation

The Duration of Systemic Disease

Amongst SSc patients developing severe interstitial lung involvement, the time of the greatest risk of progression of SSc-ILD appears to be early in the disease course. In a cohort of patients who eventually developed severe interstitial lung disease (defined as an FVC ≤50 %), a reduced FVC within 4 years of the onset of symptoms was an important predictor of the eventual development of major SSc-ILD [26]. Steen and co-workers also reported a cohort of 953 patients with dcSSc of whom 16 % went on to develop a severe restrictive ventilatory (FVC <55 %) defect associated with SSc-ILD. In this group, 62 % of patients who declined to an FVC of less than 55 % of predicted during follow-up had progressed to this stage within 5 years of the onset of symptoms [38]. In both series, symptom onset included any SSc-related symptom, not specifically a pulmonary symptom. Morgan and co-workers reported similar results in a UK population confirming an abnormal FVC early in disease course as an important predictor for eventual end-stage lung disease [39]. In summary, it appears that patients with only minor impairment in FVC after more than 5 years of disease duration are much less likely to develop severe fibrotic lung disease later in their disease course.

Baseline Disease Severity and Changes in Disease Severity with Time

In a large surgical biopsy series, Bouros and co-workers reported mortality to be more tightly linked to the degree of physiological impairment at baseline than to the histopathologic subtype of SSc-ILD [8]. In this retrospective study of 80 patients who underwent surgical lung biopsy, the 5-year survival did not differ significantly between groups with a biopsy pattern of NSIP compared with a UIP/end-stage lung (91 % vs. 82 %). However, mortality was associated with lower initial FVC and diffusing capacity for carbon monoxide levels (DLco). The recognition of this at-risk subgroup in which there is an early development of abnormalities in pulmonary function tests, often before the onset of respiratory symptoms, highlights the need for regular monitoring of PFTs early in the course of disease, i.e. within the first 5 years of disease onset.

Goh and co-workers extended these observations in the development of a staging system incorporating HRCT disease extent and FVC that offers predictive power in identifying a large patient group at greater risk of progressive SSc-ILD [16]. In this model, an extent threshold of SSc-ILD on HRCT of 20 % separated the cohort into two groups with clearly different survivals. The group with HRCT disease extent of <20 % had a 10-year survival of 67 %, whereas for the group with HRCT disease extent of >20 %, the 10-year survival was considerably poorer at 43 %. In approximately 30 % of cases where the HRCT disease extent was 'indeterminate' on rapid evaluation (i.e. could not be easily categorized), an FVC threshold of 70 % provided an adequate prognostic substitute (Fig. 24.1).

These observations were mirrored by findings in the Scleroderma Lung Study of oral cyclophosphamide treatment in SSc-ILD. The placebo-controlled treatment effect largely consisted of the prevention of disease progression in patients with greater pulmonary function impairment and more extensive fibrotic pulmonary disease on HRCT [15]. Specifically, the FVC threshold of 70 % was an accurate indicator of the likelihood of a treatment benefit, and the optimal HRCT threshold in this regard was the HRCT threshold in that study that was closest to the Goh extent threshold of 20 %.

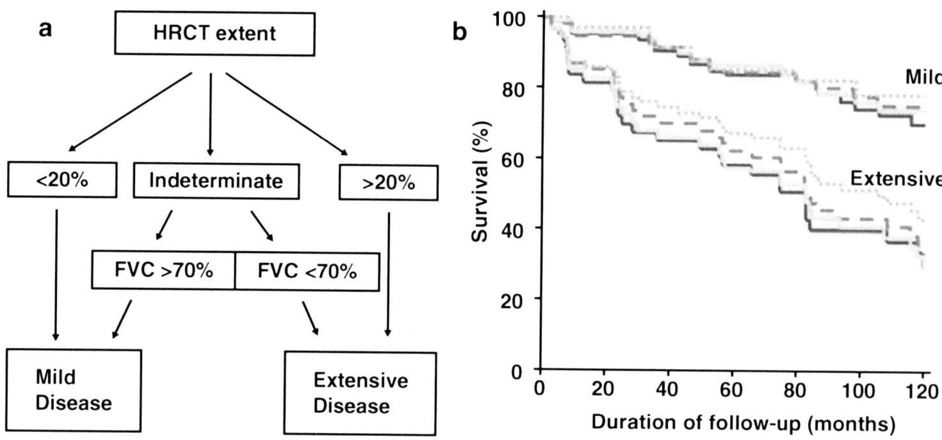

Fig. 24.1 Goh staging system + survival curves. (**a**) A staging system for scleroderma-related interstitial lung disease as devised by Goh and colleagues. When HRCT disease extent is close to 20%, SSc-ILD is defined as mild or extensive. If HRCT disease extent cannot be categorized with confidence, a forced vital capacity (FVC) of 70% predicted becomes the cutpoint for defining mild or extensive disease. (**b**) Survival outcomes in relation to mild or extensive disease based on the Goh staging system. There is a clear separation in survival when the staging system is applied by two clinicians and two radiologists experienced in interstitial lung disease

From these observations, common to both studies, it appears that a simple staging approach based upon HRCT and FVC will prove useful in clinical practice in identifying patients who require treatment. However, a further important factor has not been sufficiently studied in SSc-ILD. In idiopathic interstitial lung disease, observed deterioration in PFTs despite treatment during the first 6–12 months is the most powerful poor prognostic determinant of all: with knowledge of the treated disease course, the distinction between UIP and NSIP at biopsy confers no additional prognostic information [39]. In the management of idiopathic interstitial lung disease, it is now viewed as axiomatic that serial monitoring of PFTs at four to six monthly intervals should be instituted [40], with changes in disease severity leading to the reappraisal of management. Based upon clinical 'common sense', exactly the same approach is justifiably applied in SSc-ILD but has not been formally validated by longitudinal data. In the subset of patients undergoing a surgical lung biopsy, studied by Bouros and colleagues, gas transfer trends at 3 years were predictive of mortality [8]. However, this cohort was underpowered for the evaluation of the prognostic significance of pulmonary function trends and was necessarily subject to major selection bias, with the exclusion of patients with more advanced disease. Studies are now needed to establish the best integration in prognostic evaluation of baseline severity data and short-term pulmonary function trends for future clinical practice and for the selection of patients for treatment studies (in which a high likelihood of disease progression in control arms is required in order to detect any potential benefit of the treatment arm).

It should be stressed that in routine monitoring and in the definition of trends for prognostic purposes alike, FVC is the most useful serial PFT variable. As for prognostic evaluation, discussed above, much of the data supporting the use of serial FVC to identify the progression of SSc-ILD progression has been extrapolated from studies in the idiopathic interstitial pneumonias (IIPs). However, the same broad principles apply in SSc-ILD. The forced vital capacity is easy to perform and highly reproducible, and change is specific to interstitial lung disease. By contrast, although DLco levels correlate best with the severity of SSc-ILD on HRCT at a single point in time [41], the use of this variable to identify progression of SSc-ILD is complicated by its variability and, especially, by the confounding effects of pulmonary vascular involvement.

Precisely, what amount of serial reduction in PFTs in SSc-ILD constitutes clinically important change is not known. In idiopathic pulmonary fibrosis and non-specific interstitial pneumonia, a decline in FVC by ≥10% from baseline has been shown to predict increased mortality [40, 42, 43]. More recently, Zappala et al. demonstrated that in IPF, more marginal reductions in FVC (of 5–10% from baseline values) may be associated with similarly poor outcomes [44]. Whether or not similar marginal declines in FVC in SSc-ILD impart the same poor prognosis is not yet known, particularly given SSc-ILD generally follows a more indolent course than IPF (which is characterized by inexorable progression). However, in routine monitoring, it would seem logical to integrate symptomatic change, change on images and pulmonary function trends, with a lower threshold for suspecting deterioration in patients with marginal (5–10%) changes in FVC.

Six-Minute Walk Test (6MWT)

The 6MWT is a simple, easily performed measure of a subject's submaximal exercise capacity that measures the distance walked over a flat surface in 6 min, in addition to oxygen desaturation. The test is not only a measure of pulmonary function but also reflects the function of the multitude of other organ systems involved in exercise (including cardiac, musculoskeletal, neurological and peripheral vascular systems). In idiopathic pulmonary fibrosis (IPF), the 6-min walk distance (6MWD) is highly reproducible over short time periods (1–2 weeks) and correlates strongly with cardiopulmonary exercise test (CPET)-derived maximal oxygen uptake [45].

In pulmonary arterial hypertension (PAH), desaturation during 6MWT has been associated with increased mortality, and the 6MWT has gained widespread acceptance as a surrogate for mortality and NYHA/WHO functional classification in studies of PH therapies. In a cohort of patients with idiopathic PAH who underwent a pretreatment 6MWT, a change in arterial oxygen saturation (SaO_2) from rest to peak exercise of ≥10 % was associated with an increased mortality risk of 2.9. After adjustment for pulmonary vascular resistance (PVR), there remained a 27 % increased risk of death for each percent decrease in SaO_2 [46].

The value of the 6MWT in SSc-ILD is less certain. The Bosentan Use in Interstitial Lung Disease (BUILD) Study-2 used the 6MWT at 12 months as the primary outcome measure in a study comparing bosentan to placebo in patients with SSc-ILD [47]. No difference in effect on 6MWT was found. Whilst 6MWT was a highly reproducible test in this cohort (within-subject, inter-test correlation coefficient, 0.95; $p<0.001$), there was only weak correlation with other accepted physiological measures including FVC% ($r=0.19$) and DLco% ($r=0.06$) [48]. More importantly, the 6MWT exhibits a very major change in the longer term, despite a relative lack of change in other variables, due to the multifactorial basis for limited exercise capacity in patients with SSc. This indicates that the test is not useful in detecting specific longer-term changes in the severity of interstitial lung disease, either in clinical trials or clinical practice. Two caveats when using the 6MWT in SSc include the recognition that finger or ear oximeters often do not provide accurate data in the setting of Raynaud's phenomenon, and in such cases, a forehead oximeter is preferable; and lower extremity pain or weakness may significantly contribute to exercise limitation, thus masking any dyspnoea limitation that might otherwise exist [49].

Other Clinical Tests

Selected Biomarkers

Currently, there is an unmet need for an accurate biomarker in SSc-ILD that identifies patients at a higher risk of progression. Ideally, short-term changes in such a biomarker with treatment should identify which treatments are likely to be effective in the long term in individual patients. However, whether or not this utopian goal can be achieved, the accurate prediction of disease progression would complement attempts to stage disease severity using HRCT and PFTs. Specifically, the subset of patients with 'mild lung disease', as judged by HRCT extent and FVC levels, must necessarily include some patients with progressive disease of short duration, in whom earlier therapy would be beneficial.

Two lung glycoproteins, KL-6 and SP-D, have been studied in a number of interstitial lung diseases including SSc-ILD [50]. KL-6 (Krebs von den Lungen-6) is a lung glycoprotein belonging to the mucin 1 gene family. Mucins are either secreted at the respiratory tract surface or are membrane associated, with KL-6 belonging to the latter group (recently reviewed in [51]). Surfactant protein-D (SP-D) is one of the four surfactant proteins vital for normal respiratory function, which also plays an important role in the humoral and innate immune systems. SP-D is a member of the collagen-containing C-type lectins, or 'collectins'. Like KL-6, it is produced and secreted by type II alveolar epithelial cells and is detectable in serum especially in the setting of active interstitial lung injury (reviewed in [51]). In a Japanese study of 39 SSc patients who underwent serial KL-6 measurements, levels were higher in SSc patients with ILD compared with normal controls, and importantly, KL-6 levels increased rapidly in four patients who developed progressive interstitial lung involvement. Conversely, KL-6 levels remained stable in those patients with stable ILD [52]. Hant and colleagues in the Scleroderma Lung Study (SLS) group assessed both KL-6 and surfactant protein-D (SP-D) levels in 66 SSc patients compared with ten healthy controls. In the SSc group, 44 patients were identified with 'alveolitis' (as assessed by HRCT ground-glass change and/or BAL neutrophilia/eosinophilia), whereas 22 patients had no evidence of alveolitis. Both KL-6 and SP-D levels were elevated in SSc patients compared to controls and were higher in patients with alveolitis compared to those without alveolitis [50]. Receiver-operating characteristic curve analysis demonstrated high sensitivity and specificity of both SP-D and KL-6 for the determination of 'alveolitis' in these SSc patients. KL-6 and SP-D were positively correlated with maximum fibrosis scores, but not with maximum ground-glass opacities, on HRCT [53].

Another potential biomarker in SSc-ILD is CC chemokine ligand CCL18, also known as the pulmonary and activation-regulated chemokine (PARC). This protein is produced predominantly by alveolar macrophages (and to a lesser extent by peripheral blood monocytes, tissue macrophages and dendritic cells) which have been activated by the Th2 cytokine pathway. These so-called 'alternatively activated' macrophages result in increased collagen production by lung fibroblasts and perpetuation of the fibrotic process [54]. Kodera and co-workers demonstrated higher baseline serum CCL18 levels in patients with SSc-ILD compared to healthy controls [55]. Changes in CCL18 levels appeared to parallel changes in activity of interstitial lung involvement (as assessed by extent of ground-glass and reticular changes on HRCT, a decline in FVC or DLco, or neutrophilia/eosinophilia on BALF). In 20 of 21 patients, CCL18 levels improved in parallel with improvements in SSc-ILD, during a mean follow-up of 4.9 years. There remains considerable debate as to how best define 'alveolitis' in SSc-ILD with neither ground-glass change nor BALF cell profile being gold standard measures. Therefore, referencing biomarkers as measures of disease progression against other tests which may not accurately identify disease progression or inflammatory disease is a source of potential confusion. Nonetheless, biomarkers, including KL-6, SP-D and CCL18, warrant further study and validation against proven predictors of SSc-ILD progression.

DTPA Clearance

Another predictor of the progression of SSc-ILD is the speed of clearance of inhaled technetium-labelled diethylene triamine pentacetate (^{99m}Tc-DTPA) from the lungs. Rapid clearance of DTPA from the lungs is a marker of increased alveolar epithelial cell permeability and/or injury and has been associated with more extensive disease on HRCT in IPF [56]. More recently, rapid DTPA clearance in SSc-ILD has been associated with a shorter time to decline in FVC, independent of disease severity [57]. This latter study can be viewed as a proof of concept study, underlining the potential value of a biomarker that reflects epithelial events. The means of measuring DTPA clearance is not widely available, and the radiation burden of the test is significant, limiting its value in routine practice.

Bronchoalveolar Lavage

Until recently, BAL cellularity was viewed as an important guide to the need for treatment in patients with SSc-ILD. In a number of clinical series, the presence of a BAL neutrophilia was associated with a higher risk of disease progression. However, a BAL neutrophilia has been associated with more extensive fibrotic disease in several interstitial lung diseases, and in general, more extensive fibrotic disease is more likely to progress, as indeed was the case in the Scleroderma Lung Study of oral cyclophosphamide [15]. Thus, the possibility existed that BAL findings were associated with disease progression simply because of a linkage to a more severe disease, which can be identified in a more 'patient-friendly' fashion using PFTs and thoracic HRCT.

This hypothesis was borne out by recent studies in moderately large patient cohorts. In the BAL study from the Brompton group of Goh et al., BAL neutrophil levels were linked to measures of global disease severity and had no independent prognostic value, when evaluated against subsequent pulmonary function trends and long-term mortality [58]. This finding was mirrored by observations in the Scleroderma Lung Study in which PFT follow-up was short in duration but carried out at standardized time intervals. BAL findings were not linked to a treatment effect and did not identify the likelihood of disease progression in the placebo arm [59]. Taken in isolation, the two studies had different strengths and flaws (lack of a means to control effectively for treatment in the Brompton study, selection bias inherent in a placebo-controlled study and a short duration of follow-up in the SLS study), but the lack of added value from BAL findings was a common theme.

It is worth highlighting that BAL continues to have clinical value in certain scenarios. From time to time, patients present with disproportionate upper lobe fibrosis, leading to a suspicion of previous pulmonary tuberculosis, and negative BAL cultures for tuberculosis are highly reassuring when immunosuppressive therapy is thought to be needed for systemic or pulmonary reasons. When there is a suspicion of a coexisting disease process, such as smoking-related respiratory bronchiolitis, BAL findings may help to establish that smoking-related damage is the major pulmonary pathology. The invaluable role of the collection of BAL fluid in ongoing research should be highlighted, and if an accurate BAL biomarker is eventually disclosed, the performance of BAL may enjoy a renaissance, although a serum biomarker would be preferable. However, for the moment, BAL adds usefully to clinical evaluation only in selected patients, as discussed above, and does not make a routine contribution to diagnosis or prognostic evaluation.

Lung Microarrays

Differential gene expression in lung tissue obtained either by open lung biopsy or by lung transplantation distinguishes SSc patients with NSIP from patients with idiopathic pulmonary fibrosis (IPF) and healthy controls [60]. Expressed genes include macrophage markers, chemokines, collagen and TGF-beta- and interferon-regulated genes. Expression of several of these genes is correlated with progressive lung fibrosis by change in HRCT fibrosis scores and the change in % predicted forced vital capacity [61]. Whilst such studies are based on invasive or end-stage procedures and will, therefore, not likely be clinically useful, these studies may yield important insights in to disease pathogenesis that could suggest new biomarkers (serum, bronchoalveolar lavage, exhaled breath condensates) and future therapeutic targets.

The Role of Gastro-oesophageal Reflux

Gastro-oesophageal reflux disease (GERD) and microaspiration are increasingly recognized as a potential risk factor for the development and progression of SSc-ILD. It is hypothesized that aspirated gastric contents, with its component acid, pepsin and bile salts, may contribute to alveolar epithelial cell damage and progressive lung injury in several conditions including post-lung transplant rejection, IPF and SSc-ILD [62].

Early work in pig models in which gastric contents were instilled into the right main bronchus resulted in the development of alveolar injury followed by interstitial fibrosis. Interestingly, pretreatment with cimetidine (H2 blockers) and buffering of the gastric contents to a neutral pH did not prevent the development of fibrosis, suggesting that components of the gastric contents other than acid (e.g. pepsin, bile salts) may also contribute to lung injury [63]. In rodent models, chronic aspiration has been shown to be associated with lymphocytic pulmonary infiltrates, obliterative bronchiolitis and interstitial fibrosis [64]. These changes were associated with increased bronchoalveolar lavage (BAL) fluid levels of pro-fibrotic cytokines, transforming growth factor-β (TGF-β) and tumour necrosis factor-α (TNF-α).

In a retrospective review of 457 patients who underwent lung transplantation for end-stage lung disease, Cantu and colleagues demonstrated that patients with post-transplant GERD who underwent early surgical intervention with fundoplication had improved survival and lower rates of chronic rejection [65]. In IPF, there is increasing observational evidence that GERD may play an important role in disease development and progression in a subgroup of patients. Raghu has reported long-term disease stability in four patients with IPF treated solely with acid suppression [66]. More recently, Tcherakian and co-workers reported a series of 32 IPF patients with asymmetrical distribution of lung disease on HRCT, compared to a matched control group. The group with asymmetric disease had a significantly higher rate of GERD, more acute exacerbations (predominantly affecting the more severely involved lung), and intriguingly, the more severely affected lung was the dependent lung on falling asleep in 94 % of patients. The authors suggested that locoregional factors play an important role where IPF affects the lung in an asymmetric fashion and that GERD may be an important contributor [67].

These data are highly relevant to SSc-ILD because oesophageal involvement occurs in up to 90 % of SSc patients [68] and may lead to increased GERD via mechanisms of reduced lower oesophageal sphincter pressure and abnormal oesophageal motility. In a group of 40 patients with SSc, Savarino and co-workers reported a higher number of acid and non-acid reflux episodes and a higher number of reflux episodes reaching the proximal oesophagus in patients with SSc-ILD compared to those without significant ILD. In addition, there was a moderately strong correlation between the HRCT fibrosis extent scores and the number of distal ($r^2=0.637$) and proximal ($r^2=0.644$) reflux episodes [66]. In a recent review of the medical literature, Christmann and colleagues found reports of PFTs being related to the presence of GERD in several oesophageal functional tests (endoscopy, pH monitoring and manometric analysis) [69]. Christmann also reported a particular histopathologic pattern of centrilobular fibrosis being associated with a bronchocentric distribution and intraluminal content resembling gastric fluid [70].

There remains considerable debate as to whether the increased GERD in IPF and SSc-ILD may be as a consequence of lung disease rather than a cause. More severe lung disease is associated with reduced lung compliance and leads to greater intrathoracic pressure swings during respiration, which may promote GERD. However, based on the data summarized above, the detection and treatment of reflux have assumed increasing importance in the management of SSc-ILD.

References

1. Chifflot H, Fautzi B, Sordet C, et al. Incidence and prevalence of systemic sclerosis: a systematic literature review. Semin Arthritis Rheum. 2008;37:223–35.
2. Travis WD, Costabel U, Hansell DM, et al. An official American Thoracic Society/European Society statement: update of the international multidisciplinary classification of the idiopathic interstitial pneumonias. Am J Respir Crit Care Med. 2013;188:733–48.
3. Tyndal AJ, Banert B, Vonk M, et al. Causes and risk factors for death in systemic sclerosis: a study from the EULAR Scleroderma Trials and Research (EUSTAR) database. Ann Rheum Dis. 2010;69:1809–15.
4. Steen VD, Conte C, Owens GR, Medsger Jr TA. Severe restrictive lung disease in systemic sclerosis. Arthritis Rheum. 1994;37:1283–9.
5. Mayes MD, Lacey Jr JV, Beebe-Dimmer J, et al. Prevalence, incidence, survival, and disease characteristics of systemic sclerosis in a large US population. Arthritis Rheum. 2003;48:2246–55.
6. Reveille JD. Ethnicity and race and systemic sclerosis: how it affects susceptibility, severity, antibody genetics, and clinical manifestations. Curr Rheumatol Rep. 2003;5:160–7.
7. D'Angelo WA, Fries JF, Masi AT, Shulman LE. Pathologic observations in systemic sclerosis (scleroderma). A study of fifty-eight autopsy cases and fifty-eight matched controls. Am J Med. 1969;46:428–40.
8. Bouros D, Wells AU, Nicholson AG, et al. Histopathologic subsets of fibrosing alveolitis in patients with systemic sclerosis and their relationship to outcome. Am J Respir Crit Care Med. 2002;165:1581–6.
9. Launay D, Remy-Jardin M, Michon-Pasturel U, et al. High resolution computed tomography in fibrosing alveolitis associated with systemic sclerosis. J Rheumatol. 2006;33:1789–801.
10. De Santis M, Bosello S, La Torre G, et al. Functional, radiological and biological markers of alveolitis and infections of the lower respiratory tract in patients with systemic sclerosis. Respir Res. 2005;6:96.

11. Desai SR, Veeraraghavan S, Hansell DM, et al. CT features of lung disease in patients with systemic sclerosis: comparison with idiopathic pulmonary fibrosis and nonspecific interstitial pneumonia. Radiology. 2004;232:560–7.
12. Wells AU, Cullinan P, Hansell DM, et al. Fibrosing alveolitis associated with systemic sclerosis has a better prognosis than lone cryptogenic fibrosing alveolitis. Am J Respir Crit Care Med. 1994;149:1583–90.
13. Daniil ZD, Gilchrist FC, Nicholson AG, et al. A histologic pattern of nonspecific interstitial pneumonia is associated with a better prognosis than usual interstitial pneumonia in patients with cryptogenic fibrosing alveolitis. Am J Respir Crit Care Med. 1999;160:899–905.
14. Kocheril SV, Appleton BE, Somers EC, et al. Comparison of disease progression and mortality of connective tissue disease-related interstitial lung disease and idiopathic interstitial pneumonia. Arthritis Rheum. 2005;53:549–57.
15. Tashkin DP, Elashoff R, Clements PJ, Scleroderma Lung Study Research Group, et al. Cyclophosphamide versus placebo in scleroderma lung disease. N Engl J Med. 2006;354:2655–66.
16. Goh NS, Desai SR, Veeraraghavan S, et al. Interstitial lung disease in systemic sclerosis: a simple staging system. Am J Respir Crit Care Med. 2008;177:1248–54.
17. Walker UA, Tyndall A, Czirják L, et al. Clinical risk assessment of organ manifestations in systemic sclerosis: a report from the EULAR scleroderma trials and research group database. Ann Rheum Dis. 2007;66:754–63.
18. Freire M, Alonso M, Rivera A, Sousa A, Soto A, Gómez-Sousa JM, Baroja A, Vázquez-Triñanes C, Sopeña B. Clinical peculiarities of patients with scleroderma exposed to silica: a systematic review of the literature. Semin Arthritis Rheum. 2015. pii: S0049-0172(15)00142-0. doi:10.1016/j.semarthrit.2015.06.004. [Epub ahead of print].
19. Nihtyanova SI, Schreiber BE, Ong VH, et al. Prediction of pulmonary complications and long-term survival in systemic sclerosis. Arthritis Rheum. 2014;66:1625–35.
20. Czömpöly T, Simon D, Czirják L, Németh P. Anti-topoisomerase I autoantibodies in systemic sclerosis. Autoimmun Rev. 2009;8:692–6.
21. Briggs DC, Vaughan RW, Welsh KI, et al. Immunogenetic prediction of pulmonary fibrosis in systemic sclerosis. Lancet. 1991;14(338):661–2.
22. Gilchrist FC, Bunn C, Foley PJ, et al. Class II HLA associations with autoantibodies in scleroderma: a highly significant role for HLA-DP. Genes Immun. 2001;2:76–81.
23. Kuwana M, Kaburaki J, Mimori T, Kawakami Y, Tojo T. Longitudinal analysis of autoantibody response to topoisomerase I in systemic sclerosis. Arthritis Rheum. 2000;43:1074–84.
24. Hu PQ, Fertig N, Medsger Jr TA, Wright TM. Correlation of serum anti-DNA topoisomerase I antibody levels with disease severity and activity in systemic sclerosis. Arthritis Rheum. 2003;48:1363–73.
25. Assassi S, Sharif R, Lasky RE, McNearney TA, Estrada-Y-Martin RM, Draeger H, Nair DK, Fritzler MJ, Reveille JD, Arnett FC, Mayes MD, GENISOS Study Group. Predictors of interstitial lung disease in early systemic sclerosis: a prospective longitudinal study of the GENISOS cohort. Arthritis Res Ther. 2010;12(5):R166.
26. Reveille JD, Solomon DH, American College of Rheumatology Ad Hoc committee of immunologic testing guidelines. Evidence-based guidelines for the use of immunologic tests: anticentromere, Scl-70, and nucleolar antibodies. Arthritis Rheum. 2003;49:399–412.
27. Feghali-Bostwick C, Medsger Jr TA, Wright TM. Analysis of systemic sclerosis in twins reveals low concordance for disease and high concordance for the presence of antinuclear antibodies. Arthritis Rheum. 2003;48:1956–63.
28. Zhou X, Tan FK, Wang N, et al. Genome-wide association study for regions of systemic sclerosis susceptibility in a Choctaw Indian population with high disease prevalence. Arthritis Rheum. 2003;48:2585–92.
29. Mayes M. The genetics of scleroderma: looking into the postgenomic era. Curr Opin Rheumatol. 2012;24:677–84.
30. Sumita Y, Sugiura T, Kawaguchi Y, et al. Genetic polymorphisms in the surfactant proteins in systemic sclerosis in Japanese: T/T genotype at 1580 C/T (Thr131Ile) in the SP-B gene reduces the risk of interstitial lung disease. Rheumatology (Oxford). 2008;47:289–91.
31. Nogee LM, Dunbar 3rd AE, Wert SE, et al. A mutation in the surfactant protein C gene associated with familial interstitial lung disease. N Engl J Med. 2001;344:573–9.
32. Stock CJ, Sato H, Fonesca C, et al. Mucin 5B promoter polymorphism is associated with idiopathic pulmonary fibrosis but not with development of lung fibrosis in systemic sclerosis or sarcoidosis. Thorax. 2013;68:436–41.
33. Kawaguchi Y, Tochimoto A, Ichikawa N, et al. Association of IL1A gene polymorphisms with susceptibility to and severity of systemic sclerosis in the Japanese population. Arthritis Rheum. 2003;48:186–92.
34. Beretta L, Bertolotti F, Cappiello F, et al. Interleukin-1 gene complex polymorphisms in systemic sclerosis patients with severe restrictive lung physiology. Hum Immunol. 2007;68:603–9.
35. de Oliveira NC, dos Santos Sabbag LM, Ueno LM, et al. Reduced exercise capacity in systemic sclerosis patients without pulmonary involvement. Scand J Rheumatol. 2007;36:458–61.
36. Battle RW, Davitt MA, Cooper SM, et al. Prevalence of pulmonary hypertension in limited and diffuse scleroderma. Chest. 1996;110:1515–9.
37. Harrison NK, Myers AR, Corrin B, et al. Structural features of interstitial lung disease in systemic sclerosis. Am Rev Respir Dis. 1991;144:706–13.
38. Steen V. Severe organ involvement in systemic sclerosis with diffuse scleroderma. Arthritis Rheum. 2000;43:2437–44.
39. Morgan C, Knight C, Lunt M, Black CM, Silman AJ. Predictors of end stage lung disease in a cohort of patients with scleroderma. Ann Rheum Dis. 2003;62:146–50.
40. Latsi PI, du Bois RM, Nicholson AG, et al. Fibrotic idiopathic interstitial pneumonia: the prognostic value of longitudinal functional trends. Am J Respir Crit Care Med. 2003;168:531–7.
41. Raghu G, Collard HR, on behalf of the ATS/ERS/JRS/ALAT Committee on Idiopathic Pulmonary Fibrosis, et al. An Official ATS/ERS/JRS/ALAT statement: idiopathic pulmonary fibrosis: evidence-based guidelines for diagnosis and management. Am J Respir Crit Care Med. 2011;183:788–824.
42. Flaherty KR, Mumford JA, Murray S, et al. Prognostic implications of physiologic and radiographic changes in idiopathic interstitial pneumonia. Am J Respir Crit Care Med. 2003;168:543–8.
43. Jegal Y, Kim DS, Shim TS, et al. Physiology is a stronger predictor of survival than pathology in fibrotic interstitial pneumonia. Am J Respir Crit Care Med. 2005;171:639–44.
44. Zappala CJ, Latsi PI, Nicholson AG, et al. Marginal decline in forced vital capacity is associated with a poor outcome in idiopathic pulmonary fibrosis. Eur Respir J. 2010;35:830–6.
45. Eaton T, Young P, Milne D, Wells AU. Six-minute walk, maximal exercise tests: reproducibility in fibrotic interstitial pneumonia. Am J Respir Crit Care Med. 2005;171:1150–7.
46. Paciocco G, Martinez FJ, Bossone E, et al. Oxygen desaturation on the six-minute walk test and mortality in untreated primary pulmonary hypertension. Eur Respir J. 2001;17:647–52.
47. Seibold JR, Denton CP, Furst DE, et al. Randomized, prospective, placebo-controlled trial of bosentan in interstitial lung disease secondary to systemic sclerosis. Arthritis Rheum. 2010;62:2101–8.
48. Buch MH, Denton CP, Furst DE, et al. Submaximal exercise testing in the assessment of interstitial lung disease secondary to systemic sclerosis: reproducibility and co correlations of the 6-min walk test. Ann Rheum Dis. 2007;66:169–73.

49. Garin MC, Highland KB, Silver RM, Strange C. Limitations to the 6-minute walk test in interstitial lung disease and pulmonary hypertension in scleroderma. J Rheumatol. 2009;36(2):330–6.
50. Ohnishi H, Yokoyama A, Kondo K, et al. Comparative study of KL-6, surfactant protein-A, surfactant protein-D, and monocyte chemoattractant protein-1 as serum markers for interstitial lung diseases. Am J Respir Crit Care Med. 2002;165:378–81.
51. Hant FN, Silver RM. Biomarkers of scleroderma lung disease: recent progress. Curr Rheumatol Rep. 2011;13(1):44–50.
52. Yanaba K, Hasegawa M, Hamaguchi Y, et al. Longitudinal analysis of serum KL-6 levels in patients with systemic sclerosis: association with the activity of pulmonary fibrosis. Clin Exp Rheumatol. 2003;21:429–36.
53. Hant FN, Ludwicka-Bradley A, Wang HJ, Scleroderma Lung Study Research Group, et al. Surfactant protein D and KL-6 as serum biomarkers of interstitial lung disease in patients with scleroderma. J Rheumatol. 2009;36:773–80.
54. Prasse A, Pechkovsky DV, Toews GB, et al. A vicious circle of alveolar macrophages and fibroblasts perpetuates pulmonary fibrosis via CCL18. Am J Respir Crit Care Med. 2006;173:781–92.
55. Kodera M, Hasegawa M, Komura K, et al. Serum pulmonary and activation-regulated chemokine/CCL18 levels in patients with systemic sclerosis. Arthritis Rheum. 2005;52:2889–96.
56. Antoniou KM, Malagari K, Tzanakis N, et al. Clearance of technetium-99m-DTPA and HRCT findings in the evaluation of patients with idiopathic pulmonary fibrosis. BMC Pulm Med. 2006;6:4.
57. Goh NS, Desai SR, Anagnostopoulos C et al. Increased epithelial permeability in pulmonary fibrosis in relation to disease progression. Eur Respir J. 2011;38(1):184–90.
58. Goh NS, Veeraraghavan S, Desai SR, et al. Bronchoalveolar lavage cellular profiles in patients with systemic sclerosis-associated interstitial lung disease are not predictive of disease progression. Arthritis Rheum. 2007;56:2005–12.
59. Strange C, Bolster MB, Roth MD, Scleroderma Lung Study Research Group, et al. Bronchoalveolar lavage and response to cyclophosphamide in scleroderma interstitial lung disease. Am J Respir Crit Care Med. 2008;177:91–8.
60. Hsu E, Shi H, Jordan RM, Lyons-Weiler J, Pilewski JM, Feghali-Bostwick CA. Lung tissues in patients with systemic sclerosis have gene expression patterns unique to pulmonary fibrosis and pulmonary hypertension. Arthritis Rheum. 2011;63(3):783–94. doi:10.1002/art.30159.
61. Christmann RB, Sampaio-Barros P, Stifano G, Borges CL, de Carvalho CR, Kairalla R, Parra ER, Spira A, Simms R, Capellozzi VL, Lafyatis R. Association of Interferon- and transforming growth factor β-regulated genes and macrophage activation with systemic sclerosis-related progressive lung fibrosis. Arthritis Rheumatol. 2014;66(3):714–25. doi:10.1002/art.38288.
62. Sweet MP, Patti MG, Hoopes C, Hays SR, Golden JA. Gastro-oesophageal reflux and aspiration in advanced lung disease. Thorax. 2009;64:167–73.
63. Popper H, Juettner F, Pinter J. The gastric juice aspiration syndrome (Mendelson syndrome). Aspects of pathogenesis and treatment in the pig. Virchows Arch A Pathol Anat Histopathol. 1986;409:105–17.
64. Appel 3rd JZ, Lee SM, Hartwig MG, et al. Characterization of the innate immune response to chronic aspiration in a novel rodent model. Respir Res. 2007;8:87.
65. Cantu 3rd E, Appel 3rd JZ, Hartwig MG, Maxwell Chamberlain Memorial Paper, et al. Early fundoplication prevents chronic allograft dysfunction in patients with gastroesophageal reflux disease. Ann Thorac Surg. 2004;78:1142–51.
66. Raghu G, Yang ST, Spada C, Hayes J, Pellegrini CA. Sole treatment of acid gastroesophageal reflux in idiopathic pulmonary fibrosis: a case series. Chest. 2006;129:794–800.
67. Tcherakian C, Cottin V, Brillet PY, et al. Progression of idiopathic pulmonary fibrosis: lessons from asymmetrical disease. Thorax. 2011;66:226–31.
68. Marie I, Dominique S, Levesque H, et al. Oesophageal involvement and pulmonary manifestations in systemic sclerosis. Arthritis Rheum. 2001;45:346–54.
69. Savarino E, Bazzica M, Zentilin P, et al. Gastroesophageal reflux and pulmonary fibrosis in scleroderma: a study using pH-impedance monitoring. Am J Respir Crit Care Med. 2009;179:408–13.
70. Christmann RB, Wells AU, Capelozzi VL, Silver RM. Gastroesophageal reflux incites interstitial lung disease in systemic sclerosis: clinical, radiologic, histopathologic, and treatment evidence. Semin Arthritis Rheum. 2010;40(3):241–9.

Treatment of Interstitial Lung Disease

25

Kevin K. Brown and Vincent Cottin

Pulmonary disease is the leading disease-associated cause of hospitalizations and death in patients with systemic sclerosis (SSc) [1–3]. This chapter will discuss the management of ILD in SSc with a focus on whom to treat, and what to use, and how long to use it. Previous chapters in this textbook have discussed the pathogenesis of SSc-ILD in detail.

Natural History of ILD in SSc

Depending upon the cohort studied, up to 80 % of patients with SSc will have chest imaging evidence of interstitial lung disease (ILD) [4], and when physiologically severe or radiologically extensive disease is present, long-term survival is significantly reduced [4, 5]. While the majority of patients will have physiologically and radiographically mild and relatively stable disease, at least one in four will have clinically significant ILD [6]. In analyzing 78 Greek patients with SSc, Plastiras and colleagues showed that when patients had a normal forced vital capacity (FVC) early after the diagnosis of SSc, the clear majority remained stable and were significantly less likely to show an important decline in their FVC during subsequent follow-up when compared to those with a reduced FVC at initial testing [7]. In those patients with physiologically progressive disease as measured by a declining FVC, most of the loss of lung function appears to occur within the first 6 years of the onset of symptomatic SSc. Steen et al. [5] demonstrated that the major loss of FVC occurred within the first 4–6 years after the first symptom attributable to SSc; patients who developed severe restrictive disease (FVC ≤50 % of predicted) had lost 32 % of their FVC each year in the first 2 years, 12 % of remaining FVC in each of the next 2 years, and 3 % of remaining FVC in each of the following 2 years. However, Khanna et al. [8] found that duration of SSc prior to enrollment in the Scleroderma Lung Study placebo group was not associated with differences in the rate of decline in FVC, though it was associated with the extent of fibrosis on HRCT, and when extensive radiographic disease was present, the rate of decline of FVC was highest in those with early disease (0–2 years). With the available data, patients with significant disease as measured by HRCT or FVC, particularly those in the early years after the diagnosis of SSc, are at increased risk for early mortality and disease progression.

Who Should Be Screened?

In an analysis of 7,655 patients in the EUSTAR cohort, 52 % of patients had evidence of lung fibrosis on HRCT [9], thus the pretest probability of ILD in any one patient is high. Respiratory symptoms are uncommon in physiologically or radiographically mild ILD, and even if present, these symptoms cannot distinguish between ILD and pulmonary arterial hypertension (PAH) [10] nor can the subtype of SSc predict the presence of ILD as it occurs in both limited cutaneous (lcSSc) and diffuse cutaneous SSc (dcSSc) [11]. In the EUSTAR cohort, HRCT evidence of lung fibrosis was found in 43 % of patients with lcSSc and 64 % of those with dcSSc [9]. The probability of developing ILD is more strongly associated with the autoantibody profile than with the clinical classification of SSc. In a prospective study of 3,656 patients with SSc of EUSTAR, 60.2 % of patients with antitopoisomerase 1 antibodies (anti-Scl70) had ILD as compared to 21.3 % of those with anticentromere antibodies [12]. However, neither the clinical presentation of SSc nor the autoantibody profile is sufficient to select patients at high risk of ILD. Therefore, at the initial visit, all patients with SSc should undergo evaluation to screen for ILD with a high-resolution computed tomography (HRCT) of the chest and pulmonary function tests (PFTs).

K.K. Brown, MD (✉)
Department of Medicine, National Jewish Health, Denver, CO, USA
e-mail: brownk@njhealth.org

V. Cottin, MD, PhD
Department of Pulmonology, Reference Center for Rare Pulmonary Diseases, Louis Pradel Hospital, Lyon, France

J. Varga et al. (eds.), *Scleroderma*, DOI 10.1007/978-3-319-31407-5_25

Who Is at Increased Risk of Progressive ILD?

Pulmonary function tests are critical for the diagnosis and follow-up of lung involvement in SSc. Interstitial lung disease in SSc is physiologically manifest as a restrictive ventilatory defect with decreases in total lung capacity (TLC), FVC, and single-breath diffusing capacity of the lung for carbon monoxide (DLCO) [10]. Thirty to 40 % of patients with SSc will have a restrictive ventilatory defect at presentation [5, 9], and the presence and severity of this restriction appears to be linked to mortality and disease progression [4, 7]. Progressive loss of lung function as measured by a declining FVC is not uncommon; by 3 years after diagnosis, 25 % of patients will have experienced a 10 % decline in FVC. Similar to other forms of fibrosing ILD, the longitudinal behavior of the disease is prognostic, and serial measurements of pulmonary physiology may predict outcome, as a declining FVC is associated with poor survival [13].

Chest imaging with thoracic HRCT is a sensitive method of detecting and risk stratifying patients with SSc-ILD. Both the baseline extent of overall disease and the extent of reticular abnormalities on HRCT are independent predictors of mortality [4]. In an analysis of 215 SSc patients followed for 10 years, both baseline PFTs and chest HRCTs were predictive of mortality risk. An extent of disease on HRCT >20 % (as defined by the extent and coarseness of reticulation [fibrosis] and proportion of ground-glass opacity) was associated with increased mortality (hazard ratio [HR] 2.48, $p<0.0005$). In this same cohort, subjects with a baseline FVC <70 % also had increased mortality risk (HR 2.11, $p=0.001$). When the two modalities were combined, patients with both an HRCT extent of ≥20 % and a FVC <70 % had the highest mortality risk (HR 3.46, $p<0.0005$).

Analysis from the Scleroderma Lung Study I (SLS-I), a large multicenter randomized clinical trial of oral cyclophosphamide versus placebo in 158 patients with symptomatic SSc-ILD (see below), found that the most common HRCT findings at baseline were chest imaging features of fibrosis (reticular opacity, traction bronchiectasis, and/or bronchiolectasis [93 %]), ground-glass opacities (90 %), and honeycombing (37 %) [14]. The imaging extent of fibrotic features correlated well with pulmonary physiology. The extent of pulmonary fibrosis seen on HRCT was negatively correlated with FVC ($r=-0.22$), DLCO ($r=-0.44$), and TLC ($r=-0.36$) [15]. While the extent of fibrosis on baseline HRCT scan is predictive of the rate of decline in FVC in the placebo group, the patients with the most extensive fibrosis on baseline HRCT scans also showed the greatest response to cyclophosphamide treatment [15, 16].

Although bronchoalveolar lavage has often been used to assess ILD activity, its utility and clinical significance in SSc is in doubt. Analysis from both the SLS-1 [17] and another real-life cohort [18] showed that bronchoalveolar lavage was unable to predict either disease progression or response to cyclophosphamide.

Scleroderma-specific autoantibodies are also associated with severity of disease. The presence of a nucleolar pattern of antinuclear antibodies (representing anti-Th/To, anti-U3-RNP, and anti-PM-Scl) and anti-Scl-70 antibodies are associated with more severe SSc-ILD [19], while anti-topoisomerase antibodies appear to be associated with physiologic progression [13]. Conversely, anticentromere antibodies appear to be associated with a lower likelihood of developing severe ILD [5]. However, the relative value of autoantibody status to predict disease progression has not been compared to that of functional impairment and ILD extent at HRCT.

In Whom Should Treatment Be Considered?

Interstitial lung disease is common in patients with SSc; therefore, all patients with SSc should undergo evaluation with pulmonary function tests (including spirometry and DLCO) and an HRCT of the chest (using an ILD protocol) regardless of the pattern of skin involvement, presence or absence of respiratory symptoms, or autoantibody profile. Fortunately the majority of SSc patients with ILD will have few of any respiratory symptoms, generally mild physiologic abnormalities, and at most a modest extent of chest imaging abnormalities that remain relatively stable over time.

However, some patients will present with or develop clinically significant respiratory symptoms, pulmonary physiologic, or chest imaging abnormalities. Eligibility criteria for patients who should be offered treatment include clinically significant disease, extensive disease at chest imaging, and/or rapid decline of pulmonary function during follow-up (Table 25.1). An FVC <70 % at presentation or an overall extent of disease on HRCT of >20 % predicts early mortality, and these patients should be offered treatment [4].

Because the development and/or progression of ILD generally occurs within the first 5–6 years after a SSc diagnosis (defined from first non-Raynaud's sign or symptom attributable to SSc), in those patients with a normal FVC and DLCO and a normal HRCT, one might consider performing pulmonary physiology every 6 months for first 3–5 years after disease onset [5, 8]. In those patients with abnormal, but mild physiologic abnormalities (FVC >70 %) or mild HRCT fibrosis (extent of disease <20 %), one might consider serial pulmonary physiology every 4 months during the first 5 years after disease onset. In those patients with evidence of disease progression during follow-up (defined as declines in FVC of >5–10 % and/or DLCO of >10–15 %), treatment should be considered and offered, recognizing that isolated declines in DLCO could represent the development of pulmonary hypertension. Even if the FVC or DLCO remains in the nor-

Table 25.1 Proposed indications for patients in whom treatment or further investigation for SSc-ILD should be considered

Consider treatment in patients with limited or diffuse SSc AND
FVC% predicted of ≤70 %
Extent of ILD on baseline HRCT of >20 % at time of presentation
Decline in FVC% predicted by ≥5–10 % in the preceding 12 month
Consider further investigations
Patients with new or progressive respiratory symptoms: consider pulmonary function testing and HRCT of the chest
Patients with progressive chest imaging abnormalities: consider pulmonary function testing
Patients with an isolated decline in DLCO: consider evaluation for pulmonary hypertension

Modified from Au et al. [10]

mal range after a measurable decline (e.g., from 115 % predicted to 90 % predicted), this should be considered clinically significant. The role of serial HRCTs for the early detection of ILD is uncertain and generally not felt to be necessary. However, an HRCT is indicated when there is evidence of a significant decline in lung function to identify the underlying cause. Moreover, HRCTs are not routinely recommended to assess worsening or stabilization of ILD during treatment since the minimum clinically important change has not been established and pulmonary function tests appear to be more sensitive to change over time than chest imaging.

Though infrequent, patients may newly acquire ILD, or show disease progression late in their SSc disease course. Yearly pulmonary physiology has been recommended by the American College of Chest Physicians to monitor for pulmonary arterial hypertension [20] and may be used to assess for a change in FVC.

Table 25.1 discusses our proposed indications for patients who should be offered treatment or further evaluation.

What Should Be Used When Treatment Is Indicated?

Clinical Trials of Potential Disease-Modifying Therapies

Although a number of agents have been proposed for improving or slowing the rate of progression of SSc-ILD, few have been subjected to a rigorous randomized controlled trial (RCT). Thus, for a number of older agents, there is no evidence base to support their effectiveness or lack thereof. We will focus our attention on specific clinical trials or observational studies in SSc-ILD.

Corticosteroids

Corticosteroids (moderate-to-high dose) have been used for ILD associated with connective tissue diseases (idiopathic inflammatory myopathy, rheumatoid arthritis, etc.) based on clinical experience; however, there are no RCTs of the efficacy of this therapy in SSc-ILD. Low-to-medium doses of prednisone (25 mg daily or 20 mg every other day) have been used in the initial treatment of SSc-ILD [21, 22] and have been allowed in RCTs of SSc-ILD. However, because of the risk of renal crisis with moderate or higher doses of corticosteroids, we generally do not recommend these doses for SSc-ILD. Many centers use doses of up to 15 mg per day of prednisone in combination with other immunosuppressive therapy, although evidence is lacking.

Potentially Useful Agents

Cyclophosphamide

A variety of immunosuppressive agents have been considered as disease-modifying agents in SSc-ILD with cyclophosphamide being shown to be effective in an RCT. Previous uncontrolled trials have suggested efficacy [23, 24], and this led to a large randomized controlled trial, the Scleroderma Lung Study (SLS) [16]. The SLS was designed as a multicenter, double-blind RCT to evaluate the effectiveness and safety of oral cyclophosphamide administered for 1 year in 158 patients with symptomatic SSc-ILD who had evidence of active ILD by bronchoalveolar lavage (≥3 % neutrophils and/or ≥2 % eosinophils) and/or thoracic HRCT (any ground-glass opacification). The SLS was the first RCT to demonstrate the effectiveness of a compound in improving lung function (FVC and TLC) relative to placebo after a 1-year treatment period [16]. Although the physiologic benefits of cyclophosphamide compared to placebo were quite modest (2.53 % and 4.09 % improvements in % predicted FVC and TLC at 12 months, respectively; $p<0.03$), these results were supported by improvement in some patient-reported outcomes, including breathlessness (transition dyspnea index +1.4 and −1.5 in the cyclophosphamide and placebo groups, respectively; $p<0.001$ for the difference between the two groups) and quality of life measures [25], as well as improvement in skin thickness scores. Progression of disease over a 2-year period was modest in the placebo arm, suggesting that the population enrolled in the study did not have generally progressive SSc-ILD; a more relevant difference between cyclophosphamide and placebo might have been achieved, had a population of patients with more progressive and/or more severe disease be studied. In addition, follow-up HRCT scans revealed that the change in extent of fibrosis from baseline to 12 months was significantly worse in the placebo group ($p=0.012$), and this difference was correlated with the favorable effect of cyclophosphamide on FVC, TLC, and dyspnea [15]. Moreover, extent of fibrosis on the *baseline* HRCT scan was a significant predictor of a worsening FVC in the placebo group and of a response to cyclophosphamide in the active treatment group, as indicated by a significant interaction of fibrosis with treatment ($p=0.009$) [16]. In a retrospective analysis, the severity of reticular infiltrates on baseline HRCT and the baseline modified Rodnan skin score were also predictive of responsiveness to cyclophosphamide therapy [26]. These findings are consistent with the hypothesis that a greater extent of inflammation as compared to fibrosis *in early disease* prior to initiation of treatment may be indicative of a more rapidly progressive phenotype that is more likely to be responsive to anti-inflammatory/immunosuppressive therapy.

One of the hypotheses of the SLS was that 1 year of treatment with cyclophosphamide would be sufficient to prevent further disease progression without the need for ongoing immunosuppressive therapy, thereby obviating the risk of toxicity from ongoing treatment with cyclophosphamide [27]. During the 12 months following cessation of randomized treatment in the SLS, the beneficial effects of cyclophosphamide on lung function (FVC and TLC) continued to accrue over the first 6 months after the drug was withdrawn when compared to the placebo group [28]. These findings are consistent with the concept that suppression of inflammation for 1 year impedes progression of inflammation to fibrosis for a limited period of time beyond the year of treatment. On the other hand, after 18 months, the physiologic benefits waned so that by the end of the 2-year period, lung function in the two treatment groups was essentially the same [28], suggesting that maintenance therapy may be necessary to maintain any benefit of cyclophosphamide therapy. The second scleroderma lung study (SLS II) used 12 months of oral cyclophosphamide as a comparator arm for 24 months of mycophenolate mofetil, and the initial results of this study are discussed in the following section on mycophenolate mofetil.

In another randomized controlled trial assessing pulse intravenous cyclophosphamide, 45 patients with SSc-ILD were randomized to cyclophosphamide (600 mg/m^2) for 6 months followed by daily oral azathioprine 2.5 mg/kg/day [maximum 200 mg/day], or to placebo infusions followed by oral placebo [19]. At 12 months, a modest improvement in FVC% was seen in the actively treated group, though this did not meet statistical significance ($p=0.08$). In a retrospective study, 27 patients who presented with SSc-ILD and whose FVC and/or TLC had declined more than 10 % and/or DLCO of more than 15 % during the previous year received six monthly pulses of 0.6 mg/m^2 cyclophosphamide followed by oral azathioprine for 18 months. At 6 months, 7 (26 %) patients improved, 12 (44 %) stabilized, and 8 (30 %) worsened. At 2-year follow-up, 6 (22.2 %) had improved, 8 (29.6 %) were stable, and 13 (48.2 %) had worsened. Evolution of the slope of FVC (in % per year) varied from −15.5 prior to treatment to +3 ($p=0.004$) at 6 months and to +1 ($p<5\times10-5$) at 24 months. Although retrospective, these results suggest that intravenous cyclophosphamide followed by oral maintenance immunosuppressive therapy was associated with stable or improved pulmonary function in 70 % and 51.8 % of patients with prior worsening disease at 6 months and 2 years, respectively [29]. A RCT is under way to evaluate the benefit of cyclophosphamide in patients with rapidly progressing SSc-ILD (www.clinicaltrials.gov, NCT01570764).

Based on the above trials, EULAR/EUSTAR recommends considering cyclophosphamide for treatment of clinically significant SSc-ILD [30]. Pulse intravenous cyclophosphamide has demonstrated better tolerability (in the setting of systemic vasculitis [31]) and may be preferred to oral cyclophosphamide. Overall, both the limited magnitude and duration of benefit of cyclophosphamide and the short-term and potential long-term toxicity of treatment underscore the need for a therapeutic alternative with greater and more durable efficacy and less toxicity.

Mycophenolate Mofetil

Mycophenolate mofetil emerged as a less toxic alternative to cyclophosphamide for treating SSc-ILD, based on encouraging clinical evidence, case reports, case series, and retrospective cohort studies supporting its use. MMF inhibits inosine monophosphate dehydrogenase and has been shown to deplete guanosine nucleotides, thereby suppressing T- and B-cell proliferation and promoting apoptosis of monocytes and other inflammatory cells, resulting in inhibition of cell-mediated immunity and antibody formation [32–34]. It also inhibits proliferation of smooth muscle cells and fibroblasts. The decrease in IL-6 and TGF-β mRNA seen in renal biopsies from patients undergoing acute rejection treated with MMF [35] is also felt to be relevant to SSc, as increased TGF-β may play a central pathogenetic role. Because of its immunosuppressive and antiproliferative properties and its favorable safety profile, MMF has been used for SSc [36], and its ongoing use is supported by preliminary data from uncontrolled clinical studies and recently published retrospective analyses (summarized in Table 25.2) [36–41], which suggested that MMF may be a more effective, as well as safer, immunosuppressive agent than cyclophosphamide and may stabilize pulmonary physiology in patients with progressive disease.

Based on the results of these preliminary studies, the relative safety of MMF, and the biologic rationale for its potential efficacy in SSc-ILD, a prospective, randomized, and controlled study of mycophenolate versus cyclophosphamide was performed, Scleroderma Lung Study II (SLS II). The hypothesis was that oral MMF for 2 years would be safer, better tolerated, and at least as efficacious as cyclophosphamide in patients with SSc-ILD. While final results have not yet been published, publicly available data offers the following: 142 SSc-ILD patients from 14 sites were ran-

Table 25.2 Summary of pilot studies examining MMF for the treatment of SSc-ILD

Author	No. of patients	Disease severity	Treatment regimen	Results
Swigris (2006) [40]	28 with CTD, 9 with SSc	Mean FVC 65 % pred (range 56–76 % pred)	MMF (2 g/day) for median of 371 day, mostly after failing other drugs	Mean FVC, TLC, and DLCO improved by 2.3 %, 4.0 %, and 2.6 %, respectively
Liossis (2006) [37]	6 with SSc and active alveolitis	Mean FVC 71 % pred (range 32–80 %)	MMF 2 g/day plus low-dose prednisolone for up to 12 months	Mean ↑ in FVC from 65.6–76.2 % ($p=0.057$) and in DLCO from 64.2–75.4 % ($p = 0.033$)
Nihtyanova (2007) [36]	172 with early SSc, 109 MMF treated	Progressive ILD in 27.5 % of MMF group prior to Rx	In MMF group, MMF × 1 year (79 %) and × 12–36 months (59 %)	12 % (MMF) versus 19 % (control) developed progressive ILD ($p< 0.04$); 5-year survival 95.4 % vs. 85.7 % ($p = 0.027$)
Zamora (2008) [38]	17 with SSc-ILD	Mean FVC 72 % pred, mean DLCO 52 % pred	MMF 2 g/day for 12–24 months (9× 12 months, 8 × 24 months)	At 12 month, FVC improved by 2.6 % and DLCO by 1.4 %. At 24 month, FVC improved on ave. 2.4 %
Gerbino (2008) [39]	13 with early SSc-ILD	Mean VC 70 % pred, mean DLCO 51 % pred	MMF in a median dose of 2 g/day for median of 21 months	VC improved by a mean of 4 % pred in contrast to a *decrease* of 5 % pred during a median of 14 months prior to MMF Rx
Fischer (2013) [41]	125 including 44 with SSc	Mean FVC 66.7 pred, mean DLCO 47.4	MMF at a dose of 3 g/day in 60 % of subjects for median of 897 days	Trends toward significant improvements in FVC%, significant improvement in DLCO with MMF compared to prior MMF Rx

From Au et al. [10], modified

domized to MMF (≤1.5 g bid) for 2 years or cyclophosphamide (≤2 mg/kg/day) for 1 year followed by placebo. Patients were 18–75 years of age with a disease duration ≤7 years, an FVC of 45–80 % of predicted value, and the presence of any ground-glass opacity on HRCT. Patients with pulmonary hypertension requiring treatment, a DLCO <40 % of predicted (30–39 % of predicted if no evidence of pulmonary hypertension), FEV1/FVC <65 %, or actively smoking were excluded. Lung function and other measures were assessed every 3 months. The primary endpoint was the change in % predicted FVC over 24 months assessed using a joint longitudinal model. Of 73 patients randomized to cyclophosphamide and 69 to MMF, half of the cyclophosphamide and ~29 % of the MMF subjects failed to complete the 24-month trial. The time to treatment failure or withdrawal favored MMF ($p=0.019$; log-rank test). At 24 months, the FVC % predicted improved by 2.86 ± 0.86 ($p<0.001$) and 2.17 ± 0.85 ($p<0.01$) in the cyclophosphamide and MMF arms, respectively (between-arm difference $p=0.24$, joint model). The DLCO % predicted decreased by 2.77 ± 1.35 ($p=0.07$) in the cyclophosphamide arm and 0.53 ± 1.23 ($p=0.67$) in the MMF arm (between-arm difference favored MMF; $p<0.001$, joint model). Weight loss ($p>0.05$) and leukopenia/thrombocytopenia ($p<0.05$) occurred more often in the cyclophosphamide arm. Serious adverse events were similar between arms. Sixteen deaths (cyclophosphamide 11; MMF 5) occurred during the 2-year trial. So in this first RCT comparing MMF with cyclophosphamide in SSc-ILD, the agents had comparable efficacy, but MMF appeared to be better tolerated and had fewer treatment failures or withdrawals and fewer adverse events. The final published data is eagerly awaited, and results have so far only been published in abstract form [42a].

Azathioprine

The results of studies of azathioprine as disease-modifying therapy in SSc patients have been mixed. In a study of 11 patients with SSc-related ILD treated with azathioprine [42], 8 were able to complete more than 1 year of treatment and had either stable disease or clinical improvement at 12 months. In an unblinded randomized trial [43] of patients with early diffuse SSc receiving either cyclophosphamide or azathioprine for an 18-month treatment period (30 patients in each arm), azathioprine did not appear to prevent development of ILD. Only one patient in both cyclophosphamide and azathioprine treatment groups had x-ray findings of pulmonary fibrosis at baseline, but three more developed lung fibrosis in the azathioprine group compared to none in the cyclophosphamide arm. There was a statistically significant decline in FVC (mean decline of − 11.1, standard deviation [SD] 1.0, $p<0.001$) and DLCO (mean decline of − 11.6, SD 1.3, $p<0.001$) in patients taking azathioprine at 18 months compared to baseline. Azathioprine was also used as maintenance therapy after pulse cyclophosphamide in the study by Hoyles and colleagues, but the independent contribution of azathioprine to the outcomes in that study could not be assessed [21]. Overall, efficacy of azathioprine seems to be at best modest in SSc-ILD.

High-Dose Immunosuppressive Therapy and Hematopoietic Stem Cell Transplantation

High-dose immunosuppressive therapy (HDIT) and hematopoietic stem cell transplantation (HSCT) have been evaluated in patients with SSc, including some with severe or progressive ILD. Eligibility criteria for these studies included 65 years of age or less, early (4 years or less) diffuse SSc, and significant visceral organ involvement, including progressive pulmonary disease with a decrease of at least 15 % in FVC or DLCO in the previous 6 months with any skin involvement [44]. These eligibility criteria selected patients with a mortality risk from SSc of approximately 50 % at 5 years with conventional treatment. Nineteen patients were enrolled, with a Kaplan-Meier estimated 2-year survival rate of 79 %. Long-term follow-up of 17 of the 27 evaluable patients who survived at least 1 year after HDIT and HSCT had sustained responses at a median follow-up of 4 (range, 1–8) years with stabilization of their FVC and DLCO [45]. In another open-label, randomized, controlled phase 2 trial, autologous HSCT with a non-myeloablative regimen of cyclophosphamide and rabbit anti-thymocyte immunoglobulin in 90 patients, improvements in Rodnan skin scores were observed at 1 year (58 patients, $p<0.0001$), 2 years (42 patients, $p<0.0001$), and 3 years (27 patients, $p<0.0001$) and FVC at 1 year (58 patients, $p=0.009$), 2 years (40 patients, $p=0.02$), and 3 years (28 patients, $p=0.004$) [46]. However, TLC and DLCO were not improved significantly [46]. Five (6 %) of the 90 patients died from treatment-related causes. In a phase 3, multicenter, randomized (1:1), open-label, parallel-group, clinical trial [47], 156 patients with early diffuse cutaneous systemic sclerosis (86 % of them with significant lung involvement) were randomized to receive HDIT and autologous HSCT or intravenous pulse cyclophosphamide. Autologous HSCT was associated with increased treatment-related mortality in the first year; however, it conferred a significant long-term event-free survival benefit. Mean changes in FVC (6.3 % predicted vs. −2.8 % predicted; difference, −9.1 [95 % CI, −14.7 to −2.5]; $P=0.004$) and TLC (5.1 % predicted vs. −1.3 % predicted; difference, −6.4 [95 % CI, −11.9 to −0.9]; $P=0.02$) both favored HSCT.

Two studies are ongoing to assess HSCT and HDIT versus high-dose pulse cyclophosphamide in early diffuse cutaneous SSc with moderate-to-severe ILD: Autologous Stem Cell Transplantation in Scleroderma (ASTIS) in Europe and Scleroderma Cyclophosphamide or Transplant (SCOT) in the USA.

Newer Investigational Therapies

Other investigational agents such as endothelin-1 blocker (bosentan) [48], anti-transforming growth factor-β_1 [49], anti-IL13, and tyrosine kinase inhibitor (imatinib) [50, 51] have been either ineffective or the results of controlled trials are pending. Preliminary evidence from accumulating short series and case reports suggests that rituximab may be useful in patients with severe or refractory SSc-ILD [52–54]. However, no RCT has been conducted to evaluate its benefit to risk profile in patients with SSc-ILD, and the small potential risk of infection, hypogammaglobulinemia, progressive multifocal leukoencephalopathy, and organizing pneumonia [55] should not be overlooked.

Whether the newer antifibrotic drugs that have proved beneficial in idiopathic pulmonary fibrosis, pirfenidone and nintedanib, are also effective in patients with SSc-ILD (especially those with progressive fibrotic disease with a histologic pattern of usual interstitial pneumonia or fibrotic nonspecific interstitial pneumonia) requires RCTs. There is currently no data to support their use outside of prospective trials.

Lung Transplantation

Some patients with SSc-ILD will continue to progress despite aggressive medical therapy. In these patients, lung transplantation should be considered as this can be a life-prolonging procedure in patients with both SSc-ILD and SSc-PH. While there has been a hesitancy to transplant patients with SSc or other rheumatic diseases because of general concerns about the risks associated with the underlying systemic disease as well as early data suggesting poor outcomes, more recent data is more encouraging. Khan IY et al. [56] performed a systematic review of the available data on lung transplantation in SSc and noted posttransplant survival rates of 69–91 % at 30 days, 69–85 % at 6 months, 59–93 % at 1 year, 49–80 % at 2 years, and 46–79 % at 3 years, survival rates similar to those seen in patients who underwent lung transplantation for idiopathic pulmonary artery hypertension and ILD. Recurrence of SSc in the lung allograft has not been described. Broadly similar data was found by a recent review of the UNOS database by Bernstein et al. [57]. They compared the 1-year posttransplant survival rates of 229 patients with SSc with patients transplanted for non-SSc-pulmonary artery hypertension and ILD. While the multivariable risk of death in the SSc patients was slightly higher than that seen in ILD, it was no different than that seen in pulmonary artery hypertension.

Conclusion

In conclusion, SSc-ILD is common and associated with significant morbidity and early mortality. Evidence-based data show that patients are at risk of accelerated decline in lung function over time and that treatment with cyclophosphamide may lead to stabilization. Because of this, treatment should be considered in patients with significant impairment (as measured by PFTs and HRCT) at

Table 25.3 A potential approach to the treatment of SSc-ILD by the current authors

Pulse cyclophosphamide monthly titrated to 500–750 mg/m^2 (assuming normal renal function) for 6–12 months. Consider 2-mercaptoethane sulfonate sodium (MESNA) with each cyclophosphamide infusion
If pulse cyclophosphamide is not an option, consider oral cyclophosphamide (titrated up to 2 mg/kg/day as tolerated) for 1 year
Upon completion of cyclophosphamide infusions, switch to oral mycophenolate mofetil 2–3 g/day or azathioprine 2–3 mg/kg/day and plan to continue this treatment for several years if tolerated
In patients considered at risk for cyclophosphamide-related adverse events, mycophenolate mofetil titrated up to 1.5 g bid for 2 years or more if tolerated can be considered
Repeat PFTs every 3–4 months while on treatment to confirm a response
Chest imaging with HRCT should be performed with the development of significant respiratory symptoms and/or declines in pulmonary physiology. Do not forget about the potential development of pulmonary hypertension

Adapted from Rao and Khanna [58], modified

baseline as well as in those who show an important decline during longitudinal follow-up. Based on current available data, we recommend initiating treatment with pulse monthly intravenous cyclophosphamide for 6–12 months and then switching to MMF (or to azathioprine) for the next few years (Table 25.3). Although there is no clinical trial data on how long to continue immunosuppression, we recommend treatment with MMF or azathioprine for at least 2 years after completing the course of cyclophosphamide. In those patients unable to receive pulse intravenous cyclophosphamide, oral therapy should be considered. While the published manuscript is pending, the available data suggest that an alternative is to initiate MMF as first-line therapy in patients with clinically significant disease. Low-dose oral corticosteroid therapy (up to 15 mg/day of prednisone) may be considered in addition to immunosuppressive therapy. While patients are receiving therapy, PFTs should be performed every 3–4 months to document durable stability.

References

1. Steen VD, Medsger TA. Changes in causes of death in systemic sclerosis, 1972–2002. Ann Rheum Dis. 2007;66:940–4.
2. Tyndall AJ, Bannert B, Vonk M, Airo P, Cozzi F, Carreira PE, Bancel DF, Allanore Y, Muller-Ladner U, Distler O, Iannone F, Pellerito R, Pileckyte M, Miniati I, Ananieva L, Gurman AB, Damjanov N, Mueller A, Valentini G, Riemekasten G, Tikly M, Hummers L, Henriques MJ, Caramaschi P, Scheja A, Rozman B, Ton E, Kumanovics G, Coleiro B, Feierl E, Szucs G, Von Muhlen CA, Riccieri V, Novak S, Chizzolini C, Kotulska A, Denton C, Coelho PC, Kotter I, Simsek I, de la Pena Lefebvre PG, Hachulla E, Seibold JR, Rednic S, Stork J, Morovic-Vergles J, Walker UA. Causes and risk factors for death in systemic sclerosis: a study from the EULAR Scleroderma Trials and Research (EUSTAR) database. Ann Rheum Dis. 2010;69:1809–15.
3. Simeon-Aznar CP, Fonollosa-Pla V, Tolosa-Vilella C, Espinosa-Garriga G, Campillo-Grau M, Ramos-Casals M, Garcia-Hernandez FJ, Castillo-Palma MJ, Sanchez-Roman J, Callejas-Rubio JL, Ortego-Centeno N, Egurbide-Arberas MV, Trapiellla-Martinez L, Caminal-Montero L, Saez-Comet L, Velilla-Marco J, Camps-Garcia MT, de Ramon-Garrido E, Esteban-Marcos EM, Pallares-Ferreres L, Navarrete-Navarrete N, Vargas-Hitos JA, Torre RG, Salvador-Cervello G, Rios-Blanco JJ, Vilardell-Tarres M. Registry of the Spanish network for systemic sclerosis: survival, prognostic factors, and causes of death. Medicine (Baltimore). 2015;94:e1728.
4. Goh NS, Desai SR, Veeraraghavan S, Hansell DM, Copley SJ, Maher TM, Corte TJ, Sander CR, Ratoff J, Devaraj A, Bozovic G, Denton CP, Black CM, du Bois RM, Wells AU. Interstitial lung disease in systemic sclerosis: a simple staging system. Am J Respir Crit Care Med. 2008;177:1248–54.
5. Steen VD, Conte C, Owens GR, Medsger TA. Severe restrictive lung disease in systemic sclerosis. Arthritis Rheum. 1994;37:1283–9.
6. Steen VD, Medsger Jr TA. Severe organ involvement in systemic sclerosis with diffuse scleroderma. Arthritis Rheum. 2000;43:2437–44.
7. Plastiras SC, Karadimitrakis SP, Ziakas PD, Vlachoyiannopoulos PG, Moutsopoulos HM, Tzelepis GE. Scleroderma lung: initial forced vital capacity as predictor of pulmonary function decline. Arthritis Rheum. 2006;55:598–602.
8. Khanna D, Tseng CH, Farmani N, Steen V, Furst DE, Clements PJ, Roth MD, Goldin J, Elashoff R, Seibold JR, Saggar R, Tashkin DP. Clinical course of lung physiology in patients with scleroderma and interstitial lung disease: analysis of the Scleroderma Lung Study Placebo Group. Arthritis Rheum. 2011;63:3078–85.
9. Meier FM, Frommer KW, Dinser R, Walker UA, Czirjak L, Denton CP, Allanore Y, Distler O, Riemekasten G, Valentini G, Muller-Ladner U. Update on the profile of the EUSTAR cohort: an analysis of the EULAR Scleroderma Trials and Research group database. Ann Rheum Dis. 2012;71:1355–60.
10. Au K, Khanna D, Clements PJ, Furst DE, Tashkin DP. Current concepts in disease-modifying therapy for systemic sclerosis-associated interstitial lung disease: lessons from clinical trials. Curr Rheumatol Rep. 2009;11:111–9.
11. Clements PJ, Roth MD, Elashoff R, Tashkin DP, Goldin J, Silver RM, Sterz M, Seibold JR, Schraufnagel D, Simms RW, Bolster M, Wise RA, Steen V, Mayes MD, Connelly K, Metersky M, Furst DE. Scleroderma lung study (SLS): differences in the presentation and course of patients with limited versus diffuse systemic sclerosis. Ann Rheum Dis. 2007;66:1641–7.
12. Walker UA, Tyndall A, Czirjak L, Denton C, Farge-Bancel D, Kowal-Bielecka O, Muller-Ladner U, Bocelli-Tyndall C, Matucci Cerinic M, Co-authors E. Clinical risk assessment of organ manifestations in systemic sclerosis: a report from the EULAR scleroderma trials and research group database. Ann Rheum Dis. 2007;66:754–63.
13. Assassi S, Sharif R, Lasky RE, McNearney TA, Estrada YMRM, Draeger H, Nair DK, Fritzler MJ, Reveille JD, Arnett FC, Mayes MD. Predictors of interstitial lung disease in early systemic sclerosis: a prospective longitudinal study of the GENISOS cohort. Arthritis Res Ther. 2010;12:R166.
14. Goldin JG, Lynch DA, Strollo DC, Suh RD, Schraufnagel DE, Clements PJ, Elashoff RM, Furst DE, Vasunilashorn S, McNitt-Gray MF, Brown MS, Roth MD, Tashkin DP. High-resolution CT scan findings in patients with symptomatic scleroderma-related interstitial lung disease. Chest. 2008;134:358–67.
15. Goldin J, Elashoff R, Kim HJ, Yan X, Lynch D, Strollo D, Roth MD, Clements P, Furst DE, Khanna D, Vasunilashorn S, Li G,

Tashkin DP. Treatment of scleroderma-interstitial lung disease with cyclophosphamide is associated with less progressive fibrosis on serial thoracic high-resolution CT scan than placebo: findings from the scleroderma lung study. Chest. 2009;136:1333–40.

16. Tashkin DP, Elashoff R, Clements PJ, Goldin J, Roth MD, Furst DE, Arriola E, Silver R, Strange C, Bolster M, Seibold JR, Riley DJ, Hsu VM, Varga J, Schraufnagel DE, Theodore A, Simms R, Wise R, Wigley F, White B, Steen V, Read C, Mayes M, Parsley E, Mubarak K, Connolly MK, Golden J, Olman M, Fessler B, Rothfield N, Metersky M. Cyclophosphamide versus placebo in scleroderma lung disease. N Engl J Med. 2006;354:2655–66.
17. Strange C, Bolster MB, Roth MD, Silver RM, Theodore A, Goldin J, Clements P, Chung J, Elashoff RM, Suh R, Smith EA, Furst DE, Tashkin DP. Bronchoalveolar lavage and response to cyclophosphamide in scleroderma interstitial lung disease. Am J Respir Crit Care Med. 2008;177:91–8.
18. Goh NS, Veeraraghavan S, Desai SR, Cramer D, Hansell DM, Denton CP, Black CM, du Bois RM, Wells AU. Bronchoalveolar lavage cellular profiles in patients with systemic sclerosis-associated interstitial lung disease are not predictive of disease progression. Arthritis Rheum. 2007;56:2005–12.
19. Steen VD. Autoantibodies in systemic sclerosis. Semin Arthritis Rheum. 2005;35:35–42.
20. McGoon M, Gutterman D, Steen V, Barst R, McCrory DC, Fortin TA, Loyd JE. Screening, early detection, and diagnosis of pulmonary arterial hypertension: ACCP evidence-based clinical practice guidelines. Chest. 2004;126:14S–34.
21. Hoyles RK, Ellis RW, Wellsbury J, Lees B, Newlands P, Goh NS, Roberts C, Desai S, Herrick AL, McHugh NJ, Foley NM, Pearson SB, Emery P, Veale DJ, Denton CP, Wells AU, Black CM, du Bois RM. A multicenter, prospective, randomized, double-blind, placebo-controlled trial of corticosteroids and intravenous cyclophosphamide followed by oral azathioprine for the treatment of pulmonary fibrosis in scleroderma. Arthritis Rheum. 2006;54:3962–70.
22. Beretta L, Caronni M, Raimondi M, Ponti A, Viscuso T, Origgi L, Scorza R. Oral cyclophosphamide improves pulmonary function in scleroderma patients with fibrosing alveolitis: experience in one centre. Clin Rheumatol. 2007;26:168–72.
23. White B, Moore WC, Wigley FM, Xiao HQ, Wise RA. Cyclophosphamide is associated with pulmonary function and survival benefit in patients with scleroderma and alveolitis. Ann Intern Med. 2000;132:947–54.
24. Silver RM, Warrick JH, Kinsella MB, Staudt LS, Baumann MH, Strange C. Cyclophosphamide and low-dose prednisone therapy in patients with systemic sclerosis (scleroderma) with interstitial lung disease. J Rheumatol. 1993;20:838–44.
25. Khanna D, Yan X, Tashkin DP, Furst DE, Elashoff R, Roth MD, Silver R, Strange C, Bolster M, Seibold JR, Riley DJ, Hsu VM, Varga J, Schraufnagel DE, Theodore A, Simms R, Wise R, Wigley F, White B, Steen V, Read C, Mayes M, Parsley E, Mubarak K, Connolly MK, Golden J, Olman M, Fessler B, Rothfield N, Metersky M, Clements PJ. Impact of oral cyclophosphamide on health-related quality of life in patients with active scleroderma lung disease: results from the scleroderma lung study. Arthritis Rheum. 2007;56:1676–84.
26. Roth MD, Tseng CH, Clements PJ, Furst DE, Tashkin DP, Goldin JG, Khanna D, Kleerup EC, Li N, Elashoff D, Elashoff RM. Predicting treatment outcomes and responder subsets in scleroderma-related interstitial lung disease. Arthritis Rheum. 2011;63:2797–808.
27. Martinez FJ, McCune WJ. Cyclophosphamide for scleroderma lung disease. N Engl J Med. 2006;354:2707–9.
28. Tashkin DP, Elashoff R, Clements PJ, Roth MD, Furst DE, Silver RM, Goldin J, Arriola E, Strange C, Bolster MB, Seibold JR, Riley DJ, Hsu VM, Varga J, Schraufnagel D, Theodore A, Simms R, Wise R, Wigley F, White B, Steen V, Read C, Mayes M, Parsley E, Mubarak K, Connolly MK, Golden J, Olman M, Fessler B, Rothfield N, Metersky M, Khanna D, Li N, Li G. Effects of 1-year treatment with cyclophosphamide on outcomes at 2 years in scleroderma lung disease. Am J Respir Crit Care Med. 2007;176:1026–34.
29. Berezne A, Ranque B, Valeyre D, Brauner M, Allanore Y, Launay D, Le Guern V, Kahn JE, Couderc LJ, Constans J, Cohen P, Mahr A, Pagnoux C, Hachulla E, Kahan A, Cabane J, Guillevin L, Mouthon L. Therapeutic strategy combining intravenous cyclophosphamide followed by oral azathioprine to treat worsening interstitial lung disease associated with systemic sclerosis: a retrospective multicenter open-label study. J Rheumatol. 2008;35:1064–72.
30. Kowal-Bielecka O, Landewe R, Avouac J, Chwiesko S, Miniati I, Czirjak L, Clements P, Denton C, Farge D, Fligelstone K, Foldvari I, Furst DE, Muller-Ladner U, Seibold J, Silver RM, Takehara K, Toth BG, Tyndall A, Valentini G, van den Hoogen F, Wigley F, Zulian F, Matucci-Cerinic M. EULAR recommendations for the treatment of systemic sclerosis: a report from the EULAR Scleroderma Trials and Research group (EUSTAR). Ann Rheum Dis. 2009;68:620–8.
31. Guillevin L, Cordier JF, Lhote F, Cohen P, Jarrousse B, Royer I, Lesavre P, Jacquot C, Bindi P, Bielefeld P, Desson JF, Détrée F, Dubois A, Hachulla E, Hoen B, Jacomy D, Seigneuric C, Lauque D, Stern M, Longy-Boursier M. A prospective, multicenter, randomized trial comparing steroids and pulse cyclophosphamide versus steroids and oral cyclophosphamide in the treatment of generalized Wegener's granulomatosis. Arthritis Rheum. 1997;40:2187–98.
32. Takebe N, Cheng X, Fandy TE, Srivastava RK, Wu S, Shankar S, Bauer K, Shaughnessy J, Tricot G. IMP dehydrogenase inhibitor mycophenolate mofetil induces caspase-dependent apoptosis and cell cycle inhibition in multiple myeloma cells. Mol Cancer Ther. 2006;5:457–66.
33. Colic M, Stojic-Vukanic Z, Pavlovic B, Jandric D, Stefanoska I. Mycophenolate mofetil inhibits differentiation, maturation and allostimulatory function of human monocyte-derived dendritic cells. Clin Exp Immunol. 2003;134:63–9.
34. Andrikos E, Yavuz A, Bordoni V, Ratanarat R, De Cal M, Bonello M, Salvatori G, Levin N, Yakupoglu G, Pappas M, Ronco C. Effect of cyclosporine, mycophenolate mofetil, and their combination with steroids on apoptosis in a human cultured monocytic U937 cell line. Transplant Proc. 2005;37:3226–9.
35. Kaminska D, Tyran B, Mazanowska O, Letachowicz W, Kochman A, Rabczynski J, Szyber P, Patrzalek D, Chudoba P, Klinger M. Mycophenolate mofetil but not the type of calcineurin inhibitor (cyclosporine vs tacrolimus) influences the intragraft mRNA expression of cytokines in human kidney allograft biopsies by in situ RT-PCR analysis. Transplant Proc. 2005;37:770–2.
36. Nihtyanova SI, Brough GM, Black CM, Denton CP. Mycophenolate mofetil in diffuse cutaneous systemic sclerosis – a retrospective analysis. Rheumatology (Oxford). 2007;46:442–5.
37. Liossis SN, Bounas A, Andonopoulos AP. Mycophenolate mofetil as first-line treatment improves clinically evident early scleroderma lung disease. Rheumatology (Oxford). 2006;45:1005–8.
38. Zamora AC, Wolters PJ, Collard HR, Connolly MK, Elicker BM, Webb WR, King Jr TE, Golden JA. Use of mycophenolate mofetil to treat scleroderma-associated interstitial lung disease. Respir Med. 2008;102:150–5.
39. Gerbino AJ, Goss CH, Molitor JA. Effect of mycophenolate mofetil on pulmonary function in scleroderma-associated interstitial lung disease. Chest. 2008;133:455–60.
40. Swigris JJ, Olson AL, Fischer A, Lynch DA, Cosgrove GP, Frankel SK, Meehan RT, Brown KK. Mycophenolate mofetil is safe, well tolerated, and preserves lung function in patients with connective

tissue disease-related interstitial lung disease. Chest. 2006;130:30–6.

41. Fischer A, Brown KK, Du Bois RM, Frankel SK, Cosgrove GP, Fernandez-Perez ER, Huie TJ, Krishnamoorthy M, Meehan RT, Olson AL, Solomon JJ, Swigris JJ. Mycophenolate Mofetil improves lung function in connective tissue disease-associated interstitial lung disease. J Rheumatol. 2013;40:640–6.
42. Dheda K, Lalloo UG, Cassim B, Mody GM. Experience with azathioprine in systemic sclerosis associated with interstitial lung disease. Clin Rheumatol. 2004;23:306–9.

42a. Clements PJ, Tashkin D, Roth M, Khanna D, Furst DE, Tseng CH, Volkmann ER, Elashoff R. The Scleroderma Lung Study II (SLS II) shows that both oral Cyclophosphamide (CYC) and Mycophenolate Mofitil (MMF) are efficacious in treating progressive Interstitial Lung Disease (ILD) in patients with Systemic Sclerosis (SSc) [abstract]. Arthritis Rheumatol. 2015;67(suppl 10). Abstract no. 1075.

43. Nadashkevich O, Davis P, Fritzler M, Kovalenko W. A randomized unblinded trial of cyclophosphamide versus azathioprine in the treatment of systemic sclerosis. Clin Rheumatol. 2006;25:205–12.
44. McSweeney PA, Nash RA, Sullivan KM, Storek J, Crofford LJ, Dansey R, Mayes MD, McDonagh KT, Nelson JL, Gooley TA, Holmberg LA, Chen CS, Wener MH, Ryan K, Sunderhaus J, Russell K, Rambharose J, Storb R, Furst DE. High-dose immunosuppressive therapy for severe systemic sclerosis: initial outcomes. Blood. 2002;100:1602–10.
45. Nash RA, McSweeney PA, Crofford LJ, Abidi M, Chen CS, Godwin JD, Gooley TA, Holmberg L, Henstorf G, LeMaistre CF, Mayes MD, McDonagh KT, McLaughlin B, Molitor JA, Nelson JL, Shulman H, Storb R, Viganego F, Wener MH, Seibold JR, Sullivan KM, Furst DE. High-dose immunosuppressive therapy and autologous hematopoietic cell transplantation for severe systemic sclerosis: long-term follow-up of the US multicenter pilot study. Blood. 2007;110:1388–96.
46. Burt RK, Oliveira MC, Shah SJ, Moraes DA, Simoes B, Gheorghiade M, Schroeder J, Ruderman E, Farge D, Chai ZJ, Marjanovic Z, Jain S, Morgan A, Milanetti F, Han X, Jovanovic B, Helenowski IB, Voltarelli J. Cardiac involvement and treatment-related mortality after non-myeloablative haemopoietic stem-cell transplantation with unselected autologous peripheral blood for patients with systemic sclerosis: a retrospective analysis. Lancet. 2013;381:1116–24.
47. van Laar JM, Farge D, Sont JK, Naraghi K, Marjanovic Z, Larghero J, Schuerwegh AJ, Marijt EW, Vonk MC, Schattenberg AV, Matucci-Cerinic M, Voskuyl AE, van de Loosdrecht AA, Daikeler T, Kotter I, Schmalzing M, Martin T, Lioure B, Weiner SM, Kreuter A, Deligny C, Durand JM, Emery P, Machold KP, Sarrot-Reynauld F, Warnatz K, Adoue DF, Constans J, Tony HP, Del Papa N, Fassas A, Himsel A, Launay D, Lo Monaco A, Philippe P, Quere I, Rich E, Westhovens R, Griffiths B, Saccardi R, van den Hoogen FH, Fibbe WE, Socie G, Gratwohl A, Tyndall A. Autologous hematopoietic stem cell transplantation vs intravenous pulse cyclophosphamide in diffuse cutaneous systemic sclerosis: a randomized clinical trial. JAMA. 2014;311:2490–8.
48. Seibold JR, Denton CP, Furst DE, Guillevin L, Rubin LJ, Wells A, Matucci Cerinic M, Riemekasten G, Emery P, Chadha-Boreham H, Charef P, Roux S, Black CM. Randomized, prospective, placebo-controlled trial of bosentan in interstitial lung disease secondary to systemic sclerosis. Arthritis Rheum. 2010;62:2101–8.
49. Denton CP, Merkel PA, Furst DE, Khanna D, Emery P, Hsu VM, Silliman N, Streisand J, Powell J, Akesson A, Coppock J, Hoogen F, Herrick A, Mayes MD, Veale D, Haas J, Ledbetter S, Korn JH, Black CM, Seibold JR. Recombinant human anti-transforming growth factor beta1 antibody therapy in systemic sclerosis: a multicenter, randomized, placebo-controlled phase I/II trial of CAT-192. Arthritis Rheum. 2007;56:323–33.
50. Prey S, Ezzedine K, Doussau A, Grandoulier AS, Barcat D, Chatelus E, Diot E, Durant C, Hachulla E, de Korwin-Krokowski JD, Kostrzewa E, Quemeneur T, Paul C, Schaeverbeke T, Seneschal J, Solanilla A, Sparsa A, Bouchet S, Lepreux S, Mahon FX, Chene G, Taieb A. Imatinib mesylate in scleroderma-associated diffuse skin fibrosis: a phase II multicentre randomized double-blinded controlled trial. Br J Dermatol. 2012;167:1138–44.
51. Bosello S, De Santis M, Lama G, Spano C, Angelucci C, Tolusso B, Sica G, Ferraccioli G. B cell depletion in diffuse progressive systemic sclerosis: safety, skin score modification and IL-6 modulation in an up to thirty-six months follow-up open-label trial. Arthritis Res Ther. 2010;12:R54.
52. Keir GJ, Maher TM, Hansell DM, Denton CP, Ong VH, Singh S, Wells AU, Renzoni EA. Severe interstitial lung disease in connective tissue disease: rituximab as rescue therapy. Eur Respir J. 2012;40:641–8.
53. Daoussis D, Liossis SN, Tsamandas AC, Kalogeropoulou C, Paliogianni F, Sirinian C, Yiannopoulos G, Andonopoulos AP. Effect of long-term treatment with rituximab on pulmonary function and skin fibrosis in patients with diffuse systemic sclerosis. Clin Exp Rheumatol. 2012;30:S17–22.
54. Jordan S, Distler JH, Maurer B, Huscher D, van Laar JM, Allanore Y, Distler O. Effects and safety of rituximab in systemic sclerosis: an analysis from the European Scleroderma Trial and Research (EUSTAR) group. Ann Rheum Dis. 2015;74:1188–94
55. Liote H, Liote F, Seroussi B, Mayaud C, Cadranel J. Rituximab-induced lung disease: a systematic literature review. Eur Respir J. 2010;35:681–7.
56. Khan IY, Singer LG, de Perrot M, Granton JT, Keshavjee S, Chau C, Kron A, Johnson SR. Survival after lung transplantation in systemic sclerosis. A systematic review. Respir Med. 2013;107:2081–7.
57. Bernstein EJ, Peterson ER, Sell JL, D'Ovidio F, Arcasoy SM, Bathon JM, Lederer DJ. Survival of adults with systemic sclerosis following lung transplantation: a nationwide cohort study. Arthritis Rheumatol. 2015;67:1314–22.
58. Rao V, Khanna D. Scleroderma and fibrosing disorders: advances in management. Int J Adv Rheumatol. 2010;8:53–62.

Pathogenesis of Pulmonary Arterial Hypertension

26

Rubin M. Tuder, Markella Ponticos, and Alan Holmes

Introduction

There is hardly a field in pulmonary diseases in which mechanistic paradigms evolved so rapidly like in pulmonary hypertension. In fact, idiopathic pulmonary arterial hypertension (IPAH), the paradigmatic form of group 1 disease [1], was formally reported more than 100 years ago [2]. The disease remained largely uncharacterized, until the insights gained with the introduction of pulmonary hemodynamics allowed defining the disease in terms of pulmonary artery pressures and cardiac output, spurring investigations aimed at dissecting its pathogenesis [3]. For the past six decades, the field of pulmonary hypertension has undergone an explosion of cellular and molecular insights, which have clearly made important translational impacts, notably in novel therapies aimed at PAH [4]. The clinical importance of pulmonary hypertension is also underscored by its impact on morbidity and increased mortality; this applies not only to collagen vascular diseases but also to several of the other forms of pulmonary hypertension (PH), including when associated with interstitial lung disease [5] and chronic obstructive pulmonary diseases [6].

The group 1 pulmonary arterial hypertension (PAH) contains, in addition to IPAH (and its closely related familial/genetic counterpart), disparate diseases, including collagen vascular disease (CVD), HIV infection, anorectic and addiction-related drugs, and schistosomiasis [7], all of which have suprasystemic levels of pulmonary artery pressures and characteristic spectrum of pulmonary vascular remodeling. While all of the forms of PAH have some shared pathology, there are structural differences pertaining to pulmonary vascular remodeling, which may underlie different pathogenetic processes. For instance, while pulmonary media and intima remodeling can occur in IPAH and collagen vascular disease-associated PAH (CVD-PAH), an association with interstitial lung disease is predominantly seen in the latter. All forms of PAH have significant inflammation; however, the specific type of inflammatory cells and cytokines and how they affect pathogenesis may differ. It is becoming apparent that a TH1-/M1-driven inflammation (characterized by activation of interferon-γ, TNF-α, IL-12/IL-18) or TH2/M2 inflammation (characterized by IL-4/IL-13, TGF-β, among others) may ultimately affect how a particular cause of PAH ultimately results in pulmonary vascular disease.

Given that detailed studies in any single entity associated with PAH (including CVD-related PAH) are limited, we have to rely on the knowledge derived from shared and distinct discoveries gained from the aggregate of investigations in each disease. Despite significant insights into PAH pathogenesis [8], much remains unknown, including the molecular pathogenesis of shared or unique pathological features. Moreover, several key pathogenetic processes appear to be also shared, as most of the present investigations have centered largely on IPAH and/or derived their support from the limited scope of experimental models. In the present review, the authors chose to initially focus on key pathological features of PAH and then underscore key pathogenetic processes. These include the role of growth factors, metabolic reprogramming, and inflammation.

Pathology of Pulmonary Arterial Hypertension

The normal pulmonary circulation is structurally organized to accommodate a low-pressure/high-capacitance system. The current understanding on how this structure varies

R.M. Tuder, MD (✉)
Division of Pulmonary Science & Critical Care Medicine, Department of Medicine, University of Colorado Denver, Aurora, CO, USA
e-mail: Rubin.Tuder@ucdenver.edu

M. Ponticos, PhD
Centre for Rheumatology and Connective Tissue Disease, Royal Free Hospital (University College London), London, UK

A. Holmes, PhD
Drug Discovery Group, Translational Research Office, School of Pharmacy, University College London, London, UK

J. Varga et al. (eds.), *Scleroderma*, DOI 10.1007/978-3-319-31407-5_26

regionally, from the large pulmonary arteries to precapillary vessels, derives from casting studies in humans and a handful of animal investigations. The key structural characteristics of this system have been reviewed elsewhere; we strongly encourage the readers to access these reviews as they provide editorialized key information about the normal pulmonary circulation [9–11]. We will revisit some of these data as we discuss the pathology of PAH.

One can segregate the pathology of pulmonary vascular remodeling in PAH as based on the size of the pulmonary arteries being affected; large: between 2 mm and approximately 500–700 μm in diameter; medium: between 500/700 and 70 μm in diameter; and precapillary arteries: usually nonmuscularized, below 70 μm in diameter. Given that pulmonary arteries have well-demarcated intima, media, and adventitia, it is possible to describe pulmonary vascular remodeling in regard to the specific region of the vascular wall being compromised. Finally, as the intima, media, and adventitia compartment has different cellular components, the remodeling process can be further characterized in relation to the contribution of endothelial, smooth muscle, and fibroblasts in each of the pulmonary vascular compartments. While, historically, intima lesions have been associated with PAH (restricting pulmonary artery blood flow to a larger degree), it is apparent that each compartment/vascular cell type works in concert in the different stages of the disease, ultimately resulting in the elevation of pulmonary artery pressures. In the paragraphs below, we describe the involvement of each of these compartments (vessel segment, vascular compartment, and predominant vascular cell involved), highlighting which of the forms of group 1 PAH they appear to be involved.

Perhaps the most characteristic vascular remodeling, particularly of less than 500 μm vessels, is the intima remodeling. This can appear as occlusive lesions, largely acellular containing amorphous extracellular material or cellular, with cells organized concentrically, or forming poorly organized intravascular capillaries, known as plexiform lesions (Fig. 26.1). Given the high capacitance of pulmonary arteries, in which the luminal surface area is approximately severalfold larger than that of the vessel wall, it is intuitive that these lesions impart significant restriction to blood flow, accounting for the increase resistance in PAH (Fig. 26.2). However, as discussed previously [9], their distribution, fre-

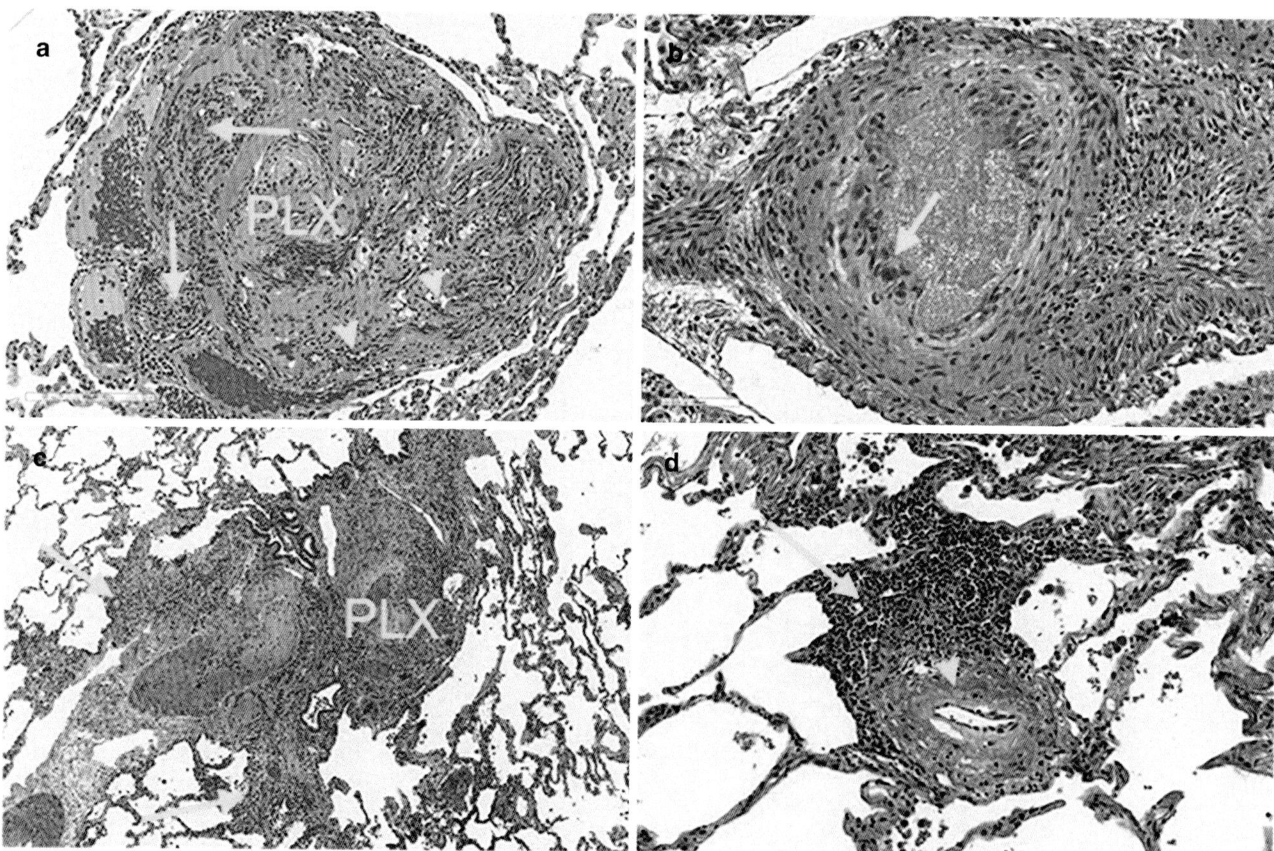

Fig. 26.1 Spectrum of complex vascular lesions in pulmonary arterial hypertension. (**a**) Plexiform lesion (PLX) with formation of poorly formed slit-like channels (*arrowheads*) surrounded by clusters of primitive cells in an organoid pattern (*arrowheads*). (**b**) Layer of endothelial cell in intima of thickened pulmonary artery (*arrow*) in PAH. (**c**) Plexiform lesion (PLX) surrounded by inflammatory cells (*arrows*). (**d**) Muscularized pulmonary artery (*arrowhead*) surrounded by inflammatory cells

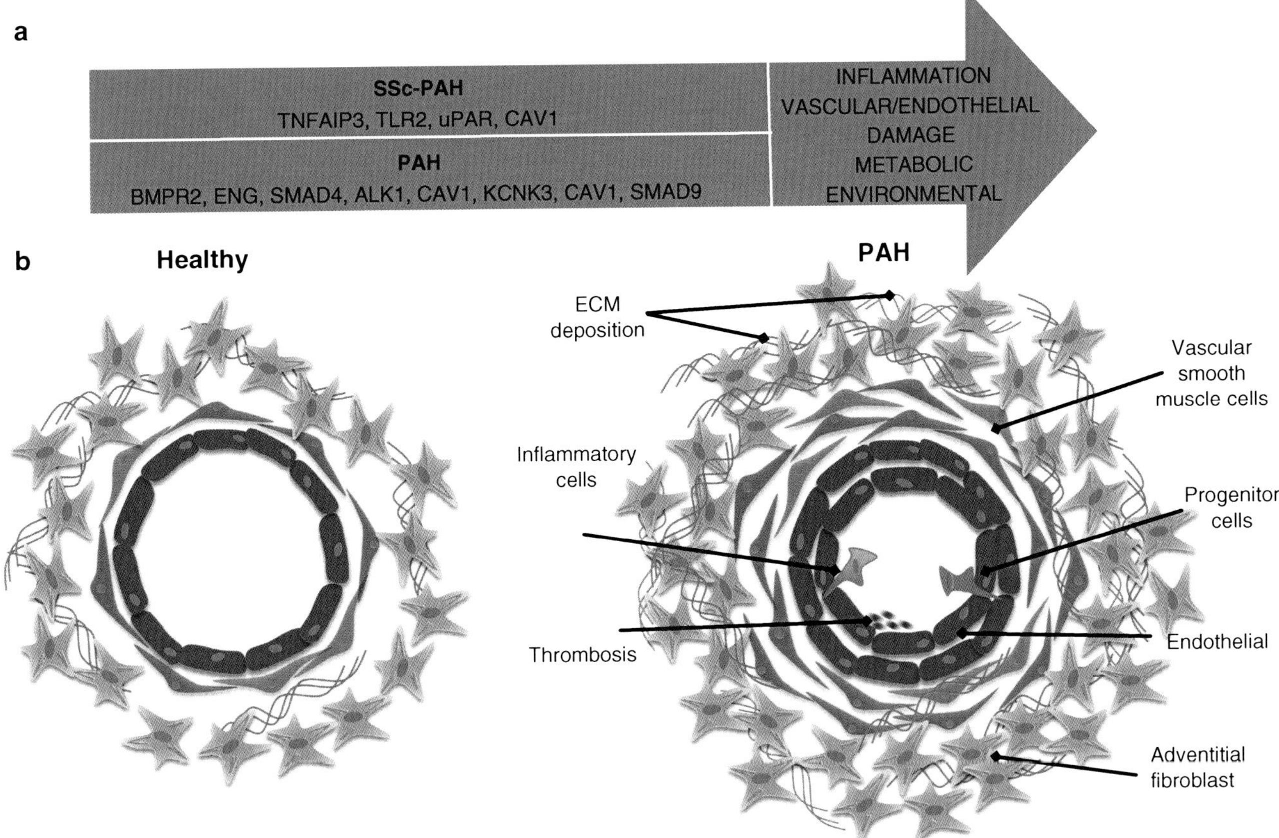

Fig. 26.2 Vascular remodeling in PAH: (**a**) A number of genes have been implicated in the development of PAH. Heritable and idiopathic PAH is strongly associated with a number of gene mutations that lead to a reduction in functional protein, whereas four polymorphisms have been identified to be associated with the development of SSc-PAH. A number of mechanism(s) have been implicated in initiation and development of PAH including inflammation vascular damage. (**b**) Vascular remodeling in PAH involves the infiltration of immune and progenitor (e.g., endothelial progenitor cells) cells, endothelial apoptosis, proliferation, and transdifferentiation. In addition expansion of smooth muscle cells and fibroblast and enhanced extracellular matrix (*ECM*) deposition

quency, and time of appearance during the natural course of disease remain unknown. These lesions are frequently seen in explanted lung in all conditions associated with group 1 PAH. There are however some more subtle differences, which have not been stringently quantified.

The relation between plexiform and intima obliterative lesions is unknown. We speculated, based on three-dimensional reconstruction studies [12], that the obliterative lesions originated as the plexiform lesions remodel in their most proximal segments, exposed to blood products and pressure waves. This is supported by the largely circumstantial evidence that both lesions – concentric and plexiform lesions – physically coexist in PAH lungs [13]. As the obliterative lesions impart the most drastic impingement on pulmonary vascular flow, even a single lesion might have a significant impact on pulmonary arterial pressure (it should be noted that a large number of lesions are required to reduce the overall reserve capacity of the pulmonary circulation). However, as mentioned above, their overall distribution, when they arise, and how these intima lesions progress overtime are not known. It is therefore conceivable that they could arise when the disease is fully established, i.e., they are not the cause of PH but rather consequence of increased pulmonary artery pressures (as suggested by Wagenvoort [14]). On the other hand, their potential importance in severe PH, including PAH, is supported by animal models of the disease, including the monocrotaline plus pneumectomy [15] and the SU5416 plus chronic hypoxia [16] models. In this particular model, endothelial cell proliferative lesions start on week 3 of PH, evolving into plexiform-like lesions within 4–6 weeks after the initiation of the model [17].

Notwithstanding the potential pathogenetic and diagnostic importance of intima lesions, it is apparent that milder intima lesions can be present in the normal lung, notably in the lungs of older individuals [18]; our report was the first demonstration that intima lesions are apparent in so-called normal lungs. It is unclear if their presence reflects a predisease state (like cardiovascular disease) or is without major consequences.

Interestingly, their impact on pulmonary vascular luminal area can be significant, well within the range seen in PAH [18]. Whether they are localized in normal lungs (and therefore of no clinical relevance) is unclear; in this case, PAH lungs would have a wider distribution of lesions leading to overall significant reduction of pulmonary artery perfusion capacity.

The pathogenesis of the intima lesions remains elusive. Based on experimental models, notably the monocrotaline and the SU+chronic hypoxia, endothelial cell death appears to be critical for subsequent intima remodeling and severe PH [16, 19]. However, a single hit – endothelial cell injury – is probably not sufficient; a second stimulus is probably required, often provided by the increase in pulmonary flow due to vasoconstriction or due to cellular signaling secondary to hypoxia-inducible growth factors. Though the lesions are contributed by cells and extracellular matrix, it is not clear if the extent of contribution of thrombi and platelets aggregates to the overall intima remodeling.

Media remodeling is largely composed by pulmonary vascular smooth muscle cells (SMCs). Though cell proliferation might contribute to the increase in media thickness, markers of proliferation are not usually detected in media SMC in lungs with established disease [20]. The contribution of media remodeling to restriction of pulmonary vascular lumen is unclear; however, it is of interest that the media mass increases as normal pulmonary arteries branch, particularly in precapillary arteries around 200 μm in diameter [9]. It is therefore conceivable that these pulmonary artery segments may further increase their overall mass. Interestingly, the extent of remodeling of media in PAH (largely in IPAH) correlated more closely with pulmonary hemodynamics than intima alone [18]. IPAH and CVD-PAH had a similar extent of media remodeling. Overall, media remodeling in PAH was significantly more pronounced than when compared with control lungs. However, an approximate 25 % of lungs of patients with PAH had media fractional thickness that was within the range seen in control lungs [18].

Non-muscularized pulmonary arteries become muscularized in PAH. The origin of these SMCs is not determined. Conceivably, these cells might arise from the peripheral extension of SMC originated from proximal segments of muscularized pulmonary arteries. Alternatively, pericytes might transdifferentiate into SMC. The specific molecular phenotype of these SMC in muscularized pulmonary arteries vs. that of cells located in more proximal arterial segments is unknown. Both vascular compartments express smooth muscle cell markers and may be responding similarly to growth and differentiation factors.

Adventitia remodeling contributes to the overall structural alterations associated with PH [21]. Though quantification of the extent of adventitia remodeling is difficult (the boundaries of adventitia is unclear as it extends toward the adjacent airway), there is growing evidence that the adventitia is a signaling hub, interfacing the systemic circulation (via the vasa vasorum in hilar structures or bronchial circulation around small airways) with the pulmonary artery compartments [10]. The intima compartment, which is normally largely composed of fibroblast, interacts with recruited inflammatory and progenitor cells, which play an inducing role of PH, as determined in animal models [22].

We have emphasized thus far overall patterns of remodeling involving the intima, media, and adventitia. These processes manifest with pathology that is shared with changes that occur in the systemic circulation and occur in most of forms of PH. However, there are some distinctive pulmonary vascular lesions in PAH, which are not shared with other groups of PH (2–5), and diseases involving the systemic circulation. Plexiform lesions are paradigmatic lesions in the lungs with PAH. They consist of an expansive intraluminal growth of poorly differentiated cells [23], forming irregular channels, which occlude the pulmonary vascular lumen. These lesions are largely seen (and initially described) in autopsy series [13]. The original identification of plexiform lesions in autopsy series [13, 24] led to the concept that these lesions occur in "terminal disease states" and are therefore of unclear pathogenetic relevance in PAH. However, it remains unclear when these lesions do appear in early or during progression of the disease. We have previously commented anecdotally that we observed plexiform lesions in diagnostic open lung biopsies of patients with PAH [25], suggesting that these lesions may appear during the course of PAH. Interestingly, the occurrence of plexiform lesions has been used as evidence for the potential inclusion of a PH-associated condition as group 1 PAH; conversely, the potential lack of well-formed plexiform lesions may have underlined the reclassification of PH associated with sickle cell disease in group 5 PH (rather than PAH group 1) [1].

Plexiform lesions are unique to PAH; they occur in all conditions listed under group 1, including conditions as disparate as schistosomiasis and HIV. Interestingly, they do not occur in other forms of PH, including severe forms of PH due to ILD and COPD; this difference underscores potential different pathogenetic processes among all PH conditions. Our impression that plexiform lesion would be less frequently detected in explanted lungs with CVD-PAH (and possibly liver cirrhosis-PAH) was not supported by our study of the modern age pathology of PAH; in fact, there were no differences in detected plexiform lesion profiles between IPAH and CVD-PAH (see below [18]).

Comparative Pathology of CVD-Associated PAH Versus Other Forms of PAH

Our recent study of explanted lungs of patients obtained after lung transplantation did not confirm our earlier overall impression that there might be categorical differences between CVD-PAH vs. other forms of PAH [18]. It should be noted that these lung samples were largely from IPAH patients ($n=48$) vs. CVD-PAH ($n=12$). The key parameters of intima, media, and adventitia fractional thicknesses were similar between these two groups. Nine of the 12 lungs with CVD-PAH had plexiform lesions; on the other hand, 35 IPAH lungs showed plexiform lesions. Interestingly, despite the lack of meaningful differences between the numbers of profiles of plexiform lesions between the two PAH subgroups, the IPAH lungs had a wider scatter of the number of lesions than in CVD-PAH. This finding further underscores the potential heterogeneity of pulmonary vascular remodeling despite the consistent elevation of pulmonary artery pressures to a suprasystemic level.

The main and categorical difference between CVD-PAH and IPAH lungs is the finding of active interstitial lung disease, including inflammation and fibrosis, in the former. How interstitial destruction affects pulmonary vascular remodeling and pulmonary artery pressures remains unknown; the same limitation applies to idiopathic pulmonary fibrosis with pulmonary hypertension [26]. Given that CVD with no PAH manifests with pulmonary fibrosis similar to the lungs with PAH, it is conceivable that there is a unique pathogenetic process restricted to the pulmonary circulation in the latter (see below).

We have proposed that plexiform lesions might represent a form of abnormal intravascular angiogenesis [27], with key properties shared with cancer growth, notably of clonal expansion of abnormal cells [28] and somatic instability [29]. Alternative views underscored that these lesions might represent a form of abnormal repair, largely due to organization of intraluminal clots [30]. In our view, plexiform lesions contain multiple layers of either endothelial or angiogenic precursor cells (Fig. 26.1), distinguishing them from the single-layer capillaries present in old clots. In this regard, plexiform lesions also depart significantly from the usual pattern of a single-layer, squamous-like, lining of larger arteries and veins. Interestingly, this unique feature also applies to normal glands (lined by single cells) vs. malignant glands or adenocarcinoma, which have layers of lining cells.

Perhaps the most compelling evidence that these lesions might occur early in severe PH and therefore contribute to the disease severity was provided by the development of the rat model based on SU5416-mediated VEGF receptor blockade combined with chronic hypoxia (CH) [16]. Endothelial cell proliferative lesions start to develop during the second and third weeks after induction of PH, progressing to lesions similar if not identical to human PAH [17]. In line with our prior suggestion that plexiform lesions can be identified in the lungs with minimal or no media remodeling [25], similar numbers of profiles of plexiform lesion were detected in quartile groups of media remodeling in our recently published observations in PAH lungs [18]. This finding, though not definitive, argues against the concept that plexiform lesions arise due to abnormal pulmonary artery pressures or abnormalities imparted by remodeling involving pulmonary vascular media [31]. An alternative explanation for this distinct lesion consists that, in IPAH, they arise from genetic instability in a selected population of endothelial cells with progenitor-like properties [28, 32].

Pathogenetic Insights of PAH

For the past six decades, the main concepts underlying the pathogenesis of PH have revolved around processes of vasoconstriction and vascular remodeling. The former has been supported by the vasoconstrictive effect of hypoxia and of relevant mediators, like endothelin (which is increased in PH [33]); loss of nitric oxide or prostacyclin would impair pulmonary vasodilation further enhancing vasoconstriction [34]. There is an important conundrum that resides on the observation that patients with PAH are largely unresponsive to vasodilators, notably calcium channel blockers, suggesting that, at least established (or advanced) disease, is largely independent of vasoconstriction.

For the past two decades, there has been a progressive focus of the pathobiological processes leading to altered pulmonary vascular remodeling. The focus on vasoconstrictors and vasodilators progressively incorporated a growing interest on how vasoconstrictors, like endothelin, and vasodilators, such as nitric oxide and prostacyclin, can double as growth factors or growth inhibitors, respectively. These insights led to two of the main therapies for PAH, based on endothelin receptor blockers or phosphodiesterase five inhibitors, respectively [4]. Investigations in the subsequent decade have focused on prototypic growth factors (with no vasodilatory function), including platelet-derived growth factor and TGF-β, among others. More recent insights into the interplay of metabolism and gene mutations have expanded considerably the scope of key pathogenetic mechanisms involved in PH. As with multiple chronic diseases, inflammation is a likely factor, promoting an interface between the pulmonary vascular compartment and growth signals affecting pulmonary vascular remodeling.

Pulmonary vascular remodeling has been largely considered within the scope of abnormal injury/repair paradigm. Interestingly, there is no clear data on how inciting events trigger the pulmonary remodeling process, notably in severe PH. In mild/moderate PH, hypoxia is a well-known trigger of pulmonary vascular remodeling. However, the triggers of severe PH, including PAH, are not delineated. The potential for endothelial cell apoptosis as the key triggering factor in severe PH is based on the SU+CH rat model of severe PH [16]; endothelial cell-toxic autoantibodies may underlie severe PH in the setting of autoimmune disease, like in SSc.

Though these potential mechanisms are well within the processes involved in injury/repair, they are also consistent with the conceptual framework that PH shares key features with malignant processes.

The concept that pulmonary vascular remodeling resembles cancer is now approximately 20 years old [35, 36]: it arouse from the finding that the expansion of endothelial cells in plexiform lesions in IPAH was monoclonal, i.e., they originated from a single progenitor cell [28, 35, 37]. This finding implied a selection process based on genetic events [32], which was subsequently validated with the findings of BMPR2 mutations [38, 39] and TGF-β receptor 2 somatic instability [29]. More recently, additional evidence of somatic genetic loss became evident when comparing primary cultures of pulmonary vascular cells from IPAH lungs with explanted lungs [40]. It is however worth mentioning that these events are restricted to IPAH; there is no current evidence that similar genetic processes affected other forms of PAH, including CVD-PAH. This difference implies that pulmonary vascular remodeling, involving pathologically similar lesions (see above), is stereotypic regardless of potentially diverse trigger factors. The concept that these lesions may arise from derepression of progenitor cells residing in the pulmonary vascular wall may well fit into this overall concept; genetic events would occur within a single cell, giving rise to a monoclonal expansion in IPAH. On the other hand, nongenetic hits would recruit multiple progenitor cells, giving rise to a polyclonal growth in PAH due to left-to-right heart shunt; whether in SSc-PAH or schistosomiasis-associated PAH plexiform lesions are monoclonal or polyclonal remains unclear. We discuss below in more depth several of these pathogenetic processes and the role of mediators of PH.

Genetic Basis of PAH

Genetic studies of heritable forms of PAH have identified a significant number of genes associated with the susceptibility to developing PH. Heralded by the identification of bone morphogenetic protein receptor type II (BMPR2) mutations in PAH patients in the early 2000s [39, 41], a number of mutations in genes associated with this receptor and the downstream signal pathway have been identified. These include the BMPR2 binding partner, ALK1, and type III receptor endoglin (CD105), as well as components of the SMAD downstream signaling pathway, SMAD4 and SMAD8 [42, 43].

By far, the most common gene associated to the development of PAH is BMPR2, which is mutated in greater than 70 % of heritable (hPAH) and at least 25 % of sporadic cases of IPAH [39, 41, 44]. Several missense, frameshifts, and nonsense mutations in this gene have subsequently been identified, collectively reducing the expression of functional BMPR2 on the cell surface [41, 43]. Functionally, BMPR2 inhibits proliferation of vascular smooth muscle cells (SMCs) while promoting the survival of pulmonary arterial endothelial cells, thereby protecting the pulmonary artery from damage and adverse inflammatory responses [43].

Genetic studies of SSc patients have identified a number of genes associated with vascular complications, including the development of PAH. Assessment of the Toll-like receptor (TLR) genes revealed a rare functional polymorphism in the TLR2 gene to be associated with anti-topoisomerase-positive SSc patients and with the development of SSc-PAH. Functionally, this polymorphism led to elevated induction of IL-6 and TNF-α by monocytes in response to TLR agonists [45]. Polymorphisms in ubiquitin-modifying enzyme TNFAIP3, a key regulator of NF-kB inflammatory signaling pathway, have also been shown to be associated with the development of SSc, notably diffuse cutaneous SSc (dcSSc), fibrosing alveolitis, and PAH [46]. In addition, a genetic variation located in the promoter region of the urokinase-type plasminogen activator receptor (uPAR) is associated with the vascular complications of SSc including digital ulceration and SSc-related PAH has been identified [47]. uPAR encodes a pleiotropic receptor, which is involved in fibrosis, immunity, angiogenesis, as well as vascular remodeling. Caveolin-1 (CAV1) is essential for the formation of caveolae and has been shown to be an inhibitor of tissue fibrosis. Recent SNP studies by Manetti and colleagues have identified a protective polymorphism associated with increased CAV1 protein expression in tissues of SSc patients. Mutations in CAV1 that lead to a reduction in protein expression have also been identified in heritable PAH patients. CAV1 appears to modify TGF-β signaling, including the reduction in BMP signaling [48]. Surprisingly, no association to members of the TGF-β superfamily of receptors, including BMPR2 and ALK1, has been detected in SSc-PAH patients [49].

Genetic studies of SSc-PAH have identified a number of genes associated with regulating inflammation including TLR2 and TNFAIP3. These findings are of interest, since the majority of genes associated with hPAH and IPAH are associated with a reduction in BMPR2/SMAD activity. Collectively this may suggest different genetic determinants of PAH between SSc-PAH and IPAH. The advent of whole genome sequencing will further assist in defining if genes associated with predisposition and progression of PAH are shared between SSc-PAH patients and other group 1 pathologies.

Pathogenic Factors and Signaling Pathways Implicated in the Development of PAH

Several proteins, gases, and lipids and their receptor- or sensor-dependent cognate signaling pathways have been implicated in the development of PAH. These include the established role of endothelin, nitric oxide, and prostacyclin; moreover, there is an increasing realization of the role of established and emerging mediators including TGF-β, platelet-derived growth factor (PDGF), serotonin, and epigenetic components such as microRNAs (miRNAs). Rather than existing in isolation, growing evidence demonstrates the interplay and cross talk between these factors/pathways in promoting the pathological cellular changes that drive PAH. We direct readers to a number of excellent reviews [50–53] and shall focus on a number of well-established and some of the key emerging mediators.

The TGF-β/BMP Axis

The TGF-β superfamily comprises more than 35 structurally related genes, which include activin, bone morphogenetic proteins (BMPs), and growth/differentiation factor. Perhaps the best known is TGF-β itself whose effects are strongly associated with promoting pro-fibrotic effects in numerous pathologies, including of course SSc [54, 55]. Although this family of growth factors has wide-ranging cellular effects, their activities are mediated through the activation of multiple but restricted set of receptors and canonical (SMAD) and noncanonical (such as members of the MAPK pathways [54, 55]). Broadly the TGF-β superfamily can be divided based upon their activation of signaling via either SMAD1, SMAD5, and SMAD8 (as in the case of BMPs) or SMAD2 and SMAD3 (as with TGF-β) [55, 56].

TGF-β has been implicated in promoting several of the cellular changes synonymous with remodeling, including SMC proliferation, matrix deposition, and alterations in cell growth, particularly of endothelial cells [57–59] (Fig. 26.2). On the other hand, BMPs play a major role in maintaining pulmonary vascular homeostasis (for excellent reviews readers are directed to [56, 60]), notably inhibiting smooth muscle cell growth and endothelial cell apoptosis.

Notwithstanding these apparently independent functions between these related but parallel signaling systems, it is apparent that they are interrelated functionally. The identification of BMPR2 mutations in hereditary PAH patients more than 15 years ago has heralded subsequent investigations that shed evidence for an imbalance in the TGF-β/BMP axis [44]. A broad body of work has documented demonstrating that the blunted activation of the BMP pathway in hPAH and IPAH due to a reduction in BMPR2 receptor expression leads to an enhancement in the activity of TGF-β and downstream pathway [61–63]. Studies in a number of preclinical models, including hypoxia and MCT-induced PH, showed a reduction in BMPR2 and an enhancement in the downstream activity of TGF-β/SMAD signaling [58, 64]; these are independent of mutations in BMPR2. While mutations in BMPR2 are not present in SSc patients, the expression of a number of proteins with a bias activity in favor of TGF-β or impaired BMP actions has been reported [65, 66]. In addition TGF-β-driven preclinical models of SSc also spontaneously develop PAH and exhibit endothelial cell damage and a pulmonary vasculopathy [67]. Gilbane et al. demonstrated that a reduction of BMPR2 levels in SSc-PAH patients [68] is associated with enhanced activity in downstream signaling components of the TGF-β pathways, including SMAD2 and MAPK [68]. As mentioned, the mechanistic link between decreased BMP signaling (due to loss of function mutations and loss of expression) may result in (and from) heightened TGF-β activity and therefore contribute to the development of PAH in SSc and provide a unifying mechanism across different forms of PAH.

The scope of forms of PAH in which TGF-β contributes to their pathogenesis is expanding. More recently, enhanced TGF-β signaling contributes to hypoxia PH [69] and to schistosomiasis-induced PH [70]; the PH and vascular remodeling in the latter involve SMAD3 signaling, while SMAD2 either does not have a prominent role or is somewhat protecting.

A number of approaches to restore the balance between BMPs and TGF-β have proven successful. For example, targeted gene delivery of BMPR2 can attenuate PAH [71], and inhibition of the TGF-β receptor ALK5 also prevents the development and progression of PAH [58, 64]. However this latter approach may prove problematic due to significant side effects [55]. More recently treatment of animals with BMP9 has been shown to reverse established PAH in preclinical models [72]. The relevance of BMP9 to SSc-PAH as yet remains unknown.

Serotonin (5-HT)

The "serotonin hypothesis of PAH" arose over 40 years ago when patients taking the anorexigen aminorex fumarate were associated with an increased risk of developing PAH. Serotonin is thought to mediate PAH by promoting both vasoconstriction and remodeling of the pulmonary vasculature [73]. Serotonin also induces proliferation of pulmonary arterial fibroblasts and SMC [74, 75]. In addition the serotonin transporter (SERT) has been implicated in both clinical and experimental PAH, functionally activating the PDGF-β receptor to induce SMC proliferation [76]. A number of studies have highlighted the dysregulation of components of the serotonin pathway in SSc [77]. In animal models and IPAH patients, PAH was found to be associated with a substantial increase in 5-HT (2B) receptor expression in the pulmonary arteries [78, 79]. Serotonin has also been shown to induce ECM synthesis in interstitial fibroblasts from SSc patients via the 5-HT (2B) receptors in a TGF-β-dependent manner [77], while the expression of 5-HT (2B) receptors in the vasculature of SSc-PAH remains unclear. A selective antagonist of S2-serotonergic receptors, ketanserin, given to 14 SSc-PAH patients led to a significant reduction in PVR, and an increase of PAP was observed in three patients, whereas two patients with mild PAH normalized both pulmonary pressure and vascular resistance [80]. Future therapeutic approaches targeting this pathway remain an attractive approach to treatment of SSc-PAH.

Platelet-Derived Growth Factor

PDGF is composed of four polypeptide chains A, B, C, and D, which form dimers in the full protein (PDGF-AA, PDGF-BB, PDGF-CC, PDGF-DD, and PDGF-AB). By far the best studied of these are PDGF-AA and PDGF-BB. Initially identified from platelets, PDGF isoforms are secreted from a number of cell types including macrophage, endothelial cells, SMC, and fibroblasts [81]. Acting as a potent mitogen and chemoattractant for fibroblasts, SMCs, and endothelial cells, PDGF has been implicated in PAH [81, 82]. Circulating levels of PDGF-BB are elevated in IPAH patients [83], but not in SSc-PAH [84]. PDGF receptor-β expression in SSc-PAH is more intense in small and postcapillary vessels compared to IPAH [85]. Autoantibodies against the PDGF receptors have also been detected in SSc patients and induce activation of ERK1/2 and ROS pathways in cells [86]. Further, serum levels of miR30b, which represses PDGFR-β expression, are reduced in SSc patients [87]. Indeed fibroblasts isolated from SSc patients exhibit enhanced IL-6 secretion in response to PDGF stimulation [88]. Growing evidence suggests antagonism of PDGF is an attractive approach to the treatment of PAH. Animal studies have shown a PDGFR-β tyrosine kinase inhibitor imatinib can reverse vascular remodeling via reduction in serotonin through inhibition of tryptophan hydroxylase 1 expression [89]. Whereas administration of imatinib to PAH patients led to the downregulation of PDGF plasma levels [90], the precise mechanism by which imatinib impacts PAH remains unclear, having inhibitory effects on a number of kinases in addition to PDGF-β receptor, including TGF-β-induced activation of c-abl and c-kit.

Extracellular Matrix (ECM)

Pulmonary vessels are highly susceptible to hypertension and to radial, axial, and circumferential strains generated by pulse pressure [91]. In PAH, the structural rearrangement of the pulmonary vessels (vascular remodeling) occurs as a result of cell proliferation and the excessive deposition of ECM resulting in vessel occlusion and stiffening of the vessel. The vascular ECM has a crucial role in conferring structural and functional integrity to normal function and diseased vessels [92]. Vascular ECM composition varies depending on vessel size and includes elastic microfibrils (elastin, fibrillins), collagens (mainly types I, III, IV, V, and VI), matricellular proteins (fibronectin, tenascin, and thrombospondin), growth factors and matrix metalloproteases sequestered in matrix, and proteoglycans [93]. Each compartment of the pulmonary vasculature (the intima, media, and adventitia) is embedded in ECM specifically composed by proteins secreted by the resident cells (vascular endothelial, SMC, and fibroblasts) (Table 26.1). The fine balance between ECM turnover, deposition, and degradation is crucial in maintaining normal vascular function, and any disturbance in this balance results in vascular remodeling and pathology such as that observed in PAH [92, 94]. Regulation of ECM turnover is performed by matrix metalloproteinases (MMPs), adamalysines (ADAM), serine elastases, and their endogenous inhibitors [95]. Metaloproteases (MMP) are a family of structurally related, zinc-dependent multifunctional proteases that are either soluble or membrane anchored and their inhibitors tissue inhibitors of metalloproteases (TIMPs).

Table 26.1 Extracellular matrix components altered in pulmonary vessels of PAH patients

Intima	Media	Adventitia
Collagen IV, VI, VIII, XV, XVIII [168]	Collagen I, III, V, VI [168, 169]	Collagen I, III, IV, V, VI [168, 169]
Aggrecan	Emlin	Decorin
Biglycan	Fibrillin-1 and -2	Elastin
BM-40	Fibronectin [170]	Fibronectin [170]
Fibronectin [170]	Fibulin-1	Fibrillin
Fibulin-1	Heparin	Laminin [171]
Laminin [171]	Hyaluronan	Lumican
Nidogen/entactin	Laminin [171]	Vitronectin
Perlecan (HSPG-2)	Lumican	
Thrombospondin-1 and -2 [172]	Microfibril	
vWF [172]	Osteopontin [173]	
Versican	Tenascin [174]	
	Vitronectin	
	Elastin	

# Denotes altered expression in PAH patients [168–174]

Although scleroderma is well described as a connective tissue disease driven by mechanisms which result in the overproduction of ECM [96], to date there has not been a comprehensive survey or comparison of the matrix components found in the pulmonary vasculature of patients with PAH and SSc-PAH.

There are many ECM components altered in PAH and the in-depth account of each component is beyond the scope of this review. The ECM structural proteins known to be most important in PAH are the fibrillar collagens. One of the features of remodeled pulmonary vessels is the deposition of collagen types I and III. In addition, collagen metabolism measured by circulating levels of N-terminal pro-peptide of type III procollagen, C-terminal telopeptide of collagen type I, MMP-9, and TIMP-1 is significantly increased in PAH and correlates with the severity of disease [97]. In addition to collagens, proteoglycans (such as hyaluronan, lumican, perlecan, versican) along with elastin also have an important role in arterial viscoelasticity in PAH [98]. Another important ECM component, tenascin-C, is upregulated in PAH and is believed to be involved in intimal hyperplasia [99]. A recent study has revealed that another key ECM component, fibronectin, is posttranslationally modified by tissue transglutaminase to form serotonylated fibronectin in pulmonary artery SMC, leading to stimulation of their proliferation and migration, hallmarks of pulmonary hypertension [100].

Several MMPs and TIMPs have been associated with vascular pathologies and PAH. In particular MMP-2, MMP-9, and MMP-14 and TIMP-1 and TIMP-2 have been shown to be important in pulmonary vascular remodeling particularly in plexiform and concentric lesions [101]. Although some studies for MMP inhibition in PAH animal models have been carried out, they have been inconclusive [94]. However, in an elegant study of human TIMP-1 overexpression in the lungs of rats exposed to monocrotaline, Vieillard-Baron et al. [102] demonstrated that TIMP-1 mediated right ventricular hypertrophy, gelatinase activity, and muscularization of peripheral pulmonary arteries, suggesting that balancing the MMP/TIMP ratio can reverse the disease.

Epigenetics

The contribution of nongenetic mechanisms to the cellular changes and the development of PAH is an emerging area of interest in the field; its relevance in the context of SSc however remains to be extensively explored. There are three main mechanisms of epigenetic regulation, which are methylation of CpG islands, mediated by DNA methyltransferases, modification to histone proteins, and microRNAs (miRNAs or miRs) [103]. In PAH a number of studies have highlighted the roles for all three epigenetic mechanisms. Histone acetylation is a key mechanism by which cell proliferation and survival are regulated. Zhao et al. demonstrated elevated protein levels of histone deacetylase (HDAC) 1 and 5 in PAH patient lungs. Administration of HDAC inhibitors reduced proliferation of PAH vascular fibroblasts and PDGF-stimulated growth of SMC [104]. In SSc microvascular endothelial cells, BMPR2 expression is repressed due to extensive CpG site methylation in the promoter region [105]. The relevance to the reduced BMPR2 expression observed in PAH-SSc fibroblasts however remains unclear [68]. The downregulation of superoxide dismutase 2 (SOD2) in PH results from methylation of CpG islands by lung DNA methyltransferases [106]. This partial silencing of SOD2 alters redox signaling, activates HIF-1-α, and leads to excessive cell proliferation, a mechanism observed also in some cancers [103].

miRs have been proposed as secreted biomarkers and mediators in the development of PAH [107, 108]. The growing relevance of miRNAs in modulating the pathogenic processes that contribute to the development of PAH is becoming more apparent in recent years. However the relevance of these miRNAs in the development and progression of SSc-PAH lags that of IPAH. Within the context of hPAH and IPAH, a number of differentially expressed miRNAs have been identified that have relevance to PAH. Expression of miR96 is reduced in PASMCs from female patients with PAH and negatively regulates the expression of the serotonin receptor 5-HT1BR. Restoration of miR96 expression reduces the development of hypoxia-induced PH in mice [109]. Hypoxia can promote broader changes in miR expression impacting cellular functions. For example, hypoxia leads to the upregulation of miR210 in SMC inhibiting apoptosis, whereas miR98, reduced in PAECs from PAH patients, is repressed by hypoxia and regulates ET-1 expression and PAEC proliferation [110, 111].

miR424 and miR503 are decreased in idiopathic PAH (IPAH); as these miRs suppress fibroblast growth factor (FGF)-2 expression, their decrease resulted in upregulation of FGF2 expression and a decrease in apelin in IPAH endothelial cells [112]. More recently, downregulated myocyte-enhancing factor 2 (MEF), which enhances endothelial cell survival, was also linked to decreased miR424/503 in PAH. Interestingly, apelin-induced upregulation of miR424/503 also relied on MEF binding to their promoter. Interestingly, MEF also increases expression of connexins 37 and 40 and KLF-2 and KLF-4, which are decreased in PAH vs. control endothelial cells [113]. Moreover, the repression of these miR family is linked to epigenetic histone acetylation/deacetylation. Pharmacological blockade of HDACIIa with MC1568 can decrease HDACs 4 and 5, causing increased expression of miR424/503. In line with these observations, in vivo administration of MC1568 reversed established rat PH caused by MCT or SU5416+chronic hypoxia treatment, which also included improved right ventricular remodeling [113].

Within the group of miRs, whose downregulation is associated with PH, miR204 has a remarkable impact on experimental PH [114]. miR204 is downregulated in IPAH serum and cells, allowing for the activation of STAT3 and HIF-1-α, which are permissive to experimental PH. The effect of mIR204 downregulation with antimiRs is pronounced, sufficing to trigger several of the key features of PH, both in SMC in vitro and in rats, in vivo.

Metabolism in PAH

Paralleling the development of the "cancer" paradigm applied to PH, early investigations zoomed in on the potential role of hypoxia-inducible factor (HIF)-1-α and (HIF)2-α in the pathogenesis of PH [115]. Indeed, mice heterozygous for both isoforms of HIF showed protection against hypoxic pulmonary hypertension [116, 117], and HIF-1-α and its partner, HIF-1-β, were demonstrated to be expressed in plexiform lesion in IPAH lungs [27]. In fact, these earlier insights were largely driven by the link between HIF's transcriptional control of gene products involved in angiogenesis, like VEGF, which were also shown to be expressed in PAH lungs [27].

The development of methods that allowed the isolation and culture of pulmonary vascular cells from PAH lungs led to experimentation that bridged pulmonary vascular remodeling, HIF signaling, and metabolism [118]. Cultured IPAH endothelial cells proliferated more and were more resistant to apoptosis than normal cells; this in vitro observations with human disease relevant cells validated earlier observations in the rat model of severe PH based on chronic hypoxia+SU5416 [16, 119]. Further investigations addressing the underpinnings of the growth advantage in IPAH endothelial cells documented that these cells were more glycolytic and had less mitochondria than control cells [120]. Parallel investigations in pulmonary SMC from models of PH have also implicated HIF-1-α signaling in the growth properties of these cells (vs. control cells) [121]. Subsequent work from the same group demonstrated that PH SMCs are indeed glycolytic (as in anaerobic glycolysis), at the expense of glucose oxidation; however, given that the lung is exposed to environmental oxygen, this likely reflects aerobic glycolysis or the Warburg effect [122]. This interface between the pulmonary vascular cell growth and metabolism has been largely underscored in cancer cells; the authors recommend that the reader refer to recent reviews in the specific area of PH research [122–124].

This paradigm was recently expanded to include adventitia fibroblast derived from hypoxic pulmonary circulation with PH [125]. These cells integrate pro-inflammatory signaling in hypoxic PH, involving reprogramming of naïve macrophages. The PH adventitia fibroblast shares some key features with those identified in hypertensive endothelial [16, 126] and SMC [127], notably aerobic glycolysis, hyperproliferation, apoptosis resistance, and pro-inflammatory properties [128]. The overall signaling is reliant on the integration of STAT3 and HIF-1-α signaling. Of note, a similar metabolic and pro-inflammatory phenotype is observed in cancer-associated fibroblasts [125], including the expression of an isoform of pyruvate kinase, PKM2, which, via its lower catalytic activity as compared with the ubiquitously expressed PKM1, can drive the pentose phosphate pathway (major cell source of ribonucleotides and reducing equivalents for fatty acid synthesis) [129, 130]. Interestingly, as discussed below (inflammation in PH), pro-remodeling macrophages appear to mirror the metabolic and pro-inflammatory phenotype of PH adventitia fibroblast. Indeed, type 1 inflammation (like that generated by lipopolysaccharide (LPS) is characterized by activation of HIF-1-α and aerobic glycolysis [131].

What is the specific growth advantage afforded by anaerobic glycolysis? Carbon flux thorough the glycolytic pathway (resulting in lactate production) promotes enhanced NADPH production via the pentose monophosphate pathway, therefore enhancing antioxidant defenses, while producing ribonucleotides for DNA synthesis. A similar benefit may derive from the single-carbon metabolism involving in serine synthesis from phosphoenolpyruvate [132, 133], which generates NADPH for antioxidant defenses.

The "metabolic shift" hypothesis of PAH has been largely centered on the concept that PAH develops by alterations in substrate utilization, with mitochondria playing a somewhat "passive" role in the development of PH. In fact, endothelial cells are normally glycolytic as means to improve O2 availability to target organs; however, they are metabolically active as indicated by the recent evidence that fatty acid oxidation (via providing acetyl Co-A intermediates via the mitochondria-β oxidation) is used to generate nucleotides in proliferating endothelial cells [134].

These insights have already generated translational insights into the human disease. Enhanced PET imaging of 18F-fluorodeoxyglucose (18F-FDG) of PAH lungs may offer new modes of assessment of pulmonary vascular remodeling, short of performing invasive hemodynamic measurements [120, 135]. This patient-based evidence has been largely supported by animal models [136]. Moreover, the dichloroacetate (DCA, used in the 1960s for mitochondria diseases) is in its first trial in patients with PAH. DCA inhibits pyruvate dehydrogenase kinase (PDK), allowing for activation of pyruvate dehydrogenase (PDH) and increased oxidation of pyruvate generated via the glycolytic pathway. DCA was highly effective in the monocrotaline model [137]; however, it has not been tested in other rodent models, including the SU+CH model.

Inflammation in PAH

Earlier pathological studies brought attention to the presence of inflammatory cells around and within the pulmonary vascular lesions in IPAH [138, 139]. More recent studies, employing a wide range of markers of specific inflammatory cells, further confirmed these earlier observations and expanded to include regulatory and Th17 lymphocytes [140]. Experimental studies addressed a potential contribution of cytokines, notably of IL-1, in monocrotaline-induced PH and IL-6 [141]. Progressively, markers of inflammation, notably cytokines, were shown to be increased in serum of patients with PAH [142]. As apparent through the discussion below, the insights on how inflammation affects pulmonary vascular disease have expanded significantly; however, some central questions related to the nature of the inflammatory process (innate vs. acquired immunity, source of potential antigens, relative contribution of cytokine networks) and its mechanistic role as a trigger, amplifier, or mere consequence of PH remain to be clarified. The presence of perivascular inflammation in PAH has been confirmed more recently in PAH lungs, from patients who have been treated with the current standards of therapy. Importantly, these studies confirmed the correlation between perivascular inflammation and pulmonary artery pressures [18].

An important overall advance in the understanding on how inflammation can affect hypoxic responses certainly impacts the field of inflammation and PH. Teleologically, both acute and chronic inflammatory processes occur in the setting of low oxygen; therefore, adaption of inflammatory cells to hypoxia is a central process to control infectious agents. As alluded in the miRNA, metabolism, and PH sections above, hypoxia and HIF appear to have an important role in these processes [115]. Hypoxia-induced PH in mice increases inflammatory cells, including macrophages [143], which, if attenuated with hemoxygenase, prevent the increase in pulmonary artery pressures. Given that both the acquired and innate immunity arms appear to be involved in PH, one might predict cross talk between HIF-1-α and NF-kB, which has been uncovered more recently [144]. Indeed, blockade of each of HIF-1-α [115] or NF-kB [145, 146] transcription factors protects against hypoxia-induced PH. Furthermore, activation of NF-AT and STAT3 may participate in the activation of the immune system in experimental PH [147, 148]. These data indicate that the innate immunity has a role in hypoxic PH and may contribute to PAH.

The role of acquired immunity in PH has been progressively addressed as it appears to bridge specific antigen triggers and pulmonary vascular remodeling. Autoantibodies directed against endothelial cell antigens may drive pulmonary vascular disease in SSc-PAH and possibly in IPAH as well [149, 150]. The presence of autoantigens might also explain the finding of tertiary follicles in explanted IPAH lungs in a French cohort of patients [151]; it is however unclear the extent that these findings apply to non-French cohorts of PAH patients, as these lymphoid follicles were not observed in a recent extensive review of North American cases of PAH [18]. Notwithstanding some degree of heterogeneity in the finding of inflammation in PAH lungs, studies in the monocrotaline model suggested that antigens derived from the lung might drive the hypertensive process [152].

Within group 1 PAH, schistosomiasis-induced PAH (Schisto-PAH) represents a paradigmatic example of acquired immunity linked to PH [153]. Schisto-PAH is caused by the parasite *Schistosoma mansoni*, when the mature worms deposit eggs in the intestinal wall that migrate to the liver and subsequently to the lung. It represents the most frequent form of PAH worldwide, involving temperate countries with large populations like Brazil and China. *S. mansoni* causes a prototypic type 2 inflammation, involving the key type 2 cytokines IL-4 and IL-13 [154]. This inflammatory response is directed toward *S. mansoni* antigens, as elimination of the adult worms with praziquantel also blocks the inflammatory process. Schisto-PH can be modeled in mice, which are permissive to the worm, allowing animal modeling of key life cycle and pathology seen in humans.

Challenge of mice with the infective larval stage of cercaria or with eggs triggers substantial pulmonary vascular remodeling and a mild form of PH [155, 156]; the cercarial infection reproduced the life cycle in humans, with liver and lung involvement after 4–5 months after initial infection. The sequential intravenous *S. mansoni* egg injection followed by intraperitoneal immunization causes pulmonary hypertension with remodeling within 21 days [70]. This modified model has led to the identification of TGF-β as the key signaling mediator of pulmonary hypertension and remodeling, acting downstream of Th2 inflammation [70]. These data have relevance to SSc-PAH, as both SSc and Schistosomiasis exhibit the characteristic feature of fibrosis, the link between TH2/TGF-β inflammation and signaling, and a similar spectrum of pulmonary vascular lesions.

However, it is apparent that inflammation in PH belies the classic immunological frameworks. A recent extensive study of cytokine expression in a large cohort of patients with PAH revealed that IL-1-β, IL-2, IL-4, IL-6, IL-8, IL-10, 12p70, TNF-α, and IL-10 were all increased when compared with controls. IL-6 levels were most notably associated with worse clinical outcome [157]. IL-6 has been linked to the development of experimental PH, while its overexpression is sufficient to cause PH in mice [158]; on the other hand, IL-6 knockouts are protected against hypoxia-induced PH [159]. Of note, despite being younger and with worse disease than patients with IPAH, patients with BMPR2 mutations had similar levels of cytokines when compared with patients with the wild-type BMPR2 genotype. The data appear to indicate that an innate response based on IL-6 levels has a significant role in the development of PH.

Macrophages, among all inflammatory cells, have a key role in PH. They are present within and concentrate around advanced vascular lesions in IPAH [139]. Recent evidence has linked IL-6 with a STAT3-driven macrophage phenotype and activated adventitia fibroblasts in PH [128]. This signaling hub is shared between the macrophages and fibroblasts, allowing a mutual feedback enhancement of a pro-inflammatory phenotype and possibly of pulmonary vascular remodeling in the cow model of hypoxic PH; these data were further validated with IPAH macrophages and fibroblasts [128]. In Schisto-PH, macrophages, shaped by IL-4/IL-13 Th2 inflammation, are the probable source of TGF-β, a key distal determinant of PH in the mouse model [70]. The precise range of phenotypes exhibited by lung macrophages in PH will require extensive investigation, as these cells are mutable, assuming diverse and transient phenotypes. These phenotypes are probably shaped by the underlying stimulus for PH (hypoxia, endothelial cell injury, cytokine overexpression, etc.) and the local inflammatory microenvironment.

The role of lymphocytic cell populations in PH is still unclear. Transfer of antibodies purified from lungs of rats with monocrotaline-induced PH increased pulmonary artery pressures, possibly reacting with adventitia fibroblasts [152]. These results imply that B and plasma cells (originated from bronchoalveolar lymphoid tissue) might be pathogenic, particularly in the monocrotaline model of PH. There is a deficiency of regulatory (reg) T cells as FoxP3-positive mononuclear cells (FoxP3 is a key transcription factor for T reg differentiation) are reduced in IPAH lungs [140]; this deficiency would further support the concept of an immunologic dysregulation in PAH lungs, a feature shared with SSc.

Mast cells have long been shown to be present in IPAH patient lungs [138]. Mast cells contain several preformed mediators, including histamine, serotonin, matrix metalloproteases, proteoglycans, and leukotriene derivatives [160]. Their activation requires FcεR1 and the growth factor c-kit, whose expression is increased in IPAH [161]. Some recent insights revealed the contribution of mast cells in venous PH due to left heart failure [162] and hypoxic PH [163]. The identification of mast cells in hypoxic rats dates back to the 1970s [164]; mast cell accumulation due to hypoxia involves increased bone marrow recruitment and possibly local proliferation [160]. However, the role of mast cells and their degranulation products in hypoxic PH are unclear since several studies (using histamine receptor blockers or rats deficient in mast cells) failed to confirm a definitive role for mast cells in hypoxic PH. Similar contradictory results were obtained with cromolyn sodium, a mast cell degranulation inhibitor.

Notwithstanding the abundant data on the presence and potential role for inflammation in PAH, the translation of these insights into clinical management remains open. There is no evidence as yet that immunosuppressive approaches that have proven so successful in autoimmune disorders offer benefit to patients with PAH. An ongoing clinical trial is testing the effect of TNF-receptor blocker rituximab in SSc-PAH (clinicaltrials.gov identifier NCT01086540; https://clinicaltrials.gov/ct2/show/NCT01086540?term=scleroderma+and+pulmonary+hypertension&rank=29). The data from this trail may represent the first clear indication of anti-inflammatory therapies in PAH.

Conclusion

PAH is a leading cause of morbidity and mortality in patients with SSc and PH adversely impacts several diseases associated with the disease. Our understanding of PH in general has grown exponentially in the recent decades, positioning PH as the leading disease research focus among pulmonary diseases. The aggregate of several decades of research in PH have provided a range of therapies and improved means to assess outcome and prognosis. The field of research and clinical care in PH is highly organized with, at the present time, five international symposia that allowed for in-depth discussion of several key aspects related to PH [165]; this effort has provided important guiding recommendations that impacted the field. Importantly, these guidelines and assessment of what we know about the disease contributed to critical advances. These are apparent in the discussion above. In fact, novel therapies are in the near horizon, including metabolic regulators like DCA (ClinicalTrials.gov Identifier: NCT01083524) and, as mentioned, immune-based therapies. There are several other candidates that have provided optimistic preclinical data, including the vascular elastase inhibitor elafin [166] and a small molecule that targets FK506 and enhances expression of BMPR2 [167]. However, disease-tailored or patient-oriented specific therapies still need to be developed. This limitation is particularly pertinent to patients with SSc-PAH.

Acknowledgments RMT was supported by; AH was supported by the Arthritis Research UK.

References

1. Simonneau G, Gatzoulis MA, Adatia I, Celermajer D, Denton C, Ghofrani A, et al. Updated clinical classification of pulmonary hypertension. J Am Coll Cardiol. 2013;62(25 Suppl):D34–41.
2. Zaiman A, Fijalkowska I, Hassoun PM, Tuder RM. One hundred years of research in the pathogenesis of pulmonary hypertension. Am J Respir Cell Mol Biol. 2005;33(5):425–31.
3. Fishman AP. A century of primary pulmonary hypertension. In: Rubin LJ, Rich S, editors. Primary pulmonary hypertension. 1st ed. New York: Macel Decker; 1997. p. 1–17.
4. Humbert M, Sitbon O, Simonneau G. Treatment of pulmonary arterial hypertension. N Engl J Med. 2004;351(14):1425–36.
5. Shorr AF, Wainright JL, Cors CS, Lettieri CJ, Nathan SD. Pulmonary hypertension in patients with pulmonary fibrosis awaiting lung transplant. Eur Respir J. 2007;30(4):715–21.
6. Cuttica MJ, Kalhan R, Shlobin OA, Ahmad S, Gladwin M, Machado RF, et al. Categorization and impact of pulmonary

hypertension in patients with advanced COPD. Respir Med. 2010;104(12):1877–82.

7. Simonneau G, Robbins IM, Beghetti M, Channick RN, Delcroix M, Denton CP, et al. Updated clinical classification of pulmonary hypertension. J Am Coll Cardiol. 2009;54(1 Suppl):S43–54.
8. Archer SL, Weir EK, Wilkins MR. Basic science of pulmonary arterial hypertension for clinicians: new concepts and experimental therapies. Circulation. 2010;121(18):2045–66.
9. Tuder RM, Stacher E, Robinson J, Kumar R, Graham BB. Pathology of pulmonary hypertension. Clin Chest Med. 2013;34(4):639–50.
10. Tuder RM, Archer SL, Dorfmuller P, Erzurum SC, Guignabert C, Michelakis E, et al. Relevant issues in the pathology and pathobiology of pulmonary hypertension. J Am Coll Cardiol. 2013;62(25 Suppl):D4–12.
11. Tuder RM. How do we measure pathology in PAH (lung and RV) and what does it tell us about the disease. Drug Discov Today. 2014;19(8):1257–63.
12. Cool CD, Stewart JS, Werahera P, Miller GJ, Williams RL, Voelkel NF, et al. Three-dimensional reconstruction of pulmonary arteries in plexiform pulmonary hypertension using cell specific markers: evidence for a dynamic and heterogeneous process of pulmonary endothelial cell growth. Am J Pathol. 1999;155(2):411–9.
13. Heath D, Edwards JE. The pathology of hypertensive pulmonary vascular disease; a description of six grades of structural changes in the pulmonary arteries with special reference to congenital cardiac septal defects. Circulation. 1958;18:533–47.
14. Wagenvoort CA. Plexogenic arteriopathy. Thorax. 1994;49(Suppl):S39–45.
15. Tanaka Y, Schuster DP, Davis EC, Patterson GA, Botney MD. The role of vascular injury and hemodynamics in rat pulmonary artery remodeling. J Clin Invest. 1996;98(2):434–42.
16. Taraseviciene-Stewart L, Kasahara Y, Alger L, Hirth P, Mc Mahon GG, Waltenberger J, et al. Inhibition of the VEGF receptor 2 combined with chronic hypoxia causes cell death-dependent pulmonary endothelial cell proliferation and severe pulmonary hypertension. FASEB J. 2001;15(2):427–38.
17. Abe K, Toba M, Alzoubi A, Ito M, Fagan KA, Cool CD, et al. Formation of plexiform lesions in experimental severe pulmonary arterial hypertension. Circulation. 2010;121:2747–54.
18. Stacher E, Graham BB, Hunt JM, Gandjeva A, Groshong SD, McLaughlin VV, et al. Modern age pathology of pulmonary arterial hypertension. Am J Respir Crit Care Med. 2012;186(3):261–72.
19. Teichert-Kuliszewska K, Kutryk MJ, Kuliszewski MA, Karoubi G, Courtman DW, Zucco L, et al. Bone morphogenetic protein receptor-2 signaling promotes pulmonary arterial endothelial cell survival: implications for loss-of-function mutations in the pathogenesis of pulmonary hypertension. Circ Res. 2006;98(2):209–17.
20. Tuder RM. Pathology of pulmonary arterial hypertension. Semin Respir Crit Care Med. 2009;30(4):376–85.
21. Chazova I, Loyd JE, Newman JH, Belenkov Y, Meyrick B. Pulmonary artery adventitial changes and venous involvement in primary pulmonary hypertension. Am J Pathol. 1995;146(2):389–97.
22. Pugliese SC, Poth JM, Fini MA, Olschewski A, El Kasmi KC, Stenmark KR. The role of inflammation in hypoxic pulmonary hypertension: from cellular mechanisms to clinical phenotypes. Am J Physiol Lung Cell Mol Physiol. 2015;308(3):L229–52.
23. Smith P, Heath D. Electron microscopy of the plexiform lesion. Thorax. 1979;34:177–86.
24. Wagenvoort CA, Wagenvoort N. Primary pulmonary hypertension. A pathologic study of the lung vessels in 156 clinically diagnosed cases. Circulation. 1970;42:1163–84.
25. Tuder RM, Zaiman AL. Pathology of pulmonary vascular disease. In: Peacock A, Rubin LJ, editors. Pulmonary circulation. 2nd ed. London: Arnold; 2004. p. 25–32.
26. Nathan SD, Noble PW, Tuder RM. Idiopathic pulmonary fibrosis and pulmonary hypertension: connecting the dots. Am J Respir Crit Care Med. 2007;175(9):875–80.
27. Tuder RM, Chacon M, Alger LA, Wang J, Taraseviciene-Stewart L, Kasahara Y, et al. Expression of angiogenesis-related molecules in plexiform lesions in severe pulmonary hypertension: evidence for a process of disordered angiogenesis. J Pathol. 2001;195(3):367–74.
28. Lee SD, Shroyer KR, Markham NE, Cool CD, Voelkel NF, Tuder RM. Monoclonal endothelial cell proliferation is present in primary but not secondary pulmonary hypertension. J Clin Invest. 1998;101(5):927–34.
29. Yeager ME, Halley GR, Golpon HA, Voelkel NF, Tuder RM. Microsatellite instability of endothelial cell growth and apoptosis genes within plexiform lesions in primary pulmonary hypertension. Circ Res. 2001;88(1):e8–11.
30. Yi ES, Kim H, Ahn H, Strother J, Morris T, Masliah E, et al. Distribution of obstructive intimal lesions and their cellular phenotypes in chronic pulmonary hypertension. A morphometric and immunohistochemical study. Am J Respir Crit Care Med. 2000;162(4):1577–86.
31. Yamaki S, Wagenvoort CA. Plexogenic pulmonary arteriopathy: significance of medial thickness with respect to advanced pulmonary vascular lesions. Am J Pathol. 1981;105(1):70–5.
32. Tuder RM, Lee SD, Cool CD. Histopathology of pulmonary hypertension. Chest. 1998;114(1 Suppl):1S–6.
33. Giaid A, Yanagisawa M, Langleben D, Michel RP, Levy R, Shennib H, et al. Expression of endothelin-1 in the lungs of patients with pulmonary hypertension. N Engl J Med. 1993;328(24):1732–9.
34. Giaid A, Saleh D. Reduced expression of endothelial nitric oxide synthase in the lungs of patients with pulmonary hypertension. N Engl J Med. 1995;333(4):214–21.
35. Voelkel NF, Cool CD, Lee SD, Wright L, Geraci MW, Tuder RM. Primary pulmonary hypertension between inflammation and cancer. Chest. 1999;114 Suppl 3:225S–30.
36. Rai PR, Cool CD, King JAC, Stevens T, Burns N, Winn RA, et al. The cancer paradigm of severe pulmonary arterial hypertension. Am J Respir Crit Care Med. 2008;178(6):558–64.
37. Tuder RM, Radisavljevic Z, Shroyer KR, Polak JM, Voelkel NF. Monoclonal endothelial cells in appetite suppressant-associated pulmonary hypertension. Am J Respir Crit Care Med. 1998;158(6):1999–2001.
38. The International PPH Consortium, Lane KB, Machado RD, Pauciulo MW, Thompson JR, Philips III JA, et al. Heterozygous germline mutations in BMPR2 encoding a TGF-B receptor cause familiar pulmonary hypertension. Nat Genet. 2000;26(1):81–4.
39. Deng Z, Morse JH, Slager SL, Cuervo N, Moore KJ, Venetos G, et al. Familial primary pulmonary hypertension (gene PPH1) Is caused by mutations in the bone morphogenetic protein receptor-II gene. Am J Hum Genet. 2000;67(3):737–44.
40. Aldred MA, Comhair SA, Varella-Garcia M, Asosingh K, Xu W, Noon GP, et al. Somatic chromosome abnormalities in the lungs of patients with pulmonary arterial hypertension. Am J Respir Crit Care Med. 2010;182(9):1153–60.
41. Lane KB, Machado RD, Pauciulo MW, Thomson JR, Phillips III JA, Loyd JE, et al. Heterozygous germline mutations in BMPR2, encoding a TGF-beta receptor, cause familial primary pulmonary hypertension. Nat Genet. 2000;26(1):81–4.
42. Ma L, Chung WK. The genetic basis of pulmonary arterial hypertension. Hum Genet. 2014;133(5):471–9.
43. Austin ED, Loyd JE. The genetics of pulmonary arterial hypertension. Circ Res. 2014;115(1):189–202.

44. Trembath RC, Thomson JR, Machado RD, Morgan NV, Atkinson C, Winship I, et al. Clinical and molecular genetic features of pulmonary hypertension in patients with hereditary hemorrhagic telangiectasia. N Engl J Med. 2001;345(5):325–34.
45. Broen JC, Bossini-Castillo L, van Bon L, Vonk MC, Knaapen H, Beretta L, et al. A rare polymorphism in the gene for toll-like receptor 2 is associated with systemic sclerosis phenotype and increases the production of inflammatory mediators. Arthritis Rheum. 2012;64(1):264–71.
46. Dieude P, Guedj M, Wipff J, Ruiz B, Riemekasten G, Matucci-Cerinic M, et al. Association of the TNFAIP3 rs5029939 variant with systemic sclerosis in the European Caucasian population. Ann Rheum Dis. 2010;69(11):1958–64.
47. Manetti M, Allanore Y, Revillod L, Fatini C, Guiducci S, Cuomo G, et al. A genetic variation located in the promoter region of the UPAR (CD87) gene is associated with the vascular complications of systemic sclerosis. Arthritis Rheum. 2011;63(1):247–56.
48. Austin ED, Ma L, LeDuc C, Berman RE, Borczuk A, Phillips III JA, et al. Whole exome sequencing to identify a novel gene (caveolin-1) associated with human pulmonary arterial hypertension. Circ Cardiovasc Genet. 2012;5(3):336–43.
49. Koumakis E, Wipff J, Dieude P, Ruiz B, Bouaziz M, Revillod L, et al. TGFbeta receptor gene variants in systemic sclerosis-related pulmonary arterial hypertension: results from a multicentre EUSTAR study of European Caucasian patients. Ann Rheum Dis. 2012;71(11):1900–3.
50. Sitbon O, Morrell N. Pathways in pulmonary arterial hypertension: the future is here. Eur Respir Rev. 2012;21(126):321–7.
51. Guignabert C, Tu L, Girerd B, Ricard N, Huertas A, Montani D, et al. New molecular targets of pulmonary vascular remodeling in pulmonary arterial hypertension: importance of endothelial communication. Chest. 2015;147(2):529–37.
52. Baliga RS, MacAllister RJ, Hobbs AJ. New perspectives for the treatment of pulmonary hypertension. Br J Pharmacol. 2011;163(1):125–40.
53. Thomas M, Ciuclan L, Hussey MJ, Press NJ. Targeting the serotonin pathway for the treatment of pulmonary arterial hypertension. Pharmacol Ther. 2013;138(3):409–17.
54. Varga J, Whitfield ML. Transforming growth factor-beta in systemic sclerosis (scleroderma). Front Biosci (Schol Ed). 2009;1:226–35.
55. Budd DC, Holmes AM. Targeting TGFbeta superfamily ligand accessory proteins as novel therapeutics for chronic lung disorders. Pharmacol Ther. 2012;135(3):279–91.
56. Upton PD, Morrell NW. The transforming growth factor-beta-bone morphogenetic protein type signaling pathway in pulmonary vascular homeostasis and disease. Exp Physiol. 2013;98(8):1262–6.
57. Good RB, Gilbane AJ, Trinder SL, Denton CP, Coghlan G, Abraham DJ, et al. Endothelial to mesenchymal transition contributes to endothelial dysfunction in pulmonary artery hypertension. Am J Pathol. 2015;185(7):1850–8.
58. Thomas M, Docx C, Holmes AM, Beach S, Duggan N, England K, et al. Activin-like kinase 5 (ALK5) mediates abnormal proliferation of vascular smooth muscle cells from patients with familial pulmonary arterial hypertension and is involved in the progression of experimental pulmonary arterial hypertension induced by monocrotaline. Am J Pathol. 2009;174(2):380–9.
59. Morrell NW, Yang X, Upton PD, Jourdan KB, Morgan N, Sheares KK, et al. Altered growth responses of pulmonary artery smooth muscle cells from patients with primary pulmonary hypertension to transforming growth factor-beta(1) and bone morphogenetic proteins. Circulation. 2001;104(7):790–5.
60. Cai J, Pardali E, Sanchez-Duffhues G, ten Dijke P. BMP signaling in vascular diseases. FEBS Lett. 2012;586(14):1993–2002.
61. Upton PD, Davies RJ, Tajsic T, Morrell NW. Transforming growth factor-beta(1) represses bone morphogenetic protein-mediated Smad signaling in pulmonary artery smooth muscle cells via Smad3. Am J Respir Cell Mol Biol. 2013;49(6):1135–45.
62. Davies RJ, Holmes AM, Deighton J, Long L, Yang X, Barker L, et al. BMP type II receptor deficiency confers resistance to growth inhibition by TGF-beta in pulmonary artery smooth muscle cells: role of proinflammatory cytokines. Am J Physiol Lung Cell Mol Physiol. 2012;302(6):L604–15.
63. Burton VJ, Ciuclan LI, Holmes AM, Rodman DM, Walker C, Budd DC. Bone morphogenetic protein receptor II regulates pulmonary artery endothelial cell barrier function. Blood. 2011;117(1):333–41.
64. Long L, Crosby A, Yang X, Southwood M, Upton PD, Kim DK, et al. Altered bone morphogenetic protein and transforming growth factor-beta signaling in rat models of pulmonary hypertension: potential for activin receptor-like kinase-5 inhibition in prevention and progression of disease. Circulation. 2009;119(4):566–76.
65. Wellbrock J, Harbaum L, Stamm H, Hennigs JK, Schulz B, Klose H, et al. Intrinsic BMP antagonist gremlin-1 as a novel circulating marker in pulmonary arterial hypertension. Lung. 2015;193(4):567–70.
66. Cahill E, Costello CM, Rowan SC, Harkin S, Howell K, Leonard MO, et al. Gremlin plays a key role in the pathogenesis of pulmonary hypertension. Circulation. 2012;125(7):920–30.
67. Derrett-Smith EC, Dooley A, Gilbane AJ, Trinder SL, Khan K, Baliga R, et al. Endothelial injury in a transforming growth factor beta-dependent mouse model of scleroderma induces pulmonary arterial hypertension. Arthritis Rheum. 2013;65(11):2928–39.
68. Gilbane AJ, Derrett-Smith E, Trinder SL, Good RB, Pearce A, Denton CP, et al. Impaired bone morphogenetic protein receptor II signaling in a transforming growth factor-beta-dependent mouse model of pulmonary hypertension and in systemic sclerosis. Am J Respir Crit Care Med. 2015;191(6):665–77.
69. Ma W, Han W, Greer PA, Tuder RM, Toque HA, Wang KK, et al. Calpain mediates pulmonary vascular remodeling in rodent models of pulmonary hypertension, and its inhibition attenuates pathologic features of disease. J Clin Invest. 2011;121(11):4548–66.
70. Graham BB, Chabon J, Gebreab L, Poole J, Debella E, Davis L, et al. Transforming growth factor-beta signaling promotes pulmonary hypertension caused by Schistosoma mansoni. Circulation. 2013;128(12):1354–64.
71. Reynolds AM, Holmes MD, Danilov SM, Reynolds PN. Targeted gene delivery of BMPR2 attenuates pulmonary hypertension. Eur Respir J. 2012;39(2):329–43.
72. Long L, Ormiston ML, Yang X, Southwood M, Graf S, Machado RD, et al. Selective enhancement of endothelial BMPR-II with BMP9 reverses pulmonary arterial hypertension. Nat Med. 2015;21(7):777–85.
73. MacLean MR, Herve P, Eddahibi S, Adnot S. 5-hydroxytryptamine and the pulmonary circulation: receptors, transporters and relevance to pulmonary arterial hypertension. Br J Pharmacol. 2000;131(2):161–8.
74. Welsh DJ, Harnett M, MacLean M, Peacock AJ. Proliferation and signaling in fibroblasts: role of 5-hydroxytryptamine2A receptor and transporter. Am J Respir Crit Care Med. 2004;170(3):252–9.
75. Lee SL, Wang WW, Lanzillo JJ, Fanburg BL. Serotonin produces both hyperplasia and hypertrophy of bovine pulmonary artery smooth muscle cells in culture. Am J Physiol. 1994;266(1 Pt 1):L46–52.
76. Ren W, Watts SW, Fanburg BL. Serotonin transporter interacts with the PDGFbeta receptor in PDGF-BB-induced signaling and mitogenesis in pulmonary artery smooth muscle cells. Am J Physiol Lung Cell Mol Physiol. 2011;300(3):L486–97.
77. Dees C, Akhmetshina A, Zerr P, Reich N, Palumbo K, Horn A, et al. Platelet-derived serotonin links vascular disease and tissue fibrosis. J Exp Med. 2011;208(5):961–72.

78. Long L, MacLean MR, Jeffery TK, Morecroft I, Yang X, Rudarakanchana N, et al. Serotonin increases susceptibility to pulmonary hypertension in BMPR2-deficient mice. Circ Res. 2006;98(6):818–27.
79. Launay JM, Herve P, Peoc'h K, Tournois C, Callebert J, Nebigil CG, et al. Function of the serotonin 5-hydroxytryptamine 2B receptor in pulmonary hypertension. Nat Med. 2002;8(10):1129–35.
80. Seibold JR, Molony RR, Turkevich D, Ruddy MC, Kostis JB. Acute hemodynamic effects of ketanserin in pulmonary hypertension secondary to systemic sclerosis. J Rheumatol. 1987;14(3):519–24.
81. Antoniu SA. Targeting PDGF pathway in pulmonary arterial hypertension. Expert Opin Ther Targets. 2012;16(11):1055–63.
82. Perros F, Montani D, Dorfmuller P, Durand-Gasselin I, Tcherakian C, Le PJ, et al. Platelet-derived growth factor expression and function in idiopathic pulmonary arterial hypertension. Am J Respir Crit Care Med. 2008;178(1):81–8.
83. Selimovic N, Bergh CH, Andersson B, Sakiniene E, Carlsten H, Rundqvist B. Growth factors and interleukin-6 across the lung circulation in pulmonary hypertension. Eur Respir J. 2009;34(3):662–8.
84. Riccieri V, Stefanantoni K, Vasile M, Macri V, Sciarra I, Iannace N, et al. Abnormal plasma levels of different angiogenic molecules are associated with different clinical manifestations in patients with systemic sclerosis. Clin Exp Rheumatol. 2011;29(2 Suppl 65):S46–52.
85. Overbeek MJ, Boonstra A, Voskuyl AE, Vonk MC, Vonk-Noordegraaf A, van Berkel MP, et al. Platelet-derived growth factor receptor-beta and epidermal growth factor receptor in pulmonary vasculature of systemic sclerosis-associated pulmonary arterial hypertension versus idiopathic pulmonary arterial hypertension and pulmonary veno-occlusive disease: a case-control study. Arthritis Res Ther. 2011;13(2):R61.
86. Baroni SS, Santillo M, Bevilacqua F, Luchetti M, Spadoni T, Mancini M, et al. Stimulatory autoantibodies to the PDGF receptor in systemic sclerosis. N Engl J Med. 2006;354(25):2667–76.
87. Tanaka S, Suto A, Ikeda K, Sanayama Y, Nakagomi D, Iwamoto T, et al. Alteration of circulating miRNAs in SSc: miR-30b regulates the expression of PDGF receptor beta. Rheumatology (Oxford). 2013;52(11):1963–72.
88. Takemura H, Suzuki H, Fujisawa H, Yuhara T, Akama T, Yamane K, et al. Enhanced interleukin 6 production by cultured fibroblasts from patients with systemic sclerosis in response to platelet derived growth factor. J Rheumatol. 1998;25(8):1534–9.
89. Ciuclan L, Hussey MJ, Burton V, Good R, Duggan N, Beach S, et al. Imatinib attenuates hypoxia-induced pulmonary arterial hypertension pathology via reduction in 5-hydroxytryptamine through inhibition of tryptophan hydroxylase 1 expression. Am J Respir Crit Care Med. 2013;187(1):78–89.
90. Hatano M, Yao A, Shiga T, Kinugawa K, Hirata Y, Nagai R. Imatinib mesylate has the potential to exert its efficacy by down-regulating the plasma concentration of platelet-derived growth factor in patients with pulmonary arterial hypertension. Int Heart J. 2010;51(4):272–6.
91. Halka AT, Turner NJ, Carter A, Ghosh J, Murphy MO, Kirton JP, et al. The effects of stretch on vascular smooth muscle cell phenotype in vitro. Cardiovasc Pathol. 2008;17(2):98–102.
92. Nakasu S, Fujisawa H, Minagawa T. Purification of characterization of gene 8 product of bacteriophage T3. Virology. 1985;143(2):422–34.
93. Bou-Gharios G, Ponticos M, Rajkumar V, Abraham D. Extra-cellular matrix in vascular networks. Cell Prolif. 2004;37(3):207–20.
94. Chelladurai P, Seeger W, Pullamsetti SS. Matrix metalloproteinases and their inhibitors in pulmonary hypertension. Eur Respir J. 2012;40(3):766–82.
95. Nagase H, Visse R, Murphy G. Structure and function of matrix metalloproteinases and TIMPs. Cardiovasc Res. 2006;69(3):562–73.
96. Denton CP, Black CM, Abraham DJ. Mechanisms and consequences of fibrosis in systemic sclerosis. Nat Clin Pract Rheumatol. 2006;2(3):134–44.
97. Safdar Z, Tamez E, Chan W, Arya B, Ge Y, Deswal A, et al. Circulating collagen biomarkers as indicators of disease severity in pulmonary arterial hypertension. JACC Heart Fail. 2014;2(4):412–21.
98. Wang Z, Lakes RS, Golob M, Eickhoff JC, Chesler NC. Changes in large pulmonary arterial viscoelasticity in chronic pulmonary hypertension. PLoS ONE. 2013;8(11), e78569.
99. Golledge J, Clancy P, Maguire J, Lincz L, Koblar S. The role of tenascin C in cardiovascular disease. Cardiovasc Res. 2011;92(1):19–28.
100. Wei L, Warburton RR, Preston IR, Roberts KE, Comhair SA, Erzurum SC, et al. Serotonylated fibronectin is elevated in pulmonary hypertension. Am J Physiol Lung Cell Mol Physiol. 2012;302(12):L1273–9.
101. Matsui K, Takano Y, Yu ZX, Hi JE, Stetler-Stevenson WG, Travis WD, et al. Immunohistochemical study of endothelin-1 and matrix metalloproteinases in plexogenic pulmonary arteriopathy. Pathol Res Pract. 2002;198(6):403–12.
102. Vieillard-Baron A, Frisdal E, Raffestin B, Baker AH, Eddahibi S, Adnot S, et al. Inhibition of matrix metalloproteinases by lung TIMP-1 gene transfer limits monocrotaline-induced pulmonary vascular remodeling in rats. Hum Gene Ther. 2003;14(9):861–9.
103. Kim GH, Ryan JJ, Marsboom G, Archer SL. Epigenetic mechanisms of pulmonary hypertension. Pulm Circ. 2011;1(3):347–56.
104. Zhao L, Chen CN, Hajji N, Oliver E, Cotroneo E, Wharton J, et al. Histone deacetylation inhibition in pulmonary hypertension: therapeutic potential of valproic acid and suberoylanilide hydroxamic acid. Circulation. 2012;126(4):455–67.
105. Wang Y, Kahaleh B. Epigenetic repression of bone morphogenetic protein receptor II expression in scleroderma. J Cell Mol Med. 2013;17(10):1291–9.
106. Archer SL, Marsboom G, Kim GH, Zhang HJ, Toth PT, Svensson EC, et al. Epigenetic attenuation of mitochondrial superoxide dismutase 2 in pulmonary arterial hypertension: a basis for excessive cell proliferation and a new therapeutic target. Circulation. 2010;121(24):2661–71.
107. Meloche J, Pflieger A, Vaillancourt M, Graydon C, Provencher S, Bonnet S. miRNAs in PAH: biomarker, therapeutic target or both? Drug Discov Today. 2014;19(8):1264–9.
108. Zhou G, Chen T, Raj JU. MicroRNAs in pulmonary arterial hypertension. Am J Respir Cell Mol Biol. 2015;52(2):139–51.
109. Wallace E, Morrell NW, Yang XD, Long L, Stevens H, Nilsen M, et al. A sex-specific microRNA-96/5-hydroxytryptamine 1B axis influences development of pulmonary hypertension. Am J Respir Crit Care Med. 2015;191(12):1432–42.
110. Kang BY, Park KK, Kleinhenz JM, Murphy TC, Green DE, Bijli KM, et al. PPARgamma activation reduces hypoxia-induced endothelin-1 expression through upregulation of miR-98. Am J Respir Cell Mol Biol. 2015;54(1):136–46.
111. Gou D, Ramchandran R, Peng X, Yao L, Kang K, Sarkar J, et al. miR-210 has an antiapoptotic effect in pulmonary artery smooth muscle cells during hypoxia. Am J Physiol Lung Cell Mol Physiol. 2012;303(8):L682–91.
112. Kim J, Kang Y, Kojima Y, Lighthouse JK, Hu X, Aldred MA, et al. An endothelial apelin-FGF link mediated by miR-424 and miR-503 is disrupted in pulmonary arterial hypertension. Nat Med. 2013;19(1):74–82.
113. Kim J, Hwangbo C, Hu X, Kang Y, Papangeli I, Mehrotra D, et al. Restoration of impaired endothelial myocyte enhancer factor 2

function rescues pulmonary arterial hypertension. Circulation. 2015;131(2):190–9.
114. Courboulin A, Paulin R, Giguère NJ, Saksouk N, Perreault T, Meloche J, et al. Role for miR-204 in human pulmonary arterial hypertension. J Exp Med. 2011;208:535–48.
115. Shimoda LA, Semenza GL. HIF and the lung: role of hypoxia-inducible factors in pulmonary development and disease. Am J Respir Crit Care Med. 2011;183(2):152–6.
116. Yu AY, Shimoda LA, Iyer NV, Huso DL, Sun X, McWilliams R, et al. Impaired physiological responses to chronic hypoxia in mice partially deficient for hypoxia-inducible factor 1 alpha. J Clin Invest. 1999;103(5):691–6.
117. Brusselmans K, Compernolle V, Tjwa M, Wiesener MS, Maxwell PH, Collen D, et al. Heterozygous deficiency of hypoxia-inducible factor-2a protects mice against pulmonary hypertension and right ventricular dysfunction during prolonged hypoxia. J Clin Invest. 2003;111(10):1519–27.
118. Comhair SA, Xu W, Mavrakis L, Aldred MA, Asosingh K, Erzurum SC. Human primary lung endothelial cells in culture. Am J Respir Cell Mol Biol. 2012;46(6):723–30.
119. Masri FA, Xu W, Comhair SA, Asosingh K, Koo M, Vasanji A, et al. Hyperproliferative apoptosis-resistant endothelial cells in idiopathic pulmonary arterial hypertension. Am J Physiol Lung Cell Mol Physiol. 2007;293(3):L548–54.
120. Xu W, Koeck T, Lara AR, Neumann D, DiFilippo FP, Koo M, et al. Alterations of cellular bioenergetics in pulmonary artery endothelial cells. Proc Natl Acad Sci U S A. 2007;104(4):1342–7.
121. Bonnet S, Michelakis ED, Porter CJ, Andrade-Navarro MA, Thebaud B, Bonnet S, et al. An abnormal mitochondrial-hypoxia inducible factor-1 alpha-Kv channel pathway disrupts oxygen sensing and triggers pulmonary arterial hypertension in fawn hooded rats – similarities to human pulmonary arterial hypertension. Circulation. 2006;113(22):2630–41.
122. Tuder RM, Davis LA, Graham BB. Targeting energetic metabolism: a new frontier in the pathogenesis and treatment of pulmonary hypertension. Am J Respir Crit Care Med. 2012;185(3):260–6.
123. Archer SL, Gomberg-Maitland M, Maitland ML, Rich S, Garcia JGN, Weir EK. Mitochondrial metabolism, redox signaling, and fusion: a mitochondria-ROS-HIF-1a}-Kv1.5 O2-sensing pathway at the intersection of pulmonary hypertension and cancer. Am J Physiol Heart Circ Physiol. 2008;294(2):H570–8.
124. Sutendra G, Michelakis ED. The metabolic basis of pulmonary arterial hypertension. Cell Metab. 2014;19(4):558–73.
125. Stenmark KR, Tuder RM, El Kasmi KC. Metabolic reprogramming and inflammation act in concert to control vascular remodeling in hypoxic pulmonary hypertension. J Appl Physiol (1985). 2015; In Press:jap.
126. Sakao S, Taraseviciene-Stewart L, Lee JD, Wood K, Cool CD, Voelkel NF. Initial apoptosis is followed by increased proliferation of apoptosis-resistant endothelial cells. FASEB J. 2005;19(9):1178–80.
127. McMurtry MS, Archer SL, Altieri DC, Bonnet S, Haromy A, Harry G, et al. Gene therapy targeting survivin selectively induces pulmonary vascular apoptosis and reverses pulmonary arterial hypertension. J Clin Invest. 2005;115(6):1479–91.
128. El Kasmi KC, Pugliese SC, Riddle SR, Poth JM, Anderson AL, Frid MG, et al. Adventitial fibroblasts induce a distinct proinflammatory/profibrotic macrophage phenotype in pulmonary hypertension. J Immunol. 2014;193(2):597–609.
129. Lunt SY, Muralidhar V, Hosios AM, Israelsen WJ, Gui DY, Newhouse L, et al. Pyruvate kinase isoform expression alters nucleotide synthesis to impact cell proliferation. Mol Cell. 2015;57(1):95–107.
130. Christofk HR, Vander Heiden MG, Harris MH, Ramanathan A, Gerszten RE, Wei R, et al. The M2 splice isoform of pyruvate kinase is important for cancer metabolism and tumour growth. Nature. 2008;452(7184):230–3.
131. Pearce EL, Pearce EJ. Metabolic pathways in immune cell activation and quiescence. Immunity. 2013;38(4):633–43.
132. Vander Heiden MG, Cantley LC, Thompson CB. Understanding the Warburg effect: the metabolic requirements of cell proliferation. Science. 2009;324(5930):1029–33.
133. Fan J, Ye J, Kamphorst JJ, Shlomi T, Thompson CB, Rabinowitz JD. Quantitative flux analysis reveals folate-dependent NADPH production. Nature. 2014;510(7504):298–302.
134. Schoors S, Bruning U, Missiaen R, Queiroz KC, Borgers G, Elia I, et al. Fatty acid carbon is essential for dNTP synthesis in endothelial cells. Nature. 2015;520(7546):192–7.
135. Zhao L, Ashek A, Wang L, Fang W, Dabral S, Dubois O, et al. Heterogeneity in lung 18FDG uptake in PAH: potential of dynamic 18FDG-PET with kinetic analysis as a bridging biomarker for pulmonary remodeling targeted treatments. Circulation. 2013;128(11):1214–24.
136. Marsboom G, Wietholt C, Haney CR, Toth PT, Ryan JJ, Morrow E, et al. Lung (1)(8)F-fluorodeoxyglucose positron emission tomography for diagnosis and monitoring of pulmonary arterial hypertension. Am J Respir Crit Care Med. 2012;185(6):670–9.
137. McMurtry MS, Bonnet S, Wu X, Dyck JR, Haromy A, Hashimoto K, et al. Dichloroacetate prevents and reverses pulmonary hypertension by inducing pulmonary artery smooth muscle cell apoptosis. Circ Res. 2004;95(8):830–40.
138. Caslin AW, Heath D, Madden B, Yacoub M, Gosney JR, Smith P. The histopathology of 36 cases of plexogenic pulmonary arteriopathy. Histopathology. 1990;16(1):9–19.
139. Tuder RM, Groves BM, Badesch DB, Voelkel NF. Exuberant endothelial cell growth and elements of inflammation are present in plexiform lesions of pulmonary hypertension. Am J Pathol. 1994;144(2):275–85.
140. Savai R, Pullamsetti SS, Kolbe J, Bieniek E, Voswinckel R, Fink L, et al. Immune and inflammatory cell involvement in the pathology of idiopathic pulmonary arterial hypertension. Am J Respir Crit Care Med. 2012;186(9):897–908.
141. Voelkel NF, Tuder RM, Bridges J, Arend WP. Interleukin-1 receptor antagonist treatment reduces pulmonary hypertension generated in rats by monocrotaline. Am J Respir Cell Mol Biol. 1994;11(6):664–75.
142. Humbert M, Monti G, Brenot F, Sitbon O, Portier A, Grangeot-Keros L, et al. Increased interleukin-1 and interleukin-6 serum concentrations in severe primary pulmonary hypertension. Am J Respir Crit Care Med. 1995;151(5):1628–31.
143. Minamino T, Christou H, Hsieh CM, Li Y, Dhawan V, Abraham, et al. Targeted expression of hemeoxygenase-1 prevents the pulmonary inflammatory and vascular responses to hypoxia. Proc Natl Acad Sci U S A. 2001;98(15):8798–803.
144. Rius J, Guma M, Schachtrup C, Akassoglou K, Zinkernagel AS, Nizet V, et al. NF-kappaB links innate immunity to the hypoxic response through transcriptional regulation of HIF-1alpha. Nature. 2008;453(7196):807–11.
145. Farkas D, Alhussaini AA, Kraskauskas D, Kraskauskiene V, Cool CD, Nicolls MR, et al. Nuclear factor kappaB inhibition reduces lung vascular lumen obliteration in severe pulmonary hypertension in rats. Am J Respir Cell Mol Biol. 2014;51(3):413–25.
146. Li L, Wei C, Kim IK, Janssen-Heininger Y, Gupta S. Inhibition of nuclear factor-kappaB in the lungs prevents monocrotaline-induced pulmonary hypertension in mice. Hypertension. 2014;63(6):1260–9.
147. Bonnet S, Rochefort G, Sutendra G, Archer SL, Haromy A, Webster L, et al. The nuclear factor of activated T cells in pulmonary arterial hypertension can be therapeutically targeted. PNAS. 2007;104(27):11418–23.

148. Paulin R, Sutendra G, Gurtu V, Dromparis P, Haromy A, Provencher S, et al. A miR-208-Mef2 axis drives the decompensation of right ventricular function in pulmonary hypertension. Circ Res. 2015;116(1):56–69.
149. Bussone G, Tamby MC, Calzas C, Kherbeck N, Sahbatou Y, Sanson C, et al. IgG from patients with pulmonary arterial hypertension and/or systemic sclerosis binds to vascular smooth muscle cells and induces cell contraction. Ann Rheum Dis. 2012;71(4):596–605.
150. Terrier B, Tamby MC, Camoin L, Guilpain P, Broussard C, Bussone G, et al. Identification of target antigens of antifibroblast antibodies in pulmonary arterial hypertension. Am J Respir Crit Care Med. 2008;177(10):1128–34.
151. Perros F, Dorfmuller P, Montani D, Hammad H, Waelput W, Girerd B, et al. Pulmonary lymphoid neogenesis in idiopathic pulmonary arterial hypertension. Am J Respir Crit Care Med. 2012;185(3):311–21.
152. Colvin KL, Cripe PJ, Ivy DD, Stenmark KR, Yeager ME. Bronchus-associated lymphoid tissue in pulmonary hypertension produces pathologic autoantibodies. Am J Respir Crit Care Med. 2013;188(9):1126–36.
153. Graham BB, Bandeira AP, Morrell NW, Butrous G, Tuder RM. Schistosomiasis-associated pulmonary hypertension: pulmonary vascular disease: the global perspective. Chest. 2010;137(6 Suppl):20S–9.
154. Wynn TA, Chawla A, Pollard JW. Macrophage biology in development, homeostasis and disease. Nature. 2013;496(7446):445–55.
155. Crosby A, Jones FM, Southwood M, Stewart S, Schermuly R, Butrous G, et al. Pulmonary vascular remodeling correlates with lung eggs and cytokines in murine schistosomiasis. Am J Respir Crit Care Med. 2010;181(3):279–88.
156. Graham BB, Mentink-Kane MM, El-Haddad H, Purnell S, Zhang L, Zaiman A, et al. Schistosomiasis-induced experimental pulmonary hypertension: role of interleukin-13 signaling. Am J Pathol. 2010;177(3):1549–61.
157. Soon E, Holmes AM, Treacy CM, Doughty NJ, Southgate L, Machado RD, et al. Elevated levels of inflammatory cytokines predict survival in idiopathic and familial pulmonary arterial hypertension. Circulation. 2010;122(9):920–7.
158. Steiner MK, Syrkina OL, Kolliputi N, Mark EJ, Hales CA, Waxman AB. Interleukin-6 overexpression induces pulmonary hypertension. Circ Res. 2009;104(2):236–44.
159. Savale L, Tu L, Rideau D, Izziki M, Maitre B, Adnot S, et al. Impact of interleukin-6 on hypoxia-induced pulmonary hypertension and lung inflammation in mice. Respir Res. 2009;10:6.
160. Maxova H, Herget J, Vizek M. Lung mast cells and hypoxic pulmonary hypertension. Physiol Res. 2012;61(1):1–11.
161. Montani D, Perros F, Gambaryan N, Girerd B, Dorfmuller P, Price LC, et al. C-kit-positive cells accumulate in remodeled vessels of idiopathic pulmonary arterial hypertension. Am J Respir Crit Care Med. 2011;184(1):116–23.
162. Hoffmann J, Yin J, Kukucka M, Yin N, Saarikko I, Sterner-Kock A, et al. Mast cells promote lung vascular remodelling in pulmonary hypertension. Eur Respir J. 2011;37(6):1400–10.
163. Novotny T, Krejci J, Malikova J, Svehlik V, Wasserbauer R, Uhlik J, et al. Mast cell stabilization with sodium cromoglycate modulates pulmonary vessel wall remodeling during four-day hypoxia in rats. Exp Lung Res. 2015;41(5):283–92.
164. Kay JM, Waymire JC, Grover RF. Lung mast cell hyperplasia and pulmonary histamine-forming capacity in hypoxic rats. Am J Physiol. 1974;226(1):178–84.
165. Galie N, Simonneau G. The Fifth World Symposium on pulmonary hypertension. J Am Coll Cardiol. 2013;62(25 Suppl):D1–3.
166. Nickel NP, Spiekerkoetter E, Gu M, Li CG, Li H, Kaschwich M, et al. Elafin reverses pulmonary hypertension via caveolin-1-dependent bone morphogenetic protein signaling. Am J Respir Crit Care Med. 2015;191(11):1273–86.
167. Spiekerkoetter E, Tian X, Cai J, Hopper RK, Sudheendra D, Li CG, et al. FK506 activates BMPR2, rescues endothelial dysfunction, and reverses pulmonary hypertension. J Clin Invest. 2013;123(8):3600–13.
168. Saker M, Lipskaia L, Marcos E, Abid S, Parpaleix A, Houssaini A et al. Osteopontin, a Key Mediator Expressed by Senescent Pulmonary Vascular Cells in Pulmonary Hypertension. Arterioscler Thromb Vasc Biol 2016;36(9):1879–90.
169. Good RB, Gilbane AJ, Trinder SL, Denton CP, Coghlan G, Abraham DJ, et al. Endothelial to Mesenchymal Transition Contributes to Endothelial Dysfunction in Pulmonary Arterial Hypertension. Am J Pathol 2015;185(7):1850–8.
170. Hoffmann J, Wilhelm J, Marsh LM, Ghanim B, Klepetko W, Kovacs G, et al. Distinct differences in gene expression patterns in pulmonary arteries of patients with chronic obstructive pulmonary disease and idiopathic pulmonary fibrosis with pulmonary hypertension. Am J Respir Crit Care Med 2014;190(1):98–111.
171. Chelladurai P, Seeger W, Pullamsetti SS. Matrix metalloproteinases and their inhibitors in pulmonary hypertension. Eur Respir J 2012;40(3):766–82.
172. Wei L, Warburton RR, Preston IR, Roberts KE, Comhair SA, Erzurum SC, et al. Serotonylated fibronectin is elevated in pulmonary hypertension. Am J Physiol Lung Cell Mol Physiol 2012 15;302(12):L1273–L1279.
173. Schumann C, Lepper PM, Frank H, Schneiderbauer R, Wibmer T, Kropf C, et al. Circulating biomarkers of tissue remodelling in pulmonary hypertension. Biomarkers 2010;15(6):523–32.
174. Geraci MW, Moore M, Gesell T, Yeager ME, Alger L, Golpon H, et al. Gene expression patterns in the lungs of patients with primary pulmonary hypertension: a gene microarray analysis. Circ Res 2001;88(6):555–62.

Clinical Assessment of Pulmonary Hypertension

27

Harrison W. Farber and Marc Humbert

Introduction

Pulmonary arterial hypertension (PAH) is primarily a disease due to pulmonary vascular remodeling predominating on pulmonary arteries of less than 500 μm of diameter. PAH is a frequent complication of systemic sclerosis (SSc) observed with a prevalence of 8–12 % [1–4]. In order to diagnose PAH, it is necessary to establish the appropriate cardiopulmonary hemodynamics: mean pulmonary artery pressure (mPAP) ≥25 mmHg, pulmonary capillary wedge pressure (PCWP) or left ventricular end-diastolic pressure ≤15 mmHg, and a pulmonary vascular resistance (PVR) >3 Wood units. Currently, the only available method for detecting and assessing these and other important cardiopulmonary hemodynamic parameters (i.e., cardiac output) is RHC. Thus, RHC should be performed in all cases in which PAH is suspected. RHC will confirm the presence of pulmonary hypertension (PH) and its pre and/or postcapillary mechanisms. RHC enables the establishment of a specific diagnosis of PAH, rules out other cardiac etiologies such as left ventricular failure, and assesses the degree of right heart dysfunction [5].

Within the last two decades, pulmonary fibrosis and PAH have become the leading causes of morbidity and mortality in SSc patients [6]. The estimated 3-year survival among patients with PAH associated with SSc (SSc-PAH) is approximately 50 % [7]. The development of PAH in SSc must be differentiated from PH due to chronic lung disease (pulmonary fibrosis) and/or hypoxia. Distinguishing PAH from PH due to pulmonary fibrosis is not always easy, especially since some patients can have both pulmonary fibrosis and a true pulmonary vasculopathy. However, if lung volumes (forced vital capacity, FVC, and/or total lung capacity, TLC) are <60 % of the predicted value and mPAP <35 mmHg at rest, PH is deemed more likely related to pulmonary fibrosis [8]. When lung volumes (CPT and/or CVF) are >70 % of the predicted value, the PH is considered more likely to be PAH. When lung volumes (CPT and/or CVF) are between 60 % and 70 % of the predicted value, the diagnosis becomes more difficult; however, if mPAP is >35 mmHg, the PH is considered severe and most probably reflects a true pulmonary artery microangiopathy. Nevertheless, as noted, PH due to hypoxia/lung fibrosis and PAH may coexist in SSc patients. In this chapter, we will mainly focus on PAH.

Epidemiology

PAH is a frequent complication of SSc [1–4]. A meta-analysis of more than 3,500 SSc patients showed that PAH prevalence in SSc, based on gold standard RHC definition, is slightly less than 10 % [4]. The incidence of SSc-PAH has been estimated in a large, multicenter cohort study of SSc patients using a revised screening algorithm for PAH diagnosis based on dyspnea and Doppler echocardiographic evaluation of tricuspid regurgitant jet velocity (TRJ) for referral of patients to RHC [9]. The overall incidence of PH was 1.37 cases per 100 patient-years [95 % confidence interval 0.74–2.00] corresponding to PAH in 0.61 cases per 100 patient-years. Postcapillary PH had a similar incidence of 0.61 cases per 100 patient-years emphasizing the importance of a complete workup to rule out left heart disease in SSc patients presenting with PH [9]. Lastly, PH due to pulmonary fibrosis had an incidence of 0.15 cases per 100 patient-years. In all cases, it should be emphasized that RHC is mandatory for PAH diagnosis, as well as excluding a diagnosis of postcapillary PH.

PAH is generally considered a late complication of SSc [10]. Previous reports of the duration between diagnosis of SSc and onset of PAH vary according to study, ranging from

H.W. Farber, MD
Pulmonary Hypertension Center, Boston University Medical Center, Boston, MA, USA

M. Humbert, MD, PhD (✉)
Department of Respiratory Medicine, Hôpital Bicêtre, Paris, France
e-mail: marc.humbert@bct.aphp.fr

J. Varga et al. (eds.), *Scleroderma*, DOI 10.1007/978-3-319-31407-5_27

9.1 ± 6.6 years [11] to 14 ± 5 years [2]. Another study showed that PAH diagnosis occurred 6.3 ± 6.6 years after the first non-Raynaud's phenomenon symptom of SSc and that PAH can occur at any time following the diagnosis of SSc (in about half of cases within the first 5 years following the first non-Raynaud's symptom) [12]. In this study, patients with early-onset PAH (within the first 5 years following the first non-Raynaud's symptom) were older at the time of SSc diagnosis, with more severe pulmonary vascular disease and with a lower cardiac index and higher PVR than in patients with late-onset PAH.

Patients with limited cutaneous SSc are generally considered at greater risk of PAH than patients with diffuse cutaneous SSc [13–15]. However, diagnosis of PAH is often not based on RHC in these studies, and therefore, false-positive diagnosis of PAH or existence of postcapillary PH cannot be excluded in a significant proportion of cases. The frequency of diffuse cutaneous SSc observed in several registries is around 25 % [2, 14], indicating that PAH should not be considered to be a specific vascular complication of limited cutaneous SSc alone.

Risk Factors

All subsets of SSc are at risk for development of PAH. However, several PAH risk factors have been shown in SSc, including the number of telangiectasias [16–18], reduced capillary nail fold density [16, 19], anticentromere antibodies, anti-topoisomerase antibodies, male gender, underlying pulmonary fibrosis, and Raynaud's phenomenon of greater than 3 years duration. SSc duration as a risk factor is more controversial, as indicated before [10–12, 16]. Other manifestations of SSc vasculopathy, such as digital ulcers, scleroderma renal crisis, and digital ischemia, have also been regarded as potential risk factors for development of PAH; however, a study of 938 SSc patients found no association between digital ulcers or digital ischemia and development of PAH [20]. The strong association of PAH with >10 telangiectasias and the lack of clear association with digital ulcers, renal crisis, and digital ischemia suggest a shared pathogenesis with microvascular rather than macrovascular manifestations of SSc.

Screening: Why Is PAH Screening Needed in Scleroderma Patients?

PAH is a progressive disease with a poor prognosis, and SSc-PAH is particularly aggressive, accounting for 30 % of deaths among SSc patients [21]. If left untreated, SSc-PAH is associated with a median survival time of 1 year following diagnosis [22, 23]. Recent advances in diagnostic techniques and the emergence of evidence-based therapies for PAH facilitate earlier detection of the disease and, thus, earlier initiation of effective treatment. Early detection of PAH and prompt initiation of effective therapy are considered an essential component of disease management, as patients diagnosed earlier in the course of the disease have a more pronounced benefit from therapy [24, 25].

The predisposition of SSc patients to develop PAH as a complication means that with regular screening, the early diagnosis of PAH may be a realistic possibility in this patient population. Without screening, data from the French National Registry have shown that the majority of patients are diagnosed in New York Heart Association (NYHA) functional class (FC) III or IV and, as such, are already severely compromised [26]. Diagnosis of PAH in NYHA FC I or II is challenging, and even when patients become symptomatic, symptoms such as dyspnea and fatigue are nonspecific, and patients remain difficult to identify. Therefore, despite the potential for earlier diagnosis, in reality SSc-PAH is still frequently identified late, with more than two-thirds of patients in NYHA FC III or IV at the time of diagnosis [9, 27, 28]. Of note, data from the French Registry have showed that, compared with patients in routine clinical practice, PAH detection programs in SSc are able to identify patients with milder forms of the disease, allowing earlier management and better outcomes: the 1-, 3-, 5-, and 8-year survival rates were 75 %, 31 %, 25 %, and 17 %, respectively, in the routine practice cohort, compared with 100 %, 81 %, 73 %, and 64 %, respectively, in the detection cohort ($p = 0.0037$) [29].

How Should PAH Screening Be Accomplished in Scleroderma Patients?

Screening is the systematic application of a test to identify individuals at sufficient risk of a specific disorder to warrant further investigation or direct preventive action, among persons who have not sought medical attention on account of symptoms of that disorder [29, 30]. Therefore, screening for PH/PAH applies to asymptomatic individuals belonging to groups in which PH/PAH is highly prevalent, such as SSc. Echocardiography is currently the most effective screening tool to suspect PAH in SSc. For example, the 2009 ESC/ERS diagnostic algorithm in SSc patients with suspected PAH is based on the maximal TRJ velocity [5]:

1. A patient with a TRJ of ≤2.8 m/s or systolic PAP (sPAP) of ≤36 mmHg (assuming mean right atrial pressure [mRA is ≤5 mmHg) is unlikely to have PH, and RHC based on these measurements is not justified.
2. A patient with a TRJ of >3.4 m/s or sPAP of >50 mmHg is likely to have PH, and RHC is indicated to confirm the diagnosis.

3. In patients with a TRJ between these extremes (i.e., 2.9–3.4 m/s), other additional indicators of PH should be considered, and clinical judgment is required as to whether RHC is warranted.

This algorithm is relatively easy to follow, and using a slight adaptation of this, it has been possible to detect PAH in SSc patients following RHC dependent upon both echocardiographic readings and the presence or absence of dyspnea. Importantly, by using this adapted algorithm, 56.3 % of patients were diagnosed in NYHA FC II [1, 9] (Fig. 27.1).

There are other structural and functional echocardiographic features that could be used to indicate the need for diagnostic RHC in addition to criteria based on TRJ velocity. These signs provide assessment of the RV size and pressure overload, pattern of blood flow velocity out of the right ventricle, diameter of the pulmonary artery, and an estimate of right atrial pressure [5]. Resting echocardiography is recommended as a screening test in asymptomatic SSc patients, followed by annual screening with echocardiography, DLCO, and biomarkers [5, 30]. Importantly, exercise echocardiography has technical and methodological limitations and is not recommended for PH/PAH screening [5].

Additional clinical information that may be indicative of PH is a diffusing capacity for carbon monoxide (DLCO) of <60 % of the predicted value in the absence of extensive interstitial lung disease (i.e., disease extent on HRCT >20 % and/or FVC <70 % of the predicted value) [30, 31]. As reported by Steen et al. [21], DLCO may be significantly decreased <60 % of normal for many years prior to the occurrence of PAH. In contrast, although one sixth of PAH-SSc patients have a DLCO >60 % at PAH diagnosis, a DLCO >80 % of the predicted value may exclude the diagnosis of PAH [12].

N-terminal pro-brain natriuretic peptide (NT-proBNP) levels are also significantly correlated with RHC results [2]. Even with a normal echocardiogram, NT-proBNP levels >3× the upper limit of normal is highly suggestive of PH. Elevated NT-proBNP levels may be predictive of PAH development in SSc patients [32], and as NT-proBNP detection is simple and noninvasive, it may be an attractive screening tool used alongside other parameters [30]. However, increased NT-proBNP levels are not specific of PAH, and elevated BNP or NT-proBNP levels do not differentiate left from right heart disease and cannot differentiate pre- from postcapillary PH. Moreover, normal NT-proBNP levels do not exclude PAH [33].

The DETECT study has proposed to refine the screening process in SSc patients at increased risk of PAH (defined as SSc patients known for >3 years and DLCO <60 % of the predicted value) [34]. These patients underwent a broad panel of noninvasive assessments followed by RHC. Of 466 SSc patients at increased risk of PAH, 87 (19 %) had RHC-confirmed PAH. PAH was NYHA FC I/II in 64 % of cases. A two-step composite score has been proposed in the DETECT study to select patients who should have a RHC [34]: six simple assessments in step 1 of the algorithm determined referral to echocardiography; then, in step 2, the step 1 prediction score and two echocardiographic variables determined referral to RHC. The DETECT algorithm recommended RHC in 62 % of patients (referral rate) and missed 4 % of PAH patients (false negatives). By comparison, applying ESC/ERS 2009 guidelines to these patients [5], 29 % of diagnoses were missed while requiring a RHC referral rate of 40 %. Long-term follow-up and outcomes have not been reported in the DETECT study [34].

RHC in SSc patients may show borderline elevations in mPAP (ranging from 21 to 24 mmHg). A recent study has

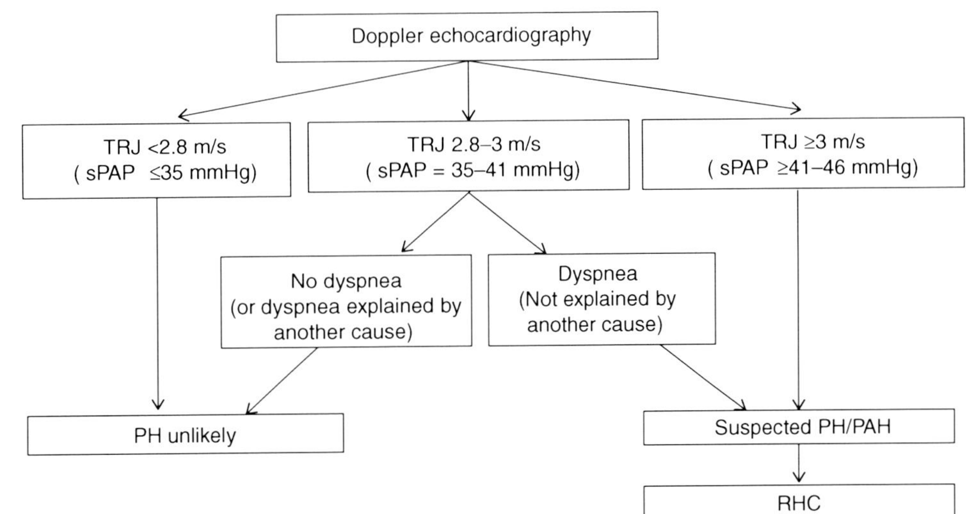

Fig. 27.1 Screening protocol for SSc patients. *TRJ* tricuspid regurgitant jet, *sPAP* systolic pulmonary arterial pressure, *PAH* pulmonary arterial hypertension, *PH* pulmonary hypertension, *RHC* right heart catheterization (Adapted from Hachulla et al. [9])

attempted to determine whether these patients are more likely to develop PH than those in whom mPAP is in the normal range [35]. Follow-up of a large monocenter cohort of SSc patients including 86 with borderline mPAP at baseline demonstrated that 29 of these patients later developed PH (of whom two cases were related to left heart disease). Patients with borderline mPAP were more likely to develop PH than patients with mPAP ≤20 mmHg (hazard ratio 3.7). A transpulmonary gradient (mPAP–PCWP) ≥11 mmHg at baseline also predicted progression to PH (hazard ratio 7.9). Of note, incident development of PAH was not benign, with a mortality of 18% within 3 years. Thus SSc patients with borderline mPAP and an elevated transpulmonary gradient are more likely to progress to PH. These patients should be monitored closely for the development of PH [35].

Diagnosis and Evaluation

Patients with SSc-PAH tend to be asymptomatic early in the disease or only have symptoms related to involvement of other organs by SSc. Clinical symptoms are nonspecific, including progressive dyspnea with exertion and fatigue which are the most common initial presentation. However, functional impairment may be confounded by overall dysfunction from SSc, concomitant musculoskeletal disease, and lack of fitness. Physical examination findings may be absent early in the disease. Clinical findings include loud pulmonic component of the second heart sound and pulmonic/tricuspid regurgitant murmur.

Signs of right ventricular dysfunction become more evident as the disease progresses. Syncope, dyspnea at rest, chest pain, jugular vein extension, peripheral edema, and ascites generally indicate the development of right heart failure (Table 27.1) [36].

Diagnosis of PAH is suggested, in part, through the exclusion of other diseases. Pulmonary function testing, including measurement of DLCO, chest X-ray, ventilation/perfusion lung scintigraphy (and CT pulmonary angiography if needed), high-resolution computed tomography (HRCT) of the chest, echocardiography, laboratory testing for underlying diseases, and ECG are all employed for further signs of PAH or to diagnose a separate underlying cause.

As indicated above, RHC is the gold standard for diagnosis of PAH, as well as providing prognostic parameters, such as cardiac index/output and right atrial pressure. Direct cardiac involvement can occur in SSc, affecting the myocardium, pericardium, and/or small intramyocardial vessels by vascular, fibrotic, and inflammatory changes. There is thus a higher prevalence of systolic left ventricular dysfunction compared with idiopathic PAH [9]. Patients with left heart disease may present with postcapillary PH (elevated PCWP). If PCWP is normal at baseline and left heart disease remains suspected, a fluid-loading test (or RHC at exercise) may be performed to identify diastolic left ventricle dysfunction which is common in patients with SSc [5, 37]. If appropriate, a left heart catheterization will allow better evaluation of an underlying left heart disease [37]. SSc-PAH patients more commonly present with pericardial effusion compared to idiopathic PAH, although it remains unknown whether the effusions are related to progressive right ventricular dysfunction or to the underlying inflammatory processes.

Pulmonary veno-occlusive disease (PVOD) is a less commonly recognized cause of precapillary PH in SSc but is not rare in SSc [38, 39]. When PVOD exists in SSc, it may lead to hydrostatic pulmonary edema without left ventricle dysfunction, frequently after treatment with pulmonary vasodilators [39]. Compared with isolated PAH, patients with PVOD often present with more severe hypoxemia and a more pronounced decrease of DLCO [39]. HRCT of the chest demonstrating centrilobular ground-glass opacities, increased septal lines, and lymph node enlargement is suggestive of PVOD in the setting of PH [39]. Similarly, occult alveolar hemorrhage on bronchoalveolar lavage in patients with PH is suggestive of PVOD. The diagnosis of PVOD is important, since pulmonary vasodilators are usually contraindicated in this form of PAH, and lung transplantation is the treatment of choice.

Table 27.1 Clinical manifestations of PAH – primary symptom is dyspnea [36]

Preclinical	Symptomatic	Declining
Few symptoms manifest or are mistaken for lack of fitness	Increasing dyspnea on exertion	Dyspnea at rest
	Decreasing exercise tolerance	Severe impairment of exercise tolerance
	Fatigue	Hypoxemia
		Syncope
		Chest pain
		Edema
		Right heart failure
NYHA functional class I	NYHA functional class II–III	NYHA functional class IV

Natural History

The natural history of SSc-PAH is subclinical progression of pulmonary vascular injury and its consequences on the right side of the heart until dyspnea results. Once PAH has been recognized, the median survival before pulmonary vasodilator therapy was available was as low as 1–3 years [22, 23]. The eventual cause of death in SSc-PAH is usually the result of right heart failure [40]. As such, the combination of interstitial lung disease and SSc-PAH portends a much worse

Table 27.2 Prognosis factors according to recommendations [29]

Better prognosis	Determinants of prognosis	Worse prognosis
No	Clinical signs of right ventricular failure	Yes
Slow	Progression	Fast
No	Syncope	Yes
I, II	NYHA functional class	IV
>500 m	Walk test 6 min	<300 m
VO_2 max >15 mL/min/kg	Cardiopulmonary function	VO_2 max <12 mL/min/kg
Normal or quasi-normal	BNP/NT-proBNP (plasma rate)	Very high and increasing
No pericardial effusion	Echocardiography	Pericardial effusion
TAPSE >2.0 cm		TAPSE <1.5 cm
RAP <8 mmHg and CI ≥2.5 L/min/m^2	Hemodynamics	RAP >15 mmHg or CI ≤2.0 L/min/m^2

BNP brain natriuretic peptide, *CI* cardiac index, *6MWT* 6-min walk test, *RAP* right atrial pressure, *TAPSE* tricuspid annular plane systolic excursion, *NYHA* New York Heart Association

prognosis than isolated SSc-PAH; indeed, two large studies have shown <50 % survival at 2 years in patients with both entities [2, 40].

Prognosis

Before specific PAH treatment era, the 3-year survival rate for patients with SSc-PAH was less than 35 % [21]. Survival in two groups of matched patients with SSc-PAH has been recently reported: those treated with conventional medical therapy and prostanoids if needed (historical control group) and those treated with oral first-line treatment (current treatment era) [41]. Survival at 1 year was 68 % in the historical control group, compared with 81 % in the current treatment era group; the 2-year survival rates were 47 % and 71 %, respectively.

Mukerjee et al. reported that the prognosis of SSc-PAH is better if mPAP is mildly elevated at diagnosis. In patients with mPAP <32 mmHg, survival rates were 93 % and 78 % at 1 and 2 years, respectively [2]. Although one cannot rule out lead-time bias, these observations, as well as those reported above from the French Registry [29], indicate that early detection of PAH may improve prognosis. Earlier diagnosis of PAH is a sine qua non condition for earlier management; however, whether earlier diagnosis is associated with increased life expectancy in SSc patients is not yet known.

Table 27.2 indicates signs and symptoms associated with prognosis and may guide clinical management.

However, these prognosis factors have been extrapolated from patients with idiopathic PAH and may not be pertinent or achievable in patients with SSc-PAH (i.e., 6-min walk test >500 m) because of associated comorbidities, muscular involvement, and lower limb ischemia [42]. Moreover, there are multiple causes of dyspnea in SSc that may mask the intensity of dyspnea due to PAH [43]. It appears therefore necessary to identify specific SSc-PAH goals. However, if a patient with SSc-PAH remains in NYHA FC I/II after 4 months of treatment, prognosis is relatively good compared with patients who have deteriorated to NYHA FC III/IV during this period ($p = 0.007$). A cardiac index >2.71 L/min/m^2 is also associated with a better prognosis than a cardiac index of <2.71 L/min/m^2 ($p = 0.03$) [44]. Therefore, monitoring RHC 4 months after initiation of PAH therapy is recommended. If dyspnea or functional class status is not improved to appropriate levels and/or if cardiac index remains low, more aggressive therapy should be considered.

Prognosis in SSc-PAH Is Worse than in Idiopathic PAH

Although the manifestations of PAH in SSc are similar to those in patients with PAH due to other etiologies, several independent studies have demonstrated increased morbidity and mortality in patients with SSc-PAH compared to patients with idiopathic PAH [7, 22]. Data from the REVEAL registry have showed that, compared to patients with idiopathic PAH and other forms of PAH, connective tissue disease-associated PAH patients had more favorable hemodynamics at right heart catheterization yet had worse 6MWD, higher BNP levels, increased likelihood of pericardial effusion, and worse 1-year survival [45]. Of the connective tissue disease-associated PAH, SSc-PAH had the worst prognosis and was associated with increased BNP levels, decreased DLCO, and increased mortality. These observations could be explained, in part, by the 50–80 % incidence of concomitant interstitial lung disease in the SSc-PAH patients. Patients with SSc are also more likely to be chronically ill, have nutritional deficiencies from gastrointestinal involvement, and often have subclinical cardiac involvement with an increased propensity to arrhythmias. Therefore, increased mortality observed in SSc-PAH is most likely a result of a combination of factors: the presence of comorbidities in SSc-PAH and/or differences in the pathogenesis of PAH leading to a more severe phenotype in SSc-PAH. Supporting the latter possibility are observations of unique gene expression profiles in patients with IPAH and SSc-PAH in both lung tissue [26, 46] and peripheral blood cells [47, 48].

References

1. Hachulla E, Gressin V, Guillevin L, et al. Early detection of pulmonary arterial hypertension in systemic sclerosis: a French nationwide prospective multicenter study. Arthritis Rheum. 2005;52:3792–800.
2. Mukerjee D, St George D, Coleiro B, et al. Prevalence and outcome in systemic sclerosis associated pulmonary arterial hypertension: application of a registry approach. Ann Rheum Dis. 2003;62:1088–93.
3. Phung S, Strange G, Chung LP, et al. Prevalence of pulmonary arterial hypertension in an Australian scleroderma population: screening allows for earlier diagnosis. Intern Med J. 2009;39:682–91.
4. Avouac J, Airo P, Meune C, Beretta L, Dieude P, Caramaschi P, Tiev K, et al. Prevalence of pulmonary hypertension in systemic sclerosis in European Caucasians and metaanalysis of 5 studies. J Rheumatol. 2010;37:2290–8.
5. Galiè N, the Task Force for Diagnosis and Treatment of Pulmonary Hypertension of European Society of Cardiology (ESC), European Respiratory Society (ERS), International Society of Heart and Lung Transplantation (ISHLT). Guidelines for the diagnosis and treatment of pulmonary hypertension. Eur Respir J. 2009;34:1219–63.
6. Steen VD, Medsger TA. Changes in causes of death in systemic sclerosis, 1972–2002. Ann Rheum Dis. 2007;66:940–4.
7. Fisher MR, Mathai SC, Champion HC, et al. Clinical differences between idiopathic and scleroderma-related pulmonary hypertension. Arthritis Rheum. 2006;54:3043–50.
8. Simonneau G, Gatzoulis MA, Adatia I, Celermajer D, Denton C, Ghofrani A, et al. Updated clinical classification of pulmonary hypertension. J Am Coll Cardiol. 2013;62:D34–41.
9. Hachulla E, de Groote P, Gressin V, et al. The three-year incidence of pulmonary arterial hypertension associated with systemic sclerosis in a multicenter nationwide longitudinal study in France. Arthritis Rheum. 2009;60:1831–9.
10. Medsger Jr TA. Natural history of systemic sclerosis and the assessment of disease activity, severity, functional status, and psychologic well-being. Rheum Dis Clin N Am. 2003;29:255–73.
11. Coral-Alvarado P, Rojas-Villarraga A, Latorre MC, et al. Risk factors associated with pulmonary arterial hypertension in Colombian patients with systematic sclerosis: review of the literature. J Rheumatol. 2008;35:244–50.
12. Hachulla E, Launay D, Mouthon L, et al. Is pulmonary arterial hypertension really a late complication of systemic sclerosis? Chest. 2009;136:1211–9.
13. Chang B, Schachna L, White B, et al. Natural history of mild-moderate pulmonary hypertension and the risk factors for severe pulmonary hypertension in scleroderma. J Rheumatol. 2006;33:269–74.
14. MacGregor AJ, Canavan R, Knight C, et al. Pulmonary hypertension in systemic sclerosis: risk factors for progression and consequences for survival. Rheumatology. 2001;40:453–9.
15. Scorza R, Caronni M, Bazzi S, et al. Post-menopause is the main risk factor for developing isolated pulmonary hypertension in systemic sclerosis. Ann N Y Acad Sci. 2002;966:238–46.
16. Cox SR, Walker JG, Coleman M, et al. Isolated pulmonary hypertension in scleroderma. Int Med J. 2005;35:28–33.
17. Robert-Thomson PJ, Mould TL, Walker JG, Smith MD, Ahern MJ. Clinical utility of telangiectasia of hands in scleroderma and other rheumatic disorders. Asian Pac J Allergy Immunol. 2002;20:7–12.
18. Shah AA, Wigley FM, Hummers LK. Telangiectases in scleroderma: a potential clinical marker of pulmonary arterial hypertension. J Rheumatol. 2010;37:98–104.
19. Ong YY, Nikoloutsopoulos T, Bond CP, Smith MD, Ahern MJ, Roberts-Thomson PJ. Decreased nailfold capillary density in limited scleroderma with pulmonary hypertension. Asian Pac J Allergy Immunol. 1998;16:81–6.
20. Khimdas S, Harding S, Bonner A, Zummer B, Baron M, Pope J. Associations with digital ulcers in a large cohort of systemic sclerosis: results from the Canadian Scleroderma Research Group registry. Arthritis Care Res. 2011;63:142–9.
21. Steen V, Medsger Jr TA. Predictors of isolated pulmonary hypertension in patients with systemic sclerosis and limited cutaneous involvement. Arthritis Rheum. 2003;48:516–22.
22. Kawut SM, Taichman DB, Archer-Chicko CL, Palevsky HI, Kimmel SE. Hemodynamics and survival in patients with pulmonary arterial hypertension related to systemic sclerosis. Chest. 2003;123:344–50.
23. Koh ET, Lee P, Gladman DD, Abu-Shakra M. Pulmonary hypertension in systemic sclerosis: an analysis of 17 patients. Br J Rheumatol. 1996;35:989–93.
24. McLaughlin VV, Shillington A, Rich S. Survival in primary pulmonary hypertension: the impact of epoprostenol therapy. Circulation. 2002;106:1477–82.
25. Sitbon O, Humbert M, Nunes H, et al. Long-term intravenous epoprostenol infusion in primary pulmonary hypertension: prognostic factors and survival. J Am Coll Cardiol. 2002;40:780–8.
26. Humbert M, Sitbon O, Chaouat A, et al. Pulmonary arterial hypertension in France: results from a national registry. Am J Respir Crit Care Med. 2006;173:1023–30.
27. Condliffe R, Kiely DG, Peacock AJ, Corris PA, Gibbs JS, Vrapi F, Das C, Elliot CA, Johnson M, DeSoyza J, Torpy C, Goldsmith K, Hodgkins D, Hughes RJ, Pepke-Zaba J, Coghlan JG. Connective tissue disease-associated pulmonary arterial hypertension in the modern treatment era. Am J Respir Crit Care Med. 2009;179:151–7.
28. Hachulla E, Carpentier P, Gressin V, et al. Risk factors for death and the 3-year survival of patients with systemic sclerosis: the French ItinérAIR-Sclérodermie study. Rheumatology (Oxford). 2009;48:304–8.
29. Humbert M, Yaici A, de Groote P, Montani D, Sitbon O, Launay D, et al. Screening for pulmonary arterial hypertension in patients with systemic sclerosis: clinical characteristics at diagnosis and long-term survival. Arthritis Rheum. 2011;63:3522–30.
30. Khanna D, Gladue H, Channick R, Chung L, Distler O, Furst DE, et al. Recommendations for screening and detection of connective-tissue disease associated pulmonary arterial hypertension. Arthritis Rheum. 2013;65:3194–201.
31. Goh NS, Desai SR, Veeraraghavan S, et al. Interstitial lung disease in systemic sclerosis: a simple staging system. Am J Respir Crit Care Med. 2008;177:1248–54.
32. Allanore Y, Borderie D, Avouac J, Zerkak D, Meune C, Hachulla E, et al. High N-terminal pro-brain natriuretic peptide levels and low diffusing capacity for carbon monoxide as independent predictors of the occurrence of precapillary pulmonary arterial hypertension in patients with systemic sclerosis. Arthritis Rheum. 2008;58:284–91.
33. Cavagna L, Caporali R, Klersy C, Ghio S, Albertini R, Scelsi L, Moratti R, Bonino C, Montecucco C. Comparison of brain natriuretic peptide (BNP) and NT-proBNP in screening for pulmonary arterial hypertension in patients with systemic sclerosis. J Rheumatol. 2010;37:2064–70.
34. Coghlan JG, Denton CP, Gruenig E, Bonderman D, Distler O, Khanna D, et al. Evidence-based detection of pulmonary arterial hypertension in systemic sclerosis: the DETECT study. Ann Rheum Dis. 2014;73:1340–9.
35. Valerio CJ, Schreiber BE, Handler CE, Denton CP, Coghlan JG. Borderline mean pulmonary artery pressure in patients with systemic sclerosis: transpulmonary gradient predicts risk of developing pulmonary hypertension. Arthritis Rheum. 2013;65:1074–84.
36. Rich S. Primary pulmonary hypertension. Prog Cardiovasc Dis. 1988;31:205.
37. Fox BD, Shimony A, Langleben D, Hirsch A, Rudski L, Schlesinger R, et al. High prevalence of occult left heart disease in scleroderma-pulmonary hypertension. Eur Respir J. 2013;42:1083–91.

38. Dorfmüller P, Humbert M, Perros F, et al. Fibrous remodeling of the pulmonary venous system in pulmonary arterial hypertension associated with connective tissue diseases. Hum Pathol. 2007;38:893–902.
39. Günther S, Jaïs X, Maitre S, Bérezné A, Dorfmüller P, Seferian A, et al. Computed tomography findings of pulmonary veno-occlusive disease in scleroderma patients presenting with precapillary pulmonary hypertension. Arthritis Rheum. 2012;64:2995–3005.
40. Mathai SC, Hummers LK, Champion HC, et al. Survival in pulmonary hypertension associated with the scleroderma spectrum of diseases: impact of interstitial lung disease. Arthritis Rheum. 2009;60:569–77.
41. Williams MH, Das C, Handler CE, et al. Systemic sclerosis associated pulmonary hypertension: improved survival in the current era. Heart. 2006;92:926–32.
42. Impens AJ, Wangkaew S, Seibold JR. The 6-minute walk test in scleroderma–how measuring everything measures nothing. Rheumatology (Oxford). 2008;47 Suppl 5:v68–9.
43. Hachulla E, Bervar JF, Launay D, Lamblin N, Perez T, Mouthon L, et al. Dyspnea upon exertion in systemic scleroderma: from symptom to etiological diagnosis. Presse Med. 2009;38:911–26.
44. Launay D, Sitbon O, Le Pavec J, et al. Long-term outcome of systemic sclerosis-associated pulmonary arterial hypertension treated with bosentan as first-line monotherapy followed or not by the addition of prostanoids or sildenafil. Rheumatology. 2010;49:490–500.
45. Chung L, Liu J, Parsons L, et al. Characterization of connective tissue disease-associated pulmonary arterial hypertension from REVEAL: identifying systemic sclerosis as a unique phenotype. Chest. 2010;138:1383–94.
46. Hsu E, Shi H, Jordan RM, Lyons-Weiler J, Pilewski JM, Feghali-Bostwick CA. Lung tissues in patients with systemic sclerosis have gene expression patterns unique to pulmonary fibrosis and pulmonary hypertension. Arthritis Rheum. 2011;63:783–94.
47. Christmann RB, Hayes E, Pendergrass S, et al. Interferon and alternative activation of macrophage/monocytes in systemic sclerosis-associated pulmonary arterial hypertension. Arthritis Rheum. 2011;63:1718–28.
48. Pendergrass SA, Hayes E, Farina G, et al. Limited systemic sclerosis patients with pulmonary arterial hypertension show biomarkers of inflammation and vascular injury. PLoS One. 2010;5(8):e12106.

The Management of Pulmonary Arterial Hypertension in the Setting of Systemic Sclerosis

28

Stephen C. Mathai and N. Nazzareno Galié

Definition and Classification of Pulmonary Hypertension in Systemic Sclerosis

Pulmonary hypertension is a chronic disease of the pulmonary vasculature characterized by pulmonary vascular injury and remodeling that leads to increased pulmonary vascular resistance, right ventricular failure, and, ultimately, death [1]. PH can develop in association with many different diseases, including connective tissue diseases (CTD) such as SSc, systemic lupus erythematosus, and mixed connective tissue disease, and can result from processes that primarily affect organ systems distinct from the pulmonary vasculature, such as the heart, lung parenchyma, liver, skin, and kidneys [2]. Direct pulmonary vascular involvement can occur from pulmonary embolism and from pulmonary vascular remodeling in response to endothelial damage without overt venous thromboembolism, known as pulmonary arterial hypertension (PAH).

PH is defined by mean pulmonary artery pressure ≥25 mmHg and thus can only be diagnosed by right heart catheterization. PH is currently classified into one of five groups based upon associated diseases and risk factors [3] (Fig. 28.1). SSc can affect multiple organ systems, and thus, PH related to CTD can be associated with any of the five groups of PH. Most commonly, PH in CTD is either group I (PAH) or group III (PH related to lung disease). PAH can occur in the absence of associated diseases or risk factors (idiopathic PAH or IPAH) or can complicate CTD (CTD-PAH), particularly SSc. Importantly, PAH refers to pulmonary vasculopathy with elevated mean pulmonary artery pressures in the absence of underlying heart or lung disease and underlying pulmonary embolism. This is an important distinction because most of the current targeted therapies are only approved for PAH; one recently has been approved for use in chronic thromboembolic PH (CTEPH) [1]. Regardless of the cause, however, the presence of PH in any form is associated with an increased risk of morbidity and mortality [4–6].

Epidemiology of PH and Impact on Outcomes

PAH occurs in about 8–14 % of patients with SSc when the diagnosis is properly established by RHC; higher estimates of PAH (up to 45 % in certain series) have overestimated the prevalence due to the use of echocardiography which has significant limitations in accuracy [7–10]. Risk factors for development of PAH within SSc populations include female sex, older age at diagnosis of SSc, longer duration of SSc, and limited disease (formerly known as the "CREST" syndrome) [2]. Because of the high risk of development of PAH in SSc, screening for PAH is recommended; an algorithm such as the one developed in the recently completed DETECT study that includes serum markers, physiologic data, and echocardiographic parameters may be employed [11]. However, whether early detection improves outcomes is unknown. Overall, outcomes in SSc-PAH are poor with worse survival than other forms of PAH such as IPAH and other forms of CTD-PAH [12–15].

SSc patients can also develop PH related to interstitial lung disease (SSc-ILD); however, there are few data describing the incidence and prevalence of PH in SSc-ILD. While the presence of ILD in SSc in the absence of PH portends a poor prognosis, survival is even worse in SSc patients with combined ILD and PH [5, 6, 16, 17]. In a cohort of 59 SSc-PH patients, 20 of whom had significant ILD (defined as

S.C. Mathai, MD, MHS (✉)
Division of Pulmonary and Critical Care Medicine, Johns Hopkins University School of Medicine, Baltimore, MD 21205, USA
e-mail: smathai4@jhmi.edu

N.N. Galié, MD
Department of Experimental, Diagnostic and Specialty Medicine-DIMES, University of Bologna,
Via Massarenti 9, Bologna 40138, Italy

J. Varga et al. (eds.), *Scleroderma*, DOI 10.1007/978-3-319-31407-5_28

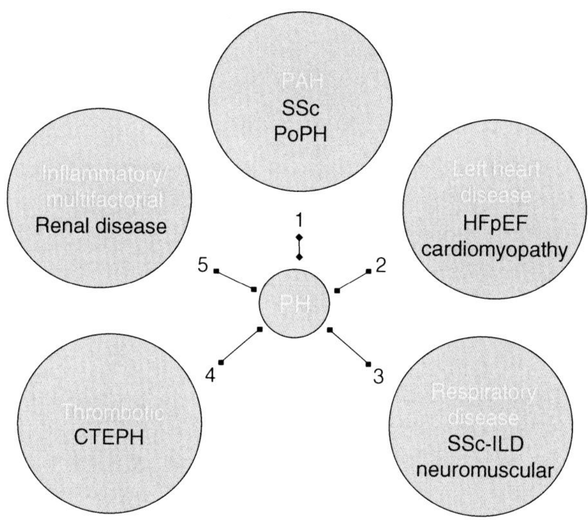

Fig. 28.1 Types of pulmonary hypertension in SSc. *PH* pulmonary hypertension, *PAH* pulmonary arterial hypertension, *PoPH* portopulmonary hypertension (related to primary biliary cirrhosis), *HFpEF* heart failure with preserved ejection fraction, *SSc-ILD* scleroderma-related interstitial lung disease, CTEPH: chronic thromboembolic pulmonary hypertension

a TLC <60 % predicted or TLC between 60 and 70 % predicted combined with moderate to severe fibrosis on high-resolution CT of the chest), the presence of ILD portended a fivefold increased risk of death compared to PAH [6]. Similar 3-year survival rates (47 %) were noted in another cohort of 47 SSc-PH-ILD patients [17]. Importantly, no randomized clinical trials have been conducted in this patient population, and no PAH-specific therapies are currently approved for treatment of PH in this group.

Therapy for CTD-PAH: Overview

While specific therapies for PAH have been studied in randomized clinical trials that have included patients with SSc-PAH, there has been only one study conducted exclusively in patients with SSc-PAH [18]. Further, the classification of the specific CTD associated with PAH is often not reported in these clinical trials (Table 28.1). When reported, response to therapy in short-term studies seems to vary between types of CTD-PAH, with patients with SSc-PAH demonstrating the poorest response among the CTD population [19, 20]. However, since specific CTD diagnosis is not adjudicated, it is possible that misclassification of CTD exists and may influence observed associations between CTD type and response to therapy. Still, observational cohort studies have consistently demonstrated poorer survival for patients with SSc-PAH compared to other forms of CTD-PAH, suggesting poorer response to therapy in this population [5, 15].

General Measures

Despite a lack of specific data for SSc-PAH, consensus guidelines recommend the use of supplemental oxygen and diuretics [1]. While anticoagulation is recommended in patients with IPAH based upon a high prevalence of in situ thrombosis in histopathologic evaluation of the lung tissue from patients with IPAH, the use of this medication is not routinely recommended in SSc-PAH [21]. A recent large retrospective study regarding the utility of anticoagulation in SSc-PAH reported a strong trend toward worse outcomes in SSc-PAH patients treated with anticoagulation compared to those not treated (HR 1.82; 95 % CI 0.94–3.54, $p=0.08$) [22]. Some experts tend not to anticoagulate SSc-PAH patients based upon concerns about increased risk of gastrointestinal bleeding from vascular ectasias that may be common in SSc [23, 24]. Furthermore, although the prevalence of in situ thrombosis in IPAH patients may be high, these lesions may be less frequent in SSc-PAH patients [25]. There is an evolving evidence base to support pulmonary rehabilitation in PAH, and based upon these studies, current guidelines recommend participation in such programs [1, 26].

Anti-inflammatory Agents

Inflammation is a key mediator in the pathogenesis of SSc and recent observations have identified the inflammatory nature of PAH. Histologically, perivascular inflammatory infiltrates are observed around plexiform lesions in PAH [27]. In SSc-PAH, inflammatory infiltrates have been described around plexiform lesions, but not around uninvolved pulmonary vessels, implicating active inflammation as a key contributor to disease pathogenesis [28]. SSc-PAH has recently been described as a prototypical inflammatory disease, characterized by autoantibody-mediated endothelial cell injury, increased cytokine release, and increased expression of genes involved in the inflammatory response. In patients with other forms of connective tissue disease-associated PAH (systemic lupus erythematosus, mixed connective tissue disease), modest numbers have responded to anti-inflammatory treatment with cyclophosphamide and prednisone, demonstrating improvement in functional class, hemodynamic indices, and survival [29].

Unfortunately, a similar response to immunosuppressive therapy has not been observed in patients with SSc-PAH. Given the lack of demonstrated benefit and potential adverse effects of high-dose or long-term immunosuppressive therapies, these are generally not used for patients with SSc-PAH. In particular, the risk of scleroderma renal crisis with high-dose steroids dampens enthusiasm for its use in this patient population [30, 31].

Table 28.1 Inclusion of SSc Patients in pivotal trials of PAH therapy

	CTD-PAH (n, overall %)	Type of CTD (n, % CTD)
Epoprostenol	111(100 %)	lcSSc: 77(69 %)
		dcSSc: 14(13 %)
		Others: 20(18 %)
Oral treprostinil	110(19 %)	NR
Oral treprostinil add-on	92(26 %)	NR
SC treprostinil	90(19 %)	lcSSc: 20(22 %)
		dcSSc: 25(28 %)
		SLE: 25(28 %)
		MCTD: 17(19 %)
		Overlap: 3(3 %)
Inhaled treprostinil	77(33 %)	NR
Inhaled iloprost (AIR)	35(17 %)	NR
Inhaled iloprost + bosentan	NR	NR
Beraprost	13(10 %)	NR
Vardenafil (EVOLUTION)	20(30 %)	NR
Tadalafil (PHIRST)	95(29 %)	NR
Sildenafil + epoprostenol (PACES)	55(21 %)	SSc: 31(56 %)
		SLE: 14(25 %)
		Other: 10(18 %)
Sildenafil (SUPER)	84(30 %)	SSc: 50(60 %)*
		SLE: 19(23 %)
		MCTD: 8(10 %)
		SjS: 4(5 %)
		RA: 1(1 %)
Bosentan (EARLY)	33(18 %)	SSc: 15(46 %)
		SLE: 11(6 %)
		MCTD: 3(9 %)
		SjS: 1(3 %)
		Other: 1(3 %)
Bosentan (study 351 + BREATHE)	66(27 %)	SSc: 52(78 %)
		SLE: 8(12 %)
		Overlap: 4(6 %)
		UCTD: 2(3 %)
Bosentan + epoprostenol (BREATHE-2)	6(18 %)	SSc: 5(83 %)
		SLE: 1(17 %)
Ambrisentan (ARIES 1 + ARIES 2)	136(35 %)	NR
Macitentan (SERAPHIN)	225 (30.5 %)	SSc 117 (52 %)
		SLE 66 (29 %)
		MCTD 42 (19 %)

Calcium Channel Blockers

Oral calcium channel blockers (nifedipine, diltiazem) given at high doses have proven to be an effective long-term therapy in a minority of IPAH patients (<7 %) who demonstrate acute vasodilatation in response to nitric oxide, epoprostenol, or adenosine during hemodynamic testing [32, 33]. Unfortunately, the vast majority of patients with PAH related to connective tissue disease (>97 %) fail to respond to acute vasodilators during hemodynamic testing [34]. Further, less than 1 % of patients with PAH related to connective tissue disease treated with CCB have sustained response at 1 year [35]. Thus, although many SSc patients receive low-dose calcium channel blockers for Raynaud symptoms, high-dose calcium channel blocker therapy is not routinely prescribed for patients with SSc-PAH.

Prostaglandins

Prostacyclin, produced by endothelial cells, is a potent vasodilator, inhibits platelet aggregation, and effectively prevents the release of growth factors from endothelial cells, platelets, and macrophages [36]. As such, prostacyclin has the capacity to inhibit many of the fundamental abnormalities in PAH. In the United States, prostacyclin analogs are available for delivery via intravenous (epoprostenol, treprostinil), subcutaneous (treprostinil), inhaled (iloprost, treprostinil), and oral (treprostinil) routes. Continuous intravenous infusion of epoprostenol has been shown to provide sustained improvements in exercise capacity, pulmonary vascular resistance, mean pulmonary artery pressure, and quality of life in patients with PAH [37–39]. In one study of IPAH patients, epoprostenol was associated with improved survival over a 12-week period when compared to controls. Although no studies have demonstrated improved long-term survival in PAH patients with epoprostenol in randomized, controlled trials, IPAH patients with New York Heart Association (NYHA) class III or IV disease have demonstrated improved survival when compared to historical controls [40, 41].

In patients with SSc-PAH, a 12-week trial of IV epoprostenol was associated with increased exercise capacity, reduced symptoms, and improved functional class when compared to controls [18]. However, no short-term mortality benefit was seen. A prospective, noncontrolled, open-label study of IV epoprostenol in SSc-PAH patients demonstrated a 1-year survival of 71 % and 3-year survival of 48 % [42]. These estimates were similar to those described in SSc-PAH patients taking various oral therapies. Further, when compared to patients with IPAH on epoprostenol, survival for SSc-PAH patients on epoprostenol also appeared worse [43]. Unfortunately, the therapy is cumbersome due to the short half-life of epoprostenol and instability at ambient temperatures. Requirements for frequent mixing and changing ice packs may be especially challenging for patients with sclerodactyly and Raynaud phenomena. Furthermore, IV epoprostenol requires continuous infusion through a dedicated indwelling central venous catheter, resulting in increased risk of thromboembolic complications and catheter-associated infections. Finally, abrupt withdrawal of the therapy can lead to immediate rebound pulmonary vasoconstriction, a potentially fatal adverse effect.

To mitigate some of these drug-related complications, treprostinil, a tricyclic benzidine analog of epoprostenol, has been developed. Treprostinil is stable at ambient temperatures and has a longer half-life than epoprostenol. Treprostinil, delivered as a continuous, subcutaneous infusion (obviating the need for an indwelling catheter), resulted in reduced dyspnea, increased exercise capacity, and improved hemodynamics during a 12-week trial in patients with various forms of PAH [44]. Ninety patients with various types of CTD-associated PAH were included in the large randomized clinical trial of SC treprostinil (Table 28.1). The response in this subset, as reported by Oudiz and colleagues, suggested clinical efficacy, with improvements in dyspnea scores, functional capacity, and hemodynamics, though thechange in 6MWD between treatment and placebo groups was of marginal statistical significance (25 m, $p = 0.055$) [49]. Unfortunately, injection site pain proved limiting for routine clinical practice. When delivered as a continuous intravenous infusion, treprostinil improved exercise capacity, symptoms, and World Health Organization functional status in a small, open-label study in PAH patients [45]. Although a central venous catheter is required, several benefits (including stability at ambient temperature and less frequent mixing) are appealing for treatment of SSc-PAH patients. Treprostinil is also available in an inhaled form. However, although patients with CTD-PAH were included in the TRIUMPH study investigating the addition of inhaled treprostinil to bosentan or sildenafil and significant improvement in functional capacity was found, no subgroup analyses on CTD-PAH patients were reported [50].

There are several other formulations of prostacyclin analogs that are currently available for use in the treatment of PAH and have been studied in CTD-PAH. Iloprost is formulated in both intravenous and inhaled versions, though only the inhaled form is approved for therapy of PAH in the United States. IV iloprost has been studied in CTD patients without PAH for treatment of peripheral vascular complications and shown to improve exercise capacity and hemodynamics compared to baseline values; however no specific data exist in patients with CTD-PAH [46, 47]. Studies of inhaled iloprost in various forms of PAH, including CTD-PAH, have demonstrated significant improvements in functional class, exercise capacity, and hemodynamics compared to placebo. However no disaggregated data for CTD-PAH are available [48].

The oral formulation of treprostinil was recently approved for use in patients with PAH based upon the results of several randomized clinical trials [51–53]. However, overall, the impact on functional capacity seems marginal and less robust than other prostacyclin formulations. Further, the impact on patients with CTD-PAH is unclear. A recent large clinical trial examining the effect of selexipag, a novel therapy targeting the prostacyclin pathway via agonism of the prostacyclin receptor, on morbidity and mortality in PAH has been completed. While preliminary results suggest efficacy of this agent in PAH overall and in the CTD-PAH population, complete results have yet to be published. Importantly, development of oral formulations of therapies active in the prostacyclin pathway is likely to be useful in patients in whom other formulations are less practical or feasible such as those with SSc-PAH.

Prostaglandins, via their acute vasodilatory effects, have the potential to precipitate acute pulmonary edema in patients with veno-occlusive disease. As the prevalence of PVOD in patients with SSc-PAH appears to be high, special consideration is required when initiating or titrating prostaglandins in this group [25, 54]. Thus, while Overall, prostaglandins provide effective symptomatic relief and improve functional capacity in patients with SSc-PAH, caution must be exercised with its use in SSc-PAH. Nevertheless, IV epoprostenol is considered first-line therapy in severe PAH (WHO functional class IV) and in some patients as a bridge or alternative to lung transplantation [1].

Endothelin Receptor Antagonists

Endothelin 1 is produced by endothelial cells and has direct vasoconstrictor and mitogenic effects on vascular smooth muscle cells. Endothelin's vasoconstrictive effects are mediated by two receptors (ERA, ERB) on pulmonary arterial smooth muscle cells. Conversely, ERB is also functional on endothelial cells, and stimulation mediates nitric oxide production and prostacyclin release, resulting in endothelial-mediated vasodilatation. Currently available endothelin receptor antagonists target both receptors (bosentan, macitentan) or selectively target ERA (ambrisentan).

The dual endothelin receptor antagonist bosentan has been shown to improve exercise capacity, functional class, hemodynamics, and dyspnea score after 12 weeks in a small, randomized, controlled trial of patients with class III PAH [55]. A subsequent larger randomized, controlled trial included a significant number of patients with SSc-PAH (22 %) and demonstrated similar improvements in exercise capacity (measured by 6-min walk distance, 6MWD) and functional class [56]. However, post hoc analysis showed no increase in 6MWD in the SSc-PAH patients. Similarly, a retrospective review of IPAH and SSc-PAH patients treated with bosentan monotherapy at a single center showed improvements in functional status only in patients with IPAH [57].

Post hoc subgroup analysis of a large randomized, controlled trial showed that patients with PAH related to connective tissue disease had improved 1- and 2-year survival when compared to historical controls [58]. However, Girgis et al. showed that SSc-PAH patients treated with bosentan monotherapy demonstrated a nonsignificant trend toward increased mortality when compared to IPAH patients [57].

Macitentan, a compound with increased receptor binding kinetics and enhanced tissue penetration, was recently studied in a large cohort of patients with PAH, including CTD-associated disease. In the Study with an Endothelin Receptor Antagonist in Pulmonary Arterial Hypertension to Improve Clinical Outcome (SERAPHIN) trial, the impact of macitentan on the novel primary outcome of morbidity and mortality was tested in 742 patients with PAH [59]. Treatment with 10 mg daily of macitentan reduced the incidence of the composite end point of death, atrial septostomy, lung transplantation, initiation of treatment with intravenous or subcutaneous prostanoids, or worsening of PAH by 45 % (HR = 0.55, 97.5 % CI 0.39–0.76; $p<0.001$). Approximately 30 % of the cohort had CTD-PAH; and the dose of 10 mg exerted the same risk reduction for the primary end point also in this subgroup as compared to the overall group [59].

In an effort to selectively limit endothelin-mediated vasoconstriction while allowing vasodilatory effects, selective ERA antagonists have been developed. Ambrisentan has been associated with improved exercise capacity in patients with PAH in a randomized, controlled trial [60]. However, improvements in 6MWD were more pronounced in patients with IPAH (50–66 m) than in patients with SSc-PAH (15–23 m). While selective inhibitors appear to hold promise for symptomatic relief in patients with SSc-PAH, they appear to be more effective for patients with IPAH.

Phosphodiesterase Inhibitors and Soluble Guanylate Cyclase Stimulators

Sildenafil enhances the effects of nitric oxide on pulmonary vascular smooth muscle cells and causes pulmonary vasodilatation by inhibiting the enzyme phosphodiesterase-5 (PDE5). PDE5 is the predominant phosphodiesterase isoform in the lung tissue and is responsible for catabolism of the nitric oxide second messenger cyclic guanosine monophosphate (cGMP). By inhibiting PDE5, sildenafil promotes accumulation of cGMP following nitric oxide stimulation, leading to smooth muscle cell relaxation and growth inhibition.

In patients with PAH, sildenafil has been shown to increase 6MWD after 12 weeks of therapy, with responses sustained after 1 year [61]. Additionally, sildenafil was associated with improved functional class and hemodynamic indices (including cardiac output), though there was no delay in the time to clinical worsening when compared to placebo. Approximately 20 % of the subjects enrolled in this trial had SSc-PAH, most with class II or III disease. A post hoc, subgroup analysis of the 84 patients enrolled with connective tissue disease-associated PAH (45 % of these with SSc-PAH) demonstrated improved 6MWD, improved hemodynamics, and a mild safety profile [62].

Tadalafil, a long-acting PDE5 inhibitor, is approved for once daily administration for PAH in the United States, A large, randomized, controlled trial (including 23 % of subjects with CTD-associated PAH) showed that daily administration of tadalafil improved 6MWD on average 20–33 m [63]. At the highest dose, tadalafil therapy was also associated with a reduced risk of clinical worsening after 16 weeks of therapy. Like sildenafil, side effects were mild, and no disaggregated data for CTD-PAH population have been yet published. Recently, the soluble guanylate cyclase (sGC) stimulator riociguat has been studied in the treatment of both PAH and CTEPH [64, 65]. This agent acts by increasing the production of nitric oxide by enhancing the response of sGC to endogenous nitric oxide to produce cyclic GMP and directly stimulating sGC independent of NO binding. Thus, it is theorized that SGC stimulators will be effective in situations where NO production is low compared to PDE5I where adequate levels of NO are required for efficacy [66]. In the pivotal clinical trial of this agent in PAH, subjects experienced improvement in symptoms and functional capacity at 12 weeks. (reference 1) Specific data regarding effects in the CTD population have yet to be reported.

Combination Therapy

As many of the agents described above work by affecting unique signaling pathways to promote pulmonary vasodilatation or inhibit pulmonary vasoconstriction, there may be additive or synergistic benefit to combining various agents in the treatment of PAH. So far, the results have been rather disappointing. Two studies have compared the addition of inhaled iloprost to placebo in patients taking bosentan monotherapy. While one study demonstrated a 30-m improvement in 6MWD, improved NYHA functional class, improved hemodynamics, and delayed time to worsening in patients receiving added iloprost, the other was stopped early due to futility, with no improvement in exercise capacity, functional class, or time to clinical worsening [67, 68]. In the multicenter PACES trial, PAH patients (11.6 % with SSc-PAH) on long-term IV epoprostenol were randomized to receive added sildenafil versus placebo for 16 weeks [69]. Those randomized to the sildenafil arm demonstrated improved exercise capacity, hemodynamics (including cardiac output), and delayed time to clinical worsening when compared to those randomized to receive placebo.

Therapy with dual oral agents appears to be a rational approach, though the current data are limited. Two small, prospective, noncontrolled studies showed improved 6MWD in IPAH patients when sildenafil was added to bosentan for clinical worsening [70, 71]. In one report, 12 patients with SSc-PAH showed no improvement in 6MWD after sildenafil was added to bosentan and increased frequency of hepatotoxicity with combination therapy [71]. Careful consideration should be given to this combination, as bosentan is a CYP3A4 inducer and sildenafil is a CYP3A4 substrate. The combination may lead to reduced levels of sildenafil and increased levels of bosentan, though the clinical significance of this interaction remains unclear [72]. A recently published randomized, controlled trial examining the impact of adding bosentan to sildenafil in over 300 PAH patients did not demonstrate reduction in the incidence of achieving a composite end point of death, hospitalization for PAH, need for IV PAH therapy, atrial septostomy, lung transplantation, or worsening PAH. Subgroup analysis did not suggest response in the CTD-PAH patients who comprised about 25 % of the study cohort [73]. However, in an open-label real-world experience, sequential combination of sildenafil with bosentan has shown favorable functional and hemodynamic results also in the PAH-CTD subgroup [74]. Preliminary data from the recently completed AMBITION study, in which treatment-naive PAH patients were randomized to receive initial therapy with both tadalafil and ambrisentan or either drug alone suggests efficacy of this combination of PDE5I and ERA in reducing time to clinical failure, both in the overall PAH group and in the CTD-PAH group alone [75].

Lung Transplantation

Although disease-specific therapy for severe PAH has reduced the referral of patients with PAH for lung transplantation, transplant remains a therapeutic option for select patients failing medical therapy [76]. Classically, the diagnosis of SSc has discouraged providers from proceeding with transplant, as frequent gastrointestinal involvement (namely, esophageal dysmotility associated with reflux) raises concern for aspiration and damage to the allograft. However, international consensus recommendations do not preclude lung transplant for patients with SSc or other connective tissue diseases, as long as additional systemic manifestations are controlled [77]. Accordingly, 2-year survival was shown to be comparable (64 %) among patients receiving lung transplant for SSc, interstitial lung disease, or IPAH [78]. An additional report from a single center recently showed that 1-year mortality, chronic rejection, infections, and pulmonary function were similar between 14 patients transplanted for pulmonary complications of SSc when compared to 38 patients with idiopathic pulmonary fibrosis [79]. Interestingly, more episodes of acute rejection were observed in SSc patients receiving transplant. A recent study using the United Network for Organ Sharing database found that while patients with SSc-ILD had a nearly 50 % increased risk of death at 1-year post-transplant compared to patient with other forms of ILD, there was no difference in 1-year survival in patients with SSc-PAH compared to those with other forms of PAH [80]. These data suggest that lung transplantation remains a viable option in carefully selected patients with SSc-PAH that proves refractory to medical management.

Summary and Future Directions

Despite the high prevalence of pulmonary involvement in SSc, including SSc-PAH and SSc-ILD-PH, and its major contribution to morbidity and mortality, treatment strategies for SSc-associated PH remain limited. Numerous clinical trials of currently available PAH-specific therapies have shown an inferior response in patients with SSc-PAH when compared to IPAH. Even less is known about SSc-ILD-PH response to currently available therapies. Accordingly, survival continues to lag behind patients with IPAH. The relative lack of efficacy in SSc-PAH when compared to IPAH may be related to fundamental differences in the pulmonary vasculopathy or in the greater incidence of intrinsic RV dysfunction observed in patients with SSc. Future investigational drug trials must continue to evaluate efficacy separately in patients with SSc-PAH.

Rituximab, a monoclonal antibody against the CD20 protein found on B cells, is currently being studied in patients with SSc-PAH (NCT01086540) and may suggest a role for immunotherapy in the treatment of pulmonary vascular disease in SSc. Hematopoietic stem cell transplantation (HSCT) has proven effective in reversing skin findings in patients with diffuse scleroderma, though safety concerns and a lack of improvement in pulmonary function limit enthusiasm for the use of HSCT in the treatment of SSc-associated PH [81, 82]. Nevertheless, it remains a future experimental consideration.

References

1. Galie N, Corris PA, Frost A, Girgis RE, Granton J, Jing ZC, et al. Updated treatment algorithm of pulmonary arterial hypertension. J Am Coll Cardiol. 2013;62(25 Suppl):D60–72.
2. Mathai SC, Hummers LK. Pulmonary hypertension associated with connective tissue disease. In: Dellaripa PF, Fischer A, Flaherty KR, editors. Pulmonary manifestations of rheumatic diseases: a comprehensive guide. 1st ed. New York: Springer; 2014. p. 139–66.
3. Simonneau G, Gatzoulis MA, Adatia I, Celermajer D, Denton C, Ghofrani A, et al. Updated clinical classification of pulmonary hypertension. J Am Coll Cardiol. 2013;62(25 Suppl):D34–41.
4. Steen VD, Medsger TA. Changes in causes of death in systemic sclerosis, 1972–2002. Ann Rheum Dis. 2007;66(7):940–4.
5. Condliffe R, Kiely DG, Peacock AJ, Corris PA, Gibbs JS, Vrapi F, et al. Connective tissue disease-associated pulmonary arterial hypertension in the modern treatment era. Am J Respir Crit Care Med. 2009;179(2):151–7.
6. Mathai SC, Hummers LK, Champion HC, Wigley FM, Zaiman A, Hassoun PM, et al. Survival in pulmonary hypertension associated with the scleroderma spectrum of diseases: impact of interstitial lung disease. Arthritis Rheum. 2009;60(2):569–77.
7. Hachulla E, Gressin V, Guillevin L, Carpentier P, Diot E, Sibilia J, et al. Early detection of pulmonary arterial hypertension in systemic sclerosis: a French nationwide prospective multicenter study. Arthritis Rheum. 2005;52(12):3792–800.
8. Mukerjee D, St George D, Coleiro B, Knight C, Denton CP, Davar J, et al. Prevalence and outcome in systemic sclerosis associated pulmonary arterial hypertension: application of a registry approach. Ann Rheum Dis. 2003;62(11):1088–93.
9. Fisher MR, Forfia PR, Chamera E, Housten-Harris T, Champion HC, Girgis RE, et al. Accuracy of Doppler echocardiography in the hemodynamic assessment of pulmonary hypertension. Am J Respir Crit Care Med. 2009;179(7):615–21.
10. Rich JD, Shah SJ, Swamy RS, Kamp A, Rich S. Inaccuracy of Doppler echocardiographic estimates of pulmonary artery pressures in patients with pulmonary hypertension: implications for clinical practice. Chest. 2011;139(5):988–93.
11. Coghlan JG, Denton CP, Grunig E, Bonderman D, Distler O, Khanna D, et al. Evidence-based detection of pulmonary arterial hypertension in systemic sclerosis: the DETECT study. Ann Rheum Dis. 2014;73(7):1340–9.
12. Fisher MR, Mathai SC, Champion HC, Girgis RE, Housten-Harris T, Hummers L, et al. Clinical differences between idiopathic and scleroderma-related pulmonary hypertension. Arthritis Rheum. 2006;54(9):3043–50.
13. Kawut SM, Taichman DB, Archer-Chicko CL, Palevsky HI, Kimmel SE. Hemodynamics and survival in patients with pulmonary arterial hypertension related to systemic sclerosis. Chest. 2003;123(2):344–50.
14. Chung L, Farber HW, Benza R, Miller DP, Parsons L, Hassoun PM, et al. Unique predictors of mortality in patients with pulmonary arterial hypertension associated with systemic sclerosis in the REVEAL registry. Chest. 2014;146(6):1494–504.
15. Chung L, Liu J, Parsons L, Hassoun PM, McGoon M, Badesch DB, et al. Characterization of connective tissue disease-associated pulmonary arterial hypertension from REVEAL: identifying systemic sclerosis as a unique phenotype. Chest. 2010;138(6):1383–94.
16. Le Pavec J, Launay D, Mathai SC, Hassoun PM, Humbert M. Scleroderma lung disease. Clin Rev Allergy Immunol. 2011;40(2):104–16.
17. Launay D, Humbert M, Berezne A, Cottin V, Allanore Y, Couderc LJ, et al. Clinical characteristics and survival in systemic sclerosis-related pulmonary hypertension associated with interstitial lung disease. Chest. 2011;140(4):1016–24.
18. Badesch DB, Tapson VF, McGoon MD, Brundage BH, Rubin LJ, Wigley FM, et al. Continuous intravenous epoprostenol for pulmonary hypertension due to the scleroderma spectrum of disease. A randomized, controlled trial. Ann Intern Med. 2000;132(6):425–34.
19. Galie N, Manes A, Negro L, Palazzini M, Bacchi-Reggiani ML, Branzi A. A meta-analysis of randomized controlled trials in pulmonary arterial hypertension. Eur Heart J. 2009;30(4):394–403.
20. Avouac J, Wipff J, Kahan A, Allanore Y. Effects of oral treatments on exercise capacity in systemic sclerosis related pulmonary arterial hypertension: a meta-analysis of randomised controlled trials. Ann Rheum Dis. 2008;67(6):808–14.
21. Pietra GG, Edwards WD, Kay JM, Rich S, Kernis J, Schloo B, et al. Histopathology of primary pulmonary hypertension. A qualitative and quantitative study of pulmonary blood vessels from 58 patients in the National Heart, Lung, and Blood Institute, Primary Pulmonary Hypertension Registry. Circulation. 1989;80(5):1198–206.
22. Olsson KM, Delcroix M, Ghofrani HA, Tiede H, Huscher D, Speich R, et al. Anticoagulation and survival in pulmonary arterial hypertension: results from the Comparative, Prospective Registry of Newly Initiated Therapies for Pulmonary Hypertension (COMPERA). Circulation. 2014;129(1):57–65.
23. Duchini A, Sessoms SL. Gastrointestinal hemorrhage in patients with systemic sclerosis and CREST syndrome. Am J Gastroenterol. 1998;93(9):1453–6.
24. Mathai SC, Hassoun PM. Pulmonary arterial hypertension in connective tissue diseases. Heart Fail Clin. 2012;8(3):413–25.
25. Overbeek MJ, Vonk MC, Boonstra A, Voskuyl AE, Vonk-Noordegraaf A, Smit EF, et al. Pulmonary arterial hypertension in limited cutaneous systemic sclerosis: a distinctive vasculopathy. Eur Respir J. 2009;34(2):371–9.
26. Mereles D, Ehlken N, Kreuscher S, Ghofrani S, Hoeper MM, Halank M, et al. Exercise and respiratory training improve exercise capacity and quality of life in patients with severe chronic pulmonary hypertension. Circulation. 2006;114(14):1482–9.
27. Tuder RM, Archer SL, Dorfmuller P, Erzurum SC, Guignabert C, Michelakis E, et al. Relevant issues in the pathology and

pathobiology of pulmonary hypertension. J Am Coll Cardiol. 2013;62(25 Suppl):D4–12.

28. Cool CD, Kennedy D, Voelkel NF, Tuder RM. Pathogenesis and evolution of plexiform lesions in pulmonary hypertension associated with scleroderma and human immunodeficiency virus infection. Hum Pathol. 1997;28(4):434–42.
29. Sanchez O, Sitbon O, Jais X, Simonneau G, Humbert M. Immunosuppressive therapy in connective tissue diseases-associated pulmonary arterial hypertension. Chest. 2006;130(1):182–9.
30. Guillevin L, Berezne A, Seror R, Teixeira L, Pourrat J, Mahr A, et al. Scleroderma renal crisis: a retrospective multicentre study on 91 patients and 427 controls. Rheumatol (Oxford). 2012;51(3):460–7.
31. Montanelli G, Beretta L, Santaniello A, Scorza R. Effect of dihydropyridine calcium channel blockers and glucocorticoids on the prevention and development of scleroderma renal crisis in an Italian case series. Clin Exp Rheumatol. 2013;31(2 Suppl 76):135–9.
32. Rich S, Kaufmann E, Levy PS. The effect of high doses of calcium-channel blockers on survival in primary pulmonary hypertension. N Engl J Med. 1992;327(2):76–81.
33. Sitbon O, Humbert M, Jais X, Ioos V, Hamid AM, Provencher S, et al. Long-term response to calcium channel blockers in idiopathic pulmonary arterial hypertension. Circulation. 2005;111(23):3105–11.
34. Humbert M, Sitbon O, Chaouat A, Bertocchi M, Habib G, Gressin V, et al. Pulmonary arterial hypertension in France: results from a national registry. Am J Respir Crit Care Med. 2006;173(9):1023–30.
35. Montani D, Savale L, Natali D, Jais X, Herve P, Garcia G, et al. Long-term response to calcium-channel blockers in non-idiopathic pulmonary arterial hypertension. Eur Heart J. 2010;31(15):1898–907.
36. Vane JR, Anggard EE, Botting RM. Regulatory functions of the vascular endothelium. N Engl J Med. 1990;323(1):27–36.
37. Barst RJ, Rubin LJ, Long WA, McGoon MD, Rich S, Badesch DB, et al. A comparison of continuous intravenous epoprostenol (prostacyclin) with conventional therapy for primary pulmonary hypertension. N Engl J Med. 1996;334(5):296–301.
38. McLaughlin VV, Genthner DE, Panella MM, Rich S. Reduction in pulmonary vascular resistance with long-term epoprostenol (prostacyclin) therapy in primary pulmonary hypertension. N Engl J Med. 1998;338(5):273–7.
39. Rubin LJ, Mendoza J, Hood M, McGoon M, Barst R, Williams WB, et al. Treatment of primary pulmonary hypertension with continuous intravenous prostacyclin (epoprostenol). Results of a randomized trial. Ann Intern Med. 1990;112(7):485–91.
40. Sitbon O, Humbert M, Nunes H, Parent F, Garcia G, Herve P, et al. Long-term intravenous epoprostenol infusion in primary pulmonary hypertension: prognostic factors and survival. J Am Coll Cardiol. 2002;40(4):780–8.
41. McLaughlin VV, Shillington A, Rich S. Survival in primary pulmonary hypertension: the impact of epoprostenol therapy. Circulation. 2002;106(12):1477–82.
42. Badesch DB, McGoon MD, Barst RJ, Tapson VF, Rubin LJ, Wigley FM, et al. Longterm survival among patients with scleroderma-associated pulmonary arterial hypertension treated with intravenous epoprostenol. J Rheumatol. 2009;36(10):2244–9.
43. Fagan KA, Badesch DB. Pulmonary hypertension associated with connective tissue disease. Prog Cardiovasc Dis. 2002;45(3):225–34.
44. Simonneau G, Barst RJ, Galie N, Naeije R, Rich S, Bourge RC, et al. Continuous subcutaneous infusion of treprostinil, a prostacyclin analogue, in patients with pulmonary arterial hypertension: a double-blind, randomized, placebo-controlled trial. Am J Respir Crit Care Med. 2002;165(6):800–4.
45. Tapson VF, Gomberg-Maitland M, McLaughlin VV, Benza RL, Widlitz AC, Krichman A, et al. Safety and efficacy of IV treprostinil for pulmonary arterial hypertension: a prospective, multicenter, open-label, 12-week trial. Chest. 2006;129(3):683–8.
46. Caravita S, Wu SC, Secchi MB, Dadone V, Bencini C, Pierini S. Long-term effects of intermittent Iloprost infusion on pulmonary arterial pressure in connective tissue disease. Eur J Intern Med. 2011;22(5):518–21.
47. Hoeper MM, Gall H, Seyfarth HJ, Halank M, Ghofrani HA, Winkler J, et al. Long-term outcome with intravenous iloprost in pulmonary arterial hypertension. Eur Respir J. 2009;34(1):132–7.
48. Olschewski H, Simonneau G, Galie N, Higenbottam T, Naeije R, Rubin LJ, et al. Inhaled iloprost for severe pulmonary hypertension. N Engl J Med. 2002;347(5):322–9.
49. Oudiz RJ, Schilz RJ, Barst RJ, Galie N, Rich S, Rubin LJ, et al. Treprostinil, a prostacyclin analogue, in pulmonary arterial hypertension associated with connective tissue disease. Chest. 2004;126(2):420–7.
50. McLaughlin VV, Benza RL, Rubin LJ, Channick RN, Voswinckel R, Tapson VF, et al. Addition of inhaled treprostinil to oral therapy for pulmonary arterial hypertension: a randomized controlled clinical trial. J Am Coll Cardiol. 2010;55(18):1915–22.
51. Tapson VF, Torres F, Kermeen F, Keogh AM, Allen RP, Frantz RP, et al. Oral treprostinil for the treatment of pulmonary arterial hypertension in patients on background endothelin receptor antagonist and/or phosphodiesterase type 5 inhibitor therapy (the FREEDOM-C study): a randomized controlled trial. Chest. 2012;142(6):1383–90.
52. Tapson VF, Jing ZC, Xu KF, Pan L, Feldman J, Kiely DG, et al. Oral treprostinil for the treatment of pulmonary arterial hypertension in patients receiving background endothelin receptor antagonist and phosphodiesterase type 5 inhibitor therapy (the FREEDOM-C2 study): a randomized controlled trial. Chest. 2013;144(3):952–8.
53. Jing ZC, Parikh K, Pulido T, Jerjes-Sanchez C, White RJ, Allen R, et al. Efficacy and safety of oral treprostinil monotherapy for the treatment of pulmonary arterial hypertension: a randomized, controlled trial. Circulation. 2013;127(5):624–33.
54. Dorfmuller P, Humbert M, Perros F, Sanchez O, Simonneau G, Muller KM, et al. Fibrous remodeling of the pulmonary venous system in pulmonary arterial hypertension associated with connective tissue diseases. Hum Pathol. 2007;38(6):893–902.
55. Channick RN, Simonneau G, Sitbon O, Robbins IM, Frost A, Tapson VF, et al. Effects of the dual endothelin-receptor antagonist bosentan in patients with pulmonary hypertension: a randomised placebo-controlled study. Lancet. 2001;358(9288):1119–23.
56. Rubin LJ, Badesch DB, Barst RJ, Galie N, Black CM, Keogh A, et al. Bosentan therapy for pulmonary arterial hypertension. N Engl J Med. 2002;346(12):896–903.
57. Girgis RE, Mathai SC, Krishnan JA, Wigley FM, Hassoun PM. Long-term outcome of bosentan treatment in idiopathic pulmonary arterial hypertension and pulmonary arterial hypertension associated with the scleroderma spectrum of diseases. J Heart Lung Transplant. 2005;24(10):1626–31.
58. Denton CP, Humbert M, Rubin L, Black CM. Bosentan treatment for pulmonary arterial hypertension related to connective tissue disease: a subgroup analysis of the pivotal clinical trials and their open-label extensions. Ann Rheum Dis. 2006;65(10):1336–40.
59. Pulido T, Adzerikho I, Channick RN, Delcroix M, Galie N, Ghofrani HA, et al. Macitentan and morbidity and mortality in pulmonary arterial hypertension. N Engl J Med. 2013;369(9):809–18.
60. Galie N, Olschewski H, Oudiz RJ, Torres F, Frost A, Ghofrani HA, et al. Ambrisentan for the treatment of pulmonary arterial hypertension: results of the ambrisentan in pulmonary arterial hypertension, randomized, double-blind, placebo-controlled, multicenter, efficacy (ARIES) study 1 and 2. Circulation. 2008;117(23):3010–9.
61. Galie N, Ghofrani HA, Torbicki A, Barst RJ, Rubin LJ, Badesch D, et al. Sildenafil citrate therapy for pulmonary arterial hypertension. N Engl J Med. 2005;353(20):2148–57.
62. Badesch DB, Hill NS, Burgess G, Rubin LJ, Barst RJ, Galie N, et al. Sildenafil for pulmonary arterial hypertension associated with connective tissue disease. J Rheumatol. 2007;34(12):2417–22.

63. Galie N, Brundage BH, Ghofrani HA, Oudiz RJ, Simonneau G, Safdar Z, et al. Tadalafil therapy for pulmonary arterial hypertension. Circulation. 2009;119(22):2894–903.
64. Ghorfrani HA, Galie N, Grimminger F et al. Riociguat for the treatment of pulmonary arterial hypertension. N Engl J Med 2013; 369:330–40.
65. Ghofrani HA, D'Armini AM, Grimminger F, et al. Riociguat for the treatment of chronic thromboembolic pulmonary hypertension. N Engl J Med 2013;369:319–29.
66. Ghofrani HA, Grimminger F. Soluble guanylate cyclase stimulation: an emerging option in pulmonary hypertension. Eur REspir Rev 2009;18:35–41.
67. McLaughlin VV, Oudiz RJ, Frost A, Tapson VF, Murali S, Channick RN, et al. Randomized study of adding inhaled iloprost to existing bosentan in pulmonary arterial hypertension. Am J Respir Crit Care Med. 2006;174(11):1257–63.
68. Hoeper MM, Leuchte H, Halank M, Wilkens H, Meyer FJ, Seyfarth HJ, et al. Combining inhaled iloprost with bosentan in patients with idiopathic pulmonary arterial hypertension. Eur Respir J. 2006;28(4):691–4.
69. Simonneau G, Rubin LJ, Galie N, Barst RJ, Fleming TR, Frost AE, et al. Addition of sildenafil to long-term intravenous epoprostenol therapy in patients with pulmonary arterial hypertension: a randomized trial. Ann Intern Med. 2008;149(8):521–30.
70. Hoeper MM, Faulenbach C, Golpon H, Winkler J, Welte T, Niedermeyer J. Combination therapy with bosentan and sildenafil in idiopathic pulmonary arterial hypertension. Eur Respir J. 2004;24(6):1007–10.
71. Mathai SC, Girgis RE, Fisher MR, Champion HC, Housten-Harris T, Zaiman A, et al. Addition of sildenafil to bosentan monotherapy in pulmonary arterial hypertension. Eur Respir J. 2007;29(3):469–75.
72. Paul GA, Gibbs JS, Boobis AR, Abbas A, Wilkins MR. Bosentan decreases the plasma concentration of sildenafil when coprescribed in pulmonary hypertension. Br J Clin Pharmacol. 2005;60(1):107–12.
73. McLaughlin V, Channick RN, Ghofrani HA, Lemarie JC, Naeije R, Packer M, et al. Bosentan added to sildenafil therapy in patients with pulmonary arterial hypertension. Eur Respir J. 2015;46:405–13.
74. Dardi F, Manes A, Palazzini M, Bachetti C, Mazzanti G, Rinaldi A, et al. Combining bosentan and sildenafil in pulmonary arterial hypertension patients failing monotherapy: real-world insights. Eur Respir J. 2015;46:414–21.
75. Galie N, Barbera JA, Frost A, Hoeper M, McLaughlin VV, Peacock A, Simonneau G, Vachiery JL, Blair C, Gillies HC, Langley J, Rubin L. AMBITION: a randomised, multicenter study of first-line ambrisentan and tadalafil combination therapy in subjects with pulmonary arterial hypertension (PAH). Munich: European Respiratory Society Congress; 2014.
76. Keogh AM, Mayer E, Benza RL, Corris P, Dartevelle PG, Frost AE, et al. Interventional and surgical modalities of treatment in pulmonary hypertension. J Am Coll Cardiol. 2009;54(1 Suppl):S67–77.
77. Orens JB, Estenne M, Arcasoy S, Conte JV, Corris P, Egan JJ, et al. International guidelines for the selection of lung transplant candidates: 2006 update – a consensus report from the Pulmonary Scientific Council of the International Society for Heart and Lung Transplantation. J Heart Lung Transplant. 2006;25(7):745–55.
78. Schachna L, Medsger Jr TA, Dauber JH, Wigley FM, Braunstein NA, White B, et al. Lung transplantation in scleroderma compared with idiopathic pulmonary fibrosis and idiopathic pulmonary arterial hypertension. Arthritis Rheum. 2006;54(12):3954–61.
79. Saggar R, Khanna D, Furst DE, Belperio JA, Park GS, Weigt SS, et al. Systemic sclerosis and bilateral lung transplantation: a single centre experience. Eur Respir J. 2010;36(4):893–900.
80. Bernstein EJ, Peterson ER, Sell JL, D'Ovidio F, Arcasoy SM, Bathon JM, et al. Survival of adults with systemic sclerosis following lung transplantation: a nationwide cohort study. Arthritis Rheumatol. 2015;67(5):1314–22.
81. Binks M, Passweg JR, Furst D, McSweeney P, Sullivan K, Besenthal C, et al. Phase I/II trial of autologous stem cell transplantation in systemic sclerosis: procedure related mortality and impact on skin disease. Ann Rheum Dis. 2001;60(6):577–84.
82. Vonk MC, Marjanovic Z, van den Hoogen FH, Zohar S, Schattenberg AV, Fibbe WE, et al. Long-term follow-up results after autologous haematopoietic stem cell transplantation for severe systemic sclerosis. Ann Rheum Dis. 2008;67(1):98–104.

Part VI

Gastrointestinal Manifestations and Management

Overview of Gastrointestinal Tract Involvement

29

Christopher P. Denton

Introduction

Gastrointestinal manifestations are the commonest internal organ complications of systemic sclerosis and are a major cause of morbidity [1]. The commonest features are gastro-oesophageal reflux and chronic constipation, both reflecting altered gut motility and contractility. However, there are many other manifestations that span the entire gastrointestinal tract. These include sicca symptoms akin to those typically observed in Sjögren's syndrome, together with all of the predictable secondary consequences of defective salivation [2]. Oesophageal dysmotility leads to dysphagia as well as reflux symptoms and this includes oesophagitis. Stomach involvement includes delayed emptying with post-prandial bloating and also vascular complications, most notably gastric astral vascular ectasia (watermelon stomach) [3]. Other vascular lesions reminiscent of cutaneous telangiectasia can occur throughout the gastrointestinal tract and may be complicated by bleeding and anaemia. Small bowel involvement also manifests as altered motility, and this can lead to episodes of ileus or pseudo-obstruction. Similar processes occur in the large bowel, and recurrent distention and pain are important clinical problems that may require hospital-based treatment. Other consequences of slow intestinal transit include small intestinal bacterial overgrowth that may lead to diarrhoea, bloating and malabsorption [4]. Malnutrition is a frequent problem in SSc. It results in part from poor nutritional intake, but pancreatic enzymes on mucosal enzyme deficiency also contribute, and altered motility and mucosal and intestinal vasculature also contribute [pancreas]. In some cases nutritional support is needed and some cases require parenteral supplementation. Finally, anorectal involvement is a very common problem leading to anorectal incontinence. There may be associated or contributory manifestations such as rectal prolapse. Taken together this range of GI manifestations contributes to the enormous personal impact of SSc and represents one of the most unmet clinical needs for SSc patients. The development of a validated assessment tool for SSc bowel complications has permitted more systematic and standardised assessment of the disease in a patient-relevant way that will hopefully help in clinical research to improve outcomes and better define and understand the disease [5]. The SCTC-UCLA Scleroderma GI Assessment tool was developed to assess burden of diseases in a relevant and measureable way and is freely available for academic and clinical use (see www.uclascleroderma.researchcore.org/pdf/git_english.pdf).

Pathogenesis

The fundamental mechanisms underlying gastrointestinal tract pathology in SSc are likely to reflect the basic disease processes of inflammation, autoimmunity, fibrosis and vasculopathy [6]. There is also compelling evidence that there are enteric neuropathic mechanisms operating. The end consequence of these processes is undoubtedly a fibrotic bowel wall with poor intestinal blood flow and altered contractility together with likely reduction in the functional microcirculation that is intrinsic to the absorptive function of the intestine [7]. Many of the manifestations of bowel involvement including bloating, pseudo-obstruction and intestinal bacterial overgrowth can be unified through these pathological processes. However the symptoms of GI scleroderma are not always well correlated with structural or histopathological severity. In one genetically determined mouse model of scleroderma that is triggered by altered TGF-beta activity, there is evidence of adventitial and mural fibrosis in the large intestine with altered smooth muscle contractility, and the use of animal models may help to dissect out the sequence of events underlying

C.P. Denton, PhD, FRCP
Division of Medicine, Department of Inflammation, Centre for Rheumatology and Connective Tissue Diseases, UCL Division of Medicine, Royal Free Hospital, London, UK
e-mail: c.denton@ucl.ac.uk

J. Varga et al. (eds.), *Scleroderma*, DOI 10.1007/978-3-319-31407-5_29

progression of GI features [8]. This suggests that cofactors such as diet, medications and other comorbidities are likely to be extremely relevant. Although traditionally thought to be one of the most irreversible aspects of the disease, there is very often a favourable clinical outcome when individual components of the disease are tackled and medical approaches that are effective in similar clinical processes occurring outside the context of SSc can be helpful. Some of these processes are considered in more detail below. The potential importance of immunological, and especially humoral, autoimmune processes is suggested by some reports of benefit from immunosuppressive treatments and especially for treatment with long-term intravenous immunoglobulin therapy [9].

Upper GI Complications

At the time of diagnosis, almost all SSc patients describe some symptoms of heartburn or dysphagia. These may be relatively mild and not always associated by patients with the other disparate symptoms of Raynaud's and skin changes that are typical of early-stage SSc. They may be treated effectively with antacid therapy, and the availability of routine proton pump inhibitors, including without prescription, has made this a much less significant issue for many patients. Although evidence for long-term benefit is sparse, it is clear from routine practice that these agents are remarkably effective and many patients find that even short-term discontinuation results in severe return of intolerable symptoms of oesophagitis [10]. However, in later stages of SSc, there are often very severe and refractory symptoms, and this may require high doses and combination of different antacid classes. It is important to treat reflux occurring in the context of lung fibrosis as it may lead to progression or worsening of lung disease or to important superadded complications such as aspiration and infection. Of the stomach complications of SSc, the most important is GAVE. This is under-recognised but can lead to recurrent severe anaemia or precipitous falls in haematocrit that may require regular transfusion. If oral iron supplementation is not sufficient or feasible, especially in the context of PPI therapy, then parenteral iron treatments may be beneficial. Photocoagulation, especially with argon plasma-based therapy, can be transformative although recurrent treatment is usually needed and the success of this can be monitored by repeat endoscopy and regular monitoring of full blood count [11]. Barrett's metaplasia is increasingly recognised in SSc and may be a consequence of chronic reflux. The management is in line with other cases of this disease with regular surveillance and individual assessment of risk and need for additional treatment [12].

Midgut Disease

Wight loss and malnutrition are common in SSc. The most frequent mechanism is inadequate oral intake, and this must be explored carefully so that patients try to maximise energy and protein consumption. This can be a real challenge due to the dental and mouth problems, dysphagia and postprandial bloating and the problems with lower bowel symptoms that may be improved when less is eaten. However oral nutritional supplements may be possible. Parenteral supplementation can be used intermittently or long-term enteral strategies with percutaneous gastrostomy or jejunostomy [13]. The latter is usually more feasible due to the problems of volume reflux associated with gastric feeding with risk of severe complications such as aspiration from reflux. Pancreatic enzyme supplements may be useful, and other comorbidities such as coeliac disease should be excluded. Interestingly many patients do report benefit from dietary modification and restriction; wheat, dairy products and red meat have all been reported to be useful in some cases. Probiotics may be useful although small intestinal bacterial overgrowth is also a common exacerbating factor that can be treated; broad spectrum antibiotics are used and can be given intermittently or if necessary in rotation with different classes of agent [14]. The most effective treatment usually is ciprofloxacin or a similar agent although many drugs are used including rifaximin when available. This has the theoretical advantage of not being absorbed and so may cause fewer systemic side effects. All SSc cases should be routinely assessed for clinically significant malnutrition, and the MUST (Malnutrition Universal Screening Tool) questionnaire provides a simple method to assess this [15]. If there is significant malnutrition, then expert input is needed, and sometimes cases need to be referred to intestinal failure specialist to be considered for parenteral nutrition. This can be given intermittently and may not be the total parenteral nutrition. Sometimes patients improve after medium-term treatment and are able to discontinue this form of feeding although these cases represent a minority.

Lower GI Complications

Up to half of patients with SSc experience lower GI complications of the disease, but these may be intermittent. In the most severe cases, there is severe constipation, sometimes leading to secondary complications such as sigmoid volvulus, diarrhoea that more often reflects midgut disease or pancreatic insufficiency and incontinence. The latter is underreported by patients but can be very debilitating. Treatments have been ineffective in part due to poor understanding of the pathology. More systematic studies have started to define better the links between investigational abnormality and symptoms, and this is central to progress. Modern imaging approaches and functional studies are shedding light on the structural pathology of anorectal SSc [16]. Interestingly, in the light of the multiple pathogenetic mechanisms that may operate, there is better correlation between altered neural function in the anorectum and structural change, and this may be important in the treatment [17]. There have been limited successes using sacral neuromodulation, and this is often a method used in severe late-stage disease. Recently preliminary data support alternative neurological approaches such as posterior tibial nerve stimulation, and this is a potential avenue for future treatment, and this may be superior to conventional sacral nerve stimulation [18]. Better engagement with other incontinence approaches can also be valuable, and some approaches such as sphincter augmentation with fillers as well as more simple approaches such as voluntary muscle strengthening exercises may be used.

Recommended Approach to Gastrointestinal Tract Complications in Systemic Sclerosis

Although it has been conventional to take an anatomical approach to the evaluation and classification of the GI manifestations of SSc, this has clear limitations since there is likely to be crossover in the mechanism and overlap in symptoms, and so it has recently been proposed that a more problem-orientated approach may be better. This emerged from a systematic exercise in defining the best practice management for the key GI complications of SSc and involved close collaboration between scleroderma specialists, gastroenterologists and nutritional experts. Pathways for the key complications have been suggested, and although these focus on UK healthcare system, they are relevant generally [19]. A focus is on the investigation and treatment together with the interface with treatment of other complications and GI comorbidities. Identifying the pointers for referral to specialist centres for investigation and treatment provides important keys to a better management. The need for close cross-speciality collaboration is highlighted and likely to become the expected standard for future treatment and better outcomes for GI scleroderma.

Concluding Remarks

Although some aspects of GI disease in SSc have been effectively related and the outcomes and complications such as stricture of the lower oesophagus and bolus obstruction are now much rarer, there remain real problems for patients related to some of the commonest aspects of SSc. Closer collaboration between specialists, a more problem-orientated approach and the use of innovative treatment strategies together will hopefully lead to more progress and better outcomes for some of the most difficult manifestations of SSc.

References

1. Thoua NM, Bunce C, Brough G, Forbes A, Emmanuel AV, Denton CP. Assessment of gastrointestinal symptoms in patients with systemic sclerosis in a UK tertiary referral centre. Rheumatology (Oxford). 2010;49(9):1770–5. doi:10.1093/rheumatology/keq147. Epub 2010 Jun 8.
2. Baron M, Hudson M, Tatibouet S, Steele R, Lo E, Gravel S, Gyger G, El Sayegh T, Pope J, Fontaine A, Masetto A, Matthews D, Sutton E, Thie N, Jones N, Copete M, Kolbinson D, Markland J, Nogueira G, Robinson D, Fritzler M, Gornitsky M. Relationship between disease characteristics and orofacial manifestations in systemic sclerosis: Canadian Systemic Sclerosis Oral Health Study III. Arthritis Care Res (Hoboken). 2015;67(5):681–90. doi:10.1002/acr.22490. PubMed PMID:25303223; PubMed Central PMCID: PMC4464822.
3. Ghrénassia E, Avouac J, Khanna D, Derk CT, Distler O, Suliman YA, Airo P, Carreira PE, Foti R, Granel B, Berezne A, Cabane J, Ingegnoli F, Rosato E, Caramaschi P, Hesselstrand R, Walker UA, Alegre-Sancho JJ, Zarrouk V, Agard C, Riccieri V, Schiopu E, Gladue H, Steen VD, Allanore Y. Prevalence, correlates and outcomes of gastric antral vascular ectasia in systemic sclerosis: a EUSTAR case-control study. J Rheumatol. 2014;41(1):99–105. doi:10.3899/jrheum.130386. Epub 2013 Dec 1.
4. Tauber M, Avouac J, Benahmed A, Barbot L, Coustet B, Kahan A, Allanore Y. Prevalence and predictors of small intestinal bacterial overgrowth in systemic sclerosis patients with gastrointestinal symptoms. Clin Exp Rheumatol. 2014;32(6 Suppl 86):S-82–7. Epub 2014 Nov 3.
5. Khanna D, Hays RD, Maranian P, Seibold JR, Impens A, Mayes MD, Clements PJ, Getzug T, Fathi N, Bechtel A, Furst DE. Reliability and validity of the University of California, Los Angeles scleroderma clinical trial consortium gastrointestinal tract instrument. Arthritis Rheum. 2009;61(9):1257–63.
6. Manetti M, Neumann E, Milia AF, Tarner IH, Bechi P, Matucci-Cerinic M, Ibba-Manneschi L, Müller-Ladner U. Severe fibrosis and increased expression of fibrogenic cytokines in the gastric wall of systemic sclerosis patients. Arthritis Rheum. 2007;56(10):3442–7.
7. Malandrini A, Selvi E, Villanova M, Berti G, Sabadini L, Salvadori C, Gambelli S, De Stefano R, Vernillo R, Marcolongo R, Guazzi G. Autonomic nervous system and smooth muscle cell involvement in systemic sclerosis: ultrastructural study of 3 cases. J Rheumatol. 2000;27(5):1203–6.
8. Thoua NM, Derrett-Smith EC, Khan K, Dooley A, Shi-Wen X, Denton CP. Gut fibrosis with altered colonic contractility in a mouse model of scleroderma. Rheumatology (Oxford). 2012;51(11):1989–98. doi:10.1093/rheumatology/kes191. Epub 2012 Aug 20.
9. Raja J, Nihtyanova SI, Murray CD, Denton CP, Ong VH. Sustained benefit from intravenous immunoglobulin therapy for gastrointestinal involvement in systemic sclerosis. Rheumatology. 2016;55(1):115–9.
10. Pakozdi A, Wilson H, Black CM, Denton CP. Does long term therapy with lansoprazole slow progression of oesophageal involvement in systemic sclerosis? Clin Exp Rheumatol. 2009;27(3 Suppl 54):5–8.

11. Kar P, Mitra S, Resnick JM, Torbey CF. Gastric antral vascular ectasia: case report and review of the literature. Clin Med Res. 2013;11(2):80–5. doi:10.3121/cmr.2012.1036. PubMed PMID: 23262190, PubMed Central PMCID: PMC3692392, Epub 2012 Dec 21. Review.
12. Wipff J, Coriat R, Masciocchi M, Caramaschi P, Derk CT, Hachulla E, Riccieri V, Mouthon L, Krasowska D, Ananyeva LP, Kahan A, Matucci-Cerinic M, Chaussade S, Allanore Y. Outcomes of Barrett's oesophagus related to systemic sclerosis: a 3-year EULAR scleroderma trials and research prospective follow-up study. Rheumatology (Oxford). 2011;50(8):1440–4. doi:10.1093/rheumatology/ker110. Epub 2011 Mar 16.
13. Bharadwaj S, Tandon P, Gohel T, Corrigan ML, Coughlin KL, Shatnawei A, Chatterjee S, Kirby DF. Gastrointestinal manifestations, malnutrition, and role of enteral and parenteral nutrition in patients with scleroderma. J Clin Gastroenterol. 2015;49(7):559–64. doi:10.1097/MCG.0000000000000334. PubMedPMID: 25992813.
14. Frech TM, Khanna D, Maranian P, Frech EJ, Sawitzke AD, Murtaugh MA. Probiotics for the treatment of systemic sclerosis-associated gastrointestinal bloating/distention. Clin Exp Rheumatol. 2011;29(2 Suppl 65):S22–5. Epub 2011 May 12.
15. Cereda E, Codullo V, Klersy C, Breda S, Crippa A, Rava ML, Orlandi M, Bonardi C, Fiorentini ML, Caporali R, Caccialanza R. Disease-related nutritional risk and mortality in systemic sclerosis. Clin Nutr. 2014;33(3):558–61. doi:10.1016/j.clnu.2013.08.010. Epub 2013 Sep 3.
16. Thoua NM, Schizas A, Forbes A, Denton CP, Emmanuel AV. Internal anal sphincter atrophy in patients with systemic sclerosis. Rheumatology (Oxford). 2011;50(9):1596–602. doi:10.1093/rheumatology/ker153. Epub 2011 Apr 18.
17. Thoua NM, Abdel-Halim M, Forbes A, Denton CP, Emmanuel AV. Fecal incontinence in systemic sclerosis is secondary to neuropathy. Am J Gastroenterol. 2012;107(4):597–603. doi:10.1038/ajg.2011.399. Epub 2011 Nov 15.
18. Butt S, Alam A, Cohen R, Krogh K, Buntzen S, Emmanuel A. Lack of effect of sacral nerve stimulation for incontinence in patients with systemic sclerosis. Colorectal Dis. 2015;17(10):903–7. doi:10.1111/codi.12969. [Epub ahead of print].
19. Hansi N, Thoua N, Carulli M, Chakravarty K, Lal S, Smyth A, Herrick A, Ogunbiyi O, Shaffer J, Mclaughlin J, Denton C, Ong V, Emmanuel AV, Murray CD. Consensus best practice pathway of the UK scleroderma study group: gastrointestinal manifestations of systemic sclerosis. Clin Exp Rheumatol. 2014;32(6 Suppl 86):S-214–21. Epub 2014 Nov 5.

Upper Gastrointestinal Tract: Manifestations of Systemic Sclerosis

30

John O. Clarke and John E. Pandolfino

Introduction

Systemic sclerosis (SSc) is a chronic connective tissue disorder with multisystem involvement. The gastrointestinal (GI) tract is affected in up to 90% of patients [1–3] and gut involvement is a leading cause of morbidity. Symptoms vary based on location of involvement and degree of impairment; however, dysphagia, reflux, nausea, vomiting, pain, diarrhea, constipation, fecal incontinence, and weight loss are all commonly reported. GI involvement severely impacts quality of life and is a major cause of mortality associated with SSc [4].

While the esophagus is the most widely described site of GI involvement, SSc can affect any site within the GI tract from the mouth to the anus. This chapter will focus on foregut manifestations of SSc, ranging from the mouth to stomach with an emphasis on both motility and bleeding. Involvement of other regions of the GI tract will be detailed in other chapters.

Oropharyngeal Cavity

Oropharyngeal manifestations of scleroderma are not well studied, with estimates of involvement ranging from 20 to 80% [5–7]. Sclerosis of the oropharyngeal mucosa, muscles associated with mastication and salivary glands, can lead to difficulty in speaking, chewing, and swallowing. Reported symptoms include head and neck numbness; tongue, hard palate, and soft palate fibrosis; microstomia; oral mucosa damage; perioral skin injury; xerostomia; periodontal ligament fibrous thickening; bone resorption; oral telangiectasia; trigeminal neuropathy; and significant dental caries. In addition, *sicca* symptoms are reported in up to 20% of SSc patients, and the associated decreased salivary gland production is typically associated with mild oropharyngeal dysphagia, due to lack of effective food bolus lubrication that impairs oropharyngeal transfer and esophageal transit. Significant perioral skin involvement can limit the mouth aperture and restrict food intake. Mixed connective tissue disorders that combine features of scleroderma with myositis may present with oropharyngeal dysphagia.

Therapeutic options are often limited to dietary modifications using small bolus size, soft foods, and increased use of liquid supplementation during meals. Close follow-up with a dentist or oral specialist is also recommended, as is optimal oral hygiene. To date, there are not good data to suggest that oropharyngeal manifestations of SSc respond to any specific medical therapy.

Esophagus

The esophagus is the most commonly affected organ in the GI tract in SSc, with involvement seen in over 90% of patients via both pathology [8] and symptom assessment [9]. Symptoms are related to dysmotility and commonly consist of dysphagia, heartburn, and regurgitation. The pathogenesis of dysfunction is still not clear and prior investigations have suggested several potential mechanisms. Sjogren proposed a progression of GI SSc involvement composed of three distinct steps: (1) vascular damage, (2) neurogenic impairment, and (3) replacement of normal smooth muscle by fibrosis and atrophy [10]. Under this model, there is loss of response to prokinetic therapy as fibrosis develops and progressive GI symptoms. However, to a certain extent, this theory remains speculative, as causal progression has never been demonstrated and other competing theories exist. Autoantibodies directed against enteric neurons have been identified in a subset of SSc patients [11]

J.O. Clarke, MD (✉)
Division of Gastroenterology & Hepatology, Johns Hopkins University, Baltimore, MD, USA
e-mail: john.clarke@jhu.edu

J.E. Pandolfino, MD, MS
Division of Gastroenterology & Hepatology, Feinberg School of Medicine, Northwestern University, Chicago, IL, USA

J. Varga et al. (eds.), *Scleroderma*, DOI 10.1007/978-3-319-31407-5_30

as have anti-muscarinic antibodies [12]. Responsiveness of the lower esophageal sphincter to exogenously administered methacholine but not pharmacologic administration of agents acting via cholinergic neurons supports the concept of a neurologic defect in SSc [13]. Autonomic dysfunction has also been posited as a potential mechanism [14]. In addition, there is contradictory data with regard to whether esophageal fibrosis is even present in these patients. A recent study using endoscopic ultrasound in patients with SSc revealed significant esophageal thickening as compared to unaffected controls [15]; however, in contrast, an autopsy study evaluating the esophagi of 74 patients with SSc showed significant atrophy (94 % of patients) but no evidence of abnormal fibrosis [8]. It is of note that the autopsy study did not demonstrate a correlation between the histopathology and disease duration. Interestingly, although the neurons within the myenteric plexus were intact, a reduction in the interstitial cells of Cajal important in modulating nerve-muscle interactions was demonstrated. In addition, no animal model for scleroderma esophageal disease exists, although there is a mouse model for colonic fibrosis [16].

Very recently, in a novel experiment, Taroni and colleagues evaluated esophageal biopsies in patients with and without scleroderma. They performed molecular characterization of gene expression combined with detailed histological analysis and identified distinct subgroups with either an inflammatory gene expression signature or a proliferative/non-inflammatory signature – and showed that these signatures appeared to be independent of traditional clinical markers of disease progression. Interestingly, similar gene expression signatures previously identified in SSc skin biopsies were recapitulated in SSc esophageal biopsies – implying that the underlying pathogenesis in individual patients may be similar in different organ systems. This study also suggested disease heterogeneity across SSc patients. Numbers evaluated in this study were small and clinical significance remains to be elucidated, but the mechanistic implications of this work are fascinating, and potentially this could lead to the development of future tissue biomarkers and recognition of molecular phenotypes with possible clinical implications [17].

Clinical Presentation and Complications

Symptoms attributable to esophageal dysfunction occur in the vast majority of patients with SSc and include heartburn, regurgitation, and dysphagia [7, 18–21]. Gastroesophageal reflux is of particular concern due to multiple contributing mechanisms, including peristaltic dysfunction, decreased lower esophageal sphincter (LES) pressure, delayed gastric emptying, autonomic dysfunction, occasional *sicca* syndrome (seen in 20 % of patients), and occasionally an associated hiatal hernia [19]. Just as important as the loss of the LES as an antireflux barrier is the loss of reflux clearance mechanisms that include secondary peristalsis and salivary bicarbonate secretion. Medications used to treat other manifestations of SSc including phosphodiesterase inhibitors and calcium channel antagonists further impair LES function and may worsen reflux. Dysphagia for solid food is related to decreased or absent esophageal peristalsis. In spite of the degree of functional impairment of esophageal motility, dysphagia is generally mild and intermittent owing to the ability of gravity to facilitate bolus transit. Furthermore, many patients, up to 40 % in some series, are asymptomatic despite well-documented esophageal dysmotility [22–25]. The clinical situation, however, can be complicated if a stricture is present due to reflux, pill-induced esophagitis, *Candida*, or other etiologies. Compensatory strategies include assuming an upright posture during meals and use of liquids between swallowing of solid food.

Esophageal dysmotility and reflux in the context of SSc can be associated with significant complications. Stricture formation is particularly prevalent and believed to be related to multiple possible etiologies, including reflux, pill-induced injury, and candidal infection. Prevalence of esophageal strictures in patients with SSc has been estimated to be as high as 29 % [26]. The frequent administration of proton pump inhibitor in SSc has, however, almost certainly reduced the prevalence of peptic strictures over the past two decades. A case-control study involving over 100,000 subjects evaluating risk factors for erosive esophagitis or esophageal stricture formation reported that a concurrent diagnosis of scleroderma was associated with an odds ratio of 6.1 for erosive esophagitis and 12.3 for stricture formation [27]. While reflux is believed to be the classic precipitant, candidal esophagitis is worth discussing given that patients with SSc typically have multiple risk factors, including chronic acid suppression, antibiotic administration, impaired esophageal motility, and use of immunosuppressive agents. One study reported colonization/infection rates of 15 % with strictures associated with all cases [28].

The prevalence of Barrett's esophagus has been reported to be as high as 37 % [29]; however, other investigators have reported significantly lower findings [26, 28], and due to this wide variation, it is not clear whether the prevalence of Barrett's esophagus in SSc patients exceeds that of the general public. Likewise, it is not clear that the risk of esophageal carcinoma is abnormal for patients with SSc [30]. It is also worth noting that most of the literature evaluating concerns for Barrett's esophagus and cancer predates widespread PPI use.

Finally, the natural history of esophageal dysmotility in SSc is not well studied; however, one recent publication evaluated patients seen over a 13-year period who had multiple esophageal scintigraphy transit studies performed. In this publication, esophageal motility worsened in 96% of patients with diffuse SSc as compared to 59% of patients with limited SSc [31].

Relationship to Pulmonary Disease

The relationship between reflux and pulmonary disease is not well established; however, reflux may contribute to pulmonary disease through two mechanisms: (1) microaspiration leading to direct injury and (2) vagal stimulation leading to bronchoconstriction. In addition, pulmonary disease may lead to increased reflux through alteration of esophageal/gastric pressure dynamics related to enhanced inspiratory force and diminished intrathoracic pressure, use of medications that decrease lower esophageal sphincter pressure (in particular bronchodilators and sildenafil), and potentially hiatal hernia formation. Given the morbidity and mortality associated with SSc lung disease, this relationship has substantial clinical importance.

Several studies have suggested a correlation between esophageal reflux and SSc lung disease [32–36]. However, this finding has not been universal as one study did not show any association [37]. Recently, this relationship has been evaluated with pH/impedance monitoring and high-resolution computed tomography, and a strong correlation was noted between interstitial lung disease and esophageal acid exposure, acid reflux numbers, nonacid reflux numbers, and proximal reflux (all with p values <0.01) [38]. Another recent study from the Canadian Scleroderma Research Group with over 1,000 patients also showed a strong correlation between symptoms of esophageal dysmotility and worsening pulmonary function (also with p values <0.01) [39]. Given this information, the relationship between the two entities appears consistent and likely genuine; however, causality has not been established, and there is no data at present to prove that treatment of reflux in patients with SSc has any effect upon long-term pulmonary function [40].

Diagnostic Evaluation

Multiple diagnostic modalities exist to evaluate esophageal function and disease in patients with SSc. If dysphagia is present, a barium esophagram is often the initial study as it provides information related to both structure and function. Dysphagia in SSc, however, is most commonly the result of dysmotility and not a structural lesion that can be visualized radiographically. On the other hand, while manometry is often considered the gold standard for esophageal function in SSc, it does not provide structural information and would not detect an esophageal stricture. Typical radiographic features include esophageal dilatation, presence of intraesophageal air, poor barium clearance, and a widely patent lower esophageal sphincter (Fig. 30.1) [41, 42]. Some authorities have recommended that a barium esophagram be the initial study for all patients with suspected scleroderma [43]; however, the sensitivity of barium studies for detection of SSc-related dysmotility has been shown to be less than manometry in several studies [43–46]. For this reason, most authorities would not recommend a barium study as the initial test for assessment of esophageal motility in the absence of significant dysphagia [19, 47].

Esophagogastroduodenoscopy (EGD) should be considered in patients presenting with esophageal symptoms related to SSc. Esophagitis has been reported in 32–77% of SSc patients undergoing endoscopy [21–23, 27, 28, 35, 43, 48–50]; however, multiple studies have shown that symptoms do not necessarily correlate with esophageal injury and that even SSc patients with no symptoms can have significant esophageal damage (Fig. 30.2) [28, 49–51]. In addition, as detailed above, *Candida* and Barrett's esophagus are clinical concerns and neither can be reliably detected without endoscopy. For these reasons, some authorities recommend early endoscopy for all patients diagnosed with SSc [49]; however, at present there are no guidelines to support that position and the decision to pursue endoscopy need to be individualized given the relative risks and benefits of the procedure. Other potential benefits of endoscopy include tissue acquisition for Barrett's esophagus to exclude dysplasia, identification of sites of upper GI hemorrhage, and ability to perform dilation of esophageal strictures.

Esophageal manometry is considered the gold standard for assessment of esophageal motility in patients with SSc [19, 47, 52]. Abnormalities are detected in up to 90% of patients, even in the absence of symptoms [53]. Typical findings on manometry include low-contraction amplitudes in the distal esophagus and, in more advanced stages, esophageal aperistalsis with decreased lower esophageal sphincter pressure (Fig. 30.3). Classically, esophageal contractile forces are maintained in the proximal esophagus, and the upper esophageal sphincter is uninvolved [54]. Defects in proximal esophageal contractile function may indicate concomitant myositis in patients with a mixed connective tissue disorder. Recently, high-resolution esophageal manometry (HRM) has entered the clinical arena, providing better quantification of peristaltic dysfunction (Fig. 30.3).

Finally, for patients with suspected reflux or continued symptoms despite medical therapy, formal reflux testing is often employed [55]. Traditional reflux testing consisted of a catheter-based pH study; however, two emerging technologies have been developed over the last decade and have changed the landscape with regard to reflux testing. Wireless pH testing eliminates the need for a catheter and records esophageal pH over a 48–96 h span. It can be combined with endoscopy, but also can be placed without endoscopic guid-

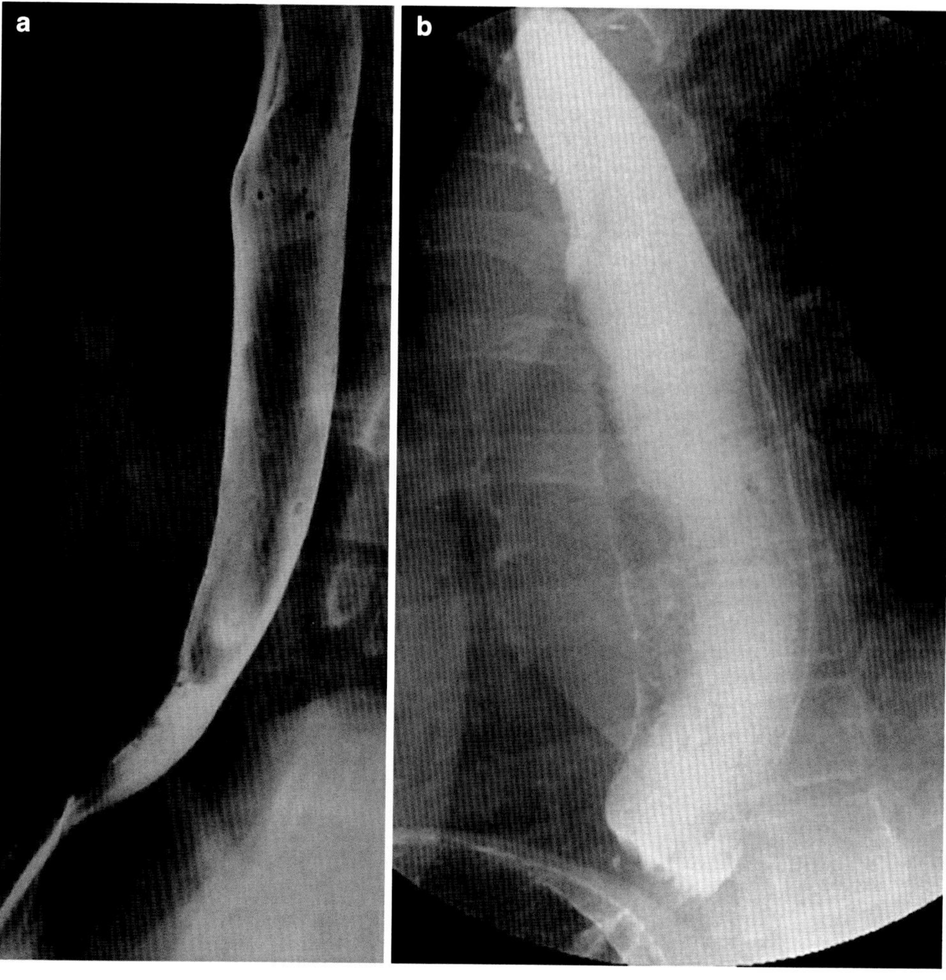

Fig. 30.1 Barium esophagram in scleroderma. Panel (**a**) depicts a normal esophagus with tapering at the esophagogastric junction. Panel (**b**) from a patient with scleroderma demonstrates pan esophageal dilatation

ance if baseline endoscopic information is known or a manometry is performed concurrently. Advantages of the wireless pH system include improve patient tolerability and prolonged recording periods that allow for increased detection of symptom-reflux correlation. The main limitation of wireless pH testing, though, is that it only looks at esophageal pH and does not allow assessment of weakly acidic or nonacidic reflux. The second emerging technology is pH impedance, which allows simultaneous measurement of bolus flow and esophageal pH, thereby allowing separation of acidic, weakly acidic, and nonacidic reflux as well as assessment of the proximal extent of reflux. While PPI therapy effectively controls esophageal acid exposure, it does not eliminate nonacid reflux which can be a major cause of morbidity in SSc patients owing to incompetency of the LES and delayed gastric emptying. Impedance technology has been studied in patients with SSc [38, 56] and does provide additional information; however, it requires an indwelling nasogastric tube for 24 h and the associated limitations therein. For clinical purposes, both modalities allow accurate assessment of reflux and can help guide clinical management in the context of ongoing reflux symptoms related to SSc [57].

Treatment

Treatment of SSc esophageal disorders can be challenging. Available therapies directed at the slowing or reversing of SSc progression including high-dose immunosuppression and stem cell transplantation have not demonstrated correction of the underlying gastrointestinal dysmotility. Nevertheless, effective therapies exist for managing the consequences of esophageal dysfunction. For those with reflux, initial treatment often consists of lifestyle modifications – including elevation of the head of the bed, avoidance of meals within 3 or more hours of lying supine, and avoidance of alcohol, caffeine, nicotine, and other known reflux exacerbants (such as tomatoes, citrus, garlic, chocolate, peppermint, onions). Care should be taken to minimize medication use that could result in esophageal inflammation or altered esophageal motility. If therapy is required for Raynaud's syndrome, diltiazem should be employed rather than other smooth muscle relaxants as it may have less effect on lower esophageal sphincter pressure [58, 59].

Acid suppressive therapy with proton pump inhibitors (PPI) is the mainstay of therapy for reflux in patients with

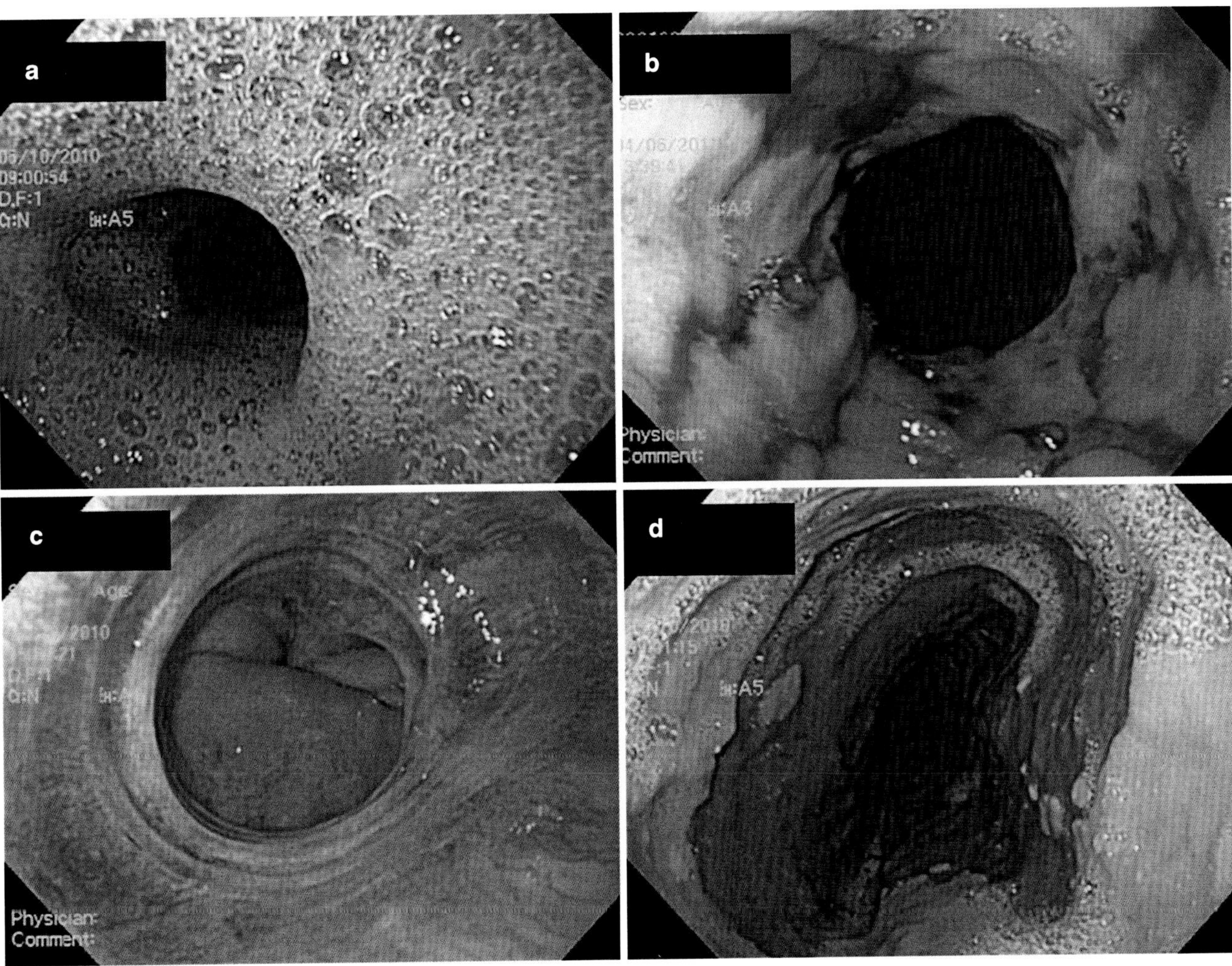

Fig. 30.2 Esophageal endoscopic findings in scleroderma. Panel (**a**) depicts retention of saliva within the esophagus. Panel (**b**) demonstrates reflux esophagitis with ulceration and stricture formation at the esophagogastric junction above a hiatal hernia. Panel (**c**) shows a peptic stricture. Panel (**d**) illustrates long segment Barrett's esophagus with small islands of squamous mucosa in a patient with scleroderma

SSc. Specific randomized controlled trials showing efficacy of PPI use in patients with SSc are lacking; however, the efficacy of PPI use in the treatment of gastroesophageal reflux in the general population is well documented, and recent expert consensus (European League against Rheumatism Scleroderma Trials and Research group, UK Scleroderma Study Group) recommends PPI use for the prevention of SSc-related reflux disease, strictures, and esophageal ulcers [60, 61]. This recommendation is supported by several small studies showing improvement in either symptoms or esophagitis with prolonged PPI use [50, 62, 63]. Despite the above recommendation, it is not clear that PPI use changes the natural history of scleroderma, and there is still some debate as to whether treatment should be based on symptoms or objective measures of esophageal acid exposure [19]. There is also data to suggest that SSc patients may require higher PPI dosages than other patients with reflux symptoms [50, 64]. This is not surprising given the impairment of multiple physiologic determinants of reflux in SSc. On the other hand, concerns exist regarding potential complications of long-term PPI therapy such as small intestinal bacterial overgrowth [65] and osteoporosis [66]. Histamine receptor blockers have also been employed with some efficacy; however, the data behind their use is less robust than with PPI use [67, 68]. One study adding ranitidine to high-dose omeprazole in SSc patients showed no change in nocturnal acid breakthrough, reflux, or quality of life [69].

If symptoms progress despite high-dose acid suppressive therapy and lifestyle change, the next step in therapy is typically the addition of a prokinetic agent. This pharmacologic category has been shown to accelerate gastric emptying and increase lower esophageal sphincter pressure. Several small randomized controlled trials demonstrated efficacy of short-term cisapride [70–74]; however, cisapride has been withdrawn from the market in the United States due to fatal, albeit rare, arrhythmias associated with long QT syndrome

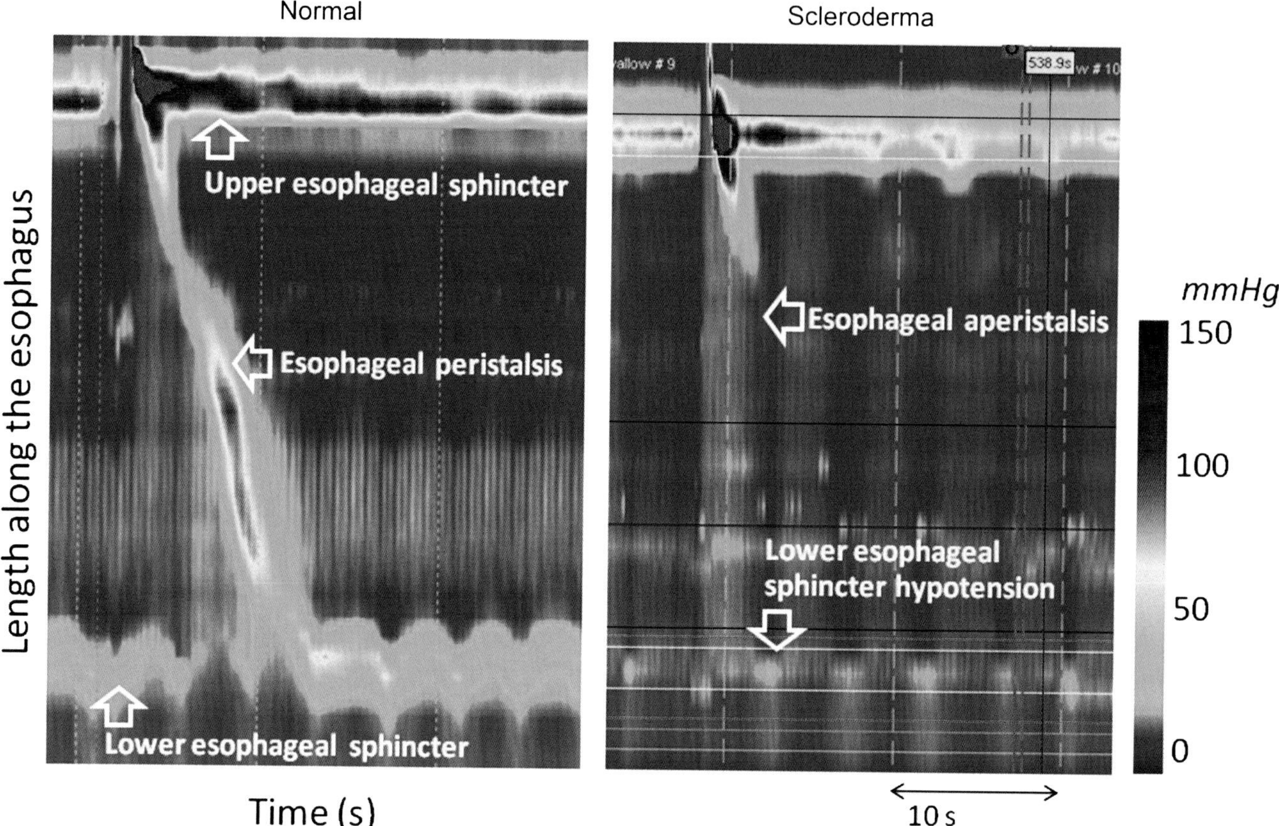

Fig. 30.3 High-resolution esophageal manometry contour plot in scleroderma. The *left* panel depicts a normal swallow with relaxation of the upper esophageal sphincter, sequential contractions in the esophageal body, and relaxation of the lower esophageal sphincter. The *right* panel from a patient with scleroderma demonstrates intact function of the upper esophageal sphincter and proximal esophagus but complete loss of contractile activity in the esophageal body and lower esophageal sphincter

and is available only in select countries or via Janssen Pharmaceutica for compassionate use. Limited data supports the use of metoclopramide in acute use [75–78]; however, long-term data demonstrating efficacy for metoclopramide is lacking, and safety concerns exist regarding long-term metoclopramide and tardive dyskinesia [79]. Limited data exist regarding erythromycin [80, 81]; however, this agent can be associated with tachyphylaxis and nausea in a substantial subset of patients and may not be ideal for long-term use. Finally, domperidone has been suggested as possible treatment [82] with less side effects than metoclopramide; however, there is limited data regarding domperidone in SSc patients, and this drug is not FDA approved in the United States. Overall, the clinical and physiologic benefits of available prokinetic agents in SSc are, at best, modest. Nevertheless, despite the limitations detailed above, a recent expert consensus recommends consideration of prokinetic drugs for the management of SSc-related symptomatic motility disturbances, including dysphagia and reflux [60].

A recent addition to the SSc dysmotility armamentarium has been buspirone, an oral 5-HT_{1A} recent agonist which is believed to exert action on receptors in the esophagus and fundus. It was recently found to reduce symptom severity in patients with dyspepsia, presumably due to enhanced fundic accommodation [83] – and also to improve esophageal peristalsis and enhance lower esophageal sphincter pressure in healthy volunteers [84]. Investigators from Greece evaluated 20 SSc patients with manometry before and after buspirone administration and found that buspirone enhanced lower esophageal sphincter pressure and improved peristalsis [85]. Clinical implications of this work remain uncertain; however, buspirone may be an option for patients who remain symptomatic despite further therapy, although more data are required to determine clinical efficacy and long-term safety.

In the event that gastroesophageal reflux cannot be controlled with medical therapy, surgical options do exist. Surgery is sometimes contemplated for relief of symptoms of heartburn or regurgitation that persist in spite of high-dose proton pump inhibition. The most common antireflux procedure performed today is the laparoscopic Nissen fundoplication; however, this can be associated with substantial dysphagia in SSc patients with severe dysmotility. The addition of even a minor degree of mechanical restriction at the esophagogastric junction in an SSc patient with absent esophageal peristalsis may result in the development of secondary achalasia. Early published series report postoperative dysphagia rates ranging from 31 to 71 % [86–89]. Because of these reports, surgical intervention has typically been reserved for severe cases. Recently, a retrospective review of 23 SSc patients undergoing antireflux surgery revealed improved reflux and dysphagia postoperative rates with laparoscopic Roux-en-Y gastric bypass as compared to fundoplication [90]. Based on these studies, surgery is an option for select patients; however, the risk of postoperative dysphagia needs to be considered, and this is typically a last resort when medical therapy has been unsuccessful.

Stomach

Gastric manifestations of SSc are highly variable and stem from both dysmotility and vascular ectasia. Symptoms of gastric dysmotility (including heartburn, regurgitation, nausea, bloating, epigastric pain, early satiety, and postprandial fullness) have been reported in approximately 50 % of patients [7, 26, 52, 91, 92]. Bleeding related to gastric antral vascular ectasia is seen far less commonly and will be discussed later in this chapter [93, 94]. The pathogenesis of gastric dysmotility remains unclear but is believed to be related to both neuropathic and fibrotic changes as detailed above. Gastric involvement is associated with worsened morbidity and mortality [2, 3].

Clinical Presentation

Symptoms associated with gastric dysmotility are seen in approximately 50 % of patients and include nausea, bloating, epigastric pain, early satiety, and postprandial fullness. In addition, gastric dysfunction also contributes to gastroesophageal reflux and may manifest only as traditional reflux symptoms, such as heartburn and regurgitation. Interestingly, the presence and severity of symptoms may not correlate with gastric dysfunction as measured by scintigraphy and electrogastrography (EGG) [92, 95, 96]; however, there is data to suggest that the presence of esophageal involvement corresponds with a higher rate of gastric involvement [7].

Multiple potential mechanisms have been hypothesized and objective studies of gastric function have recorded widely divergent findings – based on patient selection and study protocol. For example, gastric emptying has been recorded to be delayed in anywhere from 10 to 75 % of SSc patients, based on studies using scintigraphy, radio-opaque markers, C^{13}-labeled breath tests, and ultrasonography [51, 52, 78, 95–102]. Hypothesized mechanisms whereby SSc impairs gastric motility include alterations in gastric accommodation, motility patterns, gastric myoelectrical activity, and gastric emptying [92]. The relative role of each of the aforementioned mechanisms is not clearly established at this time and may vary for individual patients.

Diagnostic Evaluation

There is no consensus regarding the appropriate initial study for the evaluation of gastric dysmotility in patients with SSc. Given the high prevalence of esophageal dysmotility and the nonspecific nature of the recorded symptoms, initial evaluation often consists of a barium contrast study and/or upper endoscopy. Barium contrast radiography allows a gross evaluation of gastric motility and exclusion of mechanical obstruction. Typical findings related to gastric involvement include gastric dilatation, hypomotility, and delayed transit; however, barium contrast radiography is neither sensitive nor specific and is rarely if ever performed solely for assessment of gastric SSc involvement [42]. Similarly, upper endoscopy has utility in the evaluation of SSc and allows assessment of gastritis, peptic ulcer disease, esophagitis, and a gross assessment of pyloric contractions; however, the utility of endoscopy for SSc is primarily limited to assessment of inflammation and potential bleeding etiologies, whereas the role of endoscopy in assessment of gastric motility is limited. Retained food within the stomach during routine endoscopy is generally indicative of delayed gastric emptying as patients are instructed to fast for approximately 8 h prior to the procedure. If identified in the setting of an accurate history of meal timing, retained food may obviate the need for additional testing for gastric transit.

Gastric emptying studies have been the traditional test of choice for evaluation of gastric motility. Studies employing a variety of techniques – including scintigraphy, radio-opaque markers, C^{13} breath tests, and ultrasonography – have reported abnormalities in gastric emptying in between 10 and 75 % of SSc patients, although the bulk of the studies appear to show impairment in approximately 50 % of patients [26, 52, 78, 96, 99]. As these studies were performed in tertiary care facilities, these recorded values may overestimate the true prevalence of impaired gastric emptying in SSc. In the United States, the most commonly performed modality of gastric emptying study is scintigraphy, and normative values have been well-established [103]. However, this study is not without controversy as it can be expensive, and symptoms do not always correlate with objective emptying abnormalities, both in SSc and other unrelated conditions [99, 104]. Gastric emptying has also been assessed by other modalities, including radio-opaque marker transit [96], ultrasonography [102, 105], and breath testing [52, 106].

Recently, gastric emptying has been evaluated via a wireless capsule motility system (SmartPill) that provides prolonged recording of temperature, pH, and pressure. Whole transit is recorded over a several day period, and region transit (gastric emptying, small intestinal transit, colonic transit) can be distinguished through analysis of the pH and pressure profiles. In theory, this technology offers the ability to measure whole gut and regional transit as well as segmental motility patterns without the need for radiation exposure or catheter-based monitoring; however, data is still emerging regarding appropriate normative values and subtleties of interpretation. In addition, there is no data to date regarding the use of this technology in SSc patients. Finally, as the capsule is ingested, a theoretical risk of capsule retention does exist, and patients must be monitored to ensure the capsule has exited appropriately [107–109].

Gastric motility and myoelectrical activity can also be recorded using antroduodenal manometry (ADM) and electrogastrography (EGG). ADM consists of a manometry catheter which is passed transnasally and positioned so that pressure sensors are located in the duodenum and stomach. Prolonged pressure monitoring can be performed to allow assessment of migrating motor complex activity – in particular assessment of frequency, amplitude, and coordination of contractions. In patients with SSc, this technology can demonstrate decreased contractile amplitudes and disrupted patterns of motor activity [26, 110, 111]. EGG consists of multichannel surface recordings of gastric myoelectrical activity. The use of this technology has been largely experimental, and while abnormalities are frequently detected, it remains controversial whether EGG abnormalities correlate with either symptoms or delayed gastric emptying [99, 111, 112]. At present, both ADM and EGG are offered primarily in tertiary motility centers, and their role in routine clinical care of SSc patients remains unclear. In addition, the wireless capsule motility study has been compared directly to ADM with favorable correlation and may offer a less invasive means of obtaining similar data [107].

Treatment

Treatment of SSc-related gastric dysmotility can be challenging owing to limited treatment options. Dietary modification is typically the first line of therapy, and a gastroparesis diet, consisting of multiple, small volume, low-fat meals, is typically recommended. Liquid emptying may be preserved in certain cases, and liquid nutritional supplements and a soft diet that requires less emulsification may be of benefit, although the data behind this recommendation are limited. Enteral feeding and/or decompression via gastrostomy or jejunostomy is occasionally performed, although there are no data available regarding this approach. Similarly, limited data are available regarding the utilization of total parenteral nutrition although this is usually reserved for SSc patients with severe gastric and small bowel dysmotility.

Prokinetic agents have been the mainstay of therapy, although the data are relatively limited. Nevertheless, this approach is recommended by recent expert consensus panels [60, 61]. Metoclopramide is the only agent approved by the Food and Drug Administration in the United States for treatment of gastroparesis; however, it is associated with significant side effects including potentially irreversible tardive dyskinesia. Data regarding metoclopramide in SSc-related gastric dysmotility is largely limited to small studies evaluating short-term effects [76, 78, 110]. While short-term efficacy has been demonstrated, there is no data regarding long-term use or safety. In addition, there is a case report of one SSc patient who experienced bradycardia and cardiac arrest following metoclopramide administration [113].

Domperidone is a peripheral dopamine receptor antagonist that is believed to cross the blood-brain barrier less effectively than metoclopramide and may provide equal or superior efficacy with less side effects. There is no data regarding usage of domperidone in SSc (other than one study evaluating domperidone in esophageal dysmotility) [85]; however, there is data to support the use of domperidone in other conditions associated with impaired gastric emptying [114, 115]. At present, this medication is not approved for use in the United States; however, it can be obtained via an FDA Investigational New Drug application and is also available in at least 50 other countries. Despite the lack of data in SSc, the use of this agent can be justified based on the recent EULAR consensus recommendations [60], favorable side effect profile, and limited options available. Concern does exist for potential QT prolongation and patients must be monitored closely if this agent is employed [116].

Erythromycin is a motilin agonist and has data to support usage in both scleroderma and unrelated conditions with impaired gastric emptying. Two short-term studies demonstrated improvement in gastric emptying with erythromycin administration; one of the studies also looked at symptom response and reported improvement in early satiety, nausea, vomiting, and abdominal pain [81, 97]. A single study looked at long-term use of erythromycin (up to 48 weeks in duration) and reported benefit; however, the patients in the study were also administered octreotide concurrently, and the relative merits of each agent were not clearly elucidated [117]. Of the available agents, erythromycin has been demonstrated to have the most potent gastric prokinetic function; however, in practice it is often not as attractive as other options for several reasons. First, it is associated with tachyphylaxis. Second, side effects include cramps, nausea, diarrhea, ototoxicity, and QT interval prolongation – all limiting use [118]. Third, although erythromycin has potent prokinetic properties, a systematic review concluded that available studies do not establish efficacy of erythromycin in relieving symptoms of delayed gastric emptying [119]. For all of these reasons, erythromycin may be a less than ideal option for long-term use – although it does have the benefit of documented short-term improvement in SSc and availability in the United States.

Cisapride is a combined $5HT_4$ agonist/$5HT_3$ antagonist and is the most investigated prokinetic available for treatment of SSc-associated dysmotility. Small studies have demonstrated improvement in gastric emptying, antroduodenal motility, and symptoms with acute and chronic use [70, 92, 120]. However, cisapride was removed from the US market due to QT interval prolongation and numerous deaths related to cardiac arrhythmia. It is available on a limited basis for compassionate use; however, it should be used with caution, and close monitoring of the QT interval is required if this medication is initiated.

Alternative therapies have also been employed for SSc-associated gastric dysmotility and are worth considering given the imperfections of established therapies. Ginger has been shown to accelerate gastric emptying in normal individuals [121] and has been used to relieve pregnancy-associated nausea [122]. This has not been studied in SSc or gastroparesis; however, given the innocuous side effect profile, it is worth considering as an adjunct therapy.

Recently, there has also been research directed toward acupuncture and related entities as a potential remedy [123]. Acupressure to a specific GI-associated acupuncture site (PC6) was found to alter gastric myoelectrical activity (GMA) as assessed by EGG in patients with SSc in one small study. Interestingly, the alterations in GMA correlated with symptoms [124]. Based on this preliminary study, the same group evaluated the role of transcutaneous electrical nerve stimulation in symptomatic SSc patients for a 14-day trial. They reported improvement in heart rate variability, symptoms, and quality of life [125]. A further study by the same investigators showed improvement in GMA, decreased mean plasma VIP and motilin levels, increased IL-6 levels, and symptom improvement after a 14-day trial [126]. While further studies are needed, these preliminary investigations are encouraging.

Finally, endoscopic and surgical options have been posited and are worth discussing. Botulinum toxin has been investigated in impaired gastric emptying. The proposed mechanism is that botulinum toxin injected into the pylorus may relieve gastric outlet obstruction and accelerate gastric emptying. Early anecdotal experience supported this assumption; however, more recent randomized controlled trials have not shown a benefit for botulinum toxin in idiopathic or diabetic gastroparesis, and for this reason, it has largely fallen out of favor unless there is documented pyloric spasm [127]. There is no data regarding the use of botulinum toxin in patients with SSc; however, as the physiology of SSc often results in impaired contractions and lower contractile amplitudes, one could argue that SSc-associated gastric dysmotility may be even more unlikely to respond to this therapy than patients with impaired gastric emptying related to other conditions [118]. Surgical options have also been proposed for impaired gastric emptying, including pyloric myotomy, subtotal gastrectomy, gastric bypass, and gastric electrical stimulation. There is no data to support the use of any of these procedures in SSc-associated gastric dysmotility.

Gastric Antral Vascular Ectasia

GI hemorrhage is a known consequence of SSc and can be seen in up to 15 % of SSc patients in a tertiary care facility [128]. Gastric antral vascular ectasia (GAVE), also known as watermelon stomach, is the major gastric manifestation which may lead to bleeding. This is an uncommon vascular condition that was first described in 1984 [129]. While classically associated with SSc, it is not specific to rheumatologic disorders and can also be seen in atrophic gastritis, diabetes mellitus, cirrhosis, chronic renal failure, and heart disease – as well as autoimmune disorders. The true prevalence of GAVE is difficult to determine; however, this does appear to be relatively uncommon and the largest series to date to evaluate this issue reported a prevalence of 5.7 % (15 cases in 274 SSc patients); however, this may be an underestimation given that many patients may be asymptomatic in early stages, and the endoscopic findings of mild GAVE can be misinterpreted as antral gastritis by even experienced endoscopists [93]. A recent publication from the European League Against Rheumatism Scleroderma Trials and Research (EUSTAR) network estimated the prevalence of GAVE to be about 1 % in SSc patients [130].

The pathogenesis of GAVE remains unclear. At the moment, there are two leading hypotheses. The first theory holds that antral mucosal prolapse and abnormal gastric motility may lead to submucosal ischemia and elongation/dilatation of mucosal vessels. This theory is supported by two lines of reasoning: (1) histological evidence of both fibromuscular hyperplasia and mucosal capillary dilatation and (2) documentation of select SSc patients with high-amplitude gastric antral contractions on antroduodenal manometry [93, 129, 131, 132]. The second theory suggests that GAVE may be related to SSc-associated diffuse cutaneous telangiectasia. This theory is supported by the fact that most patients with GAVE also have telangiectasia involving other regions of the body (in particular skin) or GI tract [93]. In either case, the predilection of this vascular abnormality for the gastric antrum may be related to the distinct motility patterns that characterize the gastric antrum in distinction to other regions of the stomach.

Given the rarity of GAVE, the natural history is not well studied; however, available data suggests that the vast majority of SSc patients diagnosed with GAVE (81 %) already have an established diagnosis of SSc at the time of their endoscopic GAVE diagnosis. In an additional 8 % of patients, the diagnoses of SSc and GAVE were established concurrently, whereas in the remaining 11 %, the diagnosis of GAVE preceded the diagnosis of SSc. In patients known to have a diagnosis of GAVE, the median time between SSc diagnosis and GAVE onset was 18 months. Given this data, GAVE appears to be an early manifestation of SSc and the majority of cases were diagnosed within 5 years of diagnosis. The prevalence of GAVE also appears to be similar in diffuse and limited SSc, although diagnosis may be earlier in diffuse SSc as opposed to limited. It is unclear whether GAVE activity is associated with SSc activity or a more aggressive SSc phenotype. One review reported that in the majority of patients, GAVE activity does not parallel SSc activity, and GAVE can occur or progress even when disease activity was not active on other fronts; however, another recent publication reported that in the majority of patients with diffuse SSc diagnosed with early GAVE, there was also a rapid progression of cutaneous disease [93, 94]. Finally, a recent EUSTAR case-control study of 49 patients with SSc and GAVE reported that patients with GAVE were associated with a vascular phenotype, including anti-RNA polymerase III antibodies and a high risk of renal crisis [130].

The classic clinical presentation of GAVE is iron-deficiency anemia related to occult GI bleeding. Available data suggests that this is the case in approximately 90 % of patients, and the mean hemoglobin at time of diagnosis has been reported to be 6.7 g/dl. Other clinical presentations include overt bleeding with melena or hematemesis; however, this is present in only a minority of patients [93]. GAVE is not specific for SSc and has been described in other autoimmune disorders, hepatic cirrhosis, chronic renal failure, cardiac disease, and bone marrow transplantation. GAVE is sometimes confused with but is distinct from portal hypertensive gastropathy with the latter entity involving the mucosa of the gastric fundus and body. Histopathology of GAVE demonstrates the presence of microvascular thrombi, vascular ectasia, spindle cell proliferation, and fibrohyalinosis.

The endoscopic appearance is classically described as erythematous streaks projecting from the pylorus in radial fashion throughout the antrum (Fig. 30.4). The term "watermelon stomach" was coined as these streaks appear similar to the outside of a watermelon [129]. Another endoscopic variant that has been described is referred to as "honeycomb stomach" and consists of diffuse angiodysplastic lesions that coalesce in the antrum [133]. Finally, a third variant has been described in which there are well-demarcated round or mushroom-shaped lesions formed by a tuft of ecstatic blood vessels [134]. In addition, involvement can extend proximal to the antrum in a subset of patients [93, 94].

Treatment for GAVE remains a challenge and data is relatively limited. There are no randomized controlled trials for non-endoscopic treatments and initial therapy is often supportive. Given that the majority of GAVE patients present with occult bleeding and iron-deficiency anemia, the first step is often iron replacement therapy, optimization of bleeding parameters (if necessary), and minimization or avoidance of medications that could either promote bleeding or injure the gastric mucosa [134, 135]. Proton pump inhibitors are also usually employed to decrease any further mucosal injury that may be potentiated by gastric acid [93]. Blood transfusions are often required given the low hemoglobin at diagnosis, other comorbidities, and slow response with the above measures – and despite conservative therapy, as many as 60–70 % of patients remain transfusion dependent [134].

The number of medical therapies that have been attempted bespeaks to the inadequacies of the current options. Steroids were attempted in several early reports with moderate success. Combining those reports, 11 patients have been given steroids alone and six were reported to have complete resolution of bleeding; however, another patient had hyperglycemia and four patients had no response [134]. A case report detailed a single patient who received intravenous methylprednisolone and cyclophosphamide with complete resolution [136]. The potential benefits of steroids have to be weighed against the risks and potential caustic effect on GI mucosa.

Cyclophosphamide is also an option for refractory GAVE. In addition to the single case report detailed above using cyclophosphamide in combination with steroids, there is a recent case series describing three patients with SSc-related GAVE treated with intravenous pulse cyclophosphamide – all of whom had improvement via both clinical and endoscopic parameters [137]. However, at present this data is limited to three patients and confirmatory studies are needed.

Hormonal therapy was initially hypothesized as a treatment due to the observation that epistaxis associated with Osler-Weber-Rendu syndrome decreases during pregnancy and worsens postpartum. In an open pilot study looking at a combination of estrogen and progesterone for GAVE related to cirrhosis, four of six patients had complete cessation of bleeding; however, the endoscopic appearance was not altered, raising concern that bleeding would recur upon symptom discontinuation. In addition, the long-term risks of hormonal therapy have to be considered, and it is worth mentioning that three of the six patients treated in this study developed gynecomastia and menorrhagia [138]. A few case reports support this approach; however, data remains very limited, and this likely remains an option best suited for post-menopausal women or SSc patients judged to be too high risk for endoscopic approaches [134].

Octreotide is a third option that has been studied in cirrhotic patients with refractory vascular GI bleeding, some of whom had GAVE. However, much of this benefit may have

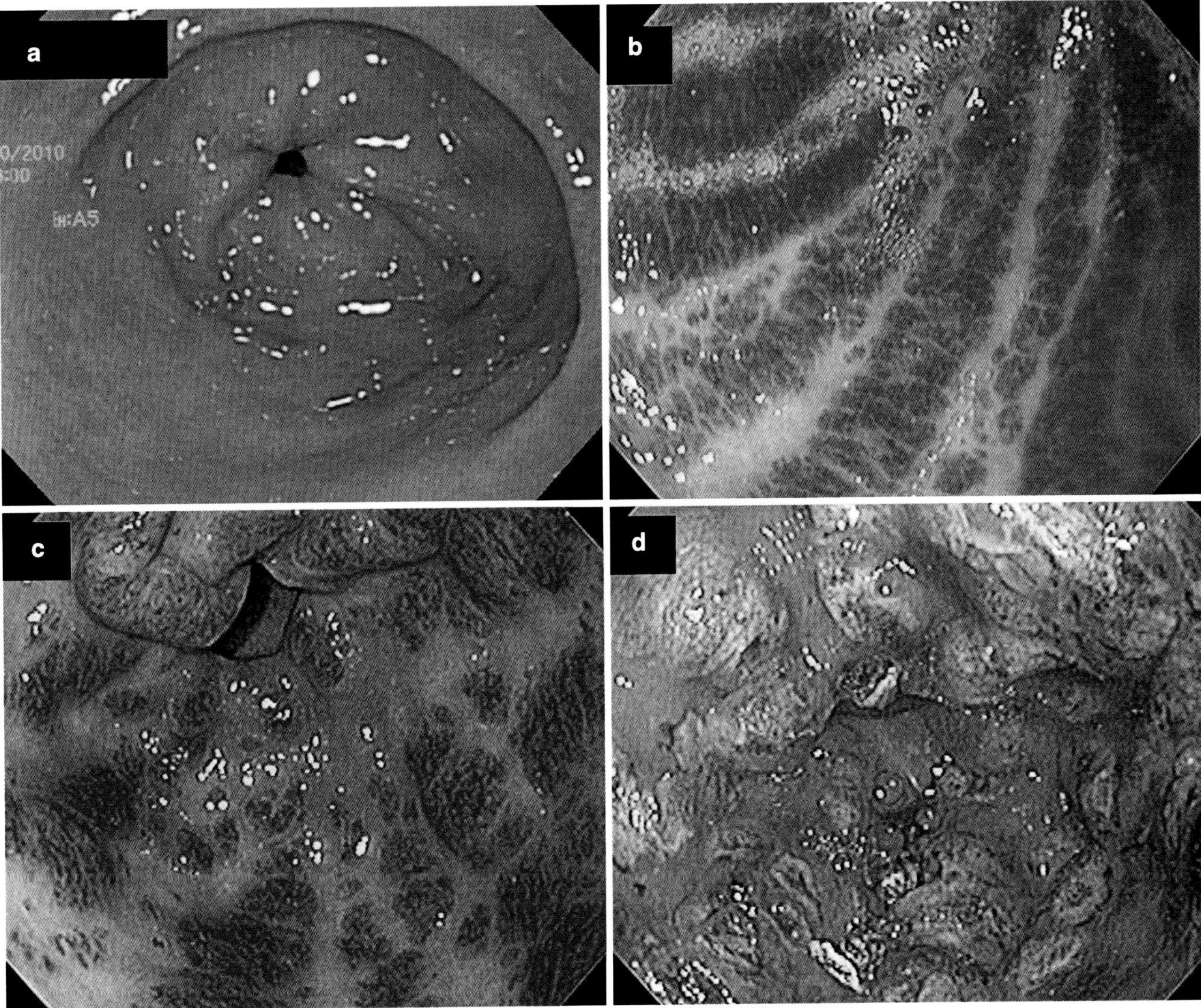

Fig. 30.4 Gastric endoscopic findings in scleroderma. Panel (**a**) shows the normal appearance to the gastric antrum. Panels (**b**, **c**) depict scleroderma patients with gastric antral vascular ectasia (GAVE) with erythematous, linear streaks along the long axis of the antrum. Panel (**d**) shows the appearance of GAVE immediately after therapy with argon plasma coagulation. The white patches represent superficial mucosal injury created by the therapy that rapidly heal and are replaced by normal gastric mucosa

been from decreased portal pressure in the context of cirrhosis, and it is unclear if the same benefit would apply to patients with SSc. A case report describes a patient with SSc who received octreotide for GAVE without benefit [93]. Finally, there are additional case reports of other medical therapies for GAVE patients without SSc, including histamine receptor antagonists, calcitonin, tranexamic acid, interferon, serotonin antagonists, and thalidomide; however, none of these have been reported for SSc-related GAVE [93, 134].

Endoscopic therapy has become the mainstay of treatment when supportive care and medical therapy is unsuccessful. Multiple endoscopic ablative modalities have been employed, including Nd:YAG laser, argon plasma coagulation (APC), bipolar electrocautery, heater probe, and argon laser. Traditionally, the mainstay of treatment was with the Nd:YAG laser system, and it has the largest literature to support use, with reported success rates of approximately 80 % over multiple treatments; however, significant complications were reported, including hyperplastic polyps, multifocal gastric neoplasia, perforation, and death [93, 134]. APC is an electrocoagulation technique which induces superficial injury to the affected tissue through a high-frequency monopolar current conducted through ionized argon gas. As compared to Nd:YAG laser, APC offers the theoretical advantages of limited penetration depth and coagulation effect to the surrounding tissue, resulting in less complications. Published success rates for APC have been similar to those for Nd:YAG laser. Due to similar efficacy and less risk, APC has become the standard of care at present for endoscopic treatment of SSc-related GAVE [3, 93, 134].

Two new endoscopic techniques have entered the clinical arena and are worth considering: cryotherapy and radiofrequency ablation (RFA). Cryotherapy consists of the endoscopic application of either nitrous oxide or carbon dioxide (based on the system employed), resulting in a controlled thermal injury to the gastric mucosa. As opposed to Nd:YAG laser or APC, cryotherapy allows treatment of large mucosal areas relatively quickly and offers the potential of shorter procedure times and technical ease with perhaps equal efficacy. This may be especially beneficial for diffuse GAVE with large areas of involvement. The first trial evaluating cryotherapy in the human GI tract was in 2003 and included seven patients with GAVE (71.4 % response) [139]. A second study employing cryotherapy specifically for 12 patients with GAVE reported a 50 % complete response rate and 50 % partial response rate; however, it is worth noting that eight of the 12 patients enrolled in the study had previously been treated unsuccessfully with APC [140]. Of note, it is unclear from both studies whether any of the affected patients had SSc. Nevertheless, given this information, cryotherapy is worth considering in patients with disease refractory to APC, in particular in those patients with diffuse involvement.

The second emerging endoscopic technology is RFA. This technology allows a focused radio-frequency energy delivery to gastric tissue and results in a controlled superficial injury with uniform depth of ablation. There is recent extensive data regarding this technology in Barrett's esophagus, showing both efficacy and safety [141]. Recently, this technology was employed in six patients with GAVE with no complications and improvement in five of the six treated [142]. While it is unclear if any of the patients in the study had SSc and this data is limited, this technology may be used more frequently in the future given the growing usage of RFA in Barrett's esophagus, presence in endoscopy units, and increasing technical proficiency of endoscopists.

Surgical management has been reserved as the final option for those patients who have failed endoscopic treatment options. Antrectomy has been the most common procedure performed; however, there is significant morbidity and mortality associated with this procedure, and one report suggested a mortality rate of 7.4 % (in all GAVE patients, not SSc-related GAVE specifically) [93, 134, 135]. Given this, antrectomy should be reserved as a last resort for SSc patients with GAVE; however, it is an option if all else fails.

References

1. LeRoy EC, Black C, Fleischmajer R, et al. Scleroderma (systemic sclerosis): classification, subsets and pathogenesis. J Rheumatol. 1988;15:202–5.
2. Clements PJ, Becvar R, Drosos AA, Ghattas L, Gabrielli A. Assessment of gastrointestinal involvement. Clin Exp Rheumatol. 2003;21:S15–8.
3. Forbes A, Marie I. Gastrointestinal complications: the most frequent internal complications of systemic sclerosis. Rheumatology (Oxford). 2009;48 Suppl 3:iii36–9.
4. Steen VD, Medsger TA. Changes in causes of death in systemic sclerosis, 1972–2002. Ann Rheum Dis. 2007;66:940–4.
5. Vitali C, Borghi E, Napoletano A, et al. Oropharyngolaryngeal disorders in scleroderma: development and validation of the SLS scale. Dysphagia. 2010;25:127–38.
6. Scardina GA, Mazzullo M, Messina P. Early diagnosis of progressive systemic sclerosis: the role of oro-facial phenomena. Minerva Stomatol. 2002;51:311–7.
7. Domsic R, Fasanella K, Bielefeldt K. Gastrointestinal manifestations of systemic sclerosis. Dig Dis Sci. 2008;53:1163–74.
8. Roberts CG, Hummers LK, Ravich WJ, Wigley FM, Hutchins GM. A case-control study of the pathology of oesophageal disease in systemic sclerosis (scleroderma). Gut. 2006;55:1697–703.
9. Thoua NM, Bunce C, Brough G, Forbes A, Emmanuel AV, Denton CP. Assessment of gastrointestinal symptoms in patients with systemic sclerosis in a UK tertiary referral centre. Rheumatology (Oxford). 2010;49:1770–5.
10. Sjogren RW. Gastrointestinal motility disorders in scleroderma. Arthritis Rheum. 1994;37:1265–82.
11. Howe S, Eaker EY, Sallustio JE, Peebles C, Tan EM, Williams Jr RC. Antimyenteric neuronal antibodies in scleroderma. J Clin Invest. 1994;94:761–70.
12. Goldblatt F, Gordon TP, Waterman SA. Antibody-mediated gastrointestinal dysmotility in scleroderma. Gastroenterology. 2002;123:1144–50.
13. Cohen S, Fisher R, Lipshutz W, Turner R, Myers A, Schumacher R. The pathogenesis of esophageal dysfunction in scleroderma and Raynaud's disease. J Clin Invest. 1972;51:2663–8.
14. Dessein PH, Joffe BI, Metz RM, Millar DL, Lawson M, Stanwix AE. Autonomic dysfunction in systemic sclerosis: sympathetic overactivity and instability. Am J Med. 1992;93:143–50.
15. Zuber-Jerger I, Muller A, Kullmann F, et al. Gastrointestinal manifestation of systemic sclerosis – thickening of the upper gastrointestinal wall detected by endoscopic ultrasound is a valid sign. Rheumatology (Oxford). 2010;49:368–72.
16. Thoua NM, Derrett-Smith EC, Khan K, Dooley A, Shi-Wen X, Denton CP. Gut fibrosis with altered colonic contractility in a mouse model of scleroderma. Rheumatology (Oxford). 2012;51:1989–98.
17. Taroni JN, Martyanov V, Huang CC, et al. Molecular characterization of systemic sclerosis esophageal pathology identifies inflammatory and proliferative signatures. Arthritis Res Ther. 2015;17:194.
18. Ostojic P, Damjanov N. Different clinical features in patients with limited and diffuse cutaneous systemic sclerosis. Clin Rheumatol. 2006;25:453–7.
19. Ebert EC. Esophageal disease in scleroderma. J Clin Gastroenterol. 2006;40:769–75.
20. Ebert EC. Esophageal disease in progressive systemic sclerosis. Curr Treat Options Gastroenterol. 2008;11:64–9.
21. Arif T, Masood Q, Singh J, Hassan I. Assessment of esophageal involvement in systemic sclerosis and morphea (localized scleroderma) by clinical, endoscopic, manometric and pH metric features: a prospective comparative hospital based study. BMC Gastroenterol. 2015;15:24.
22. Abu-Shakra M, Guillemin F, Lee P. Gastrointestinal manifestations of systemic sclerosis. Semin Arthritis Rheum. 1994;24:29–39.
23. Ling TC, Johnston BT. Esophageal investigations in connective tissue disease: which tests are most appropriate? J Clin Gastroenterol. 2001;32:33–6.
24. Kaye SA, Siraj QH, Agnew J, Hilson A, Black CM. Detection of early asymptomatic esophageal dysfunction in systemic sclerosis using a new scintigraphic grading method. J Rheumatol. 1996;23:297–301.

25. Harper RA, Jackson DC. Progressive systemic sclerosis. Br J Radiol. 1965;38:825–34.
26. Weston S, Thumshirn M, Wiste J, Camilleri M. Clinical and upper gastrointestinal motility features in systemic sclerosis and related disorders. Am J Gastroenterol. 1998;93:1085–9.
27. El-Serag HB, Sonnenberg A. Association of esophagitis and esophageal strictures with diseases treated with nonsteroidal anti-inflammatory drugs. Am J Gastroenterol. 1997;92:52–6.
28. Zamost BJ, Hirschberg J, Ippoliti AF, Furst DE, Clements PJ, Weinstein WM. Esophagitis in scleroderma. Prevalence and risk factors. Gastroenterology. 1987;92:421–8.
29. Katzka DA, Reynolds JC, Saul SH, et al. Barrett's metaplasia and adenocarcinoma of the esophagus in scleroderma. Am J Med. 1987;82:46–52.
30. Segel MC, Campbell WL, Medsger Jr TA, Roumm AD. Systemic sclerosis (scleroderma) and esophageal adenocarcinoma: is increased patient screening necessary? Gastroenterology. 1985;89:485–8.
31. Vischio J, Saeed F, Karimeddini M, et al. Progression of esophageal dysmotility in systemic sclerosis. J Rheumatol. 2012;39:986–91.
32. Denis P, Ducrotte P, Pasquis P, Lefrancois R. Esophageal motility and pulmonary function in progressive systemic sclerosis. Respiration. 1981;42:21–4.
33. Johnson DA, Drane WE, Curran J, et al. Pulmonary disease in progressive systemic sclerosis. A complication of gastroesophageal reflux and occult aspiration? Arch Intern Med. 1989;149: 589–93.
34. Lock G, Pfeifer M, Straub RH, et al. Association of esophageal dysfunction and pulmonary function impairment in systemic sclerosis. Am J Gastroenterol. 1998;93:341–5.
35. Marie I, Dominique S, Levesque H, et al. Esophageal involvement and pulmonary manifestations in systemic sclerosis. Arthritis Rheum. 2001;45:346–54.
36. Kinuya K, Nakajima K, Kinuya S, Michigishi T, Tonami N, Takehara K. Esophageal hypomotility in systemic sclerosis: close relationship with pulmonary involvement. Ann Nucl Med. 2001;15:97–101.
37. Troshinsky MB, Kane GC, Varga J, et al. Pulmonary function and gastroesophageal reflux in systemic sclerosis. Ann Intern Med. 1994;121:6–10.
38. Savarino E, Bazzica M, Zentilin P, et al. Gastroesophageal reflux and pulmonary fibrosis in scleroderma: a study using pH-impedance monitoring. Am J Respir Crit Care Med. 2009;179:408–13.
39. Zhang XJ, Bonner A, Hudson M, Canadian Scleroderma Research G, Baron M, Pope J. Association of gastroesophageal factors and worsening of forced vital capacity in systemic sclerosis. J Rheumatol. 2013;40:850–8.
40. Christmann RB, Wells AU, Capelozzi VL, Silver RM. Gastroesophageal reflux incites interstitial lung disease in systemic sclerosis: clinical, radiologic, histopathologic, and treatment evidence. Semin Arthritis Rheum. 2010;40:241–9.
41. Olive A, Juncosa S, Evison G, Maddison PJ. Air in the oesophagus: a sign of oesophageal involvement in systemic sclerosis. Clin Rheumatol. 1995;14:319–21.
42. Madani G, Katz RD, Haddock JA, Denton CP, Bell JR. The role of radiology in the management of systemic sclerosis. Clin Radiol. 2008;63:959–67.
43. Clements PJ, Kadell B, Ippoliti A, Ross M. Esophageal motility in progressive systemic sclerosis (PSS). Comparison of cine-radiographic and manometric evaluation. Dig Dis Sci. 1979;24: 639–44.
44. Weihrauch TR, Korting GW. Manometric assessment of oesophageal involvement in progressive systemic sclerosis, morphea and Raynaud's disease. Br J Dermatol. 1982;107:325–32.
45. Jayanthi V, Srinivasan V, Nayak VM, Krishnamurthi V, Victor S. Comparative evaluation of cine-esophagogram with esophageal manometry in assessing esophageal motility in progressive systemic sclerosis. Indian J Gastroenterol. 1996;15:129–31.
46. Klein HA, Wald A, Graham TO, Campbell WL, Steen VD. Comparative studies of esophageal function in systemic sclerosis. Gastroenterology. 1992;102:1551–6.
47. Lock G, Zeuner M, Straub RH, et al. Esophageal manometry in systemic sclerosis: screening procedure or confined to symptomatic patients? Rheumatol Int. 1997;17:61–6.
48. Bassotti G, Battaglia E, Debernardi V, et al. Esophageal dysfunction in scleroderma: relationship with disease subsets. Arthritis Rheum. 1997;40:2252–9.
49. Thonhofer R, Siegel C, Trummer M, Graninger W. Early endoscopy in systemic sclerosis without gastrointestinal symptoms. Rheumatol Int. 2012;32(1):165–8.
50. Marie I, Ducrotte P, Denis P, Hellot MF, Levesque H. Oesophageal mucosal involvement in patients with systemic sclerosis receiving proton pump inhibitor therapy. Aliment Pharmacol Ther. 2006;24:1593–601.
51. Wegener M, Adamek RJ, Wedmann B, Jergas M, Altmeyer P. Gastrointestinal transit through esophagus, stomach, small and large intestine in patients with progressive systemic sclerosis. Dig Dis Sci. 1994;39:2209–15.
52. Savarino E, Mei F, Parodi A, et al. Gastrointestinal motility disorder assessment in systemic sclerosis. Rheumatology (Oxford). 2013;52:1095–100.
53. Rajapakse CN, Bancewicz J, Jones CJ, Jayson MI. Pharyngo-oesophageal dysphagia in systemic sclerosis. Ann Rheum Dis. 1981;40:612–4.
54. Mainie I, Tutuian R, Patel A, Castell DO. Regional esophageal dysfunction in scleroderma and achalasia using multichannel intraluminal impedance and manometry. Dig Dis Sci. 2008;53:210–6.
55. Hirano I, Richter JE. ACG practice guidelines: esophageal reflux testing. Am J Gastroenterol. 2007;102:668–85.
56. Carlo-Stella N, Belloli L, Barbera R, et al. Gastroesophageal reflux and lung disease in systemic sclerosis. Am J Respir Crit Care Med. 2009;179:1167; author reply -8.
57. Carlson DA, Hinchcliff M, Pandolfino JE. Advances in the evaluation and management of esophageal disease of systemic sclerosis. Curr Rheumatol Rep. 2015;17:475.
58. Kahan A, Bour B, Couturier D, Amor B, Menkes CJ. Nifedipine and esophageal dysfunction in progressive systemic sclerosis. A controlled manometric study. Arthritis Rheum. 1985;28:490–5.
59. Jean F, Aubert A, Bloch F, et al. Effects of diltiazem versus nifedipine on lower esophageal sphincter pressure in patients with progressive systemic sclerosis. Arthritis Rheum. 1986;29:1054–5.
60. Kowal-Bielecka O, Landewe R, Avouac J, et al. EULAR recommendations for the treatment of systemic sclerosis: a report from the EULAR Scleroderma Trials and Research group (EUSTAR). Ann Rheum Dis. 2009;68:620–8.
61. Hansi N, Thoua N, Carulli M, et al. Consensus best practice pathway of the UK scleroderma study group: gastrointestinal manifestations of systemic sclerosis. Clin Exp Rheumatol. 2014;32:S-214–21.
62. Olive A, Maddison PJ, Davis M. Treatment of oesophagitis in scleroderma with omeprazole. Br J Rheumatol. 1989;28:553.
63. Hendel L. Hydroxyproline in the oesophageal mucosa of patients with progressive systemic sclerosis during omeprazole-induced healing of reflux oesophagitis. Aliment Pharmacol Ther. 1991;5:471–80.
64. Shoenut JP, Wieler JA, Micflikier AB. The extent and pattern of gastro-oesophageal reflux in patients with scleroderma oesophagus: the effect of low-dose omeprazole. Aliment Pharmacol Ther. 1993;7:509–13.

65. Gough A, Andrews D, Bacon PA, Emery P. Evidence of omeprazole-induced small bowel bacterial overgrowth in patients with scleroderma. Br J Rheumatol. 1995;34:976–7.
66. Reimer C. Safety of long-term PPI therapy. Best Pract Res Clin Gastroenterol. 2013;27:443–54.
67. Hendel L, Aggestrup S, Stentoft P. Long-term ranitidine in progressive systemic sclerosis (scleroderma) with gastroesophageal reflux. Scand J Gastroenterol. 1986;21:799–805.
68. Petrokubi RJ, Jeffries GH. Cimetidine versus antacid in scleroderma with reflux esophagitis. A randomized double-blind controlled study. Gastroenterology. 1979;77:691–5.
69. Janiak P, Thumshirn M, Menne D, et al. Clinical trial: the effects of adding ranitidine at night to twice daily omeprazole therapy on nocturnal acid breakthrough and acid reflux in patients with systemic sclerosis – a randomized controlled, cross-over trial. Aliment Pharmacol Ther. 2007;26:1259–65.
70. Horowitz M, Maddern GJ, Maddox A, Wishart J, Chatterton BE, Shearman DJ. Effects of cisapride on gastric and esophageal emptying in progressive systemic sclerosis. Gastroenterology. 1987;93:311–5.
71. Wehrmann T, Caspary WF. Effect of cisapride on esophageal motility in healthy probands and patients with progressive systemic scleroderma. Klin Wochenschr. 1990;68:602–7.
72. Kahan A, Chaussade S, Gaudric M, et al. The effect of cisapride on gastro-oesophageal dysfunction in systemic sclerosis: a controlled manometric study. Br J Clin Pharmacol. 1991;31:683–7.
73. Limburg AJ, Smit AJ, Kleibeuker JH. Effects of cisapride on the esophageal motor function of patients with progressive systemic sclerosis or mixed connective tissue disease. Digestion. 1991;49:156–60.
74. Wang SJ, La JL, Chen DY, Chen YH, Hsieh TY, Lin WY. Effects of cisapride on oesophageal transit of solids in patients with progressive systemic sclerosis. Clin Rheumatol. 2002;21:43–5.
75. Ramirez-Mata M, Ibanez G, Alarcon-Segovia D. Stimulatory effect of metoclopramide on the esophagus and lower esophageal sphincter of patients of patients with PSS. Arthritis Rheum. 1977;20:30–4.
76. Johnson DA, Drane WE, Curran J, et al. Metoclopramide response in patients with progressive systemic sclerosis. Effect on esophageal and gastric motility abnormalities. Arch Intern Med. 1987;147:1597–601.
77. Drane WE, Karvelis K, Johnson DA, Curran JJ, Silverman ED. Scintigraphic detection of metoclopramide esophageal stimulation in progressive systemic sclerosis. J Nucl Med. 1987;28:810–5.
78. Sridhar KR, Lange RC, Magyar L, Soykan I, McCallum RW. Prevalence of impaired gastric emptying of solids in systemic sclerosis: diagnostic and therapeutic implications. J Lab Clin Med. 1998;132:541–6.
79. Mercado U, Arroyo de Anda R, Avendano L, Araiza-Casillas R, Avendano-Reyes M. Metoclopramide response in patients with early diffuse systemic sclerosis. Effects on esophageal motility abnormalities. Clin Exp Rheumatol. 2005;23:685–8.
80. Fiorucci S, Distrutti E, Bassotti G, et al. Effect of erythromycin administration on upper gastrointestinal motility in scleroderma patients. Scand J Gastroenterol. 1994;29:807–13.
81. Folwaczny C, Laritz M, Meurer M, Endres SP, Konig A, Schindlbeck N. Effects of various prokinetic drugs on gastrointestinal transit times in patients with progressive systemic scleroderma. Z Gastroenterol. 1997;35:905–12.
82. Sjogren RW. Gastrointestinal features of scleroderma. Curr Opin Rheumatol. 1996;8:569–75.
83. Tack J, Janssen P, Masaoka T, Farre R, Van Oudenhove L. Efficacy of buspirone, a fundus-relaxing drug, in patients with functional dyspepsia. Clin Gastroenterol Hepatol. 2012;10:1239–45.
84. Di Stefano M, Papathanasopoulos A, Blondeau K, et al. Effect of buspirone, a 5-HT1A receptor agonist, on esophageal motility in healthy volunteers. Dis Esophagus. 2012;25:470–6.
85. Karamanolis GP, Panopoulos S, Karlaftis A, et al. Beneficial effect of the 5-HT1A receptor agonist buspirone on esophageal dysfunction associated with systemic sclerosis: a pilot study. U Eur Gastroenterol J. 2015;3:266–71.
86. Henderson RD, Pearson FG. Surgical management of esophageal scleroderma. J Thorac Cardiovasc Surg. 1973;66:686–92.
87. Orringer MB, Orringer JS, Dabich L, Zarafonetis CJ. Combined collis gastroplasty – fundoplication operations for scleroderma reflux esophagitis. Surgery. 1981;90:624–30.
88. Mansour KA. Surgery for scleroderma of the esophagus: a 12-year experience. Updated in 1995. Ann Thorac Surg. 1995;60:227.
89. Poirier NC, Taillefer R, Topart P, Duranceau A. Antireflux operations in patients with scleroderma. Ann Thorac Surg. 1994;58:66–72; discussion -3.
90. Kent MS, Luketich JD, Irshad K, et al. Comparison of surgical approaches to recalcitrant gastroesophageal reflux disease in the patient with scleroderma. Ann Thorac Surg. 2007;84:1710–5; discussion 5-6.
91. Szamosi S, Szekanecz Z, Szucs G. Gastrointestinal manifestations in Hungarian scleroderma patients. Rheumatol Int. 2006;26:1120–4.
92. Sallam H, McNearney TA, Chen JD. Systematic review: pathophysiology and management of gastrointestinal dysmotility in systemic sclerosis (scleroderma). Aliment Pharmacol Ther. 2006;23:691–712.
93. Marie I, Ducrotte P, Antonietti M, Herve S, Levesque H. Watermelon stomach in systemic sclerosis: its incidence and management. Aliment Pharmacol Ther. 2008;28:412–21.
94. Ingraham KM, O'Brien MS, Shenin M, Derk CT, Steen VD. Gastric antral vascular ectasia in systemic sclerosis: demographics and disease predictors. J Rheumatol. 2010;37:603–7.
95. Maddern GJ, Horowitz M, Jamieson GG, Chatterton BE, Collins PJ, Roberts-Thomson P. Abnormalities of esophageal and gastric emptying in progressive systemic sclerosis. Gastroenterology. 1984;87:922–6.
96. Marie I, Levesque H, Ducrotte P, et al. Gastric involvement in systemic sclerosis: a prospective study. Am J Gastroenterol. 2001;96:77–83.
97. Fiorucci S, Distrutti E, Gerli R, Morelli A. Effect of erythromycin on gastric and gallbladder emptying and gastrointestinal symptoms in scleroderma patients is maintained medium term. Am J Gastroenterol. 1994;89:550–5.
98. Pfaffenbach B, Adamek RJ, Hagemann D, et al. Effect of progressive systemic sclerosis on antral myoelectrical activity and gastric emptying. Z Gastroenterol. 1996;34:517–21.
99. Franck-Larsson K, Hedenstrom H, Dahl R, Ronnblom A. Delayed gastric emptying in patients with diffuse versus limited systemic sclerosis, unrelated to gastrointestinal symptoms and myoelectric gastric activity. Scand J Rheumatol. 2003;32:348–55.
100. Marycz T, Muehldorfer SM, Gruschwitz MS, et al. Gastric involvement in progressive systemic sclerosis: electrogastrographic and sonographic findings. Eur J Gastroenterol Hepatol. 1999;11:1151–6.
101. Mittal BR, Wanchu A, Das BK, Ghosh PP, Sewatkar AB, Misra RN. Pattern of gastric emptying in patients with systemic sclerosis. Clin Nucl Med. 1996;21:379–82.
102. Wedmann B, Wegener M, Adamek RJ, el Gammal S. Gastrobiliary motility after liquid fatty meal in progressive systemic sclerosis. A sonographic study. Dig Dis Sci. 1994;39:565–70.
103. Abell TL, Camilleri M, Donohoe K, et al. Consensus recommendations for gastric emptying scintigraphy: a joint report of the American Neurogastroenterology and Motility Society and the Society of Nuclear Medicine. Am J Gastroenterol. 2008;103:753–63.
104. Talley NJ. Diabetic gastropathy and prokinetics. Am J Gastroenterol. 2003;98:264–71.

105. Bortolotti M, Bolondi L, Santi V, Sarti P, Brunelli F, Barbara L. Patterns of gastric emptying in dysmotility-like dyspepsia. Scand J Gastroenterol. 1995;30:408–10.
106. Tang DM, Friedenberg FK. Gastroparesis: approach, diagnostic evaluation, and management. Dis Mon. 2011;57:74–101.
107. Cassilly D, Kantor S, Knight LC, et al. Gastric emptying of a non-digestible solid: assessment with simultaneous SmartPill pH and pressure capsule, antroduodenal manometry, gastric emptying scintigraphy. Neurogastroenterol Motil. 2008;20:311–9.
108. Kuo B, McCallum RW, Koch KL, et al. Comparison of gastric emptying of a nondigestible capsule to a radio-labelled meal in healthy and gastroparetic subjects. Aliment Pharmacol Ther. 2008;27:186–96.
109. Parkman HP. Assessment of gastric emptying and small-bowel motility: scintigraphy, breath tests, manometry, and SmartPill. Gastrointest Endosc Clin N Am. 2009;19:49–55, vi.
110. Rees WD, Leigh RJ, Christofides ND, Bloom SR, Turnberg LA. Interdigestive motor activity in patients with systemic sclerosis. Gastroenterology. 1982;83:575–80.
111. Marie I, Levesque H, Ducrotte P, et al. Manometry of the upper intestinal tract in patients with systemic sclerosis: a prospective study. Arthritis Rheum. 1998;41:1874–83.
112. McNearney TA, Sallam HS, Hunnicutt SE, et al. Gastric slow waves, gastrointestinal symptoms and peptides in systemic sclerosis patients. Neurogastroenterol Motil. 2009;21:1269–e120.
113. Tung A, Sweitzer B, Cutter T. Cardiac arrest after labetalol and metoclopramide administration in a patient with scleroderma. Anesth Analg. 2002;95:1667–8, table of contents.
114. Patterson D, Abell T, Rothstein R, Koch K, Barnett J. A double-blind multicenter comparison of domperidone and metoclopramide in the treatment of diabetic patients with symptoms of gastroparesis. Am J Gastroenterol. 1999;94:1230–4.
115. Parkman HP, Jacobs MR, Mishra A, et al. Domperidone treatment for gastroparesis: demographic and pharmacogenetic characterization of clinical efficacy and side-effects. Dig Dis Sci. 2011;56:115–24.
116. Buffery PJ, Strother RM. Domperidone safety: a mini-review of the science of QT prolongation and clinical implications of recent global regulatory recommendations. N Z Med J. 2015;128:66–74.
117. Verne GN, Eaker EY, Hardy E, Sninsky CA. Effect of octreotide and erythromycin on idiopathic and scleroderma-associated intestinal pseudoobstruction. Dig Dis Sci. 1995;40:1892–901.
118. Masaoka T, Tack J. Gastroparesis: current concepts and management. Gut Liver. 2009;3:166–73.
119. Maganti K, Onyemere K, Jones MP. Oral erythromycin and symptomatic relief of gastroparesis: a systematic review. Am J Gastroenterol. 2003;98:259–63.
120. Linke R, Meier M, Muenzing W, Folwaczny C, Schnell O, Tatsch K. Prokinetic therapy: what can be measured by gastric scintigraphy? Nucl Med Commun. 2005;26:527–33.
121. Wu KL, Rayner CK, Chuah SK, et al. Effects of ginger on gastric emptying and motility in healthy humans. Eur J Gastroenterol Hepatol. 2008;20:436–40.
122. Chaiyakunapruk N, Kitikannakorn N, Nathisuwan S, Leeprakobboon K, Leelasettagool C. The efficacy of ginger for the prevention of postoperative nausea and vomiting: a meta-analysis. Am J Obstet Gynecol. 2006;194:95–9.
123. Sallam HS, McNearney TA, Chen JD. Acupuncture-based modalities: novel alternative approaches in the treatment of gastrointestinal dysmotility in patients with systemic sclerosis. Explore (NY). 2014;10:44–52.
124. Wollaston DE, Xu X, Tokumaru O, Chen JD, McNearney TA. Patients with systemic sclerosis have unique and persistent alterations in gastric myoelectrical activity with acupressure to Neiguan point PC6. J Rheumatol. 2005;32:494–501.
125. Sallam H, McNearney TA, Doshi D, Chen JD. Transcutaneous electrical nerve stimulation (TENS) improves upper GI symptoms and balances the sympathovagal activity in scleroderma patients. Dig Dis Sci. 2007;52:1329–37.
126. McNearney TA, Sallam HS, Hunnicutt SE, Doshi D, Chen JD. Prolonged treatment with transcutaneous electrical nerve stimulation (TENS) modulates neuro-gastric motility and plasma levels of vasoactive intestinal peptide (VIP), motilin and interleukin-6 (IL-6) in systemic sclerosis. Clin Exp Rheumatol. 2013;31:140–50.
127. Friedenberg FK, Palit A, Parkman HP, Hanlon A, Nelson DB. Botulinum toxin A for the treatment of delayed gastric emptying. Am J Gastroenterol. 2008;103:416–23.
128. Duchini A, Sessoms SL. Gastrointestinal hemorrhage in patients with systemic sclerosis and CREST syndrome. Am J Gastroenterol. 1998;93:1453–6.
129. Jabbari M, Cherry R, Lough JO, Daly DS, Kinnear DG, Goresky CA. Gastric antral vascular ectasia: the watermelon stomach. Gastroenterology. 1984;87:1165–70.
130. Ghrenassia E, Avouac J, Khanna D, et al. Prevalence, correlates and outcomes of gastric antral vascular ectasia in systemic sclerosis: a EUSTAR case-control study. J Rheumatol. 2014;41:99–105.
131. Gostout CJ, Viggiano TR, Ahlquist DA, Wang KK, Larson MV, Balm R. The clinical and endoscopic spectrum of the watermelon stomach. J Clin Gastroenterol. 1992;15:256–63.
132. Suit PF, Petras RE, Bauer TW, Petrini Jr JL. Gastric antral vascular ectasia. A histologic and morphometric study of "the watermelon stomach". Am J Surg Pathol. 1987;11:750–7.
133. Chawla SK, Ramani K, Lo Presti P. The honeycomb stomach: coalesced gastric angiodysplasia. Gastrointest Endosc. 1990;36:516–8.
134. Sebastian S, O'Morain CA, Buckley MJ. Review article: current therapeutic options for gastric antral vascular ectasia. Aliment Pharmacol Ther. 2003;18:157–65.
135. Dulai GS, Jensen DM. Treatment of watermelon stomach. Curr Treat Options Gastroenterol. 2006;9:175–80.
136. Lorenzi AR, Johnson AH, Davies G, Gough A. Gastric antral vascular ectasia in systemic sclerosis: complete resolution with methylprednisolone and cyclophosphamide. Ann Rheum Dis. 2001;60:796–8.
137. Schulz SW, O'Brien M, Maqsood M, Sandorfi N, Del Galdo F, Jimenez SA. Improvement of severe systemic sclerosis-associated gastric antral vascular ectasia following immunosuppressive treatment with intravenous cyclophosphamide. J Rheumatol. 2009;36:1653–6.
138. Tran A, Villeneuve JP, Bilodeau M, et al. Treatment of chronic bleeding from gastric antral vascular ectasia (GAVE) with estrogen-progesterone in cirrhotic patients: an open pilot study. Am J Gastroenterol. 1999;94:2909–11.
139. Kantsevoy SV, Cruz-Correa MR, Vaughn CA, Jagannath SB, Pasricha PJ, Kalloo AN. Endoscopic cryotherapy for the treatment of bleeding mucosal vascular lesions of the GI tract: a pilot study. Gastrointest Endosc. 2003;57:403–6.
140. Cho S, Zanati S, Yong E, et al. Endoscopic cryotherapy for the management of gastric antral vascular ectasia. Gastrointest Endosc. 2008;68:895–902.
141. Shaheen NJ, Sharma P, Overholt BF, et al. Radiofrequency ablation in Barrett's esophagus with dysplasia. N Engl J Med. 2009;360:2277–88.
142. Gross SA, Al-Haddad M, Gill KR, Schore AN, Wallace MB. Endoscopic mucosal ablation for the treatment of gastric antral vascular ectasia with the HALO90 system: a pilot study. Gastrointest Endosc. 2008;67:324–7.

Small and Large Intestinal Involvement and Nutritional Issues

31

Elizabeth Harrison, Charles Murray, and Simon Lal

Introduction

Most patients with systemic sclerosis (SSc) develop gastrointestinal (GI) manifestations, which can involve any part of the GI tract. The small intestine, large intestine, and anorectal regions are affected in 40–80 %, 20–50 %, and 50–70 % of patients, respectively [1]. GI manifestations may increase morbidity and mortality, reduce quality of life, and result in malnutrition [2–5].

Anatomic Aspects of Intestinal Involvement

SSc-associated pathological changes are similar throughout the GI tract. The epithelial morphology and villous structure of the small intestine are preserved, except when secondary processes such as bacterial overgrowth or celiac disease are present [6–8].

The primary site for histopathological changes is the muscularis propria. There is mild chronic inflammation of the lamina propria and progressive atrophy and fragmentation of the smooth muscle, beginning in a patchy distribution. Later, with disease progression, collagen infiltration and fibrosis become more extensive [9, 10]. These changes are more marked in the circular than in the longitudinal muscle layer, and muscle atrophy exceeds fibrosis [11, 12]. In addition to fibrosis, there are decreased numbers of gap junctions between smooth muscle cells, a feature which impairs transmission of peristalsis. There is thickening and fibrosis of the serosa.

E. Harrison, MBChB (✉)
Institute of Inflammation and Repair, University of Manchester, Manchester, UK
e-mail: elizabeth.harrison-3@manchester.ac.uk

C. Murray, MA, PhD, FRCP
Department of Gastroenterology, Royal Free London NHS Trust, London, UK

S. Lal, PhD, FRCP
Intestinal Failure Unit, Salford Royal NHS Foundation Trust, Salford, UK

Vascular abnormalities include myointimal proliferation and sclerosis with narrowing and irregularity of the lumen and disruption of the internal elastic lamina of small arteries [13]. Capillary basement membranes are thickened and laminated. Large and medium arteries, as well as veins, are relatively spared.

It is not clear whether muscle atrophy is secondary to vascular ischemia or to primary nerve damage. An esophageal biopsy series reported that autonomic nerves appear normal by light and electron microscopy [14]. However, a more recent gastric biopsy series revealed subtle involvement of gastric wall nerves [10]. In addition, telocytes are lost from fibrotic sections. These are stromal cells which normally transmit signals from the gastric pacemaker [15].

Motility Aspects of Intestinal Involvement

Abnormal motility frequently affects the small (40–80 %) and large intestines. In the fasting state in healthy controls, antroduodenal motility recordings show that there is spontaneous peristalsis in the form of migrating myoelectric complexes (MMCs) or "housekeeping waves" (Fig. 31.1a). MMC is a cyclic pattern of contractile activity during the fasting state that is absent in patients with SSc and is responsible for sweeping bacteria into the colon. In patients with SSc, normal MMCs are replaced by irregular and/or low-amplitude contractile activity as seen in the antrum and small intestine (Fig. 31.1b). After eating, the uncoordinated activity may persist, but there may be no contractile response of the stomach or intestine to a meal. Both myopathic and neuropathic processes have been implicated in the pathogenesis GI involvement in patients with SSc. Neuropathic disorders are usually associated with uncoordinated contractions, whereas myopathic processes are associated with normal but low-amplitude contractions. In some instances, duodenal hyperactivity with uncoordinated activity may be seen and that abnormality is similar to that observed in individuals with diabetic neuropathy. In patients with advanced intestinal SSc, dramatic hypomotility of the stomach and small

J. Varga et al. (eds.), *Scleroderma*, DOI 10.1007/978-3-319-31407-5_31

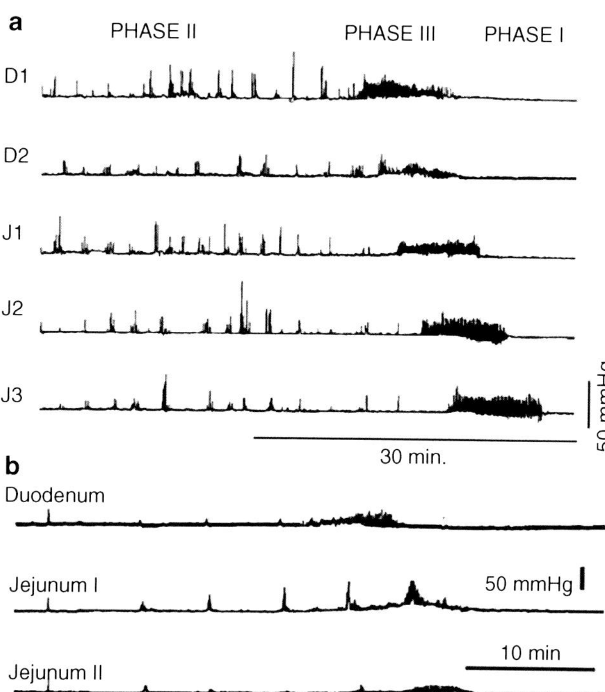

Fig. 31.1 (**a**) Small intestinal manometry taken from an ambulatory study in a fasting healthy subject. The catheter has built-in strain-gauge transducers spaced 10 cm apart (first two sensors in the duodenum and the last three in the jejunum). The tracing shows a coordinated electrical movement of a bolus through the small intestine (MMC). Phase II is a period of irregular contractions. Phase III is a period of intense phasic activity which promotes the aborally directed movement of a bolus. (**b**) Ambulatory small intestinal recording (recorded during fasting) from a patient with SSc. The catheter has three built-in strain-gauge transducers placed 15 cm apart (first sensor was in the duodenum, and the second and third were in the jejunum). Phase II of the MMC is hypoactive with low-amplitude contractions. There is one phase III of the MMC with normal migration. This patient did not have a dilated intestine but clearly demonstrated manometric abnormalities which correlated with the severity of GI symptoms (Reprinted with permission from "An Illustrated Guide to Gastrointestinal Motility," Churchill-Livingstone, 1993) (Chap. 14. Ambulatory Manometry by EE Soffer, RW Summers, Fig. 14.7, p 205)

intestine can occur which, at times, gives rise to pseudoobstruction. This pattern suggests a myopathic disorder and is often the underlying defect leading to recalcitrant intestinal pseudoobstruction. The progressive nature of intestinal hypomotility has been demonstrated. A study which serially evaluated eight patients with SSc over a 5-year period, using small intestinal manometry, showed a significant and progressive worsening of their intestinal hypomotility [16].

Hypotheses for Gastrointestinal Involvement

Vascular Hypothesis

Cohen et al. [17] and Sjogren [18] proposed that the initial GI tract lesion is injury to neural function, which is caused by arteriolar changes in the vasa nervorum and/or by collagen deposits. During the earliest phase of injury, the smooth muscle is generally still functional, and the patient is generally asymptomatic; the smooth muscle still responds to prokinetic agents. In the second phase, the smooth muscle begins to atrophy, which results in GI tract-related symptoms with reduced response to prokinetic agents. In the final phase, there is no response to prokinetic agents because the smooth muscle has completely atrophied.

Autoimmune Hypothesis

Another possible explanation for GI dysmotility is autoimmune-mediated injury. Contractile activity of the GI tract is controlled predominantly by intrinsic neurons in the myenteric plexus. Acetylcholine, acting predominantly via the muscarinic-3 receptor (M3R), is the principal excitatory neurotransmitter regulating GI tract motility.

In one study, effects on intestinal motility were assessed after rats were immunized with purified immunoglobulin G (IgG) from the sera of patients with SSc who had antimyenteric neuronal antibodies [19]. Passive immunization led to the prolongation and disruption of rat intestinal myoelectrical activity; there was no effect on the myoelectric activity when the rats were immunized with the IgG of normal healthy controls. In another study, the IgG from patients with SSc inhibited M3R activation in the smooth muscle cells of the internal anal sphincter of rats [20]. The removal of the antibodies reversed this effect. Subsequent studies of the effects of IgG from patients with SSc on healthy human smooth muscle tissue showed similar results [21].

In human studies, high-titer antibodies directed against myenteric neurons have been detected in approximately half (19/41) of patients with SSc, but not in patients with idiopathic GI dysmotility [22]. In addition, patients with SSc (within 2 years of onset) and severe GI tract involvement have higher titers of anti-M3R antibody than patients without severe GI tract involvement [23]. It remains to be seen whether these autoantibodies are pathogenetic in nature or an end result of collagenous cuffing.

Functional Denervation of GI Smooth Muscle

Cohen's work of 1972 explained, in part, what happens to the motility of the esophagus in patients with SSc [17]. His report showed functional denervation of the smooth muscle that lines the esophagus (and by extension the entire GI tract). He demonstrated that in the early stages of SSc, stimulation with edrophonium and gastrin 1 (compounds that act indirectly through stimulation of cholinergic nerves) failed to stimulate smooth muscle motility, while methacholine (a direct stimulator of smooth muscle) did. This suggests that, in the early stages of SSc, the GI smooth muscle becomes hypomotile due to denervation, but that this denervated smooth muscle remains capable of responding to direct stimulation (i.e., methacholine in the initial experiments and by extension cisapride, erythromycin, domperidone, metoclopramide, and octreotide in clinical practice). However, in patients with SSc of longer disease duration, the GI tract did not respond to direct stimulation, suggesting that the smooth muscle had atrophied. Thus, it was no longer capable of being stimulated. This may explain the process responsible for disease progression leading to intestinal pseudoobstruction.

Small Intestinal Involvement Clinical Manifestations

Intestinal dysmotility has been reported to affect 40–80 % of patients with SSc [18, 24]. Resultant clinical syndromes include small intestine bacterial overgrowth (SIBO), intestinal pseudoobstruction, malabsorption from other causes, pneumatosis cystoides intestinalis, intestinal pseudosacculations, and telangiectasias.

Small Intestinal Bacterial Overgrowth

Dysmotility/hypomotility of the smooth muscle in the small intestine (particularly loss of MMC) leads to stasis and stagnation of intestinal contents, allowing the migration of colonic bacteria up into the small intestine (ileum, jejunum, and duodenum) [18, 25]. Once there, the bacteria catabolize the bile acids rendering them unable to break down lipids, particularly triglycerides, for absorption [26].

The symptoms and signs associated with SIBO include nausea, vomiting, early satiety, postprandial bloating (what patients feel), abdominal distention (what patients see), diarrhea (including steatorrhea), excessive flatulence, fecal soilage, weight loss (or inability to gain weight), and cachexia [27]. Some of these symptoms, such as nausea, vomiting, early satiety, and postprandial bloating, may overlap with those of gastroparesis [28]. Bacteria in the small intestine metabolize sugars and carbohydrates and in the process produce gas. This gas may be incompletely reabsorbed and released as flatus. Large volumes of unabsorbed gases may contribute to abdominal pain, distention, and bloating.

Studies involving unselected patients with SSc showed 43–55 % to have SIBO on breath testing [27, 29, 30]. SIBO testing was positive in only 7 % of healthy controls [29]. In addition, in the patients with SSc, the SIBO diagnosis correlated with digestive symptoms, which improved upon

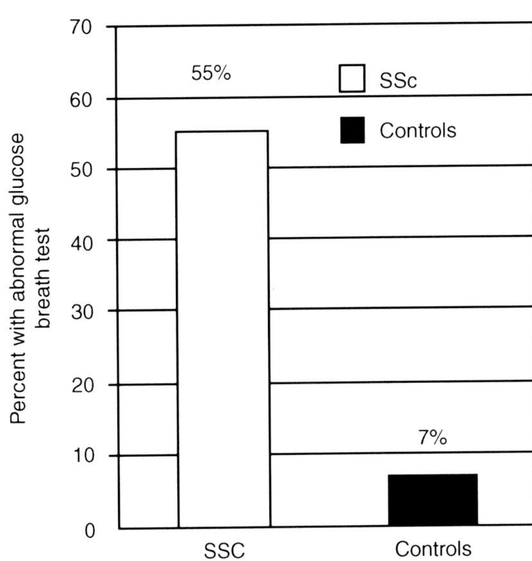

Fig. 31.2 Prevalence of positive glucose breath tests (hydrogen and methane) in SSc patients and controls [29]

eradication using either a single or multiple (rotational) antibiotics [27, 29] (Fig. 31.2).

It has been suggested that the high frequency of SIBO in patients with SSc may be, in part, linked to the use of proton pump inhibitors to control gastroesophageal reflux disease and to prevent esophageal strictures [31, 32]. However, other large series involving patients without SSc offer conflicting evidence [33].

Intestinal Pseudoobstruction

It is not uncommon for patients with SSc to have disrupted small intestinal motility. However, few patients progress to intestinal pseudoobstruction, which is characterized by the failure of the intestinal tract to propel its luminal contents in a forward direction, in the absence of any mechanical cause. In patients with SSc, this failure of forward motion is attributed to uncoordinated smooth muscle activity and intestinal wall hypomotility [34]. This failure may result in recurrent clinical episodes of obstruction which, based on their pattern of onset, may be defined as either acute or chronic (obstructive symptoms for >6 months).

Most reports of pseudoobstruction in patients with SSc are in the form of single case reports or small case series. Several larger series have reported the proportion of patients with episodes of pseudoobstruction or a malabsorption syndrome as a combined figure, thus masking the proportion with only pseudoobstruction. However, recently one center reported pseudoobstruction to affect 3.9 % (44/1120) of all their patients [35].

When present, intestinal pseudoobstruction leads to symptoms similar to those of SIBO. A recent study described 64 cases (37 unique patients) of acute intestinal pseudoobstruction in patients with SSc [36]. The most common symptoms were nausea (77 %) and abdominal pain (50 %). However, other common symptoms include constipation, diarrhea, vomiting, and distention and postprandial bloating [36, 37]. Some patients also report an inability to pass flatus and a progressively increasing abdominal girth (greater than that with SIBO). In severe cases, patients may develop nutritional complications, as evidenced by the recent series in which 17 % lost weight [36]. In this series, coexistent SIBO was diagnosed in 16 % of patients.

Patients may have abnormal small intestinal imaging. Abnormalities on contrast imaging which are suggestive of small intestinal involvement include dilated loops, pseudodiverticulae, "hidebound," or "wire spring" [6]. However, these findings do not necessarily translate to symptoms associated with delayed transit. Similarly, abnormal small intestinal manometry may not be correlated with radiological small intestinal dilation or delayed transit [34]. Findings on plain imaging suggestive of pseudoobstruction include significant small bowel dilation and the presence of air-fluid levels (Fig. 31.3).

Malabsorption

In patients with SSc, malabsorption usually results from one or more of three mechanisms [18], namely, SIBO (the most common), other intestinal absorptive surface abnormality (e.g., celiac disease), and pancreatic insufficiency.

SIBO

Conjugated bile acids are necessary for the breakdown and absorption of fats within the small intestine. Some bacteria are able to deconjugate bile acids within the small intestine [26]. Deconjugated bile acids are less able to absorb fat, leading to a calorie deficit and deficiencies of fat-soluble vitamins. Clinically, this may also result in steatorrhea. In addition, patients may experience problems related to increased gas production, due to bacteria metabolizing sugars and carbohydrates. SIBO may also result in villous atrophy, which reduces the absorptive surface area, to further reduce nutrient absorption [38].

Celiac Disease

Celiac disease is an immune-mediated gluten-dependent enteropathy. Diagnosis is based upon clinical presentation, supportive serology, and confirmatory histology (Marsh classification). Patients may develop malabsorption as a consequence of villous atrophy reducing the absorptive area of the small intestine.

Some studies suggest that patients with SSc may have an increased prevalence (8 %) of celiac disease [39]. However, more recent larger studies have not confirmed this [40, 41]. In one study, only 4 % (3/72) had supportive serology and none of those biopsied had confirmatory histology (2/2 – Marsh grade 0; 1 died pre-biopsy) [40].

Pancreatic Insufficiency

A significant reduction in pancreatic secretions is necessary to cause malabsorption. Small studies ($n = 16$; $n = 20$) suggest that it is common for patients with SSc to have a reduction in their pancreatic exocrine function [42, 43]. However, this reduction is only large enough to be considered clinically significant in a few patients.

Malabsorption may result in numerous vitamin and mineral deficiencies. Fat-soluble vitamin (A, D, E, and K) malabsorption may be caused by bacterial bile acid deconjugation or pancreatic enzyme insufficiency. However, any reduction in vitamin K levels may be partially compensated by its production by intestinal bacteria. Absorption of water-soluble vitamins may also be impaired. Vitamin B_{12} is competitively utilized by the bacteria, and this may lead to its deficiency. Iron and folic acid malabsorption, due to villous atrophy, can lead to the development of anemia. However, in cases of SIBO, any folic acid deficiency may be offset by its production by bacteria.

Pneumatosis (Cystoides) Intestinalis

Pneumatosis intestinalis is a rare, but normally benign, complication of SSc [44, 45]. It is characterized by the presence of multiple gas-filled cysts within the intestinal wall. The pathogenesis is unproven, despite several hypotheses being proposed. These include mucosal breaks from immunosuppressive agents (e.g., steroids) causing shrinkage of Peyer's patches, which disrupts mucosal integrity; bacterial carbohydrate fermentation leading to production of gaseous end products which are absorbed into the luminal wall; and SSc-related atrophy and fibrosis leading to increased wall permeability [38, 46–48].

Intestinal Pseudodiverticula

In contrast to true diverticular, which contain all the layers of the parent structure, pseudodiverticula are composed solely of mucosa projecting through a muscular wall. In patients with SSc, they are thought to be due to intestinal smooth muscle loss and gaseous products inflating the intestines, which cause weak hypomotile areas on the anti-mesenteric to dilate. These outpouchings are visible on contrast studies [6, 49].

Telangiectasia

Approximately 15 % of patients with SSc experience GI bleeding, the most common cause of which is mucosal

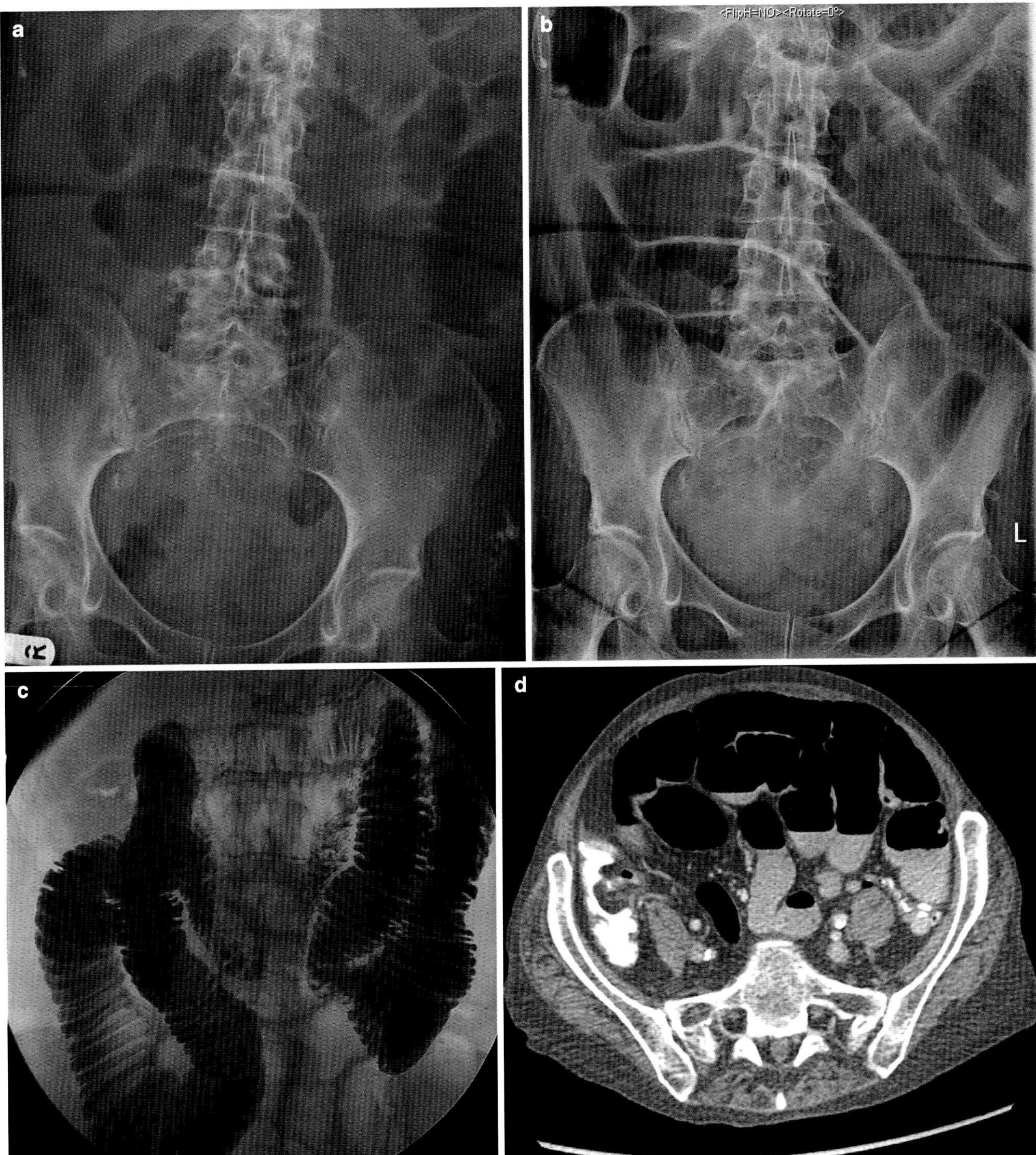

Fig. 31.3 Plain abdominal x-rays showing (**a**) air-filled, dilated small intestine with some crowding and stacking of the circular folds and (**b**) widespread dilation (up to a maximum of 6 cm) in a patient with pseudoobstruction. Barium follow-through (**c**) showing dilated loops of small intestine with tightly packed mucosal folds. CT scan (**d**) showing a moderately dilated small intestine filled and distended with air and fluid (with air-fluid levels)

telangiectasia, which may occur anywhere in the GI tract [50]. A recent video capsule endoscopy study, in unselected patients, showed small intestinal telangiectasia in 10 %, angiodysplasia in 16 %, and red spots in 8 % [51]. It is unknown how many would have bled.

Clinical Large Intestinal Involvement

SSc affects the colon and anorectum in 20–50 % and 50–70 % of patients, respectively [52, 53]. Common clinical manifestations include constipation and fecal incontinence. However, patients may also develop other manifestations, such as telangiectasia and pseudodiverticula [54, 55].

Constipation

In one study, almost 50 % of patients with SSc reported having some degree of constipation in the preceding 7 days [56]. However, in practice, fewer patients experience significant problems. Another study found that 20 % of patients reported a frequency of alternate daily or more, 12 % required manual evacuation, and 24 % took oral laxatives [57].

Colonic studies have shown evidence of smooth muscle atrophy and/or fibrosis and the absence of an increase in postprandial myoelectric activity (i.e., absent gastrocolic reflex) [12, 58]. Clinically, this leads to slow-transit constipation which may be demonstrated by radiological transit studies (e.g., sitz marker test; radionucleotide transit studies) [52, 59].

Fecal Incontinence

In one study, 33 % of patients reported incontinence with liquid stools, while 9 % reported it with solid stools [57]. However, unless specifically asked, patients may not volunteer this symptom. In addition, some patients also report rectal prolapse, which may worsen symptoms [60].

In health, continence is established by the combined functioning of the pelvic floor, rectum, and anal sphincters (internal and external). Resting anal tone is maintained by the internal anal sphincter, which is composed of smooth muscle. Its dysfunction is associated with passive fecal incontinence. In both symptomatic and asymptomatic patients, there is evidence of thinning and atrophy of the internal anal sphincter [61]. However, only patients with fecal incontinence have reduced resting anal tone [62].

The rectoanal inhibitory response, which helps to maintain continence, is the normal, transient relaxation of the internal anal sphincter in response to rectal distension. In symptomatic patients with SSc, this rectoanal inhibitory response is impaired [63].

Nutritional Issues

As their disease progresses, patients with SSc may develop a range of nutritional problems. This may result in weight loss and/or micronutrient deficiencies. These nutritional problems may develop due to difficulties in consuming or absorbing nutrients due to oral, GI, and/or other disease-related manifestations and/or increased requirements due to severe organ (e.g., severe cardiac, respiratory, or renal) involvement.

Clinically, patients with possible malnutrition may be identified by their low BMI and/or recent unintentional weight loss. Studies involving outpatients with SSc have reported 9–17 % of patients to be at high risk of malnutrition [64, 65]. Patients with severe nutritional problems, as a consequence of GI involvement, may require parenteral nutrition (PN) to survive. In one series of 586 unselected patients, 2 % required PN [64].

It is important to detect, and manage, weight loss. A low BMI has been shown to be predictive of mortality in patients with early SSc (<5 years) and to correlate with left ventricular mass [66, 67]. However, another study of unselected outpatients did not show any increased risk of mortality associated with a low BMI and/or weight loss ("MUST" ≥2) [65].

Assessment of Gastrointestinal Symptoms

Over recent years, numerous non-SSc-specific tools have been developed to facilitate patient self-assessment. To date, only two patient-reported outcome measures have been developed for GI involvement in patients with SSc. These are the University of California-Scleroderma Clinical Trial Consortium Gastrointestinal Instrument (UCLA SCTC GIT 2.0) and the National Institute of Health Patient-Reported Outcomes Measurement System (NIH PROMIS).

UCLA SCTC GIT 2.0

This is currently the best validated GI questionnaire (patient-reported outcome measure) for use in patients with SSc [68, 69]. It is a 34-item instrument available in multiple languages [70]. It is composed of seven scales, namely, reflux, distention/bloating, diarrhea, fecal soilage, constipation, emotional well-being, and social functioning and a total GI score. All scales are scored from 0 (better health-related quality of life (HRQOL)) to 3 (worse HRQOL) except diarrhea and constipation scales that range from 0 to 2 and from 0 to 2.5, respectively. It takes approximately 5–7 min to complete and is freely available online at http://uclascleroderma.researchcore.org/.

NIH PROMIS

This is a new 102-item patient-reported outcome measure. The development involved a systematic literature review, focus group consultations, a qualitative review to develop the draft version and its subsequent evaluation by quantitative psychometric testing, which involved 865 patients with GI disease and 1,177 healthy participants [71]. The resultant scale which covers eight major GI symptom domains represents a wide range of GI disorders and shows evidence of reliability. These eight domains are gastroesophageal reflux, disrupted swallowing, diarrhea, bowel incontinence/soilage, nausea and vomiting, constipation, belly pain, and gas/bloat/flatulence.

Investigations for Intestinal Involvement

When investigating GI symptoms in patients with SSc, it is important to remember that patients may also develop GI problems unrelated to SSc. In particular, attention needs to be given to the detection of any red flag symptoms which require prompt investigation to exclude malignancies.

Some symptoms that patients report are characteristic of one GI region's involvement, whereas others are nonspecific. Nonspecific symptoms may require a number of investigations, directed at the different parts of the GI tract, in order to identify the correct diagnosis or diagnoses. Best practice pathways have recently been developed for the investigation and management of GI symptoms, including gastroesophageal symptoms, abdominal pain and distension, weight loss and nutritional problems, diarrhea, incontinence, and constipation [72].

The following sections describe the investigation and management of selected SSc-related intestinal manifestations.

SIBO

Investigation and Diagnosis

SIBO may be considered in patients with any of the following symptoms and signs: nausea, vomiting, bloating, abdominal pain, abdominal distention, diarrhea, and weight loss.

The gold standard test is the culture (>10^5 colony-forming units/mL) of jejunal aspirates [27, 31, 32, 73–77]. However, this procedure is unpleasant and not widely available. Therefore, other more accessible, noninvasive methods are often employed. These include simple clinical suspicion together with a favorable response to empirical antibiotics, a glucose breath test (sensitivity of 62–90 % and specificity of 62 %) [27, 73, 75–78] and a lactulose hydrogen breath test (LBT) [29, 73, 75–79] (sensitivity of 68 % and specificity of 44 %). The sensitivity of breath tests is increased by measuring both methane and hydrogen levels, as up to 27 % of patients with SIBO are methane producers and almost half do not produce hydrogen [79].

The breath testing procedure requires the patient to provide a baseline (end-expired) breath sample and then to consume a carbohydrate-containing (usually glucose or lactulose) liquid. Following this, they provide repeat breath samples every 15 min for 2 h. Bacteria metabolize the carbohydrate and, in doing so, produce hydrogen and/or methane which is exhaled (collected in breath samples). In the absence of SIBO, a significant early rise in the percentage of hydrogen or methane exhaled is not detected. However, in the presence of SIBO, there is an early rise (usually within 1–2 h) of hydrogen and/or methane, due to the presence of small intestinal bacteria (Fig. 31.4). Another later peak often follows due to the action of colonic bacteria.

Treatment

In the first instance, a single course of empirical antibiotics is usually tried. Antibiotics to consider include ciprofloxacin, metronidazole, doxycycline, amoxicillin and clavulanic acid are combined in a single tablet in this preparation (co-amoxiclav), norfloxacin, minocycline, tetracycline, and rifaximin [80]. Rifaximin has the advantage of not being systemically absorbed, but it is more expensive. There is no consensus as to which antibiotic is most likely to be successful. In studies assessing antibiotic effectiveness in patients with SSc and SIBO, 73 % had normalization of LBT with 10 days of rifaximin [78] and 52 % (n=51) improved with rotating norfloxacin and metronidazole (7 days/month) [81]. When deciding which antibiotic to prescribe, it is important to consider potential side effect profiles and the patient's other comorbidities/medications.

In order to help gauge any clinical improvement from treatment, patients can be asked to document their daily stool and/or incontinence frequency and symptoms of abdominal bloating, pain, distention, and/or cramps. If treatment is successful, symptoms would be expected to improve. Failure of symptoms to fully resolve may indicate a failure to eradicate all the bacteria, and a second, different, antibiotic course may be considered.

Following successful antibiotic treatment, it may be possible to merely monitor for the recurrence of symptoms. When symptoms recur, the patient may then be prescribed a further course of the successful antibiotic. If the patient has infrequent relapses, this cycle of monitoring and retreating may be continued. However, if the patient frequently requires antibiotic intervention, two or three different antibiotics may be used alternately, to limit the likelihood of developing resistance. With disease progression, some patients may rapidly relapse after stopping antibiotics. In these patients, continual rotating courses of antibiotics may be considered.

Probiotics are a potential treatment for SIBO. However, to date, there have only been small studies assessing their effectiveness against antibiotics, and recommendations are complicated by the variety of preparations available [82, 83]. However, in a small study involving patients with SSc and moderate to severe symptoms of bloating, but without proven SIBO, probiotics were shown to offer symptomatic benefit [84]. Therefore, despite a lack of evidence to support their use for the treatment of SIBO, their use may be considered as they may provide some symptomatic benefit [80].

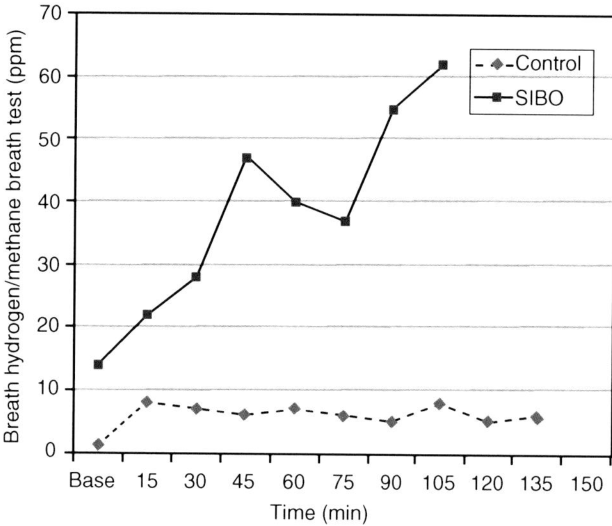

Fig. 31.4 Normal and abnormal hydrogen/methane breath tests

Other Considerations

Nutritional problems may develop as a consequence of SIBO, and thus, following diagnosis, the clinician may wish to assess the patient's nutritional status. In patients with severe dysmotility, prokinetic agents (e.g., octreotide) may be considered [80]. These are discussed in more detail in subsequent sections. In patients with diarrhea, but without evidence of SIBO, other causes of diarrhea may need to be considered, including those not associated with SSc.

Intestinal Pseudoobstruction

Investigation and Diagnosis

The diagnosis of pseudoobstruction may be thought of in patients with suggestive symptoms, such as abdominal distention, nausea, vomiting, bloating, abdominal pain, constipation, diarrhea, and weight loss. Clinically, patients may have visible abdominal distension.

If intestinal obstruction, of any cause, is suspected, a plain abdominal x-ray may be considered as the initial test. This may allow confirmation of clinically suspected obstruction and give a guide as to the extent of intestinal dilation. In the presence of obstruction, air-fluid levels (segments of the intestine containing only fluid and others containing contrast) may be visible. The next step is to exclude a true, mechanical obstruction, which may require surgical intervention. This may be achieved by means of an abdominal computed tomography (CT) scan with contrast, which can usually detect or exclude any luminal or extra-GI mechanical obstructive pathology (e.g., malignancy, volvulus). CT scans may also estimate the extent of intestinal involvement.

Treatment

Most cases of acute pseudoobstruction in patients with SSc resolve spontaneously (45/64; 70 %) [36]. In one study, common management strategies employed included keeping the patients nil by mouth (72 %); prescribing intravenous fluids (64 %), prokinetics (48 %), and antibiotics (31 %); and the use of nasogastric or nasojejunal decompression (45 %). Antibiotics may be tried, due to the possibility of coexistent SIBO.

In some cases, the use prokinetic agents, such as those listed in Table 31.1, may be considered and, when used, preferably taken 30 min before meals and at bedtime for optimal benefit. However, no one agent will be successful for every patient, and due to the nature of the GI tract involvement in patients with SSc, patients with more severe involvement are less likely to achieve a satisfactory response. When considering which agent to trial, consideration of the anatomical extent of the patient's GI involvement may be helpful as the different agents preferentially stimulate different regions of the GI tract. Erythromycin increases gastric motility, but not small intestinal motility [85]. Prucalopride increased colonic motility in case series involving patients with SSc [86]. However, larger series, not involving patients with SSc, show it has minimal effect on small intestinal mucosa [87]. Thus, neither erythromycin nor prucalopride would be the first choice agent in patients with small intestinal dysmotility, but they may be beneficial for isolated gastric or colonic dysmotility. Other agents which stimulate small intestinal motility include metoclopramide, domperidone, cisapride, and octreotide. Metoclopramide increases esophageal, gastric, and small and large intestinal activity in patients with SSc [58, 88, 89]. Domperidone acts on similar receptors to metoclopramide. It stimulates the stomach and small intestine. However, no series report its successful use in patients with SSc. Cisapride increases esophageal, gastric, and colonic motility in patients with SSc and small intestinal motility in controls [90–92]. Octreotide, which must be injected, stimulates small intestinal activity and reduces SIBO and abdominal discomfort [81, 93–95]. However, as it does not influence gastric motility, it will not benefit patients with gastroparesis-related vomiting. If successful, the octreotide short-acting formulation can be changed to the long-acting formulation.

Due to safety concerns, not all prokinetic agents are widely available. Cisapride has had its license suspended in several countries, including the UK and Canada, due to a rare risk of inducing fatal arrhythmias, but is still available in the USA, on compassionate grounds. The European Medicines Association has cautioned against the long-term use of metoclopramide, due to the risk of neurological problems. In particular, due to its inconsistent results, it advises against its use for gastroparesis. Finally, domperidone, which is associated with a small increased risk of serious cardiac side

Table 31.1 Prokinetic agents and their putative areas of action in the GI tract

Agent	GI areas stimulated
Erythromycin	Stomach
Octreotide	Small intestine
Domperidone	Stomach and small intestine
Metoclopramide	Stomach and small and large intestine
Cisapride	Stomach and small and large intestine
Prucalopride	Large intestine

effects, has had its use restricted to the relief of nausea and vomiting (not bloating or heartburn) by the European Medicines Association and is contraindicated in patients with selected underlying cardiac and severe hepatic conditions (Table 31.1).

When in bed, it may help to nurse patients with acute obstruction and vomiting at an angle of at least 30° to prevent aspiration of luminal contents. In addition, insertion of an intestinal decompression nasogastric or nasojejunal tube is recommended until the abdominal distention/pain subsides. During this period, the patient remains nil by mouth. Occasionally, a rectal tube may need to be inserted to relieve the abdominal pressure/distention. In addition, for the symptomatic management of chronic intestinal pseudoobstruction, a recent single case report describes the placement of a transgastric long tube following the insertion of a percutaneous endoscopic gastrostomy tube [96]. Based on a single case report, this cannot be recommended, but may be a consideration for future management.

In a recent series of patients with acute pseudoobstruction, 9 % proceeded to surgery [36]. However, if possible, it may be wise to try to avoid segmental bowel resections in patients with SSc-related intestinal pseudoobstruction, as GI involvement is usually diffuse. In addition, surgery could make patients prone to adhesions, which may later confuse the clinical picture.

Patients with acute or chronic intestinal pseudoobstruction are at risk of developing malnutrition. In a recent series of patients with SSc and acute intestinal pseudoobstruction, 41 % (26/64) required total parenteral nutrition (TPN) during the acute period, and of these, 62 % (16/26) subsequently required it for a prolonged period. Indeed, in some severe cases of chronic intestinal pseudoobstruction, patients require long-term, home parenteral nutrition (HPN) in order to meet their nutritional requirements [97, 98].

Malabsorption

Investigations and Diagnosis

Suggestive symptoms, which may trigger investigation for causes of malabsorption, are similar to those of SIBO (one cause of malabsorption) and pseudoobstruction. Patients may also describe steatorrhea.

The gold standard investigation for the diagnosis of malabsorption is the D-xylose test. This involves the drinking of a D-xylose-containing solution and subsequent monitoring of blood and urine concentrations. As xylose is a sugar molecule, capable of being absorbed through the intestinal luminal wall without the need for enzymatic digestion, failure to absorb indicates an abnormality of the intestinal surface, rather than an enzyme deficit.

Given the similar presentations and likelihood of coexistent disease, SIBO and pseudoobstruction are differential diagnoses to be excluded (as described earlier). Other differential diagnoses include celiac disease and pancreatic insufficiency.

Investigation for celiac disease requires serological blood tests, such as the anti-tissue transglutaminase and anti-endomysial antibodies, both of which are IgA antibodies. Thus, they may be falsely negative in patients with IgA deficiency (approximately 2 % of patients with celiac disease). Negative serology excludes celiac disease in most patients (unless seronegative celiac disease), but cannot diagnose it (high sensitivity; low specificity). It is recommended that patients with positive serology proceed to an esophagogastroduodenoscopy (EGD) with duodenal biopsy. Confirmatory findings include increased intraepithelial lymphocytosis, crypt hyperplasia, and villous atrophy (Marsh criteria). The fecal elastase test, which has a low sensitivity (especially in mild to moderate disease) and specificity, is used to investigate for pancreatic insufficiency.

Treatment

The management of SIBO and pseudoobstruction is described in the earlier sections. Patients diagnosed with celiac disease ought to commence a gluten-free diet with dietetic support. Follow-up may help to improve dietary adherence and clinical resolution. A repeat biopsy may be needed if doubt exists about clinical resolution when adherent to a gluten-free diet.

Patients with pancreatic insufficiency may be prescribed replacement pancreatic enzymes, to be taken with all fat-containing meals and snacks. Proton pump inhibitors or histamine H2 receptor antagonists, which reduce gastric acid secretion, may improve the effectiveness of pancreatic replacement preparations.

Other Considerations

Following the exclusion of the above, other causes of malabsorption (e.g., lactose intolerance) which are common in patients without SSc may be considered in patients who are still symptomatic. As discussed earlier, probiotics may be considered for the symptomatic relief of bloating [84].

Finally, if all of the above measures fail to control a patient's diarrhea, other measures can be considered for symptomatic relief. Very low, intermittent, doses of loperamide may allow patients the freedom to leave the house without worry of diarrhea or incontinence. However, their use must be considered on a case-by-case basis, given the potential risks of constipation and obstipation. Similarly, cholestyramine can be considered, but because of its binding action on other drugs, care must be taken regarding the dosing time. In addition, in the absence of constipation, where fiber supplements are not recommended, bulking agents may prove useful.

Pneumatosis (Cystoides) Intestinalis

Investigation and Diagnosis

Patients may have nonspecific abdominal symptoms. Thus, it is usually diagnosed through the incidental finding of linear, curvilinear, small bubbles, or collections of cysts in the luminal wall on a plain abdominal x-ray or CT scan.

Treatment

In patients with SSc, it is usually considered a benign complication. On occasion, the intramural air-filled cysts may rupture, releasing free air into the abdominal cavity (pneumoperitoneum), without there being a true transmural perforation [44, 99]. It is important to differentiate this from a potentially life-threatening, true bowel perforation, leading to peritonitis from the leak of luminal contents into the abdominal cavity. Coexistent SIBO may also be considered and, if detected, treated as described above. Hyperbaric oxygen may help to remove intramural gas [46, 100].

Intestinal Pseudodiverticula

Investigation and Diagnosis

This is often an incidental finding, noted on contrast studies.

Treatment

In most cases, pseudodiverticula do not require any specific treatment. However, they may predispose to SIBO, which may require treatment.

Telangiectasia

Investigation and Diagnosis

These may be found during the investigation of iron deficiency anemia or overt GI bleeding. Colonic lesions may be detected on colonoscopy. Small intestinal lesions may be seen on EGD (proximal duodenum) or video capsule endoscopy.

Treatment

Lesions which are a source of iron deficiency anemia, or bleeding, may be endoscopically cauterized [50, 54].

Slow-Transit Constipation

Investigation and Diagnosis

A careful history may help to identify any associated symptoms suggestive of non-colonic pathology. For instance, constipation may be reported by patients with SIBO (especially methane producers) and, to a lesser extent, small intestinal pseudoobstruction and true obstruction and by patients with disordered defecation [101]. In addition, the effects of contributory medications (e.g., opiates), diet, and lifestyle and of other conditions common to patients without SSc may be considered.

Slow-transit constipation may be demonstrated by means of transit studies. The most commonly clinically used transit study is the sitz marker test. This involves patients swallowing a capsule containing radiopaque markers on day 0 and attending for a plain abdominal x-ray on day 5, by which time >80 % of the markers would be expected to have been passed in patients with normal transit.

Treatment

Symptoms can often be managed by careful dietary modification and laxative use. However, when considering the nature of any dietary modification and the laxative formulation to prescribe, one must remember that in patients with slow-transit constipation, which is the predominant form in patients with SSc-related colonic involvement, high-fiber diets and bulk-forming laxatives can exacerbate symptoms [102]. Thus, stimulant laxatives (e.g., senna, bisacodyl, lubiprostone) and/or osmotic laxatives (e.g., polyethylene glycol, lactulose) may be considered, both of which require liberal fluid ingestion. There is recent evidence to suggest that little harm will result from their long-term use [103]. In addition, consideration may be given to whether alternatives can be prescribed for any constipating medications.

When these measures fail to improve symptoms, promotility agents may be considered. The effectiveness of these may diminish with disease progression. Unfortunately, cisapride and tegaserod, which have been shown to increase colonic motility, are no longer widely available [90]. In patients with slow-transit constipation but without SSc, prucalopride accelerates colonic transit [104]. In patients with SSc, it has been shown to offer some benefit in small ($n=2$) case series [86]. However, prucalopride is currently only licensed for the treatment of chronic constipation in women for whom other laxatives have failed.

Fecal Incontinence and Rectal Prolapse

Investigation and Diagnosis

Symptoms may be aggravated by coexistent diarrhea which, if present, can be addressed as described earlier. Anorectal investigations are important to confirm, and to assess, the extent of any SSc involvement and to exclude other causes unrelated to SSc. In patients with SSc, anorectal manometry will show reduced resting pressures and ultrasound will show thinning of the sphincters [105].

Treatment

Biofeedback involves teaching the patient to control their anal sphincter and pelvic floor muscle, with the assistance of computer-assisted biofeedback equipment. In patients without SSc, it has been successfully used in the management of fecal incontinence due to anorectal involvement [106]. No studies exist to support its use in patients with SSc; however, it is often tried.

Sacral nerve stimulation requires the insertion of an implantable pulse generator, under local anesthesia, by a surgeon. The procedure is associated with minimal morbidity. In patients with SSc ($n=3$), the short- and medium-term responses (median follow-up 24 months; range 6–60) were very encouraging, with a decrease in episodes of fecal incontinence and marked improvement in quality of life [107]. However, larger, longer-term studies are still needed.

Surgical intervention is usually needed to correct persistently prolapsed rectal mucosa. In patients without SSc, correction improves continence and quality of life [108]. However, in a small series of patients with SSc ($n=3$), although rectal prolapse did not recur after surgery, incontinence did after a period (1 week to 7 years) [60]. This may be reflective of underlying SSc-related anorectal dysfunction.

Assessment of Nutritional Issues

Nutritional problems are common in all patients with SSc. However, those patients with severe GI involvement may be at increased risk of acute and/or chronic problems. For instance, dysphagia may lead to the avoidance of textured foods; severe dyspepsia, uncontrolled gastroparesis, untreated SIBO, and/or pseudoobstruction associated with nausea/vomiting may limit all intake (acute or chronic); acute pseudoobstruction is managed by a period nil by mouth; any cause of small intestinal malabsorption will result in a failure to absorb luminal nutrients. In addition, the patient may face additional nutritional challenges unrelated to their GI involvement, including acute illness/sepsis, severe cardiac, renal or respiratory disease, depression, and impaired mobility and/or manual dexterity. Thus, it is vital that clinicians actively monitor for signs of emerging nutritional problems, both in the outpatient and ward settings.

Numerous different screening tools have been developed, in order to help clinicians to identify nutritional problems. However, the tool which has been applied most commonly to patients with SSc is "Malnutrition Universal Screening Tool" (MUST) [65, 80, 109–113]. "MUST" uses BMI, any recent (3–6 months) weight loss and acute disease effect (defined as "acutely ill and has been or is likely to be no nutritional intake for >5 days") to divide patients into low-, medium-, and high-risk groups. For patients at medium or high risk of malnutrition, "MUST" recommends referral for further nutritional assessment.

Nutritional assessment may include a review by a dietitian, who will determine the patient's current micro- and macronutrient intake and target requirements, by using a combination of predictive calculations, clinical judgment, detailed anthropometric assessments, and a dietary history. Target requirements are based on existing nutritional status, current activity level, and any disease-related nutritional implications. In addition, when a patient is identified as having nutritional problems, the clinician may wish to consider any contributory factors, which may be amenable to treatment (e.g., medical optimization of GI, cardiac, respiratory, or renal manifestations; social or cognitive support for functional problems or depression).

Serum albumin is not regarded to be a screening marker for malnutrition, as it may remain well within normal ranges in patients at high risk of malnutrition [114]. In patients with SSc, a low serum prealbumin has been associated with malnutrition [115]. Prealbumin has a much shorter (approximately 2 days) half-life than albumin and is thus more indicative of recent dietary intake than overall nutritional status. However, concentrations also fall in acute illness (negative acute phase response).

Consideration may be given to screening patients with malnutrition, or those with newly diagnosed malabsorption, for evidence of micronutrient deficiencies. The clinician may wish to consider checking hematinics (iron, folic acid, and vitamin B_{12}) in patients with anemia [80]. Malabsorption may lead to fat-soluble vitamin deficiency (A, D, E, and K). Reduced serum carotene, a vitamin A precursor, has been noted in patients with SSc and severe esophageal dysmotility, which may reflect more extensive GI involvement [116]. Thus, it may be appropriate to check serum carotene or vitamin A in patients with malnutrition related to severe GI dysfunction. Vitamin D insufficiency/deficiency is common in patients with SSc, but may be related to reduced production (sunlight and skin thickness) rather than fat malabsorption [112, 117–119]. Due to the metabolic consequences from deficiency, biochemical screening may be considered. Severe malabsorption may also result in other micronutrient deficiency, such as magnesium which, when severe, may result in arrhythmias and seizures. Thus, care must be taken to screen at-risk patients for deficiencies, and once corrected, serum levels ought to be monitored and maintained. Patients at nutritional risk may benefit from a general micronutrient supplement (e.g., Forceval).

Management of Nutritional Issues

A range of different methods of support may be considered to help a patient to optimize their nutritional status. These include dietary fortification, dietary supplementation, enteral tube feeding, and PN. Some patients require a combination of these. The simplest measures may be considered first, taking into account each patient's current nutritional status, the likely duration and nature of any barriers to nutrition (e.g., acute illness vs. chronic manifestation), and their wishes.

Diet Modification

In a recent study, patients with SSc and malnutrition ("MUST"≥1), who received tailored dietary advice (including two-ninths commenced on oral nutritional supplements), maintained or increased their body weight and increased (not significantly) their protein and energy intake [112]. No specific dietary advice exists for patients with SSc. General advice exists for patients with xerostomia, microstomia, poor oral health, dysphagia, and delayed gastric emptying. However, for patients with SSc, this advice may be complicated by the fact that they often have more than one problem. Simple suggestions for people with dysphagia include maintaining an upright position during and after a meal and altering food consistency (e.g., pureed). Patients with early satiety or fatigue are advised to eat multiple small meals/snacks throughout the day and to avoid filling up with fluids while eating. Finally, patients without malabsorption may be educated about food fortification techniques. This involves the inclusion of calorie dense everyday foods (e.g., cream, butter, milk powder, full-fat rather than low-fat products) in the diet, so that nutritional content may be increased without the need to increase portion size.

When these measures fail, dietitians may recommend adding commercial nutritional supplements to the diet, the variety of which can be tailored to the patient. Available supplements differ in their textures (e.g., powders, semisolids, liquids), calorie densities (1–2 kcal/ml), compositions (e.g., elemental), and levels of nutritional completeness.

Enteral Support

Patients with swallowing difficulty may benefit from enteral tube feeding. In the short-term, this may be delivered via a nasoenteric tube (nasogastric or nasojejunal) and in the long-term via a percutaneous tube which terminates in either the stomach or jejunum. However, due to the possibility of patients with SSc having extensive GI involvement, it may be advisable for patients to have passed a nasoenteric trial before the placement of a percutaneous tube. The type of tube inserted may need careful consideration. Gastric feeding may be appropriate in patients with isolated pharyngeal or esophageal dysphagia, but may lead to the exacerbation of symptoms in patients with delayed gastric emptying [120–123]. In these patients, a post-pyloric feeding (jejunostomy) may be beneficial, provided that the patient does not have small intestinal dysmotility [123].

Parenteral Nutrition

PN is the delivery of tailored liquid nutrients via a central or peripheral vein. It may be considered for patients who are unable to meet their nutritional requirements enterally (oral ± tube feeding). It may be used in the short term while overcoming an acute illness, such as acute pseudoobstruction, and stopped following the successful reintroduction of oral nutrition following symptom resolution [36]. Alternatively, PN may be required long term (HPN) due to severe, uncontrolled GI involvement resulting in intestinal failure. The decision to commence HPN involves an assessment of patient suitability by a multidisciplinary team and careful patient counseling about the risks versus the benefits.

To date, several case reports and small series (largest 25 cases) have described the use of HPN in patients with SSc [123–129]. In patients receiving HPN, solutions are instilled via a dedicated tunneled catheter or implanted port. Possible complications, which may affect any patient on HPN, include catheter-related complications (sepsis, thrombosis, occlusion, and fracture), metabolic complications, and hepatic dysfunction. Typically, volumes of 2–3 l are instilled over a period of 12 h. However, some patients with SSc-related cardiac involvement may experience problems tolerating these large volumes [124].

Most patients who require HPN are trained to care for their own catheter and instill their own fluids. In order to minimize the risk of catheter-related sepsis, patients require significant manual dexterity. Thus, patients with SSc with sclerodactyly, contractures, finger ulcers, or multiple amputations may be unable to do this [124, 129]. Instead, they will be reliant on the support of specialist nurses at the start and end of their feed. However, despite these additional considerations, in patients with SSc and severe GI involvement resulting in intestinal failure, HPN is still a viable option to maintain a patient's nutritional status.

References

1. Clements PJ, Becvar R, Drosos AA, Ghattas L, Gabrielli A. Assessment of gastrointestinal involvement. Clin Exp Rheumatol. 2003;21(3 Suppl 29):S15–8.
2. Omair MA, Lee P. Effect of gastrointestinal manifestations on quality of life in 87 consecutive patients with systemic sclerosis. J Rheumatol. 2012. doi:10.3899/jrheum.110826. jrheum.110826 [pii].
3. Rubio-Rivas M, Royo C, Simeon CP, Corbella X, Fonollosa V. Mortality and survival in systemic sclerosis: systematic review and meta-analysis. Semin Arthritis Rheum. 2014. doi:10.1016/j.semarthrit.2014.05.010.

4. Bodukam V, Hays RD, Maranian P, Furst DE, Seibold JR, Impens A, Mayes MD, Clements PJ, Khanna D. Association of gastrointestinal involvement and depressive symptoms in patients with systemic sclerosis. Rheumatology. 2011;50(2):330–4. doi:10.1093/rheumatology/keq296.
5. Jewett LR, Razykov I, Hudson M, Baron M, Thombs BD, Canadian Scleroderma Research G. Prevalence of current, 12-month and lifetime major depressive disorder among patients with systemic sclerosis. Rheumatology. 2013;52(4):669–75. doi:10.1093/rheumatology/kes347.
6. Bluestone R, Macmahon M, Dawson JM. Systemic sclerosis and small bowel involvement. Gut. 1969;10(3):185–93.
7. Marguerie C, Kaye S, Vyse T, Mackworth-Young C, Walport MJ, Black C. Malabsorption caused by coeliac disease in patients who have scleroderma. Br J Rheumatol. 1995;34(9):858–61.
8. Schuffler MD, Kaplan LR, Johnson L. Small-intestinal mucosa in pseudoobstruction syndromes. Am J Dig Dis. 1978;23(9):821–8.
9. Manetti M, Neumann E, Milia AF, Tarner IH, Bechi P, Matucci-Cerinic M, Ibba-Manneschi L, Muller-Ladner U. Severe fibrosis and increased expression of fibrogenic cytokines in the gastric wall of systemic sclerosis patients. Arthritis Rheum. 2007;56(10):3442–7. doi:10.1002/art.22940.
10. Manetti M, Milia AF, Benelli G, Messerini L, Matucci-Cerinic M, Ibba-Manneschi L. The gastric wall in systemic sclerosis patients: a morphological study. Ital J Anat Embryol Arch Ital Anat Embriol. 2010;115(1–2):115–21.
11. Stafford-Brady FJ, Kahn HJ, Ross TM, Russell ML. Advanced scleroderma bowel: complications and management. J Rheumatol. 1988;15(5):869–74.
12. D'Angelo WA, Fries JF, Masi AT, Shulman LE. Pathologic observations in systemic sclerosis (scleroderma). A study of fifty-eight autopsy cases and fifty-eight matched controls. Am J Med. 1969;46(3):428–40.
13. Campbell PM, LeRoy EC. Pathogenesis of systemic sclerosis: a vascular hypothesis. Semin Arthritis Rheum. 1975;4(4):351–68.
14. Atkinson M, Summerling MD. Oesophageal changes in systemic sclerosis. Gut. 1966;7(4):402–8.
15. Manetti M, Rosa I, Messerini L, Guiducci S, Matucci-Cerinic M, Ibba-Manneschi L. A loss of telocytes accompanies fibrosis of multiple organs in systemic sclerosis. J Cell Mol Med. 2014;18(2):253–62. doi:10.1111/jcmm.12228.
16. Marie I, Ducrotte P, Denis P, Hellot MF, Levesque H. Outcome of small-bowel motor impairment in systemic sclerosis – a prospective manometric 5-yr follow-up. Rheumatology. 2007;46(1):150–3. doi:10.1093/rheumatology/kel203.
17. Cohen S, Fisher R, Lipshutz W, Turner R, Myers A, Schumacher R. The pathogenesis of esophageal dysfunction in scleroderma and Raynaud's disease. J Clin Invest. 1972;51(10):2663–8. doi:10.1172/JCI107084.
18. Sjogren RW. Gastrointestinal motility disorders in scleroderma. Arthritis Rheum. 1994;37(9):1265–82.
19. Eaker EY, Kuldau JG, Verne GN, Ross SO, Sallustio JE. Myenteric neuronal antibodies in scleroderma: passive transfer evokes alterations in intestinal myoelectric activity in a rat model. J Lab Clin Med. 1999;133(6):551–6.
20. Singh J, Mehendiratta V, Del Galdo F, Jimenez SA, Cohen S, DiMarino AJ, Rattan S. Immunoglobulins from scleroderma patients inhibit the muscarinic receptor activation in internal anal sphincter smooth muscle cells. Am J Physiol Gastrointest Liver Physiol. 2009;297(6):G1206–13. doi:10.1152/ajpgi.00286.2009.
21. Singh J, Cohen S, Mehendiratta V, Mendoza F, Jimenez SA, Dimarino AJ, Rattan S. Effects of scleroderma antibodies and pooled human immunoglobulin on anal sphincter and colonic smooth muscle function. Gastroenterology. 2012;143(5):1308–18. doi:10.1053/j.gastro.2012.07.109.
22. Howe S, Eaker EY, Sallustio JE, Peebles C, Tan EM, Williams Jr RC. Antimyenteric neuronal antibodies in scleroderma. J Clin Invest. 1994;94(2):761–70. doi:10.1172/JCI117395.
23. Kawaguchi Y, Nakamura Y, Matsumoto I, Nishimagi E, Satoh T, Kuwana M, Sumida T, Hara M. Muscarinic-3 acetylcholine receptor autoantibody in patients with systemic sclerosis: contribution to severe gastrointestinal tract dysmotility. Ann Rheum Dis. 2009;68(5):710–4. doi:10.1136/ard.2008.096545.
24. Marie et al - manometry of the upper intestinal tract in patients with SSc 1998 Arthritis and Rheum - 41:10:1874–1883
25. Bures J, Cyrany J, Kohoutova D, Forstl M, Rejchrt S, Kvetina J, Vorisek V, Kopacova M. Small intestinal bacterial overgrowth syndrome. World J Gastroenterol WJG. 2010;16(24):2978–90.
26. Shindo K, Machida M, Koide K, Fukumura M, Yamazaki R. Deconjugation ability of bacteria isolated from the jejunal fluid of patients with progressive systemic sclerosis and its gastric pH. Hepatogastroenterology. 1998;45(23):1643–50.
27. Marie I, Ducrotte P, Denis P, Menard JF, Levesque H. Small intestinal bacterial overgrowth in systemic sclerosis. Rheumatology. 2009;48(10):1314–9. doi:10.1093/rheumatology/kep226.
28. Marie I, Levesque H, Ducrotte P, Denis P, Hellot MF, Benichou J, Cailleux N, Courtois H. Gastric involvement in systemic sclerosis: a prospective study. Am J Gastroenterol. 2001;96(1):77–83. doi:10.1111/j.1572-0241.2001.03353.x.
29. Parodi A, Sessarego M, Greco A, Bazzica M, Filaci G, Setti M, Savarino E, Indiveri F, Savarino V, Ghio M. Small intestinal bacterial overgrowth in patients suffering from scleroderma: clinical effectiveness of its eradication. Am J Gastroenterol. 2008;103(5):1257–62. doi:10.1111/j.1572-0241.2007.01758.x.
30. Savarino E, Mei F, Parodi A, Ghio M, Furnari M, Gentile A, Berdini M, Di Sario A, Bendia E, Bonazzi P, Scarpellini E, Laterza L, Savarino V, Gasbarrini A. Gastrointestinal motility disorder assessment in systemic sclerosis. Rheumatology. 2013. doi:10.1093/rheumatology/kes429.
31. Gough A, Andrews D, Bacon PA, Emery P. Evidence of omeprazole-induced small bowel bacterial overgrowth in patients with scleroderma. Br J Rheumatol. 1995;34(10):976–7.
32. Thorens J, Froehlich F, Schwizer W, Saraga E, Bille J, Gyr K, Duroux P, Nicolet M, Pignatelli B, Blum AL, Gonvers JJ, Fried M. Bacterial overgrowth during treatment with omeprazole compared with cimetidine: a prospective randomised double blind study. Gut. 1996;39(1):54–9.
33. Ratuapli SK, Ellington TG, O'Neill MT, Umar SB, Harris LA, Foxx-Orenstein AE, Burdick GE, Dibaise JK, Lacy BE, Crowell MD. Proton pump inhibitor therapy use does not predispose to small intestinal bacterial overgrowth. Am J Gastroenterol. 2012;107(5):730–5. doi:10.1038/ajg.2012.4.
34. Sjolund K, Bartosik I, Lindberg G, Scheja A, Wildt M, Akesson A. Small intestinal manometry in patients with systemic sclerosis. Eur J Gastroenterol Hepatol. 2005;17(11):1205–12.
35. Muangchan C, Canadian Scleroderma Research G, Baron M, Pope J. The 15% rule in scleroderma: the frequency of severe organ complications in systemic sclerosis. A systematic review. J Rheumatol. 2013;40(9):1545–56. doi:10.3899/jrheum.121380.
36. Mecoli C, Purohit S, Sandorfi N, Derk CT. Mortality, recurrence, and hospital course of patients with systemic sclerosis-related acute intestinal pseudo-obstruction. J Rheumatol. 2014;41(10):2049–54. doi:10.3899/jrheum.131547.
37. Zapatier JA, Ukleja A. Intestinal obstruction and pseudo-obstruction in patients with systemic sclerosis. Acta Gastroenterol Latinoam. 2013;43(3):227–30.
38. Cobden I, Rothwell J, Axon AT, Dixon MF, Lintott DJ, Rowell NR. Small intestinal structure and passive permeability in systemic sclerosis. Gut. 1980;21(4):293–8.
39. Rosato E, De Nitto D, Rossi C, Libanori V, Donato G, Di Tola M, Pisarri S, Salsano F, Picarelli A. High incidence of celiac disease in patients with systemic sclerosis. J Rheumatol. 2009;36(5):965–9. doi:10.3899/jrheum.081000.
40. Forbess LJ, Gordon JK, Doobay K, Bosworth BP, Lyman S, Davids ML, Spiera RF. Low prevalence of coeliac disease in patients with systemic sclerosis: a cross-sectional study of a regis-

try cohort. Rheumatology. 2013;52(5):939–43. doi:10.1093/rheumatology/kes390.
41. Nisihara R, Utiyama SR, Azevedo PM, Skare TL. Celiac disease screening in patients with scleroderma. Arq Gastroenterol. 2011;48(2):163–4.
42. Hendel L, Worning H. Exocrine pancreatic function in patients with progressive systemic sclerosis. Scand J Gastroenterol. 1989;24(4):461–6.
43. Cobden I, Axon AT, Rowell NR. Pancreatic exocrine function in systemic sclerosis. Br J Dermatol. 1981;105(2):189–93.
44. Devgun P, Hassan H. Pneumatosis cystoides intestinalis: a rare benign cause of pneumoperitoneum. Case Rep Radiol. 2013;2013:353245. doi:10.1155/2013/353245.
45. Balbir-Gurman A, Brook OR, Chermesh I, Braun-Moscovici Y. Pneumatosis cystoides intestinalis in scleroderma-related conditions. Intern Med J. 2012;42(3):323–9. doi:10.1111/j.1445-5994.2011.02557.x.
46. Sequeira W. Pneumatosis cystoides intestinalis in systemic sclerosis and other diseases. Semin Arthritis Rheum. 1990;19(5):269–77.
47. Keyting WS, McCarver RR, Kovarik JL, Daywitt AL. Pneumatosis intestinalis: a new concept. Radiology. 1961;76:733–41. doi:10.1148/76.5.733.
48. Yale CE, Balish E, Wu JP. The bacterial etiology of pneumatosis cystoides intestinalis. Arch Surg. 1974;109(1):89–94.
49. Rohrmann Jr CA, Ricci MT, Krishnamurthy S, Schuffler MD. Radiologic and histologic differentiation of neuromuscular disorders of the gastrointestinal tract: visceral myopathies, visceral neuropathies, and progressive systemic sclerosis. AJR Am J Roentgenol. 1984;143(5):933–41. doi:10.2214/ajr.143.5.933.
50. Duchini A, Sessoms SL. Gastrointestinal hemorrhage in patients with systemic sclerosis and CREST syndrome. Am J Gastroenterol. 1998;93(9):1453–6. doi:10.1111/j.1572-0241.1998.00462.x.
51. Marie I, Antonietti M, Houivet E, Hachulla E, Maunoury V, Bienvenu B, Viennot S, Smail A, Duhaut P, Dupas JL, Dominique S, Hatron PY, Levesque H, Benichou J, Ducrotte P. Gastrointestinal mucosal abnormalities using videocapsule endoscopy in systemic sclerosis. Aliment Pharmacol Ther. 2014;40(2):189–99. doi:10.1111/apt.12818.
52. Wang SJ, Lan JL, Chen DY, Chen YH, Hsieh TY, Lin WY. Colonic transit disorders in systemic sclerosis. Clin Rheumatol. 2001;20(4):251–4.
53. Sallam HS, McNearney TA, Chen JZ. Anorectal motility and sensation abnormalities and its correlation with anorectal symptoms in patients with systemic sclerosis: a preliminary study. ISRN Gastroenterol. 2011;2011:402583. doi:10.5402/2011/402583.
54. Jharap B, Koudstaal LG, Neefjes-Borst EA, Van Weyenberg SJ. Colonic telangiectasias in progressive systemic sclerosis. Endoscopy. 2012;44 Suppl 2 UCTN:E42-43. doi:10.1055/s-0031-1291521.
55. Govoni M, Muccinelli M, Panicali P, La Corte R, Nuccio Scutellari P, Orzincolo C, Pazzi P, Trotta F. Colon involvement in systemic sclerosis: clinical-radiological correlations. Clin Rheumatol. 1996;15(3):271–6.
56. Thoua NM, Bunce C, Brough G, Forbes A, Emmanuel AV, Denton CP. Assessment of gastrointestinal symptoms in patients with systemic sclerosis in a UK tertiary referral centre. Rheumatology. 2010;49(9):1770–5. doi:10.1093/rheumatology/keq147.
57. Franck-Larsson K, Graf W, Ronnblom A. Lower gastrointestinal symptoms and quality of life in patients with systemic sclerosis: a population-based study. Eur J Gastroenterol Hepatol. 2009;21(2):176–82. doi:10.1097/MEG.0b013e32831dac75.
58. Battle WM, Snape Jr WJ, Wright S, Sullivan MA, Cohen S, Meyers A, Tuthill R. Abnormal colonic motility in progressive systemic sclerosis. Ann Intern Med. 1981;94(6):749–52.
59. Basilisco G, Barbera R, Vanoli M, Bianchi P. Anorectal dysfunction and delayed colonic transit in patients with progressive systemic sclerosis. Dig Dis Sci. 1993;38(8):1525–9.
60. Leighton JA, Valdovinos MA, Pemberton JH, Rath DM, Camilleri M. Anorectal dysfunction and rectal prolapse in progressive systemic sclerosis. Dis Colon Rectum. 1993;36(2):182–5.
61. Thoua NM, Schizas A, Forbes A, Denton CP, Emmanuel AV. Internal anal sphincter atrophy in patients with systemic sclerosis. Rheumatology. 2011;50(9):1596–602. doi:10.1093/rheumatology/ker153.
62. Fynne L, Worsoe J, Laurberg S, Krogh K. Faecal incontinence in patients with systemic sclerosis: is an impaired internal anal sphincter the only cause? Scand J Rheumatol. 2011;40(6):462–6. doi:10.3109/03009742.2011.579575.
63. Thoua NM, Abdel-Halim M, Forbes A, Denton CP, Emmanuel AV. Fecal incontinence in systemic sclerosis is secondary to neuropathy. Am J Gastroenterol. 2012;107(4):597–603. doi:10.1038/ajg.2011.399.
64. Baron M, Hudson M, Steele R, Canadian Scleroderma Research G. Malnutrition is common in systemic sclerosis: results from the Canadian scleroderma research group database. J Rheumatol. 2009;36(12):2737–43. doi:10.3899/jrheum.090694.
65. Cereda E, Codullo V, Klersy C, Breda S, Crippa A, Rava ML, Orlandi M, Bonardi C, Fiorentini ML, Caporali R, Caccialanza R. Disease-related nutritional risk and mortality in systemic sclerosis. Clin Nutr. 2014;33(3):558–61. doi:10.1016/j.clnu.2013.08.010.
66. Rosato E, Gigante A, Gasperini ML, Molinaro I, Di Lazzaro Giraldi G, Afeltra A, Amoroso D, Salsano F, Rossi Fanelli F, Laviano A. Nutritional status measured by BMI is impaired and correlates with left ventricular mass in patients with systemic sclerosis. Nutrition. 2014;30(2):204–9. doi:10.1016/j.nut.2013.07.025.
67. Assassi S, Del Junco D, Sutter K, McNearney TA, Reveille JD, Karnavas A, Gourh P, Estrada YMRM, Fischbach M, Arnett FC, Mayes MD. Clinical and genetic factors predictive of mortality in early systemic sclerosis. Arthritis Rheum. 2009;61(10):1403–11. doi:10.1002/art.24734.
68. Khanna D, Furst DE, Maranian P, Seibold JR, Impens A, Mayes MD, Clements PJ, Getzug T, Hays RD. Minimally important differences of the UCLA Scleroderma Clinical Trial Consortium Gastrointestinal Tract Instrument. J Rheumatol. 2011;38(9):1920–4. doi:10.3899/jrheum.110225.
69. Khanna D, Hays RD, Maranian P, Seibold JR, Impens A, Mayes MD, Clements PJ, Getzug T, Fathi N, Bechtel A, Furst DE. Reliability and validity of the University of California, Los Angeles scleroderma clinical trial consortium gastrointestinal tract instrument. Arthritis Rheum. 2009;61(9):1257–63. doi:10.1002/art.24730.
70. Bae S, Allanore Y, Coustet B, Maranian P, Khanna D. Development and validation of French version of the UCLA scleroderma clinical trial consortium gastrointestinal tract instrument. Clin Exp Rheumatol. 2011;29(2 Suppl 65):S15–21.
71. Spiegel BM, Hays RD, Bolus R, Melmed GY, Chang L, Whitman C, Khanna PP, Paz SH, Hays T, Reise S, Khanna D. Development of the NIH patient-reported outcomes measurement information system (PROMIS) gastrointestinal symptom scales. Am J Gastroenterol. 2014. doi:10.1038/ajg.2014.237.
72. Hansi N, Thoua N, Carulli M, Chakravarty K, Lal S, Smyth A, Herrick A, Ogunbiyi O, Shaffer J, McLaughlin J, Denton C, Ong V, Emmanuel AV, Murray CD. Consensus best practice pathway of the UK scleroderma study group: gastrointestinal manifestations of systemic sclerosis. Clin Exp Rheumatol. 2014;32(6 Suppl 86):S-214–21.
73. Corazza GR, Menozzi MG, Strocchi A, Rasciti L, Vaira D, Lecchini R, Avanzini P, Chezzi C, Gasbarrini G. The diagnosis of

small bowel bacterial overgrowth. Reliability of jejunal culture and inadequacy of breath hydrogen testing. Gastroenterology. 1990;98(2):302–9.
74. Kaye SA, Lim SG, Taylor M, Patel S, Gillespie S, Black CM. Small bowel bacterial overgrowth in systemic sclerosis: detection using direct and indirect methods and treatment outcome. Br J Rheumatol. 1995;34(3):265–9.
75. Romagnuolo J, Schiller D, Bailey RJ. Using breath tests wisely in a gastroenterology practice: an evidence-based review of indications and pitfalls in interpretation. Am J Gastroenterol. 2002;97(5):1113–26. doi:10.1111/j.1572-0241.2002.05664.x.
76. Khoshini R, Dai SC, Lezcano S, Pimentel M. A systematic review of diagnostic tests for small intestinal bacterial overgrowth. Dig Dis Sci. 2008;53(6):1443–54. doi:10.1007/s10620-007-0065-1.
77. Simren M, Stotzer PO. Use and abuse of hydrogen breath tests. Gut. 2006;55(3):297–303. doi:10.1136/gut.2005.075127.
78. Pimentel M, Chow EJ, Lin HC. Normalization of lactulose breath testing correlates with symptom improvement in irritable bowel syndrome. a double-blind, randomized, placebo-controlled study. Am J Gastroenterol. 2003;98(2):412–9. doi:10.1111/j.1572-0241.2003.07234.x.
79. Di Baise JK. Nutritional consequences of small intestinal bacterial overgrowth. Pract Gastroenterol. 2008;69:15–28.
80. Baron M, Bernier P, Cote LF, Delegge MH, Falovitch G, Friedman G, Gornitsky M, Hoffer J, Hudson M, Khanna D, Paterson WG, Schafer D, Toskes PP, Wykes L. Screening and therapy for malnutrition and related gastro-intestinal disorders in systemic sclerosis: recommendations of a North American expert panel. Clin Exp Rheumatol. 2010;28(2 Suppl 58):S42–6.
81. Nikou GC, Toumpanakis C, Katsiari C, Charalambopoulos D, Sfikakis PP. Treatment of small intestinal disease in systemic sclerosis with octreotide: a prospective study in seven patients. J Clin Rheumatol Pract Rep Rheum Musculoskelet Dis. 2007;13(3):119–23. doi:10.1097/RHU.0b013e3180645d2a.
82. Soifer LO, Peralta D, Dima G, Besasso H. Comparative clinical efficacy of a probiotic vs. an antibiotic in the treatment of patients with intestinal bacterial overgrowth and chronic abdominal functional distension: a pilot study. Acta Gastroenterol Latinoam. 2010;40(4):323–7.
83. Barrett JS, Canale KE, Gearry RB, Irving PM, Gibson PR. Probiotic effects on intestinal fermentation patterns in patients with irritable bowel syndrome. World J Gastroenterol WJG. 2008;14(32):5020–4.
84. Frech TM, Khanna D, Maranian P, Frech EJ, Sawitzke AD, Murtaugh MA. Probiotics for the treatment of systemic sclerosis-associated gastrointestinal bloating/ distention. Clin Exp Rheumatol. 2011;29(2 Suppl 65):S22–5.
85. Folwaczny C, Laritz M, Meurer M, Endres SP, Konig A, Schindlbeck N. Effects of various prokinetic drugs on gastrointestinal transit times in patients with progressive systemic scleroderma. Z Gastroenterol. 1997;35(10):905–12.
86. Boeckxstaens GE, Bartelsman JF, Lauwers L, Tytgat GN. Treatment of GI dysmotility in scleroderma with the new enterokinetic agent prucalopride. Am J Gastroenterol. 2002;97(1):194–7. doi:10.1111/j.1572-0241.2002.05396.x.
87. Bouras EP, Camilleri M, Burton DD, McKinzie S. Selective stimulation of colonic transit by the benzofuran 5HT4 agonist, prucalopride, in healthy humans. Gut. 1999;44(5):682–6.
88. Johnson DA, Drane WE, Curran J, Benjamin SB, Chobanian SJ, Karvelis K, Cattau Jr EL. Metoclopramide response in patients with progressive systemic sclerosis. Effect on esophageal and gastric motility abnormalities. Arch Intern Med. 1987;147(9):1597–601.
89. Rees WD, Leigh RJ, Christofides ND, Bloom SR, Turnberg LA. Interdigestive motor activity in patients with systemic sclerosis. Gastroenterology. 1982;83(3):575–80.
90. Wang SJ, Lan JL, Lan JL, Chen DY, Chen YH, Hsieh TY, Lin WY. Effects of cisapride on colonic transit in patients with progressive systemic sclerosis. Clin Rheumatol. 2002;21(4):271–4. doi:10.1007/s100670200072.
91. Horowitz M, Maddern GJ, Maddox A, Wishart J, Chatterton BE, Shearman DJ. Effects of cisapride on gastric and esophageal emptying in progressive systemic sclerosis. Gastroenterology. 1987;93(2):311–5.
92. Evans PR, Bak YT, Kellow JE. Effects of oral cisapride on small bowel motility in irritable bowel syndrome. Aliment Pharmacol Ther. 1997;11(5):837–44.
93. Soudah HC, Hasler WL, Owyang C. Effect of octreotide on intestinal motility and bacterial overgrowth in scleroderma. N Engl J Med. 1991;325(21):1461–7. doi:10.1056/NEJM199111213252102.
94. Verne GN, Sninsky CA. Chronic intestinal pseudo-obstruction. Dig Dis. 1995;13(3):163–81.
95. Perlemuter G, Cacoub P, Chaussade S, Wechsler B, Couturier D, Piette JC. Octreotide treatment of chronic intestinal pseudoobstruction secondary to connective tissue diseases. Arthritis Rheum. 1999;42(7):1545–9.doi:10.1002/1529-0131(199907)42:7<1545::AID-ANR30>3.0.CO;2-T.
96. Nunokawa T, Yokogawa N, Ohtsuka H, Shimada K, Sugii S. Transgastric long tube placement following percutaneous endoscopic gastrostomy for severe chronic intestinal pseudo-obstruction related to systemic sclerosis. Modern Rheumatol Jpn Rheum Assoc. 2013. doi:10.3109/14397595.2013.844385.
97. Amiot A, Joly F, Alves A, Panis Y, Bouhnik Y, Messing B. Long-term outcome of chronic intestinal pseudo-obstruction adult patients requiring home parenteral nutrition. Am J Gastroenterol. 2009;104(5):1262–70. doi:10.1038/ajg.2009.58.
98. Ishikawa M, Okada J, Kondo H. Five cases of systemic sclerosis with associated with intestinal pseudo-obstruction. Ryumachi [Rheum]. 1999;39(5):768–73.
99. Vischio J, Matlyuk-Urman Z, Lakshminarayanan S. Benign spontaneous pneumoperitoneum in systemic sclerosis. J Clin Rheumatol Pract Rep Rheum Musculoskelet Dis. 2010;16(8):379–81. doi:10.1097/RHU.0b013e3181ffeb49.
100. Satoh A, Hoshina Y, Shimizu H, Morita K, Uchiyama M, Moriuchi J, Takaya M, Ichikawa Y. Systemic sclerosis with various gastrointestinal problems including pneumoperitoneum, pneumatosis cystoides intestinalis and malabsorption syndrome. Ryumachi [Rheum]. 1995;35(6):927–33.
101. Chatterjee S, Park S, Low K, Kong Y, Pimentel M. The degree of breath methane production in IBS correlates with the severity of constipation. Am J Gastroenterol. 2007;102(4):837–41. doi:10.1111/j.1572-0241.2007.01072.x.
102. Gough A, Sheeran T, Bacon P, Emery P. Dietary advice in systemic sclerosis: the dangers of a high fibre diet. Ann Rheum Dis. 1998;57(11):641–2.
103. Wald A. Is chronic use of stimulant laxatives harmful to the colon? J Clin Gastroenterol. 2003;36(5):386–9.
104. Emmanuel A, Cools M, Vandeplassche L, Kerstens R. Prucalopride improves bowel function and colonic transit time in patients with chronic constipation: an integrated analysis. Am J Gastroenterol. 2014;109(6):887–94. doi:10.1038/ajg.2014.74.
105. Franck-Larsson K, Graf W, Eeg-Olofsson KE, Axelson HW, Ronnblom A. Physiological and structural anorectal abnormalities in patients with systemic sclerosis and fecal incontinence. Scand J Gastroenterol. 2014;49(9):1076–83. doi:10.3109/00365521.2014.913188.
106. Miner PB, Donnelly TC, Read NW. Investigation of mode of action of biofeedback in treatment of fecal incontinence. Dig Dis Sci. 1990;35(10):1291–8.
107. Kenefick NJ, Vaizey CJ, Nicholls RJ, Cohen R, Kamm MA. Sacral nerve stimulation for faecal incontinence due to systemic sclerosis. Gut. 2002;51(6):881–3.

108. Winiarski M, Jozwiak D, Pusty M, Dziki A. Satisfaction with life after rectal prolapse surgery. Pol Przegl Chir. 2013;85(1):29–34. doi:10.2478/pjs-2013-0005.
109. Stratton RJ, Hackston A, Longmore D, Dixon R, Price S, Stroud M, King C, Elia M. Malnutrition in hospital outpatients and inpatients: prevalence, concurrent validity and ease of use of the 'malnutrition universal screening tool' ('MUST') for adults. Br J Nutr. 2004;92(5):799–808.
110. Malnutrition Universal Screening Tool. BAPEN (British Association for Enteral & Parenteral Nutrition). 2003. www.bapen.co.uk.
111. Murtaugh MA, Frech TM. Nutritional status and gastrointestinal symptoms in systemic sclerosis patients. Clin Nutr. 2012. doi:10.1016/j.clnu.2012.06.005.
112. Ortiz-Santamaria V, Puig C, Soldevillla C, Barata A, Cuquet J, Recasens A. Nutritional support in patients with systemic sclerosis. Reumatol Clin. 2014;10(5):283–7. doi:10.1016/j.reuma.2013.12.011.
113. Weekes CE, Elia M, Emery PW. The development, validation and reliability of a nutrition screening tool based on the recommendations of the British Association for Parenteral and Enteral Nutrition (BAPEN). Clin Nutr. 2004;23(5):1104–12. doi:10.1016/j.clnu.2004.02.003.
114. Baron M, Hudson M, Steele R, Canadian Scleroderma Research G. Is serum albumin a marker of malnutrition in chronic disease? The scleroderma paradigm. J Am Coll Nutr. 2010;29(2):144–51.
115. Caporali R, Caccialanza R, Bonino C, Klersy C, Cereda E, Xoxi B, Crippa A, Rava ML, Orlandi M, Bonardi C, Cameletti B, Codullo V, Montecucco C. Disease-related malnutrition in outpatients with systemic sclerosis. Clin Nutr. 2012. doi:10.1016/j.clnu.2012.02.010.
116. Lundberg AC, Akesson A, Akesson B. Dietary intake and nutritional status in patients with systemic sclerosis. Ann Rheum Dis. 1992;51(10):1143–8.
117. Caramaschi P, Dalla Gassa A, Ruzzenente O, Volpe A, Ravagnani V, Tinazzi I, Barausse G, Bambara LM, Biasi D. Very low levels of vitamin D in systemic sclerosis patients. Clin Rheumatol. 2010;29(12):1419–25. doi:10.1007/s10067-010-1478-3.
118. Vacca A, Cormier C, Piras M, Mathieu A, Kahan A, Allanore Y. Vitamin D deficiency and insufficiency in 2 independent cohorts of patients with systemic sclerosis. J Rheumatol. 2009;36(9):1924–9. doi:10.3899/jrheum.081287.
119. Arnson Y, Amital H, Agmon-Levin N, Alon D, Sanchez-Castanon M, Lopez-Hoyos M, Matucci-Cerinic M, Szucs G, Shapira Y, Szekanecz Z, Shoenfeld Y. Serum 25-OH vitamin D concentrations are linked with various clinical aspects in patients with systemic sclerosis: a retrospective cohort study and review of the literature. Autoimmun Rev. 2011;10(8):490–4. doi:10.1016/j.autrev.2011.02.002.
120. Fynne L, Kruse A, Borre M, Sondergaard K, Krogh K. Percutaneous endoscopic gastrostomy in patients with systemic sclerosis. Scand J Rheumatol. 2010;39(3):266–8. doi:10.3109/03009740903468990.
121. Das L, Bowden A, Cooper RG, Mitchell W, O'Sullivan M, Herrick AL. Percutaneous endoscopic gastrostomy feeding – a life-saving intervention in SSc-myositis overlap with pharyngeal dysfunction. Rheumatology. 2012;51(8):1518–20. doi:10.1093/rheumatology/kes020.
122. Abell TL, Bernstein RK, Cutts T, Farrugia G, Forster J, Hasler WL, McCallum RW, Olden KW, Parkman HP, Parrish CR, Pasricha PJ, Prather CM, Soffer EE, Twillman R, Vinik AI. Treatment of gastroparesis: a multidisciplinary clinical review. Neurogastroenterol Motil Off J Eur Gastrointest Motil Soc. 2006;18(4):263–83. doi:10.1111/j.1365-2982.2006.00760.x.
123. Grabowski G, Grant JP. Nutritional support in patients with systemic scleroderma. JPEN J Parenter Enter Nutr. 1989;13(2):147–51.
124. Brown M, Teubner A, Shaffer J, Herrick AL. Home parenteral nutrition – an effective and safe long-term therapy for systemic sclerosis-related intestinal failure. Rheumatology. 2008;47(2):176–9. doi:10.1093/rheumatology/kem329.
125. Ng SC, Clements PJ, Berquist WE, Furst DE, Paulus HE. Home central venous hyperalimentation in fifteen patients with severe scleroderma bowel disease. Arthritis Rheum. 1989;32(2):212–6.
126. Levien DH, Fiallos F, Barone R, Taffet S. The use of cyclic home hyperalimentation for malabsorption in patients with scleroderma involving the small intestines. JPEN J Parenter Enter Nutr. 1985;9(5):623–5.
127. Lyons JM, Falkenbach L, Cerra FB. Home parenteral nutrition with full-time home care nurses. JPEN J Parenter Enter Nutr. 1981;5(6):528–30.
128. Jawa H, Fernandes G, Saqui O, Allard JP. Home parenteral nutrition in patients with systemic sclerosis: a retrospective review of 12 cases. J Rheumatol. 2012. doi:10.3899/jrheum.110896.
129. Harrison E, Herrick AL, Dibb M, McLaughlin JT, Lal S. Long-term outcome of patients with systemic sclerosis requiring home parenteral nutrition. Clin Nutr. 2014. doi:10.1016/j.clnu.2014.11.002.

Part VII

Skin, Musculoskeletal and Other Complications

Calcinosis

32

Antonia Valenzuela and Lorinda Chung

Introduction

Calcinosis cutis is the deposition of calcium in the skin and subcutaneous tissues. It is a manifestation of several autoimmune connective tissue diseases (ACTDs) including systemic sclerosis (SSc). Calcinosis has a substantial impact on quality of life as it is often associated with pain, recurrent episodes of local inflammation, and functional impairment. Complications of calcinosis include infection and ulceration. Herein, we review the most current knowledge regarding pathogenesis of calcinosis, associated clinical factors, diagnostic approach, and treatment options.

Definition and Classification of Calcinosis

Calcinosis cutis is a disorder characterized by calcium deposition in the skin and subcutaneous tissues [1] (Fig. 32.1). It is associated with autoimmune connective tissue diseases (ACTDs) including systemic sclerosis (SSc), dermatomyositis (DM), mixed connective tissue diseases (MCTDs), and, more rarely, systemic lupus erythematosus (SLE) [2].

The most updated classification system for calcinosis cutis includes four categories [1,3]: dystrophic calcification, metastatic calcification, calciphylaxis, and idiopathic or iatrogenic. Dystrophic calcification is the most common type and is defined as the deposition of calcified material in damaged tissues in the presence of normal serum calcium and phosphate levels [4]. Tissue ischemia is thought to play a role in the tissue damage that serves as a nidus for dystrophic calcification. It is associated with ACTD, heritable disorders (Ehlers-Danlos syndrome), benign and malignant cutaneous neoplasms, infections, and trauma [5]. In contrast, metastatic calcification is the deposition of calcium in normal cutaneous or subcutaneous tissue as a result of a defect in metabolism of calcium and/or phosphate [4,5]. Calciphylaxis also results from disturbances of calcium and phosphate metabolism, but affects the small vessels of the dermis or subcutaneous fat. It may cause secondary ischemia and necrosis and predominates in patients with end-stage renal disease (ESRD) [6]. These patients have decreased phosphate clearance that leads to hyperphosphatemia, decreased intestinal calcium absorption that causes hypocalcemia, and secondary hyperparathyroidism, which in turn increases bone resorption, and efflux of calcium and phosphate into the serum. However, the pathogenic role of these metabolic changes is controversial [7], and calciphylaxis is thought to occur in previously sensitized tissue by a specific calcifying factor (i.e., parathyroid hormone) when challenged with a specific inciting agent (local trauma, steroids) [6,8]. Idiopathic or iatrogenic calcification is not associated with any underlying tissue damage or metabolic disorder and occurs in otherwise healthy individuals [3].

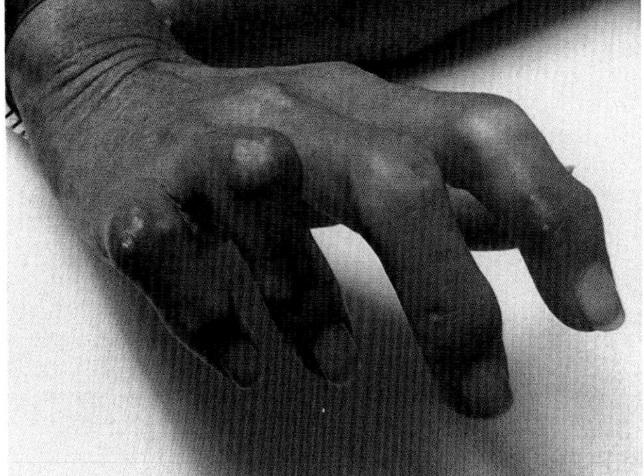

Fig. 32.1 Calcinosis of the fingers

A. Valenzuela, MD, MS
Department of Medicine, Stanford University, Palo Alto, CA, USA

L. Chung, MD, MS (✉)
Department of Medicine and Dermatology (Immunology and Rheumatology Division), Stanford University School of Medicine, Palo Alto, CA, USA

Palo Alto VA Hospital, Palo Alto, CA, USA
e-mail: shauwei@stanford.edu; lorindachung@hotmail.com

J. Varga et al. (eds.), *Scleroderma*, DOI 10.1007/978-3-319-31407-5_32

Epidemiology and Clinical Associations of Calcinosis in Systemic Sclerosis

Calcinosis is not uncommon in SSc, especially in the limited cutaneous SSc (lcSSc) subtype. An international multicenter cohort study that included 7,056 SSc patients reported an overall frequency of calcinosis of 22 % (17 % in patients with diffuse cutaneous SSc (dcSSc), 25 % in patients with lcSSc, and 28 % in patients with scleroderma sine sclerosis (ssSSc) [9]. Calcinosis is known to be a long-term complication in SSc and presents after a mean disease duration from the first non-Raynaud's symptom of 9–13 years [9,10].

Several clinical features have been found to be associated with calcinosis (Table 32.1). One study of 103 consecutively recruited patients with SSc found that male gender and digital ulcers were significant independent predictive factors for radiological progression of calcinosis (HR 3.99, 95 % CI 1.45–12.13, and HR 3.16, 95 % CI 1.22–9.43, respectively) [11]. The latter finding was also reported by Koutaissoff et al. in a study that included hand radiographs of 167 SSc patients matched with 168 hand radiographs of patients without SSc, showing that patients with terminal tuft calcinosis had more digital ulcerations (28 % vs. 11 %, $p=0.03$) and pitting scars (64 % vs. 38 %, $p=0.03$) [12]. Similar to SSc, we found in a cross-sectional study of 126 patients with DM (11 % with calcinosis) that those patients with calcinosis were significantly more likely to suffer from fingertip ulcers than patients without calcinosis (50.0 % vs. 9.3 %, $p<0.001$) [13]. Additionally, a retrospective study of 101 patients with SSc in whom hand radiographs were available reported that patients with moderate or severe acro-osteolysis (resorption of the distal bony phalanges thought to be related to digital ischemia) were more likely to have severe calcinosis (33 % vs. 13 %), although this did not reach statistical significance after adjustment for potential confounders [14].

In one study that included 95 patients with lcSSc, patients with positive anti-centromere antibody (ACA) were more likely to have calcinosis than those with negative ACA (55 % vs. 22 % in the fingers only and 60 % vs. 26 % in any location, p-value<0.0001) [15]. Calcinosis also was positively associated with the presence of the anti-PM/Scl antibody in a Canadian study of 763 SSc patients (58 % in patients with positive anti-PM/Scl antibody vs. 30 % in patients with negative anti-PM/Scl antibody, $p=0.04$) [16].

We recently confirmed several of these clinical associations in a retrospective multicenter international cohort study of 5,280 patients with SSc in which 24 % had calcinosis. In this study, when compared with patients without calcinosis, patients with calcinosis were older and more likely to be female and had a higher modified Rodnan skin score at baseline and longer disease duration from the first non-Raynaud's phenomenon symptom. In addition, they were more likely to have digital ulcers, acro-osteolysis and telangiectasias, cardiac disease, pulmonary hypertension, gastrointestinal involvement, and arthritis, but less likely to have myositis. Autoantibodies independently associated with the presence of calcinosis included ACA, anti-PM/Scl antibody, and anticardiolipin antibodies. Interestingly, a novel association between calcinosis and osteoporosis was found, but this needs further exploration (unpublished data).

Table 32.1 Clinical features associated with calcinosis in systemic sclerosis

Demographics:
Longer disease duration
Limited cutaneous SSc subtype
Male gender
Physical findings:
Digital ulcerations
Pitting scars
Acro-osteolysis
Autoantibodies:
Positive anti-centromere antibody
Positive anti-PM/Scl antibody

SSc systemic sclerosis

Pathophysiology of Calcinosis

The detailed pathophysiology of calcinosis cutis remains poorly understood and varies among the different subtypes [2]. Calcium deposits are made of calcium hydroxyapatite crystals and contain calcium, hydroxides, and phosphates. It has been proposed that dystrophic calcinosis cutis occurs when calcium precipitates in tissue damaged by local trauma, chronic inflammation, or vascular hypoxia [1].

Given the association between digital ulcers and calcinosis in ACTD, vascular ischemia is thought to play an important role in the pathogenesis of calcinosis. Davies et al. demonstrated increased expression of the hypoxia-associated glucose transporter molecule (GLUT-1) by immunohistochemistry in skin biopsies of patients with dcSSc and lcSSc-associated calcinosis, indicating that hypoxia is a possible contributing factor [17]. Similarly, the same group evaluated the expression of recognized markers of oxidative stress, the advanced glycation/lipoperoxidation end products (AGEs) and their receptor (RAGE), and concluded that it was greater in the dermis of patients with SSc, especially in those with calcinosis, when compared to healthy controls [18].

The role of inflammation in the subsequent development of calcinosis is unclear. Juvenile DM patients with calcinosis have been found to have elevated serum IL-1 levels. In addition, the presence of interleukin (IL)-6, IL-1α, and tumor necrosis factor (TNF)-α in the "milk of calcium" (calcium-laden fluid collections) of JDM patients [19] supports a role for activated macrophages and inflammation at least in a subset of patients with calcinosis.

An imbalance between various mediators that cause increased calcium influx into cells has also been suggested as a contributing factor [20]. Membrane damage is hypothesized to lead to abnormally high mitochondrial calcium and phosphate levels, which creates a more acidic environment that interferes with inhibitors of calcification [4,5,21]. On the other hand, osteonectin, a promoter of calcification, has been found to be increased in endothelial cells and fibroblasts of SSc patients, particularly in those with calcinosis compared with those without calcinosis [18]. High levels of the calcium-binding amino acid (CBAA) and gamma-carboxyglutamic acid (GCGA) have also been found in subcutaneous calcifications from patients with DM or SSc [22]. These amino acids were discovered in vitamin K-dependent clotting factors, but are also present in proteins from mineralized tissues, as the bone and dentin (osteocalcin), and are probably implicated in the deposition of calcium [23].

More studies are necessary to better define the roles of hypoxia, inflammation, and metabolic derangements in the pathogenesis of calcinosis and to identify other mechanisms that may be involved.

Diagnostic Approach

Calcinosis in SSc presents as subcutaneous nodules or lumps of variable size and shape, typically at sites of recurrent microtrauma. Small pebble-sized lesions can sometimes come to the surface and extrude and may be associated with white, milky fluid. Other morphologies that can be observed in ACTD but are less frequent in SSc include deeper nodules, tumor-like lesions in the dermis or subcutaneous tissue, or diffuse deposits along myofascial planes that can rarely form an extensive exoskeleton [3,24]. The most frequent body sites involved in SSc are the hands (particularly the fingers) and feet. Other common areas that can be affected include the elbows and knees, arms and legs, trunk, and face, in order of frequency. This is consistent with a retrospective study performed at Mayo Clinic, including 78 patients with ACTD and calcinosis assessed by physical examination or imaging studies, including 24 with lcSSc. In this study, 18 lcSSc patients had calcinosis in the hands or feet, 13 in the extremities, three on the head, and one on the trunk. This differed from patients with DM in whom calcinosis most commonly affected the extremities [25]. Although calcinosis in the hands clearly affects the quality of life for patients with SSc, calcinosis of the foot is also common, affecting 18 % of 50 patients with SSc assessed by a podiatrist [26].

In cases where the calcinosis is not clearly palpable or visible on physical examination, imaging studies may be helpful. In addition, the extent and severity of calcinotic lesions can be evaluated. Plain radiography is recommended for the initial imaging evaluation of calcinosis in patients with ACTD [27], and a "wet cotton-wool appearance" may be observed [28] (Fig. 32.2). In collaboration with the Scleroderma Clinical Trial Consortium, a novel radiographic scoring system was recently developed for potential use in clinical trial testing agents for the treatment of calcinosis. This scoring system provides an estimate of the calcinosis burden affecting the hands in patients with SSc, taking into account the area coverage, density, number, and anatomic location of calcinotic lesions (Fig. 32.3). This scoring system has excellent reliability (inter-rater reliability

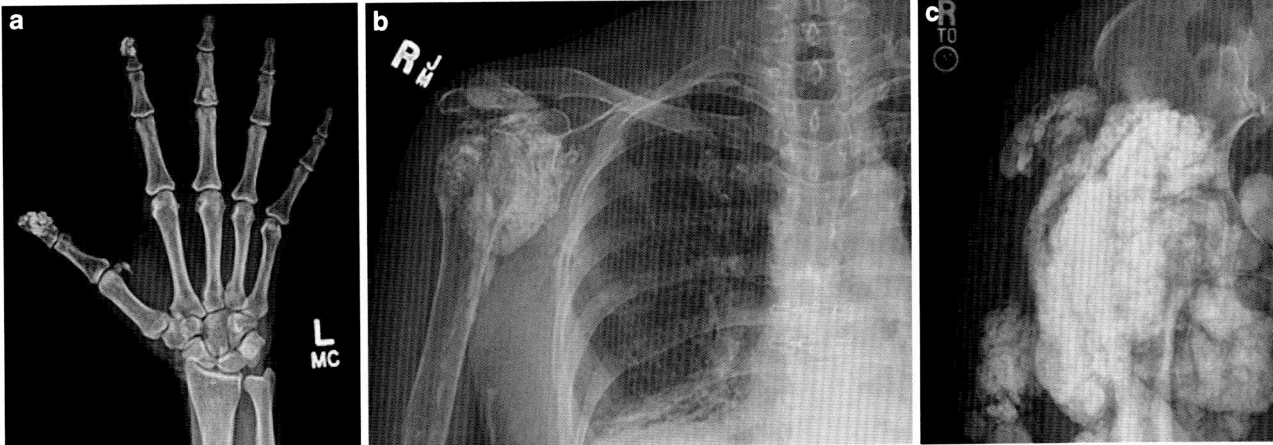

Fig. 32.2 (**a**) "Wet cotton-wool appearance" of calcinosis on radiography of the hands. (**b**) Anteroposterior radiograph of the right shoulder in a 58-year-old female with long-standing scleroderma demonstrates calcinosis around the glenohumeral and acromioclavicular joints, with calcification extending distally along the bicipital groove. Linear opacities are seen at the right lung base compatible with the underlying interstitial lung disease related to scleroderma. (**c**) Frontal radiograph of the right hip in a 57-year-old female with scleroderma demonstrates extensive calcinosis around the hip, hemipelvis, and proximal thigh

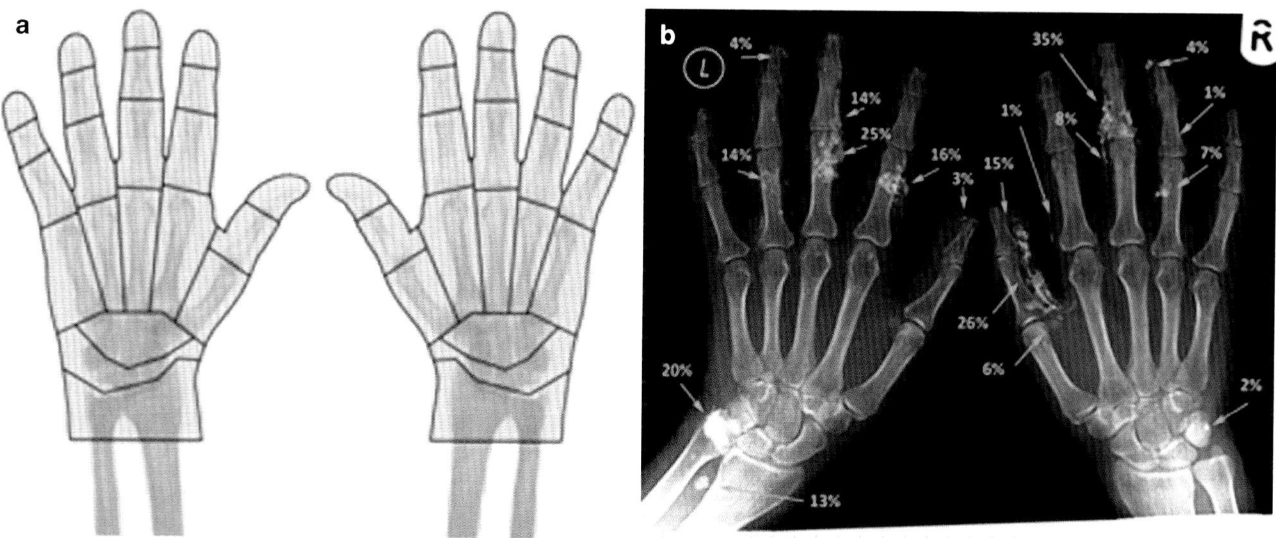

Fig. 32.3 (**a**) Anatomic regions of hand x-rays for radiographic scoring system. (**b**) Examples of % areal coverage for radiographic scoring system (Reproduced with permission from Chung L et al. *Arthritis Care and Research*. 2015;67(3))

ICC = 0.89, 95 % CI 0.86–0.92, and intra-rater reliability ICC = 0.89, 95 % CI 0.8–0.97) but requires further validation with respect to sensitivity to change [29]. Conventional computed tomography (CT) scans may be useful in the assessment of lesions involving the trunk, or plaque-like lesions. Likewise, magnetic resonance imaging (MRI) can be helpful in visualizing these lesions, but this technique has variable contrast resolution and fails to identify small calcifications [30].

More experimental diagnostic studies include ultrasonography (US), multidetector computed tomography (MDCT), and dual-energy computed tomography (DECT). One cross-sectional study investigated hand features by US in 52 consecutive SSc patients and found no significant difference between US and radiography in detecting calcinosis (40 % vs. 36 %, $p = 0.8$) [31]. A case-control study that included 44 SSc patients found calcinosis in 17 patients (39 %) with US of the hands and wrists and estimated a sensitivity of 89 % [32]. MDCT has greater contrast resolution and can provide three-dimensional images (Figs. 32.4 and 32.5) which may provide a more accurate assessment of the extent of calcinotic lesions [30]. DECT is a modern technique used for assessing monosodium urate deposits in soft tissue from patients with gout, which has recently been proposed as a useful modality to evaluate SSc-calcinosis of the hands [33]. DECT scan was performed in two dcSSc patients and successfully showed calcinosis deposits in the subcutaneous fat pads of the fingertips, along the tendon sheaths, within the carpal tunnel, and adjacent to the muscles (Fig. 32.6). Further studies are necessary to determine whether US, MDCT, and/or DECT might be more useful in the assessment and measurement of calcinosis burden than plain radiography.

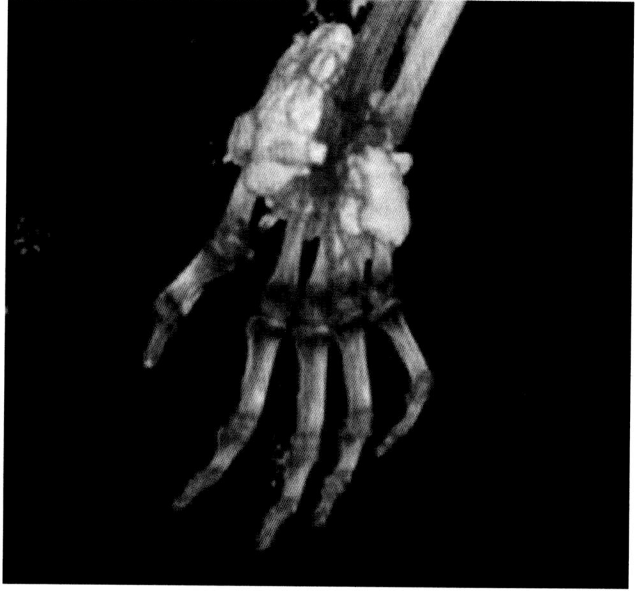

Fig. 32.4 MDCT image with multiplanar 3D of calcinosis of the hand (Courtesy of Pr Allanore)

Complications of Calcinosis

Common complications of calcinosis are ulceration at the site of lesions (Fig. 32.7), infection, pain, impaired function, and compression of nerves. Pain may be related to calcinosis over pressure areas or to associated inflammation. In the Mayo Clinic study, from the total of 78 patients with calcinosis cutis and ACTD, 43 patients (55 %) had ulcer formation in the context of calcinosis cutis, and 54 patients (69 %) had pain associated with calcinosis cutis [25]. Infection of calcinosis in SSc is an underreported complication, but may also

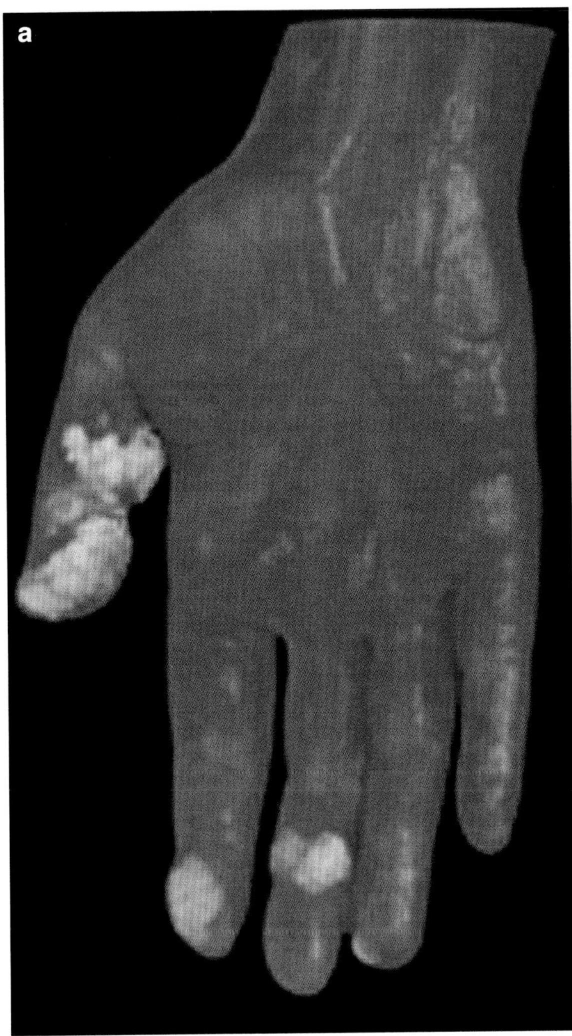

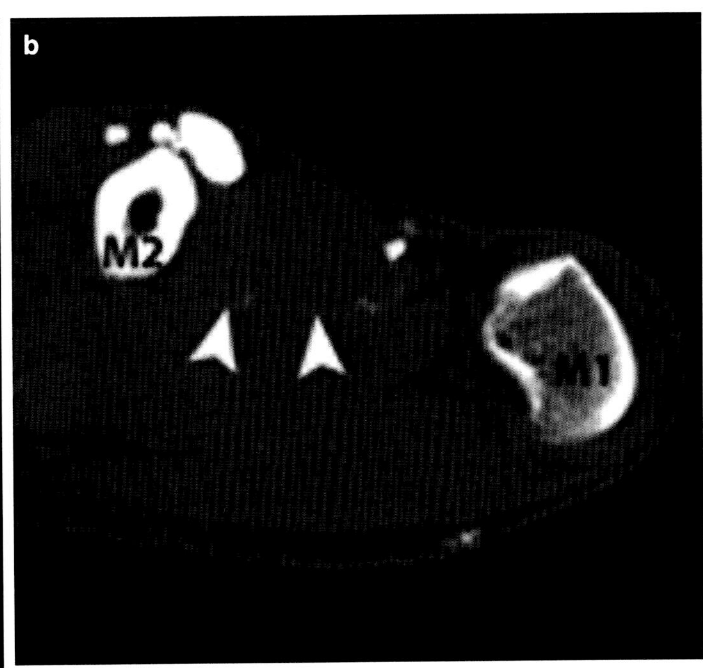

Fig. 32.5 (**a**) Volume-rendered MDCT image of the left hand displays calcinosis involving the thumb, the index, and the middle finger. (**b**) Axial-unenhanced MDCT image of the left hand depicts the thin linear distribution of calcinosis in the intermuscular plane of the first commissure (*arrowheads*). *M1* first metacarpal, *M2* second metacarpal (Reprinted with permission from Freire V et al. *Radiology*. 2013;269(3))

cause pain and, potentially, septicemia [34]. Spreading redness and thick green/yellow discharge from a lesion are signs of infection and warrant antibiotic therapy. When cultured, the most frequent organism identified has been *Staphylococcus aureus* [34–36].

Treatment of Calcinosis

General Measures

Treatment of dystrophic calcification is a major clinical challenge. General measures to improve blood flow to the extremities, such as avoiding trauma, smoking, stress and cold exposure, are of crucial importance. Given its relation to hypoxia, medical treatment of Raynaud's phenomenon and digital ulcers may play a role in prevention and treatment of calcinosis. Supportive therapies such as antibiotics for infections, pain medications, and wound care are also key. An antibiotic should be prescribed if there is suspicion of superinfection of a calcinotic lesion with clinical features as described above. Appropriate empirical treatment is oral antibiotics with good coverage for *Streptococci* and *Staphylococci*, such as cephalexin, dicloxacillin, or clindamycin. If pain is present, acetaminophen and nonsteroidal anti-inflammatory agents can help; however narcotics may be necessary for adequate pain control. If calcinosis becomes ulcerated, hydrocolloid membranes such as DuoDerm may be useful.

Corticosteroid injections are well tolerated and palliative and may be effective in reducing secondary inflammation from calcinosis. In one published case of a patient with SSc and calcinosis, injection of the margins of the lesion with 20 mg/mL of triamcinolone acetonide suspension at 4- to 8-week intervals resulted in healing at 12 months [37].

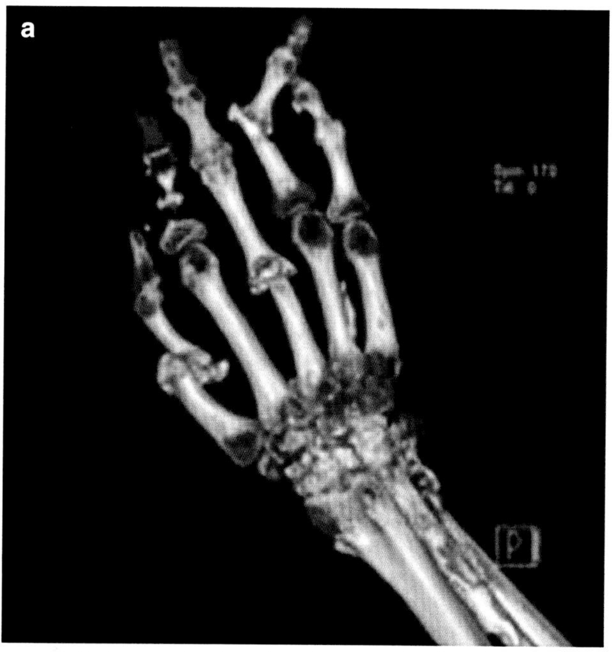

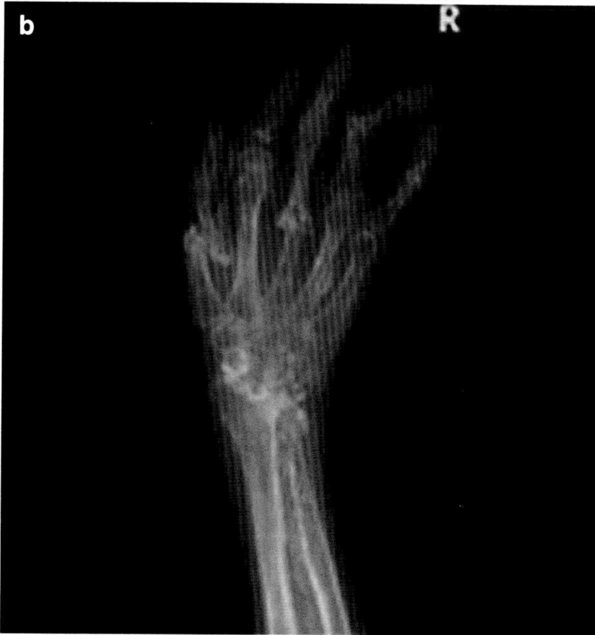

Fig. 32.6 Calcinosis in dual-energy computed tomography. Two views of the right hand with extensive calcinosis seen throughout the fingers and carpal bones and surrounding the remaining waist of the proximal second phalanx. (**a**) Dual-energy computed tomography. (**b**) Hand radiography (Reprinted with permission from Hsu V et al. *J Rheumatol*. 2015;42(2))

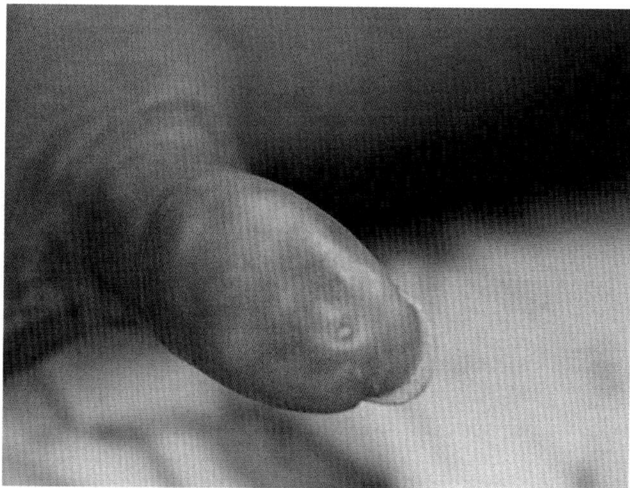

Fig. 32.7 Ulceration related to calcinosis. Calcium has come to the surface and is extruding from a small ulceration in the skin

Medical Therapies

Several pharmacologic therapies have been tried for the treatment of calcinosis, as monotherapy or in combination, with variable results (Table 32.2). None have received regulatory approval; since until recently, there have not been any validated outcome measures to study these agents in randomized clinical trials. In addition, clinical impact of these agents requires a prolonged observation period.

Warfarin

By antagonizing vitamin K, warfarin inhibits the production of gamma-carboxyglutamic acid, which has calcium-binding properties, and has been found to be increased in patients with calcinosis [52]. In a double-blind placebo-controlled study of seven patients with SSc or DM and evidence of substantial and multiple subcutaneous calcifications, three patients received warfarin 1 mg/day for 18 months, and four patients received placebo. Two patients in the treatment arm showed decreased extraskeletal uptake on a whole-body bone scintigraphy with injection of technetium 99 m-diphosphonate compared with none in the placebo arm [38]. Another case series of three patients with SSc found that two patients had complete resolution of their disseminated calcinosis evaluated at physical examination after 1 year of treatment with low-dose warfarin. The nonresponding patient had larger and longer-standing calcinosis [39]. However, conflicting data on the efficacy of warfarin for calcinosis has been published. Five of six patients with extensive and long-standing calcinosis (one with SSc) treated with low-dose warfarin for a mean of 14.6 months had clinical and radiological worsening of calcinosis [55]. In the Mayo Clinic study, of 19 patients with calcinosis and ACTD, four received warfarin for conditions other than calcinosis, without differences in response compared with the group that did not receive warfarin [25]. Although several studies suggest that warfarin may be effective for small calcified deposits [56], evidence supporting the use of warfarin in calcinosis is conflicting, and its use is not widely accepted.

Table 32.2 Pharmacologic therapies for calcinosis in systemic sclerosis

Drug	Suggested dosing	Proposed mechanism of action	Supportive evidence
Warfarin	1 mg/day PO	Antagonizes vitamin K, inhibiting the production of gamma-carboxyglutamic acid	Berger et al.[38] Cukierman et al.[39]
Bisphosphonate		Inhibits macrophage pro-inflammatory cytokine production and reduces calcium turnover	Rabens et al.[40] Fujii et al.[41]
Etidronate	10–20 mg/kg/day PO		
Risedronate	35 mg/week PO		
Diltiazem	240–480 mg/day PO	Alters intracellular calcium levels, lowering the ability for calcium nidus formation and crystallization	Palmieri et al.[42] Dolan et al.[43] Farah et al. [44]
Ceftriaxone	2 g/day for 20 days IV	Binds calcium ions and forms insoluble calcium complexes	Reiter et al.[45]
Colchicine	1 mg/day PO	Induces anti-inflammatory effects by inhibiting microtubule polymerization and disrupting leukocyte chemotaxis and phagocytosis	Fuchs et al.[46] Vereecken et al.[47]
Minocycline	50 or 100 mg/d PO in cyclic long-term use	Anti-inflammatory effect and calcium-binding properties	Robertson et al. [48]
Probenecid	Up to 500 mg three times daily PO	Increases renal phosphate clearance, decreasing the serum phosphate level and reducing the calcification process	Eddy et al.[49]
Aluminum hydroxide	30 ml four times daily PO	Decreases serum phosphate levels by decreasing intestinal absorption	Hudson et al. [50]
Infliximab	3 mg/kg at 0, 2, and 6 weeks, and every 8 weeks IV	Anti-inflammatory effect	Tosounidou et al.[51]
Rituximab	Four weekly infusions of 375 mg/m^2 each IV	Anti inflammatory effect	Daoussi et al.[52] De Paula et al.[53]
Intravenous immunoglobulin	2 g/day for 4 days IV	Anti-inflammatory effect, possibly related to suppression of activated macrophages	Schanz et al.[54]

PO oral, *IV* intravenous

Bisphosphonates

Bisphosphonates may be useful in reversing the calcification process by inhibiting macrophage pro-inflammatory cytokine production and reducing calcium turnover. As with warfarin, conflicting reports regarding the effect of bisphosphonates on calcinosis have been published. A report of six patients with dystrophic calcinosis associated with DM or SSc treated with etidronate for a mean of 10 months demonstrated little success and moreover showed that all three patients with SSc had clinical and radiological progression of calcinotic lesions [57]. However, another SSc patient with extensive calcinosis seen on clinical and radiological examination was treated with etidronate for 1 year and had functional improvement and partial regression of lesions [40]. A more recent case report described clinical and radiological resolution of calcinosis in one lcSSc patient after 6 months of treatment with risedronate for glucocorticoid-induced osteoporosis [41]. Given the paucity of evidence, the efficacy of bisphosphonates in calcinosis treatment remains unclear. In addition, studies using newer and/or intravenous forms of bisphosphonates have not yet been performed.

Diltiazem

This calcium channel blocker alters intracellular calcium levels, thereby lowering the ability for calcium nidus formation and crystallization. Numerous case studies have reported positive results with diltiazem from 240 to 480 mg/day for calcinosis in SSc patients [42–44]. In contrast, one larger retrospective study of 23 patients with SSc and calcinosis on x-ray treated with a lower dose of 180 mg/day of diltiazem showed only a slight regression of lesions in three patients that was not clinically significant [58].

Ceftriaxone

This third-generation cephalosporin is able to bind calcium ions and form insoluble calcium complexes [56]. There is one report of a patient with morphea and multiple calcinosis deposits who experienced significant regression of lesions and no new lesions with ceftriaxone (2 g/day) intravenously for 20 days [45].

Colchicine

Colchicine induces anti-inflammatory effects by inhibiting microtubule polymerization and hence disrupting leukocyte chemotaxis and phagocytosis. Since inflammation often accompanies calcinosis and may be involved in resultant ulceration, colchicine has been used for the treatment of these lesions, but only a few reports in patients with SSc have been published [2]. One patient with SSc and prepatellar calcinosis received 1 mg/day of oral colchicine and had regression of the associated local inflammation and healing of associated skin ulcers after 2 months of follow-up [46]. Another patient with linear scleroderma and ulcerated cutaneous calcinosis was treated with colchicine 1 mg/day, with healing of the ulcerations after 4 months [47].

Minocycline

This tetracycline antibiotic has anti-inflammatory and calcium-binding properties. Nine patients with SSc-associated calcinosis causing pain and/or ulceration were treated with 50 or 100 mg/d of minocycline for a mean of 3.5 years. Eight patients who were able to tolerate the therapy experienced reduction in ulceration and inflammation associated with calcinosis, with a modest decrease in the size of deposits assessed clinically and radiographically. Patients had recurrence of calcinosis when the treatment was stopped, so the authors recommended cyclic long-term use of minocycline (treatment for 4–8 weeks followed by discontinuation for 3–4 months) [48].

Probenecid

Probenecid increases renal phosphate clearance and therefore decreases the serum phosphate level, reducing the calcification process. Although not studied in SSc, one patient with JDM and extensive calcinosis who was treated with probenecid up to 500 mg three times daily showed clinical and radiographic improvement after 7 months [49].

Aluminum Hydroxide

Aluminum hydroxide also decreases serum phosphate levels by decreasing intestinal absorption. Aluminum hydroxide has been used successfully as a treatment for calcinosis in SLE and several DM patients, with softening and size reduction of calcinosis deposits [3,59]. One case report of treatment with aluminum hydroxide 30 ml four times daily for calcinosis has been published in an SSc patient, showing good response [50].

Antitumor Necrosis Factor-α Therapies

Given the potential role of inflammation and TNF-α in calcinosis, there may be a role for anti-TNF agents in the treatment of calcinotic lesions, particularly those with clinical evidence of associated inflammation. A patient with SSc-myositis overlap and refractory calcinosis was treated with infliximab 3 mg/kg infused at 0, 2, and 6 weeks and every 8 weeks thereafter. Calcinosis evolution was monitored with serial pelvic CT imaging at baseline, 7 and 41 months after infliximab was initiated. Imaging confirmed reduction in size of calcifications with no new deposits [51].

Rituximab

This chimeric anti-CD20 antibody may be another promising therapy to treat calcinosis in patients with SSc, although conflicting experiences have been published. One lcSSc patient with extensive, frequently ulcerating and painful calcinotic lesions was treated with two courses of rituximab (four weekly infusions of 375 mg/m^2 each) 18 months apart. Twelve months after the therapy was initiated, she experienced reduction in size of multiple lesions as assessed by physical examination, and her pain improved substantially [52]. Another recent case report of a female with lcSSc using the same regimen of rituximab to treat interstitial lung disease and arthritis showed complete resolution of calcinosis in her hands after 7 months of the first infusion [53]. In both cases, the effect of rituximab on calcinosis was rather unexpected, and authors did not suggest any specific mechanism of action other than its anti-inflammatory properties. In contrast, Hurabielle et al. reported the case of a female SSc patient with calcinosis on her right wrist, who received two infusions of rituximab (1 g each) at a 2-week interval and then every 6 months, for interstitial lung disease and arthritis. This patient experienced remarkable worsening of the number and size of calcifications revealed by x-ray [54].

Intravenous Immunoglobulins

The use of intravenous immunoglobulins (IVIGs) in the treatment of calcinosis is limited and has shown mixed results. Only one case report in SSc-associated calcinosis treated with IVIG has been published by Schanz et al. They reported that a patient with lcSSc and disabling calcinosis of the left index finger was free of symptoms after 5 months of IVIG [60]. The authors hypothesize that this effect was based on its anti-inflammatory properties, possibly related to suppression of activated macrophages. There is conflicting data on DM-associated calcinosis with positive [61] and negative [62] results.

Novel Therapies

Potential future medical therapies for calcinosis in SSc and other ACTD include more powerful vasodilatory therapies such as phosphodiesterase-5 inhibitors and prostacyclins. Preliminary observations in the Pulmonary Hypertension Assessment and Recognition of Outcomes in Scleroderma (PHAROS) registry have found that two patients with SSc-PAH and calcinosis treated with subcutaneous treprostinil for PAH simultaneously experienced approximately 50 % radiographic improvement in their calcinotic lesions after 6 months of therapy (Shapiro et al. unpublished data). Other anti-inflammatory and immunomodulatory agents such as calcineurin inhibitors, other anti-TNF agents, anakinra (IL-1 receptor inhibitor), or tocilizumab (monoclonal antibody to IL-6) may potentially have an effect on calcinosis. These treatments will need evaluation in prospective studies and randomized controlled trials.

Nonmedical Therapies

Carbon Dioxide Laser Vaporization

The carbon dioxide (CO) laser-tissue vaporization procedure is a bloodless technique that allows excellent visualization and vaporization of calcium deposits and has been used as an alternative to surgery. Bottomley et al. treated five patients with lcSSc and calcinosis and found that after a median follow-up time of 20 months after the procedures, three patients were pain-free, and two had partial relief of pain. However, two patients had recurrence within 3–4 months [63]. In a second case report, six affected digits in an lcSSc patient received a single treatment with CO laser vaporization, with complete healing after 6 weeks [64].

Extracorporeal Shock Wave Lithotripsy

Extracorporeal shock wave lithotripsy (ESWL) is a minimally invasive, safe, and well-tolerated technique that may offer effective remission of symptoms and healing of ulcerations related to calcinosis. Sparsa et al. described the case of an lcSSc patient with calcinosis and extensive secondary ulcerations that was successfully treated by ESWL [65]. One prospective study of nine patients (three with SSc) with progressive calcinosis found that after three ESWL sessions at 3-week intervals, there was a reduction in the median area of calcinosis from 3.1 to 1.9 cm^2. In addition, visual analog scale pain scores (range 0–10) decreased from 7 to 2 after 6 months [66].

Surgical Excision

Despite potential risks and frequent recurrence, surgical excision of calcium deposits can be helpful in reducing pain and disability associated with calcinosis, with improvement soon after the procedure is performed. Surgery is reserved for localized or large lesions, with success in the majority of cases, and partial response in almost all. In the Mayo Clinic study of ACTD patients with calcinosis, all 11 patients who underwent surgical excision alone responded (eight with complete response), as well as 16 out of 17 patients who received medical and surgical therapy (14 with complete response). In contrast, only 7 of 19 patients treated with medical therapy alone had any response (one with complete response) [25].

Potential risks of surgical excision are slow wound healing, which may lead to skin necrosis, infection, and decreased range of motion [67,68]. Other less-invasive surgical approaches have been attempted to decrease complications. A retrospective study of nine SSc patients who underwent a debulking procedure using a high-speed micro-burr to soften calcinosis affecting the digits showed a high degree of patient satisfaction and lower disabilities scores (measured by the Disabilities of the Arm, Shoulder, and Hand Questionnaire and the Michigan Hand Questionnaire). However, no patients reported complete resolution of calcinosis, and seven patients had recurrence [69]. Saddic et al. proposed curettage as a less-invasive, potential procedure for treatment of localized painful fingertip lesions. They reported excellent clinical outcomes, including decreased pain and short healing times, in one patient with lcSSc who underwent curettage of calcinosis on the tip of his left third finger [70].

Conclusions

Calcinosis is a common problem affecting almost one quarter of patients with SSc. It most commonly affects the hands, particularly the fingers, and is related to trauma and hypoxia. Common and potentially debilitating complications include pain, local inflammation, ulceration, and infection. Surgery remains the mainstay for the treatment of calcinosis, but a combination of medical and surgical therapies may yield the best outcomes. Randomized controlled trials using novel outcome measures are necessary to test the efficacy of future treatments.

References

1. Chander S, Gordon P. Soft tissue and subcutaneous calcification in connective tissue diseases. Curr Opin Rheumatol. 2012;24(2):158–64. Epub 2012/01/10. eng.
2. Gutierrez Jr A, Wetter DA. Calcinosis cutis in autoimmune connective tissue diseases. Dermatol Ther. 2012;25(2):195–206. Epub 2012/06/30. eng.
3. Boulman N, Slobodin G, Rozenbaum M, Rosner I. Calcinosis in rheumatic diseases. Semin Arthritis Rheum. 2005;34(6):805–12. Epub 2005/06/09. eng.
4. Reiter N, El-Shabrawi L, Leinweber B, Berghold A, Aberer E. Calcinosis cutis: part I. Diagnostic pathway. J Am Acad Dermatol. 2011;65(1):1–12; quiz 3–4. Epub 2011/06/18. eng.
5. Walsh JS, Fairley JA. Calcifying disorders of the skin. J Am Acad Dermatol. 1995;33(5 Pt 1):693–706; quiz 7–10. Epub 1995/11/01. eng.
6. Wilmer WA, Magro CM. Calciphylaxis: emerging concepts in prevention, diagnosis, and treatment. Semin Dial. 2002;15(3):172–86. Epub 2002/07/09. eng.
7. Budisavljevic MN, Cheek D, Ploth DW. Calciphylaxis in chronic renal failure. J Am Soc Nephrol JASN. 1996;7(7):978–82. Epub 1996/07/01. eng.
8. Khafif RA, DeLima C, Silverberg A, Frankel R. Calciphylaxis and systemic calcinosis. Collective review. Arch Intern Med. 1990;150(5):956–9. Epub 1990/05/01. eng.
9. Valenzuela A, Cuomo G, Sutton E, Gordon J, Spiera R, Rodriguez-Reyna T, et al. Frequency of calcinosis in a multi-center international cohort of patients with systemic sclerosis: a Scleroderma Clinical Trials Consortium Study (abstract). 13th international workshop on scleroderma research, August 2013, Boston, 2013.

10. Valenzuela A, Baron M, the Canadian Scleroderma Research Group, Herrick A, Proudman S, Stevens W, the Australian Scleroderma Interest Group, Rodriguez-Reyna T, Vacca A, Medsger TA, Fiorentino D, Chung L. Calcinosis is associated with digital ulcers and osteoporosis in patients with Systemic Sclerosis: A Scleroderma Clinical Trials Consortium Study. Accepted for publication in Seminars in Arthritis and Rheumatism.
11. Avouac J, Mogavero G, Guerini H, Drape JL, Mathieu A, Kahan A, et al. Predictive factors of hand radiographic lesions in systemic sclerosis: a prospective study. Ann Rheum Dis. 2011;70(4):630–3. Epub 2010/12/07. eng.
12. Koutaissoff S, Vanthuyne M, Smith V, De Langhe E, Depresseux G, Westhovens R, et al. Hand radiological damage in systemic sclerosis: comparison with a control group and clinical and functional correlations. Semin Arthritis Rheum. 2011;40(5):455–60. Epub 2010/09/25. eng.
13. Valenzuela A, Chung L, Casciola-Rosen L, Fiorentino D. Identification of clinical features and autoantibodies associated with calcinosis in dermatomyositis. JAMA Dermatol. 2014;150(7): 724–9. Epub 2014/05/30. eng.
14. Johnstone EM, Hutchinson CE, Vail A, Chevance A, Herrick AL. Acro-osteolysis in systemic sclerosis is associated with digital ischaemia and severe calcinosis. Rheumatology (Oxford). 2012;51(12):2234–8. Epub 2012/08/28. eng.
15. Steen VD, Ziegler GL, Rodnan GP, Medsger Jr TA. Clinical and laboratory associations of anticentromere antibody in patients with progressive systemic sclerosis. Arthritis Rheum. 1984;27(2):125–31. Epub 1984/02/01. eng.
16. D'Aoust J, Hudson M, Tatibouet S, Wick J, Mahler M, Baron M, et al. Clinical and serologic correlates of anti-PM/Scl antibodies in systemic sclerosis: a multicenter study of 763 patients. Arthritis Rheumatol (Hoboken NJ). 2014;66(6):1608–15. Epub 2014/03/01. eng.
17. Davies CA, Jeziorska M, Freemont AJ, Herrick AL. The differential expression of VEGF, VEGFR-2, and GLUT-1 proteins in disease subtypes of systemic sclerosis. Hum Pathol. 2006;37(2):190–7. Epub 2006/01/24. eng.
18. Davies CA, Herrick AL, Cordingley L, Freemont AJ, Jeziorska M. Expression of advanced glycation end products and their receptor in skin from patients with systemic sclerosis with and without calcinosis. Rheumatology (Oxford). 2009;48(8):876–82. Epub 2009/06/23. eng.
19. Mukamel M, Horev G, Mimouni M. New insight into calcinosis of juvenile dermatomyositis: a study of composition and treatment. J Pediatr. 2001;138(5):763–6. Epub 2001/05/09. eng.
20. Nitsche A. Raynaud, digital ulcers and calcinosis in scleroderma. Reumatol Clin. 2012;8(5):270–7. Epub 2012/07/28. eng.
21. Touart DM, Sau P. Cutaneous deposition diseases. Part II. J Am Acad Dermatol. 1998;39(4 Pt 1):527–44; quiz 45–6. Epub 1998/10/20. eng.
22. Lian JB, Skinner M, Glimcher MJ, Gallop P. The presence of gamma-carboxyglutamic acid in the proteins associated with ectopic calcification. Biochem Biophys Res Commun. 1976;73(2):349–55. Epub 1976/11/22. eng.
23. Lian JB, Pachman LM, Gundberg CM, Partridge RE, Maryjowski MC. Gamma-carboxyglutamate excretion and calcinosis in juvenile dermatomyositis. Arthritis Rheum. 1982;25(9):1094–100. Epub 1982/09/01. eng.
24. Ngo S, Vandhuick T, Janvresse A, Levesque H, Marie I. Pseudotumoral calcinosis. La Revue de medecine interne/fondee par la Societe nationale francaise de medecine interne. 2011;32(4):251–2. Epub 2010/10/05. Des calcifications pseudotumorales. fre.
25. Balin SJ, Wetter DA, Andersen LK, Davis MD. Calcinosis cutis occurring in association with autoimmune connective tissue disease: the Mayo Clinic experience with 78 patients, 1996–2009. Arch Dermatol. 2012;148(4):455–62. Epub 2011/12/21. eng.
26. Sari-Kouzel H, Hutchinson CE, Middleton A, Webb F, Moore T, Griffin K, et al. Foot problems in patients with systemic sclerosis. Rheumatology (Oxford). 2001;40(4):410–3. Epub 2001/04/20. eng.
27. Shahi V, Wetter DA, Howe BM, Ringler MD, Davis MD. Plain radiography is effective for the detection of calcinosis cutis occurring in association with autoimmune connective tissue disease. Br J Dermatol. 2014;170(5):1073–9. Epub 2013/12/18. eng.
28. Madani G, Katz RD, Haddock JA, Denton CP, Bell JR. The role of radiology in the management of systemic sclerosis. Clin Radiol. 2008;63(9):959–67. Epub 2008/08/23. eng.
29. Chung L, Valenzuela A, Fiorentino D, Stevens K, Li S, Harris J, et al. Validation of a novel radiographic scoring system for calcinosis affecting the hands of patients with systemic sclerosis. Arthritis care & research. 2015 Mar;67(3):425–30.
30. Freire V, Becce F, Feydy A, Guerini H, Campagna R, Allanore Y, et al. MDCT imaging of calcinosis in systemic sclerosis. Clin Radiol. 2013;68(3):302–9. Epub 2012/09/11. eng.
31. Elhai M, Guerini H, Bazeli R, Avouac J, Freire V, Drape JL, et al. Ultrasonographic hand features in systemic sclerosis and correlates with clinical, biologic, and radiographic findings. Arthritis Care Res. 2012;64(8):1244–9. Epub 2012/03/17. eng.
32. Freire V, Bazeli R, Elhai M, Campagna R, Pessis E, Avouac J, et al. Hand and wrist involvement in systemic sclerosis: US features. Radiology. 2013;269(3):824–30. Epub 2013/09/07. eng.
33. Hsu V, Bramwit M, Schlesinger N. Dual-energy computed tomography for the evaluation of calcinosis in systemic sclerosis. J Rheumatol. 2015;42(2):345–6. Epub 2015/02/03. eng.
34. Hughes M, Freemont TJ, Denton J, Herrick AL. Infected calcinosis of the knee in limited cutaneous systemic sclerosis. J Rheumatol. 2012;39(10):2043–4. Epub 2012/10/03. eng.
35. Pando J, Nashel DJ. Clinical images: progressive calcifications and draining lesions following staphylococcal infection in a patient with limited scleroderma. Arthritis Rheum. 1998;41(2):373. Epub 1998/03/04. eng.
36. Bussone G, Berezne A, Mouthon L. Infectious complications of systemic sclerosis. Presse Medicale (Paris, France: 1983). 2009;38(2):291–302. Epub 2008/12/09. Complications infectieuses de la sclerodermie systemique. fre.
37. Hazen PG, Walker AE, Carney JF, Stewart JJ. Cutaneous calcinosis of scleroderma. Successful treatment with intralesional adrenal steroids. Arch Dermatol. 1982;118(5):366–7. Epub 1982/05/01. eng.
38. Berger RG, Featherstone GL, Raasch RH, McCartney WH, Hadler NM. Treatment of calcinosis universalis with low-dose warfarin. Am J Med. 1987;83(1):72–6. Epub 1987/07/01. eng.
39. Cukierman T, Elinav E, Korem M, Chajek-Shaul T. Low dose warfarin treatment for calcinosis in patients with systemic sclerosis. Ann Rheum Dis. 2004;63(10):1341–3. Pubmed Central PMCID: PMC1754769, Epub 2004/09/14. eng.
40. Rabens SF, Bethune JE. Disodium etidronate therapy for dystrophic cutaneous calcification. Arch Dermatol. 1975;111(3):357–61. Epub 1975/03/01. eng.
41. Fujii N, Hamano T, Isaka Y, Ito T, Imai E. [Risedronate: a possible treatment for extraosseous calcification]. Clin Calcium. 2005;15 Suppl 1:75–8; discussion 8–9. Epub 2005/11/08. jpn.
42. Palmieri GM, Sebes JI, Aelion JA, Moinuddin M, Ray MW, Wood GC, et al. Treatment of calcinosis with diltiazem. Arthritis Rheum. 1995;38(11):1646–54. Epub 1995/11/01. eng.
43. Dolan AL, Kassimos D, Gibson T, Kingsley GH. Diltiazem induces remission of calcinosis in scleroderma. Br J Rheumatol. 1995;34(6):576–8. Epub 1995/06/01. eng.
44. Farah MJ, Palmieri GM, Sebes JI, Cremer MA, Massie JD, Pinals RS. The effect of diltiazem on calcinosis in a patient with the CREST syndrome. Arthritis Rheum. 1990;33(8):1287–93. Epub 1990/08/01. eng.

45. Reiter N, El-Shabrawi L, Leinweber B, Aberer E. Subcutaneous morphea with dystrophic calcification with response to ceftriaxone treatment. J Am Acad Dermatol. 2010;63(2):e53–5. Epub 2010/07/17. eng.
46. Fuchs D, Fruchter L, Fishel B, Holtzman M, Yaron M. Colchicine suppression of local inflammation due to calcinosis in dermatomyositis and progressive systemic sclerosis. Clin Rheumatol. 1986;5(4):527–30. Epub 1986/12/01. eng.
47. Vereecken P, Stallenberg B, Tas S, de Dobbeleer G, Heenen M. Ulcerated dystrophic calcinosis cutis secondary to localised linear scleroderma. Int J Clin Pract. 1998;52(8):593–4. Epub 2000/01/06. eng.
48. Robertson LP, Marshall RW, Hickling P. Treatment of cutaneous calcinosis in limited systemic sclerosis with minocycline. Ann Rheum Dis. 2003;62(3):267–9. Pubmed Central PMCID: PMC1754479, Epub 2003/02/21. eng.
49. Eddy MC, Leelawattana R, McAlister WH, Whyte MP. Calcinosis universalis complicating juvenile dermatomyositis: resolution during probenecid therapy. J Clin Endocrinol Metab. 1997;82(11):3536–42. Epub 1997/11/14. eng.
50. Hudson PM, Jones PE, Robinson TW, Dent CE. Extensive calcinosis with minimal scleroderma: treatment of ectopic calcification with aluminum hydroxide. Proc R Soc Med. 1974;67(11):1166–8. Pubmed Central PMCID: PMC1645999, Epub 1974/11/01. eng.
51. Tosounidou S, MacDonald H, Situnayake D. Successful treatment of calcinosis with infliximab in a patient with systemic sclerosis/myositis overlap syndrome. Rheumatology (Oxford). 2014;53(5):960–1. Epub 2013/11/21. eng.
52. Daoussis D, Antonopoulos I, Liossis SN, Yiannopoulos G, Andonopoulos AP. Treatment of systemic sclerosis-associated calcinosis: a case report of rituximab-induced regression of CREST-related calcinosis and review of the literature. Semin Arthritis Rheum. 2012;41(6):822–9. Epub 2012/01/10. eng.
53. de Paula DR, Klem FB, Lorencetti PG, Muller C, Azevedo VF. Rituximab-induced regression of CREST-related calcinosis. Clin Rheumatol. 2013;32(2):281–3. Epub 2012/11/28. eng.
54. Hurabielle C, Allanore Y, Kahan A, Avouac J. Flare of calcinosis despite rituximab therapy. Semin Arthritis Rheum. 2014;44(2):e5–6. Epub 2014/05/21. eng.
55. Lassoued K, Saiag P, Anglade MC, Roujeau JC, Touraine RL. Failure of warfarin in treatment of calcinosis universalis. Am J Med. 1988;84(4):795–6. Epub 1988/04/01. eng.
56. Reiter N, El-Shabrawi L, Leinweber B, Berghold A, Aberer E. Calcinosis cutis: part II. Treatment options. J Am Acad Dermatol. 2011;65(1):15–22; quiz 3–4. Epub 2011/06/18. eng.
57. Metzger AL, Singer FR, Bluestone R, Pearson CM. Failure of disodium etidronate in calcinosis due to dermatomyositis and scleroderma. N Engl J Med. 1974;291(24):1294–6. Epub 1974/12/12. eng.
58. Vayssairat M, Hidouche D, Abdoucheli-Baudot N, Gaitz JP. Clinical significance of subcutaneous calcinosis in patients with systemic sclerosis. Does diltiazem induce its regression? Ann Rheum Dis. 1998;57(4):252–4. Pubmed Central PMCID: PMC1752566, Epub 1998/08/26. eng.
59. Park YM, Lee SJ, Kang H, Cho SH. Large subcutaneous calcification in systemic lupus erythematosus: treatment with oral aluminum hydroxide administration followed by surgical excision. J Korean Med Sci. 1999;14(5):589–92. Pubmed Central PMCID: PMC3054452, Epub 1999/11/27. eng.
60. Schanz S, Ulmer A, Fierlbeck G. Response of dystrophic calcification to intravenous immunoglobulin. Arch Dermatol. 2008;144(5):585–7. Epub 2008/05/21. eng.
61. Penate Y, Guillermo N, Melwani P, Martel R, Hernandez-Machin B, Borrego L. Calcinosis cutis associated with amyopathic dermatomyositis: response to intravenous immunoglobulin. J Am Acad Dermatol. 2009;60(6):1076–7. Epub 2009/05/27. eng.
62. Kalajian AH, Perryman JH, Callen JP. Intravenous immunoglobulin therapy for dystrophic calcinosis cutis: unreliable in our hands. Arch Dermatol. 2009;145(3):334; author reply 5. Epub 2009/03/18. eng.
63. Bottomley WW, Goodfield MJ, Sheehan-Dare RA. Digital calcification in systemic sclerosis: effective treatment with good tissue preservation using the carbon dioxide laser. Br J Dermatol. 1996;135(2):302–4. Epub 1996/08/01. eng.
64. Chamberlain AJ, Walker NP. Successful palliation and significant remission of cutaneous calcinosis in CREST syndrome with carbon dioxide laser. Dermatol Surg Off Publ Am Society Dermatol Surg [et al]. 2003;29(9):968–70. Epub 2003/08/22. eng.
65. Sparsa A, Lesaux N, Kessler E, Bonnetblanc JM, Blaise S, Lebrun-Ly V, et al. Treatment of cutaneous calcinosis in CREST syndrome by extracorporeal shock wave lithotripsy. J Am Acad Dermatol. 2005;53(5 Suppl 1):S263–5. Epub 2005/10/18. eng.
66. Sultan-Bichat N, Menard J, Perceau G, Staerman F, Bernard P, Reguiai Z. Treatment of calcinosis cutis by extracorporeal shock-wave lithotripsy. J Am Acad Dermatol. 2012;66(3):424–9. Epub 2011/07/13. eng.
67. Bogoch ER, Gross DK. Surgery of the hand in patients with systemic sclerosis: outcomes and considerations. J Rheumatol. 2005;32(4):642 8. Epub 2005/04/01. eng.
68. Yang JH, Kim JW, Park HS, Jang SJ, Choi JC. Calcinosis cutis of the fingertip associated with Raynaud's phenomenon. J Dermatol. 2006;33(12):884–6. Epub 2006/12/16. eng.
69. Lapner MA, Goetz TJ. High-speed burr debulking of digital calcinosis cutis in scleroderma patients. J Hand Surg. 2014;39(3):503–10. Epub 2014/02/25. eng.
70. Saddic N, Miller JJ, Miller 3rd OF, Clarke JT. Surgical debridement of painful fingertip calcinosis cutis in CREST syndrome. Arch Dermatol. 2009;145(2):212–3. Epub 2009/02/18. eng.

Evaluation and Management of Skin Disease

33

Noëlle S. Sherber and Fredrick M. Wigley

The term "scleroderma" originates from the Greek "sklerosis," meaning hardness, and "derma," meaning skin. The skin hardening in diffuse, limited, and localized forms of scleroderma is the most clinically evident aspect of the disease and creates significant functional and emotional challenges for patients. The dermal fibrosis that causes hardening of the skin in these diseases is also associated with distressing disfigurement, dyspigmentation, and dysregulation of normal skin functions such as sweating and oil production. The sclerotic areas of skin can develop ulcerations, infection, or calcifications that can lead to significant morbidity.

Physicians use the skin findings in scleroderma as key determinants of diagnosis, as classification of patients into diffuse, limited, and localized scleroderma is largely based on the dermatologic exam. While details of categorization of patients into these disease subsets, the pathogenesis of skin fibrosis, Raynaud's phenomenon and skin ulcerations, nail fold microscopy, and the use of systemic disease modifying drugs are discussed elsewhere in this book, this chapter will review details on skin-directed evaluation and management with the focus on clinical manifestations and options for topical therapies [1].

Localized Scleroderma

Localized scleroderma occurs as focal cutaneous fibrosis without systemic disease. It is discussed in detail elsewhere in this text. Disease involvement is classified by the morphology and distribution of skin fibrosis into unilesional morphea, generalized morphea (several lesions), linear morphea, linear scleroderma (affecting deeper subcutaneous structures than linear morphea), keloidal morphea, bullous morphea, and rare cases of pansclerotic morphea and deep morphea (involving the fasciae). Indurated plaques of morphea typically have geographic morphology with a lilac-hued advancing edge of violaceous erythema that represents active inflammation. The inflamed areas tend to resolve after several months to years, leaving a sclerotic plaque with associated postinflammatory pigmentary changes. The rare variant of localized scleroderma, pansclerotic morphea, can present with plaques on nearly any skin surface, mimicking the cutaneous fibrosis of systemic sclerosis. Pansclerotic morphea can also present with a pattern of fibrosis unique to this condition that involves the upper "v" of the chest and the torso with axillary sparing that has been described as "the tank top sign" (Fig. 33.1) [2].

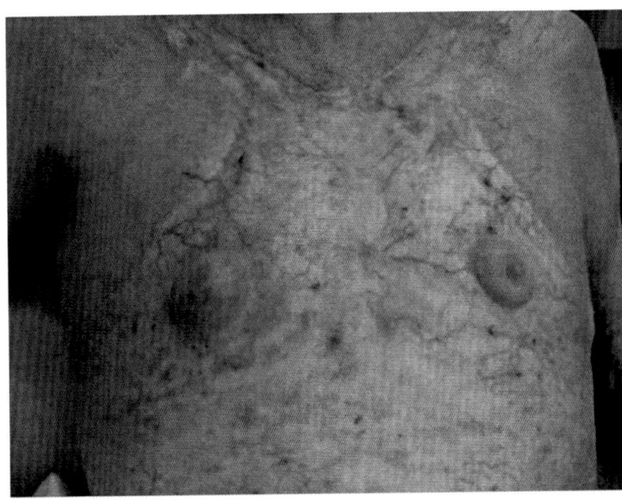

Fig. 33.1 The "tank top sign" in pansclerotic morphea (Courtesy of F.M. Wigley)

N.S. Sherber, MD
Scleroderma Center, Johns Hopkins Hospital, Baltimore, MD, USA

F.M. Wigley, MD (✉)
Department of Medicine/Rheumatology, The Johns Hopkins University School of Medicine, Baltimore, MD, USA
e-mail: fwig@jhmi.edu

J. Varga et al. (eds.), *Scleroderma*, DOI 10.1007/978-3-319-31407-5_33

Limited Scleroderma

In limited scleroderma, the skin thickening does not extend proximal to the elbows or knees. The most common subset of these patients has only face and finger involvement. Cutaneous features of limited scleroderma include numerous telangiectasias and an increased tendency to develop subcutaneous calcinosis. The CREST syndrome is considered by some to be a subtype of limited scleroderma. Other subtype limited scleroderma into patients with no skin disease (systemic sclerosis sine scleroderma), type 1 (scleroderma limited to face and fingers), and type 2 (scleroderma extending above the fingers and toes but not above the elbows or knees and not involving the trunk). Patients with limited skin disease rarely transition into diffuse skin disease, and skin changes are generally constant for a lifetime.

Diffuse Scleroderma

In diffuse scleroderma, fibrosis is widespread; although it is often most pronounced in the distal extremities, it has several characteristic features. The degree of involvement can vary among patients, and it can change in severity and distribution with time in an individual patient. Typically, diffuse skin disease is distributed over the fingers, hands, arms and legs, face, low back, and flanks, with sparing of the mid-back. The typical course is for skin changes to begin in the fingers and face and to progress to involve the hands and forearms over weeks to months.

The earliest manifestation of diffuse skin disease is an active inflammatory phase in which there is pronounced non-pitting edema of the affected areas that progresses to erythematous warm induration (Fig. 33.2) Dramatic edema of the lower legs can mimic fluid overload, and often this phase is confused with other causes of tissue edema, or with inflammatory skin diseases. The edema can cause local tissue compression. For example, in the wrist area, the patient is often diagnosed with carpal tunnel syndrome to explain hand and wrist discomfort. In association with the erythema, pruritus or pain can be pronounced as a result of inflammation. The pain often resembles the discomfort of sunburned skin, with tenderness and occasional "pricking" sensations. For some, it can even be similar to neuropathic pain with a "pins and needles" feeling. The disease process leads to loss of skin appendages including decreased hair growth and loss of sweat glands and exocrine glands; thus skin surface becomes dry and uncomfortable.

On the face, fibrosis of the perioral skin and mucous membranes leads to vertical rhytids (Fig. 33.3), loss of the vermillion border of the lip (Fig. 33.4), recession of the gums, pinching of the nose, and diminished oral aperture (Fig. 33.5). On the neck, a palpable horizontal furrow over the platysma on head extension, termed the scleroderma neck sign, can be observed (Fig. 33.6) [3].

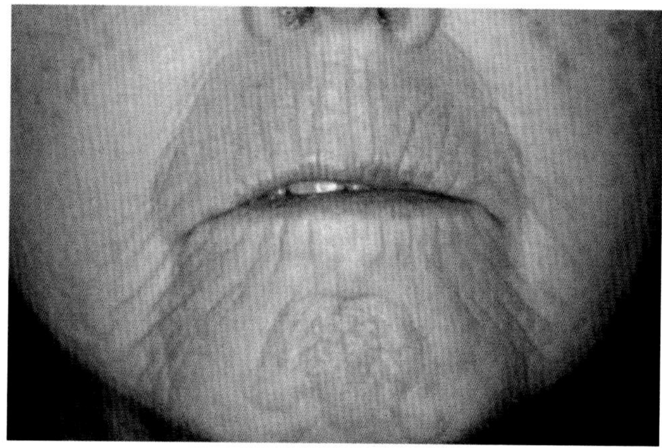

Fig. 33.3 Pronounced vertical perioral rhytids in diffuse scleroderma (Courtesy of F.M. Wigley)

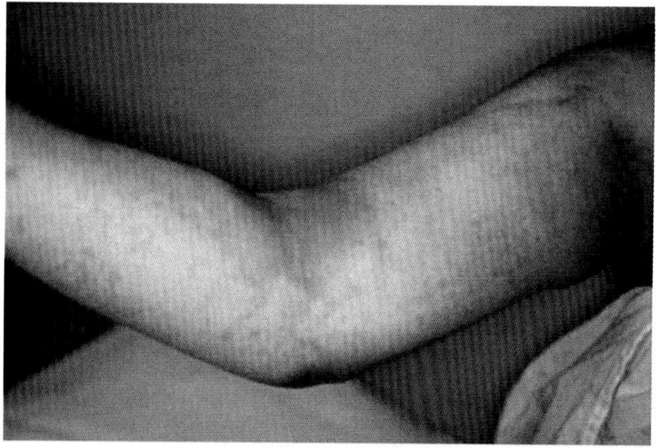

Fig. 33.2 Early active inflammatory phase of diffuse scleroderma with erythema and edema (F.M. Wigley)

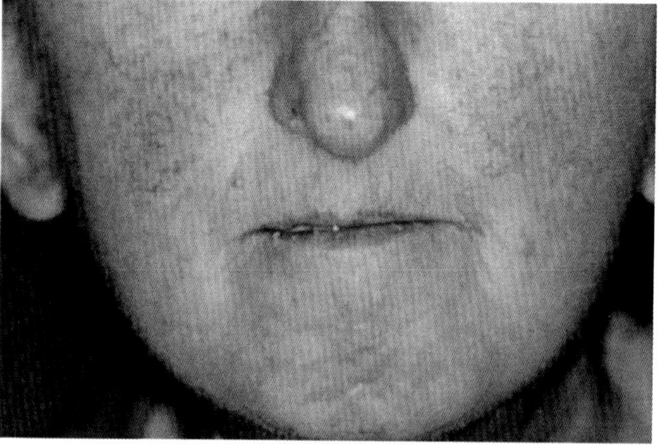

Fig. 33.4 Loss of vermillion border of the lip in diffuse scleroderma (Courtesy of F.M. Wigley)

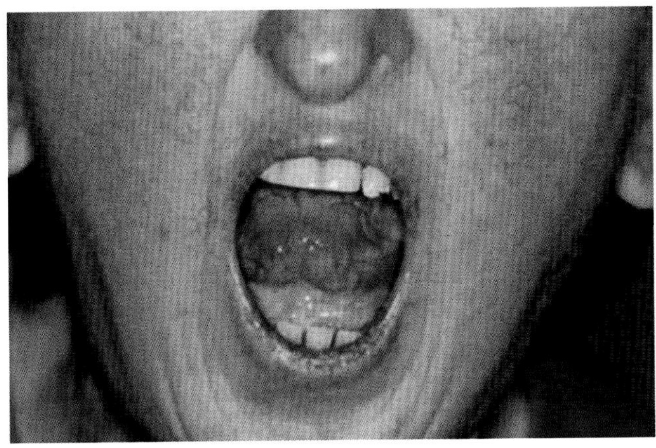

Fig. 33.5 Diminished oral aperture in diffuse scleroderma (Courtesy of F.M. Wigley)

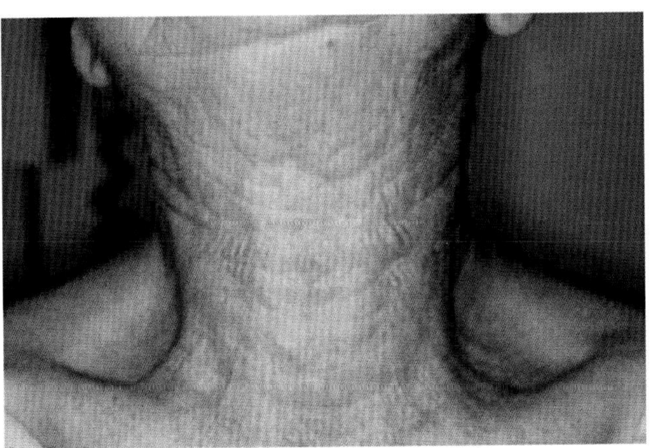

Fig. 33.6 Scleroderma neck sign (Courtesy of F.M. Wigley)

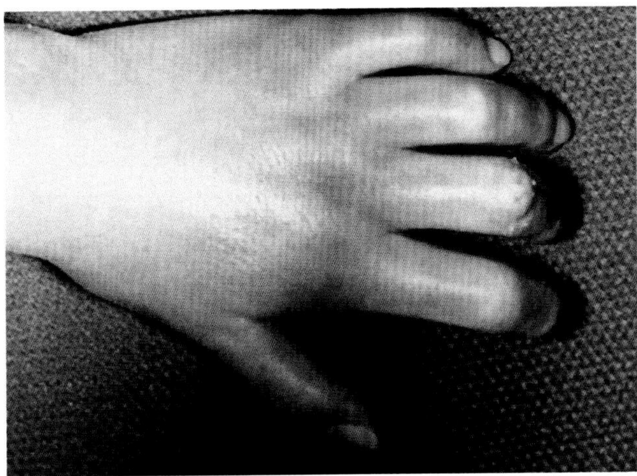

Fig. 33.7 Shiny appearance of epidermal atrophy and dermal fibrosis in diffuse scleroderma (Courtesy of F.M. Wigley)

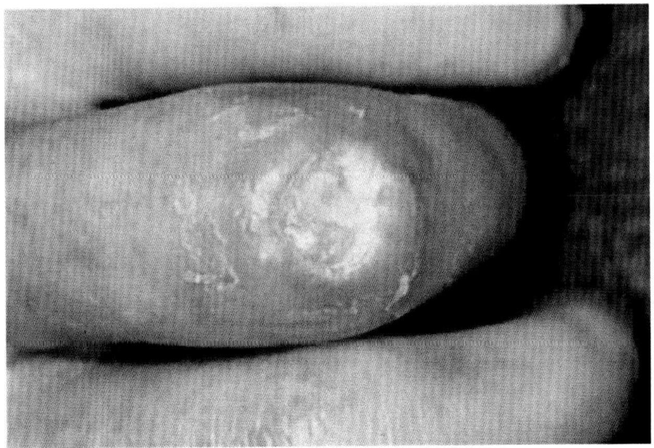

Fig. 33.8 Traumatic ulceration in a finger with sclerodactyly (Courtesy of F.M. Wigley)

Ankle and foot involvement usually begin soon after the finger changes, and then extend from the ankle to the proximal leg. The skin changes of the chest, abdomen, and lower flanks are often less intense and may not be noticed by the patient. The edematous phase continues for several weeks but eventually gives way to a fibrotic stage, with continued activity that may last months or years. As the inflammatory phase resolves, the erythema subsides and the skin becomes inflexible. Dermal fibrosis is accompanied by epidermal atrophy in late-stage disease, giving the skin a shiny appearance (Fig. 33.7). During the fibrotic phase, acute inflammation is clinically less obvious, but excessive collagen and other extracellular material produced in the dermis thickens the skin. Fibrosis extends beyond the dermis into the subcutaneous layers with loss of subcutaneous adipose tissue (lipodystrophy). The eventual loss of subcutaneous fat and deeper tissue fibrosis causes joint contractures and loss of function in the fingers, wrists, elbows, ankles, and larger joints. This combination of deep induration and superficial atrophy predisposes the skin to fragility and breakdown, and ulcerations may appear at sites of contractures (Fig. 33.8). This is especially true at the proximal interphalangeal joints, the metacarpophalangeal joints of the fingers, and the extensor surface of the elbows. Skin fibrosis is associated with microvascular disease and skin hypoperfusion with tissue hypoxia, particularly in the distal limbs and digits, which may potentiate progressive fibrosis [4]. The attenuated blood flow to the skin and the tissue fibrosis leads to ischemic changes that include a tendency for traumatic and ischemic ulcerations, fissures, and subcutaneous calcifications.

Fibrosis will often demarcate with intense thickening over the forearm with relative sparing of the antecubital fossa. Similarly, there is sparing of the axillary region and upper pectoral area of the chest compared to the central chest over the sternum. Relative sparing of the skin of the areolas is also seen. Cobblestoning of the skin (small monomorphic firm dome-shaped papules against a background of fibrotic skin) may represent lesions of prurigo nodularis from scratching, although the resemblance to elephantiasis nostra seen in lymphedema suggests that lymphatic obstruction may play a role. Cobblestoning is more commonly seen on the distal upper limbs in particular (Fig. 33.9). In the late stages of disease, skin atrophies and takes on a non-inflammatory bound-down appearance. Hypopigmentation (vitiligo-like) and hyperpigmentation of the skin ("salt-and-pepper" appearance) are typical especially on the face, arms, and trunk. A general tanning of the skin can also be seen even without sun exposure.

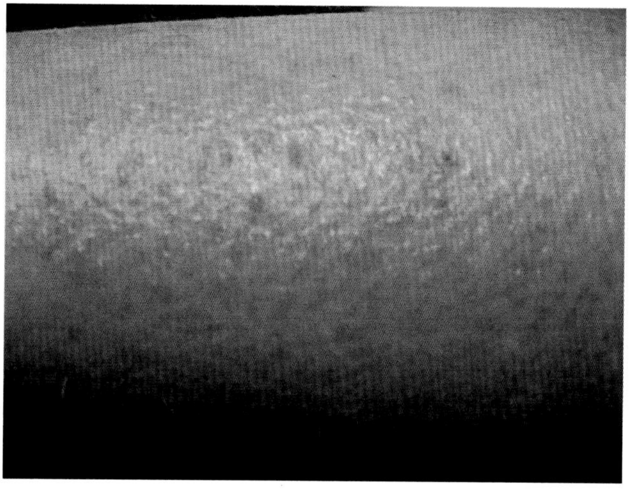

Fig. 33.9 Cobblestoning of the forearm in diffuse scleroderma (Courtesy of F.M. Wigley)

The degree of skin fibrosis in diffuse scleroderma is commonly quantified using the validated modified Rodnan skin score (MRSS) (Fig. 33.10) [5]. In the MRSS, the skin is pinched in 17 standardized areas (fingers, hands, forearms, arms, feet, legs, thighs, face, chest, and abdomen) and is scored on a scale of 0–3, where 0 is no thickening, 1 is mild thickening, 2 is moderate thickening, and 3 is severe thickening. The total MRSS can thus range from 1 to 51.

While the MRSS is an excellent method to score the severity or extent of skin disease, it does not capture a patient's current level of disease activity or inactivity. Change in MRSS over serial observations is used to define disease course and response of the skin to therapy. The natural history of the MRSS, as it would appear through studies tracking it longitudinally, is to increase for the 1–3 years following onset of disease, and then not to change for weeks to months, followed by a general tendency to decrease slowly. During this recovery phase, new robust hair growth is seen, particularly on the forearms, and itching and pain disappear, consistent with spontaneous resolution of inflammatory disease activity. The pace of MRSS decline generally seems to accelerate over time [6]. However, a flare of skin disease can occur after a period of resolution. Proximal areas of the body can return to normal texture over some extended time, but similar resolution of the more intensely affected skin of the fingers and distal limbs is unlikely. While skin texture can resolve, changes in skin pigmentation often persist.

Modified Rodnan Skin Score (MRSS)

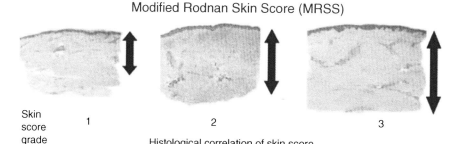

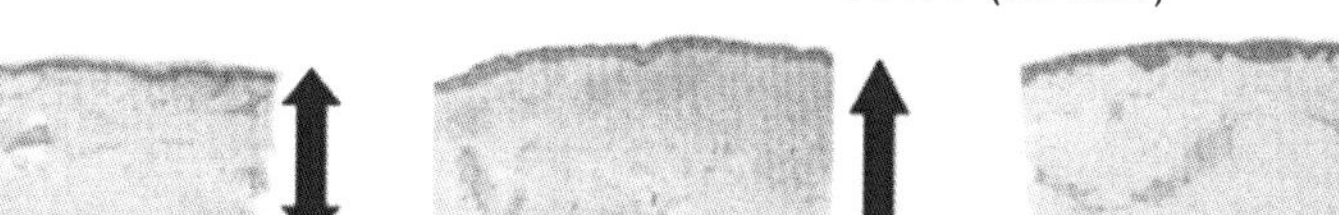

Skin score grade 1 2 3

Histological correlation of skin score

Low power full thickness biopsies taken from dcSSc skin sites with different skin score grades. Original magnification x2.5. H & E stain.

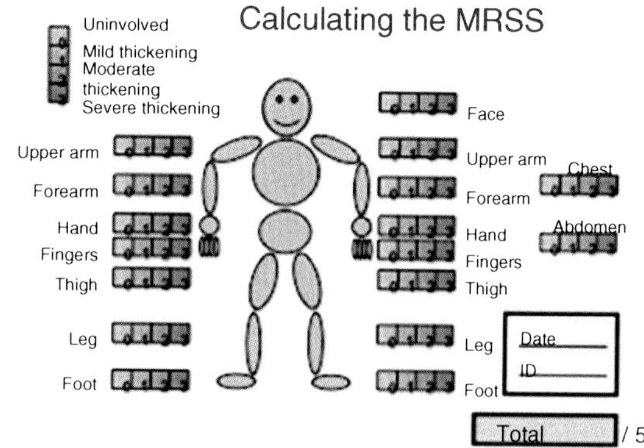

Fig. 33.10 Modified Rodnan skin score. Each area is scored from *0* = normal, *1* = mild thickening, *2* = moderate thickening, and *3* = severe thickening. Score 17 areas for maximum score of 51

Table 33.1 Clinical questions to help determine the level of skin disease activity

Have you noticed any new areas of skin thickening?				
☐ Yes ☐ No				
Then each of the following five questions is scored to help define changes in scleroderma skin disease:				
☐	☐	☐	☐	☐
A lot	A little	Same	A little	A lot
Better	Better		Worse	Worse
Global assessment: Is the skin disease overall better, the same, or worse?				
Pain: Is your pain better, the same, or worse?				
Itching: Is the itching in the skin better, the same, or worse?				
Softening: Is your skin softer in some areas, the same, or harder (worse)?				
Flexibility: Is your body more flexible (e.g., arms, hands) the same, better, or worse?				

Treatment

There are a variety of systemic drugs being used to treat diffuse scleroderma skin disease including immunosuppressive therapy and potential anti-fibrotic agents; these are discussed elsewhere in this book.

No one disease-modifying agent has been proven to be effective in the treatment of diffuse scleroderma skin disease. Many approaches used previously (including D-penicillamine, colchicine, para-aminobenzoic acid, minocycline, relaxin, oral collagen, or photopheresis) have fallen out of favor among experts in the field due to unfavorable clinical responses or lack of evidence-based efficacy.

Anti-inflammatory or low-dose immunosuppression therapies have not yielded dramatic improvements but are now commonly used, and in particular are recommended by many in the acute edematous phase of skin disease; once the skin is fibrotic, and certainly in late-stage disease, this approach is unlikely to confer a positive impact on the skin disease. Low-dose methotrexate, mycophenolate mofetil, cyclophosphamide, azathioprine, antithymocyte globulin, and corticosteroids are the most prevalent agents now being used for early active diffuse scleroderma skin disease. The EULAR recommendations are to use methotrexate first [7]; others prefer instead to use mycophenolate mofetil in the setting of active skin disease without lung disease; others use antithymocyte globulin with mycophenolate mofetil. The full treatment effect from mycophenolate mofetil takes 3 months, but if no response is noted in 6–9 weeks, we increase the dose from 1,000 to 1,500 mg BID and consider a change in therapy. Some experts recommend using corticosteroids (alone or as an adjunct) in the early active phase of the skin disease, but we generally do not use corticosteroids for skin disease alone. When corticosteroids are used, they should be limited to dosing to 20–30 mg daily due to the risk of triggering a scleroderma renal crisis at higher doses; especially in patients with severe diffuse skin disease. The impact of corticosteroids on advancing skin disease needs further study to determine its role.

If patients are not responding to mycophenolate mofetil as determined by frequent clinical assessment (Table 33.1), we attempt novel therapy with intravenous gamma globulin with or without mycophenolate. Cyclophosphamide (monthly IV or daily 2 mg/kg orally) is used in severe cases not responding to intravenous gamma globulin. Methotrexate is used for localized scleroderma when topical therapy is ineffective. Emerging avenues of therapy include intense immunoablation with or without stem cell rescue, targeted immunomodulators or anti-inflammatory agents (such as the anti-CD20 B cell therapy rituximab), anti-interferon, anti-cytokines (tocilizumab) and intravenous gamma globulin. New agents have potential to affect fibrosis directly such as tyrosine kinase inhibitors and anti-TGF beta, but none has demonstrated significant reproducible results in the acute phase of scleroderma skin disease. Study of novel therapies in well-designed clinical trials is imperative. Currently, the best practice for care of these patients remains interdisciplinary collaborative care and referral to scleroderma specialty centers.

This section will review topical therapies for localized, limited, and diffuse scleroderma skin disease. However, no topical treatment of fibrosis has yet been proven to be dramatically and reproducibly effective. Achieving high dermal concentration of an active ingredient through a topical preparation is difficult given the fibrosis of the target lesions.

Topical Therapy of Localized Skin Disease

High-potency topical steroids, such as clobetasol propionate 0.05 % ointment, can potentially be employed to treat the early active inflammatory phase of localized scleroderma, but cause treatment-limiting epidermal atrophy and skin fragility. Intralesional steroid injections are used to treat morphea, but this approach is often problematic in treating these fibrotic plaques in that the steroid solution tracks through locus minoris resistentiae and tends to infiltrate the surrounding skin, causing worsened epidermal atrophy and telangiectasias. As a steroid-sparing alternative for focal treatment of fibrosis, topical vitamin D analogs such as calcipotriene have a body of anecdotal literature to support their use, but in clinical practice, the response to this class of treatment is disappointing. More recently, better data surrounding the use of topical tacrolimus 0.1 % ointment (Protopic®) has emerged, as it has been shown in small studies to be effective in reducing the induration in plaques of localized scleroderma. The best data to support its use are those from a randomized double-blind vehicle-controlled study, in which two active lesions of localized scleroderma per subject were studied and a statistically and clinically significant difference was noted between the two plaques [8]. While there is a black box warning on the prescription regarding risk of lymphoma and nonmelanoma skin cancer from data that relate to its oral formulation, dermatologists prescribe this medication widely (particularly in children with atopic dermatitis, its FDA-approved indication) and do not consider that the topical formulation carries risk comparable to that of the oral form as there is no systemic accumulation of the drug through topical use [9]. Another steroid-sparing therapy reported to be effective clinically and histologically in improving fibrosis of localized scleroderma lesions is topical imiquimod 5 % cream (Aldara®), which is mechanistically appealing, since it induces local interferon-gamma production and should in turn inhibit TGF-beta [10]. When Aldara® is used to treat genital warts, actinic keratoses, or superficial basal cell carcinoma (its FDA-approved indications), it induces significant inflammation that results in pruritus, tenderness, or oozing. These symptoms limit treatment adherence.

Phototherapy

Phototherapy and photochemotherapy are often considered in the therapeutic ladder of treating fibrosis. Successful treatments of both localized skin disease and diffuse scleroderma are reported, but few controlled data are available. UVB (290–320 nm) is considered to have too short a wavelength to effect a significant change in scleroderma skin, even in targeted sources such as the 308-nm excimer laser. UVA wavelengths are longer (320–400 nm) and therefore penetrate more deeply into the skin. While direct comparisons of UVB and UVA in the scleroderma literature are rare, one study randomized patients with active morphea to receive narrowband UVB (NBUVB) (311 nm), low-dose UVA1, or medium-dose UVA1 in the treatment of localized scleroderma and found medium-dose UVA1 to be significantly the most effective as measured by ultrasound thickness measurement, visual analog scale, and histopathologic evaluation, although some improvement was detected in each group (which may in part relate to small sample size and the lack of internal control as active morphea may remit spontaneously) [11].

Because UVA treatments would be prohibitively time-consuming without a photosensitizing agent to decrease treatment time, methoxsalen (Oxsoralen Ultra®) is used routinely with UVA (psoralen + UVA is termed PUVA). Treatment is initiated with at least twice-weekly sessions, and the starting UVA dose is determined based on the minimum phototoxic dose (MPD) for that patient. Oral Oxsoralen is dosed at 0.4 mg/kg 1 h before treatment, and can cause nausea, prolonged photosensitivity, and a potential associated risk of cataract development. The medication should be taken with the same type of meal with each dose and is best taken with some sort of fat such as cheese, as the fatty content of food will slow its absorption and minimize nausea. If a patient develops significant nausea, then the dose of Oxsoralen can be decreased. If persistent erythema or pruritus develops, this can be an indication of phototoxicity, and treatment should be discontinued until symptom resolution and then resumed at a lower dose.

The pathophysiologic basis for the response of fibrosis in systemic sclerosis to PUVA is not supported by extensive research, but a recent serologic study of nine patients who received PUVA and three who received topical PUVA demonstrated a statistically significant increase in circulating TNF-alpha in 8/12 subjects that was accompanied by a clinically significant improvement in the Rodnan score in 11/12 subjects [12]. Larger studies are certainly indicated, but extensive observational literature exists to suggest that PUVA can produce some softening of fibrosis. The challenge in treating fibrosis with PUVA is that it is often difficult to define a treatment endpoint. The potential risk of skin cancers such as squamous cell carcinoma and melanoma limits its appropriateness for long-term treatment, particularly in patients with light constitutive pigmentation [13].

Topical PUVA treatments have been reported to be effective in open trials evaluating their role in the treatment of localized scleroderma. The mechanism of action probably relates both to increased apoptosis of T cells in the skin and upregulation of collagen-degrading matrix metalloproteinases. PUVA-cream phototherapy offers more precise focal treatment than bath PUVA and has been described to confer clinical and histologic benefit in localized scleroderma, although not in a vehicle-controlled study [14]. There is a form of Oxsoralen lotion currently approved by the FDA, but it is very costly and produces prolonged photosensitization. PUVA cream and bath PUVA often rely therefore on compounds incorporating the contents of Oxsoralen capsules, a formulation that does not have FDA approval. This is questionable, since phototoxic erythema is a well-known risk with any form of PUVA, but if it develops in the setting of use of a non-FDA-approved topical photosensitizer, the medicolegal implications are more severe. Whether through topical or systemic PUVA photochemotherapy, 40–100 treatments at twice-weekly to three-times-weekly intervals are generally required for the treatment of localized scleroderma, with 3 months of maintenance therapy of decreasing frequency required following clinical resolution of induration [15]. Postinflammatory hyperpigmentation develops in prior areas of erythema and persists for several months following the discontinuation of treatment. Postinflammatory hyperpigmentation is most pronounced and persistent in patients with Fitzpatrick skin type III or greater, and those patients should be counseled that they will develop brown pigmentation in any areas of morphea that were previously pink and that this will take approximately a year to resolve.

UVA-1 treatment (340–400 nm) has the advantage of generating high irradiation levels that do not require a photosensitizing agent, but UVA-1 light boxes are difficult for many patients to find close to home, as they are large lie-down units (as opposed to stand-up design for UVB and PUVA) that are costly for providers to purchase and to maintain. UVA-1 also causes deep tanning, which can worsen postinflammatory hyperpigmentation. Reported treatment regimens have been highly variable, ranging from three times weekly to bimonthly treatment. High-dose (~130 J/cm^2), medium-dose (~50–60 J/cm^2), and low-dose (~10–30 J/cm^2) UVA-1 regimens have been studied, with improvement in scleroderma skin having been reported in each group. However, a study of split body treatment as an internal control in nine patients failed to demonstrate any significant difference in acrosclerosis between treated and untreated hands with 40 J/cm^2 UVA-1 treatment three times weekly for 14 weeks [16]. Clearly larger-scale randomized controlled trials are needed for further evaluation. While unproven, the mechanism of treatment efficacy in UVA-1 therapy has been studied histologically, and an increase in CD34+ dendritic cells has been observed [17].

Laser Therapy

Laser treatment of localized scleroderma using low-fluence pulsed dye laser at settings used to treat hypertrophic scarring has been published in a single case report [18], and further study is underway. There is an extensive body of literature on laser and light-based therapy of hypertrophic and atrophic scarring, and devices ranging from intense pulsed light, to low-fluence pulsed dye, to Nd:YAG, to fractionated non-ablative and ablative lasers have all been described as achieving variable degrees of functional and esthetic improvement.

Skin Changes in Fibrotic Areas of Limited and Diffuse Scleroderma

Xerosis

Since scleroderma skin thickening causes loss of periadnexal fat, the adnexa (hair follicles, sebaceous glands, eccrine glands) can be compressed resulting in frequent loss of skin appendages. This translates clinically to reduced sebum production and consequent xerosis and is often accompanied by alopecia and hypohidrosis. As skin softens, the alopecia sometimes dramatically reverses with hypertrichosis (Fig. 33.11). Scleroderma skin is often rough and slightly erythematous, resembling an eczematous dermatitis. This dermatitis can produce varying degrees of pruritus. Small papules of prurigo nodularis can arise in areas of chronic rubbing or excoriation, giving the skin a "cobblestoned" appearance (as mentioned previously, there may be a component of elephantiasis nostra-type change relating to lymphatic obstruction that plays a role in the development of cobblestoning, as well) (Fig. 33.9). Even larger collagenous nodules can develop against a background of scleroderma skin, some of which are classified as keloidal morphea and some as nodular scleroderma based on their histologic characteristics (Fig. 33.12) [19].

Treatment

In patients in whom pruritus is pronounced, a short course of super potent topical steroids (such as clobetasol propionate 0.05 % ointment, or cream if ointment cannot be tolerated) to decrease the inflammation and pruritus is often required. For those patients with milder pruritus, a mid-potency topical steroid compounded 1:1 with a rich emollient (such as triamcinolone acetonide 0.1 % cream 1:1 with Eucerin or CeraVe cream) is a better first-line treatment. In patients with skin fragility in whom topical steroids would be inadvisable, topical calcineurin inhibitors such as tacrolimus ointment are an excellent alternative. Patients should be advised that these can cause a very warm sensation in the skin when first applied that should not be confused with an allergic reaction and that this subsides by about 1 week into use. Refrigerating the topical calcineurin inhibitors can help to limit this sensation of warmth on application.

For patients with a more pronounced eczematous dermatitis, narrowband UVB treatment (NBUVB, 311 nm)

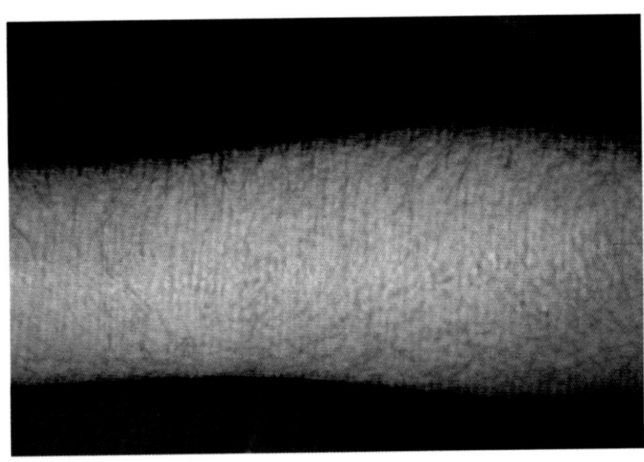

Fig. 33.11 Hypertrichosis in the setting of skin softening (Courtesy of F.M. Wigley)

can be extraordinarily helpful as a steroid-sparing treatment strategy. Three times weekly treatment is needed to achieve optimal clearance, and then it should be tapered to twice-weekly treatment for 4 weeks, followed by weekly treatment for 4 weeks. NBUVB is not as effective for weekly maintenance therapy as PUVA, so if a patient is clear at that point, treatment can be discontinued with the understanding that it will be resumed should the dermatitis flare significantly.

Systemic antipruritics can be helpful, but not uniformly so. Fexofenadine 180 mg (Allegra®) can be an effective first-line antihistamine, but patients must be instructed to take it every 24 h precisely, whether or not their skin is itchy at the time they are meant to take the next dose. The added decongestant found in some formulations is unnecessary and should be avoided. A more potent antihistamine choice would be hydroxyzine (Atarax®), but this can be highly sedating and should be taken with caution with regard to driving a car or operating machinery, until it is established that the patient is not becoming sedated. An antidepressant with H1/H2 antihistamine activity, doxepin, can be very helpful in some patients. It should be taken every 24 h and timed for several hours before bed so that the peak effect occurs during deep sleep.

For maintenance once pruritus is controlled, patients must concentrate on maintaining the hydration and moisturization of their skin. Cleansing agents should have petrolatum among the first ingredients, and antibacterial soaps (particularly those containing triclosan) should be avoided apart from instances in which they are necessary. Moisturizing lotions that are thin enough to be dispensed through a pump contain too much water to be sufficiently moisturizing for scleroderma skin. Instead, creams that are dispensed in a jar (as tubes can be difficult to use with sclerodactyly) are ideal, and ceramides as found in CeraVe Moisturizing Cream can help to strengthen the epidermal barrier to prevent internal water loss and external irritation. Exfoliants such as alpha hydroxy acids should be avoided in the areas of xerosis and dermatitis, as these can be excessively irritating.

Alopecia

Much as loss of skin appendages can result in xerosis, it can also result in alopecia. There can be follicular drop out in areas of fibrosis, but non-scarring alopecia with preservation of follicles can also be observed in areas of inflammation. Hair breakage can be seen secondary to excoriation, as well. Once the inflammatory phase has subsided, areas of previously inflamed sclerotic skin may develop paradoxical robust terminal hair growth that is often particularly evident on the forearms (Fig. 33.10).

Treatment

Topical minoxidil preparations (such as Rogaine®) can be effective in promoting terminal hair growth in areas of non-scarring alopecia that are of cosmetic significance. Minoxidil can be found in generic unscented forms that are often less irritating than the fragranced versions, and the foam vehicle is often easier to apply than the solution if a patient has sclerodactyly and is applying it to his or her scalp. Bimatoprost ophthalmic solution 0.03 % (Latisse) is FDA approved to treat hypotrichosis of the eyelashes, but is now starting to be used off-label to increase terminal hair growth in other areas. Until a version for the scalp comes to market, the bottles available for eyelash use are a maximum of 5 mL in volume and are costly since not covered by insurance, but this treatment works very well on focal areas such as eyebrows, and in clinical practice, it has become a frequent recommendation to mix Latisse into a bottle of minoxidil solution and apply to the scalp daily for a synergistic effect.

Telangiectasias

Telangiectasias (also termed telangiectases) are a hallmark of scleroderma skin disease. They blanch on diascopy and represent dilated postcapillary venules without evidence of inflammation or neovascularization [20]. They can be seen in both limited and diffuse forms of scleroderma and are more evident in patients with lighter skin. Interestingly, the number of telangiectasias increases with disease duration, even in cases when the skin and other manifestations of the disease seem clinically quiescent. The lesions are apparent first on the fingers, palms, face, and mucous membranes, and then later in the disease course appear on the arms and trunk (chest and back); rarely, they are seen on the legs and feet. It is hypothesized that they may arise due to decreased oxygen tension in the skin and are a clinical biomarker of microvascular pathology as the extent of telangiectasias has been shown to correlate with increased right ventricular systolic pressure and the development of pulmonary hypertension in scleroderma patients [21].

Stellate telangiectasias, which are more linear, can be seen in any form of scleroderma. Geometric mat telangiectasias are most prominently seen in limited scleroderma, but are also a component of diffuse disease. They can also be seen concurrently, with mat telangiectasias against a background of less prominent stellate telangiectasias (Fig. 33.13). Mat telangiectasias are often evident on the lips (Fig. 33.14) and, as a presenting sign can be confused with Osler-Weber-Rendu disease (hereditary hemorrhagic telangiectasia, HHT). However, recurrent epistaxis is pathognomonic of HHT rather than scleroderma; HHT patients often have arteriovenous malformations in the lungs and other organs that are not seen in scleroderma, and HHT does not have associated skin fibrosis. As compared to generalized essential telangiectasia, a disease characterized by numerous telangiectasias on the skin without associated systemic disease, the telangiectasias occur on acral skin (Fig. 33.14) and mucous membranes more commonly in scleroderma. Rarely, cutaneous telangiectasias can bleed, most commonly on thin mucous membranes such as the lip and nasal mucosa.

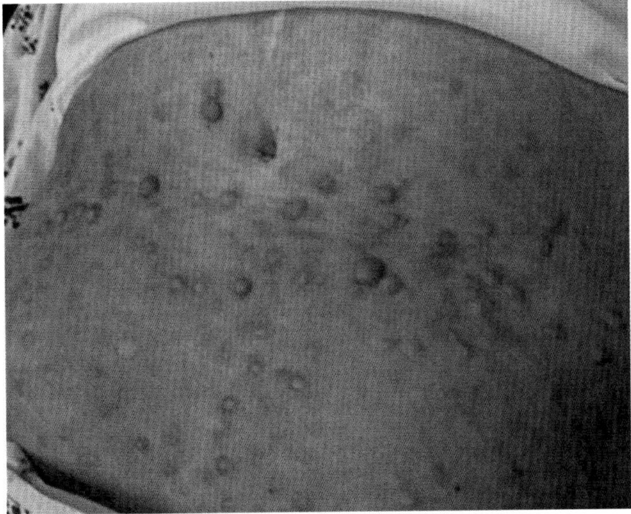

Fig. 33.12 Collagenous nodules in a patient with diffuse scleroderma (Courtesy of F.M. Wigley)

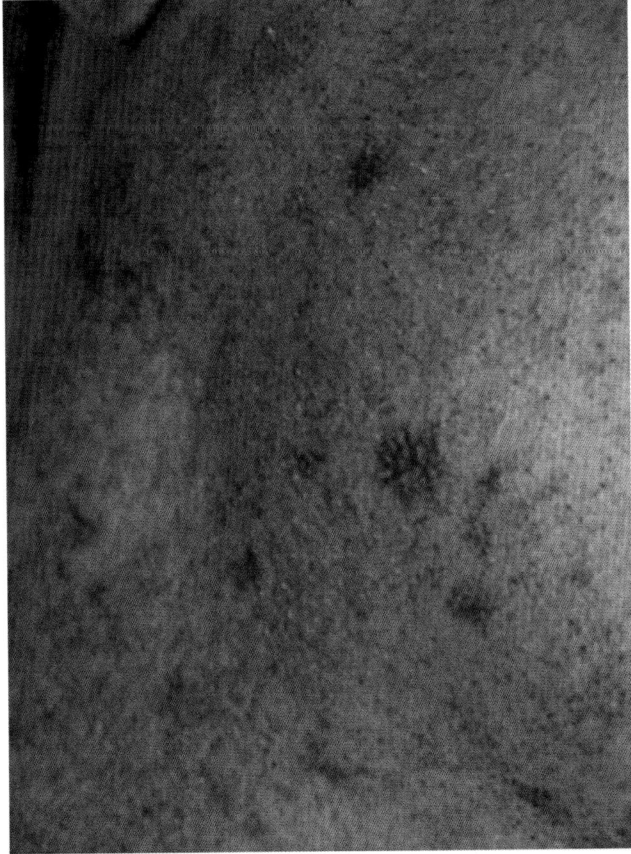

Fig. 33.13 Mat telangiectasias adjacent to stellate telangiectasias (Courtesy of F.M. Wigley)

Treatment

Telangiectasias can be treated safely and effectively with laser therapy. Either intense pulsed light with a 560 nm or similar filter depending on the device, the 585-nm or 595-nm pulsed dye laser, or the 1,064-nm Nd:YAG laser are effective modalities. Usually, several treatments are needed for optimal result, although improvement is achieved with each treatment. Since these laser treatments are non-ablative (do not disrupt the integrity of the epidermis), there is no risk for infection or scarring unless blistering results from excessive energy delivered from the laser. With appropriate settings, this is a rare complication. Posttreatment purpura is common, and associated discomfort is brief and minimal. In more darkly pigmented skin, a test spot should be performed before an entire area is treated. Laser treatment is often possible in darker skin types by decreasing the fluence and increasing the pulse width, with caution not to cause depigmentation. Telangiectasias tend to reaccumulate over time, generally making repeated treatments necessary; this may pose a problem for patients because insurance companies often deem treatment to be cosmetic and may not cover its cost.

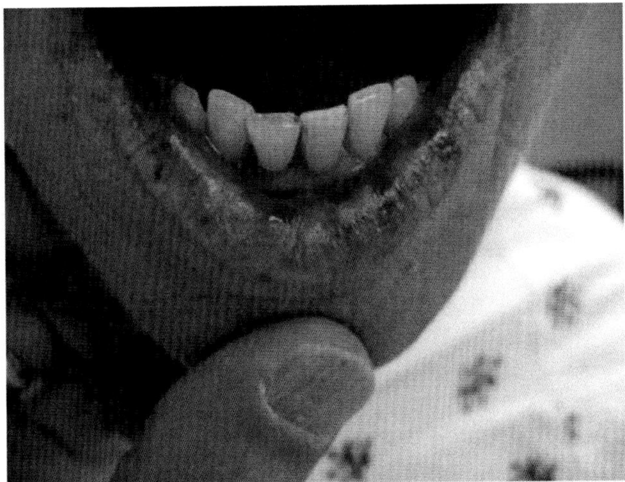

Fig. 33.14 Mat telangiectasias on the lips (Courtesy of F.M. Wigley)

Dyspigmentation

Salt and pepper leukoderma is frequently seen in association with the diffuse form of systemic sclerosis, more commonly than in the limited or localized forms. It manifests as patches of depigmentation with preserved perifollicular pigmentation. This results in a speckled appearance resembling salt and pepper (Fig. 33.15a, b). By contrast, vitiligo – which can also be seen in the setting of scleroderma – is characterized by islands of depigmentation without perifollicular sparing (Fig. 33.16). Vitiligo typically favors the fingertips, genitalia, and perioral skin. A Wood's lamp examination can demonstrate whether depigmentation (total loss of pigment) versus hypopigmentation (partial loss of pigment) has occurred, as depigmentation will fluoresce with a brighter blue-white than will hypopigmentation. Occasionally, trichrome vitiligo can occur in which both depigmentation and hypopigmentation are present concurrently.

The pathogenesis of salt and pepper leukoderma is unclear but probably relates to an autoimmune assault on melanocytes, with the perifollicular sparing reflecting sites of comparative immune privilege. Vitiligo also remains idiopathic, but humoral and cellular immune activity against melanocytes is hypothesized.

Postinflammatory dyspigmentation is seen commonly in scleroderma. After an inflammatory phase has resolved, hypopigmentation or hyperpigmentation may remain in that area for at least a year. A Wood's lamp examination (320–400 nm) can be helpful in determining whether true depigmentation has occurred – as would be seen in vitiligo – in that areas of depigmentation will demonstrate blue-white fluorescence, in contrast to hypopigmentation that will not demonstrate the same bright fluorescence. Postinflammatory dyspigmentation is often more ill-defined than the pigmentary change seen in vitiligo or salt and pepper leukoderma. In some cases of systemic sclerosis, patients will develop a diffusely tanned hyperpigmentation. The pathogenesis of this is not understood, but probably falls in the spectrum of postinflammatory change.

Treatment

Salt and pepper leukoderma does not respond as well to narrowband UVB phototherapy or PUVA (psoralen + UVA) photochemotherapy as does vitiligo. However, these are reasonable treatments to consider if a patient is very concerned with the appearance of dyspigmentation, as the photons may stimulate matrix metalloproteinases that can help to soften fibrosis. NBUVB would be the first-line phototherapy

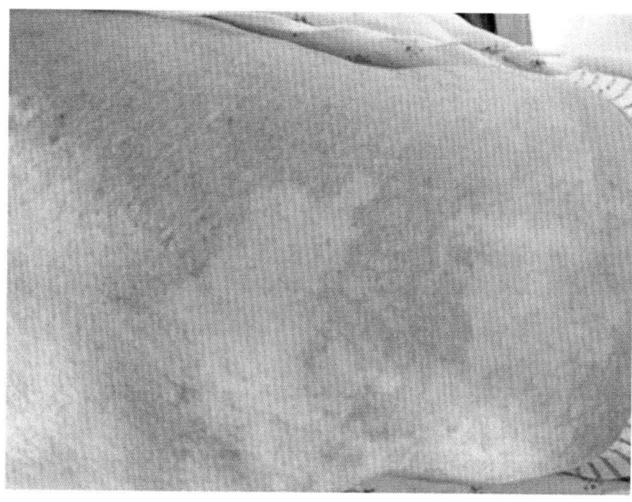

Fig. 33.16 Vitiligo in diffuse scleroderma (Courtesy of F.M. Wigley)

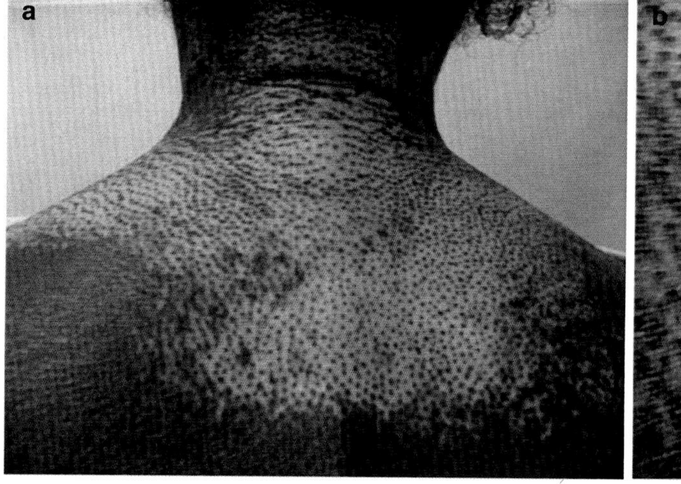

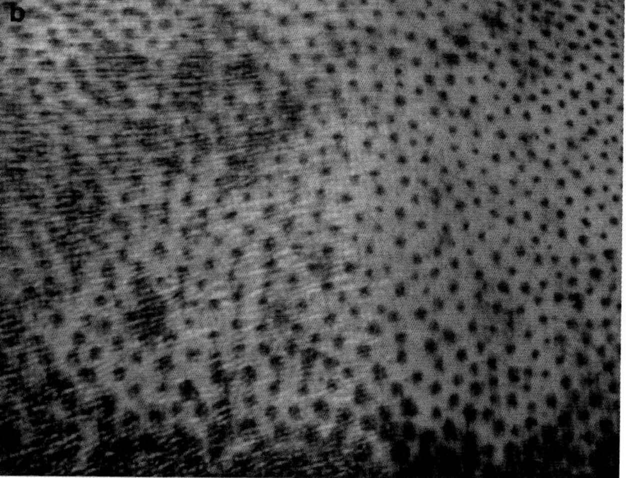

Fig. 33.15 (**a**) Salt and pepper leukoderma. (**b**) Preservation of perifollicular pigmentation in salt and pepper leukoderma (Courtesy of F.M. Wigley)

approach, but patients who have not improved with 50 treatments (25 treatments for facial skin) should progress to PUVA photochemotherapy. The excimer laser (308 nm) offers targeted UVB treatment of vitiligo so that non-lesional skin does not get unnecessary UV exposure, and adjunct treatment with topical vitamin D derivatives may augment its efficacy per a left/right comparative single-blinded clinical trial [22].

Repigmentation in vitiligo occurs perifollicularly first, giving an appearance similar to salt and pepper leukoderma. For either condition, if no significant improvement is noted after 3 months of dose- and frequency-optimized phototherapy, it should be discontinued as perpetual intense UV exposure can increase the risk of skin cancer, particularly squamous cell carcinoma.

Since vitiligo is a cosmetic concern and not a dangerous condition, the long-term use of high-potency topical steroids is inadvisable, particularly in scleroderma, as it can cause significant epidermal atrophy with prominent telangiectasias. Topical steroids can promote regimentation in vitiligo, but have not been well studied in salt and pepper leukoderma. Topical calcineurin inhibitors have been shown to be effective in the treatment of vitiligo and do not carry with them a similar risk. A randomized, double-blind, head-to-head study on two similar lesions with subjects serving as an internal control revealed nearly as high a repigmentation rate for the tacrolimus (41.3 %) as compared to clobetasol (49.3 %) when used in 20 children for 2 months. Of note, three clobetasol-treated lesions developed atrophy during the study and three developed telangiectasias [23]. Calcineurin inhibitors have not been studied in salt and pepper leukoderma, but it would be reasonable to try them in this condition or to speed the resolution of postinflammatory dyspigmentation.

Postinflammatory hyperpigmentation can be challenging to treat in scleroderma skin, as commonly prescribed hydroquinone compounds may provoke treatment-limiting inflammation. Hydroquinone, a tyrosinase inhibitor, needs to be compounded with a steroid, a retinoid, and an antioxidant for optimal pigment lightening effect, but increasing the steroid level to prevent inflammation of scleroderma skin that can be easily sensitized from the hydroquinone and retinoid can lead to skin atrophy. Nonprescription skin brighteners that are very effective against postinflammatory hyperpigmentation have emerged, such as Elure Advanced Brightening Lotion which uses lignin peroxidase as an alternative to a tyrosinase inhibitor and does not cause treatment-related inflammation, thus making it suitable for sensitive or sensitized skin. In combination with mineral sunscreens applied rigorously in sun-exposed areas, these topical skin brighteners can improve postinflammatory hyperpigmentation significantly.

Calcinosis Cutis

Calcinosis cutis, or dystrophic calcification, is a common complication in scleroderma. This problem is covered in another chapter of the book.

Ulcerations

Ulcerations can be related to several etiologies in scleroderma. Ischemic skin ulcers are covered in another section of this book. Traumatic ulcerations occur readily in the setting of sclerodactyly, particularly over the interphalangeal joints (Fig. 33.8), and often occur on the ears, elbows, and ankle areas. Ulcerations on the distal fingertips can be secondary to trauma, but often are ischemic in origin (Fig. 33.16). A clue to this is surrounding pale cool skin. Shallow ulcers can also be seen in the setting of skin fragility. Ulcers that are monomorphic and linear are likely the result of excoriations, while those that are more ill-defined and shoddy probably relate more to associated xerosis and dermatitis. Other reported causes of skin ulcerations in scleroderma patients include complications of calcinosis cutis or paronychia, cutaneous vasculitis, atrophie blanche with livedoid vasculopathy (see below), and, rarely, bullous pemphigoid or pyoderma gangrenosum.

Treatment

Fingertip ulcers must be protected from trauma and infection. Keeping an ulcer moist greatly aids in wound healing. For ulcers with surrounding erythema, edema, warmth, or tenderness, a curette culture should be the first step to assess whether an ulcer is infected and whether systemic antibiotics are needed. For infected ulcers, silver-containing dressings

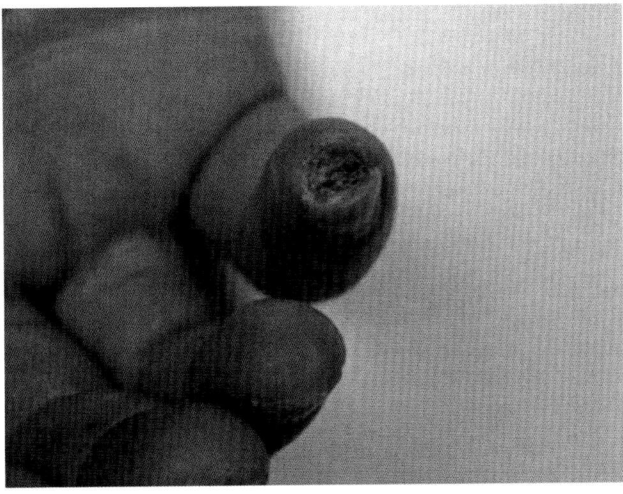

Fig. 33.17 Ischemic fingertip ulceration (Courtesy of F.M. Wigley)

are optimal for their antimicrobial benefits. Since the silver ions confer the antimicrobial effect, a moist wound bed is essential for those dressings to be effective. For infected ulcers with exudate, or for noninfected ulcers with exudate in which you want to prevent secondary infection, silver-containing hydrofiber dressings like Aquacel Ag (now available without a prescription) are an ideal choice as they absorb drainage, protect the skin, and prevent infection. For infected ulcers without exudate, mupirocin 2 % ointment can be used to moisten the wound bed before application of the silver-containing dressing. Of note, many silver-containing dressings contain sulfa and should be used with caution in sulfa-allergic patients. For noninfected ulcers without exudate, the healing area should be kept moist with Vaseline or Aquaphor and should be protected from trauma with gel blister pads or similar cushioned bandage. Wet-to-dry dressings are not optimal as they tend to pull viable tissue away from the wound bed with each dressing change and therefore slow the healing process.

Pain can be a treatment challenge in the management of digital ulcers. Topical anesthetics such as ELMA or lidocaine ointment should be avoided as they commonly provoke skin irritation and contact dermatitis that can be difficult to distinguish from signs of infection and can slow wound healing. Appropriate wound dressings are a better solution for pain management and can reduce pain to a far greater degree than topical anesthetics are able. Additionally, wound dressings shield the healing skin from trauma. For a painful dry ulcer that is noninfected, a hydrogel dressing like Curagel keeps the wound moist and reduces pain significantly by decreasing nerve impulses that transmit the sensation of pain. Hydrogels donate moisture to the wound for an optimal healing environment, but must be applied under Adaptiq or other Vaseline-impregnated gauze as a secondary dressing to maintain moisture. Hydrogels should not be used on tunneled ulcers as they can form a gelatinous mass that is difficult to remove completely. Hydrogel dressings should be changed daily. If this is difficult for a particular patient due to sclerodactyly or other concerns, hydrocolloid dressings can be left in place for up to 7 days. To avoid skin tearing after prolonged wear of a hydrocolloid dressing, patients should be cautioned to lift a corner of the dressing and stretch it parallel to the skin before attempting to remove it, so that the adhesive bonds break for easier removal [24]. For painful noninfected ulcers with exudate, a silver-containing hydrofiber dressing similarly reduces wound pain as a hydrogel or hydrocolloid does in dry wounds.

If an ulcer heals with excess granulation tissue, topical in-office application of silver nitrate is very effective treatment. Several treatments may be needed, and patients should be advised that the treated tissue will look gray or black and that this is not a cause for alarm but rather the result of silver transferring onto the skin.

Topical antibiotics can be useful in preventing secondary infection or treating mild superficial infection, but over-the-counter options such as Neosporin and bacitracin frequently incite an allergic or irritant contact dermatitis when used on compromised skin such as the site of an ulcer. Even if a patient has used these topical antibiotics previously without a reaction, mupirocin 2 % ointment (Bactroban) is a better choice for ulcer treatment since it very rarely causes dermatitis on wounds and protects against MRSA, which is increasingly common in wounds of patients with frequent hospital contact as often occurs with scleroderma patients.

To clean the ulcerated area between dressing changes, a dilute vinegar solution is gentle and effective at treating bacterial and fungal colonization. This solution can be prepared at home by mixing one teaspoon of plain white vinegar with two cups of water. To use, patients should dip a clean, soft cloth into the vinegar solution, place the wet cloth against the affected area gently pressing to ensure that the vinegar solution wets the skin, and then rinse and repeat for 10–15 min. The antibiotic ointment or gelatinous residue from a hydrogel dressing should be readily removed through this soaking process without any rubbing of the skin needed. Bleach soaks are another good option for wound cleaning in between dressing changes, but should not exceed 0.025 % in concentration.

Wound care can be discontinued when an ulcer reepithelializes completely. In general, it is not advisable to let ulcers develop an eschar as this will slow healing. However, for very small punctate ulcers that will heal quickly by secondary intention, this may be reasonable management.

Onychodystrophy

Although chapters are devoted to nail fold capillaroscopy and Raynaud's phenomenon elsewhere in this text, the nail changes that accompany scleroderma pathology of the nail matrix merit separate discussion. Prolonged tissue ischemia can lead to fibrosis of the matrix that manifests with beaking as a form of pseudo-clubbing of the nails (Fig. 33.18). Inflammation of the matrix can lead to pitting (Fig. 33.19) or beading – larger teardrop-shaped indentations in the nail plate – as can also be seen in rheumatoid arthritis. While distal splinter hemorrhages may appear secondary to trauma (Fig. 33.20), proximal splinter hemorrhages reflect vascular injury. The periungual skin can become hyperkeratotic due to xerosis and inflammation, leading to ragged cuticles (Fig. 33.21). Pterygium inversum unguium, in which the distal nail groove is obliterated by an aberrant connection between the nail plate and the hyponychium, can result from ischemia [25].

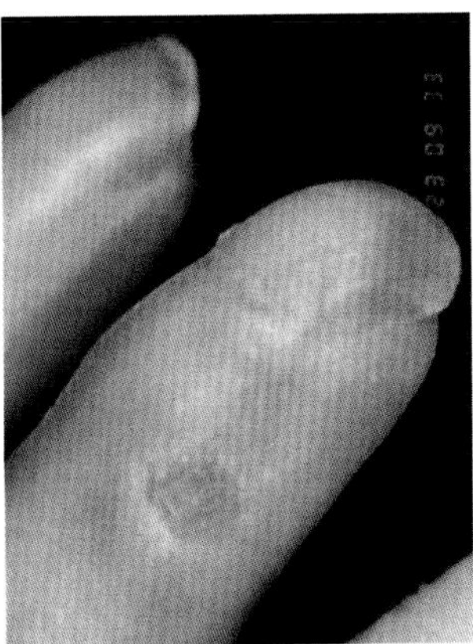

Fig. 33.18 Beaking of the nails (Courtesy of F.M. Wigley)

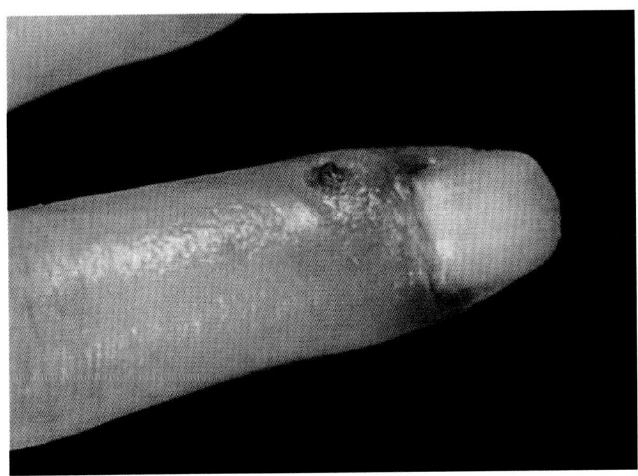

Fig. 33.19 Nail plate pitting (Courtesy of F.M. Wigley)

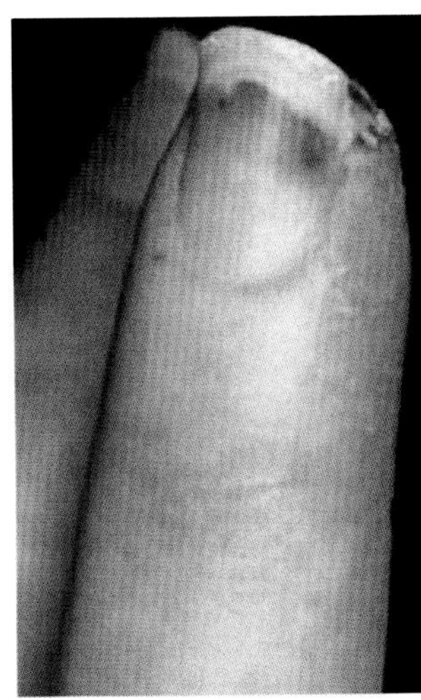

Fig. 33.20 Distal splinter hemorrhages secondary to trauma (Courtesy of F.M. Wigley)

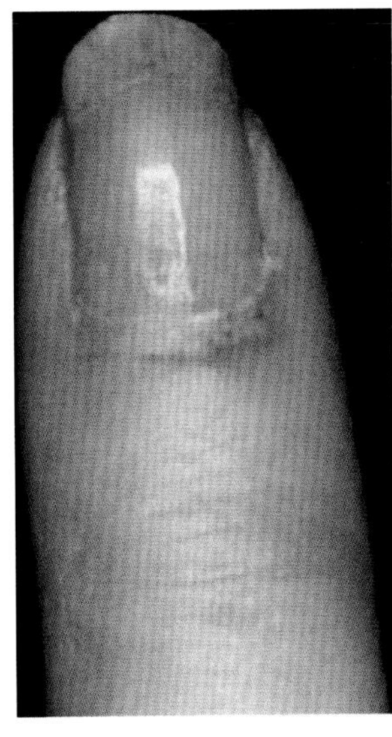

Fig. 33.21 Ragged cuticles (Courtesy of F.M. Wigley)

Treatment

Topical agents penetrate the nail plate poorly, so the inflammatory forms of onychodystrophy are generally difficult to treat topically. For ragged cuticles, a steroid-containing nongreasy treatment such as Locoid Lipocream® (hydrocortisone butyrate 0.1 % cream) is generally well tolerated at bedtime for flare-ups. For the daytime, barrier creams such as MimyX® can work very well to minimize xerosis of the skin of the hands and periungual area when used every morning. Additionally, there are cuticle creams available over the counter that work very well to keep this area moisturized and can be reapplied throughout the day, such as Eve Lom Cuticle Cream or Dior Creme d'Abricot.

Lipodystrophy

Lipodystrophy overlying inflammatory lesions such as plaques of localized scleroderma is well described. The most frequently encountered cosmetically significant forms of this are generally linear scleroderma, especially when presenting in the en coup de sabre form affecting the face, and the Parry-Romberg variant of linear scleroderma in which there is associated progressive hemifacial atrophy. Additionally, there can be prominent fat loss on the limbs or trunk in association with cutaneous fibrosis in systemic sclerosis. Since the subcutaneous fat often recovers as skin softens, the adipocytes are likely compressed by the tight fibrotic dermis rather than destroyed.

Treatment

Noninvasive treatment of facial lipodystrophy is often preferred by patients when feasible, as opposed to surgical approaches such as microvascular free tissue transfer. With

10 years of treatment efficacy established in HIV-associated lipoatrophy, and now being used widely for esthetic facial revolumization, poly-L-lactic acid (Sculptra®, PLLA) is a good option for these patients. Typically, a series of at least three treatments is needed, with each entailing topical anesthetic in addition to 1 % lidocaine without epinephrine mixed into the injected material. The viscous suspension is injected into the areas of volume deficiency using a crosshatch linear threading technique in combination with depot injections where necessary. No active inflammation should be present at the time of treatment for an optimal result, as PLLA has the potential to produce inflammatory nodules. In a paper describing PLLA treatment of four patients with linear scleroderma of the face and two with Parry-Romberg syndrome, two developed subcutaneous nodules [26]. While this is a known potential complication of PLLA treatment, a more dilute preparation than used in those cases has improved outcomes. The other filler with FDA approval for the treatment of HIV-associated lipoatrophy is Radiesse®, which consists of calcium hydroxylapatite microspheres suspended in an aqueous gel carrier. Because the microspheres can be seen on X-rays or CT scans, it should not be injected in areas that may require monitoring with those modalities. Hyaluronic acid injectable dermal fillers such as Juvéderm Voluma XC® and Juvéderm Ultra Plus XC® may be suitable for revolumizing in scleroderma patients since they are used widely to treat age-related volume loss and do not carry as high a risk of nodule formation as does PLLA, plus they can be dissolved with hyaluronidase if need be.

Atrophie Blanche

Stellate ivory sclerotic plaques with surrounding hyperpigmentation are often seen on the distal extremities, particularly the lower legs, of scleroderma patients; this morphology has been termed atrophie blanche (Fig. 33.22). These plaques result from ulcerations. While scars of similar morphology can develop following traumatic excoriation, and atrophie blanche can develop in association with several vasculitides, an etiology for lesions morphologically consistent with atrophie blanche that should be evaluated is livedoid vasculopathy. In this condition, luminal thrombi lead to ischemia and ulceration. When seen in association with autoimmune disease such as scleroderma, it may be related to a hypercoagulable state induced by inflammation rather than a true vasculitis. A recent retrospective review of 45 patients with livedoid vasculopathy revealed antiphospholipid antibody syndrome (APS) as the most common associated form of thrombophilia, followed by factor V Leiden syndrome. Other underlying conditions reported were lupus anticoagulant, protein C or S deficiency, prothrombin mutation, and hyperhomocysteinemia [27]. Ulcers of livedoid vasculopathy are characteristically intensely painful, and can generally be differentiated from ulcers of venous insufficiency given that they more commonly affect the bilateral malleoli and arise in the absence of significant background edema that would suggest venous disease.

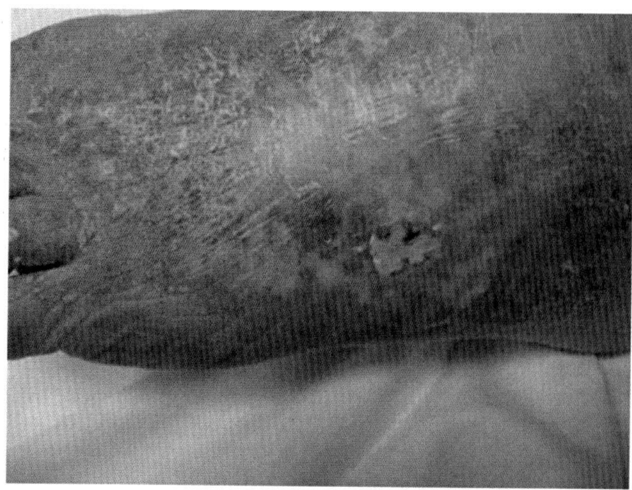

Fig. 33.22 Healing ulceration of atrophie blanche due to livedoid vasculopathy (Courtesy of F.M. Wigley)

An associated finding with thrombophilia, livedo reticularis has been observed in the setting of scleroderma. It should prompt an evaluation for underlying antiphospholipid antibody syndrome (APS). Although livedo is not a specific finding, it is commonly seen in the setting of APS. When livedo reticularis is seen in conjunction with atrophie blanche or livedoid vasculopathy, the index of suspicion for APS should increase [28].

Treatment

For established lesions of atrophie blanche, treatment is cosmetic. For patients with no new ulcerations or evidence of active inflammation, treatment of cosmetically sensitive areas could be undertaken with fractionated ablative or nonablative lasers as these work well to improve the appearance of hypopigmented atrophic scars and background dyspigmentation. In scleroderma patients, fractionated nonablative photothermolysis is preferable to an ablative treatment technique since it does not have the potential for infectious complications that accompanies disruption of the epidermis [29].

If the lesions of atrophie blanche are due to livedoid vasculopathy, diagnosis and treatment of underlying thrombophilia with anticoagulation is crucial to cessation of disease activity. Successful treatment has been described variously with anticoagulants, fibrinolytics, and antiplatelet therapies.

Future Directions

The next steps forward in skin-directed therapy of scleroderma will capitalize on the progress in drug delivery systems for topical therapies and new developments in selective photothermolysis for light and laser treatments. Additionally, advances in autologous tissue transfer are emerging as a means of inducing tissue remodeling. As an example, a study published in 2015 of 20 women with systemic sclerosis demonstrated that 2 mL of autologous fat transfer to the perioral area resulted in an increase in interincisal distance and oral perimeter, neovascularization of the tissue as assessed by video capillaroscopy and skin biopsies, and skin structural improvement as defined by flattening of the dermal-epidermal junction histologically [30]. This constellation of changes suggests a functional and structural improvement posttreatment, and using autologous fat transfer to induce beneficial tissue remodeling in areas of fibrosis is an area of promising investigation. While improved cosmesis was not a primary endpoint, this emerging research may also give hope for patients who are living longer with quiescent scleroderma than ever before, thanks to innovations in therapy and want to reduce the appearance of perioral scleroderma skin changes that have been very difficult to treat with injectable dermal fillers and laser treatments.

A boon in the treatment of scleroderma skin disease is that the esthetic medicine and cosmeceutical realms are highly invested in developing topical and light-/laser-based therapies that will reach the dermis to induce collagen remodeling with the goal of antiaging. While the goal in scleroderma skin disease is instead anti-fibrosis, these technologies may be able to be translated into meaningful progress in scleroderma treatment, as improved drug delivery to the dermis can be paired with novel pharmacologic agents, and light and laser technologies may conceivably be employed to mitigate fibrosis. The ability to treat the cutaneous manifestations of scleroderma without systemic morbidities stemming from immunosuppression or immunomodulation will be a pathbreaking advance in the field of treating these patients and offers the exciting opportunity to mollify what has to date been one of the most problematic areas of scleroderma disease management.

References

1. Weedon D. Skin pathology. 2nd ed. Philadelphia: Elsevier Health; 2005. p. 347–50.
2. Sherber NS, Boin F, Hummers LK, et al. The "tank top sign" – a unique pattern of skin fibrosis seen in pansclerotic morphea. Ann Rheum Dis. 2009;68:1511–2.
3. Barnett AJ. The "neck sign" in scleroderma. Arthritis Rheum. 1989;32:209–11.
4. Beyer C, Schett G, Gay S, et al. Hypoxia. Hypoxia in the pathogenesis of systemic sclerosis. Arthritis Res Ther. 2009;11:220.
5. Clements P, Lachenbruch P, Seibold J, et al. Inter- and intraobserver variability of total skin thickness score (modified Rodnan TSS) in systemic sclerosis. J Rheumatol. 1995;22:1281–5.
6. Amjadi S, Maranian P, Furst DE, et al. Course of the modified Rodnan skin thickness score in systemic sclerosis clinical trials: analysis of three large multicenter, double-blind, randomized controlled trials. Arthritis Rheum. 2009;60:2490–8.
7. Kowal-Bielecka O, Landewé R, Avouac J, et al. EULAR recommendations for the treatment of systemic sclerosis: a report from the EULAR Scleroderma Trials and Research group (EUSTAR). Ann Rheum Dis. 2009;68:620–8.
8. Kroft EB, Groeneveld TJ, Seyger MM, et al. Efficacy of topical tacrolimus 0.1% in active plaque morphea: randomized, double-blind, emollient-controlled pilot study. Am J Clin Dermatol. 2009;10:181–7.
9. McCollum AD, Paik A, Eichenfield LF. The safety and efficacy of tacrolimus ointment in pediatric patients with atopic dermatitis. Pediatr Dermatol. 2010;27:425–36.
10. Keuter A, Hyun J, Stucker M, et al. A randomized controlled study of low-dose UVA1, medium-dose UVA1, and narrowband UVB phototherapy in the treatment of localized scleroderma. J Am Acad Dermatol. 2006;54:440–7.
11. Dytoc M, Ting PT, Man J, et al. First case series on the use of imiquimod for morphoea. Brit J Dermatol. 2005;153:815–20.
12. Usmani N, Murphy A, Veale D, et al. Photochemotherapy for systemic sclerosis: effect on clinical and molecular markers. Clin Exp Dermatol. 2010;35:608–13.
13. Patel RV, Clark LN, Lebwohl M, et al. Treatments for psoriasis and the risk of malignancy. J Am Acad Dermatol. 2009;60:1001–7.
14. Grundmann-Kollmann M, Ochsendorf F, Zollner TM, et al. PUVA-cream photochemotherapy for the treatment of localized scleroderma. J Am Acad Dermatol. 2000;43:675–8.
15. Morison W. Phototherapy and photochemotherapy of skin disease. 3rd ed. Boca Raton: Taylor & Francis; 2005. p. 225.
16. Durand F, Staumont D, Bonnevalle A, et al. Ultraviolet A1 phototherapy for treatment of acrosclerosis in systemic sclerosis: controlled study with half-side comparison analysis. Photodermatol Photoimmunol Photomed. 2007;23:215–21.
17. Camacho NR, Sanchez JE, Martin RF, et al. Medium-dose UVA1 phototherapy in localized scleroderma and its effect in CD34-positive dendritic cells. J Am Acad Dermatol. 2001;45:697–9.
18. Eisen D, Alster T. Use of a 585-nm pulsed dye laser for the treatment of morphea. Dermatol Surg. 2002;28:615–6.
19. Rencic A, Brinster N, Nousari CH. Keloid morphea and nodular scleroderma: two distinct clinical variants of scleroderma? J Cutan Med Surg. 2003;7:20–4.
20. Braverman IM, Ken-Yen A. Ultrastructure and three-dimensional reconstruction of several macular and papular telangiectases. J Invest Dermatol. 1983;81:489–97.
21. Shah AA, Wigley FM, Hummers LK. Telangiectases in scleroderma: a potential clinical marker of pulmonary arterial hypertension. J Rheumatol. 2010;37:98–104.
22. Goldinger SM, Dummer R, Schmid P, et al. Combination of 308-nm xenon chloride Excimer laser and topical calcipotriol in vitiligo. J Eur Acad Dermatol Venereol. 2007;21:504–8.
23. Lepe V, Moncada B, Castanedo-Cazares JP, et al. A double-blind randomized trial of 0.1% tacrolimus vs 0.05% clobetasol for the treatment of childhood vitiligo. Arch Dermatol. 2003;139:581–5.
24. Lee JC, Kandula S, Sherber NS. Beyond wet-to-dry: a rational approach to treating chronic wounds. Eplasty. 2009;9:e14.
25. Sherber NS, Wigley FM, Scher RK. Autoimmune disorders: nail signs and therapeutic approaches. Dermatol Ther. 2007;20:17–30.

26. Onesti MG, Troccola A, Scuderi N. Volumetric correction using poly-L-lactic acid in facial asymmetry: Parry Romberg syndrome and scleroderma. Dermatol Surg. 2009;35:1368–75.
27. Hairston BR, Davis MDP, Pittelkow MR, et al. Livedoid vasculopathy: further evidence for procoagulant pathogenesis. Arch Dermatol. 2006;142:1413–8.
28. Weinstein S, Piette W. Cutaneous manifestations of antiphospholipid antibody syndrome. Hematol Oncol Clin North Am. 2008;22:67–77.
29. Tierney EP, Hancke CW. Review of the literature: treatment of dyspigmentation with fractionated resurfacing. Dermatol Surg. 2010;36:1499–508.
30. Del Papa N, Caviggioli F, Sambataro D, et al. Autologous fat grafting in the treatment of fibrotic perioral changes in patients with systemic sclerosis. Cell Transplant. 2015;24:63–72.

34 Assessment and Management of Progressive Skin Involvement in Diffuse Scleroderma

Robert W. Simms

This chapter will cover the assessment and management of progressive skin disease in scleroderma with the principle focus on the diffuse subset of the disease, for which progression of skin involvement is much more likely than in the limited phenotype. Before discussing the management of progressive skin involvement in a patient with diffuse scleroderma, it is important to discuss the initial assessment needed to inform decisions about appropriate treatment. The initial evaluation of this patient's skin involvement had several key points to emphasize: (1) the assessment of the scleroderma phenotype (i.e., diffuse vs. limited), (2) establishing the chronology or time course of the skin and extra-cutaneous organ involvement, and (3) the semiquantitative overall extent of skin involvement by the modified Rodnan skin score (MRSS), the standardized skin assessment tool.

Assessment of Skin Disease/Phenotype

Rodnan initially developed a semiquantitative skin score to measure skin thickness by palpation, which correlated with skin biopsy specimen weight, reflecting in turn the increased collagen content [1]. The modified Rodnan skin score (MRSS) is a simplification of Rodnan's initial semiquantitative method to assess the extent of skin involvement. It has been shown to be reliable, valid, and responsive to change, although it has been found to have a substantial interobserver variability [2, 3]. The disease phenotype of scleroderma is determined by the extent and specific distribution of skin thickening or sclerosis and is divided into the two principle categories of systemic sclerosis: limited cutaneous systemic sclerosis (lcSSc) and diffuse cutaneous systemic sclerosis (dcSSc). Skin involvement of the trunk and proximal extremities indicates the diffuse phenotype (diffuse scleroderma or dcSSc), whereas acral skin thickening involving the distal extremities only signifies the limited phenotype formerly termed CREST syndrome (for the acronym of **c**alcinosis **R**aynaud's phenomenon, **e**sophageal dysmotility, and **t**elangiectasia) now termed limited scleroderma or lcSSc. The facial skin may be involved in both phenotypes. These phenotypic categories appear to hold true over time and tend to be associated with distinctive antibody markers and disease manifestations. Thus, the diffuse phenotype tends to be more likely to be associated with scleroderma renal crisis and more rapid pulmonary involvement and has a higher mortality risk than lcSSc. Diffuse scleroderma is typically seen in association with scleroderma-specific antibodies to Scl 70 or topoisomerase, RNA polymerase III, and UI RNP. Limited scleroderma (formally termed CREST syndrome) is associated with acral skin involvement, and is more often associated with pulmonary hypertension and calcinosis. LcSSc is typically seen in association with antibodies to centromere antigen. These phenotypic clinical characteristics and antibody associations are quite but not absolutely specific, and occasional patients are difficult to characterize or demonstrate clinical and/or serologic features which are overlapping. While the two group classification into limited and diffuse scleroderma is conventional and generally accepted, others have suggested other subtyping including systemic sclerosis sine scleroderma and splitting the limited patients into those with finger involvement alone and an intermediate group with forearm and distal leg but not trunk involvement [4].

In the physical examination of the skin in a patient with known or suspected scleroderma, it is absolutely critical in the phenotypic assessment to determine the presence or absence of involvement of the trunk and proximal skin sclerosis. This may require attention to subtle changes in the skin appearance on the trunk, especially around the clavicles in particular which may develop a shiny quality before more obvious changes in skin thickness (Fig. 34.1). Repeated assessments may be required. Important is also the technique of assessing skin thickness or sclerosis and should not be confused with tightening or tethering of the skin (tightness

R.W. Simms, MD
Rheumatology Section, Boston Medical Center and Boston University School of Medicine, Boston, MA, USA
e-mail: rsimms@bu.edu

J. Varga et al. (eds.), *Scleroderma*, DOI 10.1007/978-3-319-31407-5_34

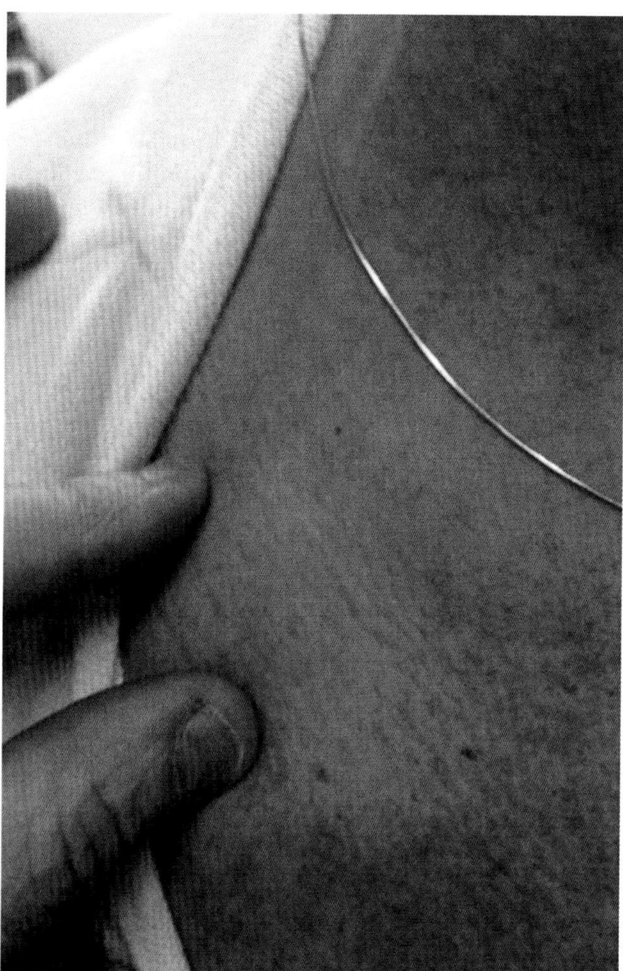

Fig. 34.1 Assessment of skin thickness on the chest. Modified Rodnan Skin Score of 3

without skin thickness or sclerosis) which is common over the digits in long-standing disease, often with contractures. Here the skin is tightened or stretched but is importantly not thickened, a critical determinant of the MRSS. In the author's experience, using the tips of both thumbs or thumb and forefinger in a gradual rolling motion on the skin surface moving the thumbs or thumb and forefinger tip together is the optimal approach to assess the degree of skin thickness or sclerosis (Fig. 34.1). Skin surface which can be pinched in this manner together to 1 mm or less is typically normal or scores zero on the MRSS (Fig. 34.1). The skin which can be pinched together close to but not 1 mm (typically about 2–5 mm) is considered MRSS score of 1. The skin which can still be pinched together or rolled between the fingers but not as closely or as easily as MRSS score of 1 (typically about 5–15 mm) is considered a MRSS score of 2 (Fig. 34.2a). The skin which cannot be pinched together or rolled under the fingers at all is considered a MRSS score of 3 (Fig. 34.2b). Tethered skin, typically seen in long-standing disease where the skin is atrophic but taught, typically because it is stretched tightly over the fingers, should not be confused with thickened skin and should be given a skin score of zero.

Assessment of Skin Disease: The Modified Rodnan Skin Score

The total MRSS is a compilation of 17 total body areas added numerically where each area is scored with 1 number assessment from 0 to 3 with the patient assessed in the sitting position. The areas assessed are the fingers (distal to the metacarpal phalangeal joints, but proximal to the proximal

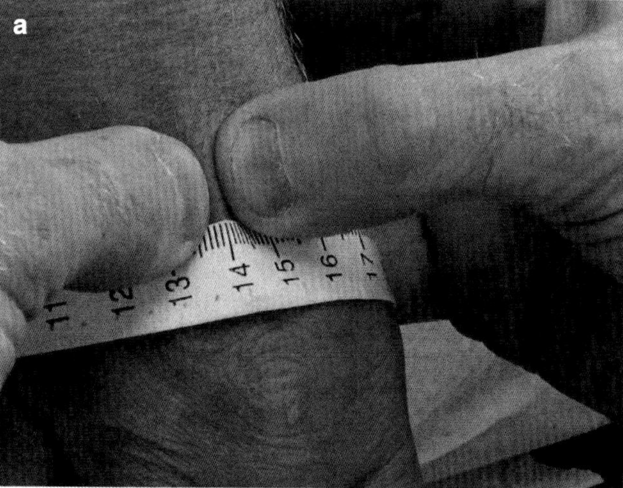

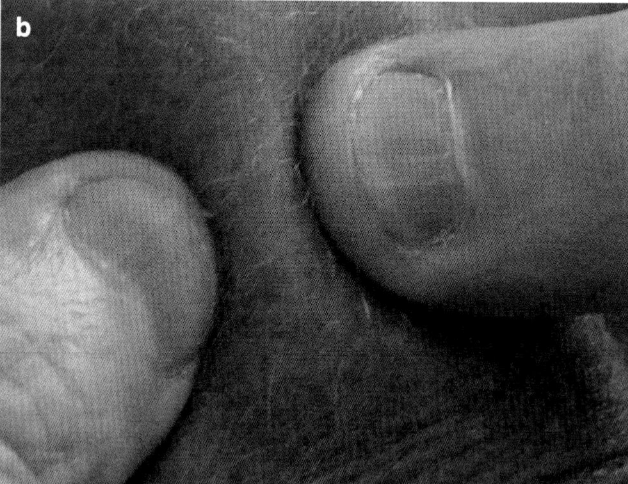

Fig. 34.2 (**a**) Assessment of skin thickness. Skin sclerosis with a modified Rodnan skin score of 2. (**b**) Assessment of skin thickness, normal skin

interphalangeal joints), the dorsum of the hands, the forearms (from wrist to elbows), the upper arm along the lateral aspect, the face (especially at the malar area or zygoma), the anterior chest (especially just below the clavicles), the abdomen, the anterior thighs, and the lower legs and feet. The examiner should be careful to avoid confusion of skin sclerosis with excess subcutaneous fat, especially on the face (the cheeks) and the anterior thighs. Often a larger body area will have skin in some regions of the same area which differs in the score: for example, the distal forearm may be scored as 3 with extensive skin thickening, but be normal more proximally in the forearm. Expert examiners in this situation will frequently "average" the score of this body to a score of 2 or give the area the maximal score of 3. Consistency in the repeated examination of the same patient is required by the examiner to be either an "averager" or "maximizer." Most scorers use the averaging method (Dan Furst MD, personal communication).

Investigators have explored other modalities in an attempt to more objectively measure skin involvement in scleroderma (Table 34.1).

Rodnan's initial description of the extent of skin thickness correlating with collagen content was extended by Verrechia et al.'s observation that the histological extent of skin fibrosis correlated closely with the MRSS. Interestingly, both skin fibrosis and MRSS were associated with the extent of TGFβ signaling in SSc skin fibroblasts and reduced in parallel following treatment with immunoablation followed by ASCT [1, 11].

Several investigators have assessed the utility of durometry in scleroderma skin. The durometer is a pressure gauge which measures surface hardness and was developed for industrial applications. It does seem to correlate with extent of skin induration and the MRSS as well as change in MRSS, but it may also be difficult to assess in certain anatomic locations, especially in the upper extremities, where its reliability and interobserver variability were problematic [10]. Ultrasound has also been evaluated in scleroderma skin as a method to assess skin thickness. Moore et al. found that this technique at 17 anatomic sites had good measurement precision, and inter- as well as intra-observer variability, but it was not correlated with change nor with the MRSS. Balbir-Gurman used a suction device to measure skin elasticity in patients with lcSSc and dcSSc as well as normal controls and found skin extensibility reduced in patients with dcSSc compared to lcSSc and normal controls, and while the observed changes correlated with the MRSS, these findings were not studied over time to determine sensitivity to change [8].

Serial skin biopsies with assessment of gene microarrays and proteomics are increasingly viewed as an important assessment tool for measuring disease outcomes in clinical trials, but currently have no clear utility in the routine diagnosis and management of individual patients. It is possible that in the future, skin biopsy assessment of one's genomic profile may assist in prognosis and selection of specific treatments [12].

Tendon Friction Rubs

In addition to assessing the distribution and extent of skin sclerosis, the initial evaluation should include assessment of oral aperture (in millimeter, from incisor to incisor), recording the location and extent of contractures and the presence or absence of tendon friction rubs. Tendon friction rubs (TFRs) are thought to represent the inflammatory changes in the tenosynovium which occur in progressive skin involvement early in the diffuse phenotype [13]. They occur most commonly in the wrists and ankles, but also may occur at the knees, elbows, and shoulders. Originally described by Westphal in 1876 and further by Shulman in 1961, they were characterized as grating sensations due to fibrinous deposits on the surface of tendon sheaths and overlying fascia during movement of affected extremity [14]. Steen and Medsger further noted the "leathery crepitus" characterizing TFRs at the knees, wrists, fingers, and ankles [13]. Steen et al. described TFRs in a large US cohort and found that these were associated with extensive skin involvement, joint contractures, cardiac and renal involvement, and poor survival. In multiple regression analyses, the presence of one or more tendon friction rubs was one of the best predictors of both evolution to diffuse scleroderma and reduced survival [13].

Table 34.1 Measurement techniques of the skin: correlates of the MRSS

Modality	References
Biochemical: collagen content and skin thickness	Rodnan et al. [5]
Durometry: skin hardness	Falanga and Bucalo [6] and Merkel et al. [7]
Elastometry: biomechanical properties of the skin	Balbir-Gurman [6, 8]
Ultrasound: skin thickness	Moore et al. [9]
Histological correlates: myofibroblasts and hyalinized collagen; immunostaining for TGFβ	Kissin et al. [10]
	Verrachia et al. [11]

Khanna et al. examined data from the D-penicillamine trial to determine the relationship between TFRs and changes in MRSS, HAQ-disability index. Of 134 patients enrolled in the trial, 49 (37 %) had TFR at baseline, and in regression analyses, changes in TFR over 6 and 12 months were found to predict changes in MRSS and HAQ-DI over 12 and 24 months, respectively [15].

Dore and colleagues studied 287 early dcSSc patients at the University of Pittsburgh Scleroderma Center between 1980 and 2006 who had palpable TFRs and matched them with 287 dcSSc patients without TFRs. They found that early dcSSc patients with ≥1 TFR had a >twofold risk of developing renal crisis, cardiac, or gastrointestinal complications [16]. In a large prospective cohort analysis, TFRs appear to independently predict disease progression in early SSc. Avouac and colleagues examined the large EUSTAR prospective cohort that included 1,301 patients with disease duration of <3 years at inclusion and follow-up of at least 2 years [17]: TFRs (HR 1.32, 95 % CI 1.03–1.70), joint synovitis (HR: 1.26, 95 % CI 1.01–1.59), diffuse cutaneous subset (HR: 1.30, 95 % CI 1.05–1.61), and the presence of anti-topoisomerase antibodies (HR: 1.25, 95 % CI 1.02–1.53).

Time Course of Skin Involvement and Assessment of Duration

Critical in the evaluation of all scleroderma patients is determining disease chronology or duration for two principle reasons: (1) adequate staging for trial inclusion and (2) appropriate management. Disease duration or chronology is important especially in skin disease, because of the time-dependent nature of spontaneous skin improvement. Rapid progression of skin involvement (and other organ involvement) predominately occurs in the earlier stages of disease, especially in the diffuse phenotype [18]. Conversely, in late-stage disease, skin fibrosis typically remains quite stable. Other manifestations of the disease may also stabilize in a time-dependent manner, for example, pulmonary fibrosis [19]. Decisions about treatment thus are best informed by an attempt to gauge the duration of disease. Late-stage or long-standing disease may therefore not change with time and not require nor benefit from aggressive intervention.

Measurement of extent of skin involvement may be used as a surrogate measure of disease severity and mortality in patients with dcSSc – an increase in skin thickening is associated with involvement of internal organs and increased mortality. Spontaneous improvement in skin score is associated with other improved outcomes [18]. Thus, an improvement of >25 % of peak skin score and a rate of change of at least 5 units/year have been shown to have improved survival (90 %) at 5 and 10 years compared to diffuse scleroderma patients who do not meet this threshold (77 %) for improvement in the skin [18]. In patients with dcSSc, the natural history of skin fibrosis is rapid initial increase, followed by stabilization and then gradual improvement. Within this general pattern, however, is substantial individual variability [18, 20].

The time course of skin involvement progression and regression is relatively well established but may differ between that reported in cohort studies compared to clinical trials. Amjadi and colleagues analyzed the course of the modified Rodnan skin score in three large negative multicenter trials (the D-penicillamine, human recombinant relaxin, and oral bovine type I collagen clinical trials) [21]. Since the course or natural history of MRSS may change depending on how disease onset is defined, Amjadi et al. evaluated the course of MRSS in these three trials of therapy by two methods: (1) by disease duration defined at baseline by the date of onset of the first non-Raynaud's symptom characteristic of SSc and (2) by disease duration defined at baseline by the date of onset of Raynaud's phenomenon [21]. Data were pooled across trials and analyzed independent of treatment assignment. MRSS was found to improve irrespective of the SSc disease duration (defined either from the first non-Raynaud's sign or from the first symptom including Raynaud's phenomenon). Interestingly, on average, having early disease was not associated with worsening of the MRSS during the trials as previously reported in natural history cohorts [21]. It is possible that patients who had experienced worsening skin disease declined to participate in these trials or that "regression to mean" occurred, i.e., patients who participate in trials tend to do so when their disease is at its worst and therefore tend to improve on average statistically.

Individual body sites within the MRSS appear to differ with respect to sensitivity to change over time. Kaldas and colleagues examined data from two large randomized controlled trials which tested either recombinant human relaxin or type I oral collagen in dcSSc [22]. They determined the magnitude of effect size and its mean change in each body site used in the total MRSS. The total MRSS was found to have a large effect size in each of the two studies; the chest, forearms, and hands had moderated effect size, whereas the lower extremities, face, abdomen, and fingers had small effect size. The authors argued that exclusion of relatively static body sites might improve the sensitivity of the overall MRSS to change [22].

In general, chronology or duration is determined from the date of onset of the first non-Raynaud's symptom. Utilizing the onset of Raynaud's phenomenon has been criticized because of the observation that some patients may experience the phenomenon for many years prior to other symptoms more clearly attributable to fibrotic manifestations. This seems especially true in patients with lcSSc. The vast majority of recent clinical trials have utilized this method of staging [23–26]. Medsger has argued, however, that this approach may confound estimating the disease duration by long enough to allow some "early disease" patients to be included in trials after their skin disease has already reached its peak or maximum MRSS (see Chap. 4). A recent longitudinal analysis of skin scores in a dcSSc cohort may support Medsger's opinion. Shand et al. studied a large, single-center cohort of 225 patients with dcSSc, for whom serial clinical information was available within 24 months of the onset of the first non-Raynaud's symptom of SSc [27]. End points assessed included death and heart, lung, kidney, and gastrointestinal tract involvement. Linear trajectory modeling was applied to identify patients with similar trajectory of MRSS over the first 3 years of follow-up. Three subgroups were identified: high baseline/nonimprover, high baseline/improver, low baseline/improver. Importantly, there was no low baseline/nonimprover group. Survival was lowest in the subgroup of patients who had a high baseline skin score and little improvement during follow-up (high baseline/nonimprovers) [27]. These patients had a mean initial MRSS of 42 and a mortality almost three times greater than the other two groups. Patients who had high baseline score but improved (high baseline/improvers) had similar survival to those who had low baseline scores and improved (low baseline/improved) [27]. Interestingly, the highest frequency of major internal organ-based complications was seen in the high baseline/improver group, suggesting that survival may not be directly attributable to the number of internal organs involved, but be associated with the severity of internal organ complications, and may be reflected in the nonimproving organ score [27].

To define predictive parameters of progressive skin fibrosis in dcSSc, Maurer and colleagues studied the EUSTAR dataset and identified 637 patients who had dcSSc, MRSS documented at first visit ≥7, and adequate data for MRSS at follow-up in 12 months [28]. Approximately, 10 % had progressive skin disease at the 12-month follow-up defined as an increase in MRSS >5 and ≥25 % from baseline to second visit (considered clinically meaningful changes). The association of joint synovitis, short disease duration, and low MRSS at baseline was found to be most predictive factors in a subsequently evaluated validation cohort for progressive skin disease [28].

In a prospective cohort study of 1,301 patients with SSc from the EUSTAR database with disease duration <3 years at entry and at least 2 years of follow-up, joint synovitis and tendon friction rubs were independently predictive of worsening of MRSS. TFRs were also confirmed to be an independent predictor of scleroderma renal crisis (HR 2.33, 95 % CI 1.03–6.19) [17].

Treatment of Skin Disease

At this time there is a paucity of effective therapy of skin disease in SSc. Chapter 33 reviews topical care of skin disease, while the main focus of this chapter is systemic therapy. Many different approaches have been attempted including immunosuppressive and immunoablative therapies and biologic agents. The reader is referred to Chaps. 41 and 42 for an extensive review of these approaches with respect to overall disease management. The discussion below will focus on the specific findings with respect to the skin.

Initial therapy of progressive skin disease frequently includes symptomatic treatment of severe pruritus. Recent studies suggest that pruritus is the result of small fiber neuropathy, and gabapentin may thus have a therapeutic role [29, 30]. The reader is referred to Chaps. 20, 32, and 33, for a discussion of topical skin care, therapy of digital ulcers, and approach to calcinosis.

Over the last two decades, immunomodulation and most recently immunoablation or myeloablation followed by autologous hematopoietic stem cell (HSC) transplantation have been evaluated as therapeutic strategies in systemic sclerosis. The reader is referred to Chaps. 41 and 42 for additional details on the pharmacology and trial design utilizing these approaches.

Immunomodulation in the context of placebo-controlled trials appears to confer modest benefit with respect to skin disease, but there has been only one reported controlled trial to date establishing the efficacy of immunomodulation or immunosuppression, either at conventional or high doses, in which skin disease has been the primary outcome [31] (Table 34.2).

Two randomized, placebo-controlled trials have examined methotrexate (MTX) in scleroderma with skin assessment via MRSS as a primary outcome. Den Hoogen evaluated

Table 34.2 Randomized, controlled therapeutic trials with MRSS as the primary outcome

Agent	MRSS treatment effect vs. placebo	Notes
Methotrexate	Pope et al.: small benefit Den Hoogen: not significant	Seen only in between group differences with intention to treat analysis
Relaxin	No benefit	
D-penicillamine	No benefit (high- vs. low dose)	
Oral collagen	No benefit	

intramuscular MTX at a dose of 15 mg weekly in a small study of dcSSc ($n = 11$) and lcSSc ($n = 18$) of less than 3 years duration for 24 weeks [32]. An intention to treat analysis showed a trend toward improvement in MRSS in MTX-treated patients compared to placebo ($p = 0.06$). A multicenter trial of methotrexate versus placebo, with MRSS as the primary outcome, showed a trend toward improvement in the methotrexate arm [31]. Seventy-one patients with dcSSc (disease duration <3 years) were randomized to MTX (15–17.5 mg orally per week) or placebo for 12 months. MTX had a favorable effect on group differences in the change in MRSS over the course of the trial (−4.3 in the MTX group vs. +1.8 in the placebo group, $p < 0.009$), but the difference was small and close to the threshold of a clinically meaningful benefit, and physician global assessment was not significantly different [31]. Pope and colleagues using a Bayesian reanalysis of their original trial data concluded that the probability that treatment with MTX results in better mean outcomes was 94 % for MRSS and that 96 % probability that at least two of three primary outcomes were better on treatment [33]. Based on these findings and expert opinion, EULAR and EUSTAR MTX is recommended for treatment of skin manifestations of early dcSSc [34]. Others in the USA recommend MTX with a dose of 15–25 mg once weekly for skin disease in the absence of lung disease [35]. In the author's opinion, MTX may be a reasonable choice of therapy for patients with mild skin involvement with dcSSc, i.e., MRSS <30 and no significant ILD.

Mycophenolate mofetil (MMF, CellCept) and mycophenolate sodium (MS, Myfortic) are hydrolyzed after absorption to the active drug mycophenolic acid. Mycophenolic acid inhibits the conversion of inosine monophosphate to guanosine monophosphate, thereby inhibiting lymphocyte activation. MMF or MS is widely used in autoimmune disease as a steroid-sparing agent and has been shown to be equivalent in efficacy to IV cyclophosphamide in SLE-associated diffuse proliferative nephritis [36]. It is currently undergoing evaluation in a randomized controlled trial in SSc-associated ILD (Scleroderma Lung Study II) in comparison with oral cyclophosphamide, but only open-label trials in small numbers of patients are published with skin disease as a primary outcome. These generally reinforce the observation that long-term therapy is tolerated well for most patients at up to 3 g per day and show modest improvements in the MRSS [35]. In the author's opinion, mycophenolate is a more potent immunosuppressive agent than methotrexate and may have a higher infection risk potential [37, 38]. Its benefits in skin disease alone appear to be modest and therefore should be used with caution in patients with moderate skin involvement (i.e., MRSS <30).

Other randomized, controlled studies of immunosuppressive therapy in scleroderma include the Scleroderma Lung Study 1 (SLS-1) which compared oral placebo to oral cyclophosphamide over a 12-month period in which the primary outcome was change in FVC over the course of the trial in a total of 84 patients. MRSS change was one of several secondary outcome variables. The results of SLS-1 showed a statistically significant, albeit modest benefit in lung function parameters (FVC) in the experimental arm [39]. In the dcSSc subgroup of SLS-1 accounting for approximately 40 % of the studied patients, and therefore eligible for MRSS evaluation, modest improvement in MRSS occurred in the cyclophosphamide arm, although the magnitude of improvement did not meet the MRSS >5 clinically meaningful threshold [39].

In the author's experience, intravenous cyclophosphamide may occasionally be associated with significant improvement in the skin score and therefore should be considered as first-line therapy in patients with severe skin involvement or rapidly progressive skin involvement who are not considered candidates for clinical trials. Its infection risk potential is likely to be similar to mycophenolate and certainly higher than methotrexate. Intravenous cyclophosphamide also has additional risks of hemorrhagic cystitis, bladder malignancy, and bone marrow suppression (see additional discussion of toxicities elsewhere in this text) [40].

While intravenous immunoglobulin therapy (IVIG) is commonly used to treat other autoimmune diseases [2], its effects on patients with SSc remain unclear. Thirty patients were treated with adjunctive IVIG (2 g/kg/month) for refractory, active dcSSc. The mean baseline mRSS of our cohort was 29.6 ± 7.2, and this significantly decreased to 24.1 ± 9.6 ($n = 29$, $p = 0.0011$) at 6 months, 22.5 ± 10.0 ($n = 25$, $p = 0.0001$) at 12 months, 20.6 ± 11.8 ($n = 23$, $p = 0.0001$) at 18 months, and 15.3 ± 6.4 ($n = 15$, $p < 0.0001$) at 24 months [41]. Takehara et al. reported the use of IVIG in a randomized, double-blind, placebo-controlled trial of 63 patients with diffuse SSc. In this trial, participants were administered a single cycle of IVIG or placebo infusions. At 12 weeks, there were no differences in change in mRSS between the two groups. Participants whose skin score did not improve by at least five points at 12 weeks were given an additional cycle of IVIG. Those who received two IVIG treatments had greater improvements in skin score over time than those who initially received placebo followed by a later IVIG infusion. These data suggest that IVIG may be a beneficial adjunctive therapy for patients with active dcSSc who are unresponsive to more traditional immunosuppressive treatments, but further studies are necessary to affirm these findings [41].

High-dose immunosuppression with autologous hematopoietic stem cell transplantation (HSCT) has recently been studied in patients with early diffuse scleroderma and poor prognosis in which the MRSS was evaluated as a secondary outcome. The ASSIST trial was an open-label, randomized, phase II trial, in which patients with dcSSc and pulmonary involvement were treated with intravenous cyclophosphamide followed by either HSC transplantation (treatment arm) or monthly pulse intravenous cyclophosphamide (control arm). At 12 months follow-up, all ten patients who received HSC transplantation showed improvement in skin score (mRSS decrease by at least 25%), and in lung function (increase of at least 10% in FVC) compared with none of the nine patients in the control arm [42].

Results from the Autologous Stem Cell Transplantation International Scleroderma (ASTIS) trial, a multicenter European trial, recently showed that high-dose immunosuppressive therapy and autologous HSC transplantation in patients with early dcSSc, who had poor prognosis (most of whom had either interstitial lung disease or a history of scleroderma renal crisis), experienced a survival benefit over conventional immunosuppression. In this study, 156 patients were randomly assigned to either conventional immune suppression with monthly intravenous cyclophosphamide or to high-dose cyclophosphamide followed by autologous HSC transplantation (ASCT), with event-free survival as the primary outcome [43]. At baseline the mean MRSS was 24.8 ± 8.1 in ASCT arm and 25.8± in the control arm. At a median of 5.8 years of follow-up, there was a significant event-free survival (death or irreversible organ failure) benefit in the transplantation group. Area under the curve analysis of MRSS showed significant improvement from baseline to 2-year follow-up in the ASCT arm (−19.9) compared to the control group (−8.8) (difference, 11.1 [95% CI, 7.3–15.0]). This approach, while clearly of benefit for patients with a poor prognosis, is not for all patients – the 10% treatment-related mortality occurred with stem cell transplantation.

Thus, although conventional doses of immunosuppressive therapy appear to have modest benefit on skin disease, high-dose immunosuppression followed by autologous hematopoietic stem cell transplantation may have potentially even greater efficacy with respect to skin disease. Nevertheless, the latter approach remains risky and thus highly controversial for patients without significant extra-dermal involvement given the high potential treatment-associated mortality.

Biologic Therapies for Skin Disease

Currently, there are several ongoing or recently completed studies of biologic therapies, both open label and randomized in which the skin in the form of MRSS or a gene expression biomarker in the skin is a primary outcome. Biologic therapies for skin disease alone should be considered experimental, and administration of these therapies is thus best conducted in the context of a clinical trial.

Anti-transforming Growth Factor β (TGFβ)

Fresolimumab is a first in class human IgG4 kappa recombinant monoclonal antibody capable of neutralizing all mammalian isoforms of TGFβ [44]. It appears to have higher affinity for TGFβ than its predecessor CAT-192 which showed no efficacy in early dcSSc [25]. In a phase I study in patients with advanced malignant melanoma or renal cell cancer, it demonstrated acceptable safety and preliminary evidence of antitumor activity [45]. It is currently undergoing evaluation in early dcSSc (MRSS >15 without significant ILD or history of SRC) with a skin biomarker to detect TGFβ-responsive gene expression and MRSS as primary outcomes (Table 34.3).

Anti-type 1 Interferon

Peripheral blood cells from SSc and SLE patients share a similar IFN-inducible gene expression pattern [46]. In particular, a subset of SSc patients shows a "lupus-like" high IFN-inducible phenotype that correlates with the presence of anti-topoisomerase-1 and anti-U1RNA antibodies [46]. Furthermore, IFNa has been reported to induce TLR3 in dermal fibroblasts, and stimulation with poly I:C resulted in increased production of the profibrotic cytokine IL-6, and increased expression of type I IFN-induced genes and proteins is found in the blood and skin or patients with SSc [46]. Also, IFN therapy appeared to exacerbate SSc [47]. A phase I, open-label dose-escalation trial of MEDI-546, an anti-type interferon monoclonal anti-

Table 34.3 Ongoing trials or recently completed of biologic therapy with MRSS or skin biomarkers as the primary outcome

Agent	Target	Design	NIH#
Fresolimumab	TGFβ	Phase I, open label	NCT01284322
Anti-type I interferon	Type 1 interferon	Phase I, open label	NCT00930683
Rilonacept	IL-1	Phase II, randomized, placebo controlled	NCT01538719
Tocilizumab	IL-6	Phase II/III randomized, double-blind placebo controlled	NCT01532869
Abatacept	T cell co-stimulation	Phase II randomized, double-blind placebo controlled	NCT02161406

body, was evaluated in patients with predominately dcSSc (94.1 %) who had a MRSS of at least two on an area amenable to repeat biopsy [48]. MEDI-546 is a human IgG kappa monoclonal antibody directed against the heterodimeric type I IFNa receptor. Following a 28-day screening period, subjects were enrolled to receive either escalating single or multiple intravenous doses of MEDI-546. Of 34 subjects, 32 completed treatment. Four treatment emergent serious adverse events occurred including a skin ulcer, osteomyelitis, vertigo, and chronic myelogenous leukemia (CML). Only CML was considered possibly treatment related [48]. Peak inhibition of the type 1 IFN signature occurred in whole blood within 1 day and in the skin after 7 days. In patients with positive baseline skin signatures for type 1 IFN-inducible genes (15 of the total, 11 in the single-dose groups, 4 in the multiple-dose groups), there was a reduction in type 1 IFN-inducible genes in the skin seen at day 7 and day 28, respectively [48]. Further studies will be needed to determine if any meaningful clinical improvement will result from anti-type interferon monoclonal antibody therapy.

Anti-interleukin 1 (Anti-IL1)

Animal models of fibrosis suggest that IL-1 plays a key role [49]. The mechanism linking IL-1 to fibrosis involves both TGFβ- and smad3-dependent stimulation. TGFβ, IL-1, and IL-6 participate in Th17 cell priming and are increased in the tissues and serum of SSc patients [49]. Rilonacept is a dimeric fusion protein, consisting of the ligand-binding domains of the extracellular portions of the human IL-1 receptor accessory protein linked to the Fc portion of human IgG1 [50]. It is designed to attach to and neutralize IL-1 before IL-1 can bind to cell surface receptors and generate signals that trigger inflammation. Rilonacept has been shown to be effective in auto-inflammatory syndromes characterized by high levels of IL-1 such as CAPS (cryopyrin-associated periodic syndromes), DIRA (deficiency of IL-1 receptor antagonist), and systemic juvenile idiopathic arthritis (JIA) [50, 51]. Rilonacept is currently undergoing evaluation in a short-term (8 week) randomized, placebo-controlled trial with a biomarker of skin-based primary outcome (Table 34.3).

Tocilizumab (Anti-interleukin 6 (Anti-IL 6))

IL-6 is a pleiotropic pro-inflammatory multifunctional cytokine produced by a variety of cell types including lymphocytes, monocytes, and fibroblasts [52]. It was originally identified as a hepatocyte growth factor and as a B cell stimulatory factor that induces the final maturation of B cells into antibody-producing cells [52]. Its secretion is stimulated by IL-1 b, IL-2, and TNF-α [52]. IL-6 is also involved in the differentiation of B and T cells and is a T cell migration factor. IL-6 dysregulation appears to occur in SSc and may play a prominent role in pathogenesis. IL-6 is elevated early in the course of dcSSc, and fibroblasts from lesional skin constitutively produce higher levels of IL-6 than non-lesional or healthy skin [53]. Tocilizumab is a humanized monoclonal anti-IL-6 receptor antibody, and thus there is substantial biologic rationale to consider tocilizumab, an IL-6 antagonist in scleroderma. Neves et al. reported three patients with refractory SSc and ILD who appeared to improve or stabilize with tocilizumab [54]. Shima and colleagues treated two patients with dcSSc at 8 mg/kg monthly for 6 months and showed significant reduction in the MRSS [55]. The results of a phase II/III multicenter, randomized, double-blind placebo 48-week-controlled trial of tocilizumab in SSc (Table 34.1) remain pending.

Role of T Cell Activation Inhibition (Anti-cytotoxic T-Lymphocyte-Associated Protein) (Anti-CTL4)

Twenty patients with refractory polyarthritis and seven with refractory myopathy in the setting of SSc and treated with either abatacept (a fusion protein that inhibits CLT4) or tocilizumab were evaluated in the EUSTAR dataset [56]. Fifteen received tocilizumab, and 12 abatacept. After 11 months treatment of patients with abatacept, joint parameters improved significantly with 6/11 patients fulfilling EULAR good-response criteria [57]. Abatacept did not improve muscle outcome measures in SSc myopathy. No significant change was seen for skin or lung fibrosis in the different groups [57].

Conclusions

At this time, there is meager definitive proof of effective therapy in diffuse skin involvement in scleroderma. While there is definite proof of effectiveness of the most aggressive approach to immunosuppression/immune ablation in overall disease management, it is the author's view that patients with skin involvement with a MRSS <30, and no significant extra-dermal disease, should not currently receive this therapy because of the high treatment-associated mortality. For patients such as those with MRSS <30 without serious extra-dermal organ involvement, the author encourages entry into promising experimental therapy. The alternatives to enrollment in a clinical trial includes the use of methotrexate, mycophenolate, or intravenous cyclophosphamide.

References

1. Rodnan GP, Lipinski E, Luksick J. Skin thickness and collagen content in progressive systemic sclerosis and localized scleroderma. Arthritis Rheum. 1979;22(2):130–40.
2. Furst DE, Clements PJ, Steen VD, et al. The modified Rodnan skin score is an accurate reflection of skin biopsy thickness in SSc. J Rheumatology. 1998;25:84–8.
3. Clements P, Lachenbruch P, Seibold J, et al. Inter- and intraobserver variability of total skin thickness score (modified Rodnan TSS) in systemic sclerosis. J Rheumatol. 1995;22:1281–5.
4. Cottrell TR, Wise RA, Wigley FM, et al. The degree of skin involvement identifies distinct lung disease outcomes and survival in systemic sclerosis. Ann Rheum Dis. 2014;73(6):1060–6.
5. Rodnan GP, Lipinski E, Lukesick J. Skin thickness and collagen content in progressive SSc. Arthritis Rheum. 1979;22:130–40.
6. Falanga V, Bucalo B. Use of a durometer to assess skin hardness. J Am Acad Dermatol. 1993;29(1):47–51.
7. Merkel PA, Silliman NP, Denton CP, et al. Validity, reliability, and feasibility of durometer measurements of scleroderma skin disease in a multicenter treatment trial. Arthritis Rheum. 2008;59(5):699–705.
8. Balbir-Gurman A, Denton CP, Nichols B, et al. Noninvasive measurement of biomechanical skin properties in systemic sclerosis. Ann Rheum Dis. 2002;61(3):237–41.
9. Moore TL, Lunt M, McManus B, et al. Seventeen-point dermal ultrasound scoring system – a reliable measure of skin thickness in patients with systemic sclerosis. Rheumatology (Oxford). 2003;42(12):1559–63.
10. Kissin EY, Schiller AM, Gelbard RB, et al. Durometry for the assessment of skin disease in systemic sclerosis. Arthritis Rheum. 2006;55(4):603–9.
11. Verrecchia F, Laboureau J, Verola O, et al. Skin involvement in scleroderma – where histological and clinical scores meet. Rheumatology (Oxford). 2007;46(5):833–41.
12. Varga J, Robertson E. Genomic advances in systemic sclerosis: it is time for precision. Arthritis Rheum. 2015;67(11):2801–5.
13. Steen VD, Medsger Jr TA. The palpable tendon friction rub: an important physical examination finding in patients with systemic sclerosis. Arthritis Rheum. 1997;40(6):1146–51.
14. Shulman LE, Kurban AK, Harvey AM. Tendon friction rubs in progressive system sclerosis (scleroderma). Trans Assoc Am Phys. 1961;74:378–88.
15. Khanna PP, Furst DE, Clements PJ, et al. Tendon friction rubs in early diffuse systemic sclerosis: prevalence, characteristics and longitudinal changes in a randomized controlled trial. Rheumatology (Oxford). 2010;49(5):955–9.
16. Dore A, Lucas M, Ivanco D, et al. Significance of palpable tendon friction rubs in early diffuse cutaneous systemic sclerosis. Arthritis Care Res. 2013;65(8):1385–9.
17. Avouac J, Walker UA, Hachulla E, et al. Joint and tendon involvement predicts disease progression in systemic sclerosis: a EUSTAR prospective study. Ann Rheum Dis. 2016;75:103–9.
18. Steen VD, Medsger Jr TA. Improvement in skin thickening in systemic sclerosis associated with improved survival. Arthritis Rheum. 2001;44(12):2828–35.
19. Herzog EL, Mathur A, Tager AM, et al. Review: interstitial lung disease associated with systemic sclerosis and idiopathic pulmonary fibrosis: how similar and distinct? Arthritis Rheumatol. 2014;66(8):1967–78.
20. Perera A, Fertig N, Lucas M, et al. Clinical subsets, skin thickness progression rate, and serum antibody levels in systemic sclerosis patients with anti-topoisomerase I antibody. Arthritis Rheum. 2007;56(8):2740–6.
21. Amjadi S, Maranian P, Furst DE, et al. Course of the modified Rodnan skin thickness score in systemic sclerosis clinical trials: analysis of three large multicenter, double-blind, randomized controlled trials. Arthritis Rheum. 2009;60(8):2490–8.
22. Kaldas M, Khanna PP, Furst DE, et al. Sensitivity to change of the modified Rodnan skin score in diffuse systemic sclerosis – assessment of individual body sites in two large randomized controlled trials. Rheumatology (Oxford). 2009;48(9):1143–6.
23. Clements PJ, Furst DE, Wong WK, et al. High-dose versus low-dose D-penicillamine in early diffuse systemic sclerosis: analysis of a two-year, double-blind, randomized, controlled clinical trial. Arthritis Rheum. 1999;42:1194–203.
24. Seibold J, Korn J, Simms R, et al. Recombinant human relaxin in the treatment of scleroderma: a randomized, double-blind, placebo-controlled trial. Ann Intern Med. 2000;132:871–9.
25. Denton CP, Merkel PA, Furst DE, et al. Recombinant human anti-transforming growth factor beta1 antibody therapy in systemic sclerosis: a multicenter, randomized, placebo-controlled phase I/II trial of CAT-192. Arthritis Rheum. 2007;56(1):323–33.
26. Postlethwaite AE, Wong WK, Clements P, et al. A multicenter, randomized, double-blind, placebo-controlled trial of oral type I collagen treatment in patients with diffuse cutaneous systemic sclerosis: I. oral type I collagen does not improve skin in all patients, but may improve skin in late-phase disease. Arthritis Rheum. 2008;58(6):1810–22.
27. Shand L, Lunt M, Nihtyanova S, et al. Relationship between change in skin score and disease outcome in diffuse cutaneous systemic sclerosis: application of a latent linear trajectory model. Arthritis Rheum. 2007;56(7):2422–31.
28. Maurer B, Graf N, Michel BA, et al. Prediction of worsening of skin fibrosis in patients with diffuse cutaneous systemic sclerosis using the EUSTAR database. Ann Rheum Dis. 2015;74:1124–31.
29. Brenaut E, Marcorelles P, Genestet S, et al. Pruritus: an underrecognized symptom of small-fiber neuropathies. J Am Acad Dermatol. 2015;72(2):328–32.
30. Maciel AA, Cunha PR, Laraia IO, et al. Efficacy of gabapentin in the improvement of pruritus and quality of life of patients with notalgia paresthetica. An Bras Dermatol. 2014;89(4):570–5.
31. Pope JE, Bellamy N, Seibold JR, et al. A randomized, controlled trial of methotrexate versus placebo in early diffuse scleroderma. Arthritis Rheum. 2001;44(6):1351–8.
32. Van den Hoogen FHJ, Boerbooms AMT, Van de Putte LBA. Methotrexate treatment in scleroderma. Am J Med. 1989;87:116–7.
33. Johnson SR, Feldman BM, Pope JE, et al. Shifting our thinking about uncommon disease trials: the case of methotrexate in scleroderma. J Rheumatol. 2009;36(2):323–9.
34. Walker KM, Pope J. Expert agreement on EULAR/EUSTAR recommendations for the management of systemic sclerosis. J Rheumatol. 2011;38(7):1326–8.
35. Frech TM, Shanmugam VK, Shah AA, et al. Treatment of early diffuse systemic sclerosis skin disease. Clin Exp Rheumatol. 2013;31(2 Suppl 76):166–71.
36. Appel GB, Contreras G, Dooley MA, et al. Mycophenolate mofetil versus cyclophosphamide for induction treatment of lupus nephritis. J Am Soc Nephrol: JASN. 2009;20(5):1103–12.
37. Danza A, Ruiz-Irastorza G. Infection risk in systemic lupus erythematosus patients: susceptibility factors and preventive strategies. Lupus. 2013;22(12):1286–94.
38. Subedi A, Magder LS, Petri M. Effect of mycophenolate mofetil on the white blood cell count and the frequency of infection in systemic lupus erythematosus. Rheumatol Int. 2015;35:1687–92.
39. Tashkin DP, Elashoff R, Clements PJ, et al. Cyclophosphamide versus placebo in scleroderma lung disease. N Engl J Med. 2006;354(25):2655–66.

40. Cavallasca JA, Costa CA, Maliandi MD, et al. Severe infections in patients with autoimmune diseases treated with cyclophosphamide. Reumatol Clin. 2014;11:221–3.
41. Poelman CL, Hummers LK, Wigley FM, et al. Intravenous immunoglobulin may be an effective therapy for refractory, active diffuse cutaneous systemic sclerosis. J Rheumatol. 2015;42(2):236–42.
42. Burt RK, Shah SJ, Dill K, et al. Autologous non-myeloablative haemopoietic stem-cell transplantation compared with pulse cyclophosphamide once per month for systemic sclerosis (ASSIST): an open-label, randomised phase 2 trial. Lancet. 2011;378(9790): 498–506.
43. van Laar JM, Farge D, Sont JK, et al. Autologous hematopoietic stem cell transplantation vs intravenous pulse cyclophosphamide in diffuse cutaneous systemic sclerosis: a randomized clinical trial. JAMA. 2014;311(24):2490–8.
44. Trachtman H, Fervenza FC, Gipson DS, et al. A phase 1, single-dose study of fresolimumab, an anti-TGF-beta antibody, in treatment-resistant primary focal segmental glomerulosclerosis. Kidney Int. 2011;79(11):1236–43.
45. Morris JC, Tan AR, Olencki TE, et al. Phase I study of GC1008 (fresolimumab): a human anti-transforming growth factor-beta (TGFbeta) monoclonal antibody in patients with advanced malignant melanoma or renal cell carcinoma. PLoS One. 2014;9(3): e90353.
46. Wu M, Assassi S. The role of type 1 interferon in systemic sclerosis. Frontiers Immunol. 2013;4:266.
47. Black CM, Silman AJ, Herrick AI, et al. Interferon-alpha does not improve outcome at one year in patients with diffuse cutaneous scleroderma: results of a randomized, double-blind, placebo-controlled trial. Arthritis Rheum. 1999;42:299–305.
48. Goldberg A, Geppert T, Schiopu E, et al. Dose-escalation of human anti-interferon-alpha receptor monoclonal antibody MEDI-546 in subjects with systemic sclerosis: a phase 1, multicenter, open label study. Arthritis Res Ther. 2014;16(1):R57.
49. Brembilla NC, Chizzolini C. T cell abnormalities in systemic sclerosis with a focus on Th17 cells. Eur Cytokine Netw. 2012;23(4): 128–39.
50. Jesus AA, Goldbach-Mansky R. IL-1 blockade in autoinflammatory syndromes. Annu Rev Med. 2014;65:223–44.
51. Lovell DJ, Giannini EH, Reiff AO, et al. Long-term safety and efficacy of rilonacept in patients with systemic juvenile idiopathic arthritis. Arthritis Rheum. 2013;65(9):2486–96.
52. Alten R, Maleitzke T. Tocilizumab: a novel humanized anti-interleukin 6 (IL-6) receptor antibody for the treatment of patients with non-RA systemic, inflammatory rheumatic diseases. Ann Med. 2013;45(4):357–63.
53. Barnes TC, Anderson ME, Moots RJ. The many faces of interleukin-6: the role of IL-6 in inflammation, vasculopathy, and fibrosis in systemic sclerosis. Int J Rheumatol. 2011;2011:721608.
54. Fernandes das Neves M, Oliveira S, Amaral MC, et al. Treatment of systemic sclerosis with tocilizumab. Rheumatology (Oxford). 2015;54(2):371–2.
55. Shima Y, Kuwahara Y, Murota H, et al. The skin of patients with systemic sclerosis softened during the treatment with anti-IL-6 receptor antibody tocilizumab. Rheumatology (Oxford). 2010;49(12):2408–12.
56. Elhai M, Meunier M, Matucci-Cerinic M, et al. Outcomes of patients with systemic sclerosis-associated polyarthritis and myopathy treated with tocilizumab or abatacept: a EUSTAR observational study. Ann Rheum Dis. 2013;72(7):1217–20.
57. Elhai M, Meunier M, Matucci-Cerinic M, et al. Outcomes of patients with systemic sclerosis-associated polyarthritis and myopathy treated with tocilizumab or abatacept: a EUSTAR observational study. Ann Rheum Dis. 2013;72:1217–20.

Skeletal Muscle Involvement

35

Andrew L. Mammen

Prevalence and Clinical Features

Although Westphal first described a case of skeletal muscle involvement in scleroderma in 1876 [1], it was considered to be a relatively rare manifestation of the disease until 1968 when Medsger and colleagues systematically evaluated muscle involvement in a cohort of scleroderma patients [2]. They found that out of 53 subjects, 6 (11 %) had "marked," 10 (19 %) had "severe," 18 (34 %) had "moderate," and 9 (17 %) had "minimal" weakness on physical exam; proximal muscle weakness was found in 20 of 38 patients (53 %). Surprisingly, despite the prevalence of weakness on exam, only 20 % of patients complained of subjective weakness.

Numerous smaller studies have documented a frequency of skeletal myopathy in scleroderma patients ranging from 14 to 96 %, depending on the diagnostic criteria used [3–9]. In one of the larger studies to date [10], 1,095 patients with scleroderma were assessed for skeletal myopathy as defined by the presence of proximal muscle weakness as well as one or more of the following: elevated serum CK level, myopathic features on electromyography (EMG), and/or muscle biopsy showing evidence of inflammation, myofiber degeneration, and myofiber necrosis (at least two of these features were required). One hundred eighty-three (17 %) patients fulfilled these criteria.

While most of the studies investigating the prevalence of myopathy in scleroderma have been cross-sectional or retrospective, Toledano and colleagues recently published a prospective study to identify incident cases [11]. From among 137 patients enrolled and followed over an average of 45 months, 9 (6.6 %) patients developed persistent proximal muscle weakness. Of particular interest, these authors also identified elevated serum aldolase levels as a predictive marker for developing myopathy. Specifically, they found that an entry aldolase level of 9 IU/L or higher had 89 % sensitivity and 67 % specificity for predicting which patients would develop persistent muscle weakness within the next 3 years.

Most scleroderma patients with skeletal myopathy have symmetric proximal limb weakness that is indistinguishable from that seen in patients with isolated dermatomyositis or polymyositis. Although distal weakness may be present, it can be difficult to distinguish myopathic weakness from the limitation of movement due to skin sclerosis and the fibrosis of underlying tissues. While rare, several recent reports have described scleroderma patients presenting with profound neck extensor weakness [12–14]. In four of the cases described, prominent neck weakness occurred in the context of mild to moderate weakness of proximal arm and leg muscles with significantly elevated CK levels. However, in one case, a patient was found to have isolated "dropped head syndrome" with intact limb strength and normal serum muscle enzyme levels. Similarly, two sclerodermas presenting with "bent spine" (i.e., camptocormia) due to weakness of the paraspinal muscles also had some weakness of the proximal limb muscles with mildly elevated CK levels [14].

In 1981, West and colleagues reported an association between myositis and myocarditis in patients with scleroderma [5]. A subsequent large study revealed that the prevalence of myocardial disease was significantly higher in scleroderma patients with skeletal myopathy (21 %) compared to those without skeletal myopathy (10 %) [10]. Several recent studies have confirmed this finding [9, 15, 16]. In addition to cardiac involvement, Mimura and colleagues have reported that scleroderma patients with skeletal myopathy also have an increased prevalence of phalangeal contracture, diffuse pigmentation of the skin, and pulmonary fibrosis [9].

Although most reports of myopathy have been reported in patients with systemic sclerosis, patients with localized scleroderma may also have skeletal muscle involvement. A review by Zivkovic and associates summarizes the

A.L. Mammen, MD, PhD
National Institutes of Health, National Institutes of Arthritis and Skin and Musculoskeletal Diseases, Bethesda, MD, USA
e-mail: andrew.mammen@nih.gov; amammen@jhmi.edu

J. Varga et al. (eds.), *Scleroderma*, DOI 10.1007/978-3-319-31407-5_35

12 published cases of inflammatory myopathy occurring in the context of localized scleroderma [17]. The onset of weakness or pain occurred at a mean age of 19 years. Typically, muscle disease occurred in the same region as the skin involvement, most commonly in the arms. Muscle enzyme levels were normal or only mildly elevated and muscle biopsies often revealed perivascular inflammation. Of note, four patients with the "en coup de sabre" variant had hemifacial atrophy and coexisting tongue hemiatrophy, headaches, and/or diplopia.

Muscle Biopsy Features

The histological features of muscle biopsies from patients with scleroderma–myopathy are heterogeneous. These include myofiber necrosis, which is seen in 29–63 % of scleroderma–myopathy cases [2, 18, 19], as well as (a) interstitial fibrosis, (b) microvascular abnormalities, and (c) inflammation. One of the most common abnormalities appears to be increased fibrosis in the perimysium and epimysium, similar to the excessive collagen deposition seen in other tissues from scleroderma patients. Among the 36 biopsy specimens reviewed by Medsger and colleagues, fibrosis was found in 13 (36 %) [2]. Similarly, Thompson reported that 7 of 12 (58 %) biopsies included increased fibrous tissue [3], and Ringel and coworkers described increased endomysial and/or perimysial connective tissue in 5 of 14 (36 %) cases of scleroderma–myopathy [18]. In the studies described above, the analyzed biopsies came either from unselected patients [2, 3] or those with weakness as the sole entry criteria [18]. In a more recent study requiring muscle weakness, myalgia, or elevated CK along with either EMG or muscle biopsy evidence of muscle involvement, only 8 of 35 (23 %) scleroderma–myopathy subjects had increased fibrosis on muscle biopsy [19]. Most recently, Bhansing and colleagues reported that fibrosis was present in 3 of 10 (30 %) biopsies from scleroderma patients with myopathy compared to 2 of 24 (8 %) biopsies from polymyositis patients [20]; the trend for increased fibrosis in overlap patients was not statistically significant.

Vascular changes observed in the muscle tissue of patients with scleroderma–myopathy include endothelial cell swelling [6], thickening of vascular walls [2, 18], basement membrane lamination [3, 6], intimal hypertrophy [18], and loss of capillary density [6, 21]. A small minority of muscle biopsies also show evidence of vasculitis [18, 19]. There is a marked variation in the reported prevalence of one or more of these pathologic changes in biopsies from patients with typical scleroderma–myopathy, ranging from 14 % [2] to 74 % [6, 18, 19]. Interestingly, all five of the muscle biopsies from scleroderma patients presenting with prominent dropped head or camptocormia included notable vascular abnormalities [14].

Although a single report found no evidence of acute inflammation in seven weak scleroderma patients [6], a majority of studies have found a significant degree of inflammation, ranging from 22 % [2] to 63 % [18, 19], in subjects with scleroderma–myopathy. In a large study evaluating 35 muscle biopsies, Ranque reported perimysial inflammation in 31 %, perimysial infiltrates in 20 %, and endomysial infiltrates in 14 % [19]. All six reported cases scleroderma with either dropped head or camptocormia were found to have endomysial and/or perivascular inflammation [13, 14].

Bhansing and colleagues compared clinical and muscle biopsy features of 25 patients with scleroderma–myopathy overlap to those with polymyositis ($n = 40$) or scleroderma ($n = 397$) alone [20]. These investigators found that pulmonary fibrosis was more common in those with overlap disease than in those with just polymyositis or scleroderma. They also found that 96 % of biopsies from scleroderma–myopathy overlap patients had necrotic muscle fibers on biopsy, whereas only 67 % of polymyositis biopsies had this feature. The prevalence of inflammation (79 % vs. 75 %), MHC class I upregulation (92 % vs. 67 %), and membrane attack complex staining (50 % vs. 39 %) was similar in biopsies from patients with overlap and polymyositis alone, respectively.

Precise characterization of the cellular infiltrates in scleroderma–myopathy patients has rarely been reported. In one detailed analysis of 11 scleroderma muscle biopsy specimens by Ahahata and Engel, CD8+ and CD4+ cells were found in roughly equal numbers at sites of perivascular inflammation, whereas CD8+ cells predominated in the perimysium [22]. In the recent study by Ranque et al. [19], three out of four biopsy specimens included CD4+ T cells, B cells, and complement deposition on vascular walls, suggesting that complement-fixing antibodies might be the cause of endothelial injury; the other biopsy specimen included mostly CD8+ T cells suggestive of a cell-mediated immune response. In addition, these investigators reported upregulation of MHC I on the surface of 11 out of 17 (65 %) cases studied.

Autoantibodies

As in other rheumatic diseases, in scleroderma, there is a strong association of unique autoantibodies with distinct clinical phenotypes. Although the mechanisms underlying these associations are not understood, several autoantibodies are preferentially found in patients with scleroderma associated with skeletal muscle disease. Autoantibodies recognizing the nuclear protein "PM-1" were first detected by Wolfe and colleagues in 1977 [23]. Several years later, this antigen was named "PM/Scl" when two separate groups described the presence of these autoantibodies in patients who had features consistent with an overlap between PM and scleroderma [24, 25]. Shortly thereafter, two distinct PM/Scl autoantigens were identified, PM/Scl-75 [26] and PM/Scl-100 [27, 28]. Each of these proteins was subsequently shown to be a component of the human exosome, a complex of proteins involved with ribosomal RNA processing and the degradation of messenger RNA [29].

The clinical features of patients with anti-PM/Scl autoantibodies have been described in numerous reports. Mahler and Raijmakers performed a meta-analysis of relevant studies and calculated that 31 % of patients with scleroderma and either polymyositis or dermatomyositis (i.e., PM/SSc patients) were anti-PM/Scl positive [30]. By comparison, patients with isolated DM, PM, and scleroderma were positive at frequencies of 11 %, 8 %, and 2 %, respectively. In a similar analysis of eight studies published between 1984 and 2006 [25, 31–37], the same authors calculated that 80 out of 139 (59 %) anti-PM/Scl-positive patients were diagnosed with PM/SSc overlap; most of the rest had SSc, PM, or DM alone [30]. In the largest sample of scleroderma patients from the Pittsburgh Scleroderma Databank, the majority (58 %) of PM/Scl-positive patients had inflammation on muscle biopsy [38]. In addition to skeletal myopathy, patients with anti PM/Scl frequently have arthritis, Raynaud's phenomenon, lung disease, kidney disease, and mechanic's hands (Fig. 35.1). In a paper from 2012, Koschik and colleagues tested for anti-PM/Scl autoantibodies in 2,425 patients with scleroderma evaluated at the University of Pittsburgh between 1980 and 2004 [39]. They found 76 (3 %) were anti-PM/Scl positive and among these 33 (1.4 %) had inflammatory myositis. Compared to scleroderma patients without anti-Pm/Scl antibodies, antibody-positive subjects had a significantly increased prevalence of muscle disease (51 % vs. 14 %; $P<0.0001$). Similarly, D'Aoust reported that 55 of 763 (7.2 %) Canadian scleroderma patients were anti-PM/Scl positive [40]. Skeletal muscle disease (along with calcinosis and inflammatory arthritis) was more common in those with PM/Scl reactivity.

Interestingly, certain immunogenetic backgrounds predispose individuals to developing anti-PM/Scl. For example, patients with specific MHC alleles (i.e., HLA-DRB1*0301 (DR3), HLA-DQB1*02, and HLA-DQA1*0501) are predisposed to mounting an anti-PM/Scl response [35, 41]. In contrast, the presence of other MHC alleles (i.e., HLA-DQA1*0101 and HLA-DRB*15/HLA-DRB*16) is protective [42]. The fact that none of the 275 Japanese patients with scleroderma were found to have anti-PM/Scl [43] further underscores importance of genetic factors in the production of these autoantibodies.

As explained above, two different proteins are recognized by anti-PM/Scl autoantibodies, PM/Scl-75 and PM/Scl-100. In a recent study, Hanke and colleagues screened 280 sera from scleroderma patients and found that the serum of 29 (10 %) recognized PM/Scl-75, 19 (7 %) recognized PM/Scl-100, and 13 (5 %) recognized both proteins [44]. Anti-PM/Scl-75-positive patients had increased rates of digital ulceration, lung involvement, contractures, and GI symptoms compared to patients without these antibodies. In contrast, patients with anti-PM/Scl-100 autoantibodies had less gastrointestinal involvement compared to those without these antibodies. Patients with either of the antibodies had an increased risk of skeletal myopathy as defined by CK elevation. However, double-positive patients with both anti-PM/Scl-75 and anti-PM/Scl-100 antibodies had a lower rate of CK elevation compared to those with just one of these antibodies.

In addition to PM/Scl-75 and PM/Scl-100, several other human exosome-associated proteins have been identified as targets of the immune system in scleroderma [45]. The most frequently targeted protein is C1D, a nucleolar protein which is required for ribosomal RNA processing by the exosomal enzyme complex. Anti-C1D autoantibodies were detected in 7 of 30 (23 %) patients with PM/scleroderma overlap but in only 4.5 % of patients with isolated polymyositis. The antibodies were not found in patients with isolated scleroderma, DM, multiple sclerosis, rheumatoid arthritis, or systemic lupus erythematosus. In 5 PM/scleroderma overlap patients, C1D autoreactivity was found in patients who also had antibodies recognizing both PM/Scl proteins. However, in two cases, anti-C1D autoantibodies were found in PM/scleroderma patients without anti-PM/Scl autoantibodies. Importantly, including the anti-C1D antibodies with the anti-PM/Scl antibodies increased the frequency of PM/scleroderma antibodies in this patient population from 30 to 37 %. In this study, antibodies recognizing the exosome-associated proteins hMtr4 and hSki8 were also found in patients with scleroderma and myopathy but only in 6.7 % and 3.3 % of patients, respectively.

Another study found that 1.9 % of scleroderma sera recognize a complex including RuvBL1 and RuvBL2, which serve as nuclear scaffolding proteins [46]. These antibodies were found only very rarely in patients with polymyositis, dermatomyositis, lupus, or other connective tissue diseases. RuvBL1/RuvBL2-positive scleroderma patients were older and had increased rates of myositis and diffuse skin thickening compared to scleroderma patients without this immunospecificity.

In a recent case-control study, scleroderma patients with anti-Ku autoantibodies (representing 2.2 % of all scleroderma patients) were found to have a significantly increased prevalence of muscle weakness, CK elevation, and myopathic EMG features compared to anti-Ku-negative patients [47]. As in the case of patients with anti-PM/Scl autoantibodies and scleroderma–myopathy overlap [38], most anti-Ku-positive patients with these features had limited cutaneous scleroderma rather than diffuse scleroderma.

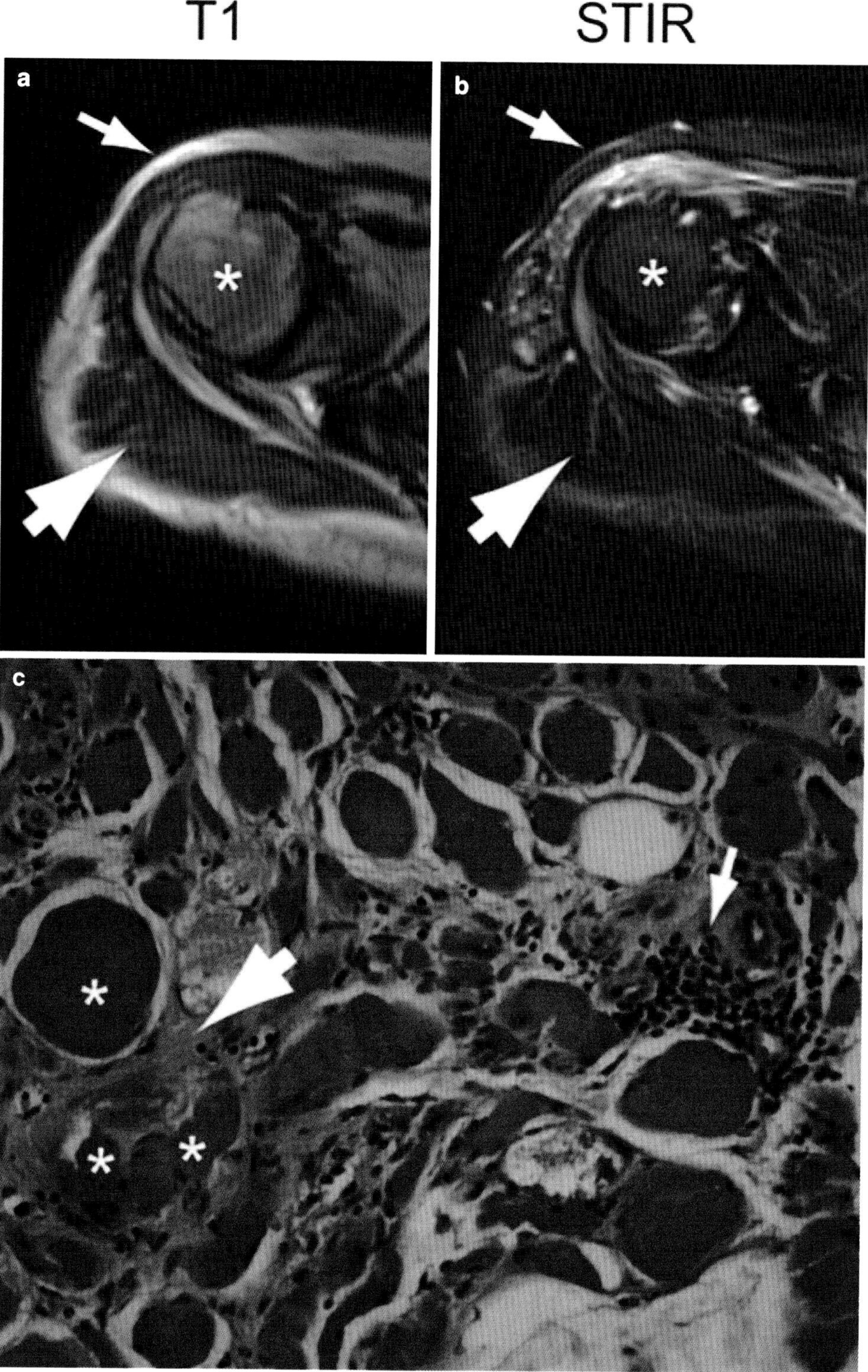

Fig. 35.1 A previously healthy 45-year-old man developed bilateral hand swelling, Raynaud's phenomenon, and proximal muscle weakness. Laboratory testing revealed a CK of ~2,000 IU/L and anti-PM/Scl autoantibodies. Four months from the onset of symptoms, a right shoulder MRI was performed (the humeral head is shown with an asterisk in these axial cuts). The T1 imaging (panel **a**) reveals muscle tissue (*gray*) and subcutaneous fat (*white*) but no fatty replacement of muscle tissue. The STIR imaging (panel **b**) reveals high signal intensity (*white*) in the anterior deltoid (*small arrow*) but not the posterior deltoid (*large arrow*). The patient underwent a right anterior deltoid muscle biopsy. The H&E-stained paraffin sections (panel **c**) revealed both a moderately large focus of inflammatory cells adjacent to a blood vessel (*small arrow*) and dramatically increased fibrosis (*large arrow*) between individual, mostly atrophic, myofibers (labeled with *asterisks*)

In contrast to the positive associations detailed above, Mimura and colleagues reported that none of the 43 patients with scleroderma and skeletal myopathy had anticentromere antibodies, while 32 % of 302 scleroderma patients without myopathy were positive for this antibody [9].

Evaluation of the Patient with Myopathy

Given the prevalence of myopathy in this population, all patients with scleroderma should be screened for muscle involvement. As part of the history, patients should be asked about symptoms suggestive of proximal muscle weakness such as difficulty washing one's hair, trouble rising from a low chair, and problems ascending stairs. On physical exam, neck extensor and flexor strength should be carefully assessed; patients with normal strength are able to resist at least moderate pressure exerted by the examiner. Evidence of deltoid weakness can be ascertained by having the patient fully abduct the arms; it should require significant effort by the examiner to overcome the deltoids with pressure applied at the elbows. Hip flexor strength should be assessed with the patient lying supine and the leg flexed to at least 45°; using one hand just proximal to the knee, the examiner should not be able to push the leg down to the table. Additionally, patients may be asked to sit on a 6-in.-high stool and rise to a standing position without using their arms; inability to do so may reveal more subtle hip flexor weakness. It should be noted that in scleroderma patients, contractures may make assessing muscle strength particularly challenging.

When the history or physical exam suggests the possibility of proximal muscle weakness, additional testing is indicated. EMG and nerve conduction studies are extremely valuable in establishing the presence of a myopathic process and excluding the possibility that a neuropathic process may be contributing to a patient's weakness. When possible, EMG should be performed only on one side, preserving the other for biopsy. Laboratory testing should include serum CK and aldolase levels as elevations of one or both are a characteristic of an underlying myopathic process. When available, testing for scleroderma–myopathy-associated autoantibodies such as anti-PM/Scl should be considered. However, negative testing for these antibodies does not preclude the presence of myopathy.

Some clinicians elect to empirically treat patients with immunosuppressive therapy when the history, physical exam, and laboratory testing support a diagnosis of myopathy. However, in almost all cases, a muscle biopsy should be performed to establish the diagnosis and, importantly, to determine whether there is inflammation or necrosis since patients with these features are most likely to respond to immunosuppression (see below). The biopsy should be obtained from the deltoid, biceps, or quadriceps muscles. Ideally, the biopsy should be taken from a mildly to moderately weak muscle (i.e., 4/5 on the MRC scale); severely weak muscles may appear histologically "end stage" without more defining features.

MRI is often performed during the evaluation of patients with suspected muscle disease. In a recent study, Schanz and colleagues studied 18 scleroderma subjects with musculoskeletal symptoms who underwent whole body MRI [48]. These investigators found that muscle weakness was correlated with perifascial enhancement and muscular edema. However, since this study did not include scleroderma subjects without musculoskeletal symptoms, it is unclear how specific these MRI features are for patients with muscle disease. Consequently, the role of MRI in diagnosing myopathy in scleroderma patients remains to be established. Nonetheless, in the author's experience, this imaging modality can be helpful in guiding the surgeon to an affected muscle for biopsy. Of note, muscles that have recently had needles inserted for vaccination or EMG study should be avoided.

Since scleroderma patients with skeletal muscle involvement have an increased risk of myocardial disease, an echocardiogram and EKG should be considered. In some instances, cardiac involvement is suspected based on the presence of an elevated CK–MB fraction. However, the CK–MB fraction may be released from damaged skeletal muscle in the absence of cardiac muscle damage. In contrast, troponin I is not released from damaged skeletal muscle in patients with inflammatory myopathies, and elevated levels of this enzyme should raise concern about cardiac disease [49].

Treatment and Prognosis

One report found that patients with scleroderma–myopathy do not seem to have a significantly increased risk of mortality compared to those scleroderma patients without myopathy [15]. In contrast, another study found that survival was reduced in scleroderma patients with CK elevations [50]. Specifically, 1-, 3-, and 10-year survival rates for those with elevated CK were 96.1, 92.9, and 84.0 % compared to 99.9, 97.7, and 93.9 % in those with normal CK. The patients with CK elevations tended to be younger, male, and have early diffuse disease, interstitial lung disease, and autoantibodies recognizing topoisomerase 1 or RNP. Independent of mortality, muscle weakness can be severely debilitating, and defining optimal treatment strategies is of significant importance.

To date, there have been no prospective studies evaluating which patients with scleroderma–myopathy are most likely to benefit from treatment and no studies revealing which treatments are most effective. However, retrospective analysis by Clements suggested there may be two groups of patients with distinct clinical courses and responses to therapy [4]. In this study, a group of scleroderma patients with "simple myopathy" was defined as those with proximal muscle weakness, mild CK elevation, a non-irritable myopathy on EMG, and muscle biopsies with fibrosis but no inflammation. These patients appeared to have a relatively stable disease course even when left untreated. A second group of scleroderma patients with "complicated myopathy" had muscle weakness, very high CK levels, an irritable myopathy on EMG, and an inflammatory myopathy as typically seen in patients with PM or DM. In contrast to those with simple myopathy, the majority of these patients experienced dramatic improvement with corticosteroid treatment.

A recent retrospective study of 35 scleroderma–myopathy patients by Ranque and colleagues confirms that these individuals can be divided into two groups, one with a more favorable response to immunosuppressive therapy [19]. However, these investigators found that the distinction between good and poor responders could be made based solely upon histopathological features of the muscle biopsy. Specifically, in patients without inflammation or necrosis on muscle biopsy, only 13 % had a favorable response to therapy. In contrast, those with necrosis, inflammation, or necrosis and inflammation had an 89 %, 90 %, and 100 % chance of favorable response to treatment, respectively.

There is no validated, evidence-based approach to treating patients with scleroderma–myopathy. However, based on personal experience and the findings described above, a cautious approach to treatment may be appropriate in those without necrosis or inflammation on biopsy since in these patients, the risks of the medications are more likely to outweigh the expected benefits. However, this author would recommend a more aggressive approach to treating patients who have necrosis and/or inflammation on biopsy. This would usually include oral steroids as the first-line therapy of choice (although scleroderma patients may need careful monitoring for the development of renal crisis). In order to taper steroids, most patients require a steroid-sparing agent such as methotrexate. Mycophenolate mofetil and azathioprine may also be considered in these patients. Intravenous gamma globulin is an alternative that has been used effectively by the author and may be considered even in those patients who do not have a good response to other medications. Interestingly, a recent observational study examined the efficacy of abatacept in treating seven scleroderma patients with refractory myopathy [51]. In each patient treated with this medication, which downregulates T-cell activation, disease activity decreased by more than 50 %. However, this trend for improvement did not reach statistical significance, and further studies are needed to confirm the efficacy of the biologic agent.

Summary

Skeletal muscle disease is known to be a relatively common manifestation of scleroderma and is associated with an increased risk of myocardial involvement. Most patients with skeletal myopathy have proximal muscle weakness on exam, and about 40 % have one of the scleroderma–myopathy-associated autoantibodies (i.e., anti-PM/Scl-75, anti-PM/Scl-100, or anti-CD1). Although fibrosis is a common muscle biopsy feature in these patients, other histopathological findings are highly variable. Importantly, those subjects with prominent inflammation and/or necrosis on muscle biopsy are most likely to benefit from immunosuppressive therapy. In contrast, those patients without either inflammation or necrosis are significantly less likely to have a favorable response to immunosuppressive therapy. Future studies are needed to identify optimal treatment strategies and to define the pathologic mechanisms underlying the different forms of scleroderma–myopathy.

References

1. Westphal C. Zwei Falle von Scleerodermie. Charite-Ann (Berlin). 1876;3:341–60.
2. Medsger Jr TA, Rodnan GP, Moossy J, Vester JW. Skeletal muscle involvement in progressive systemic sclerosis (scleroderma). Arthritis Rheum. 1968;11(4):554–68.
3. Thompson JM, Bluestone R, Bywaters EG, Dorling J, Johnson M. Skeletal muscle involvement in systemic sclerosis. Ann Rheum Dis. 1969;28(3):281–8.
4. Clements PJ, Furst DE, Campion DS, et al. Muscle disease in progressive systemic sclerosis: diagnostic and therapeutic considerations. Arthritis Rheum. 1978;21(1):62–71.
5. West SG, Killian PJ, Lawless OJ. Association of myositis and myocarditis in progressive systemic sclerosis. Arthritis Rheum. 1981;24(5):662–8.
6. Russell ML, Hanna WM. Ultrastructure of muscle microvasculature in progressive systemic sclerosis: relation to clinical weakness. J Rheumatol. 1983;10(5):741–7.
7. Averbuch-Heller L, Steiner I, Abramsky O. Neurologic manifestations of progressive systemic sclerosis. Arch Neurol. 1992;49(12):1292–5.
8. Hietaharju A, Jaaskelainen S, Kalimo H, Hietarinta M. Peripheral neuromuscular manifestations in systemic sclerosis (scleroderma). Muscle Nerve. 1993;16(11):1204–12.
9. Mimura Y, Ihn H, Jinnin M, Asano Y, Yamane K, Tamaki K. Clinical and laboratory features of scleroderma patients developing skeletal myopathy. Clin Rheumatol. 2005;24(2):99–102.
10. Follansbee WP, Zerbe TR, Medsger Jr TA. Cardiac and skeletal muscle disease in systemic sclerosis (scleroderma): a high risk association. Am Heart J. 1993;125(1):194–203.
11. Toledano C, Gain M, Kettaneh A, Baudin B, Johanet C, Cherin P, Riviere S, Cabane J, Tiev KP. Aldolase predicts subsequent myopathy occurrence in systemic sclerosis. Arthritis Res Ther. 2012;14(3):R152.
12. Rosato E, Rossi C, Salsano F. Dropped head syndrome and systemic sclerosis. Joint Bone Spine. 2009;76(3):301–3.
13. Garcin B, Lenglet T, Dubourg O, Mesnage V, Levy R. Dropped head syndrome as a presenting sign of scleromyositis. J Neurol Sci. 2010;292(1–2):101–3.
14. Rojana-Udomsart A, Fabian V, Hollingsworth PN, Walters SE, Zilko PJ, Mastaglia FL. Paraspinal and scapular myopathy associated with scleroderma. J Clin Neuromuscul Dis. 2010;11(4):213–22.
15. Ranque B, Berezne A, Le-Guern V, et al. Myopathies related to systemic sclerosis: a case-control study of associated clinical and immunological features. Scand J Rheumatol. 2010;39(6):498–505.
16. Allanore Y, Meune C, Vonk MC, et al. Prevalence and factors associated with left ventricular dysfunction in the EULAR Scleroderma Trial and Research group (EUSTAR) database of patients with systemic sclerosis. Ann Rheum Dis. 2010;69(1):218–21.
17. Zivkovic SA, Freiberg W, Lacomis D, Domsic RT, Medsger TA. Localized scleroderma and regional inflammatory myopathy. Neuromuscul Disord: NMD. 2014;24(5):425–30.
18. Ringel RA, Brick JE, Brick JF, Gutmann L, Riggs JE. Muscle involvement in the scleroderma syndromes. Arch Intern Med. 1990;150(12):2550–2.

19. Ranque B, Authier FJ, Le-Guern V, et al. A descriptive and prognostic study of systemic sclerosis-associated myopathies. Ann Rheum Dis. 2009;68(9):1474–7.
20. Bhansing KJ, Lammens M, Knaapen HK, van Riel PL, van Engelen BG, Vonk MC. Scleroderma-polymyositis overlap syndrome versus idiopathic polymyositis and systemic sclerosis: a descriptive study on clinical features and myopathology. Arthritis Res Ther. 2014;16(3):R111.
21. Scarpelli M, Montironi R, Tulli D, et al. Quantitative analysis of quadriceps muscle biopsy in systemic sclerosis. Pathol Res Pract. 1992;188(4–5):603–6.
22. Arahata K, Engel AG. Monoclonal antibody analysis of mononuclear cells in myopathies. I: quantitation of subsets according to diagnosis and sites of accumulation and demonstration and counts of muscle fibers invaded by T cells. Ann Neurol. 1984;16(2):193–208.
23. Wolfe JF, Adelstein E, Sharp GC. Antinuclear antibody with distinct specificity for polymyositis. J Clin Invest. 1977;59(1):176–8.
24. Treadwell EL, Alspaugh MA, Wolfe JF, Sharp GC. Clinical relevance of PM-1 antibody and physiochemical characterization of PM-1 antigen. J Rheumatol. 1984;11(5):658–62.
25. Reichlin M, Maddison PJ, Targoff I, et al. Antibodies to a nuclear/nucleolar antigen in patients with polymyositis overlap syndromes. J Clin Immunol. 1984;4(1):40–4.
26. Alderuccio F, Chan EK, Tan EM. Molecular characterization of an autoantigen of PM-Scl in the polymyositis/scleroderma overlap syndrome: a unique and complete human cDNA encoding an apparent 75-kD acidic protein of the nucleolar complex. J Exp Med. 1991;173(4):941–52.
27. Bluthner M, Bautz FA. Cloning and characterization of the cDNA coding for a polymyositis-scleroderma overlap syndrome-related nucleolar 100-kD protein. J Exp Med. 1992;176(4):973–80.
28. Ge Q, Frank MB, O'Brien C, Targoff IN. Cloning of a complementary DNA coding for the 100-kD antigenic protein of the PM-Scl autoantigen. J Clin Invest. 1992;90(2):559–70.
29. Schilders G, van Dijk E, Raijmakers R, Pruijn GJ. Cell and molecular biology of the exosome: how to make or break an RNA. Int Rev Cytol. 2006;251:159–208.
30. Mahler M, Raijmakers R. Novel aspects of autoantibodies to the PM/Scl complex: clinical, genetic and diagnostic insights. Autoimmun Rev. 2007;6(7):432–7.
31. Reimer G, Scheer U, Peters JM, Tan EM. Immunolocalization and partial characterization of a nucleolar autoantigen (PM-Scl) associated with polymyositis/scleroderma overlap syndromes. J Immunol. 1986;137(12):3802–8.
32. Genth E, Mierau R, Genetzky P, et al. Immunogenetic associations of scleroderma-related antinuclear antibodies. Arthritis Rheum. 1990;33(5):657–65.
33. Oddis CV, Okano Y, Rudert WA, Trucco M, Duquesnoy RJ, Medsger Jr TA. Serum autoantibody to the nucleolar antigen PM-Scl. Clinical and immunogenetic associations. Arthritis Rheum. 1992;35(10):1211–7.
34. Marguerie C, Bunn CC, Copier J, et al. The clinical and immunogenetic features of patients with autoantibodies to the nucleolar antigen PM-Scl. Medicine (Baltimore). 1992;71(6):327–36.
35. Hausmanowa-Petrusewicz I, Kowalska-Oledzka E, Miller FW, et al. Clinical, serologic, and immunogenetic features in polish patients with idiopathic inflammatory myopathies. Arthritis Rheum. 1997;40(7):1257–66.
36. Vandergheynst F, Ocmant A, Sordet C, et al. Anti-pm/scl antibodies in connective tissue disease: clinical and biological assessment of 14 patients. Clin Exp Rheumatol. 2006;24(2):129–33.
37. Selva-O'Callaghan A, Labrador-Horrillo M, Solans-Laque R, Simeon-Aznar CP, Martinez-Gomez X, Vilardell-Tarres M. Myositis-specific and myositis-associated antibodies in a series of eighty-eight Mediterranean patients with idiopathic inflammatory myopathy. Arthritis Rheum. 2006;55(5):791–8.
38. Steen VD. Autoantibodies in systemic sclerosis. Semin Arthritis Rheum. 2005;35(1):35–42.
39. Koschik RW, Fertig N, Lucas MR, Domsic RT, Medsger Jr TA. Anti-PM-Scl antibody in patients with systemic sclerosis. Clin Exp Rheumatol. 2012;30(71):S12–6.
40. D'Aoust J, Hudson M, Tatibouet S, Wick J, Canadian Scleroderma Research Group, Mahler M, Baron M, Fritzler MJ. Clinical and serologic correlates of anti-PM/Scl antibodies in systemic sclerosis: a multicenter study of 763 patients. Arthritis Rheumatol (Hoboken, NJ). 2014;66(6):1608–15.
41. Chinoy H, Salway F, Fertig N, et al. In adult onset myositis, the presence of interstitial lung disease and myositis specific/associated antibodies are governed by HLA class II haplotype, rather than by myositis subtype. Arthritis Res Ther. 2006;8(1):R13.
42. O'Hanlon TP, Carrick DM, Targoff IN, et al. Immunogenetic risk and protective factors for the idiopathic inflammatory myopathies: distinct HLA-A, -B, -Cw, -DRB1, and -DQA1 allelic profiles distinguish European American patients with different myositis autoantibodies. Medicine (Baltimore). 2006;85(2):111–27.
43. Kuwana M, Kaburaki J, Okano Y, Tojo T, Homma M. Clinical and prognostic associations based on serum antinuclear antibodies in Japanese patients with systemic sclerosis. Arthritis Rheum. 1994;37(1):75–83.
44. Hanke K, Bruckner CS, Dahnrich C, et al. Antibodies against PM/Scl-75 and PM/Scl-100 are independent markers for different subsets of systemic sclerosis patients. Arthritis Res Ther. 2009;11(1):R22.
45. Schilders G, Egberts WV, Raijmakers R, Pruijn GJ. C1D is a major autoantibody target in patients with the polymyositis-scleroderma overlap syndrome. Arthritis Rheum. 2007;56(7):2449–54.
46. Kaji K, Fertig N, Medsger Jr TA, Satoh T, Hoshino K, Hamaguchi Y, Hasegawa M, Lucas M, Schnure A, Ogawa F, Sato S, Takehara K, Fujimoto M, Kuwana M. Autoantibodies to RuvBL1 and RuvBL2: a novel systemic sclerosis-related antibody associated with diffuse cutaneous and skeletal muscle involvement. Arthritis Care Res. 2014;66(4):575–84.
47. Rozman B, Cucnik S, Sodin-Semrl S, et al. Prevalence and clinical associations of anti-Ku antibodies in patients with systemic sclerosis: a European EUSTAR-initiated multi-centre case-control study. Ann Rheum Dis. 2008;67(9):1282–6.
48. Schanz S, Henes J, Ulmer A, Kotter I, Fierlbeck G, Claussen CD, Horger M. Magnetic resonance imaging findings in patients with systemic scleroderma and musculoskeletal symptoms. Eur Radiol. 2013;23(1):212–21.
49. Aggarwal R, Lebiedz-Odrobina D, Sinha A, Manadan A, Case JP. Serum cardiac troponin T, but not troponin I, is elevated in idiopathic inflammatory myopathies. J Rheumatol. 2009;36(12):2711–4.
50. Jung M, Bonner A, Hudson M, Baron M, Pope JE, Canadian Scleroderma Research Group (CSRG). Myopathy is a poor prognostic feature in systemic sclerosis: results from the Canadian Scleroderma Research Group (CSRG) cohort. Scand J Rheumatol. 2014;43(3):217–20.
51. Elhai M, Meunier M, Matucci-Cerinic M, Maurer B, Riemekasten G, Leturcq T, Pellerito R, Von Muhlen CA, Vacca A, Airo P, Bartoli F, Fiori G, Bokarewa M, Riccieri V, Becker M, Avouac J, Muller-Ladner U, Distler O, Allanore Y, EUSTAR (EULAR Scleroderma Trials and Research group). Outcomes of patients with systemic sclerosis-associated polyarthritis and myopathy treated with tocilizumab or abatacept: a EUSTAR observational study. Ann Rheum Dis. 2013;72(7):1217–20.

Tendons, Joints, and Bone

36

Jérôme Avouac, Maya H. Buch, and Yannick Allanore

While tethering of the skin is the clinical hallmark of SSc, many patients may develop musculoskeletal symptoms as an early sign of the disease (up to 20 % of patients with SSc report joint symptoms as early as 1 year or more prior to diagnosis and a third within the same year of diagnosis) and/or during the course of their illness [1]. Manifestations may include varying degrees of rheumatic complaints ranging from carpal tunnel syndrome and arthralgia to frank inflammatory arthritis or bony lesions. Joint symptoms have been reported to be present in 66 % of patients with SSc and muscular symptoms in half of the patients, the latter with a predominance of muscle weakness and myalgia [2]. Musculoskeletal involvement has been shown to strongly contribute to disability and impaired quality of life in SSc, reducing the performance of everyday occupation [1, 3–6]. Indeed, several cross-sectional studies have been reported over the recent years all highlighting the major impact of musculoskeletal involvement on the quality of life in SSc. One report examined patients' beliefs and investigated the relationship between these beliefs, symptom reports, and clinical/demographic variables. This study included a total of 49 patients (7 males, 42 females) who underwent clinical examination and completed the Revised Illness Perception Questionnaire. The symptoms patients most frequently associated with SSc were stiff joints (79 %), pain (75 %), and fatigue (75 %), all relating to musculoskeletal involvement. More than 96 % of patients believed that their condition would be chronic and 78 % believed that the condition had serious consequences on their lives. Patients with diffuse cutaneous SSc reported more significant consequences of the condition and less personal control of their SSc compared with patients with limited cutaneous disease [7]. Another study focused on the ability to perform daily activities and analyzed in details hand function. Data from 30 patients showed that dexterity was on average reduced to 68–80 % and grip force to 46–65 % compared with values for healthy persons. Finger flexion and extension were the most impaired aspects of hand mobility. Activities building on hand and arm function were harder to perform than activities depending on lower limb function. Stiffness, grip force, and dexterity had the highest strength of association with difficulties of daily living activities after Raynaud's phenomenon, which was the master symptom [8]. A study focusing on impairment of hand function suggested that it could be similar or even higher than in rheumatoid arthritis or digital osteoarthritis: the authors showed the reliability and validity of Duruöz Hand Index in SSc and found a mean (SD) total score of 21.10 ± 19.25 (0–66), whereas mean scores of about 17 (SD) or 19 (SD) have been reported in series of patients with rheumatoid arthritis or osteoarthritis [4].

The objective of this chapter is to provide an overview of the spectrum of tendon, joint, bone, and soft tissue involvement in SSc to further highlight the multisystem nature of this condition and to review the different therapeutic approaches of the underlying pathologies.

Carpal Tunnel Syndrome

The wrist is surrounded by a band of fibrous tissue that normally functions as a support for the joint. The tight space between this fibrous band and the wrist bone is called the carpal tunnel. The median nerve passes through the carpal tunnel to send off digital cutaneous branches to common palmar digital branch and proper palmar digital branch of the median nerve, which supply the (radial) three and a half digits on the

J. Avouac, MD (✉)
Rheumatology A Department, Cochin Hospital, Paris Descartes University, Sorbonne Paris Cité, Paris, France
e-mail: jerome.avouac@cch.aphp.fr

M.H. Buch, MBChB, FRCP, PhD
Leeds Institute of Rheumatic & Musculoskeletal Medicine, University of Leeds and Leeds Musculoskeletal Biomedical Research Unit, Leeds Teaching Hospitals NHS Trust, Leeds, UK

Y. Allanore, MD
Service de Rhumatologie A, Hôpital Cochin, Université Paris Descartes, Paris, France

J. Varga et al. (eds.), *Scleroderma*, DOI 10.1007/978-3-319-31407-5_36

palmar side and index, middle, and ring finger on dorsum of the hand. The median nerve also supplies motor innervation to the first and second lumbricals of the hand. All conditions that cause swelling or soft tissue deposit within the carpal tunnel can irritate the median nerve. Nerve injury in this manner can cause tingling and numbness of the thumb, the index, and the middle fingers. Occasionally, sharp shooting pains may be felt in the forearm. In the case of chronicity, patients may develop a burning sensation, cramping, and even weakness of the hand with atrophy of the hand muscles. Carpal tunnel syndrome is commonly seen in early diffuse SSc although no large study has precisely looked at its prevalence. One electrophysiological study investigated the characteristics of the canalicular passage nerve involvement in SSc including 34 patients of less than 5 years disease duration. Fourteen (44 %) patients showed a decrement of the median nerve terminal latency index and seven (22 %) of either the median or the ulnar nerve, without severe lesions. Indeed, carpal tunnel syndrome is often the symptom that brings the patient to a physician. Therefore, all physicians should be aware of its association with SSc; in particular the co-occurrence of Raynaud's syndrome together with carpal tunnel syndrome should trigger further investigation for a potential connective tissue disorder.

In a controlled study that included 64 asymptomatic SSc patients and 30 controls, median nerve was measured using high-resolution real-time ultrasound of the carpal tunnel. The median nerve cross-sectional area, the transverse (major axis), and the flattening ratio (FR) (defined as the ratio of the nerve's major to minor axis) diameters appeared to be increased in SSc patients compared to controls, whereas the anteroposterior (minor axis) was similar. All SSc measures were higher than controls in all phases of disease and independently of duration of SSc, extent of skin involvement, cutaneous subset (limited or diffuse), and phase of skin involvement (edematous, atrophic, fibrotic) [9]. It is noteworthy that this study failed to identify any link between friction rubs, flexor tenosynovitis or radiocarpal synovitis, and median nerve involvement. This may suggest that carpal tunnel syndrome is not a consequence of compression mechanisms but raises the hypothesis, as already suggested that ischemia of *vasa nervorum*, following vasospasm, may contribute to the pathogenesis. Another report of a smaller sample size also showed data that support this hypothesis of a vascular dependent neuropathy in SSc rather than a compressive mechanism or an autoimmune-dependent neuropathy [10]. However, more data are needed before drawing any firm conclusion. The choice of treatment depends on the severity of the symptoms and any underlying disease that might be driving the symptoms. Initial treatment usually includes rest and immobilization of the wrist in a splint. Those whose occupations aggravate the symptoms may modify their activities. Ergonomic modification, for example, adjustment of computer keyboards and chair height, may optimize comfort. Similarly, nonsteroidal anti-inflammatory drugs (NSAIDs) are sometimes offered for decreasing inflammation and reducing pain, but their side effects in SSc are a major concern. Thus, corticosteroids are frequently injected directly into the carpal tunnel. This usually brings rapid relief of the symptoms with minimal side effects and can be repeated with symptom recurrence. Most patients with carpal tunnel syndrome improve with conservative measures and medications. Corticosteroid-resistant, continuous symptoms justify surgical decompression. Occasionally, chronic lesions of the median nerve can result in persistent numbness and weakness; surgical treatment may be considered although improvement at this stage is questionable. In summary, however, surgical carpal tunnel release is usually very effective in symptomatic and refractory patients [11]. However, despite thickening of the skin, subcutaneous deposits, and tenosynovitis, symptoms of numbness in the median nerve are much less frequent in SSc in comparison, for example, to rheumatoid arthritis. This further supports a vascular component in SSc.

Tendon Involvement

Clinical Presentations

Tendon abnormalities were first described in 1876 by Westphal, who noticed "coarse cracking and crepitus of finger and knees" in a 23-year-old woman with diffuse cutaneous SSc. In 1961, Shulman et al. attributed these grating sensations to fibrinous deposits on the surface of tendon sheaths and overlying fascia. Rodnan and Medsger described this finding as "leathery crepitus" on palpation of the knees, wrists, fingers, and ankles during motion in 19 of 53 patients [12]. In the leg, tendon rubs are usually localized to the tibialis anterior, or less frequently, the peroneus muscles. In the forearm the source of this rub is usually the tendons of the flexor or extensor muscles, immediately proximal to the wrist. Median nerve compression with carpal tunnel syndrome may occur, the result, presumably of changes in the tendon sheaths beneath the transverse carpal ligament. In advanced disease, fibrous deposits within the tendon sheaths might be responsible for a cracking noise during joint movements. The bursae may also be affected especially at the trochanteric or olecranon regions, with sometimes recurrent bursitis with or without associated regional arthritis. An example of magnetic resonance imaging (MRI) illustrating trochanteric bursitis associated with hip synovitis in a patient with diffuse cutaneous SSc is presented on Fig. 36.1. The inflammatory proliferative tenosynovitis may lead in rare cases to tendon rupture, which is illustrated in Fig. 36.2a–f [13]. Pathologic examination of biopsies and of tissue obtained at necropsy has revealed thickening of the tendon

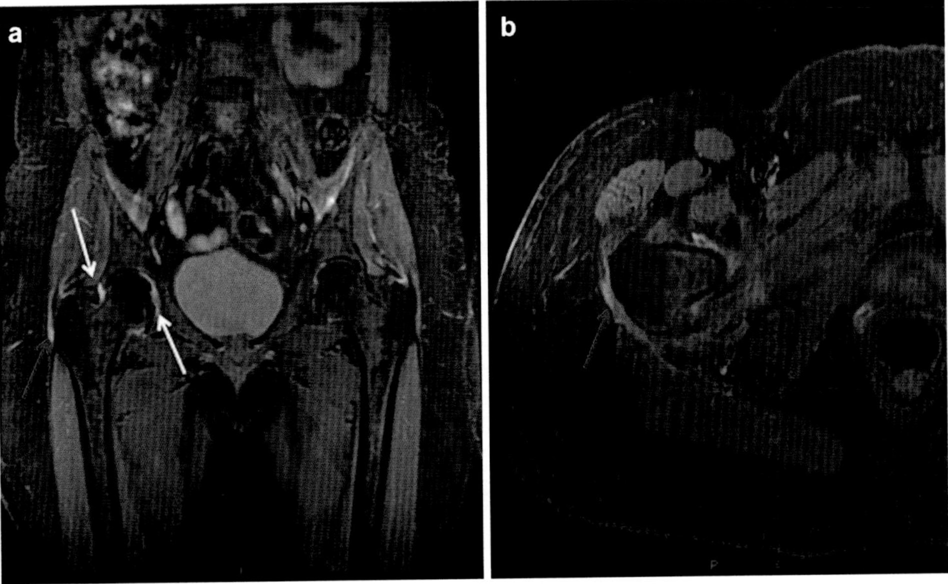

Fig. 36.1 Magnetic resonance imaging (*MRI*) showing an association of trochanteric bursitis (*white arrow*) with hip synovitis (*red arrow*) in a patient with diffuse cutaneous systemic sclerosis

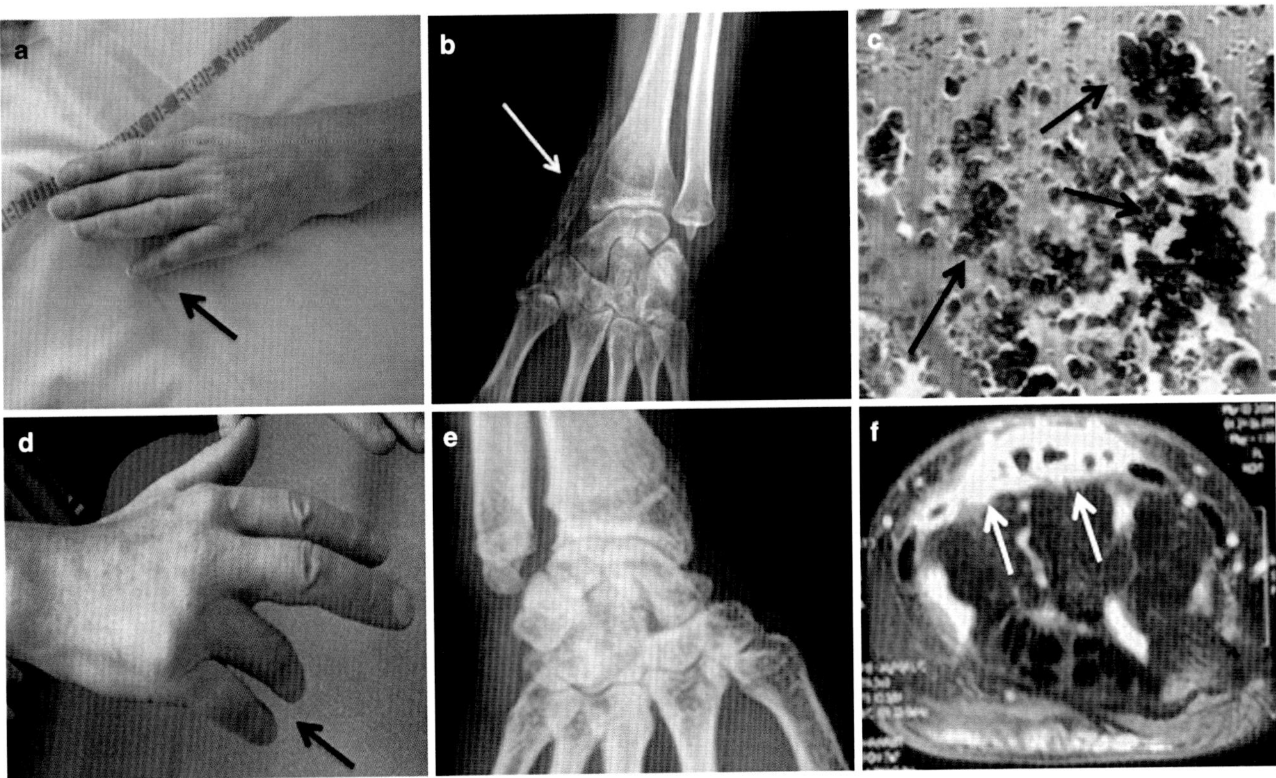

Fig. 36.2 (**a–f**) Tendon rupture in two patients with diffuse cutaneous systemic sclerosis. (**a–c**) Spontaneous rupture of the fifth extensor tendon (**a**). The X-ray did not show any cause of tendon rupture but revealed calcifications of the extensor carpi radialis longus tendon (**b**). Histology obtained after surgical reinsertion of the tendon showed large calcium and fibrin deposits (*black arrow*) on the surface of the sheaths (**c**). (**d–f**) Spontaneous rupture of the fourth and fifth extensor tendons (**d**). The X-ray showed radiocarpal joint space narrowing and radioulnar erosion (**e**). MRI revealed extensor tenosynovitis (*white arrows*) (**f**) and radioulnar joint synovitis

sheath and deposits of fibrin on the surface of the sheaths and tendons that are similar to those in the case of synovium of the suprapatellar bursa. There appears to be relatively little inflammatory reaction.

Prevalence and Correlation with SSc Features

Tendon involvement is not uncommon in SSc. In a recent study, tendon involvement was observed in 10 of 98 patients

Table 36.1 Prevalence of clinical tendon involvement

	Clements et al. [93] (*n* = 134 diffuse SSc)	Ostojic et al. [94] (*n* = 105)	Ostojic et al. [95] (*n* = 60)	Avouac et al. [19] (*n* = 7286)	Steen and Medsger [15] (*n* = 1305)
Frequency of tendon involvement, *n* (%)	48 (36 %)	16 (15 %)	9 (15 %)	802 (11 %)	368 (28 %)

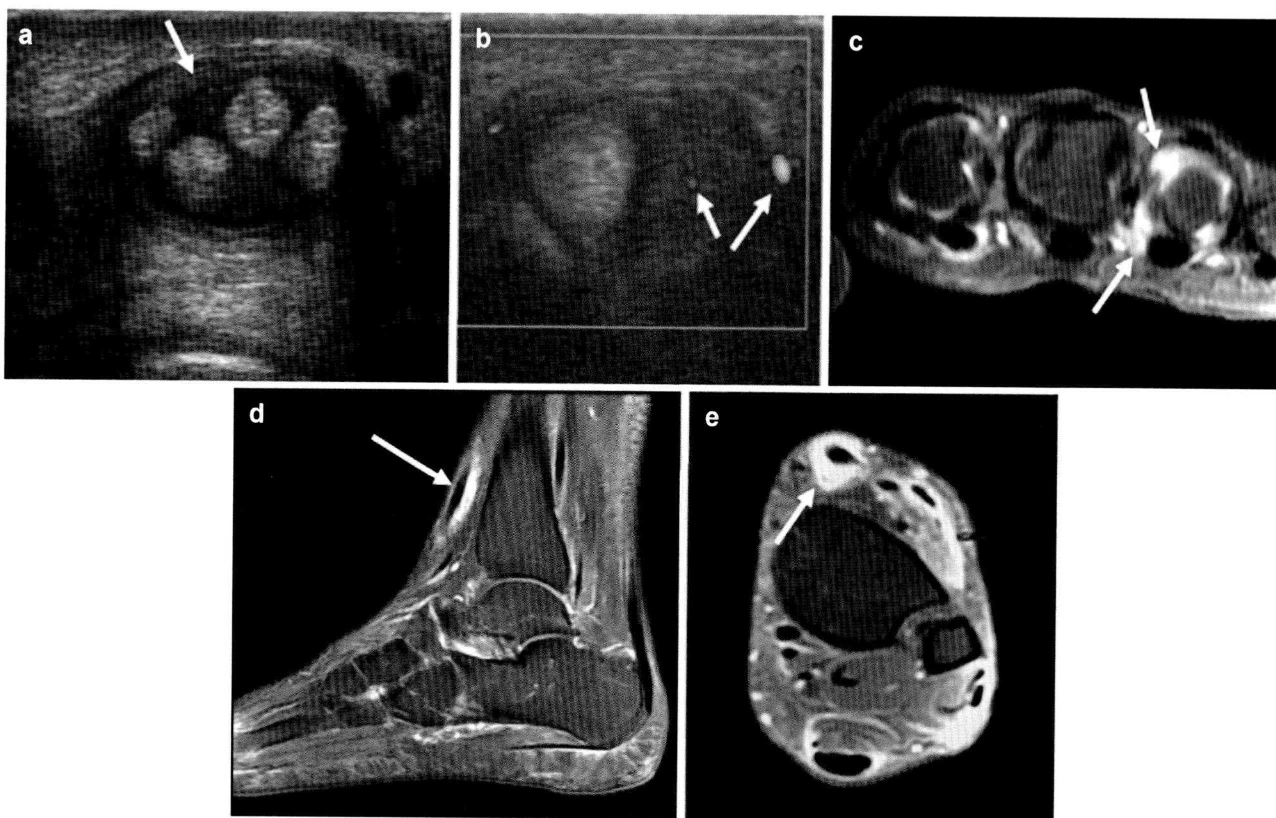

Fig. 36.3 (**a**, **b**) Fibrotic tenosynovitis of extensor digitorum communis (**a**) and inflammatory tenosynovitis of extensor carpi ulnaris (**b**), assessed by ultrasonography. (**c**–**e**) MRI showing hand flexor and extensor (**c**) and tibialis anterior (**d**, **e**) inflammatory tenosynovitis

in the leg and 23/98 in the forearm [14]. In the EUSTAR (EULAR Scleroderma Trials and Research) database, the point prevalence of tendon friction rubs, defined as a leathery, rubbing, "squeaking" sensation detected as the tendon was moved actively or passively, was 11 % (802/7,286 patients). Their prevalence was lower than previously reported in a large American study including 1,305 SSc patients. In this study, rubs were found in 28 % (368/1,305) of SSc patients [15]. This different point prevalence could be partly explained by the higher proportion of patients with the diffuse cutaneous subset in the American study (49 % vs. 33 %). The prevalence of tendon involvement in SSc is provided in Table 36.1.

The prevalence of tendon involvement has been assessed by MRI in a preliminary study performed on 17 patients; 8 had tenosynovitis, either of flexor (*n* = 7) or extensor (*n* = 3) tendons [16]. The frequency of tendon involvement has been assessed by ultrasound in two recent studies [17, 18], which found a point prevalence of 27 % (14/52 patients and 12/44 patients, respectively). Interestingly, ultrasonography detected inflammatory or fibrotic changes in tenosynovitis. Thus, ultrasound and MRI might be useful to discriminate tenosynovitis secondary to fibrous deposits on the surface of the tendon sheaths (Fig. 36.3a) from the changes of inflammatory tenosynovitis (Fig. 36.3b–e). Of note, a layered pattern (similar to the appearance of an artichoke heart) of tenosynovitis was seen commonly in SSc patients.

Tendon involvement is more prevalent in patients with the diffuse cutaneous subset and early disease. It is also associated with signs of severe vascular, muscular, and renal involvement and decreased survival [15, 19]. In particular, the data from the EUSTAR database highlighted the independent association in multivariate analysis between tendon friction rubs and digital ulcerations (odds ratio, OR: 1.21, 95 % confidence interval, 95 % CI: 1.01–1.44), muscle weakness (OR: 1.42, 95 % CI: 1.18–1.70), pulmonary fibrosis on plain chest X-ray (OR: 1.22, 95 % CI: 1.02–1.46), and proteinuria detected with a urinalysis dipstick (OR: 1.38, 95 % CI: 1.02–1.87). As recently shown, tendon friction rubs are associated with active disease [20]. The recent prospective analysis of the EUSTAR database has also confirmed that tendon friction rub is an independent predictor of skin progression and of the further occurrence of scleroderma renal crisis [21]. These results highlight that tendon friction rubs are an important physical finding, as they often precede widespread skin thickening and can be considered a poor prognostic marker. In patients with recent onset of Raynaud's phenomenon and swollen fingers, the finding of palpable tendon friction rubs should lead to a suspicion of SSc. Thus, searching for friction rub should be a routine part of the physical examination, since they are of predictive value regarding classification, severity, and progression.

Treatment

The treatment of tendon involvement is usually symptomatic and supportive, since their evolution is usually favorable after the first years of the disease course. For the most part, tenosynovitis will respond to NSAIDs and low dose of corticosteroids. Surgery may be required in the very rare cases of tendon rupture, as illustrated by the two cases presented Fig. 36.2, who required surgical reinsertion of their extensor tendons.

Joint Involvement

Clinical Presentations

Arthralgia is among the most frequent presenting symptom of SSc. At an early stage of the disease, confusion with rheumatoid arthritis is not uncommon but Raynaud's phenomenon and skin involvement are major signs indicating a connective tissue disorder and SSc. In very early diffuse cutaneous SSc, arthralgia may be difficult to assess because of rapidly progressing skin involvement leading to skin tethering and pain. However, generalized arthralgias with slight pain and stiffness are the usual presentations; although, true joint inflammation may occur and be the source of initial diagnostic confusion. The onset may be acute or insidious, oligoarticular, or polyarticular in pattern. The same joints are generally affected repeatedly and arthralgia is not migratory. Virtually, all joints may be affected with the fingers (in particular the metacarpophalangeal (MCP) and proximal interphalangeal (PIP) joints), wrists, and ankles predominating.

There is range of motion limitation or loss in all planes of wrist motion, MCP flexion, PIP extension, and thumb abduction, opposition, and flexion. The distal interphalangeal (DIP) joint may become fixed in midrange flexion. The result is a claw-type deformity with MCP extension, PIP flexion, thumb adduction, and the wrist in neutral position.

The course of the joint manifestations is either intermittent or chronic remittent. As the cutaneous involvement progresses, there is an inexorable tethering and contracture of the underlying joints with impairment of movement and function.

Clinical findings are often minimal at the onset, aside from features that may betray the presence of early SSc. Some patients may exhibit localized joint tenderness or swelling, and joint effusion may be detectable although they are usually mild. Bowing of the fingers has been suggested as a useful early diagnostic sign [22].

The presence of synovitis may be related to an overlap with rheumatoid arthritis or, more probably, to the existence of primary arthropathy specific to SSc [23–26]. Recent data supports that overlap of SSc and rheumatoid arthritis is very unusual. The prevalence of SSc-rheumatoid arthritis overlap seems close to 1–5 % and its incidence is 5 % [27]. Moreover, one study from our group showed in a population of 120 SSc patients a point prevalence of radiographic erosive arthritis of 18 %, whereas only two SSc patients (2 %) with erosive arthritis fulfilled the ACR criteria for classical rheumatoid arthritis [23]. In a study with a larger sample size ($n = 7{,}286$), much lower values for the prevalence of synovitis have been reported with synovitis affecting only one in eight patients with SSc [19]. These data are supported by the low frequency of antibodies against cyclic citrullinated peptide (anti-CCP) in SSc, which have the highest specificity for the diagnosis of rheumatoid arthritis [28–30]. The clinical and laboratory features of 15 patients with SSc-RA overlap suggest a distinct entity based on characteristic features: generalized skin fibrosis, severe seropositive erosive polyarthritis, pulmonary fibrosis, anti-topoisomerase-I antibodies, and HLA haplotype DR4. None of the reported patients had destructive DIP involvement [31].

Multicenter interventional trials have measured the presence of synovitis as a "modified Ritchie index" whereby the presence of swelling and tenderness of the MCP joints, wrists, elbows, and knees have been recorded. The DAS-28 has been recommended as a core assessment tool for inflammatory arthritis in patients with SSc [1].

Laboratory Findings

Rheumatoid factor positivity may occur in about 30 % of SSc patients [23, 32]. This test seems nonspecific however and does not serve to distinguish patients with SSc with musculoskeletal manifestations from those without [23]. However, in a series of 34 patients with a current or past history of articular symptoms selected from 300 consecutive

Table 36.2 Point prevalence of anti-CCP antibodies in systemic sclerosis

	Avouac et al. [23] (n=120)	Morita et al. [29] (n=114)	Generini et al. [37] (n=55)	Marrone et al. [30] (n=60)	Ingegnoli et al. [36] (n=75)	Ueda-Hayakawa et al. [38] (n=146)	Payet et al. [96] (n=44)
Prevalence of anti-CCP, n (%)	2 (1.5 %)	3 (2.6 %)	4 (7 %)	5 (8 %)	8 (11 %)	18 (12 %)	7 (16 %)
Sensitivity of anti-CCP for the diagnosis of associated rheumatoid arthritis	100 %	86 %	50 %	83 %	75 %	64 %	Not available

patients with SSc, a distinctive subset of 10 patients with deforming arthritis was characterized. These patients more frequently had limited cutaneous subtype, anti-centromere antibody, and also positive rheumatoid factor (80 % vs. 13 %; $P<0.05$). Seven out of these ten fulfilled rheumatoid arthritis classification criteria but anti-CCP status was not known at this time [33]. Rheumatoid factor may also be seen in patients with SSc-associated secondary Sjogren's syndrome, which is common in SSc and occurs more frequently in patients with the limited cutaneous subset and positive anti-centromere antibody [33, 34]. Detection of anti-CCP antibodies might be of great help in the identification of the uncommon cases of SSc-RA overlap [28]. Different cross-sectional studies that estimated the point prevalence of anti-CCP antibodies in patients with SSc ranged from 1 to 15 % (Table 36.2). These studies also suggested the potential diagnostic value of this test to identify patients with SSc also having RA, with a sensitivity ranging from 50 to 100 % and a specificity of about 95 % [28–30, 35–38]. However, the presence of rheumatoid factor or anti-CCP antibodies does not seem to correlate with the clinical or radiographic pattern of arthritis, including the subset of patients with erosions on X-ray, which supports the existence of a primary inflammatory and erosive arthropathy in SSc independent of RA [23].

The cross-sectional analysis of the EUSTAR database has revealed that the presence of synovitis is associated with increased levels of acute-phase reactants, markers of severe vascular disease, and muscle weakness. The presence of raised acute-phase reactants indicates systemic inflammation and has a strong association with synovitis [19].

Increased serum levels of YKL-40 (human cartilage glycoprotein-39) have recently been found in SSc. These increased levels were associated with joint involvement, suggesting a relationship with cartilage and/or fibroblast activity [39]. Anti-Ku antibodies are found in a wide spectrum of connective tissue diseases, including overlap syndromes with SSc and myositis. Synovitis and joint contractures have been found to be associated with anti-Ku antibodies in patients with SSc. A strong association has also been identified between these antibodies and the presence of muscle weakness/atrophy and muscle enzyme elevation [40].

Analysis of the synovial fluid generally reveals normal or modestly increased leukocyte concentrations of less than 2,000 cells/mm^3 and a predominantly mononuclear infiltrate [41]. Rarely, frankly inflamed synovial fluid with inclusion-containing cells indistinguishable from the ragocytes (leukocytes with peripheral cytoplasmic inclusions) of RA has been reported [42]. Immunocytologic studies have revealed that these inclusion bodies contain large amounts of fibrin and/or fibrin breakdown products as well as the immunoglobulins (Ig) G and IgM. Synovial biopsies from SSc joints have demonstrated histological evidence of inflammation in the synovial membrane, as well as inflammatory infiltrates in the subsynovium and perivascular tissues, with lymphocytic and plasma cell infiltration; these features are associated with superficial fibrin deposition and focal microvascular obliteration [41, 43, 44]. In contrast to RA, however, the usual proliferation of synovial hyperplasia and pannus formation typical of RA does not occur in the SSc. Instead, fibrin accumulation in the synovial lining cells, with atrophy of the synovial cells leading to a fibrosis is observed, similar to that present in the dermis.

Prevalence

Joint involvement has been described as an initial manifestation in 12–65 % of SSc patients with SSc and as an eventual manifestation in up to 46–97 % of patients [1, 45]. A systematic study on articular manifestations of 38 patients with SSc detected tenderness, stress pain, or effusions in approximately 61 % of patients. Ten patients had small effusions confined to the knees, with the exception of one PIP joint. The pattern was symmetrical polyarticular in 61 %, oligoarticular in 22 %, and monoarticular in 17 % of patients. A retrospective analysis of 100 patients investigating the clinical features of hand and foot involvement in SSc identified foot arthralgia and arthritis in 23 % and 14 % of patients respectively, and hand arthralgia and arthritis in 9 % and 11 % of patients respectively [14, 46]. The systematic cross-sectional examination of the EUSTAR registry, which included more than 7,000 patients, identified synovitis in 16 % (1,191/7,286) of patients with SSc, indicating synovial

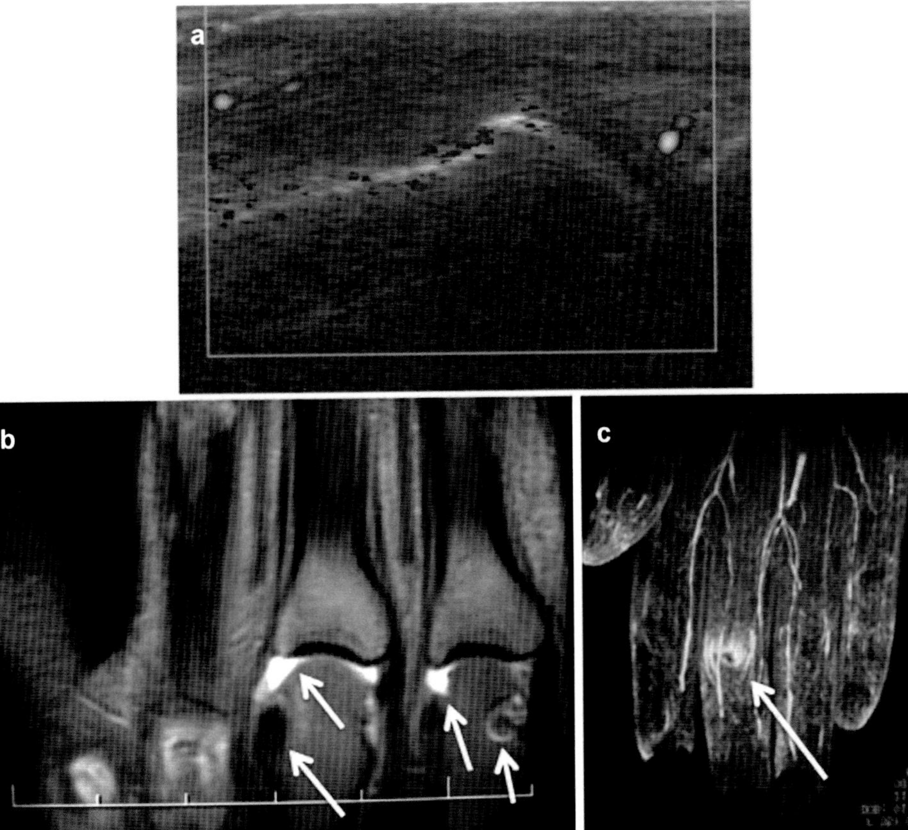

Fig. 36.4 (**a**) Ultrasonography with power Doppler imaging revealing synovitis of the second MCP joint. (**b**) MRI showing synovitis of and erosions of the third and fourth MCP joints (*white arrow*). (**c**) Magnetic resonance angiography revealing a synovitis of the third PIP joint (*white arrow*)

involvement may be a common feature in SSc [19]. The point prevalence of joint contracture, resulting from joint destruction turning into ankylosis and fibrotic changes in the skin, was 31 % (2,264/7,286) from this dataset.

We have learned from the management of rheumatoid arthritis that musculoskeletal ultrasound is very useful for detecting synovitis that is "subclinical." Sonography shows synovitis as abnormal hypoechoic (relative to subdermal fat) intra-articular tissue that is poorly compressible and that exhibits Doppler signal with color or power Doppler imaging (Fig. 36.4a). One can speculate that it may be even more useful in SSc in which swelling can be subtle, especially in the fingers and hands. Furthermore, since ultrasound can detect inflammatory activity, the monitoring of inflammatory activity with power Doppler ultrasonography could be very valuable.

An Italian study that included 45 consecutive patients with SSc assessed articular involvement using ultrasonography (Fig. 36.3) [47]. Joint effusion and synovial proliferation were found in 22 (49 %) and 19 (42 %) of the SSc patients, respectively (Table 36.3); synovial proliferation was associated with increased intra-articular power Doppler signals in 11 patients. The prevalence of synovitis detected with ultrasound (i.e., effusion and/or synovial proliferation) was significantly higher than that found by clinical examination (i.e., tenderness and/or swelling) (26 vs. 15 of 45 cases; $p=0.03$). Some correlation between synovitis and acute-phase reactants was also observed.

A second recent study has assessed ultrasonographic hand features in 52 patients with SSc [17] (Table 36.3). This study confirmed the more frequent detection of synovitis with ultrasound than with clinical examination (46 % vs. 15 %; $p<0.01$), although 57 % of patients had borderline mildly inflammatory activity with mostly Doppler grade 1.

A recent study performed on 44 patients with SSc also demonstrated the utility of ultrasonography in the assessment of hand and wrist involvement in SSc, particularly for the detection of synovitis, which was detected in 12 patients (27 %) [18] (Table 36.3).

MRI is also a very promising research tool to detect synovitis (Table 36.3). MRI reveals proliferative synovitis as thickening of the synovial membrane that appears as rapid enhancement after the administration of gadolinium; it is also well shown on fat-suppressed gadolinium-enhanced T1-weighted image (Fig. 36.4b). Hand inflammatory joint disease has been assessed by MRI in 17 patients with history of joint pain or swelling [16]. Ten patients had inflammatory MRI findings with synovitis ($n=8$), joint effusion ($n=7$), or tenosynovitis ($n=8$). In another series of 17 patients with SSc and arthralgia but no overt inflammatory arthritis, while

Table 36.3 Prevalence of joint involvement with ultrasonography and MRI

	Ultrasonography			MRI	
	Cuomo et al. [48] (n=45)	Elhai et al. [17] (n=52)	Freire et al. [18] (n=44)	Low et al. [16] (n=17)	Allanore et al. [68] (n=38)
Frequency of synovitis, n (%)	22 (49 %) 19 (42 %) with synovial proliferation	24 (46 %) 68 regions explored: 33 (48 %) power Doppler grade 1 6 (9 %) power Doppler grade 2 or 3	17 (39 %) 52 regions explored: 28/52 (54 %) power Doppler grade 1 5/52 (10 %) power Doppler grade 2 or 3	19 (50 %)	8 (47 %)
Frequency of joint space narrowing, n (%)	8 (18 %) MCP: 8 (100 %) PIP: 2 (25 %)	No data	No data	No data	No data
Frequency of erosions, n (%)	5 (11 %) Wrist: 1 (20 %) MCP: 4 (80 %)	No data	No data	7 (41 %) Wrist: 2 (29 %) MCP: 5 (71 %) PIP: 2 (29 %)	No data

both MRI and ultrasound were useful for characterizing synovial inflammation in SSc, MRI appeared clearly more sensitive than US in this setting [48]. Another recent study has compared MRI and ultrasonography to detect inflammatory arthropathy in SSc patients with hand arthralgia [49]. MRI and ultrasonography were both shown to be useful to characterize synovial inflammation, but MRI was also found more sensitive in this setting.

With regard to the burden of the vasculopathy in SSc, magnetic resonance angiography (MRA) has appeared as an appealing technique to assess hand vascular involvement. MRA can indeed be used to identify and quantitatively characterize the vascular disease in SSc fingers. We have described in a cross-sectional study the major arterial and venous involvement that can be identified using MRA. In addition, micro-MRA has also been used to focus on fingers, and non-enhanced MR angiography has also been used to improve the evaluation of the hand vasculature in vasospastic disorders [50, 51]. MRA also enables detection of synovitis, and in our study evaluating hand MRA in 38 SSc patients, 19 patients had one or more synovitis and 4 one or more tenosynovitis (Fig. 36.4c) [52].

Joint Involvement as a Correlate of Prognosis in SSc

Only a few studies to date have looked for an association between the subsets of SSc and a higher risk of developing arthritis. Analysis of the EUSTAR database revealed that synovitis was present in SSc patients at all disease stages. However, patients with synovitis and early disease (date of first non-Raynaud's symptom <5 years) were more likely to experience diffuse cutaneous thickening (Fig. 36.5).

This observation raises the question of the prognostic value of synovitis in patients with early SSc to identify those with potential risk of developing the diffuse cutaneous subset, which has a more fulminant course. The likelihood of severe vascular (elevated systolic pulmonary artery pressure above 40 mmHg) and muscular (muscle weakness) involvement was higher in patients with synovitis, regardless of their cutaneous subset or disease duration. Thus, synovitis could be viewed as a risk factor of poor prognosis in SSc.

Two recent prospective cohort studies including one from the EUSTAR database have identified joint synovitis as a predictor of disease progression. The first study included 1,301 patients with SSc with disease duration ≤3 years at inclusion and with a follow-up of at least 2 years (mean follow-up: 4.5±2.2 years) [21]. Joint synovitis, detected by clinical examination, was independently predictive of the worsening of the modified Rodnan skin score (≥30 % and ≥5 points) and of the further occurrence of new ischemic digital ulcers and decreased left ventricular ejection fraction. The second study was performed on 637 SSc patients with the diffuse cutaneous subset [53]. Joint synovitis was also identified in univariate and multivariate analysis as a predictor for progressive skin fibrosis. Using a second validation cohort of 188 patients with diffuse cutaneous SSc, joint synovitis was confirmed as an independent predictor of progressive skin fibrosis within 1 year. Taken together, the results of these two studies support that synovitis, an easily detected clinical marker, may be useful in the risk stratification of SSc patients.

The examination of the EUSTAR database also identified a strong association between synovitis and elevation of acute-phase reactants (erythrocyte sedimentation rate ≥28 mm (first hour) and C-reactive protein ≥10 mg/l), reflecting systemic inflammation. This suggests that joint involvement has a close relationship with systemic inflammation in SSc [23].

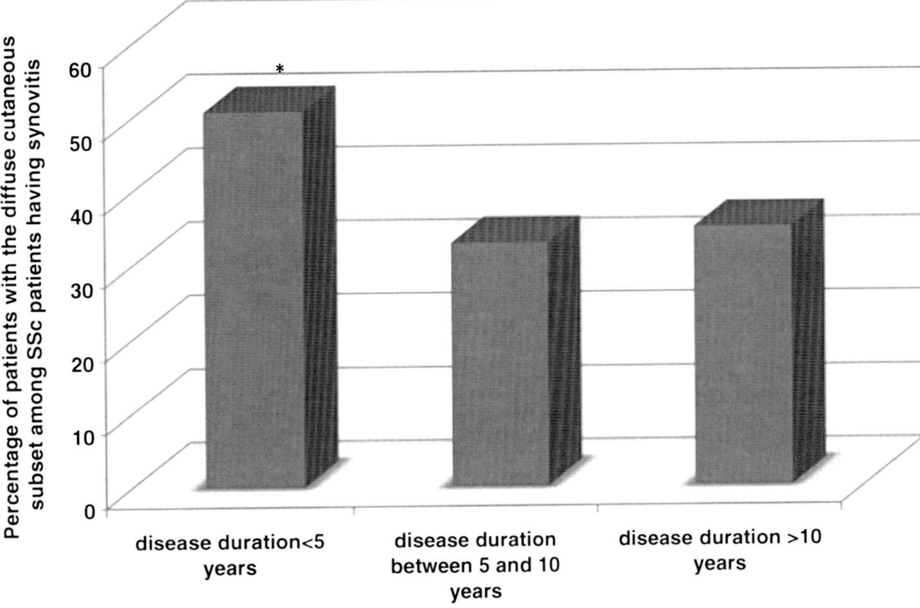

Fig. 36.5 Patients with synovitis and early disease (date of first non-Raynaud's symptom <5 years) are more likely to experience diffuse cutaneous thickening. $*P<0.05$ vs. patients with disease duration >5 years

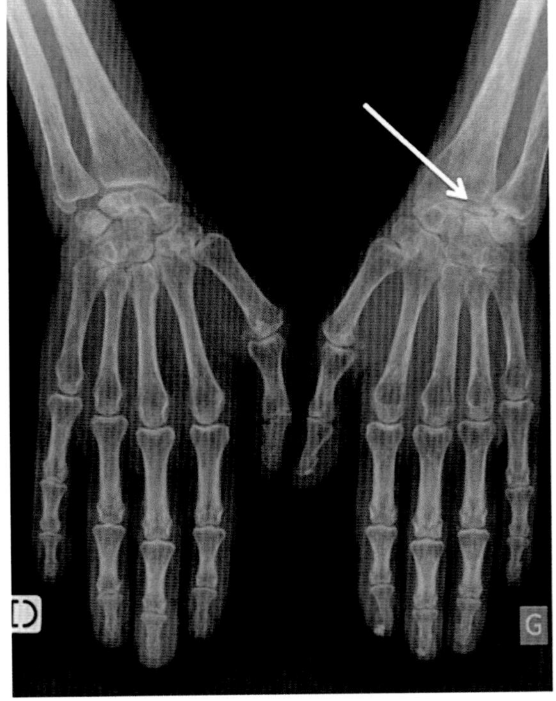

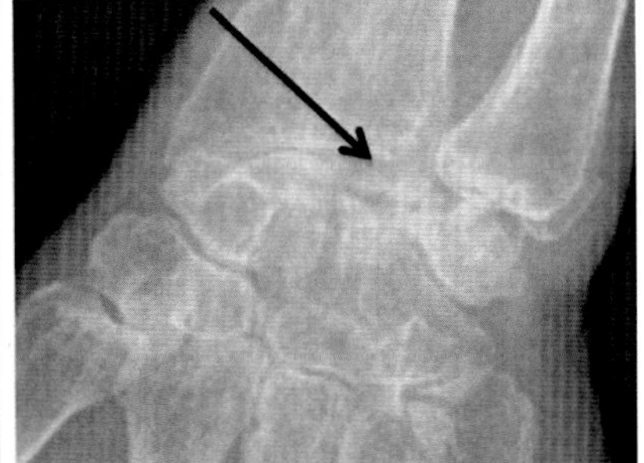

Fig. 36.6 Resorption of the left lunate in a patient with diffuse cutaneous systemic sclerosis

This is supported by the infiltration of inflammatory cell in SSc synovial biopsies [41]. Further studies are warranted to determine if joint involvement is the main contributor to systemic inflammation in SSc, as is observed in rheumatoid arthritis.

Radiologic Features: Structural Osteoarticular Lesions

Many distinctive radiographic abnormalities have been recognized in patients with SSc. A spectrum of articular and nonarticular changes have been described. Articular lesions from juxta-articular osteoporosis and joint space narrowing to frank erosions have been reported throughout the MCP, PIP, and DIP joints, as well as the wrist. Selective involvement of the first carpometacarpal phalangeal joint might be a distinctive feature of SSc. The described abnormalities include bilateral resorption of the trapezium (Fig. 36.6) and adjacent metacarpal bone along with intra-articular calcification and erosions [54]. The detection of pencil-in-cup deformity in hands and feet, considered to be relatively specific for psoriasis arthropathy, has also been reported [46]. The

Table 36.4 Prevalence of hand radiographic lesions in systemic sclerosis

	Avouac et al. [23] (n=120)	Baron et al. [1] (N=38)	La Montagna et al. [14] (N=51)	La Montagna et al. [46] (N=76)	Brun et al. [91] (N=41)	Koutaissoff et al. [55] (N=167)	Bassett et al. [32] (N=55)	Ingegnoli et al. [36] (N=75)	Erre et al. [92] (N=41)
Joint involvement, n (%):									
Erosion	25 (21)	15 (40)	10 (20)	8 (10.5)	9 (21)	30 (18)	12 (22)	11 (16)	8 (19)
Joint space narrowing	35 (28)	13 (34)	17 (33)	31 (41)	10 (24)	102 (61)	n.d.	n.d.	29 (71)
Bone involvement, n (%):									
Radiological demineralization	28 (23)	16 (42)	32 (63)	12 (16)	7 (17)	n.d.	n.d.	17 (23)	4 (10)
Acro-osteolysis	26 (22)	14 (37)	25 (55)	22 (29)	11 (27)	41 (25)	28 (51)	13 (17)	7 (17)
Soft tissue involvement, n (%):									
Flexion contracture	32 (27)	n.d.	n.d.	31 (41)	n.d.	n.d.	45 (82)	n.d.	11 (27)
Calcinosis	28 (23)	19 (50)	18 (35)	45 (59)	18 (44)	25 (15)	14 (25)	19 (25)	12 (29)

n.d. no data available

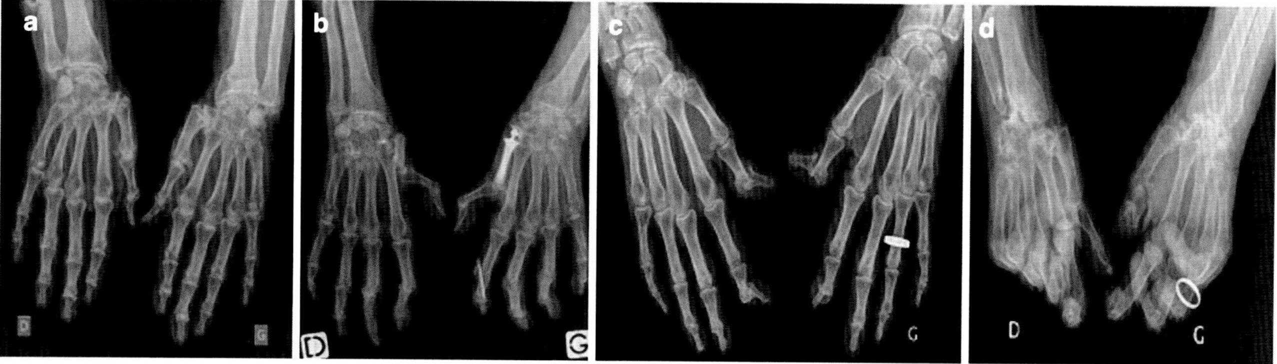

Fig. 36.7 (**a**–**d**) Four cases of erosive radiographic arthritis characterized by erosions and joint space narrowing involving the wrist, MCP, PIP, and/or DIP joints

frequency of hand radiographic erosions is estimated between 5 and 40% (Table 36.4) [1, 23, 32, 46, 55]. Joint space narrowing is not uncommon in SSc; its point prevalence on X-ray has been reported to be about 30%, with a predominant involvement of DIP joints (Table 36.4) [1, 23, 32, 46, 55]. Joint space narrowing has been found with ultrasonography in 8/45 (18%) SSc patients.

Modern techniques such as ultrasound and magnetic resonance have also been used to describe structural articular lesions. Point prevalence of erosions assessed by ultrasonography on 45 SSc patients was 11% (5/45 patients) [47]. In the two studies using MRI, hand erosions were detected in 16% (6/38 patients) and 41% (7/17 patients) [16, 52] (Fig. 36.4b). It is noteworthy that the predictive value of erosions detected by MRI is not known and remains to be determined. The pathogenesis of erosions is still unknown, although several hypotheses have been raised on the mechanisms underlying their formation. Erosions might arise secondary to inflammatory synovitis, or they might represent focal resorptive changes resulting from the continuous traction of tendons underlying demineralized bone, or they might represent a localized manifestation of an unexplained, more widespread osseous resorptive phenomenon recognized to affect various regions of the skeleton [1]. In the feet, the presence of erosions in the MTP joints could be due to an increase in plantar foot pressures identified in patients with SSc, similar to the association of erosions and abnormal plantar pressures that has been reported in patients with RA [46, 56, 57].

In a recent controlled study involving 120 patients, erosive arthritis, as defined by the occurrence of both erosions and joint space narrowing, was found in 22 (18%) SSc patients [23] (Fig. 36.7a–d). The 5-year longitudinal follow-up of these patients, with a systematic examination of dual time-point X-rays, showed a total radiographic progression of erosive arthritis in 24 (23%) patients with SSc. Among these, 10 had developed incident erosive arthritis, defined by the occurrence on the second X-ray of at least 1 erosion and joint space narrowing, and 14 experienced worsening of their baseline lesions, defined by the occurrence on the second X-ray of at least 1 new erosion and/or joint space narrowing [58]. The presence of erosive arthritis was not associated at baseline with any SSc characteristics or with the presence of rheumatoid factor or anti-CCP2 antibodies. This is in

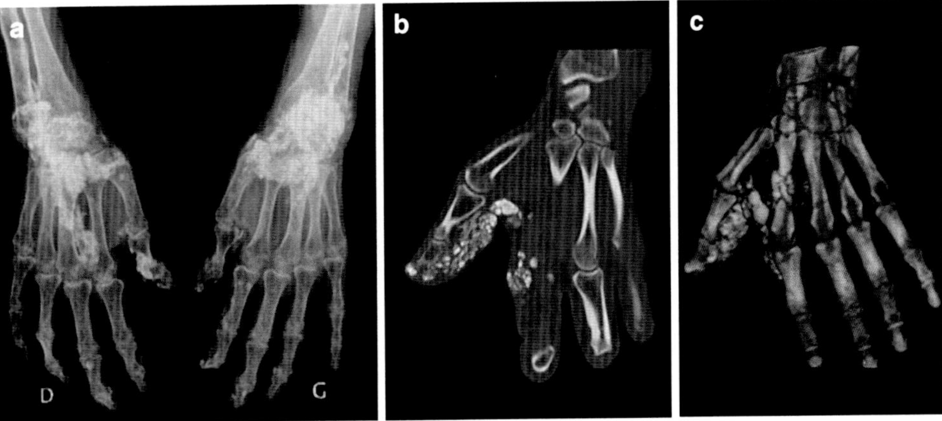

Fig. 36.8 (**a–c**) Severe hand calcinosis assessed by conventional X-ray (**a**) and CT scan without (**b**) and with 3D reconstruction (**c**)

accordance with previous studies that failed to show correlation between erosive arthritis and clinical or laboratory variables [1, 32].

Despite its high frequency in this cohort, we did not identify any independent predictor of the progression of erosive arthritis in SSc. This lack of predictive factor for erosive arthritis might be related to the multifactorial aspects of SSc arthropathy. An overlap with RA should be considered but was found only in two patients with erosive arthritis at baseline and in one patient with worsened erosive arthritis. The possibility of erosive osteoarthritis should also be considered, particularly in light of the nature of the erosions [56], the low frequency of persistent clinical synovitis in patients with development of erosive arthritis (5/24, 21 %), the high frequency of DIP joint involvement, and the large proportion in our sample of postmenopausal women. Finally, erosive arthropathy could also be as a direct result of SSc and considered as an integral feature of this disease.

There is thus a need to clarify the precise nature of the arthropathy observed in SSc in order to further identify valid predictors of the progression of erosive arthritis directly related to SSc. As reliable predictors of the future course of erosive arthritis are still unknown, patients should be followed up regularly, with clinical examination and regular X-rays. Moreover, this lack of valid predictors may significantly limit the use of potentially effective drugs. Recent developments of new imaging techniques in SSc should allow an early detection of erosive arthritis, before being detected on X-rays, and likely increase the chance of defining accurate predictors [16, 47, 52].

Nonarticular abnormalities are prominent in SSc and sometimes very specific. Indeed, subcutaneous calcifications may be seen as a hallmark of SSc in comparison to other connective tissue disorders (Fig. 36.8a–c). Recent studies using consecutive X-rays or ultrasonography have allowed clarification of its point prevalence, which is about 20–30 % (Table 36.4) [23, 47, 55]. The incidence of radiographic calcinosis after a median duration of 5 years was 14 % in a recent study from our group [58]. Calcinosis may also occur

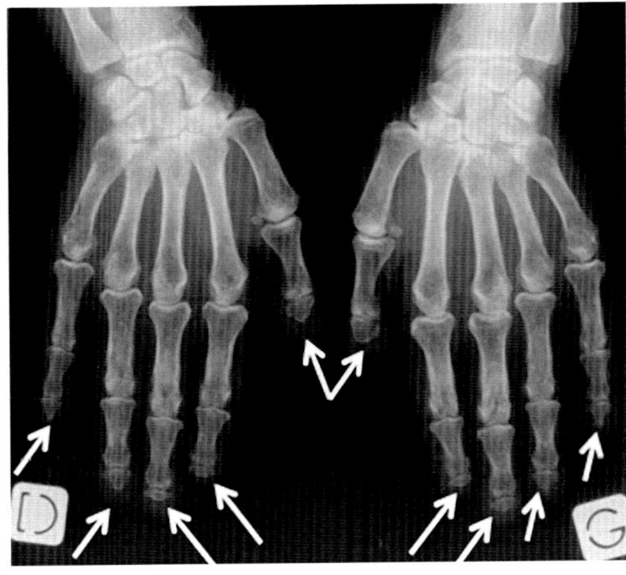

Fig. 36.9 Acro-osteolysis involving all the terminal phalanges (*white arrows*)

in other locations such as feet, knees, and legs. It is noteworthy that it predominates at sites of repetitive stress or pressure, suggesting that trauma and/or ischemia may contribute to its pathogenesis as this is well known for shoulder calcifications. This has been strengthened by recent cross-sectional series showing a link between calcinosis and digital ulcerations [23]. Calcinosis has also been found to be independently associated with the late nail fold videocapillaroscopy pattern and especially with severe capillary loss, which strengthens the link between these radiographic lesions and digital destructive vasculopathy [59]. In addition, digital ulcers have recently been identified as independent predictors of radiographic progression of calcinosis (Hazard Ratio, HR: 3.16, 95 % CI 1.22–9.43) [58].

Osseous resorption is another common finding and acro-osteolysis occurs in about 20 % of the patients [23, 46, 55] (Fig. 36.9). Furthermore, other locations may be involved such as the carpal bones, radius, ulna, ribs, mandible, clavicle, humerus, and cervical spine [60]. In a group of 134 Mediterranean patients, the incidence of vitamin D deficiency appeared to be 42 %, and secondary hyperparathyroidism was surprisingly high at 22 %. The authors observed some correlation between these abnormalities and the occurrence of acro-osteolysis and calcinosis [61]. In another study performed in two European countries, we also found that vitamin D insufficiency and deficiency rates were very high and comparable between the two populations: 74/90 (82 %) versus 57/66 (86 %) for insufficiency and 29/90 (32 %) versus 15/66 (23 %) for deficiency, in the French and Italian patient groups, respectively, [62]. The cohorts were not influenced by vitamin D supplementation, which was not statistically different in the two groups. In the combined populations, a significant negative correlation was found between low vitamin D levels and European Disease Activity Score, and an even more significant correlation was found with acute-phase reactants. Low levels of vitamin D were associated with the systolic pulmonary artery pressure estimated by echocardiography. No association was observed with calcinosis or acro-osteolysis and hyperparathyroidism. In multivariate analysis, vitamin D deficiency was associated with sPAP ($P=0.02$). This suggests that common vitamin D supplementation does not correct the deficiency in SSc patients and that a higher dose is probably needed, especially in those with high inflammatory activity or severe disease. In line, with the above results, calcinosis (HR: 6.17, 95 % CI 1.16–47.23) and digital ulcers (HR: 12.43, 95 % CI 1.97–88.40) were recently identified as independent predictors of the radiographic progression of acro-osteolysis [58]. These data suggest that patients with severe digital vasculopathy are at higher risk of sustaining radiographic progression of bone resorption and further support the role of vascular injury playing a critical role in such lesions, possibly due to repeated vasospasm, as previously suggested [63]. The association of acro-osteolysis and severe capillary loss observed with nail fold videocapillaroscopy also supports these findings. Severe acro-osteolysis is more likely to occur with neoangiogenesis (defined as irregular enlargement of the capillaries, disorganization of the normal capillary array, and ramified/bushy capillaries), which may suggest an attempt to compensate bone resorption [59].

Treatment

The management of articular involvement is essentially supportive and symptomatic. Symptomatic therapies or disease-modifying antirheumatic drugs have not yet been systematically evaluated for the treatment of articular involvement in SSc by randomized controlled trials. For the most part, the minor rheumatic symptoms of SSc, such as arthralgia, will respond to simple nonsteroidal anti-inflammatory drug treatment. Caution should be exercised, however, with this class of drugs because of the enhanced risk of gastroesophageal abnormalities or bleeding and impaired renal function in this group of patients. Low-dose corticosteroids (<10 mg/day) may also have some value for the symptomatic treatment of inflammatory arthritis or tenosynovitis. Employing a similar approach to RA, methotrexate is usually used for the treatment of inflammatory arthritis. Subcutaneous or intramuscular routes could be used to prevent reduced digestive absorption. Secondary analyses of the scleroderma lung study did not show any significant effects on articular outcomes of cyclophosphamide. In particular, there was no significant difference between placebo and cyclophosphamide groups for joint swelling and joint tenderness at 12 and 24 months [64].

A recent, small, pilot study of 6 months of intravenous immunoglobulin therapy in seven women with SSc and severe, refractory inflammatory joint involvement reported reduction in joint pain and tenderness, together with improvement of quality of life. However, this is an extremely small case series from which any reliable conclusion can be drawn. The costs of immunoglobulins might limit their use only to patients with very severe and refractory articular involvement, who failed disease-modifying antirheumatic drugs [65].

The introduction of biologic DMARDs has led to a new era in the treatment of inflammatory rheumatic conditions and is of increasing interest in SSc-related arthritis. The efficacy of tumor necrosis factor (TNF) inhibitors on inflammatory joint symptoms was suggested in a retrospective study performed on 18 patients treated with etanercept over a period of 2–66 months [66]. Fifteen of these 18 patients had "positive responses" (not defined in the "letter to the editor" report), with apparent significant decrease in signs of inflammation or synovitis on follow-up examination and complete resolution of joint symptoms in some patients. Mean HAQ Disability Index (HAQ-DI) scores also decreased with therapy, paralleling the improvement in joint disease. Despite these promising preliminary results, no other study has assessed the potential efficacy of TNF-inhibitors in SSc-related arthritis. This may be due to concerns about the safety of this therapeutic class in SSc. One case of fatal exacerbation of fibrosing alveolitis has been reported in a patient with SSc following adalimumab treatment [67]. However, other very rare cases of fatal exacerbation of pulmonary fibrosis while on treatment with TNF-inhibitors have also been described in patients with RA [68]. Nevertheless, in a 26-week open-label pilot study performed on 16 patients that aimed to assess the safety of infliximab in diffuse cutaneous SSc, 127 adverse events (10 severe) occurred in 16 patients. Of these, 19 adverse events were directly related to infliximab treatment. Moreover, infusion reactions directly related to infliximab led to early treatment discontinuation in 8/16 patients [69]. Separately, infliximab did not show a clear overall benefit at week 26, although articular involvement was not included as an outcome measure. Thus, these data may limit the further use of these drugs in SSc-related arthritis to a formal randomized clinical trial.

A three-round Delphi exercise was recently performed among EUSTAR centers to obtain expert consensus on the use of TNF-inhibitors in SSc [70]. Most EUSTAR experts recommended the use of TNF-inhibitors only as part of randomized controlled clinical trials and discouraged off-label use in individual patients outside of clinical trials. Arthritis was considered a manifestation that might respond to TNF-inhibitors, and the group recommended that the response of SSc arthritis to TNF-inhibitors should be investigated in more detail. In contrast, other manifestations of SSc, such as fibrosis, were not anticipated to benefit from treatment with TNF-inhibitors. Thus, it seems reasonable to await consistent, controlled trials regarding the safety and efficacy of TNF-α inhibitors for joint symptoms in patients with SSc.

Rituximab, a chimeric monoclonal antibody against the protein CD20 that has demonstrated efficacy and been extremely successful in RA, might also be potentially beneficial for the treatment of SSc arthritis. However, no study has yet formally assessed this drug for this specific indication. Open-label trials seem promising regarding the potential efficacy of rituximab for the treatment of skin and pulmonary manifestations in SSc, although articular involvement was not evaluated in any of these studies [71–73]. Further research assessing the efficacy of rituximab in SSc-related joint disease is now warranted before this treatment is recommended.

The EUSTAR group collected observations that revealed a trend toward articular improvement in cases of polyarthritis following tocilizumab in refractory SSc without, however, favorable signs of dermatologic or pulmonary involvement but rather with a weak decline [74]. There was decrease in the Disease Activity Score (DAS)-28 of 1.8 ± 1.5 (2.8 ± 0.6 before the last infusion administered at 6 months versus 4.6 ± 1.0 at the beginning, $p = 0.02$) with a decrease in the painful joint count of 5 (4.2 ± 4.3 versus 9.2 ± 8.6) and in the swollen joint count of 0.5 (3.0 ± 4.4 versus 3.5 ± 3). A good EULAR response was observed in three out of five patients. The preliminary results of a phase III study called FaSScinate has recently been presented [75]. It evaluated the efficacy of tocilizumab on SSc cutaneous involvement in recent and evolving diffuse cutaneous form. Favorable trends in skin score for tocilizumab were detected though the primary skin score end point was not met. In addition, encouraging changes in FVC were noted. The ongoing double-blind and open-label phases of this trial will provide additional information, especially on inflammatory joint involvement.

The EUSTAR group has also collected observations on the effects of abatacept on articular involvement in SSc [74]. Like tocilizumab, favorable effects on inflammatory articular involvement were obtained after 11 months of treatment with abatacept with a good EULAR response in 6 out of 11 patients. However, no modification in cutaneous and pulmonary involvement was observed. A phase II multicenter study called ASSET (A Study of Subcutaneous Abatacept to Treat Diffuse Cutaneous Systemic Sclerosis) on the early diffuse cutaneous form is ongoing and will evaluate the safety and the efficacy of abatacept primarily on skin involvement. Positive or negative change on 28 tender/swollen joint counts will be also assessed as a secondary outcome.

Thus, tocilizumab and abatacept seem to be safe and preliminary data suggest that they may improve joint involvement after 3–6 months in refractory SSc arthritis patients. These encouraging first reports suggest that biologic DMARDs may open major opportunities in SSc-related arthritis.

The current literature on rehabilitation techniques in SSc consists of studies evaluating the effectiveness of paraffin wax treatment, hand and face stretching exercises, connective tissue massage and joint manipulation, splints, aerobic exercise, and resistance training. The data seem promising, except for splints, for the improvement in joint motion, hand function, and cardiopulmonary endurance. However, except for four randomized controlled trials, the majority of studies involved small sample sizes and no control groups. Thus, larger randomized controlled studies are needed to fully determine the effectiveness of rehabilitation techniques for persons with SSc [76].

Surgery of the hand for SSc is generally considered for pain reduction, severe fixed deformities with functional limitations, ulceration, and calcinosis. The goals of surgery are limited and include pain relief, repositioning the digits, providing a functional position of fusion, and in some cases modest mobilization through resection arthroplasty, to marginally improve finger function for patients with marked preexisting limitations. Surgical reconstruction of severely flexed PIP joints by straightening and fusing them is quite successful if the MCP joints are mobile. This procedure may increase function and reduce the frequency of dorsal skin ulceration. Some rigid, deformed digits benefit from MCP joint resection to overcome contracture, reposition the digits, and introduce a small range of mobility. Local or regional anesthesia should be preferred for patients who present cardiac or pulmonary manifestations of SSc. Moreover, severe perioral involvement can result in difficulty with orotracheal intubation. Surgical wounds generally heal well following fusion of the PIP or DIP joints [77].

Despite many attempts, there is still a lack of efficient treatment of calcinosis [78–81]. The natural course and strong heterogeneity of calcinosis are very challenging and have prevented until now the performance of clinical trials. The results of our prospective study suggest that the treatment of calcinosis should primarily target SSc vasculopathy. This may be supported by data reported on shoulder tendinitis in which calcinosis usually appears close to tendon ischemic site [82]. Nevertheless, no robust data confirmed that calcium channel blockers have a positive effect on calcinosis. The effects of other treatments, including bisphosphonates, warfarin, and minocycline, remain controversial and were obtained through small series [83–85]. Surgical excision of calcinosis provides moderate results with respect to pain relief and function. However, the procedure requires extensive incisions and carries a risk of slower wound healing [77].

Bone Involvement

Many studies have established an increased risk of bone loss and fracture in individuals with chronic inflammatory conditions. These patients are at increased risk for osteoporosis for many reasons: the glucocorticoid medications often prescribed for the treatment can trigger significant bone loss. In addition, pain and loss of joint function caused by the disease can result in inactivity, further increasing osteoporosis risk. Studies also show that bone loss in rheumatoid arthritis may occur as a direct result of the inflammatory disease. By contrast, it is still unknown whether osteoporosis is truly increased in SSc or whether this association has been observed in some studies as a result of other confounding risk factors. Indeed, small sample size and clinical heterogeneity of SSc study samples have lead to underpowered and unprecise estimates of the risk for the development of osteoporosis [86]. In a series of 43 postmenopausal SSc patients and 47 healthy postmenopausal women, excluding severe SSc, a higher frequency of osteoporosis in the lumbar spine (32.5 %) and femoral neck (51.1 %) was observed in SSc patients when compared to controls (14.8 % vs. 19.1 %; $p<0.01$). Multiple linear regression analysis revealed an association between the presence of SSc and low bone mineral density. Lean mass was an important factor related to osteoporosis [87]. In another recent cross-sectional study including 71 SSc, 139 rheumatoid arthritis (RA), and 227 healthy women, the prevalence of osteoporosis and fracture was similar in SSc and RA and was for both higher than in healthy controls (osteoporosis: 30 % in SSc, 32 % in RA, and 11 % in controls; fracture: 35 % in SSc, 33 % in RA, and 10 % in controls) [88]. Multivariate analysis identified disease duration as a risk factor of osteoporosis in SSc. Age and low 25(OH)D levels were recognized as risk factors of fracture in SSc. Thus, these results support the performance of BMD measurements together with vitamin D supply in patients with SSc. In another report, 27/61 SSc patients presented osteopenia and 14/61 osteoporosis. Bone mineral density results in fertility, and postmenopausal SSc patients were independent of the SSc clinical variants, race, and previous use of corticosteroids and cyclophosphamide. However, a low density was associated with a low body mass index [89]. Some other series were less demonstrative and therefore there is no strong evidence in the literature for consistently lower bone mineral density scores in SSc [90]. Premature menopause, corticosteroid use, major disability, or other factors secondary to SSc (malabsorption, low weight, or sometimes systemic inflammation) may be causal factors or confounders in SSc. Therefore, more work is needed to determine the precise risk or the lack of specific risk of osteoporosis in SSc patients and to define adapted management.

Conclusion and Perspectives

Skeletal involvement is frequent in SSc and represents a heavy burden. It is multifaceted and injury of several structures, such as tendon, joint, bone, or soft tissue, can occur. Recent clinical and radiographic studies with large sample size have allowed a better estimation of the frequency of joint involvement and identified subsets of SSc patients with the higher risk of developing joint, bone, or soft tissue involvement. In addition, prospective studies have recently identified joint and tendon involvement as predictors of disease progression. Several pilot studies have underlined the potential interest of new imaging techniques, such as ultrasonography, MRI, or MRA, for the early detection of articular, tendon, or soft tissue involvement. Larger studies are now needed to confirm these promising results and validate these tools in clinical practice and estimate their predictive value. Finally, although the understanding of osteoarticular pathogenesis has significantly increased these last years, optimal treatments of inflammatory joint disease, tenosynovitis, bone resorption, and calcinosis remain to be determined and remain a major challenge for improving SSc morbidity.

References

1. Baron M, Lee P, Keystone EC. The articular manifestations of progressive systemic sclerosis (scleroderma). Ann Rheum Dis. 1982;41:147–52.
2. Hietaharju A, Jaaskelainen S, Kalimo H, Hietarinta M. Peripheral neuromuscular manifestations in systemic sclerosis (scleroderma). Muscle Nerve. 1993;16:1204–12.
3. Mau W, Listing J, Huscher D, Zeidler H, Zink A. Employment across chronic inflammatory rheumatic diseases and comparison with the general population. J Rheumatol. 2005;32:721–8.
4. Brower LM, Poole JL. Reliability and validity of the Duruoz Hand Index in persons with systemic sclerosis (scleroderma). Arthritis Rheum. 2004;51:805–9.
5. Poole JL, Gallegos M, O'Linc S. Reliability and validity of the Arthritis Hand Function Test in adults with systemic sclerosis (scleroderma). Arthritis Care Res. 2000;13:69–73.

6. Poole JL, Steen VD. The use of the Health Assessment Questionnaire (HAQ) to determine physical disability in systemic sclerosis. Arthritis Care Res. 1991;4:27–31.
7. Richards HL, Herrick AL, Griffin K, Gwilliam PD, Loukes J, Fortune DG. Systemic sclerosis: patients' perceptions of their condition. Arthritis Rheum. 2003;49:689–96.
8. Sandqvist G, Eklund M, Akesson A, Nordenskiold U. Daily activities and hand function in women with scleroderma. Scand J Rheumatol. 2004;33:102–7.
9. Bandinelli F, Kaloudi O, Candelieri A, Conforti ML, Casale R, Cammarata S, et al. Early detection of median nerve syndrome at the carpal tunnel with high-resolution 18 MHz ultrasonography in systemic sclerosis patients. Clin Exp Rheumatol. 2010;28:S15–8.
10. Tagliafico A, Panico N, Resmini E, Derchi LE, Ghio M, Martinoli C. The role of ultrasound imaging in the evaluation of peripheral nerve in systemic sclerosis (scleroderma). Eur J Radiol. 2009;77:377–82.
11. Machet L, Vaillant L, Machet MC, Esteve E, Muller C, Khallouf R, et al. Carpal tunnel syndrome and systemic sclerosis. Dermatology. 1992;185:101–3.
12. Rodnan GP, Medsger TA. The rheumatic manifestations of progressive systemic sclerosis (scleroderma). Clin Orthop Relat Res. 1968;57:81–93.
13. Rosenbaum LH, Swartz WM, Rodnan GP, Medsger Jr TA. Wrist drop in progressive systemic sclerosis (scleroderma): complete rupture of the extensor tendon mechanism. Arthritis Rheum. 1985;28:586–9.
14. La Montagna G, Baruffo A, Tirri R, Buono G, Valentini G. Foot involvement in systemic sclerosis: a longitudinal study of 100 patients. Semin Arthritis Rheum. 2002;31:248–55.
15. Steen VD, Medsger Jr TA. The palpable tendon friction rub: an important physical examination finding in patients with systemic sclerosis. Arthritis Rheum. 1997;40:1146–51.
16. Low AH, Lax M, Johnson SR, Lee P. Magnetic resonance imaging of the hand in systemic sclerosis. J Rheumatol. 2009;36:961–4.
17. Elhai M, Guerini H, Bazeli R, Avouac J, Freire V, Drapé JL, et al. Ultrasonographic hand features in systemic sclerosis and correlates with clinical, biologic, and radiographic findings. Arthritis Care Res (Hoboken). 2012;64:1244–9.
18. Freire V, Bazeli R, Elhai M, Campagna R, Pessis E, Avouac J, et al. Hand and wrist involvement in systemic sclerosis: US features. Radiology. 2013;269:824–30.
19. Avouac J, Walker U, Tyndall A, Kahan A, Matucci-Cerinic M, Allanore Y, et al. Characteristics of joint involvement and relationships with systemic inflammation in systemic sclerosis: results from the EULAR Scleroderma Trial and Research Group (EUSTAR) database. J Rheumatol. 2010;37:1488–501.
20. Khanna PP, Furst DE, Clements PJ, Maranian P, Indulkar L, Khanna D. Tendon friction rubs in early diffuse systemic sclerosis: prevalence, characteristics and longitudinal changes in a randomized controlled trial. Rheumatology (Oxford). 2010;49:955–9.
21. Avouac J, Walker UA, Hachulla E, Riemekasten G, Cuomo G, Carreira PE, et al. Joint and tendon involvement predict disease progression in systemic sclerosis: a EUSTAR prospective study. Ann Rheum Dis. 2016;75:103–9.
22. Palmer DG, Hale GM, Grennan DM, Pollock M. Bowed fingers. A helpful sign in the early diagnosis of systemic sclerosis. J Rheumatol. 1981;8:266–72.
23. Avouac J, Guerini H, Wipff J, Assous N, Chevrot A, Kahan A, et al. Radiological hand involvement in systemic sclerosis. Ann Rheum Dis. 2006;65:1088–92.
24. Cohen MJ, Persellin RH. Coexistence of rheumatoid arthritis and systemic sclerosis in four patients. Scand J Rheumatol. 1982;11: 241–5.
25. Armstrong RD, Gibson T. Scleroderma and erosive polyarthritis: a disease entity? Ann Rheum Dis. 1982;41:141–6.
26. Baron M, Srolovitz H, Lander P, Kapusta M. The coexistence of rheumatoid arthritis and scleroderma: a case report and review of the literature. J Rheumatol. 1982;9:947–50.
27. Avouac J, Airò P, Dieude P, Caramaschi P, Tiev K, Diot E, et al. Associated autoimmune diseases in Systemic Sclerosis define a subset of patients with milder disease: results from two large cohorts of European Caucasian patients. J Rheumatol. 2010;37: 608–14.
28. Avouac J, Gossec L, Dougados M. Diagnostic and predictive value of anti-cyclic citrullinated protein antibodies in rheumatoid arthritis: a systematic literature review. Ann Rheum Dis. 2006;65: 845–51.
29. Morita Y, Muro Y, Sugiura K, Tomita Y. Anti-cyclic citrullinated peptide antibody in systemic sclerosis. Clin Exp Rheumatol. 2008;26:542–7.
30. Marrone M, Chiala A, Tampoia M, Iannone F, Raho L, Covelli M, et al. Prevalence of anti-CCP antibodies in systemic sclerosis. Reumatismo. 2007;59:20–4.
31. Horiki T, Moriuchi J, Takaya M, Uchiyama M, Hoshina Y, Inada K, et al. The coexistence of systemic sclerosis and rheumatoid arthritis in five patients. Clinical and immunogenetic features suggest a distinct entity. Arthritis Rheum. 1996;39:152–6.
32. Blocka KL, Bassett LW, Furst DE, Clements PJ, Paulus HE. The arthropathy of advanced progressive systemic sclerosis. A radiographic survey. Arthritis Rheum. 1981;24:874–84.
33. Misra R, Darton K, Jewkes RF, Black CM, Maini RN. Arthritis in scleroderma. Br J Rheumatol. 1995;34:831–7.
34. Avouac J, Sordet C, Depinay C, Ardizonne M, Vacher-Lavenu MC, Sibilia J, et al. Systemic sclerosis-associated Sjogren's syndrome and relationship to the limited cutaneous subtype: results of a prospective study of sicca syndrome in 133 consecutive patients. Arthritis Rheum. 2006;54:2243–9.
35. Santiago M, Baron M, Miyachi K, Fritzler MJ, Abu-Hakima M, Leclercq S, et al. A comparison of the frequency of antibodies to cyclic citrullinated peptides using a third generation anti-CCP assay (CCP3) in systemic sclerosis, primary biliary cirrhosis and rheumatoid arthritis. Clin Rheumatol. 2008;27:77–83.
36. Ingegnoli F, Galbiati V, Zeni S, Meani L, Zahalkova L, Lubatti C, et al. Use of antibodies recognizing cyclic citrullinated peptide in the differential diagnosis of joint involvement in systemic sclerosis. Clin Rheumatol. 2007;26:510–4.
37. Generini S, Steiner G, Miniati I, Conforti ML, Guiducci S, Skriner K, et al. Anti-hnRNP and other autoantibodies in systemic sclerosis with joint involvement. Rheumatology (Oxford). 2009;48:920–5.
38. Ueda-Hayakawa I, Hasegawa M, Kumada S, Tanaka C, Komura K, Hamaguchi Y, et al. Usefulness of anti-cyclic citrullinated peptide antibody and rheumatoid factor to detect rheumatoid arthritis in patients with systemic sclerosis. Rheumatology (Oxford). 2010;49:2135–9.
39. La Montagna G, D'Angelo S, Valentini G. Cross-sectional evaluation of YKL-40 serum concentrations in patients with systemic sclerosis. Relationship with clinical and serological aspects of disease. J Rheumatol. 2003;30:2147–51.
40. Rozman B, Cucnik S, Sodin-Semrl S, Czirjak L, Varju C, Distler O, et al. Prevalence and clinical associations of anti-Ku antibodies in patients with systemic sclerosis: a European EUSTAR-initiated multi-centre case-control study. Ann Rheum Dis. 2008;67:1282–6.
41. Schumacher Jr HR. Joint involvement in progressive systemic sclerosis (scleroderma): a light and electron microscopic study of synovial membrane and fluid. Am J Clin Pathol. 1973;60:593–600.
42. Hollander JL, McCarty Jr DJ, Astorga G, Castro-Murillo E. Studies on the pathogenesis of rheumatoid joint inflammation. I. The "R.A. Cell" and a working hypothesis. Ann Intern Med. 1965;62: 271–80.

43. Barry M, Katz L, Cooney L. An unusual articular presentation of progressive systemic sclerosis. Arthritis Rheum. 1983;26:1041–3.
44. Clark JA, Winkelmann RK, McDuffie FC, Ward LE. Synovial tissue changes and rheumatoid factor in scleroderma. Mayo Clin Proc. 1971;46:97–103.
45. Tuffanelli DL, Winkelmann RK. Systemic scleroderma, a clinical study of 727 cases. Arch Dermatol. 1961;84:359–71.
46. La Montagna G, Sodano A, Capurro V, Malesci D, Valentini G. The arthropathy of systemic sclerosis: a 12 month prospective clinical and imaging study. Skeletal Radiol. 2005;34:35–41.
47. Cuomo G, Zappia M, Abignano G, Iudici M, Rotondo A, Valentini G. Ultrasonographic features of the hand and wrist in systemic sclerosis. Rheumatology (Oxford). 2009;48:1414–7.
48. Chitale S, Ciapetti A, Hodgson R, Grainger A, O'Connor P, Goodson NJ, et al. Magnetic resonance imaging and musculoskeletal ultrasonography detect and characterize covert inflammatory arthropathy in systemic sclerosis patients with arthralgia. Rheumatology (Oxford). 2007;49:2357–61.
49. Abdel-Magied RA, Lotfi A, AbdelGawad EA. Magnetic resonance imaging versus musculoskeletal ultrasonography in detecting inflammatory arthropathy in systemic sclerosis patients with hand arthralgia. Rheumatol Int. 2013;33:1961–6.
50. Wang J, Yarnykh VL, Molitor JA, Nash RA, Chu B, Wilson GJ, et al. Micro magnetic resonance angiography of the finger in systemic sclerosis. Rheumatology (Oxford). 2008;47:1239–43.
51. Sheehan JJ, Fan Z, Davarpanah AH, Hodnett PA, Varga J, Carr JC, et al. Nonenhanced MR angiography of the hand with flow-sensitive dephasing-prepared balanced SSFP sequence: initial experience with systemic sclerosis. Radiology. 2011;259:248–56.
52. Allanore Y, Seror R, Chevrot A, Kahan A, Drape JL. Hand vascular involvement assessed by magnetic resonance angiography in systemic sclerosis. Arthritis Rheum. 2007;56:2747–54.
53. Maurer B, Graf N, Michel BA, Muller-Ladner U, Czirjak L, Denton CP, et al. Prediction of worsening of skin fibrosis in patients with diffuse cutaneous systemic sclerosis using the EUSTAR database. Ann Rheum Dis. 2015;74:1124–31.
54. Resnick D, Greenway G, Vint VC, Robinson CA, Piper S. Selective involvement of the first carpometacarpal joint in scleroderma. AJR Am J Roentgenol. 1978;131:283–6.
55. Koutaissoff S, Vanthuyne M, Smith V, De Langhe E, Depresseux G, Westhovens R, et al. Hand radiological damage in systemic sclerosis: comparison with a control group and clinical and functional correlations. Semin Arthritis Rheum. 2010;40:455–60.
56. Allali F, Tahiri L, Senjari A, Abouqal R, Hajjaj-Hassouni N. Erosive arthropathy in systemic sclerosis. BMC Public Health. 2007;7:260.
57. van der Leeden M, Steultjens M, Dekker JH, Prins AP, Dekker J. Forefoot joint damage, pain and disability in rheumatoid arthritis patients with foot complaints: the role of plantar pressure and gait characteristics. Rheumatology (Oxford). 2006;45:465–9.
58. Avouac J, Mogavero G, Guerini H, Drape JL, Mathieu A, Kahan A, et al. Predictive factors of hand radiographic lesions in systemic sclerosis: a prospective study. Ann Rheum Dis. 2011;70:630–3.
59. Morardet L, Avouac J, Sammour M, Kahan A, Feydy A, Allanore Y. Nail fold videocapillaroscopy patterns associated with calcinosis and acro-osteolysis in systemic sclerosis. Arthritis Rheumatol. 2014;66:847.
60. Mugino H, Ikemura K. Progressive systemic sclerosis with spontaneous fracture due to resorption of the mandible: a case report. J Oral Maxillofac Surg. 2006;64:1137–9.
61. Braun-Moscovici Y, Furst DE, Markovits D, Rozin A, Clements PJ, Nahir AM, et al. Vitamin D, parathyroid hormone, and acroosteolysis in systemic sclerosis. J Rheumatol. 2008;35:2201–5.
62. Vacca A, Cormier C, Piras M, Mathieu A, Kahan A, Allanore Y. Vitamin D deficiency and insufficiency in 2 independent cohorts of patients with systemic sclerosis. J Rheumatol. 2009;36:1924–9.
63. Scharer L, Smith DW. Resorption of the terminal phalanges in scleroderma. Arthritis Rheum. 1969;12:51–63.
64. Au K, Mayes MD, Maranian P, Clements PJ, Khanna D, Steen VD, et al. Course of dermal ulcers and musculoskeletal involvement in systemic sclerosis patients in the scleroderma lung study. Arthritis Care Res (Hoboken). 2010;62:1772–8.
65. Nacci F, Righi A, Conforti ML, Miniati I, Fiori G, Martinovic D, et al. Intravenous immunoglobulins improve the function and ameliorate joint involvement in systemic sclerosis: a pilot study. Ann Rheum Dis. 2007;66:977–9.
66. Lam GK, Hummers LK, Woods A, Wigley FM. Efficacy and safety of etanercept in the treatment of scleroderma-associated joint disease. J Rheumatol. 2007;34:1636–7.
67. Allanore Y, Devos-Francois G, Caramella C, Boumier P, Jounieaux V, Kahan A. Fatal exacerbation of fibrosing alveolitis associated with systemic sclerosis in a patient treated with adalimumab. Ann Rheum Dis. 2006;65:834–5.
68. Ostor AJ, Crisp AJ, Somerville MF, Scott DG. Fatal exacerbation of rheumatoid arthritis associated fibrosing alveolitis in patients given infliximab. BMJ. 2004;329:1266.
69. Denton CP, Engelhart M, Tvede N, Wilson H, Khan K, Shiwen X, et al. An open-label pilot study of infliximab therapy in diffuse cutaneous systemic sclerosis. Ann Rheum Dis. 2009;68:1433–9.
70. Distler JH, Jordan S, Airo P, Alegre-Sancho J, Allanore Y, Balbir Gurman A, et al. Is there a role for TNFα antagonists in the treatment of SSc? EUSTAR expert consensus development using the Delphi technique. Clin Exp Rheumatol. 2011;29:S40–5.
71. Lafyatis R, Kissin E, York M, Farina G, Viger K, Fritzler MJ, et al. B cell depletion with rituximab in patients with diffuse cutaneous systemic sclerosis. Arthritis Rheum. 2009;60:578–83.
72. Smith V, Van Praet JT, Vandooren B, Van der Cruyssen B, Naeyaert JM, Decuman S, et al. Rituximab in diffuse cutaneous systemic sclerosis: an open-label clinical and histopathological study. Ann Rheum Dis. 2010;69:193–7.
73. Daoussis D, Liossis SN, Tsamandas AC, Kalogeropoulou C, Kazantzi A, Sirinian C, et al. Experience with rituximab in scleroderma: results from a 1-year, proof-of-principle study. Rheumatology (Oxford). 2009;49:271–80.
74. Elhai M, Meunier M, Matucci-Cerinic M, Maurer B, Riemekasten G, Leturcq T, et al. Outcomes of patients with systemic sclerosis-associated polyarthritis and myopathy treated with tocilizumab or abatacept: a EUSTAR observational study. Ann Rheum Dis. 2013;72:1217–20.
75. Khanna D, Denton CP, van Laar J, Jahreis A, Cheng S, Spotswood H, et al. Safety and efficacy of subcutaneous tocilizumab in adults with systemic sclerosis: week 24 data from a phase 2/3 trial. Arthritis Rheumatol. 2014;66:386.
76. Poole JL. Musculoskeletal rehabilitation in the person with scleroderma. Curr Opin Rheumatol. 2010;22:205–12.
77. Bogoch ER, Gross DK. Surgery of the hand in patients with systemic sclerosis: outcomes and considerations. J Rheumatol. 2005;32:642–8.
78. Vayssairat M, Hidouche D, Abdoucheli-Baudot N, Gaitz JP. Clinical significance of subcutaneous calcinosis in patients with systemic sclerosis. Does diltiazem induce its regression? Ann Rheum Dis. 1998;57:252–4.
79. Farah MJ, Palmieri GM, Sebes JI, Cremer MA, Massie JD, Pinals RS. The effect of diltiazem on calcinosis in a patient with the CREST syndrome. Arthritis Rheum. 1990;33:1287–93.
80. Dolan AL, Kassimos D, Gibson T, Kingsley GH. Diltiazem induces remission of calcinosis in scleroderma. Br J Rheumatol. 1995;34:576–8.
81. Palmieri GM, Sebes JI, Aelion JA, Moinuddin M, Ray MW, Wood GC, et al. Treatment of calcinosis with diltiazem. Arthritis Rheum. 1995;38:1646–54.

82. Matsumoto I, Ito Y, Tomo H, Nakao Y, Takaoka K. Case reports: ossified mass of the rotator cuff tendon in the subacromial bursa. Clin Orthop Relat Res. 2005;437:247–50.
83. Metzger AL, Singer FR, Bluestone R, Pearson CM. Failure of disodium etidronate in calcinosis due to dermatomyositis and scleroderma. N Engl J Med. 1974;291:1294–6.
84. Cukierman T, Elinav E, Korem M, Chajek-Shaul T. Low dose warfarin treatment for calcinosis in patients with systemic sclerosis. Ann Rheum Dis. 2004;63:1341–3.
85. Robertson LP, Marshall RW, Hickling P. Treatment of cutaneous calcinosis in limited systemic sclerosis with minocycline. Ann Rheum Dis. 2003;62:267–9.
86. Loucks J, Pope JE. Osteoporosis in scleroderma. Semin Arthritis Rheum. 2005;34:678–82.
87. Souza RB, Borges CT, Takayama L, Aldrighi JM, Pereira RM. Systemic sclerosis and bone loss: the role of the disease and body composition. Scand J Rheumatol. 2006;35:384–7.
88. Avouac J, Koumakis E, Toth E, Meunier M, Maury E, Kahan A, et al. Increased risk of osteoporosis and fracture in women with systemic sclerosis: a comparative study with rheumatoid arthritis. Arthritis Care Res (Hoboken). 2012;64:1871–8.
89. Sampaio-Barros PD, Costa-Paiva L, Filardi S, Sachetto Z, Samara AM, Marques-Neto JF. Prognostic factors of low bone mineral density in systemic sclerosis. Clin Exp Rheumatol. 2005;23: 180–4.
90. Neumann K, Wallace DJ, Metzger AL. Osteoporosis – less than expected in patients with scleroderma? J Rheumatol. 2000;27: 1822–3.
91. Brun B, Serup J, Hagdrup H. Radiological changes of the hands in systemic sclerosis. Acta Derm Venereol. 1983;63(4):349–52.
92. Erre GL, Marongiu A, Fenu P, Faedda R, Masala A, Sanna M, et al. The "sclerodermic hand": a radiological and clinical study. Joint Bone Spine. 2008;75(4):426–31.
93. Khanna PP, Furst DE, Clements PJ, Maranian P, Indulkar L, Khanna D; D-Penicillamine Investigators. Tendon friction rubs in early diffuse systemic sclerosis: prevalence, characteristics and longitudinal changes in a randomized controlled trial. Rheumatology (Oxford). 2010;49:955–9.
94. Ostojić P, Damjanov N.Different clinical features in patients with limited and diffuse cutaneous systemic sclerosis. Clin Rheumatol. 2006;25:453–7.
95. Ostojic P, Damjanov N. Indices of the Scleroderma Assessment Questionnaire (SAQ) can be used to demonstrate change in patients with systemic sclerosis over time. Joint Bone Spine. 2008;75:286–90.
96. Payet J, Goulvestre C, Bialé L, Avouac J, Wipff J, Job-Deslandre C, et al. Anticyclic citrullinated peptide antibodies in rheumatoid and nonrheumatoid rheumatic disorders: experience with 1162 patients. J Rheumatol. 2014;41:2395–402.

Cancer in Systemic Sclerosis

37

Ami A. Shah and Masataka Kuwana

Increased Cancer Risk in Systemic Sclerosis

Many epidemiologic studies have demonstrated that patients with scleroderma have an increased age- and gender-adjusted risk of cancer compared to the general population (SIRs or RR ranging from 1.4 to 3.2) [1–10]. In two recent systematic reviews and meta-analyses, investigators summarized this risk increase and examined whether patients with scleroderma were at higher risk for particular tumor types. The first conducted by Bonifazi and colleagues [2] pooled 16 original studies with more than 7,000 scleroderma patients. Patients with scleroderma had an increased cancer risk overall (summary RR 1.75, 95 % CI 1.41, 2.18) and were noted to have a higher risk of lung cancer (summary RR 4.35, 95 % CI 2.08, 9.09) and hematologic neoplasms (summary RR 2.24, 95 % CI 1.53, 3.29) in particular. While there was insufficient data to perform a meta-analysis for liver and esophageal cancers, an increased risk of these tumor types was also noted in most of the original studies that examined these cancer sites.

Onishi and colleagues [7] performed another high-quality systematic review and meta-analysis of cancer risk in scleroderma. They evaluated six studies with over 6,600 scleroderma patients. In this review, the pooled SIR for all cancers was 1.41 (95 % CI 1.18, 1.68), and they noted that there was an increased risk of lung (pooled SIR 3.18, 95 % CI 2.09, 4.85), bladder (in women only, pooled SIR 2.80, 95 % CI 1.36, 5.76), hematologic (pooled SIR 2.57, 95 % CI 1.79, 3.68), liver (pooled SIR 4.36, 95 % CI 2.0, 9.51), and non-melanoma skin (in men only, pooled SIR 2.34, 95 % CI 1.25, 4.59) cancers in scleroderma patients compared to the general population. Overall the risk of malignancy was higher in male patients with scleroderma (pooled SIR 1.85, 95 % CI 1.49, 2.31), and the authors postulated that this may be related to more smoking among men compared to women. The risk of cancer was also higher in the 12 months following a scleroderma diagnosis (SIR 2.79) than >12 months after diagnosis (SIR 1.40, $p=0.003$), suggesting that there may be a biological link between cancer and scleroderma or that there is a cancer detection bias among patients with new-onset disease.

Other studies have also demonstrated that patients with scleroderma have an increased risk of head and neck [5, 11] cancers. In one US study, scleroderma patients had a 25-fold increased incidence of tongue cancer and a 9.6-fold increased risk of oropharyngeal carcinomas (all squamous cell carcinomas) [11], whereas in a Taiwanese population scleroderma patients had a 3.67-fold increased risk of cancers of the oral cavity and pharynx [5]. Numerous investigators have probed whether there is a higher risk of gender-specific tumor types, such as breast, cervical, ovarian, uterine, prostate, or testicular cancers. These studies have not demonstrated conclusively that there is an increased risk of these cancer sites. However, breast cancer is often diagnosed around the time of scleroderma onset raising the question of whether there is a biological link between these two diagnoses [12, 13].

Potential Risk Factors and Mechanisms That May Explain the Increased Cancer Risk

It remains unclear whether particular scleroderma characteristics are risk factors for cancer in scleroderma. While the Onishi meta-analysis did not detect a difference in cancer risk by scleroderma cutaneous subtype [7], other studies have suggested that the risk of cancer may be higher in patients with diffuse scleroderma than those with limited

A.A. Shah, MD, MHS (✉)
Division of Rheumatology, Johns Hopkins University School of Medicine, Baltimore, USA
e-mail: Ami.Shah@jhmi.edu

M. Kuwana, MD, PhD
Department of Allergy and Rheumatology, Nippon Medical School Graduate School of Medicine, Tokyo, Japan

J. Varga et al. (eds.), *Scleroderma*, DOI 10.1007/978-3-319-31407-5_37

scleroderma [4]. Patients who are older when they develop the first clinical signs of scleroderma are also at higher risk of cancer [1, 14, 15].

Many investigations have suggested that chronic inflammation and damage from scleroderma itself may predispose patients to the development of malignancy. It has been hypothesized that lung cancers may develop in the context of pulmonary scar [16, 17] or that fibrosis may develop in the lung as a host response to an underlying lung neoplasm. In scleroderma, the data are controversial with some studies suggesting a higher risk of lung cancer in patients with interstitial lung disease [1, 18, 19] and others contradicting this [7, 20]. Similarly, the risk of esophageal cancer may be greater in patients with severe gastroesophageal reflux disease who develop Barrett's esophagus [21]. Patients with an overlap syndrome with primary biliary cirrhosis, particularly those with advanced histologic findings or biochemical nonresponse to ursodeoxycholic acid therapy, may have a higher risk of hepatocellular carcinoma [22, 23].

Another concern is that cytotoxic or immunosuppressive therapies employed to treat scleroderma may trigger the development of malignancy. This is a complicated issue as there is often a problem of confounding by indication; patients who are treated with cyclophosphamide for interstitial lung disease in scleroderma may have a higher risk of lung cancer, although whether this is related to the drug or damage from the disease itself is unclear. However, it is well established that patients treated with cyclophosphamide for other diseases have a higher risk of bladder and hematologic neoplasms, especially with exposure to higher cumulative doses or smoking [24, 25]. It remains controversial whether other immunosuppressive therapies employed to treat scleroderma are associated with an increased cancer risk. Mycophenolate mofetil is being employed more commonly in scleroderma to treat severe cutaneous disease, interstitial lung disease, and overlap syndromes with inflammatory myositis. While cancer risk with mycophenolate use has not been well studied in scleroderma, data from the transplant literature are conflicting as to whether or not there is an increased risk of lymphoma and nonmelanoma skin cancers with mycophenolate use [26–29]. It is difficult to draw inferences from the transplant population as these patients are often on multiple concomitant immunosuppressive therapies, a practice that is less common in scleroderma.

While immunosuppressive therapies employed to treat scleroderma and severe disease itself may be risk factors for the development of cancer, cancer therapies themselves may also increase the risk of developing scleroderma or scleroderma-like disease. For example, bleomycin, paclitaxel, gemcitabine, and carboplatin have been reported to trigger skin sclerosis and development or exacerbation of Raynaud's phenomenon and ischemic digits [30–35]. Immunotherapies that prime and amplify host immune responses to destroy neoplasms have also been reported to trigger new-onset autoimmune disease or exacerbate previously quiescent rheumatic disease [36]. Lastly, radiation therapy may trigger severe skin thickening patients with preexisting scleroderma [37, 38] or development of localized scleroderma in patients without an antecedent history of a connective tissue disease [39].

Another potential mechanism that may explain the increased risk of cancer among scleroderma patients includes a shared genetic susceptibility for both cancer and autoimmunity. A common inciting environmental exposure, such as silica, could also trigger the development of scleroderma and cancer [40, 41].

Data Suggesting That a Subset of Systemic Sclerosis Is a Paraneoplastic Disease

While all of these mechanisms likely play a role in the cancer-scleroderma relationship, a recent accumulation of data strongly suggests that scleroderma may be a paraneoplastic disease in some patients. As in dermatomyositis, a subset of patients with scleroderma is diagnosed with cancer within a short interval of the first clinical signs of scleroderma [1, 12, 13, 42–45]. This has been most striking in patients with breast cancer [12, 13, 43], where breast cancer diagnoses are often detected within 2 years of scleroderma onset. However, the temporal clustering of cancer diagnosis with the first clinical signs of scleroderma likely extends to multiple other tumor types. In a large US scleroderma cohort, it was detected that cancer diagnoses peaked around scleroderma onset (Fig. 37.1) with 22.7% of cancer diagnoses developing within 2 years of the first non-Raynaud's scleroderma symptom [15]. Anecdotal reports of cancer therapy halting the scleroderma disease process also raise the question of whether scleroderma is a paraneoplastic disease in some patients [46, 47].

An initial investigation of 23 scleroderma patients with cancer was performed to examine whether unique clinical or serologic features associated with a close temporal relationship between cancer diagnosis and scleroderma onset [45]. In this study, scleroderma patients with cancer and anti-RNA polymerase III autoantibodies had a unique clustering of cancer with scleroderma onset that was not detected among patients with anti-topoisomerase I or anticentromere antibodies. Interestingly, these patients also had unique nucleolar RNA polymerase III expression in their cancerous tissues (Fig. 37.2), in spite of nucleoplasmic expression of RNA polymerase III in normal cells. This suggests that ectopic expression of scleroderma autoantigens in cancer cells may associate with scleroderma-specific immune responses.

The clustering of cancer with scleroderma onset among patients with anti-RNA polymerase III autoantibodies has

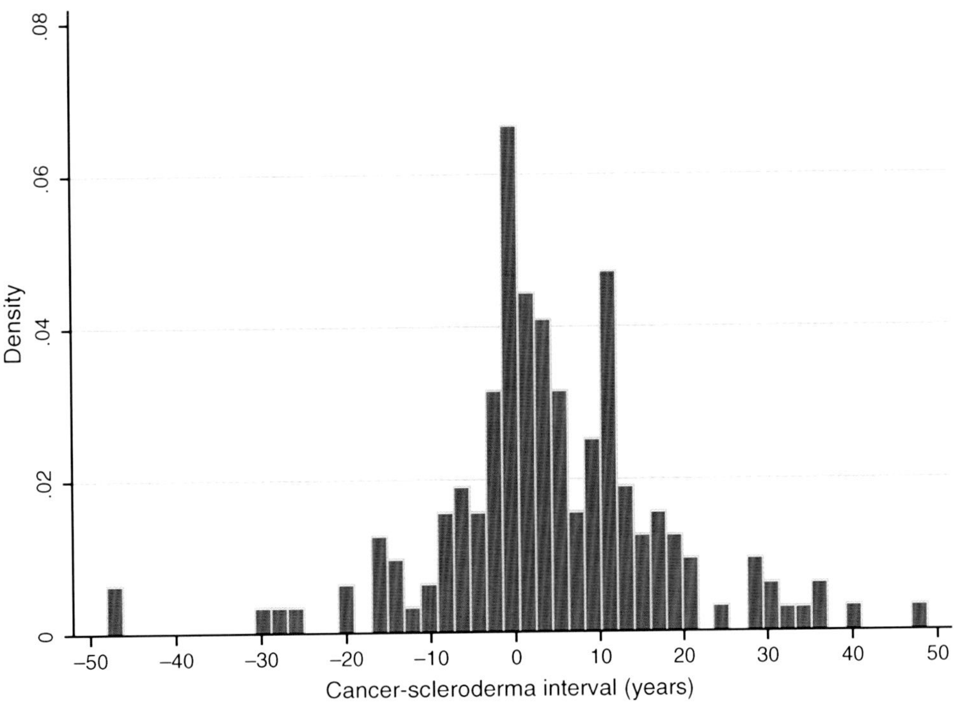

Fig. 37.1 Distribution of cancer-scleroderma interval (years) from the Johns Hopkins Scleroderma Center cohort. *Negative values* indicate that cancer diagnosis preceded scleroderma onset, whereas *positive values* indicate cancer diagnosis following scleroderma onset (From Shah et al. [15]; with permission)

since been confirmed in four other investigations. In an Italian scleroderma cohort, patients with anti-RNA polymerase III antibodies had a higher prevalence of cancer (43.8 % vs. 10.9 % among patients with anti-topoisomerase I antibodies and 8.6 % for those with anticentromere antibodies; $p<0.001$) and were more likely to have cancer synchronous with scleroderma onset (18.8 % in anti-RNA polymerase III positive patients vs. 0 % in anti-topoisomerase I and 0.4 % in anti-centromere patients; $p<0.001$) than patients in other autoantibody groups [48]. However, this study had a relatively low prevalence of anti-RNA polymerase III positivity (16/360 patients), and only 7 patients with anti-RNA polymerase III antibodies had a cancer diagnosis. An Australian scleroderma group studied 451 patients and detected that patients with anti-RNA polymerase III antibodies had a 4.2-fold increased odds of cancer within 5 years of scleroderma onset [14]. In contrast to the Italian group, they did not detect a higher prevalence of cancer in patients with anti-RNA polymerase III antibodies compared to those who were anti-RNA polymerase III negative (~13 % in both groups). A UK scleroderma cohort examined 2,177 patients and identified a higher prevalence of cancer among patients with anti-RNA polymerase III antibodies (14.2 %) compared to patients with anti-topoisomerase I (6.3 %, $p<0.0001$) or anticentromere (6.8 %, $p<0.001$) antibodies [49]. When they restricted their analyses to patients who were diagnosed with cancer within 3 years of scleroderma onset, the majority of patients were positive for anti-RNA polymerase III antibodies (55.3 % vs. 13.6 % for anti-topoisomerase I, $p<0.002$ and 23.5 % for anti-centromere, $p<0.008$). A US scleroderma cohort examined 1,044 patients, 168 of whom had cancer [15]. In this investigation, patients with anti-RNA polymerase III autoantibodies did not have a higher risk of cancer overall but had a striking 5.1-fold increased odds of cancer within 2 years of scleroderma onset. While it remains unclear whether patients with scleroderma and anti-RNA polymerase III antibodies have an increased risk of cancer overall, all of these investigations demonstrate that patients with anti-RNA polymerase III antibodies have a significantly increased risk of cancer within a short interval of scleroderma onset, suggesting that these patients may benefit from rigorous cancer screening at the time of diagnosis.

While the observation of a short cancer-scleroderma interval is most striking among patients with anti-RNA polymerase III autoantibodies, all of these cohorts had patients with a clustering of cancer with scleroderma onset among other autoantibody specificities. In the US investigation, this was most evident in patients who developed scleroderma at an older age, particularly among those with anti-topoisomerase I antibodies or those who were ANA positive but negative for the three most common scleroderma antibodies (anti-RNA polymerase III, anti-topoisomerase I, and anticentromere) (Fig. 37.3) [15]. These data suggest that older patients developing scleroderma may have paraneoplastic disease, whereas younger patients developing scleroderma may have cancers arise from damage from disease itself or as a consequence of immunosuppressive therapies [15]. Alternatively, aging may affect the quality of immunosurveillance of malignancies. Younger individuals may have a more robust immune response that allows cancers to be eradicated or held in equilibrium until the cancer finally escapes, thereby resulting in a long cancer-scleroderma

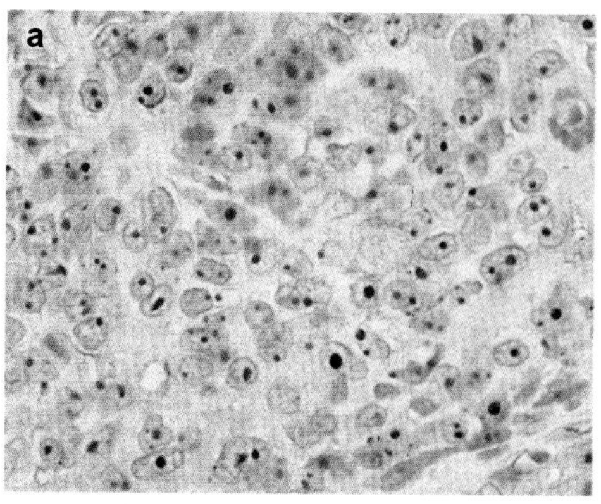

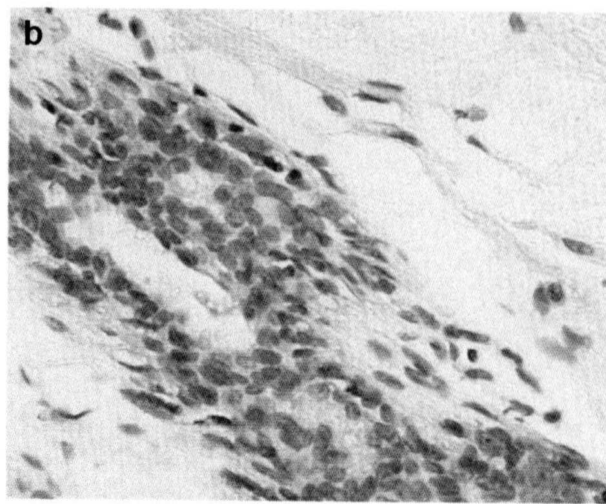

Fig. 37.2 Nucleolar RNA polymerase III expression is prominent in cancerous tissue from scleroderma patients with RNA polymerase III autoantibodies. Paraffin sections from cancerous breast tissue from a scleroderma patient with anti-RNA polymerase III antibodies (*left panel*) and from normal breast tissue (*right panel*). Tissue sections were stained with antibodies against RNA polymerase III. *Brown* shows RNA polymerase III staining, and *blue* (Mayer's hematoxylin counterstain) shows nuclei. Original magnification ×40 (From Shah et al. [45]; with permission)

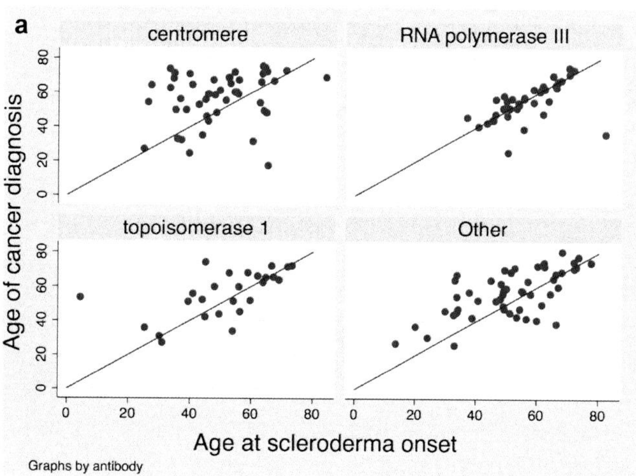

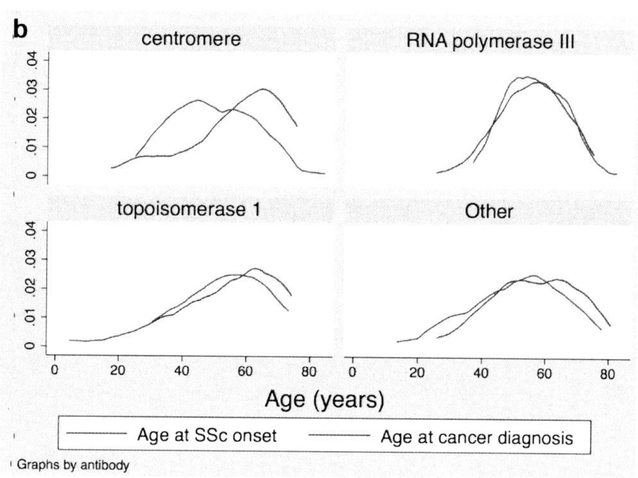

Fig. 37.3 Relationship between age of cancer diagnosis and age at scleroderma (SSc) onset by autoantibody status. Panel (**a**) the *red line* in each autoantibody group identifies the set of points at which the cancer-scleroderma interval is zero. Panel (**b**) a kernel density function demonstrates the distributions of age at scleroderma onset and age at cancer diagnosis. Patients with RNA polymerase III antibodies and cancer almost uniformly have a short cancer-scleroderma interval. In contrast, patients with anti-centromere antibodies rarely have a short cancer-scleroderma interval. Among patients with topoisomerase 1 antibodies and those who are ANA positive but negative for RNA polymerase III, topoisomerase 1 and centromere antibodies (the Other group), the cancer-scleroderma interval shortens with older age at scleroderma onset (From Shah et al. [15]; with permission)

interval [15, 50]. In contrast, older individuals may not be able to mount a potent antitumor immune response, resulting in a short cancer-scleroderma interval [15, 50]. These data also raise the question of whether cancer may be an important trigger of the immune response more broadly among scleroderma patients, especially since centromere proteins and topoisomerase I may play a key role in cancer fitness [50]. This hypothesis is supported by one investigation in which two patients with scleroderma and late lung cancer diagnoses had significant increases in anti-topoisomerase 1 antibody levels at the time of lung cancer diagnosis [51]. Furthermore, study of longitudinal serum samples revealed that these patients' sera reacted with new, previously unrecognized epitopes of the topoisomerase 1 molecule after lung cancer diagnosis [51]. These data further support the possibility that cancers may be an antigen source that drives rheumatic disease [45, 51].

Genetic Alteration of Autoantigens in Malignancies May Be an Antigen Source That Triggers Scleroderma

The data demonstrating unique nucleolar RNA polymerase III expression in cancerous tissues from scleroderma patients with anti-RNA polymerase III antibodies raised the question of whether autoimmunity may be triggered by structural

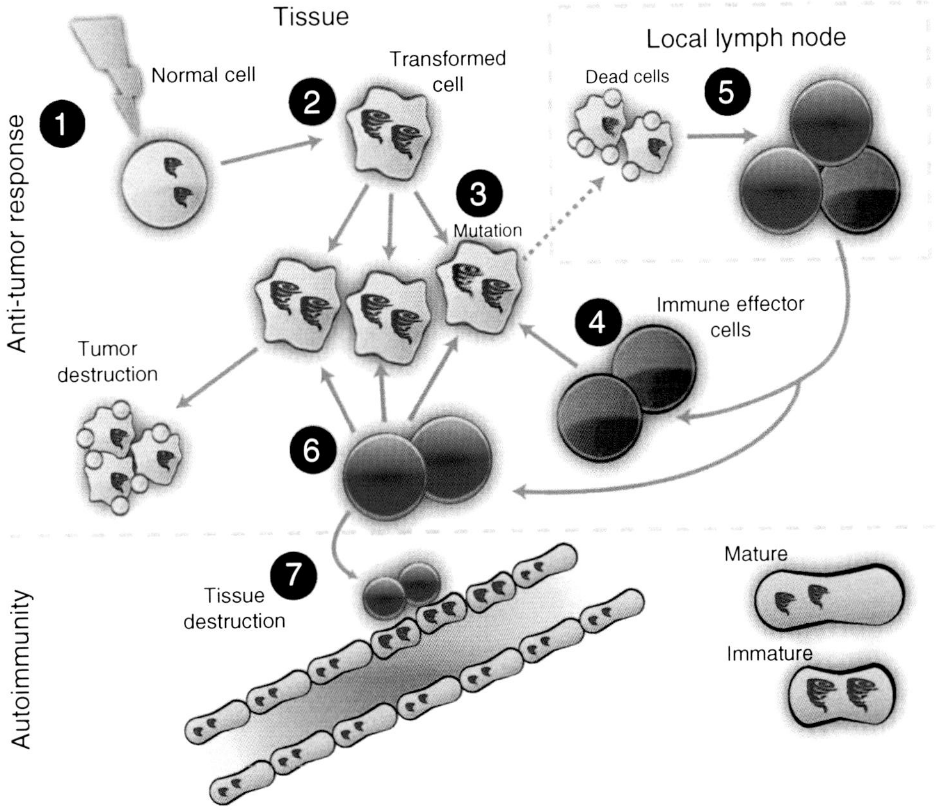

Fig. 37.4 Paraneoplastic model. Transformation of normal cells (*1*) may result in gene expression patterns that resemble immature cells involved in tissue healing (*2*). Occasionally, autoantigens become mutated (*3*); these are not driver mutations, and not all cancer cells have them. The first immune response is directed against the mutated form of the antigen (*4*) and may spread to the wild-type version (*5*). Immune effector cells directed against the mutant (depicted in *red*) delete exclusively cancer cells containing the mutation (*6*). Immune effector cells directed against the wild type (depicted in *blue*) delete cancer cells without the mutation and also cross-react with the patient's own tissues (particularly immature cells expressing high levels of antigen, found in damaged/repairing tissue) (*7*). Once autoimmunity has been initiated, the disease is self-propagating. Immature cells (expressing high antigen levels) that repair the immune-mediated injury can themselves become the targets of the immune response, sustaining an ongoing cycle of damage/repair that provides the antigen source that fuels the autoimmune response (From Shah et al. [50]; with permission)

alterations of RNA polymerase III in cancers from these patients, thereby resulting in recognition as a "foreign antigen" by immune system [52]. To address this possibility, a group of investigators searched for missense mutations in the *POLR3A* gene, which encodes the largest subunit of RNA polymerase III, in cancers from 16 scleroderma patients, 8 with anti-RNA polymerase III antibodies and 8 with anti-topoisomerase I or anticentromere antibodies [52]. Three of the eight patients with anti-RNA polymerase III antibodies had evidence of somatic, missense variants in *POLR3A*. Each of these three patients had a different mutation resulting in a single amino acid change, and two of these three patients exhibited mutation-specific T-cell immune responses. There was evidence that the immune response that may have been initiated against mutated subunit of RNA polymerase III spread to the wild-type version, as autoantibodies that cross-reacted with both wild-type and mutant RNA polymerase III were detected. In addition to somatic mutations in *POLR3A*, loss of heterozygosity at the *POLR3A* locus was also detected in five of the eight patients with anti-RNA polymerase III autoantibodies (two of whom also had somatic mutations). In contrast, no genetic alterations were detected in the *POLR3A* locus in tumors from patients with anti-topoisomerase I or anticentromere antibodies [52].

These data provided further evidence to support a paraneoplastic model of disease pathogenesis, wherein mutated autoantigens result in the generation of T-cell responses specific to mutant proteins and B-cell responses cross-reactive with both mutant and wild-type proteins (Fig. 37.4) [50]. Due to subsequent antibody-mediated uptake of wild-type proteins by antigen-presenting cells, T-cell responses may then be directed against to the wild-type molecule [50]. These immune effector cells may cross-react with self-tissue, resulting in target tissue damage [50]. It has been shown that myositis autoantigens are detectable in immature, regenerating myoblasts in myositis muscle, and this antigen source may sustain and propagate the autoimmune response [53]. Data regarding a causal relationship between autoantibody responses and pathogenic process are limited in scleroderma, although it has been reported that immunization of topoisomerase I in conjunction with adjuvant induces scleroderma-like skin sclerosis and lung fibrosis in mice [54]. Alternatively, autoantibody production and scleroderma development may be independent consequences, both of which result from cancer development. In this regard, development of scleroderma-like skin lesions was reported in patients with cancer, which produces a large amount of fibrogenic factors, including TGF-β [55–57].

Implications for Cancer Screening and Scleroderma Therapeutics

The optimal approach for cancer screening in scleroderma remains unknown. The recent data supporting a model of cancer-induced autoimmunity among patients with anti-RNA polymerase III autoantibodies suggests that aggressive malignancy screening may be warranted at the clinical onset of scleroderma. In particular, these data raise the question of whether early cancer diagnosis and treatment could play a significant role in achieving scleroderma remission.

It is the authors' practice to perform comprehensive, age- and gender-appropriate cancer screening in all new patients with scleroderma according to guidelines established in the United States. In women, we recommend pelvic exams and Pap smears every 3 years starting at age 21 or every 5 years if HPV testing has been performed, with shorter intervals if there have been prior abnormal results [58]. While Pap smears are typically not recommended beyond the age of 65, we suggest that this be done once in older patients with new-onset scleroderma. While the current recommendations for mammography screening in the US general population are controversial, it is our practice to follow a more aggressive screening protocol with annual mammography starting at age 40. For men younger than age 40, we recommend an annual testicular examination, and for older gentleman, we discuss the risks and benefits of digital rectal examination and prostate-specific antigen testing given the controversies of this test for prostate cancer screening. We initiate colonoscopy screening for colon cancer at the age of 50 with testing every 10 years if the baseline study is normal. While it is not recommended that colonoscopies be performed in individuals above the age of 75 due to anticipated life expectancy, in older patients with new-onset scleroderma, we recommend this test to ensure there is not an underlying colonic malignancy that may drive disease.

Further testing should be considered if particular risk factors are present. Patients who have refractory gastroesophageal reflux disease despite high-dose proton pump inhibitor therapy are referred for upper endoscopy, and sequential screenings are performed in those with (1) Barrett's esophagus at 1–3-year intervals depending on the presence of dysplasia or (2) severe erosive esophagitis at intervals suggested by the evaluating gastroenterologist [59]. Low-dose chest computed tomography (CT) is now recommended for patients aged 55–74 with a 30+ pack year smoking history if they continue to smoke or have quit in the last 15 years [60]. We also recommend a baseline high-resolution chest CT scan in scleroderma patients who are at high risk for interstitial lung disease, including African Americans, those with topoisomerase I antibodies or diffuse cutaneous disease, and those with a restrictive ventilatory defect or forced vital capacity decline greater than 10 % of predicted. For patients with cirrhosis from primary biliary cirrhosis, the American Association for the Study of Liver Diseases recommends cross-sectional imaging with or without alpha fetoprotein levels at 6–12 month intervals [61]. Patients with dysphagia that persists without an identifiable cause (such as severe xerostomia, pharyngeal muscle weakness, or esophageal stricture) may require further examination by an otolaryngologist for evaluation of head and neck cancers. Serum protein electrophoresis, serum immunofixation, and peripheral blood flow cytometry may be useful initial tests in the evaluation of new cytopenias not otherwise explained by immunosuppressive therapies, and consultation with a hematologist and bone marrow biopsy may be required. It is also important to carefully evaluate patients with current or antecedent immunosuppressive exposure to monitor for long-term cancer risks. Annual urinalysis and urine cytology are recommended in patients with prior cyclophosphamide exposure, and full skin examination is suggested in patients treated with mycophenolate mofetil.

Lastly, we consider more aggressive cancer surveillance in select patients who are considered to be at particularly elevated risk of cancer including patients with: (1) RNA polymerase III autoantibodies; (2) an older age of scleroderma onset; (3) atypical, aggressive, or treatment unresponsive disease; (4) profound weight loss or other constitutional features out of proportion with disease severity; or (5) patients with a personal or striking family history of cancer. While there are no established trials of cancer screening in these patients, further evaluation with CT of the chest, abdomen, and pelvis or whole body PET-CT and serum tumor markers may be warranted.

Summary

The relationship between scleroderma and malignancy is complex, with many potential explanations for the increased risk of cancer in patients with scleroderma. Recent data suggest that a subset of scleroderma patients, such as those with RNA polymerase III autoantibodies or an older age of scleroderma onset, may have paraneoplastic disease. Careful malignancy screening should be considered in patients with new-onset scleroderma, and further study is required to understand whether cancer therapy may be effective treatment for scleroderma.

References

1. Abu-Shakra M, Guillemin F, Lee P. Cancer in systemic sclerosis. Arthritis Rheum. 1993;36(4):460–4.
2. Bonifazi M, Tramacere I, Pomponio G, Gabrielli B, Avvedimento EV, La Vecchia C, Negri E, Gabrielli A. Systemic sclerosis (scleroderma) and cancer risk: systematic review and meta-analysis of observational studies. Rheumatology. 2013;52(1):143–54.
3. Derk CT, Rasheed M, Artlett CM, Jimenez SA. A cohort study of cancer incidence in systemic sclerosis. J Rheumatol. 2006;33(6):1113–6.
4. Hill CL, Nguyen AM, Roder D, Roberts-Thomson P. Risk of cancer in patients with scleroderma: a population based cohort study. Annals Rheum Dis. 2003;62(8):728–31.
5. Kuo CF, Luo SF, Yu KH, Chou IJ, Tseng WY, Chang HC, Fang YF, Chiou MJ, See LC. Cancer risk among patients with systemic sclerosis: a nationwide population study in Taiwan. Scand J Rheumatol. 2012;41(1):44–9.
6. Olesen AB, Svaerke C, Farkas DK, Sorensen HT. Systemic sclerosis and the risk of cancer: a nationwide population-based cohort study. Br J Dermatol. 2010;163(4):800–6.
7. Onishi A, Sugiyama D, Kumagai S, Morinobu A. Cancer incidence in systemic sclerosis: meta-analysis of population-based cohort studies. Arthritis Rheum. 2013;65(7):1913–21.
8. Rosenthal AK, McLaughlin JK, Gridley G, Nyren O. Incidence of cancer among patients with systemic sclerosis. Cancer. 1995;76(5):910–4.
9. Siau K, Laversuch CJ, Creamer P, O'Rourke KP. Malignancy in scleroderma patients from south west England: a population-based cohort study. Rheumatol Int. 2011;31(5):641–5.
10. Zhang JQ, Wan YN, Peng WJ, Yan JW, Li BZ, Mei B, Chen B, Yao H, Yang GJ, Tao JH, et al. The risk of cancer development in systemic sclerosis: a meta-analysis. Cancer Epidemiol. 2013;37(5):523–7.
11. Derk CT, Rasheed M, Spiegel JR, Jimenez SA. Increased incidence of carcinoma of the tongue in patients with systemic sclerosis. J Rheumatol. 2005;32(4):637–41.
12. Forbes AM, Woodrow JC, Verbov JL, Graham RM. Carcinoma of breast and scleroderma: four further cases and a literature review. Br J Rheumatol. 1989;28(1):65–9.
13. Launay D, Le Berre R, Hatron PY, Peyrat JP, Hachulla E, Devulder B, Hebbar M. Association between systemic sclerosis and breast cancer: eight new cases and review of the literature. Clin Rheumatol. 2004;23(6):516–22.
14. Nikpour M, Hissaria P, Byron J, Sahhar J, Micallef M, Paspaliaris W, Roddy J, Nash P, Sturgess A, Proudman S, et al. Prevalence, correlates and clinical usefulness of antibodies to RNA polymerase III in systemic sclerosis: a cross-sectional analysis of data from an Australian cohort. Arthritis Res Ther. 2011;13(6):R211.
15. Shah AA, Hummers LK, Casciola-Rosen L, Visvanathan K, Rosen A, Wigley FM. Examination of autoantibody status and clinical features associated with cancer risk and cancer-associated scleroderma. Arthritis Rheumatol. 2015;67(4):1053–61.
16. Bobba RK, Holly JS, Loy T, Perry MC. Scar carcinoma of the lung: a historical perspective. Clin Lung Cancer. 2011;12(3):148–54.
17. Yu YY, Pinsky PF, Caporaso NE, Chatterjee N, Baumgarten M, Langenberg P, Furuno JP, Lan Q, Engels EA. Lung cancer risk following detection of pulmonary scarring by chest radiography in the prostate, lung, colorectal, and ovarian cancer screening trial. Arch Intern Med. 2008;168(21):2326–32; discussion 2332.
18. Peters-Golden M, Wise RA, Hochberg M, Stevens MB, Wigley FM. Incidence of lung cancer in systemic sclerosis. J Rheumatol. 1985;12(6):1136–9.
19. Kang KY, Yim HW, Kim IJ, Yoon JU, Ju JH, Kim HY, Park SH. Incidence of cancer among patients with systemic sclerosis in Korea: results from a single centre. Scand J Rheumatol. 2009;38(4):299–303.
20. Pontifex EK, Hill CL, Roberts-Thomson P. Risk factors for lung cancer in patients with scleroderma: a nested case-control study. Annals Rheum Dis. 2007;66(4):551–3.
21. Wipff J, Allanore Y, Soussi F, Terris B, Abitbol V, Raymond J, Chaussade S, Kahan A. Prevalence of Barrett's esophagus in systemic sclerosis. Arthritis Rheum. 2005;52(9):2882–8.
22. Trivedi PJ, Lammers WJ, van Buuren HR, Pares A, Floreani A, Janssen HL, Invernizzi P, Battezzati PM, Ponsioen CY, Corpechot C, et al. Stratification of hepatocellular carcinoma risk in primary biliary cirrhosis: a multicentre international study. Gut. 2016;65(2):321–9.
23. Cavazza A, Caballeria L, Floreani A, Farinati F, Bruguera M, Caroli D, Pares A. Incidence, risk factors, and survival of hepatocellular carcinoma in primary biliary cirrhosis: comparative analysis from two centers. Hepatology. 2009;50(4):1162–8.
24. Faurschou M, Sorensen IJ, Mellemkjaer L, Loft AG, Thomsen BS, Tvede N, Baslund B. Malignancies in Wegener's granulomatosis: incidence and relation to cyclophosphamide therapy in a cohort of 293 patients. J Rheumatol. 2008;35(1):100–5.
25. Monach PA, Arnold LM, Merkel PA. Incidence and prevention of bladder toxicity from cyclophosphamide in the treatment of rheumatic diseases: a data-driven review. Arthritis Rheum. 2010;62(1):9–21.
26. Brewer JD, Colegio OR, Phillips PK, Roenigk RK, Jacobs MA, Van de Beek D, Dierkhising RA, Kremers WK, McGregor CG, Otley CC. Incidence of and risk factors for skin cancer after heart transplant. Arch Dermatol. 2009;145(12):1391–6.
27. Marcen R, Galeano C, Fernandez-Rodriguez A, Jimenez-Alvaro S, Teruel JL, Rivera M, Burgos FJ, Quereda C. Effects of the new immunosuppressive agents on the occurrence of malignancies after renal transplantation. Transplant Proc. 2010;42(8):3055–7.
28. Bichari W, Bartiromo M, Mohey H, Afiani A, Burnot A, Maillard N, Sauron C, Thibaudin D, Mehdi M, Mariat C, et al. Significant risk factors for occurrence of cancer after renal transplantation: a single center cohort study of 1265 cases. Transpl Proc. 2009;41(2):672–3.
29. Robson R, Cecka JM, Opelz G, Budde M, Sacks S. Prospective registry-based observational cohort study of the long-term risk of malignancies in renal transplant patients treated with mycophenolate mofetil. Am J Rranspl: Off J Am Soc Transpl Am Soc Transpl Surg. 2005;5(12):2954–60.
30. Berger CC, Bokemeyer C, Schneider M, Kuczyk MA, Schmoll HJ. Secondary Raynaud's phenomenon and other late vascular complications following chemotherapy for testicular cancer. Eur J Cancer. 1995;31A(13–14):2229–38.
31. Bessis D, Guillot B, Legouffe E, Guilhou JJ. Gemcitabine-associated scleroderma-like changes of the lower extremities. J Am Acad Dermatol. 2004;51(2 Suppl):S73–6.
32. Clowse ME, Wigley FM. Digital necrosis related to carboplatin and gemcitabine therapy in systemic sclerosis. J Rheumatol. 2003;30(6):1341–3.
33. Cohen IS, Mosher MB, O'Keefe EJ, Klaus SN, De Conti RC. Cutaneous toxicity of bleomycin therapy. Arch Dermatol. 1973;107(4):553–5.
34. Finch WR, Rodnan GP, Buckingham RB, Prince RK, Winkelstein A. Bleomycin-induced scleroderma. J Rheumatol. 1980;7(5):651–9.

35. De Angelis R, Bugatti L, Cerioni A, Del Medico P, Filosa G. Diffuse scleroderma occurring after the use of paclitaxel for ovarian cancer. Clin Rheumatol. 2003;22(1):49–52.
36. Ioannou Y, Isenberg DA. Current evidence for the induction of autoimmune rheumatic manifestations by cytokine therapy. Arthritis Rheum. 2000;43(7):1431–42.
37. Varga J, Haustein UF, Creech RH, Dwyer JP, Jimenez SA. Exaggerated radiation-induced fibrosis in patients with systemic sclerosis. JAMA. 1991;265(24):3292–5.
38. Abu-Shakra M, Lee P. Exaggerated fibrosis in patients with systemic sclerosis (scleroderma) following radiation therapy. J Rheumatol. 1993;20(9):1601–3.
39. Colver GB, Rodger A, Mortimer PS, Savin JA, Neill SM, Hunter JA. Post-irradiation morphoea. Br J Dermatol. 1989;120(6):831–5.
40. Lacasse Y, Martin S, Gagne D, Lakhal L. Dose-response meta-analysis of silica and lung cancer. Cancer Causes Control: CCC. 2009;20(6):925–33.
41. McCormic ZD, Khuder SS, Aryal BK, Ames AL, Khuder SA. Occupational silica exposure as a risk factor for scleroderma: a meta-analysis. Int Arch Occup Environ Health. 2010;83(7):763–9.
42. Duncan SC, Winkelmann RK. Cancer and scleroderma. Arch Dermatol. 1979;115(8):950–5.
43. Lee P, Alderdice C, Wilkinson S, Keystone EC, Urowitz MB, Gladman DD. Malignancy in progressive systemic sclerosis – association with breast carcinoma. J Rheumatol. 1983;10(4):665–6.
44. Roumm AD, Medsger Jr TA. Cancer and systemic sclerosis. An epidemiologic study. Arthritis Rheum. 1985;28(12):1336–40.
45. Shah AA, Rosen A, Hummers L, Wigley F, Casciola-Rosen L. Close temporal relationship between onset of cancer and scleroderma in patients with RNA polymerase I/III antibodies. Arthritis Rheum. 2010;62(9):2787–95.
46. Hasegawa M, Sato S, Sakai H, Ohashi T, Takehara K. Systemic sclerosis revealing T-cell lymphoma. Dermatology. 1999;198(1):75–8.
47. Juarez M, Marshall R, Denton C, Evely R. Paraneoplastic scleroderma secondary to hairy cell leukaemia successfully treated with cladribine. Rheumatology. 2008;47(11):1734–5.
48. Airo P, Ceribelli A, Cavazzana I, Taraborelli M, Zingarelli S, Franceschini F. Malignancies in Italian patients with systemic sclerosis positive for anti-RNA polymerase III antibodies. J Rheumatol. 2011;38(7):1329–34.
49. Moinzadeh P, Fonseca C, Hellmich M, Shah AA, Chighizola C, Denton CP, Ong VH. Association of anti-RNA polymerase III autoantibodies and cancer in scleroderma. Arthritis Res Ther. 2014;16(1):R53.
50. Shah AA, Casciola-Rosen L, Rosen A. Review: cancer-induced autoimmunity in the rheumatic diseases. Arthritis Rheumatol. 2015;67(2):317–26.
51. Kuwana M, Fujii T, Mimori T, Kaburaki J. Enhancement of anti-DNA topoisomerase I autoantibody response after lung cancer in patients with systemic sclerosis. A report of two cases. Arthritis Rheum. 1996;39(4):686–91.
52. Joseph CG, Darrah E, Shah AA, Skora AD, Casciola-Rosen LA, Wigley FM, Boin F, Fava A, Thoburn C, Kinde I, et al. Association of the autoimmune disease scleroderma with an immunologic response to cancer. Science. 2014;343(6167):152–7.
53. Casciola-Rosen L, Nagaraju K, Plotz P, Wang K, Levine S, Gabrielson E, Corse A, Rosen A. Enhanced autoantigen expression in regenerating muscle cells in idiopathic inflammatory myopathy. J Exp Med. 2005;201(4):591–601.
54. Yoshizaki A, Yanaba K, Ogawa A, Asano Y, Kadono T, Sato S. Immunization with DNA topoisomerase I and Freund's complete adjuvant induces skin and lung fibrosis and autoimmunity via interleukin-6 signaling. Arthritis Rheum. 2011;63(11):3575–85.
55. Bielefeld P. Systemic scleroderma and malignant diseases. A review of the literature. La Rev Med Interne/Fondee Soc Natl Fr Med Interne. 1991;12(5):350–4.
56. Fujii T, Mimori T, Kimura N, Satoh S, Hirakata M. Pseudoscleroderma associated with transforming growth factor beta1-producing advanced gastric carcinoma: comment on the article by Varga. Arthritis Rheum. 2003;48(6):1766–7; author reply 1767–8.
57. Querfeld C, Sollberg S, Huerkamp C, Eckes B, Krieg T. Pseudoscleroderma associated with lung cancer: correlation of collagen type I and connective tissue growth factor gene expression. Br J Dermatol. 2000;142(6):1228–33.
58. Sawaya GF, Kulasingam S, Denberg T, Qaseem A. Cervical cancer screening in average-risk women: best practice advice from the clinical guidelines committee of the American College of Physicians. Annals Intern Med. 2015;162(12):851–9.
59. Shaheen NJ, Weinberg DS, Denberg TD, Chou R, Qaseem A, Shekelle P, Clinical Guidelines Committee of the American College of P. Upper endoscopy for gastroesophageal reflux disease: best practice advice from the clinical guidelines committee of the American College of Physicians. Annals Intern Med. 2012;157(11):808–16.Pubmed ID-25928075
60. National Lung Screening Trial Research T, Aberle DR, Adams AM, Berg CD, Black WC, Clapp JD, Fagerstrom RM, Gareen IF, Gatsonis C, Marcus PM, et al. Reduced lung-cancer mortality with low-dose computed tomographic screening. New England J Med. 2011;365(5):395–409.
61. Lindor KD, Gershwin ME, Poupon R, Kaplan M, Bergasa NV, Heathcote EJ, American Association for Study of Liver D. Primary biliary cirrhosis. Hepatology. 2009;50(1):291–308.

Overlooked Manifestations

38

Edward V. Lally, Ami A. Shah, and Fredrick M. Wigley

Systemic sclerosis (SSc) is a heterogeneous disease with well-described traditional clinical manifestations, such as Raynaud's phenomenon, dermal sclerosis, esophageal dysmotility, calcinosis, and telangiectasia. Because the clinical presentation can be complex and involve multiple organ systems, there are several other manifestations that often go unrecognized but cause significant morbidity. This chapter discusses a few such manifestations, including neurologic and audiovestibular disease, oral complications, thyroid dysfunction, liver disease, bladder dysfunction, avascular necrosis of the bone, and erectile dysfunction.

Neurological Manifestations

In 1898, Steven described a patient with "cerebrovascular scleroderma" [1]. Arteries in the pons, medulla, and cord were surrounded by a thick homogeneous material. However several decades went by before more comprehensive review articles on neurological manifestations of SSc appeared. The incidence of primary neurological manifestations in SSc reported in several early papers was very low. Leinwand and colleagues [2], in 1954, reported on over 150 cases of SSc and did not include any mention of neurologic abnormalities. In 1955, Piper and Hellwig [3] reported foci of ischemic necrosis in 3 of 17 SSc brains at autopsy, but no clinical correlations were reported. Tuffanelli and Winkler [4] reported on a large series of 727 SSc patients and described 2 patients with grand mal seizures and 4 with minimal seizure activity. In a comprehensive review of 130 patients with SSc by Gordon and Silverstein [5], 24 patients were found to have a total of 28 neurological manifestations but none were felt to be definitely related to the SSc process itself. At the time of that review, parenchymal central nervous system (CNS) findings with features of other involved organs had not been reported in SSc. In a study of 58 autopsy cases and 58 matched control, D'Angelo and colleagues [6] did not report any pathologic cases of nervous system involvement in SSc. However, later studies began to recognize neurological manifestations of SSc. Lee and colleagues [7] reported on 125 patients with SSc who were studied prospectively. Seven (5.6%) were found to have defined neurologic lesions, four with carpal tunnel syndrome, and one each with trigeminal neuralgia, mononeuritis multiplex, and peripheral neuropathy. More recently, an exhaustive literature search that was reported by Amaral and colleagues [8] revealed a variety of neurological manifestations in SSc. CNS involvement (headache, seizures, cognitive impairment), depression and anxiety, myopathy, trigeminal neuropathy, peripheral sensory motor polyneuropathy, and carpal tunnel syndrome were the most frequent manifestations. Chronic neuropathy was also found commonly in patients with SSc as was autonomic neuropathy.

Since SSc is a profound vasculopathic disorder, it might be expected that typical CNS vascular disease would be seen with SSc. There have been isolated reports of CNS arteritis [9–11] and cerebritis [12]. Vascular changes of hypertension and atherosclerosis would be expected to be seen in SSc but are not unique to this phenotype. Recent studies have suggested more specific vascular brain involvement in SSc patients [13–15]. These were noted as calcifications of cerebral arteries on computed tomography (CT) scans [14] and white matter lesions (WMLs) on magnetic resonance imaging (MRI) [15]. Subsequent to these studies, Terrier and colleagues [16] studied 63 patients with SSc. Severe cerebrovasculopathy was identified on CT scan in 22 patients and on MRI in 38 patients. SSc patients with severe

E.V. Lally, MD (✉)
Division of Rheumatology, Rhode Island Hospital, Providence, RI, USA
e-mail: elally@lifespan.org

A.A. Shah, MD, MHS
Department of Medicine/Rheumatology, Johns Hopkins Scleroderma Center, Baltimore, MD, USA

F.M. Wigley, MD
Department of Medicine/Rheumatology, The Johns Hopkins University School of Medicine, Baltimore, MD, USA

J. Varga et al. (eds.), *Scleroderma*, DOI 10.1007/978-3-319-31407-5_38

cerebrovasculopathy were more likely to have pulmonary arterial hypertension and showed a tendency to have scleroderma renal crisis. In another MRI study, 30 female SSc patients and 30 age-matched controls underwent brain MRIs [17]. CNS involvement in the form of white matter hyperintense foci was found more commonly in SSc patients. CNS lesions in these patients correlated with clinical features including headaches, depression, and peripheral vascular disease. Cerebrovascular abnormalities in SSc patients may be more common than previously recognized.

The vasculopathy of SSc may rarely affect the eye. Maclean and Guthrie [18] and Farkas and colleagues [19], in postmortem studies, showed abnormalities of the choroidal vasculature as well as exudates in the retina. Grennan and Foster [20] investigated the choroidal and retinal vasculature in a group of patients with early as well as advanced SSc using routine funduscopic examination, screening for keratoconjunctivitis sicca (KCS), and fluorescein angiograms. Two of the ten SSc patients had KCS, similar to the incidents found in other series [21]. Fluorescein angiography, demonstrated abnormalities of perfusion which affected the choriocapillaris and small choroidal arterioles. All but one of the patients was normotensive. Retinopathy [22, 23] and central retinal vein occlusion [24] have also been described in SSc.

Migraine headaches are vasospastic phenomena which have been studied in large reviews of SSc. Christianson and colleague [25] showed a significant association between limited cutaneous SSc and migraine headache (46 of 223 cases) in a retrospective study of 22,000 patients with the diagnosis of migraine headache seen at the Mayo Clinic between 1950 and 1975. Goldberg and colleagues [26] found 16 cases with well-documented SSc and migraine phenomena. Migraine is a frequent symptom in the general population and the coincidence noted in this study could be expected by chance. Pal and colleagues [27] noted migraines in 32 % of SSc patients studied. Headaches occurred in 23.7 % of patients in a large systematic literature review [8].

Cranial nerve involvement with SSc has been reported infrequently. Beighton and colleague [28] first reported trigeminal sensory neuropathy in a patient who later developed SSc. Ashworth and Tait [29] reported this sensory deficit in five patients classified as having SSc, but two of the five had features of systemic lupus erythematosus. Teasdall and colleague [30] described ten patients with SSc who developed cranial nerve involvement. Trigeminal neuropathy was a presenting feature in five patients; the glossopharyngeal nerve was involved in one patient. Taste was impaired in one patient and tongue fasciculations were noted in another. Tinnitus was described in three patients and facial weakness was present in five. The trigeminal lesions appeared to be peripheral since the sensory deficits were more pronounced over those parts of the face innervated by distal branches of the trigeminal nerve. The microangiopathy of SSc was felt to be responsible for the neurologic deficit with secondary deposition of fibrous tissue contributing to the process by nerve compression. Farrell and Medsger [31] noted trigeminal neuropathy in 16 of 442 consecutive patients (4 %) with SSc evaluated at the University of Pittsburgh between 1972 and 1980.

The incidence of sclerodermatous infiltration of the peripheral nervous system is unclear. Richter [32] reported a patient with quadriparesis and peripheral neuropathy who, at autopsy, was found to have visceral scleroderma with involvement of the spinal cord roots. Peripheral nerve histopathology revealed epi- and perineural fibrosis with demyelination and axonal degeneration. In a study of the nerve network of the skin, Pawlowski and Warsaw [33] documented fragmentation of the nerve fibers of the skin in SSc patients. Fleischmajer and colleague [34] also found cellular infiltrates in the perineurium of patients with diffuse cutaneous SSc. In a review of 130 patients with SSc, Gordan and Silverstein [5] were unable to demonstrate any clinical manifestations of peripheral neuropathy. Very few studies have reported the use of electrodiagnostic testing as a means of delineating the existence of peripheral neurologic involvement in SSc. Christopher and Robinson [35] performed electrodiagnostic studies including determination of conduction velocities in motor and sensory nerves on 17 patients with SSc who were also studied for other possible causes of peripheral neuropathy. A control group of 22 patients without peripheral neuropathy was studied as well. A statistically significant reduction in values of mean conduction velocity was found in ulnar and median sensory nerve of the upper extremities in SSc patients. Only the peroneal nerve of the lower extremity revealed decreased conduction velocity. These authors postulated that the significant reduction in mean values for conduction velocity in all sensory nerves studied, but only a reduction in one of the motor nerve studied, argued for early-stage neuropathy in the SSc patients, as the sensory peripheral nerves are more sensitive to disease or injury than are motor nerves. These findings have been questioned because the SSc patient group and control group did not match in age distribution and the neuropathic changes have not been confirmed by other studies. However, Poncelet and Connolly [36] studied 14 SSc patients who underwent a complete neurologic examination, nerve conduction studies (NCS), and quantitative sensory testing (QST). Neurologic examination revealed reduced vibrations or pinprick sensation in the upper extremity, focal muscle atrophy or proximal weakness, and decreased deep tendon reflexes. NCS showed reduced sensory nerve action potentials in one patient and carpal tunnel syndrome in another. QST of the upper and lower extremity revealed increased cold or vibration detection threshold in 8 of 14 patients. The authors conclude that peripheral neuropathy occurs at a higher frequency in SSc than was previously appreciated.

Compression neuropathies have been described in SSc patients and may be a presenting symptom on occasion. Carpal tunnel syndrome and tarsal tunnel syndrome have been described in SSc [37–40].

Impaired vibratory perception is one of the early signs of peripheral neuropathy. The amplitude of these vibrations, however, is markedly influenced by the viscoelastic properties of the skin and subcutaneous tissue. This is particularly important in SSc in which thickened fibrotic skin may be elevating vibratory perception thresholds and may be mistakenly interpreted as indicating peripheral neuropathy. Dahlgaard and colleagues [41] measured the vibratory perception threshold in patients with diffuse cutaneous SSc but no clinical evidence of peripheral neuropathy. The vibratory perception threshold was significantly elevated on sclerotic test loci but remained normal on loci with normal skin. The pattern of elevated vibratory perception threshold differed from that of peripheral neuropathy, and it was concluded that the sclerodermatous skin caused a damping effect on external vibration. This finding was later confirmed by Poncelet and Connolly [36].

Autonomic nervous system (ANS) dysfunction has been described clinically in SSc and may be responsible, in part, for some of the pathogenetic manifestations of the disease. It has been well recognized that one of the fundamental pathophysiologic abnormalities in SSc involves the microcirculation and is characterized by endothelial damage [41–45]. The current controversy centers on the exact cause of the blood vessel abnormalities and whether these are primary events or whether a more basic lesion, such as vascular neurogenic control, is the putative mechanism. Vasomotor integrity is controlled, in part, by the sympathetic and parasympathetic nervous system. It is reasonable to suspect that aberrations of ANS function may be important in SSc. In addition to the vascular lesions of SSc, several other clinical features of the disease are commonly seen in patients with autonomic insufficiency. These include diminished/absent peristalsis of the body of the esophagus, reduced lower esophageal sphincter pressure, delayed gastric emptying, abnormal colonic motility, anal rectal sphincter incompetence [44, 46, 47], and impotence [48]. Indirect evidence for ANS involvement in SSc was initially found in a study of five patients with spinal cord injuries above T-6 and autonomic hyperreflexia who developed dermal fibrosis suggestive of a SSc variant disorder [49].

Until recently, there had been relatively few studies on ANS function in SSc and these initially failed to demonstrate any characteristic abnormalities. Early studies focused on either direct measurements of circulating catecholamines or on the morphologic assessment of autonomic nerve endings or plexuses in the skin. Peacock [50] found elevated levels of epinephrine and norepinephrine in the plasma of patients with Raynaud's phenomenon before and after cold stimulation. However, this demonstration could not be reproduced by Kontos and Wasserman [51] and the assays used for catecholamine determination were not felt to be reliable. In 1972, Sapira and colleague [52] reported on resting venous plasma catecholamine concentrations and urinary catecholamine excretion patterns in patients with Raynaud's and SSc and could find no evidence of catecholamine excess. Pawlowski and Warsaw [33] had studied the nerve network of the skin in SSc and has found characteristic morphologic changes (degeneration and regeneration) in the nerve ending in various stages of the disease. It is not clear whether such changes were primary or secondary phenomenon. A study by Fries in 1969 [53], using electrical skin resistance and digital skin temperature recordings, failed to show evidence of sympathetic overactivity in Raynaud's phenomenon or SSc. In addition, although sympathectomy has provided some benefit in individual patients with SSc, Raynaud's, and digital ulcers [54–58], there has been no consistent evidence that sympathetic blockade has a beneficial effect on vascular perfusion.

It is worth briefly considering some clinical parallels between SSc and diabetes mellitus (DM) which might lend further support to the concept of ANS dysfunction in SSc. Both diseases manifest abnormalities to the microvascular circulation, characteristic gastrointestinal changes (delayed gastric emptying, colonic hypomotility, anal sphincter dysfunction) [59–63], and erectile dysfunction [63]. Furthermore, previous studies have demonstrated an intriguing relationship between DM and characteristic abnormalities of cutaneous and vascular connective tissue which may parallel changes seen in SSc [64–70]. Autonomic neuropathy occurs frequently in diabetics [63, 71, 72] and may contribute to the gastrointestinal lesions as well as male erectile failure. However, in diabetes, autonomic neuropathy is felt to be a phenomenon secondary to either vascular disease or metabolic abnormalities. It is not unreasonable to postulate that similar ANS dysfunction occurs in SSc.

Sonnex and colleague [73] described a case of SSc with sympathetic and parasympathetic neuropathy. These authors also performed detailed autonomic testing in six additional SSc patients. Of these six patients, three showed early parasympathetic damage. The presence of ANS dysfunction in these three patients did not correlate with the presence or severity of Raynaud's phenomenon. Suarez-Almazor and colleague [74] studied 16 consecutive patients with diffuse cutaneous systemic sclerosis (dcSSc) and performed standard noninvasive clinical and electrocardiographic procedures for the detection of cardiovascular autonomic insufficiency. A significant difference between patients and controls was observed only in the heart rate and blood pressure response to standing. The authors concluded that cardiovascular autonomic insufficiency did not appear to be a significant feature in the patients with SSc that were studied. Dessein and Gledhill [75] also studied cardiovascular autonomic function in eight patients with SSc. Compared with healthy volunteers matched by age, sex, and race, six of the eight patients had abnormal values for one or more of the ANS test performed; autonomic involvement was "severe" in four of the six patients. Autonomic neuropathy was also evaluated by Klimiuk and colleagues [76] in 25 patients with SSc and 10 patients with primary Raynaud's phenomenon. These patients were compared to 13 normal healthy subjects. Significant abnormalities were found in cardiovascular reflexes in SSc (limited cutaneous systemic sclerosis (lcSSc) and dcSSc). These authors demonstrated both sympathetic and parasympathetic dysfunction. In 1992, Dessein and colleagues [77] further evaluated autonomic function in 34 patients with SSc using five noninvasive cardiovascular autonomic function tests as well as sequential plasma catecholamine estimations at rest during standing and during sustained handgrip. Autonomic testing in these patients revealed autonomic dysfunction in each patient, while neurologic symptoms were experienced in 33 of the 34 patients. They concluded that ANS dysfunction is extremely common in SSc. It is characterized by parasympathetic impairment and marked sympathetic overactivity. Such changes were more prominent in early disease. A subsequent study by Hermosillo and colleagues [78] observed patients with lcSSc (eight patients) and with dcSSc (nine patients) and 17 age- and sex-matched healthy controls. These authors noted a decreased parasympathetic control of heart rate in patients with lcSSc which is significantly different from those with dcSSc. Twenty-five patients with SSc (13 lcSSc, 12 dcSSc) were studied, using five standard cardiovascular autonomic function tests as well as esophageal manometry, by Stacher and colleagues [79]. They noted definite cardiovascular autonomic dysfunction in five patients and borderline in seven patients. These changes correlated with esophageal motor dysfunction which was also associated with the presence of anti-topoisomerase I and anti-U1snRNP autoantibodies. Lock and colleagues [80] noted evidence of ANS dysfunction in 12 of 77 SSc patients who also had manometric changes of esophageal dysmotility. Using 24 h heart rate period variability, Morrelli and colleagues [81] showed reduction of low-frequency and high-frequency values in SSc patients compared to controls. Other authors have noted an association between ANS dysfunction in SSc and interrenal arterial stiffness [82] and preclinical cardiac involvement [83]. From an ultrastructural perspective, axonal degeneration and cytoskeletal abnormalities in the bundles of unmyelinated fibers were demonstrated in three SSc patients with recent onset of lcSSc [84].

During a recent comprehensive systemic literature review of neurologic involvement in SSc [8], ANS dysfunction was found to be common and typically involved cardiovascular and gastrointestinal systems.

Compared to more well-known visceral organ involvement with SSc, neurological manifestations are less common but are being recognized with increased frequency in recent years. The degree of CNS involvement is not well defined by robust case-control studies, but headache, cerebritis, and neurocognitive impairment have been reported. These presentations may be due to a non-scleroderma process or comorbid conditions. On the other hand, evidence for cranial neuropathies, particularly trigeminal neuropathy, is more compelling. On detailed electrodiagnostic testing, peripheral nervous system involvement may be demonstrated as sensorimotor or entrapment neuropathies. There has been increased attention focused on ANS dysfunction in SSc which may also play a role in contributing to pathogenetic mechanisms in this disease.

Audiovestibular Disease

Sensorineural hearing loss (SNHL) and other auditory symptoms may be more prevalent than previously recognized, with studies reporting involvement in 20–77 % of patients depending on subject selection criteria [85–88]. Sensorineural hearing loss involves the inner ear, cochlea, or the auditory nerve. In an initial report detailing cranial nerve involvement in ten SSc patients, three patients were noted to have tinnitus and two patients had hearing loss [89]. Subsequently, high-frequency SNHL has been demonstrated in many reports, and pathology in one case suggests a middle and inner ear vasculopathy may be responsible [90]. Histologic findings are characterized by enlarged and thickened blood vessels, perivascular fibrosis, and reduced numbers of outer hair cells. A case-control study showed that 33 % of SSc patients had vestibular impairment [91]. Patients with vestibular dysfunction showed significant association with both nailfold capillary patterns and a vascular severity score ($p = 0.049$ and $p = 0.046$, respectively) suggesting that microvascular disease may account for the dysfunction.

Berrettini and colleagues studied 31 unselected SSc patients, 62 % of whom reported audiovestibular symptoms [86]. Objective hearing loss was detected in 14 patients (10 with SNHL, 4 with mixed sensorineural and conductive hearing loss), and in all cases, the site of the lesion was cochlear. Four patients had abnormal vestibular function, and one patient had calcification of the tympanic membrane. In another study, complete ENT examination and audiological evaluation with pure tone, impedance, and speech audiometry were performed in 34 SSc patients and 45 age-matched healthy subjects [87]. Sensorineural hearing loss was detected in 20 % of SSc patients, and a quarter of patients had hearing loss affecting the middle and mainly high frequencies. Speech audiometry identified word recognition scores compatible with cochlear disease. There were no differences in age, systemic manifestations, disease duration, autoantibody profile, or drug therapy comparing patients with and without hearing loss. Interestingly, a patulous Eustachian tube was identified in three patients; the authors postulated that this finding could be secondary to an inflammatory myopathy affecting major muscles surrounding the Eustachian tube, microvascular abnormalities resulting in chronic ischemia, or fibrosis causing tendon dysfunction. A third study focused on 35 patients with limited cutaneous scleroderma and anti-centromere protein B antibodies and compared them to 59 age-, sex-, and ethnically matched controls [85]. While 54 % of SSc patients reported subjective hearing loss compared to 0 % of controls, objective hearing loss on audiogram was detected in 77 % of SSc patients compared to 26 % of controls ($p<0.001$). Hearing loss was bilateral in most cases and was attributed to asymmetric SNHL in 11 patients and symmetric SNHL in 13 patients. The audiometric curve was flat in 13 patients with high-frequency hearing loss in 14 patients. Scleroderma subjects had a higher prevalence of abnormal tympanograms, absent stapedius reflexes, abnormal oculocephalic responses, head-shaking nystagmus, and abnormal caloric tests and clinical tests of sensory integration and balance compared to controls. Overall, these findings provided strong evidence of inner and middle ear compromise resulting in auditory and vestibular dysfunction.

In another study of 42 SSc patients (35 with limited disease and anti-centromere protein B antibodies, 7 with diffuse disease) and 74 age-, sex-, and ethnically matched controls, these same authors performed Dix-Hallpike maneuvers, cephalic rotational tests, and clinical tests of sensory integration and balance [92]. Seven patients (17 %) fulfilled criteria for benign paroxysmal positional vertigo (BPPV) compared to zero controls ($p<0.001$). BPPV was related to the posterior semicircular canal in two patients with limited SSc and to the horizontal semicircular canal in five patients (three limited, two diffuse). Twenty SSc patients (48 %) had abnormal postural control, largely vestibular in origin, compared to 10 % of controls ($p<0.0001$). Because of the predominance of peripheral vestibular abnormalities, the authors postulated an ischemic etiology or an intralabyrinthine autoimmune process as potential triggers of disease.

A careful medical history probing for the use of ototoxic medications (e.g., sildenafil, high-dose nonsteroidal anti-inflammatory drugs or aspirin, loop diuretics, aminoglycoside antibiotics) is essential in scleroderma patients with audiovestibular symptoms. Patients with hearing loss should be referred for otolaryngology evaluation and audiometry, and tests of vestibular function should be considered in patients with dizziness, vertigo, and poor balance. If the onset of hearing loss, aural fullness, or tinnitus is sudden or rapid, this constitutes an otologic emergency until proven otherwise. Urgent referral to an otolaryngologist for audiometry and confirmation of sensorineural hearing loss is necessary, as prompt institution of either oral or intratympanic corticosteroids may improve or restore hearing [93]. Therapeutic options for SNHL and other audiovestibular manifestations in SSc have not been studied in great depth. In one case report of a patient who presented with bilateral SNHL as the first manifestation of SSc, hearing improved with high doses of methotrexate and intravenous immunoglobulin [94]. Similarly, Abou-Taleb and colleagues reported a woman with bilateral mixed hearing loss in the context of long-standing SSc who had improved hearing and speech discrimination after cyclophosphamide therapy [90]. Lastly, a cochlear implant was used to treat one woman with SSc, double-stranded DNA antibodies, and an auditory neuropathy [95]. Further investigation of therapeutic options, including the use of immunosuppressive therapy, is warranted.

Oral Manifestations

Oral complications frequently plague patients with scleroderma, but management of these life-altering symptoms are often overlooked Among patients with diffuse scleroderma, facial changes are prominent with decreased oral aperture, thin and retracted lips, perioral wrinkling, and skin sclerosis resulting in an altered, often grimaced appearance. Telangiectasia often develops on oral mucous membranes in patients with limited or diffuse disease, yet these lesions often go unnoticed and rarely rupture and bleed. In addition to psychological distress from these cosmetic changes [96], alterations in facial architecture can contribute to malnutrition due to fatigue with chewing and reduced capacity to eat large boluses of solid food. Xerostomia and periodontal disease are prevalent complications. A scale has been developed to measure disability [97]. Three major factors accounted for the disability: a reduced oral aperture, sicca syndrome, and cosmetic concerns [97].

Microstomia has been reported in up to 80 % of patients with scleroderma [98], and decreased oral mobility and strength significantly impairs quality of life [99]. The reduced oral aperture makes daily oral hygiene and dental treatment more complex and challenging, and at times, patients are denied dental care altogether because of restricted access to the oral cavity [100]. A narrowed oral aperture correlates with poorer oral hygiene and with increased numbers of dental caries [101]. Commissurotomy has been described in case reports but is infrequently used to treat microstomia due to concerns about poor wound healing. Two studies have demonstrated, however, that simple oral exercise regimens may be effective treatments for microstomia. In the first, Naylor and colleagues performed a

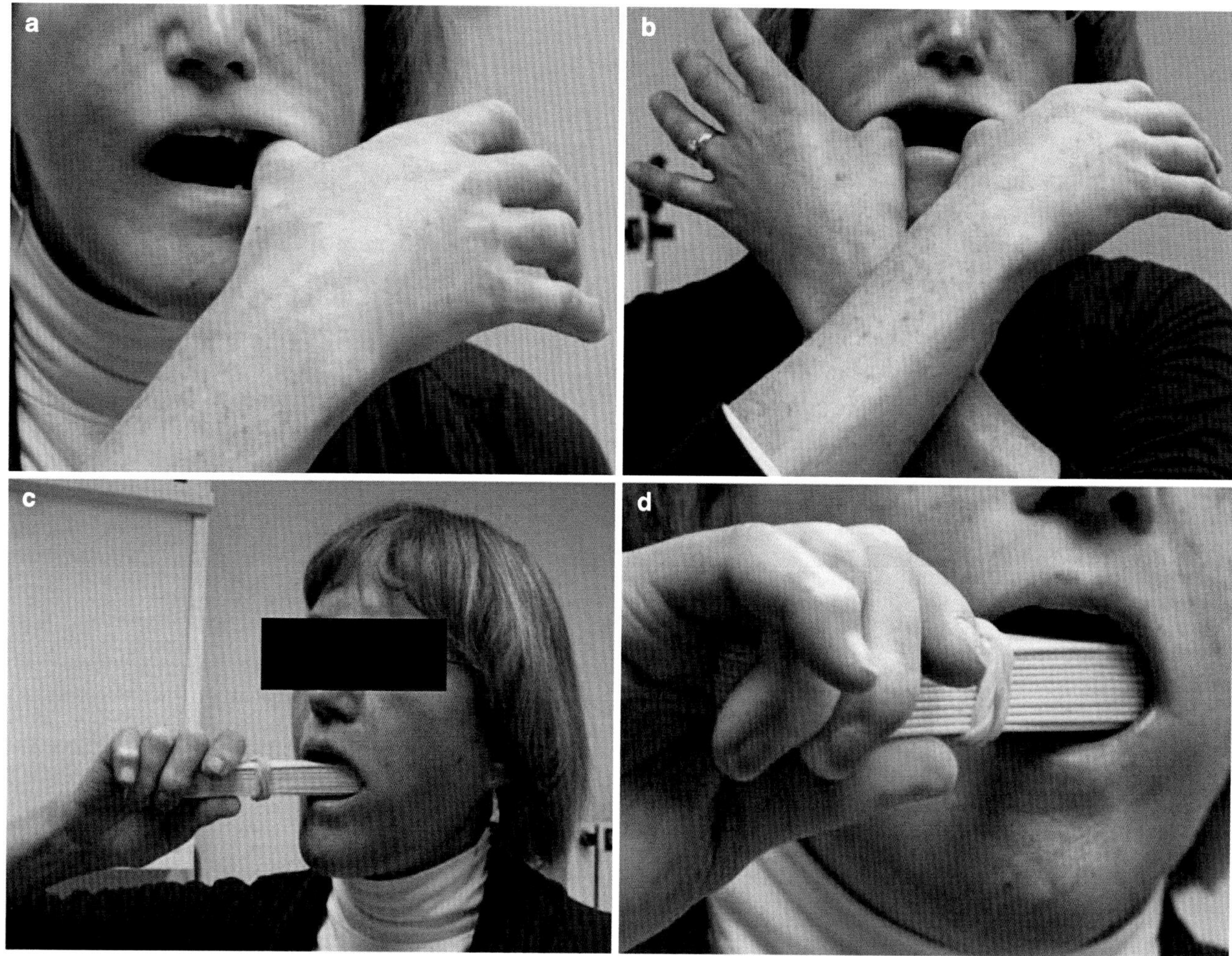

Fig. 38.1 Sample exercises to maximize oral opening. (**a**) The patient places the right thumb in the corner of the left side of the mouth and stretches for 10–15 s. Then, the patient places the left thumb in the corner of the right side of the mouth and stretches (not shown). (**b**) After doing each side, the patient stretches both sides simultaneously. Steps (**a**) and (**b**) should be repeated five to ten times. (**c**) A stack of tongue depressors bound by a rubber band is inserted into the mouth from the front middle teeth to the back molars on one side. The patient uses as many tongue depressors as necessary to stretch the facial skin and musculature. After holding the pose for several minutes, the contralateral side is stretched in the same manner (not shown). Repetitions and gradually increasing the number of tongue depressors used are encouraged. (**d**) A closer view of the angle of insertion

6-month clinical trial of nine scleroderma patients comparing two different exercise programs [102]. While the control group performed facial grimacing exercises, the experimental group did three mouth stretching exercises plus an oral augmentation exercise using tongue depressors. The mouth stretching exercises consisted of placing the right thumb in the corner of the left side of the mouth and stretching, placing the left thumb in the right side of the mouth and stretching, and then doing both sides simultaneously. Three sets of five stretches were performed. Patients then used tongue depressors placed diagonally across the posterior teeth to open the oral cavity by stretching the facial skin and musculature. After holding this pose for several minutes, repetitions were encouraged with brief rest periods. Patients were encouraged to gradually increase the number of tongue depressors used. The experimental group in this study achieved a 5.6 mm increase in vertical oral opening compared to a 3 mm increase in the control group. In 2003, Pizzo and colleagues studied a similar but slightly modified exercise regimen over an 18-week period [103]. They noted a mean increase in oral opening of 10.7 mm. By the end of the study, all patients noted greater ease eating, speaking, and maintaining oral hygiene, and denture insertion was easier in edentulous patients. These simple exercises can easily be taught to scleroderma patients in both rheumatologists and dentists' offices and may improve quality of life (Fig. 38.1). An effort to use simple facial grimacing and opening the mouth as wide as possible failed to show improvement in 6 months in part due to lack of compliance with the program [104]. The use of assistive devices including power toothbrush and

Reach Access Flosser along with oral-facial exercises improved gingival inflammation [105].

Xerostomia is a common problem in scleroderma, occurring in up to 70 % of scleroderma patients [106–108], and concomitant Sjogren's syndrome may occur in 12–21 % of patients depending on which Sjogren's diagnostic criteria are used [108–110]. A study using diagnostic criteria of the American-European Concensus Group (AECG) found grade 3 and/or grade 4 sialoadenitis in 33.9 % of 74 patients with sicca symptoms suggesting that Sjogren's syndrome was common among patients' scleroderma [111]. Xerostomia may be secondary to salivary gland fibrosis involving capillary walls and excretory ducts [108, 109, 112, 113], a pathological finding that is distinct and more common than the lymphocytic infiltrates generally seen in Sjogren's syndrome. Unstimulated salivary flow rates correlate with glandular sclerosis [112]. One survey found that low saliva production was associated with specific Sjogren's autoantibodies (Ro52/TRIM21, SSA/Ro60, or SSB/La) [114]. Salivary flow contributes to dysphagia, which may also be limited in scleroderma due to tongue fibrosis and limited tongue mobility [100, 115]. Increased dental caries and *Candida* infections are also complications [115]. Treatment of xerostomia is challenging and requires a multifaceted approach including the use of sugarless candies and mints, lozenges, saliva substitutes, pharmacological agents to stimulate salivary flow, small sips of water throughout the day, and frequent oral hygiene visits [115]. Avoidance of aggravating medications, such as anticholinergic agents, that dry mucous membranes is critical.

A survey of the oral health of 163 patients with scleroderma compared to 231 healthy controls found that patients had more missing teeth, more periodontal disease, less saliva production, and overall poorer quality of oral health [116]. A second study by the same investigators found that oral health measures associated with global quality of life but not with various measures of disease severity [117]. A third survey found that tooth loss was associated with poor upper extremity function, gastrointestinal reflux disease, and decreased saliva [114]. Periodontal disease has been reported in up to 95 % of scleroderma patients, and the most common finding is periodontal ligament distension [98, 106, 107, 118, 119]. Increased periodontal disease may not be solely due to poor oral hygiene; in one study, patients with scleroderma had more periodontal disease but similar plaque and calculus scores compared to controls [106]. In the same study, the width of tooth roots was not increased as well, suggesting that a wide periodontal ligament may occur at the expense of adjacent socket bone [106]. Tooth mobility may result, occurring in 62 % of scleroderma patients in one study [98, 106]. In our center's experience, tooth mobility is infrequent but may benefit from tooth stabilization procedures. Bony resorption of the mandibular angle, coronoid process, condylar head, and digastric region [98, 106] may contribute to reduced oral strength and mobility in scleroderma, and in one study, mandibular erosions were associated with the presence of periodontal membrane thickening [106]. Because an obliterative vasculopathy of small blood vessels has been observed in a thickened periodontal ligament from a scleroderma patient [120], it has been suggested that poor perfusion in scleroderma may increase susceptibility to periodontal disease [106].

Table 38.1 Summary of management options for oral manifestations and barriers to good oral hygiene

Clinical finding	Management options
1. Microstomia	Daily oral exercises (see Fig. 37.1) to maximize oral aperture
	Child-sized toothbrushes with only two rows of bristles to enhance cleaning of cheek sides of the teeth
	Education re: eating smaller parcels of food
2. Dental decay and caries	Early referral to an experienced dentist or dental specialist for preventive and regular dental and periodontal care
	Frequent fluoride treatments (every 3 months)
	Encourage flossing; specific floss brands for various clinical situations are provided in reference 29
3. Xerostomia	Eliminate medications that dry mucous membranes
	Treat with stimulators of muscarinic cholinergic receptors (pilocarpine, cevimeline)
	Sugarless candies/mints
	Saliva substitutes
	Nonalcoholic mouth washes
	Frequent dental hygiene visits
4. Hand contractures	Referral to hand occupational therapy for assistive devices to aid in dental care
	Mold custom grip on toothbrush handle with dental acrylic
	Consider electric toothbrushes with soft brush filaments

Limited hand dexterity and joint range of motion correlate with increased decayed surfaces and dental caries [101]. Worse gingival inflammation has been associated with poor hand dexterity and decreased flossing habits [121]. A low-cost solution to this problem may be to have the dentist mold a custom grip on the toothbrush handle with dental acrylic [122]. If this is ineffective, an electric toothbrush may need to be considered [122].

A summary of SSc oral manifestations and management options is provided in Table 38.1. An excellent patient guide on basic oral hygiene is available through the Scleroderma Foundation [122] and can be found online at http://www.scleroderma.org/medical/dental_articles/Nauert_1999.shtm. In addition to recommending child-sized toothbrushes with wide flat handles, the author suggests that patients with microstomia have a second toothbrush with all but the end two rows of bristles tweezed out to clean the cheek sides of the upper and lower teeth. Specific oral exercises, toothbrush brands, floss types, fluoride agents, and products to treat xerostomia are recommended in a concise format that is easy for patients to digest. It is notable that a survey found that depression and difficulty performing flossing decreased dental care [123]. In the setting of tooth loss, implants may be considered in those with adequate bone levels [115]. If dentures are required, frequent dental visits should be continued for denture adjustments and evaluation of the oral mucosa's ability to withstand pressure without atrophy [115]. In addition, collapsible dentures have been designed for patients with microstomia [124].

Thyroid Dysfunction

Examination for thyroid dysfunction is important in scleroderma as many symptoms of hypothyroidism and hyperthyroidism overlap with scleroderma features and are incorrectly attributed to scleroderma when treatments for thyroid disease are readily available [125]. Thyroid fibrosis, autoimmune thyroiditis resulting in hypothyroidism, and hyperthyroidism from Graves' disease are frequent and often unsuspected findings in scleroderma. Autoimmune thyroid disease should especially be sought in patients with primary biliary cirrhosis, CREST features, and Sjogren's syndrome as there are reports of overlap of all of these conditions [126, 127].

In autopsy studies, thyroid gland fibrosis is more prevalent in scleroderma patients than in matched controls [128, 129], and in one study, all hypothyroid scleroderma patients had glandular fibrosis [129]. Lymphocytic infiltration characteristic of Hashimoto's thyroiditis was infrequent [129] despite a strong association between hypothyroidism and high serum titers of antithyroid antibodies.

In one study of 719 scleroderma patients, 38 % had autoimmune thyroid disease, and 9 % of patients had a first-degree relative with autoimmune thyroid disease [130]. In a Hungarian population, the prevalence of Hashimoto's thyroiditis and Graves' disease was 220-fold higher and 102-fold higher, respectively, in scleroderma patients than in the general population [131]. In particular, antithyroid peroxidase (TPO) antibodies are more commonly observed in scleroderma than in controls [132–135], and it has been suggested that anti-TPO antibodies may identify the subset of patients at risk for subsequent thyroid dysfunction [132]. Scleroderma patients with normal basal thyroid function often have an exaggerated thyroid-stimulating hormone (TSH) response to thyrotropin-releasing hormone consistent with subclinical hypothyroidism [136, 137]. Antonelli and colleagues assessed the prevalence of clinical and subclinical thyroid disorders in 202 scleroderma patients compared to 404 controls matched on age and gender [133]. The authors specifically assessed for thyroid disease in a population that had a similar iodine intake. Among females, there were significantly increased relative odds of thyroid disease among scleroderma patients compared to controls including subclinical hypothyroidism [OR 3.2 (95 % CI 1.8, 5.7)], clinical hypothyroidism [OR 14.5 (95 % CI 2.3, 90.9)], anti-TPO positivity [OR 2.7 (95 % CI 1.8, 4.1)], thyroid ultrasound hypoechoic pattern [OR 3.2 (95 % CI 2.2, 4.7)], thyroid autoimmunity [OR 3.7 (95 % CI 2.6, 5.4)], and for small thyroid volumes <6 mL [1.8 (95 % CI 2.2, 52.4)]. The relative odds of having thyroid autoimmunity was also higher in male scleroderma patients compared to male controls. Mean TSH values were higher in scleroderma women and anti-TPO titers were higher in scleroderma patients in general than in controls. Three female scleroderma patients had Graves' disease compared to no female controls. Scleroderma patients with thyroid autoimmunity had a longer scleroderma disease duration than scleroderma patients without thyroid autoimmunity. A follow-up study by the same investigators showed a high incidence of thyroid disorders including hypothyroidism, thyroid dysfunction, anti-thyroperoxidase antibody positivity, and appearance of a hypoechoic thyroid pattern [138]. Another study found an increased prevalence of anti-TPO antibodies was identified in patients with limited SSc compared to healthy controls but not diffuse scleroderma [139]. These data suggest that assessment of thyroid function and anti-TPO antibodies should be incorporated in routine clinical evaluations of patients with scleroderma.

Liver Disease

Although the liver is generally spared as a primary target organ in scleroderma, the relative risk of chronic liver disease is 2.5–4.3 times higher in patients with scleroderma compared to the general population [140]. Abnormal liver function tests are often encountered in the routine care of these patients and require further evaluation. Initial considerations include hepatotoxic medications or coincident viral hepatitis, but primary biliary cirrhosis (PBC), autoimmune hepatitis (AIH), nodular regenerative hyperplasia (NRH), steatosis, primary sclerosing cholangitis (PSC), and idiopathic portal hypertension may develop in scleroderma in isolation or at times together [141, 142]. A study investigating the prevalence of antimitochondrial antibody (AMA), antismooth muscle antibodies (SMAs), and liver-kidney microsomal (LKM-1) autoantibody in a cohort of 63 scleroderma patients compared to 100 healthy controls found an increase in liver autoantibodies among scleroderma patients [143].

Primary biliary cirrhosis is a chronic and progressive inflammatory obliteration of intrahepatic biliary ducts leading to fibrosis and cholestatic symptoms of pruritis and jaundice.

Cholestatic liver function tests, such as an elevated total bilirubin and/or alkaline phosphatase, are often detected. The overlap of PBC with scleroderma is well established and at times is referred to by the eponym Raynaud's syndrome [144]. The prevalence of PBC among patients with scleroderma is about 2–2.5 % [145–147], and it has been estimated that 3.9–15 % of patients with PBC have scleroderma [148–150]. Primary biliary cirrhosis may develop years before or after the diagnosis of scleroderma [147, 148], though concurrent onset has been reported. Prior epidemiological studies have demonstrated that although PBC may develop in patients with limited or diffuse scleroderma, it is much more common among the limited subset, particularly in patients with anticentromere antibodies (ACAs) [145–147]. Many investigators have compared patients with both PBC and scleroderma to either patients with PBC alone or patients with scleroderma alone. These studies have demonstrated that patients with a PBC-scleroderma overlap (a) are more likely to be ACA positive than either of the other groups [151, 152], (b) are older and have a longer scleroderma disease duration than those with scleroderma alone [145], and (c) have more Sjogren's syndrome than those with limited scleroderma alone [152]. Indeed, in one study 91 % of patients with a PBC-scleroderma overlap had keratoconjunctivitis sicca such that the authors suggested using the acronym PACK (**P**BC, **A**CA, **C**REST, **K**eratoconjunctivitis sicca) syndrome to remember the key features of the disease [148].

Anti-centromere antibodies occur in up to 30 % of patients with PBC [153–155] and up to 90 % of patients with PBC and scleroderma [156]. The antimitochondrial antibodies (AMAs), which are classically associated with PBC, may occur in up to 25 % of patients with scleroderma [145, 157–159]. Antimitochondrial antibodies are highly correlated to the presence of ACA [146, 157] and increased pruritis in scleroderma [157]. Although there is a strong correlation between ACA and AMA, patients with PBC who are AMA negative are more likely to have a secondary autoimmune disease, such as scleroderma or Sjogren's syndrome, than those who are AMA positive [149, 160]. When PBC is suspected in a scleroderma patient, it is important to consider both assay methodology and the need for additional autoantibody testing. In a recent large study of 817 patients with scleroderma, 16 patients (2 %) had confirmed PBC [145]. Testing for AMA by indirect immunofluorescence had a sensitivity of only 43.8 % with a specificity of 98.9 %. When AMAs were assessed by ELISA using an M2-enhanced (MIT3) assay, the sensitivity increased to 81.3 % with only a slight decrease in specificity (94.6 %). When the authors combined the testing for AMA by ELISA with another autoantibody that is highly specific for PBC (sp100), sensitivity increased to 100 % with a specificity of 92.6 %. The authors suggested performing sp100 autoantibody testing in patients who have a persistent cholestatic picture, but are AMA negative, to improve detection of PBC. Testing for this autoantibody also has prognostic value, as sp100-positive patients progress more rapidly from early- to late-stage PBC [161].

Liver biopsy is not routinely required to diagnose PBC in the appropriate clinical setting, including an elevated alkaline phosphatase level, positive antimitochondrial antibody, elevated IgM fraction, and exclusion of extrahepatic biliary obstruction. However, biopsy should be considered in patients where the differential diagnosis remains broad: concern for granulomatous liver disease, drug toxicity, steatosis in an obese subject, autoimmune hepatitis due to an atypical laboratory profile (positive ANA, elevated IgG fraction, transaminitis out of proportion to alkaline phosphatase elevation), or nodular regenerative hyperplasia due to the presence of noncirrhotic portal hypertension or a hepatic vascular insult. Liver biopsy is not routinely performed to stage the severity of PBC because sampling error may affect results, and therapeutic management is the same regardless of stage.

Early detection of PBC and institution of ursodeoxycholic acid (UDCA) therapy improve hepatic biochemical parameters [162] and may reduce mortality [163, 164]. Therefore, it is imperative that rheumatologists consider PBC in the differential diagnosis of scleroderma patients with pruritis or abnormal liver function tests. Treatment with UDCA (typically 300 mg thrice daily) usually results in improved liver function tests within the first 6 months of treatment [66]. Normalization of alkaline phosphatase values is associated with an improved prognosis, and liver function tests should continue to be monitored in these patients two to three times per year. Treatment with bile acid sequestrants such as cholestyramine or colestipol may be helpful for pruritis [165]. In patients with PBC and scleroderma, surveillance for metabolic bone disease is also essential.

The hepatic prognosis of scleroderma patients with PBC may be better than those with PBC alone. In a study from the United Kingdom, 43 patients with PBC and scleroderma were matched on serum bilirubin concentration at initial visit to 86 patients with PBC alone [147]. Overall survival was similar between the groups, but the risk of liver transplantation was significantly lower in the PBC-scleroderma group (16 %) than in the PBC alone group (26 %) due to less severe liver disease. The rate of bilirubin increase, a marker of severity, was less in the PBC-scleroderma group than those with PBC alone. Although there were fewer liver-related deaths in the scleroderma group, this was offset by an increase in nonliver deaths due to scleroderma, and therefore overall survival did not differ between the two groups. Interestingly, hepatic complications were not different between the groups except the incidence of first occurrence of spontaneous bacterial peritonitis and septicemia, which were higher in PBC patients with scleroderma than in those without scleroderma.

In addition to PBC, autoimmune hepatitis may develop in limited scleroderma and can overlap with PBC in the same patient [142, 166–171]. Autoimmune hepatitis is characterized by liver inflammation on biopsy including interface hepatitis, hypergammaglobulinemia, and autoantibodies (ANA, antismooth muscle, anti-liver-kidney microsome type 1, anti-soluble liver antigen) [172, 173]. In our center's experience, affected patients have limited cutaneous disease and respond to immunosuppressive therapy [167]. Therefore, liver biopsy and evaluation of histology may be critical in identifying this subset of patients.

Nodular regenerative hyperplasia (NRH) of the liver may also be seen in varied rheumatic diseases and is also known as noncirrhotic portal hypertension, diffuse nodular hyperplasia, or nodular transformation of the liver [173, 174]. This condition is characterized by transformation of hepatic parenchyma into nodules consisting of hyperplastic hepatocytes without significant fibrosis [173]. It is thought that hepatic ischemia either due to alterations in hepatic perfusion or direct hepatic vascular bed injury may contribute to the pathogenesis of this condition. Nodular regenerative hyperplasia may present incidentally during the evaluation of abnormal liver function tests, with chronic abdominal pain, or as portal hypertension with signs of hepatosplenomegaly, bleeding esophageal varices, or ascites [173]. Nodular regenerative hyperplasia may also occur concurrent with PBC and scleroderma [141]. Diagnosis requires histologic examination, and it has been suggested that liver biopsy should be obtained in patients with rheumatic diseases who have persistently abnormal liver function tests, hepatosplenomegaly, or a risk factor for thrombosis (e.g., antiphospholipid antibodies) [173].

Other hepatic findings in scleroderma may include steatosis, where fatty liver may account for 20 % of liver disturbance in scleroderma [166], primary sclerosing cholangitis [175], or idiopathic portal hypertension [166, 176, 177]. These findings are reported primarily in case reports, however, and it is difficult to conclude whether these conditions are related to or associated with scleroderma.

Given the risk of these hepatic complications, the rheumatologist should screen all patients with scleroderma, particularly those with the limited subtype, with basic labs including transaminases and an alkaline phosphatase. If elevated transaminases are detected, a search for hepatic and nonhepatic causes, including inflammatory myopathies, should be performed. Although antimitochondrial antibodies may be detected years before onset of PBC, routine screening with these antibodies is controversial, as many of these patients may never develop symptomatic or clinically relevant liver disease. In the scleroderma patient with a classic constellation of findings for PBC (elevated alkaline phosphatase, positive antimitochondrial antibody, elevated IgM fraction, and exclusion of extrahepatic biliary obstruction), liver biopsy may not be required. If the alkaline phosphatase does not normalize with UDCA treatment or if the differential diagnosis remains broad, liver biopsy should be performed given that these conditions may overlap with one another and therefore impact therapy.

Bladder Dysfunction

In the few studies and case reports that have examined lower urinary tract involvement in scleroderma, urologic symptoms such as increased urinary frequency, nocturia, hesitancy, decreased stream, suprapubic pain, and hematuria have been reported [178–184]. Urodynamic assessment and bladder histology demonstrate that autonomic dysfunction, bladder fibrosis, and vascular disease may be contributing factors.

In a study comparing 21 female scleroderma patients to 15 age- and gender-matched controls, Kucharz and colleagues detected a large variation in premictional bladder volume and reduced bladder emptying in scleroderma patients (89.8 ± 13.1 % bladder emptying in scleroderma patients vs. 97.4 ± 4.1 % in controls) [178]. Twenty-nine percent of patients had bladder volumes more than two standard deviations (SDs) above the mean for controls, and 33 % of patients had bladder volumes more than two SDs below the mean for controls. Patients with long-standing scleroderma (>14 years) had higher bladder volumes, and the authors postulated that bladder fibrosis might result in decreased distensibility and contractility of the bladder.

In another study, urodynamic testing, autonomic nervous system assessments, and bladder pathology were examined in 23 female patients with scleroderma [179]. Five patients had frequent daytime urination, one had urge incontinence, and the remaining patients were asymptomatic. Urodynamic alterations were detected in only three patients, but signs of parasympathetic dysfunction were identified in 13 cases, 9 of whom also had sympathetic dysfunction. Two patients with autonomic dysfunction had urinary symptoms, and three had bladder dysfunction. Interestingly, abnormal bladder pathology was common: 78 % of patients had increased connective tissue in the lamina propria and interstitial fibrosis separating smooth muscle bundles (12 patients with mild fibrosis, 4 moderate, 2 severe), and 7 patients had proliferative changes in small arteries. There was no correlation between urinary symptoms and urodynamic features with the severity of bladder fibrosis.

In a third study, the authors detected functional bladder alterations with failed detrusor activity in four of nine patients [180]. These abnormalities did correlate with histologic findings. Three patients with detrusor areflexia had collagen accumulation in the small arteries of the detrusor along with tortuous, enlarged capillary loops and areas of capillary loss. Two patients with detrusor areflexia had fibrotic replacement of the bladder smooth muscle.

Scleroderma patients with urinary symptoms should undergo a formal urological evaluation including urodynamic testing and cystoscopy. In patients with hematuria, cystoscopy should be performed to evaluate for bladder telangiectasia in addition to malignancy. Severe gross hematuria from bladder telangiectasia requiring blood transfusions has been reported, and in one case, this was successfully treated with diathermocoagulation [184]. There are no formal treatment studies for bladder dysfunction in scleroderma, although a surgical intervention has been reported to help one patient with a thickened, poorly distensible bladder who suffered from dysuria, frequency, and urinary incontinence [183].

Avascular Necrosis of Bone

Avascular necrosis of the carpal scaphoid bone and lunate of the wrist is reported in scleroderma [185–188]. This can occur in the absence of steroid use or specific trauma to the wrist. Patients present with wrist pain with minimal, if any, signs of inflammation. One case series reported avascular necrosis of the lunate bone in patients with limited scleroderma with severe Raynaud's suggesting that vascular disease was the causative factor [186]. It may be underdiagnosed and mistaken for arthritis or tendonitis. Treatment includes attempts at placing a vascularized bone graft or surgical removal of the damaged bone and stabilization of the wrist to reduce pain and disability.

Erectile Dysfunction

Erectile dysfunction (ED) in SSc was first described in 1981 [48]. These authors described five male SSc patients who presented with impotence as a significant initial feature of their disease. Endocrinologic, urological, and psychiatric evaluations failed to reveal an alternative cause for impotence. None of the patients were taking medications known to alter sexual function. All of these patients had preservation of libido throughout their illness, but absent or greatly diminished erectile function. None had evidence for large-vessel vascular disease. Subsequently, Nowlin and colleagues [189] performed a study of ten SSc patients who were evaluated for sexual function. Five of these reported complete impotence and three partial impotence. Endocrinologic evaluation, including measurements of serum testosterone, prolactin, estradiol, follicle-stimulating hormone, and luteinizing hormones, was normal in all patients.

Since these early reports, several other descriptions of ED in male patients with SSc have been reported [190–195]. In most of these reports, comprehensive evaluations for other causes of impotence were not uncovered and ED was felt to be attributed directly to SSc. The prevalence of ED in SSc has varied from 27 to 81 % [189, 191, 196].

More recently ED was studied in 130 SSc men by the EULAR Scleroderma Trial and Research (EUSTAR) group [197]. Of the 130 men studied, only 17.7 % had normal erectile function scores. ED in these patients occurred earlier in the disease and was associated with severe cutaneous, muscular or renal involvement of SSc, elevated pulmonary pressures, and restrictive lung disease. The authors concluded that severe ED is a common and early symptom in men with SSc.

In order to determine if ED is more common in SSc than in other chronic rheumatic diseases, Hong and colleagues [196], in a case-control study, evaluated men with SSc and rheumatoid arthritis (RA). The authors found that 81 % of men with SSc had ED. ED occurred in SSc three times more commonly than in RA. In both SSc and RA, ED was associated with the presence of Raynaud's phenomenon (80 % of men with RP vs. 50 % of men without RP). The authors report that ED frequently developed within the first 3 years of disease onset and was a prominent symptom in these involved patients. The association with ED with RP in both of these patient populations suggest to these authors microvascular involvement of the penis was responsible for this symptom.

Rosato and colleagues [198] investigated ED in 20 SSc patients using color Doppler ultrasound examination in the cavernous arteries and correlated these changes with disease severity and digital vascular damage. They further evaluated these patients using nailfold videocapillaroscopy, Sexual Health Inventory for Men (SHIM), and Medsger Disease Severity Scale (DSS). In all SSc patients studied, a reduction in SHIM was present. Greater vascular damage was correlated with low SHIM scores. The authors concluded that the degree of ED in the patients correlated with the severity of the vascular damage. Using more sophisticated methodologies for measuring genital blood flow, these authors confirmed their previous observation [199]. However, Keck and colleagues [200] studied 86 men with SSc with and without ED and performed nailfold capillaroscopy. These authors noted that either the presence or absence of abnormal nailfold findings was associated with the coexistence of ED in these patients. They also could not find a correlation based on the stage or duration of SSc.

Pathogenesis of ED in the General Population: Penile erection is a neurovascular phenomenon, which depends on neural integrity, a functional vascular system, and healthy corporal tissues. Normal erectile function involves three synergistic and simultaneous processes: (1) neurologically mediated increase in penile arterial inflow, (2) relaxation of corporal smooth muscle, and (3) restriction of venous outflow from the penis. The corpus cavernosum of the penis is composed of a meshwork of interconnected smooth muscle cells lined by vascular endothelium. Of note, the small resistance helicine arteries that supply blood to the corpus cavernosum during penile tumescence are also lined by endothelial cells and underlying smooth muscle. Pathological alteration in the anatomy of the penile vasculature or impairment of any combination of neurovascular processes can result in ED [197]. The severity of ED is associated with vascular risk factors such as atherosclerosis, hypertension, hypercholesterolemia, diabetes mellitus, and cigarette smoking. Recent clinical and basic science investigations on aging, diabetes, hypercholesterolemia, and hypertension have shown that endothelial dysfunction is a major contributing factor to penile vascular pathology [201, 202]. Endothelial dysfunction can impair penile blood flow into the penis and thus cause ED. ED associated with SSc is thought to be due to underlying vasculopathic (endothelial and penile arterial dysfunction) and fibrotic changes in the penile vascular bed [203]. Pathological findings suggest penile arterial alterations such as increased collagen to smooth muscle density in the small helicine arteries of the penis as well as increased collagen deposition in the corporal sinusoids [203]. These pathological findings are associated with arteriogenic and veno-occlusive ED.

Pathogenesis of ED in SSc: Since both fibrosis and microvasculopathy occur as prominent features of SSc, it is possible that either one of these, or both, contribute to the pathogenesis of ED. In general, since tissue fibrosis occurs later in the course of SSc and since ED has been described as an early and often presenting symptom of SSc, it would be reasonable to implicate microvascular disease in the etiology of ED. In SSc, small arteries, arterioles, and capillaries undergo proliferative and sclerotic changes. Such microvascular damage in the circulation of the penis may impede the distending pressure required for penile erection. In addition, autonomic nervous system alterations may interfere with neurogenic control of penile vascular tone and contribute to ED. Autonomic dysfunction has been described in SSc [77, 81, 84]. The association of impotence with the autonomic neuropathy of diabetes mellitus has been well described. Penile fibrosis, although a late finding in SSc, could contribute to the inability to obtain sufficient distending pressure to achieve an erection. In order to investigate these various hypotheses, researchers have focused on noninvasive methods to evaluate penile blood flow. In the early report by Nowlin et al. [189], penile blood flow, evaluated by Doppler, was normal in all five impotent and one partially potent patient. Of the age-matched controls with RA, none had impotence or reduced penile blood flow. Aversa and colleagues studied the penile vasculature in SSc using the duplex ultrasound technique in 15 male patients with SSc [204]. Nine of the 15 patients had moderate to severe ED. Severely impaired mean peak systolic velocities in the presence of mild venous leakage were found in these patients. Granchi and colleagues [205] reported that penile smooth muscle cells synthesized endothelin-1 (ET-1), one of the main regulators of microvascular contractility. In general patients with SSc-associated ED are younger and have rapidly progressive decline in erectile function [204].

Reports of fibrosis of penile structures in the development of ED have emerged over the years. Pathologic examinations have shown greater than normal connective tissue infiltration of the testes and other genital organs in patients with SSc [206]. Rossman and Zorgniotti [195] described three male patients with SSc and impotence in whom the corpus cavernosum had been extensively replaced with connective tissue components. These authors postulated that extensive fibrosis resulted in limited blood flow and the inability of the venous sinusoids to distend appropriately. In a clinicopathological study by Nehra and colleagues [203], hemodynamic testing on a patient who underwent a penile implant revealed diffuse corporeal veno-occlusive dysfunction. The excised corporeal tissue demonstrated severe fibrosis. Pro-fibrotic cytokines including transforming growth factor beta and platelet-derived growth factor are overexpressed in the corpora cavernosa under various hypoxic conditions [207, 208]. Under similar hypoxic conditions, penile smooth muscle cells release ET-1 which may stimulate fibroblast proliferation. It is likely that ED in SSc has a multifactorial etiology [209, 210]. In summary, based on available data, it is likely that pathogenesis of ED and SSc is complex and develops due to both microvascular abnormalities and penile fibrosis.

Evaluation and Treatment of ED in SSc: Evaluation of patients with SSc and ED should systematically include attention to occupational exposure, medications known to be associated with ED, symptoms of depression, and assessment of comorbidities including smoking, diabetes mellitus, hypertension, and peripheral vascular disease. An endocrinologic evaluation should also be carried out including serum testosterone levels which may contribute to ED in some patients with SSc. Referral to a urologist should be initiated in order to perform a penile duplex Doppler ultrasound evaluation of the penis in order to determine the penile vascular status which can help manage both medical and surgical therapy [210]. If the duplex Doppler ultrasound of the penis shows severe penile fibrosis with poor arterial inflow to the corpora cavernosa of the penis after pharmacostimulation, then this may warrant placement of a penile prosthesis [203, 204, 210].

Treatment pharmacologic management of ED and SSc has received little attention. In small series, there does not appear to be support for calcium channel blockers or other vasodilators in treating this condition. Certainly, PDEIs should be considered as the first-line ED therapy in SSc [210–212]. However, on demand PDEIs generally have been ineffective in improving erectile function in most case series [209]. Medications in this category, given on a nearly daily basis, might improve symptoms although this has not been specifically studied.

Either sildenafil (50 mg qd) or tadalafil (10 mg qd) on a daily basis for a period of 2–3 weeks is recommended. Extrapolating from the general population, sildenafil can be increased to 100 mg and tadalafil to 20 mg daily. Inability to achieve satisfactory erections during this trial period should be considered a failure of these agents. Given the role of endothelin in the abnormalities of penile vasculature, it is possible that endothelin receptor antagonist may have a role to play in such patients, although these have not been studied either. Finally, if patients do not respond to medications in these categories, they should be referred to a urologist for other treatments including duplex Doppler ultrasound of the penis, intracavernous injection therapy with vasoactive agents, and possible placement of an inflatable penile prosthesis.

SSc patients are considered a hard-to-treat ED population of patients secondary to the severe fibrosis and endothelial dysfunction that occurs in the penile vasculature. Duplex Doppler ultrasound of the penis shows that men with SSc have severe penile fibrosis and impaired penile arterial smooth muscle relaxation [203, 210]. If the penile ultrasound shows an intact penile vascular bed with good response to pharmacostimulation with vasoactive agents such as prostaglandin E1, phentolamine, and papaverine, then most SSc men will continue with local intracavernous injection therapy. However, if there is a poor response to pharmacostimulation, then most men will proceed to placement with a penile prosthesis. During the time of prosthesis placement, Nehra and colleagues have shown that excision of severely fibrotic corporal tissue is necessary to place an inflatable penile prosthesis [203]. The published data suggest that experts can place inflatable penile prostheses in SSc patients without undue complication such as infection or penile erosion [209, 210]. However, there is limited experience with the use of penile prosthesis in SSc and the duration of benefit and long-term safety is not well defined.

Summary

Systemic sclerosis is a complex human disease resulting in tissue fibrosis likely triggered by an inflammatory autoimmune process. Although Raynaud's phenomenon, skin sclerosis, and dysfunction of gastrointestinal, cardiopulmonary, and musculoskeletal systems are widely recognized clinical manifestations, several important clinical problems of this multisystem disease are often overlooked and result in significant morbidity (see Table 38.1 for listing of these and other uncommon clinical manifestations that are discussed throughout this text). Awareness of these neglected manifestations, including neurologic audiovestibular, oral, thyroid, liver, lower urinary tract disease, avascular necrosis of bone, and erectile dysfunction, will help in the design of appropriate management strategies and hopefully improve clinical outcomes.

References

1. Steven JL. Case of scleroderma with pronounced hemi-atrophy of the face, body and extremities- death from ovarian tumor-account of the post-mortem examination: a sequel. Glasgow Med J. 1898;50:401.
2. Leinwand I, Duryee W, Richter MN. Scleroderma based on a study of over 150 cases. Ann Intern Med. 1954;41:1003–41.
3. Piper WN, Helwig EB. Progressive systemic sclerosis; visceral manifestations in generalized scleroderma. AMA Arch Dermatol. 1955;72:535–46.
4. Tuffanelli DL, Winklemann RK. Systemic scleroderma, a clinical study of 727 cases. AMA Arch Dermatol. 1961;84:357–71.
5. Gordon RM, Silverstein A. Neurologic manifestations in progressive systemic sclerosis. Arch Neurol. 1970;20:126–34.
6. D'Angelo WA, Fries J, Masi AT, et al. Pathologic observations in systemic sclerosis, scleroderma. A study of fifty-eight autopsy cases and fifty-eight matched controls. Am J Med. 1969;46:428–40.
7. Lee P, Bruni J, Sukenik S. Neurologic manifestations in systemic sclerosis. J Rheumatol. 1984;1:480–3.
8. Amaral TN, Peres FA, Lapa AT, et al. Neurologic involvement in scleroderma: a systematic review. Semin Arthritis Rheum. 2013;43:335–47.
9. Lee JE, Haynes JM. Carotid arteritis and cerebral infarction due to scleroderma. Neurology. 1967;17:18–22.
10. Estey E, Lieberman A, Pinto R, et al. Cerebral arteritis in scleroderma. Stroke. 1979;10:595–7.
11. Abers MS, Iluonakhamhe EK, Goldsmith G, et al. Central nervous system vasculitis secondary to systemic sclerosis. J Clin Neurosci. 2013;20:1168–70.
12. Wise TN, Ginzler EM. Scleroderma Cerebritis, an unusual manifestation of progressive systemic sclerosis. Dis Nerv Syst. 1975; 36:30–62.
13. Heron E, Fornes P, Rance A, et al. Brain involvement in scleroderma: two autopsy cases. Stroke J Am Heart Assoc. 1998;29: 719–21.
14. Heron E, Hernigou A, Chatellier G, et al. Intracerebral calcification in systemic sclerosis. Stroke J Am Heart Assoc. 1999;30: 2183–5.
15. Sardanelli F, Cotticelli B, Losacco C, et al. White matter hyperintensities on brain magnetic resonance in systemic sclerosis. Ann Rheum Dis. 2006;64:777–9.
16. Terrier B, Charbonneau F, Touze E, et al. Cerebral vasculopathy is associated with severe vascular manifestations in systemic sclerosis. J Rheumatol. 2009;36:1486–94.
17. Hamdy R, Mohammed A, Sabry Y, Nasef. Brain mri screening showing evidences of early central nervous system involvement in patients with systemic sclerosis. Rheumatol Int. 2011;31:667–71.
18. Maclean H, Guthrie W. Retinopathy in scleroderma. Trans Opthamol Soc UK. 1969;89:209–20.
19. Farkas TG, Sylvester V, Archer D. The choroidopathy of progressive systemic sclerosis (scleroderma). Am J Ophthalmol. 1972; 74:875–86.
20. Grennan D, Forrester J. Involvement of the eye in sle and scleroderma. Ann Rheum Dis. 1977;36:152–6.
21. Alarcon-Segovia D, Ibaniez G, Hernandez-Ortiz J, et al. Sjögren's syndrome in progressive systemic sclerosis (Scleroderma). Am J Med. 1974;57:78–85.
22. Ashton N, Comes N, Garner A, et al. Retinopathy due to progressive systemic sclerosis. J Pathol Bacteriol. 1968;96:259–68.
23. Kraus A, Guerra-Bautista G, Espinoza G, et al. Defects of the retinal pigment epithelium in scleroderma. Br J Rheumatol. 1991;30:112–4.
24. Littlejohn G, Urowitz MB, Palvin CJ. Case report: central retinal vein occlusion and scleroderma: implications for sclerodermatous vascular disease. Ann Rheum Dis. 1981;40:96–9.

25. Christianson HB, Dorsey CS, O'Leary PA, et al. Localized scleroderma. A clinical study of 235 cases. Arch Dermatol. 1956;74:629–39.
26. Goldberg NC, Duncan SC, Winkelmann RK. Migraine and systemic scleroderma. Arch Dermatol. 1978;114:550–1.
27. Pal B, Gibson C, Passmore J, et al. A study of headaches and migraine in Sjögren's syndrome and other rheumatic disorders. Ann Rheum Dis. 1989;48:312–6.
28. Beighton P, Gumpel JM, Cornes NG. Prodromal trigeminal sensory neuropathy in progressive systemic sclerosis. Ann Rheum Dis. 1968;27:367–9.
29. Ashworth B, Tait GB. Trigeminal neuropathy in connective tissue disease. Neurology. 1971;21:609–14.
30. Teasdall RD, Frayha RA, Shulman LE. Cranial nerve involvement in systemic sclerosis (scleroderma): a report of 10 cases. Medicine. 1980;59:149–59.
31. Farrell DA, Medsger TA. Trigeminal neuropathy in progressive systemic sclerosis. Am J Med. 1982;73:57–61.
32. Richter R. Peripheral neuropathy and connective tissue disease. J Neurol Pathol Exp Neurol. 1954;13:168–80.
33. Pawlowski A, Warsaw P. The nerve network of the skin in diffuse scleroderma and clinically similar conditions. Arch Dermatol. 1963;88:868–73.
34. Fleischmajer R, Perlish JS, Reeves JR. Cellular infiltrates in scleroderma skin. Arthritis Rheum. 1977;20:975–84.
35. Christopher RP, Robinson H. Studies of nerve conduction in patients with scleroderma. South Med J. 1972;65:668–72.
36. Poncelet AN, Connolly K. Peripheral neuropathy in scleroderma. Muscle Nerve. 2003;28:330–5.
37. Alonso-Ruiz A, Leiva-Santana C. Carpal tunnel syndrome in scleroderma-like syndromes. J Rheumatol. 1985;12:1030.
38. Machel L, Machet MC, Khallouf R, et al. Carpal tunnel syndrome and systemic sclerosis. Dermatology. 1992;185:101–3.
39. Bandinelli F, Kaloudi O, Candelieri A, et al. Early detection of median nerve syndrome at the carpal tunnel with high-resolution 18 MHz ultrasonography in systemic sclerosis patients. Clin Exp Rheumatol. 2010;28:S15–8.
40. Mondelli M, Romano C, Della-Porta P, et al. Electrophysiological evidence of "nerve entrapment syndromes and subclinical peripheral neuropathy in progressive systemic sclerosis (scleroderma). J Neurol. 1995;242:185–94.
41. Dahlgaard T, Kamp-Nielsen V, Kjeldstrup-Kristensen J. Vibratory perception in patients with generalized scleroderma. Acta Dermatovenerol (Stockholm). 1980;60:119–22.
42. Campbell PM, LeRoy EC. Pathogenesis of systemic sclerosis: a vascular hypothesis. Semin Arthritis Rheum. 1975;4:351–68.
43. Kahaleh MB, Sherer GK, LeRoy EC. Endothelial injury in scleroderma. J Exp Med. 1979;149:1326–35.
44. Gabrielli A, Avvedimento EV, Krieg T. Mechanisms of disease scleroderma. N Engl J Med. 2009;360:1989–2003.
45. Matucci-Cerinic M, Kahaleh B, Wigley F. Evidence that systemic sclerosis is a vascular disease. Arthritis Rheum. 2013;65:1953–62.
46. Sjögren R. Gastrointestinal motility disorders in scleroderma. Arthritis Rheum. 1994;9:1265–82.
47. Abu-Shakara M, Guillemin F, Lee P. Gastro manifestations of systemic sclerosis. Semin Arthritis Rheum. 1994;24:29–39.
48. Lally EV, Jimenez S. Impotence in progressive systemic sclerosis. Ann Intern Med. 1981;95:150–3.
49. Stover SL, Gay RE, Koopman W, et al. Dermal fibrosis in spinal cord injury patients. Arthritis Rheum. 1980;23:1312–7.
50. Peacock JH. Peripheral venous blood concentrations of epinephrine and norepinephrine in primary raynaud's disease. Circ Res. 1959;7:821–7.
51. Kontos HA, Wasserman AJ. Effect of reserpine in raynaud's phenomenon. Circulation. 1961;39:259–64.
52. Sapira JD, Rodnan GP, Scheib ET, et al. Studies of endogenous catecholamines in patients with raynaud's phenomenon secondary to progressive systemic sclerosis (scleroderma). Am J Med. 1972;52:330–6.
53. Fries JF. Physiologic studies in systemic sclerosis (scleroderma). Arch Intern Med. 1969;123:22–5.
54. Drake DB, Kesler RW, Morgan RF. Digital sympathectomy for refractory Raynaud's phenomenon in adolescent. J Rheumatol. 1992;19:1286–8.
55. Wasserman A, Brahn E. Systemic sclerosis: bilateral improvement of Raynaud's phenomenon with unilateral digital sympathectomy. J Semin Arthritis. 2009;40:137–46.
56. Tamaiho MM, Goitz RJ, Medsger TA. Surgery for ischemic pain and Raynaud's phenomenon in scleroderma: a description of treatment protocol and evaluation of results. Microsurgery. 2001;21:75–9.
57. Matsumoto Y, Ueyama T, Endo M, et al. Endoscopic thoracic sympathectomy for Raynaud's phenomenon. J Vasc Surg. 2002;36:57–61.
58. Kotsis SV, Chung KC. A systematic review of the outcomes of digital sympathectomy for treatment of chronic distal ischemia. J Rheumatol. 2003;30:1788–92.
59. Feldman M, Schiller LR. Disorders of gastrointestinal motility associated with diabetes mellitus. Ann Intern Med. 1983;98:378–84.
60. Yang R, Arem R, Chan L. Gastrointestinal tract complication of diabetes mellitus. Arch Intern Med. 1984;144:1251–6.
61. Schiller LR, Santa Ana CA, Schmulen C, et al. Pathogenesis of fecal incontinence in diabetes mellitus: evidence for internal-anal-sphincter dysfunction. N Engl J Med. 1982;307:1666–71.
62. Camilleri M. Diabetic gastroparesis. N Engl J Med. 2007;356:820–30.
63. Nathan DM. Long-term complications of diabetes mellitus. N Engl J Med. 1993;328:1676–86.
64. Rosenbloom AL, Silverstein JH, Lezotte DC, et al. Limited joint mobility in childhood diabetes mellitus indicates increased risk for microvascular disease. N Engl J Med. 1981;305:191–4.
65. Elizondo-Garza MA, Diaz-Jouanen E, Franco-Casique J, et al. Joint contractures and scleroderma-like skin changes in the hands of insulin-dependent juvenile diabetics. J Rheumatol. 1983;10:797–800.
66. Fitzcharles MA, Duby S, Waddell WR, Banks E. Limitation of joint mobility (cheiroarthropathy) in adult noninsulin-dependent diabetic patients. Ann Rheum Dis. 1984;43:251–7.
67. Starkman HS, Gleason RE, Rand LI, et al. Limited joint mobility (LJM) of the hand in patients with diabetes mellitus: relation to chronic complications. Ann Rheum Dis. 1986;45:130–5.
68. Schulte L, Roberts MS, Zimmerman C, et al. A quantitative assessment of limited joint mobility in patients with diabetes. Arthritis Rheum. 1993;36:1429–43.
69. Seibolds JR, Uitto J, Dorwart BB, Prockop DJ. Collagen synthesis and collagenase activity in dermal fibroblasts from patients with diabetes and digital sclerosis. J Lab Clin Med. 1985;105:664–7.
70. Burner TW, Rosenthal AK. Diabetes and rheumatic diseases. Curr Opin Rheumatol. 2009;20:50–4.
71. O'Brien IAD, O'Hare JP, Lewin IG, et al. The prevalence of autonomic neuropathy in insulin- dependent diabetes & mellitus: a controlled study based on heart rate variability. Q J Med. 1986;61:957–67.
72. Watkins PJ. Diabetic autonomic neuropathy. N Engl J Med. 1990;322:1078–9.
73. Sonnex C, Paice E, White AG. Autonomic neuropathy in systemic sclerosis: a case report and evaluation of six patients. Ann Rheum Dis. 1986;45:957–60.
74. Suarez-Almazor ME, Bruera E, Russel AS. Normal cardiovascular autonomic function in patients with systemic sclerosis (CREST variant). Ann Rheum Dis. 1988;47:672–4.

75. Dessein PH, Gledhill RF. More on autonomic neuropathy in systemic sclerosis. Ann Rheum Dis. 1988;47:261–3.
76. Klimiuk PS, Taylor L, Baker RD, Jayson MI. Autonomic neuropathy in systemic sclerosis. Ann Rheum Dis. 1988;47:542–5.
77. Dessein PH, Joffe BI, Metz R, et al. Autonomic dysfunction in systemic sclerosis: sympathetic overactivity and instability. Am J Med. 1992;93:143–50.
78. Hermosillo AG, Ortiz R, DaBague J, Casanova JM, Martinez-Lavin M. Autonomic dysfunction in diffuse scleroderma vs crest: an assessment by computerized heart rate variability. J Rheumatol. 1994;21:1849–54.
79. Stacher G, Merio R, Budka C, et al. Cardiovascular autonomic function, autoantibodies, and esophageal motor activity in patients with systemic sclerosis and mixed connective tissue disease. J Rheumatol. 2000;27:692–7.
80. Lock G, Straub RH, Zeuner M, et al. Association of autonomic nervous dysfunction and esophageal dysmotility in systemic sclerosis. J Rheumatol. 1998;25:1330–5.
81. Morelli S, Piccirillo G, Fimongnari F, Screccia A, et al. Twenty-four hour heart period variability in systemic sclerosis. J Rheumatol. 1996;23:643–5.
82. Gigante A, Rosato E, Liberatori M, et al. Autonomic dysfunction in patients with systemic sclerosis: correlation with intrarenal arterial stiffness. Int J Cardiol. 2014;177:578–80.
83. Othman KM, Assaf NY, Farouk HM, Hassan Aly IM. Autonomic dysfunction predicts early cardiac affection in patients with systemic sclerosis. Clin Med Insights Arthritis Musculoskelet Disord. 2010;3:45–54.
84. Malandrini A, Selvi F, Villanove M, Berti G, et al. Autonomic nervous system and smooth muscle cell involvement in systemic sclerosis: ultrastructural study of 3 cases. J Rheumatol. 2000;27:1203–6.
85. Amor-Dorado JC, Arias-Nunez MC, Miranda-Filloy JA, et al. Audiovestibular manifestations in patients with limited systemic sclerosis and centromere protein-B (CENP-B) antibodies. Medicine (Baltimore). 2008;87:131–41.
86. Berrettini S, Ferri C, Pitaro N, et al. Audiovestibular involvement in systemic sclerosis. ORLO J Otorhinolaryngol Relat Spec. 1994;56:195–8.
87. Kastanioudakis I, Ziavra N, Politi EN, et al. Hearing loss in progressive systemic sclerosis patients: a comparative study. Otolaryngol Head Neck Surg. 2001;124:522–5.
88. Tosti A, Patrizi A, Veronesi S. Audiologic involvement in systemic sclerosis. Dermatologica. 1984;168:206.
89. Teasdall RD, Frayha RA, Shulman LE. Cranial nerve involvement in systemic sclerosis (scleroderma): a report of 10 cases. Medicine (Baltimore). 1980;59:149–59.
90. Abou-Taleb A, Linthicum Jr FH. Scleroderma and hearing loss: (histopathology of a case). J Laryngol Otol. 1987;101:656–62.
91. Bassyouni IH, Emad Y, Rafaat HA, et al. Relationship between nailfold capillary abnormalities and vestibular dysfunction in systemic sclerosis. Joint Bone Spine. 2011;78:266–9.
92. Amor-Dorado JC, Barreira-Fernandez MP, Arias-Nunez MC, et al. Benign paroxysmal positional vertigo and clinical test of sensory interaction and balance in systemic sclerosis. Otol Neurotol. 2008;29:1155–61.
93. Rauch SD. Clinical practice. Idiopathic sudden sensorineural hearing loss. N Engl J Med. 2008;359:833–40.
94. Deroee AF, Huang TC, Morita N, et al. Sudden hearing loss as the presenting symptom of systemic sclerosis. Otol Neurotol. 2009; 30:277–9.
95. Santarelli R, Scimemi P, Dal Monte E, et al. Auditory neuropathy in systemic sclerosis: a speech perception and evoked potential study before and after cochlear implantation. Eur Arch Otorhinolaryngol. 2006;263:809–15.
96. Van Lankveld WG, Vonk MC, Teunissen H, et al. Appearance self-esteem in systemic sclerosis-subjective experience of skin deformity and its relationship with physician-assessed skin involvement, disease status and psychological variables. Rheumatology (Oxford). 2007;46:872–6.
97. Mouthon I, Rannou F, Bérezné A, et al. Development and validation of a scale for mouth handicap in systemic sclerosis: the Mouth Handicap in Systemic Sclerosis Scale. Ann Rheum Dis. 2007; 66:1651–5.
98. Marmary Y, Glaiss R, Pisanty S. Scleroderma: oral manifestations. Oral Surg Oral Med Oral Pathol. 1981;52:32–7.
99. Vitali C, Borghi E, napoletano A, et al. Oropharyngolaryngeal disorders in scleroderma: development and validation of the SLS scale. Dysphagia. 2010;25:127–38.
100. Eversole LR, Jacobsen PL, Stone CE. Oral and gingival changes in systemic sclerosis (scleroderma). J Periodontol. 1984;55: 175–8.
101. Poole JL, Brewer C, Rossie K, et al. Factors related to oral hygiene in persons with scleroderma. Int J Dent Hyg. 2005;3:13–7.
102. Naylor WP, Douglass CW, Mix E. The nonsurgical treatment of microstomia in scleroderma: a pilot study. Oral Surg Oral Med Oral Pathol. 1984;57:508–11.
103. Pizzo G, Scardina GA, Messina P. Effects of a nonsurgical exercise program on the decreased mouth opening in patients with systemic scleroderma. Clin Oral Investig. 2003;7:175–8.
104. Yuen HK, Marlow NM, Reed SG, et al. Effect of orofacial exercises on oral aperture in adults with systemic sclerosis. Disabil Rehabil. 2012;34:84–9.
105. Yuen HK, Weng Y, Bandyopadhyay D, et al. Effect of a multi-faceted intervention on gingival health among adults with systemic sclerosis. Clin Exp Rheumatol. 2011;29 Suppl 65:526–32.
106. Wood RE, Lee P. Analysis of the oral manifestations of systemic sclerosis (scleroderma). Oral Surg Oral Med Oral Pathol. 1988;65: 172–8.
107. Rout PG, Hamburger J, Potts AJ. Orofacial radiological manifestations of systemic sclerosis. Dentomaxillofac Radiol. 1996;25: 193–6.
108. Avouac J, Sordet C, Depinay C, et al. Systemic sclerosis-associated Sjögren's syndrome and relationship to the limited cutaneous subtype: results of a prospective study of sicca syndrome in 133 consecutive patients. Arthritis Rheum. 2006;54: 2243–9.
109. Drosos AA, Andonopoulos AP, Costopoulos JS, et al. Sjögren's syndrome in progressive systemic sclerosis. J Rheumatol. 1988; 15:965–8.
110. Avouac J, Airo P, Dieude P, et al. Associated autoimmune diseases in systemic sclerosis define a subset of patients with milder disease: results from 2 large cohorts of European Caucasian patients. J Rheumatol. 2010;37:608–14.
111. Kobak S, Oksel F, Aksu K, et al. The frequency of sicca symptoms and Sjögren's syndrome in patients with systemic sclerosis. Int J Rheum Dis. 2013;16:88–92.
112. Hebbar M, Janin A, Huglo D, et al. Xerostomia in systemic sclerosis: systematic evaluation by salivary scintigraphy and lip biopsy in thirty-four patients. Arthritis Rheum. 1994;37:439–41.
113. Janin A, Gosselin B, Gosset D, et al. Histological criteria of Sjögren's syndrome in scleroderma. Clin Exp Rheumatol. 1989; 7:167–9.
114. Baron M, Hudson M, Tatibouet S, et al. The Canadian systemic sclerosis oral health study III: relationship between disease characteristics and oro-facial manifestations in systemic sclerosis. Arthritis Care Res (Hoboken). 2015;67(5):681–90. [Epub ahead of print].
115. Fischer DJ, Patton LL. Scleroderma-oral manifestations and treatment challenges. Spec Care Dentist. 2000;20:240–4.
116. Baron M, Hudson M, Tatibouet S, et al. The Canadian systemic sclerosis oral health study: orofacial manifestations and oral health-related quality of life in systemic sclerosis compared with the general population. Rheumatology. 2014;53:1386–94.

117. Baron M, Hudson M, Tatibouet S, et al. The Canadian systemic sclerosis oral health study II: the relationship between oral and global health-related quality of life in systemic sclerosis. Rheumatology. 2015;54(4):692–6. [Epub ahead of print].
118. Rowell NR, Hopper FE. The periodontal membrane in systemic sclerosis. Br J Dermatol. 1977;96:15–20.
119. Alexandridis C, White SC. Periodontal ligament changes in patients with progressive systemic sclerosis. Oral Surg Oral Med Oral Pathol. 1984;58:113–8.
120. Gores RJ. Dental characteristics associated with acrosclerosis and diffuse scleroderma. J Am Dent Assoc. 1957;54:755–9.
121. Yuen HK, Weng Y, Reed SG, et al. Factors associated with gingival inflammation among adults with systemic sclerosis. Int J Dent Hygiene. 2014;12:55–61.
122. Nauet PL. Scleroderma and dental health. Scleroderma Found. 1999;2:14–5.
123. Yuen HK, Hant FN, Hatfield C, et al. Factors associated with oral hygiene practices among adults with systemic sclerosis. Int J Dent Hygiene. 2014;12:180–6.
124. Tűrk AG, Ulusoy M. A collapsible partial denture for a patient with limited mouth opening induced by scleroderma: a clinical report. J Prosthodont. 2015;24(4):334–8. [Epub ahead of print].
125. Nicholson D, White S, Lipson A, et al. Progressive systemic sclerosis and graves' disease report of three cases. Arch Intern Med. 1986;146:2350–2.
126. Nakamura T, Higashi S, Tomoda K, et al. Primary biliary cirrhosis (PBC)-CREST overlap syndrome with coexistence of Sjögren's syndrome and thyroid dysfunction. Clin Rheumatol. 2007;26: 596–600.
127. Horita M, Takahashi N, Seike M, et al. A case of primary biliary cirrhosis associated with hashimoto's thyroiditis, scleroderma and Sjögren's syndrome. Intern Med. 1992;31:418–21.
128. D'Angelo WA, Fries JF, Masi AT, et al. Pathologic observations in systemic sclerosis (scleroderma). A study of fifty-eight autopsy cases and fifty-eight matched controls. Am J Med. 1969;46:428–40.
129. Gordon MB, Klein I, Dekker A, et al. Thyroid disease in progressive systemic sclerosis: increased frequency of glandular fibrosis and hypothyroidism. Ann Intern Med. 1981;95:431–5.
130. Hudson M, Rojas-Villarraga A, Coral-Alverado P, et al. Polyautoimmunity and familial autoimmunity in systemic sclerosis. J Autoimmun. 2008;31:156–9.
131. Biro E, Szekanecz Z, Czirjak L, et al. Association of systemic and thyroid autoimmune diseases. Clin Rheumatol. 2006;25:240–5.
132. Marasini B, Ferrari PA, Solaro N, et al. Thyroid dysfunction in women with systemic sclerosis. Ann N Y Acad Sci. 2007;1108: 305–11.
133. Antonelli A, Ferri C, Fallahi P, et al. Clinical and subclinical autoimmune thyroid disorders in systemic sclerosis. Eur J Endocrinol. 2007;156:431–7.
134. Lippi G, Caramaschi P, Montagnana M, et al. Thyroid status in patients with systemic sclerosis. J Clin Rheumatol. 2006;12: 322–4.
135. Innocencio RM, Romaldini JH, Ward LS. Thyroid autoantibodies in autoimmune diseases. Medicina (B Aires). 2004;64:227–30.
136. Kahl LE, Medsger Jr TA, Klein I. Prospective evaluation of thyroid function in patients with systemic sclerosis (scleroderma). J Rheumatol. 1986;13:103–7.
137. De Keyser L, Narhi DC, Furst DE, et al. Thyroid dysfunction in a prospectively followed series of patients with progressive systemic sclerosis. J Endocrinol Invest. 1990;13:161–9.
138. Antonelli A, Fallahi P, Ferrari SM, et al. Incidence of thyroid disorders in systemic sclerosis: results from a longitudinal follow-up. J Clin Endocrinol Metab. 2013;98:E1198–202.
139. Danielides S, Mavragani CP, Katsakoulas I, et al. Increased prevalence of anti-thyroid antibodies in patients with limited scleroderma. Scand J Rheumatol. 2011;40:299–303.
140. Robinson Jr D, Eisenberg D, Nietert PJ, et al. Systemic sclerosis prevalence and comorbidities in the US, 2001–2002. Curr Med Res Opin. 2008;24:1157–66.
141. McMahon RF, Babbs C, Warnes TW. Nodular regenerative hyperplasia of the liver, CREST syndrome and primary biliary cirrhosis: an overlap syndrome? Gut. 1989;30:1430–3.
142. Efe C, Ozasian E, Nasiroglu N, et al. The development of autoimmune hepatitis and primary biliary cirrhosis overlap syndrome during the course of connective tissue diseases: report of three cases and review of the literature. Dig Dis Sci. 2010;55:2417–21.
143. Skare TL, Nisihara RM, Haideer O, et al. Liver autoantibodies in patients with scleroderma. Clin Rheumatol. 2011;30:129–32.
144. Reynolds TB, Denison EK, Frankl HD, et al. Primary biliary cirrhosis with scleroderma, Raynaud's phenomenon and telangiectasia, new syndrome. Am J Med. 1971;50:302–12.
145. Assassi S, Fritzler MJ, Arnett FC, et al. Primary biliary cirrhosis (PBC), PBC autoantibodies, and hepatic parameter abnormalities in a large population of systemic sclerosis patients. J Rheumatol. 2009;36:2250–6.
146. Jacobsen S, Halberg P, Ullman S, et al. Clinical features and serum antinuclear antibodies in 230 Danish patients with systemic sclerosis. Br J Rheumatol. 1998;37:39–45.
147. Rigamonti C, Shand LM, Feudjo M, et al. Clinical features and prognosis of primary biliary cirrhosis associated with systemic sclerosis. Gut. 2006;55:388–94.
148. Powell FC, Schroeter AL, Dickson ER. Primary biliary cirrhosis and the CREST syndrome: a report of 22 cases. Q J Med. 1987;62:75–82.
149. Watt FE, James OF, Jones DE. Patterns of autoimmunity in primary biliary cirrhosis patients and their families: a population-based cohort study. QJM. 2004;97:397–406.
150. Abraham S, Begum S, Isenberg D. Hepatic manifestations of autoimmune rheumatic diseases. Ann Rheum Dis. 2004;63: 123–9.
151. Akimoto S, Ishikawa O, Takagi H, et al. Immunological features of patients with primary biliary cirrhosis (PBC) overlapping systemic sclerosis: a comparison with patients with PBC alone. J Gastroenterol Hepatol. 1998;13:897–901.
152. Akimoto S, Ishikawa O, Muro Y, et al. Clinical and immunological characterization of patients with systemic sclerosis overlapping primary biliary cirrhosis: a comparison with patients with systemic sclerosis alone. J Dermatol. 1999;26:18–22.
153. Agmon-Levin N, Shapira Y, Selmi C, et al. A comprehensive evaluation of serum autoantibodies in primary biliary cirrhosis. J Autoimmun. 2010;34:55–8.
154. Nakamura M, Kondo H, Bori T, et al. Anti-gp210 and anti-centromere antibodies are different risk factors for the progression of primary biliary cirrhosis. Hepatology. 2007;45:118–27.
155. Gao L, Tian X, Liu B, et al. The value of antinuclear antibodies in primary biliary cirrhosis. Clin Exp Med. 2008;8:9–15.
156. Liberal R, Grant CR, Sakkas L, et al. Diagnostic and clinical significance of anti-centromere antibodies in primary biliary cirrhosis. Clin Res Hepatol Gastroenterol. 2013;37:572–85.
157. Gupta RC, Seibold JR, Krishnan MR, et al. Precipitating autoantibodies to mitochondrial proteins in progressive systemic sclerosis. Clin Exp Immunol. 1984;58:68–76.
158. Norman GL, Bialek A, Encabo S, et al. Is prevalence of PBC underestimated in patients with systemic sclerosis? Dig Liver Dis. 2009;41:762–4.
159. Pope JE, Thompson A. Antimitochondrial antibodies and their significance in diffuse and limited scleroderma. J Clin Rheumatol. 1999;5:206–9.
160. Sakauchi F, Mori M, Zeniya M, et al. Antimitochondrial antibody negative primary biliary cirrhosis in Japan: utilization of clinical data when patients applied to receive public financial aid. J Epidemiol. 2006;16:30–4.

161. Zuchner D, Sternsdorf T, Szostecki C, et al. Prevalence, kinetics, and therapeutic modulation of autoantibodies against Sp100 and promyelocytic leukemia protein in a large cohort of patients with primary biliary cirrhosis. Hepatology. 1997;26:1123–30.
162. Goulis J, Leandro G, Burroughs AK. Randomised controlled trials of ursodeoxycholic-acid therapy for primary biliary cirrhosis: a meta-analysis. Lancet. 1999;354:1053–60.
163. Floreani A, Caroli D, Variola A, et al. A 35-year follow-up of a large cohort of patients with primary biliary cirrhosis seen at a single centre. Liver Int. 2011;31:361–8.
164. Jones DE, Al-Rifai A, Frith J, et al. The independent effects of fatigue and UDCA therapy on mortality in primary biliary cirrhosis: results of a 9 year follow-up. J Hepatol. 2010;53:911–7.
165. Nishio A, Neuberger J, Gershwin ME. Management of patients with primary biliary cirrhosis: a practical guide. BioDrugs. 1999;12:159–73.
166. Kojima H, Uemura M, Sakurai S, et al. Clinical features of liver disturbance in rheumatoid diseases: clinicopathological study with special reference to the cause of liver disturbance. J Gastroenterol. 2002;37:617–25.
167. Shah AA, Wigley FM. Often forgotten manifestations of systemic sclerosis. Rheum Dis Clin North Am. 2008;34:221–38.
168. Ishikawa M, Okada J, Shibuya A, et al. CREST syndrome (calcinosis cutis, raynaud's phenomenon, sclerodactyly, and telangiectasia) associated with autoimmune hepatitis. Intern Med. 1995;34:6–9.
169. Marie I, Levesque H, Tranvouez JL, et al. Autoimmune hepatitis and systemic sclerosis: a new overlap syndrome? Rheumatology (Oxford). 2001;40:102–6.
170. Yabe H, Noma K, Tada N, et al. A case of CREST syndrome with rapidly progressive liver damage. Intern Med. 1992;31:69–73.
171. West M, Jasin HE, Medhekar S. The development of connective tissue diseases in patients with autoimmune hepatitis: a case series. Semin Arthritis Rheum. 2006;35:344–8.
172. Friedman LS, Gee MS, Misdraji J. Case records of the Massachusetts General Hospital, case 39-2010. A 19-year-old woman with nausea, jaundice, and pruritus. N Engl J Med. 2010; 23:2548–57.
173. Perez Ruiz F, Orte Martinez FJ, Zea Mendoza AC, et al. A nodular regenerative hyperplasia of the liver in rheumatic diseases: report of seven cases and review of the literature. Semin Arthritis Rheum. 1991;21:47–54.
174. Kaburaki J, Kuramochi S, Fujii T, et al. Nodular regenerative hyperplasia of the liver in a patient with systemic sclerosis. Clin Rheumatol. 1996;15:613–6.
175. Fraile G, Rodriguez-Garcia JL, Moreno A. Primary sclerosing cholangitis associated with systemic sclerosis. Postgrand Med J. 1991;67:189–92.
176. Moschos J, Leontiadis GI, Kelly C, et al. Idiopathic portal hypertension complicating systemic sclerosis: a case report. BMC Gastroenterol. 2005;26:5–16.
177. Kogawa H, Migita K, Ito M, et al. Idiopathic portal hypertension associated with systemic sclerosis and Sjögren's syndrome. Clin Rheumatol. 2005;24:544–7.
178. Kucharz EJ, Jonderko G, Rubisz-Brzezinska J, et al. Premictional volume and contractility of the urinary bladder in patients with systemic sclerosis. Clin Rheumatol. 1996;15:118–20.
179. Minervini R, Morelli G, Minervini A, et al. Bladder involvement in systemic sclerosis: urodynamic and histological evaluation in 23 patients. Eur Urol. 1998;34:47–52.
180. Lazzeri M, Beneforti P, Benaim G, et al. Vesical dysfunction in systemic sclerosis (scleroderma). J Urol. 1995;153:1184–7.
181. Raz S, Boxer R, Waisman J, et al. Scleroderma of lower urinary tract. Urology. 1977;9:682–3.
182. Lally EV, Kaplan SR, Susset JG, et al. Pathologic involvement of the urinary bladder in progressive systemic sclerosis. J Rheumatol. 1985;12:778–81.
183. La Civita L, Fiorentini L, Tognetti A, et al. Severe urinary bladder involvement in systemic sclerosis: case report and review of the literature. Clin Exp Rheumatol. 1998;16:591–3.
184. De Luca A, Terrone C, Tirri E, et al. Vesical telangiectasias as a cause of macroscopic hematuria in systemic sclerosis. Clin Exp Rheumatol. 2001;19:93–4.
185. Rennie C, Britton J, Rouse P. Bilateral avascular necrosis of the lunate in a patient with server Raynaud's phenomenon and scleroderma. J Clin Rheumatol. 1999;5:165–8.
186. Matsumoto AK, Moore R, Alli P, et al. Three cases of osteonecrosis of the lunate bone of the wrist in scleroderma. Clin Exp Rheumatol. 1999;17:730–2.
187. Agus B. Bilateral aseptic necrosis of the lunate in systemic sclerosis. Clin Exp Rheumatol. 1987;5:155–7.
188. Kawai H, Tsuyuguchi Y, Yonenobu K, et al. Avascular necrosis of the carpal scaphoid associated with progressive systemic sclerosis. Hand. 1983;15:270–3.
189. Nowlin NS, Brick JE, Weaver DJ, et al. Impotence in scleroderma. Ann Intern Med. 1986;104:794–8.
190. Klein LE, Posner MS. Progressive systemic sclerosis and impotence. Letter to the Editor. Ann Intern Med. 1981;95:658.
191. Lally EV, Jimenez SA. Impotence in progressive systemic sclerosis. Letter to the Editor. Ann Intern Med. 1982;96:125.
192. Nowlin NS, Brick JE, Weaver DJ, et al. Impotence in scleroderma. Letter to the Editor. Ann Intern Med. 1987;106:910.
193. Nowlin NS, Brick JE, Weaver DJ, et al. Impotence in scleroderma. Letter to the Editor. Ann Intern Med. 1988;109:148.
194. Sukenik S, Abarbanel JM, Buskila D, et al. Impotence, carpal tunnel syndrome and peripheral neuropathy as presenting symptoms in progressive systemic sclerosis. Letter to the Editor. J Rheumatol. 1987;14(3):641–3.
195. Rossman B, Zorgniotti AW. Progressive systemic sclerosis (scleroderma) and impotence. Urology. 1989;33:189–92.
196. Hong P, Pope JE, Ouimet JM, et al. Erectile dysfunction associated with scleroderma: a case-control study of men with scleroderma and rheumatoid arthritis. J Rheumatol. 2004;31: 508–13.
197. Foocharoen C, Tyndall A, Hachulla E, et al. Erectile dysfunction is frequent in systemic sclerosis and associated with severe disease: a study of EULAR Scleroderma Trial and Research group. Arthritis Res Therapy. 2012;14:R37.
198. Rosato E, Aversa A, Molinaro I, et al. Erectile dysfunction of sclerodermic patients correlates with digital vascular damage. Eur J Intern Med. 2011;22:318–21.
199. Rosato E, Barbano B, Gigante A, et al. Erectile dysfunction, endothelium dysfunction and microvascular damage in patients with systemic sclerosis. J Sex Med. 2013;10:1380–8.
200. Keck A, Foocharoen C, Rosato E, et al. Nailfold capillary abnormalities in erectile dysfunction of systemic sclerosis. A EUSTAR group analysis. Rheumatology. 2014;53:639–43.
201. Bivalacqua TJ, Usta MF, Champion HC, et al. Endothelial dysfunction in erectile dysfunction: role of the endothelium in erectile physiology and disease. J Androl. 2003;24: S17–37.
202. Burnett AL. Metabolic syndrome, endothelial dysfunction, and erectile dysfunction: association and management. Curr Urol Rep. 2005;6:470–5.
203. Nehra A, Hall SJ, Basile G, et al. Systemic sclerosis and impotence: a clinicopathological correlation. J Urol. 1995;53: 1140–6.
204. Aversa A, Proietti M, Bruzziches R, et al. The penile vasculature in systemic sclerosis: a duplex ultrasound study. J Sex Med. 2006;3:554–8.
205. Granchi S, Vannelli GB, Vignozzi L, et al. Expression and regulation of endothelin-1 and its receptors in human penile smooth muscle cells. Mol Hum Reprod. 2002;8:1053–64.

206. Varga J, Lally E, Jimenez S. Endocrinopathy and other visceral organ involvement in progressive systemic sclerosis. Systemic sclerosis: scleroderma, New York; Wiley. 1988. p. 267–78.
207. Aversa A, Basciani S, Visca P, et al. Platelet-derived growth factor (PDGF) and PDGF receptors in rat corpus cavernosum: changes in expression after transient in vivo hypoxia. J Endocrinol. 2001;170:395–402.
208. Faller DV. Endothelial cell responses to hypoxic stress. Clin Exp Pharmacol Physiol. 1999;26:74–84.
209. Walker UA, Tyndall A, Ruszat R. Erectile dysfunction in systemic sclerosis. Ann Rheum Dis. 2009;68:1083–5.
210. Aversa A, Bruzziches R, Francomano D, et al. Penile involvement in systemic sclerosis: new diagnostic and therapeutic aspects. Int J Rheum. 2010;2010:708067.
211. Proietti M, Aversa A, Letizia C, et al. Erectile dysfunction in systemic sclerosis: effects of long term inhibition of phosphodiesterase type-5 on erectile function and plasma endothelin-1 levels. J Rheumatol. 2007;34:1712–7.
212. Aversa A, Caprio M, Rosano GM, et al. Endothelial effects of drugs designed to treat erectile dysfunction. Curr Pharm Des. 2008;14:3768–78.

Pregnancy

39

Eliza F. Chakravarty and Virginia Steen

Systemic sclerosis (scleroderma, SSc) is a connective tissue disease that occurs in women three to five times more frequently than men. Clinical manifestations include fibrosis of the skin and visceral organs, as well as a noninflammatory, progressive vasculopathy. With the mean age of onset of SSc symptoms in the early 40s, almost half of women with this illness have the potential of becoming pregnant after the onset of their illness. Years ago, most women would have completed their pregnancies prior to this age, but more recently, women are frequently delaying pregnancy. Thus, there is an increased likelihood for a concurrent pregnancy in women who develop SSc early in their adult life. The interrelationships of SSc and pregnancy are important from both the effects of SSc on pregnancy and the effects pregnancy may have on underlying maternal SSc. This chapter reviews the literature relating to fertility, pregnancy, and pregnancy outcomes in women with SSc. The management of these high-risk pregnancies, the effects of pregnancy on SSc problems, and recommendations for managing medications in the pregnant SSc patient will be discussed. The use of this information in planned, well-supervised pregnancies should increase the likelihood of both the success of the pregnancy and the birth of a healthy infant and the stability of the mother.

Sexuality in Women with Systemic Sclerosis

As SSc can have a profound effect on a woman's life, a significant component of pregnancy is whether women feel well enough for sexual activity. The physical limitations of pulmonary, cutaneous, articular, and vascular disease, the changes in appearance, and the emotional effects of the disease all potentially impact sexuality and interpersonal relationships. After controlling for age and marital status, Canadian women ($n=730$) with SSc were significantly less likely to be sexually active (odds ratio (OR) 0.34, 95 % confidence interval (CI) 0.28–0.41) and more likely to report sexual impairment (OR 1.88, 95 % CI 1.42–2.49) than women in the general population [1]. Pain and lubrication were the main components of sexual impairment in this cohort of SSc women. A smaller study of 46 SSc women compared to 46 healthy women from Italy found that women with SSc had lower desire than controls, but other scales of sexual function (arousal, lubrication, orgasm, satisfaction, and pain) were indistinguishable between groups [2]. Vaginal dryness and pain as well as hand function and pain were more common among SSc women than controls. However, in spite of these many physical and psychological difficulties, a study of 101 American SSc patients found the majority (60 %) of women were sexually active. Of women who were not sexually active, only 17 % attributed their sexual inactivity to SSc [3]. Consistent with other studies, the classification of disease, i.e., diffuse or limited SSc, did not appear to have an effect on whether or not a patient was sexually active. Age, personal choice, and lack of partner were the major reasons for sexual inactivity. A few even stated their partner's health prevented sexual activity.

These studies also looked at the patients' responses to a standardized sexual function questionnaire (IPSP) and the medical outcome study questionnaire (SF-36). The results suggested that sexual dysfunction in those patients was not correlated with age, disease duration, or physical problems. It appeared to be primarily correlated with general mental health. In the American study, most patients felt that fatigue (60 %) was the primary symptom that affected their sexual function. Body pain (40 %) and vaginal dryness (42 %) were also common concerns. Others have also reported dyspareunia (37–56 %) in SSc patients [1–4], as well as vaginal discomfort, but it was difficult to separate vaginal dryness (42–71 %) from vaginal tightness. However, 5/60 patients

E.F. Chakravarty, MD, MS (✉)
Department of Arthritis and Clinical Immunology, Oklahoma Medical Research Foundation, Oklahoma City, OK, USA
e-mail: chakravartye@omrf.org; Eliza-Chakravarty@omrf.org

V. Steen, MD
Department of Medicine, Rheumatology, Clinical Immunology, and Allergy, Georgetown University Hospital, Washington, DC, USA

J. Varga et al. (eds.), *Scleroderma*, DOI 10.1007/978-3-319-31407-5_39

reported vaginal tightness or constricted introitus as the cause of dyspareunia. Surprisingly, even Raynaud's phenomenon, hand pain, and digital ulcers affect an SSc patients' ability to participate in and enjoy a sexual relationship. Other symptoms from physical problems, shortness of breath, heartburn, and emotional difficulties from cosmetic appearances and depression also played a significant role in some patients. Comparing the IFSF sexual function index in patients with and without a particular symptom, vaginal dryness (or discomfort), Raynaud's phenomenon, and depression were the features that caused the most problems [5]. Patients can, in many situations, adapt to some of the problems and anticipate difficulties by being more prepared. Attention to symptoms of depression, keeping warm, and using vaginal lubricants may be simple but important interventions.

Fertility

The issue of fertility in women with SSc is difficult to determine because many factors, both physical and psychological, affect the ability and desire to be sexually active and to consider pregnancy. Prior to the 1980s, there were frequent references to the rarity of the concomitant pregnancies in patients with established SSc. The implication was that fertility was decreased in SSc. However, it must be kept in mind that the mean age of onset of SSc is 43 years, and as recent as 20 years ago, most women had completed all their pregnancies before they developed symptoms of SSc. Englert specifically studied the occurrence of pregnancies prior to the onset of SSc [6]. In this series, there was an increased incidence of women who had a delay in conception or who had never conceived compared with population controls, but not compared with women with primary Raynaud's phenomenon who had similar findings. Prior studies did not identify decreased overall fertility, but little attempt was made to relate the timing of pregnancy to the onset of SSc [7, 8].

Steen surveyed 214 SSc patients, 167 rheumatoid arthritis patients, and 105 normal controls with questions about the occurrence of pregnancy and any delays in conception [9]. There was a significantly larger number of women with SSc and rheumatoid arthritis (RA) who had never been pregnant (21 % SSc, 23 % RA, compared to 12 % healthy controls, $p<0.05$). When this was adjusted for factors such as the number of women who had never married, who were sexually inactive, or who had chosen not to have children, there were no differences between the three groups. Only 2–5 % of patients in each group had ever attempted to become pregnant but were unsuccessful. Also, the percentage of women with at least a 1-year delay in conception was not significantly different in the three groups (12–15 %). During infertility evaluations, SSc patients were more likely to be told of possible causes of infertility such as fallopian tube obstruction or endometriosis. However, there were no unique findings causing infertility that could be attributed specifically to SSc. Curiously, the SSc patients' partners were more likely to have fertility problems than the controls' partners. The overall successful pregnancy rate in those patients with a prior period of infertility was similar in all three groups, 37 %, 40 %, and 43 %, respectively.

Pregnancy Outcomes

The reported outcomes of pregnancy in women with SSc are quite variable. Early literature is filled with case reports of concomitant pregnancy and SSc that resulted in negative outcomes to the mother and/or the baby. These have been summarized in recent reviews [10–12].

Miscarriage

Miscarriages were increased in Slate and Graham's series [13]. However, this series primarily included low-income patients at an inner-city hospital, who had other inherent risks for miscarriage. Several other case–control studies identified an increased frequency of miscarriages per pregnancy [8, 14] or in women prior to the onset of SSc [6, 14–16]. Englert and Silman found increased miscarriages before disease onset and hypothesized that these blighted pregnancies could result in transplacental transfer of cells leading to a type of chronic graft-versus-host disease; a biological process which has been discussed as a potential mechanism of disease pathogenesis in SSc [6]. In a retrospective case–control study of women with SSc, the frequency of miscarriage was only 9 % which was not different than the 7.5 % of the pregnancies seen in the healthy controls [9]. SSc patients were more likely to have miscarriages after disease onset than before (15 % vs. 8 %), but there was not a significant risk of miscarriages in SSc patients either before or after the onset of SSc.

There has been only one prospective SSc pregnancy study which included 91 pregnancies in 59 women [17]. The patients were divided into the SSc subsets, i.e., limited and diffuse SSc as well as early and late disease (less than or greater than 4 years of symptoms). Miscarriage occurred with similar frequency to the historical controls except in the group of patients with late diffuse SSc. These patients had a surprisingly high frequency of miscarriages, 42 % of the 15 women with late diffuse disease compared to 13 % in all of the other groups. Renal insufficiency and severe gastrointestinal malabsorption were present in two of the seven women who had miscarriages. Only one woman, with limited SSc, never had a healthy child. She was a habitual aborter, experiencing four miscarriages (two after SSc onset). Thus, although the data are somewhat mixed, it appears that patients with certain subsets of disease (late diffuse) may have higher risks of miscarriage than other subsets. Therefore, pregnancy counseling may be aided by this ability to stratify risk by disease subset.

Premature Delivery

Premature delivery is defined as delivery prior to 37 completed weeks of gestation. Although prematurity was not specifically addressed in many studies, several early series noted more than the expected number of premature infants [10, 12]. Steen's retrospective series identified an increase in the frequency of premature infants in SSc patients and rheumatoid arthritis patients compared to healthy controls [9]. Interestingly, in this series, prematurity was more common in SSc patients before the onset of their illness compared to after the disease. Fortunately, the premature infants in this study did well. They were small and had the usual prematurity complications, but there was only one fetal death related to prematurity. It is likely that having a chronic disease, i.e., SSc or rheumatoid arthritis, is the common denominator for the increased occurrence of prematurity.

In Steen's prospective study, prematurity again was much increased compared with controls, 29 % versus 5 % in historical controls [17]. In 65 % of the pregnancies in women with early diffuse SSc, the pregnancy ended before 38 weeks (the American Obstetrical Associations definition of premature births). In 13 of the 23 preterm births, the babies were born at 36 or 37 weeks and weighed a mean of 5.7 lb. Eight of these 13 pregnancies were artificially induced for nonmedical issues. There was only one neonatal death which was in a 25-week fetus, although several quite small babies required prolonged hospital stays. Thus, although the frequency of premature infants was increased, the overall success rate, i.e., a live birth, was 84 % in limited SSc women and 77 % in diffuse SSc women, compared with 84 % in the historical healthy controls.

Chung and colleagues reported outcomes of 18 pregnancies among women with SSc (ten pregnancies) and mixed connective tissue disease (eight pregnancies) followed at a single institution [18]. Although the sample size was small, premature delivery occurred in 37–40 % of pregnancies.

An analysis of 109 pregnancies in 99 women with SSc from a multicenter group in Italy found an increase in preterm delivery overall (25 % SSc vs. 12 % in the general population) as well as an increase in deliveries <34 weeks of gestation (10 % compared to 5 %) [19]. Multivariable analysis found only the use of corticosteroids was associated with preterm delivery (OR 3.63, 95 % CI 1.12–11.78); interestingly, in this study, the presence of SCL-70 antibodies was associated with a reduced risk of preterm delivery (OR 0.26, 95 % CI 0.08–0.85). While it is easy to speculate that corticosteroid use itself or as a marker of advanced, internal organ disease may increase risks of pregnancy complications, the association between autoantibody status and preterm delivery remains unclear. Of note, this group of investigators is currently conducting a large, multicenter, prospective observational study of pregnancy in SSc (International Multicentric Study on PREgnancy in Systemic Sclerosis, IMPRESS).

Small for Gestational Age Infants

Steen's retrospective case–control study of pregnancies of SSc patients prior to 1987, small (<5.5 lb) full-term infants occurred significantly more frequently in SSc patients than either the RA patients or normal controls (10 % vs. 4 % vs. 2 %, respectively) [9]. In the Italian experience, 6 % of SSc women had small-for-gestational-age infants compared to 1 % in the healthy population [19]. Similar findings were seen in patients with primary Raynaud's phenomenon as well as another case–control study of SSc patients [6, 20]. Much higher rates were reported (50–63 %) in Chung's relatively small study [18].

Data suggest an increase in intrauterine growth restriction even among women who later develop SSc (13.7 % of pregnancies in pre-SSc women compared to 3.9 % of healthy women) [16]; however, it is difficult to ascertain whether pregnancy complications may be very early manifestations of SSc in otherwise asymptomatic women or a risk factor for the future development of SSc [21].

Interestingly, unlike the retrospective study from Steen, none of the full-term babies in her prospective study were small for dates and the mean birth weight was 7.1 lb [22]. However, a recent analysis of hospital discharges of 504 SSc pregnancies found an increased risk of intrauterine growth retardation (OR 3.74, 95 % CI 1.51–9.28) [23].

Neonatal Mortality

Infant deaths were quite common in the individual case reports. In Chung's series, two of ten pregnancies in patients with SSc ended in fetal loss in the third trimester: In both of these cases, women were found to have comorbid coagulopathies [18]. Other cases were associated with the acute exacerbation of SSc complications in the mother. Neonatal deaths occasionally were noted in the series and case–control studies including our own, but no one found a statistically or clinically excessive number compared with controls.

Placental Pathology

Given the widespread vasculopathy present in SSc patients, there are concerns that the same pathophysiologic changes may also occur in the placental vasculature [24]. Most studies of pregnancy outcomes did not examine placental tissue, thus not allowing for direct correlation between placental vascular abnormalities and adverse pregnancy outcomes. Histopathologic examinations of placentas from a limited number of SSc pregnancies are reported; all found normal placenta weight for gestational age [25–27]. One study of three placentas from SSc patients (gestational age at delivery between 34 and 38 weeks) found evidence of decidual vasculopathy with stromal fibrosis and infarcts in chronic villi despite normal, healthy clinical outcomes [25]. In another case, an SSc patient with intrauterine growth restriction was found to have increased resistance in the umbilical artery by Doppler examination at 31 weeks of gestational age. Examination of the placenta after delivery at 37 weeks found numerous placental infarcts, placental mesenchymal dysplasia, decreased vascularity, and stromal fibrosis, all consistent with changes secondary to decidual vasculopathy [26]. In the largest study to date, 13 placentas from SSc patients were examined and correlated with perinatal outcomes [27]. Five of the 13 placentas demonstrated marked decidual vasculopathy, four of which were associated with intrauterine fetal demise between weeks 16 and 30. Chorioamnionitis and accelerated placental maturation complicated the majority of other placentas. These findings are similar to what is seen in pregnancies complicated by pregnancy-induced hypertension. Thus, placental abnormalities may be present in SSc pregnancies, even in the absence of clinical perinatal complications, and these the more severe manifestations of placental vasculature may contribute to intrauterine growth restriction, preterm delivery, and death.

The overall adverse pregnancy outcome rate in SSc is increased in most of the case–control studies. In some of the studies, however, the increase was from miscarriages, and in others, it was from preterm births or small full-term infants. Thus, although women with SSc may have increased risks of miscarriage or premature infants, these risks are not so excessive as to discourage women from becoming pregnant. Recent studies from Spain, India, Italy, and Brazil have confirmed these findings in their SSc patients [4, 19, 28, 29].

Effects of Pregnancy on Systemic Sclerosis

The above studies show that the risks for a successfully completed pregnancy in most women with SSc are quite acceptable. It is equally important to consider the effect that pregnancy may have upon the disease itself (Table 39.1). Once again, the early literature described individual cases of extremely poor maternal outcomes, particularly regarding renal crisis [24, 30]. In both the retrospective and prospective studies by Steen, the effects of pregnancy on the course of SSc and its symptoms were carefully evaluated [9, 17]. It is difficult to determine the definite changes that pregnancy has on SSc because so many pregnancy symptoms are similar to SSc symptoms (e.g., edema, arthralgias, dyspnea, and gastrointestinal reflux). The consensus of reports describing overall effects of pregnancy on SSc is that there are no significant changes in the disease status during pregnancy [10, 12]. There were no reported changes in skin disease during pregnancy in any of the studies. Steen found that the disease was stable in 61 % of pregnancies, 20 % experienced some improvement, and 20 % experienced some worsening. The 10-year cumulative survival for women with SSc with and without a pregnancy was similar [17]. The Italian study described four women who experienced worsening of SSc within the 12 months following delivery: all were SCL-70 positive, and three had early disease (<3 years), a period where SSc is often rapidly progressive even in the absence of pregnancy [19].

Table 39.1 Effects of pregnancy on systemic sclerosis

SSc involvement	Change during pregnancy
Overall	Disease generally stable
Raynaud's phenomenon	Improved during pregnancy, worse after or during complicated deliveries
Skin	Can have onset during pregnancy and some diffuse SSc have progression of skin postpartum
Joints	More arthralgias, similar to nonscleroderma pregnancy
Gastrointestinal	More reflux, similar to nonscleroderma pregnancy
Cardiopulmonary	Shortness of breath from scleroderma problems aggravated as in other diseases and managed as they would be in any pregnancy with compromised cardiopulmonary status
	Women with pregestational pulmonary artery hypertension have a high maternal mortality rate, particularly during delivery, and are strongly advised against pregnancy
Kidney	Renal crisis occurs during early diffuse scleroderma with or without pregnancy. Management must be with ACE inhibitors in spite of risks to baby

Renal Disease

Renal crisis is the most serious complication of SSc and the cause of the most maternal deaths in SSc pregnancies. Pregnancy itself has been hypothesized to be a precipitant of renal crisis. The appearance of hypertension and proteinuria related to preeclampsia of pregnancy can be easily confused with renal crisis. More recent pregnancy series and case–control studies found far fewer episodes of renal crises than were seen in the individual anecdotal case reports.

In Steen's retrospective series, two cases developed classic renal crisis during pregnancy [9]. Both had early diffuse SSc (the highest risk subtype of SSc) and thus were considered at high risk for renal crisis independent of their pregnancy. Comparing these pregnant SSc patients with a subset of women with early diffuse SSc patients without a pregnancy, Steen's study was unable to identify any increased occurrence of renal crisis in the pregnant patients. Prior to ACE inhibitors, one of two patients in the Steen series and her premature infant survived following nephrectomy. The other mother died during the renal crisis, but the premature infant survived. In the 91 prospectively followed SSc pregnancies in Steen's study, there were three early diffuse SSc patients who developed renal crisis during pregnancy. All had early disease (mean 2.2 years). This is similar to the 10–20% of diffuse SSc patients who develop renal crisis independent of pregnancy [31]. One patient required an elective abortion at 20 weeks to control the renal crisis. In the other two cases, renal crisis was treated successfully with ACE inhibitors, although each woman required dialysis for a short time. These two women had premature infants (29 and 34 weeks) who survived, although they had prolonged hospitalizations.

Several recent cases of renal crisis occurring during pregnancy that were successfully treated with ACE inhibitors have been reported [32–35]. Systematic reviews of ACE inhibitor or angiotensin receptor blocker (ARB) exposure during pregnancy confirm a high occurrence of fetal renin–angiotensin system blockade syndrome, manifesting as oligohydramnios, intrauterine death, and renal failure in the newborn [36]. Interestingly, this syndrome was seen more commonly with second and third trimester exposure to ARBs over ACE inhibitors. Captopril exposure was associated with a lower incidence of fetal renal complications. The association of other congenital malformations with first trimester exposure is more controversial. These drugs have dramatically changed the outcome of renal crisis in the nonpregnant patient [37, 38]. As no other therapies currently exist for the treatment of scleroderma renal crisis, ACE inhibitors (particularly captopril) must be considered for treating renal crisis in the pregnant woman despite risks to the fetus.

Musculoskeletal and Gastrointestinal Disease

Other pregnancy symptoms are frequently seen in SSc patients. Musculoskeletal complaints in pregnancy in general are common, including carpal tunnel syndrome [39], muscle leg cramps [40], arthralgias, and back pain [41]. SSc patients are not immune to any of these problems, and it is difficult to determine whether they occur more than expected in this population. Likewise, gastrointestinal symptoms, particularly esophageal reflux and constipation, occur with increased frequency in both SSc and during normal pregnancy [42]; it is not surprising that SSc patients during pregnancy complain of increased pyrosis, early satiety, or constipation. It is also likely that patients may not report mild-to-moderate increases in these symptoms as they may consider them to be changes related to pregnancy rather than the underlying disease. In fact, during any normal pregnancy, the tone of the lower half of the esophagus becomes profoundly depressed during the last two trimesters contributing to increased reflux [43, 44].

Raynaud's Phenomenon and Digital Ulceration

Many SSc patients volunteer that their Raynaud's phenomenon is noticeably improved during pregnancy, only to worsen after pregnancy. This may possibly be attributed to the increased blood volume and decreased systemic vascular resistance that may improve peripheral blood flow [24]. Fortunately, there are only a few cases reported of acute gangrenous changes developing late in pregnancy: These were usually associated with the use of beta-blockers or with other problems including complicated deliveries and sepsis [45, 46]. Only one patient in Chung's series experienced worsening of Raynaud's phenomenon and increased digital ulceration during pregnancy; this coincided with increased systemic hypertension diagnosed in the second trimester of pregnancy [18].

Cardiopulmonary Disease

Women with SSc do not seem to have greater adverse outcomes from cardiopulmonary problems than one would expect from other pregnant patients with similar underlying cardiopulmonary issues [47–50]. All are at high risk. Other than increased shortness of breath (typical in most pregnant women due to increased basal oxygen consumption and alveolar ventilation), there is no evidence that pregnancy increases the severity of SSc pulmonary fibrosis. SSc patients may have undetected myocardial damage, and this could, in theory, cause cardiac dysfunction and compromise during the cardiovascular stress of pregnancy. Although not well documented, these patients may be a particular risk during usual treatment of preterm labor with beta-agonist [51].

Pulmonary Arterial Hypertension

Pulmonary arterial hypertension (PAH) is a serious complication which usually occurs in anti-centromere-positive, limited SSc patients who have long-standing disease and who often have the onset of the SSc in an older age [52]. However, PAH also occurs in younger patients, particularly with anti-U1 RNP or a nucleolar pattern ANA, so there is the potential for concomitant PAH and pregnancy to occur. Any woman with PAH who becomes pregnant is at extremely high risk for severe hemodynamic complications during pregnancy because of the low reserve of the pulmonary arterioles to reduce vascular resistance to accommodate the increased blood volume and cardiac output that occurs during pregnancy. Reports estimate a 36–50 % maternal death rate in women with PAH. Delivery appears to be the most vulnerable period for cardiovascular collapse and maternal death in the pregnant PAH patient because of the acute increase in cardiac output during the second stage of labor with the return of uterine blood back to the maternal systemic vascular beds [24, 53, 54]. A more recent study showed a slightly lower but still unacceptable maternal death rate of 17–33 % [55]. Pregnant women with underlying primary pulmonary hypertension are at extremely high risk for acute hospitalization during pregnancy (OR 4.67, 95 % CI 2.88–7.57), developing hypertensive disorders of pregnancy (OR 5.62, 95 % CI 2.60–12.15), and increased length of hospital stay [23]. Women who carry a diagnosis of PAH should be strongly counseled to avoid pregnancy as it remains a condition associated with high risks for maternal and fetal morbidity and mortality.

New Onset of SSc During Pregnancy

There are reports of the new onset of SSc symptoms during pregnancy [12, 19, 56] or worsening of the disease after pregnancy [19]. In Steen's prospective pregnancy study, five of the 59 women had onset of SSc symptoms during pregnancy, but this was only five of more than 400 nonpregnant women who were seen at the University of Pittsburgh during that time period. Given the small number of pregnancy events in SSc, it is impossible to determine if SSc develops more frequently during pregnancy than expected. A few diffuse SSc patients have had worsening cutaneous disease after a period of stable disease both before and during pregnancy. Whether this was related to the postpartum status or another factor such as the fact that they had discontinued previous therapy prior to the pregnancy cannot be determined. No assurances can be given, but in general, progressive cutaneous disease during or after pregnancy was uncommon.

Pregnancy Management

All pregnancies in women with SSc should be considered to be at high risk for pregnancy morbidity including premature and small full-term infants as well as disease-related complications. In addition to a rheumatologist familiar with SSc, pregnant patients should be followed closely by an obstetrician experienced in high-risk pregnancies. At the onset of pregnancy, an SSc patient should be carefully evaluated to determine the type of disease, duration of symptoms, as well as the extent and severity of visceral involvement. Women with less than 4 years of SSc symptoms, those who have diffuse cutaneous SSc, or those who have anti-topoisomerase or RNA polymerase III antibodies are at greater risk of having more active, aggressive disease than are those who have long-standing disease with anti-centromere antibody [22]. When organs are severely damaged, that is, in cases of severe cardiomyopathy (ejection fraction <30 %), pulmonary hypertension, severe restrictive lung disease (forced vital capacity <50 % of predicted), malabsorption, or renal insufficiency, the decision to terminate the pregnancy may have to be considered depending on the risks to the mother and the infant. This decision should be made based on the specific abnormalities found and independent of the fact that SSc is the cause of the problem. Patient, partner, and all physicians involved in her care will need to make this difficult decision together.

The high risk of preterm labor necessitates special management throughout the pregnancy, as described in Table 39.2. The complete spectrum of pregnancy complications has been reported in SSc, including preeclampsia, abruptio placentae, premature rupture of membranes, placenta previa, and excessive bleeding [12]. However, none of the retrospective or prospective studies found an increased frequency of any pregnancy complications nor any specific SSc-related problems as a clear etiology for prematurity [9, 17]. In most cases, no specific explanation other than premature labor could be identified. Although several studies have not found a significant increase in preeclampsia in SSc patients [12, 17], a recent population-based study of pregnancy outcomes utilizing an administrative hospital discharge database found an increased risk of hypertensive disorders including preeclampsia [23]. It can be very difficult to distinguish between preeclampsia and renal crisis in pregnant SSc patients, and management is extremely difficult (see below).

Management of Renal Crisis During Pregnancy

It is unknown whether SSc patients have a true increase in renal crisis during pregnancy (Table 39.3). However, patients with diffuse SSc in particular should have their blood pressure monitored very closely. The standard of care for the management of SSc renal crisis is the use of angiotensin-converting enzyme (ACE) inhibitors. Prior to the availability of ACE inhibitors, nearly all SSc patients (with or without pregnancy) died within the first year. Thus, its early use can make the difference between life and death for both the mother and the infant.

SSc renal crisis has many similar features of preeclampsia, and it can be a real challenge to distinguish between these two entities. Elevation in uric acid and liver function are more frequent in preeclampsia, and progressive increases in serum creatinine are more common in renal crisis. There are some new biomarkers of preeclampsia, placenta growth factor (PlGF), and soluble fms-like tyrosine kinase-1 (sFlt-1) which may identify preeclampsia very early [57] and are not likely to be seen in renal crisis, so eventually they should be helpful. The treatment of preeclampsia is very different than treatment of renal crisis and does not include ACE inhibitors.

However, there are major difficulties in the decision to use ACE inhibitors during pregnancy, since ACE inhibitors can cause significant fetal abnormalities including anhydramnios, renal atresia, pulmonary hypoplasia, and fetal death, particularly when used in the latter half of pregnancy [58]. However, the frequency of this deadly problem or fetopathy, as it is called, is unknown [59]. In one series, non-SSc pregnant women with refractory hypertension were given low dose (total 25 mg/day) which improved their blood pressure and cardiac function, and there were no fetal or neonatal complications noted in ten patients [60]. Burrows reviewed clinical experience in the literature (85 patients) and 20 prospective patients of their own who were given ACE inhibitors [61]. The frequency of renal complications in the fetuses was very high, but was quite variable. Twenty-one percent of patients in series with less than ten patients had complications, but it was only present in 1.4 % in a series with larger numbers of patients including their own prospective study. No abnormal events occurred with the use of ACE inhibitors early in pregnancy. In contrast to other teratogenic medications, all complications associated with ACE inhibitors were after exposure in the second and third trimesters [61]. Successful use of captopril or other ACE inhibitors during pregnancy has been documented in SSc as well [17, 32–35].

Table 39.2 Management of scleroderma patients during pregnancy, labor, and delivery

Preterm
1. Early evaluation of extent of scleroderma organ involvement and autoantibody analysis, including echocardiogram and pulmonary function if necessary
2. Discontinue use of disease-remitting drugs with teratogenic potential (i.e., mycophenolate mofetil, methotrexate, etc.) before pregnancy
3. High-risk obstetric care
4. Reassurance that there is no significant worry for hereditary neonatal scleroderma
5. Minimal use of proton pump inhibitors, histamine blockers, or calcium channel blockers for gastrointestinal and vascular problems
6. Avoidance of corticosteroids
7. More frequent monitoring of fetal size and uterine activity
8. Frequent blood pressure monitoring
9. Aggressive treatment of any hypertension (preeclampsia or others)
10. Close observation and treatment for premature labor (avoid beta-adrenergic agonists)
Labor and delivery
1. Epidural anesthesia is preferred
2. Special warming of delivery room, intravenous fluids, patients themselves (e.g., extra blankets, thermal socks, gloves)
3. Venous access before delivery
4. Careful attention to the episiotomy and Cesarean section incisions, which generally heal without difficulty
Post delivery
1. Continued careful monitoring postpartum, with early reinstitution of medication and aggressive treatment of hypertension, if it is present (do not assume it will resolve following delivery)

Table 39.3 Management of renal crisis during pregnancy in scleroderma

1. New-onset hypertension must be taken seriously
2. Search for evidence of increased creatinine, proteinuria, or microangiopathic hemolytic anemia, elevated liver function and uric acid
3. Do not assume it is preeclampsia
4. Try to control blood pressure with other medications, but if not controlled or if creatinine increases, add small doses of an ACE inhibitor
5. Controlling blood pressure may be lifesaving to the mother and baby even with the risks of fetopathy from ACE inhibitor toxicity

Captopril is perhaps the best choice in the setting of pregnancy as it can be easily and quickly titrated, and it appears to be associated with lower risk of fetopathy than other ACE inhibitors or ARBs [36].

In patients with diffuse SSc and particularly those with a new onset of SSc, the authors recommend home monitoring at least three to five times a week. The presence of even a slight elevation in blood pressure compared with previous levels should be considered potentially very serious. A search for evidence of elevated serum creatinine levels, proteinuria, microangiopathic hemolytic anemia, and uric acid should be done promptly. If the serum creatinine is increasing in this setting, particularly in the setting of microangiopathy and the absence of increased liver function tests, then a diagnosis of SSc renal crisis must be assumed. It is possible to try non-ACE inhibitors to control blood pressure early on, but they may not successfully control the renal crisis process. If the blood pressure is not easily and rapidly controlled with other medications, then ACE inhibitors may be necessary. If the blood pressure remains high, the high risk to the mother may outweigh the risk of toxicity to the fetus where the adequately controlled blood pressure could be lifesaving to the fetus as well. In the opinion of the authors, delay in starting an ACE inhibitor for fear of fetal complications increases risks for both mother and fetus. If elective C-section is planned, one should begin an ACE inhibitor and not assume the blood pressure will improve after delivery.

Management of Pregnancy in Mothers with Prior Renal Crisis

The management of SSc during pregnancy is challenging, but it is particularly challenging for women who have survived renal crisis and wish to become pregnant. In general, after an episode of renal crisis, ACE inhibitors are required to maintain blood pressure control and renal function indefinitely. Patients have had successful pregnancy outcomes while on ACE inhibitors [62]; however, as discussed above, the use of these drugs during the third trimester of pregnancy is associated with an increased risk of serious kidney problems in the baby.

Ten women from our SSc cohort have had 12 pregnancies after an episode of renal crisis [63]. Five healthy babies were born to four women who remained on ACE inhibitors throughout the pregnancy. Two other women discontinued ACE inhibitors prior to or early in pregnancy, and their blood pressures were successfully managed with other medications including calcium channel blockers. None of these infants had any significant evidence of ACE inhibitor toxicity.

Pregnancy in patients after renal crisis may be successful, but potential disastrous outcomes both to the mother as well as the infant are possible. There are several possible approaches that a patient can take if she desires a pregnancy after renal crisis, but they each contain significant risk. If the patient discontinues the ACE inhibitor and the blood pressure is not controlled with other antihypertensive medications, then the ACE inhibitor must be reinstituted. Otherwise, she is likely to experience severe deterioration in renal function and potential harm to the fetus as well. In the above small series of patients, the worst outcomes occurred in patients who had very poor blood pressure control. In patients with prior renal crisis who are contemplating pregnancy, they should consider a trial of ACE inhibitors prior to pregnancy to see if there is any chance of successful blood pressure control without ACE inhibitors. Another possible way of managing the pregnancy would be to use a small dose of ACE inhibitor along with non-ACE inhibitor medication to control blood pressure along with close monitoring of oligohydramnios or other signs of fetal abnormalities. In any situation, the patient and her spouse have to seriously consider a variety of options and potential outcomes before deciding whether to become pregnant or continue a pregnancy. This is a very high-risk situation, without any easy answers.

Management of Pulmonary Hypertension During Pregnancy

Analogous to SSc renal crisis, pulmonary hypertension may have devastating effects on both the mother and infant as there is significantly less reserve in the pulmonary arterioles to reduce vascular resistant to accommodate the increased blood volume and cardiac output that is required to maintain a normal pregnancy. If a woman with PAH discovers a pregnancy and wishes to continue with the pregnancy or if PAH is diagnosed during an established pregnancy, careful hemodynamic monitoring and comanagement with pulmonologists experienced with PAH are essential. The use of pulmonary function studies with carbon monoxide to assess diffusion capacity is considered safe during pregnancy [24]. Case reports have described successful use of epoprostenol and sildenafil during pregnancy [53–55, 64, 65]. Anticoagulation with low-molecular-weight heparin is recommended to reduce the risk of thromboembolism, and some have suggested the use of supplemental oxygen to maintain a PO2 greater than 70 mmHg. Inhaled NO has been used in extreme circumstances during labor and delivery.

Management of Delivery

The pregnant SSc patient is an anesthetic challenge that needs to be carefully considered and discussed before delivery [50, 66, 67]. SSc presents several mechanical difficulties due to thickening skin and secondary tissue contractures.

This may make it difficult to get easy venous access, obtain accurate vital signs, or position the limbs for delivery. Regional anesthesia, particularly an epidural block, allows the most benefit during delivery. It not only provides adequate anesthesia but also provides peripheral vasodilatation and increased skin perfusion of lower extremities [50, 66]. Eisele suggests using smaller-than-normal doses of regional anesthesia because SSc patients may exhibit prolonged motor and sensory blockade after delivery. General anesthesia should be avoided because of the difficulty in intubation in SSc patients with reduced oral aperture as well as concerns about aspiration. Venous access, even if it requires a central line and consideration of a Swan–Ganz catheter, may be necessary if cardiopulmonary compromise, hypertension, or renal dysfunction are present.

Other measures that could prevent problems related to Raynaud's phenomenon during delivery should be routinely used, including warming the delivery room, warm intravenous fluids, thermal socks, and warm external compresses [12]. There should be no hesitation to perform a Cesarean section if medically necessary because even the tightest abdominal skin usually heals if care is taken in the surgical repair of the incision.

Postnatal care should include continued attentiveness to monitoring disease activity, particularly progressive skin changes, new signs of cardiopulmonary disease, or new hypertension, so therapeutic intervention can begin immediately. There are no data on postpartum depression being greater in SSc than in any pregnancy, but given the complexity of the situation, one should be on the alert for emotional distress. For example, if the pregnancy was stressful, the baby is particularly fussy, or the mother has more difficulty caring for the infant than she anticipated, then she may be at greater risk for depression. Close observation for physical or emotional disease and early therapeutic intervention are indicated. Necessary medications that had been disrupted specifically because of the pregnancy should be reinstituted promptly, provided they are not contraindicated during breastfeeding, or the patient decides against breastfeeding.

Summary

Pregnancy in systemic sclerosis may be uneventful with both good maternal and fetal outcomes. SSc is a multisystem disease and complications do occur, and, thus, careful antenatal evaluations, discussion of potential problems, and participation in a high-risk obstetric monitoring program are very important to optimize the outcome. Women with diffuse SSc are at a greater risk for developing serious cardiopulmonary and renal problems early in the disease, so they should be encouraged to delay pregnancy until the disease stabilizes. Women with moderate-to-severe PAH should be counseled about the high rates of maternal and fetal morbidity and mortality during the perinatal period. All patients who become pregnant during this high-risk time should be monitored extremely carefully particularly for renal crisis.

Although there have been some suggestions that infertility and miscarriages are increased in SSc patients, recent studies show that these issues do not have major impact in women with established SSc. The high risk of premature and small infants may be minimized with specialized obstetric and neonatal care. Renal crisis in SSc is the only truly unique aspect of these pregnancies. The malignant hypertension in SSc patients must be treated aggressively, and if it is not controlled with other hypertensive medications, then ACE inhibitors must be used, irrespective of potential fetopathy that may occur with ACE inhibitors. It may be lifesaving to the mother. Other pregnancy problems may not be as unique to SSc, but because it is a chronic illness, any complication carries higher risks for both mother and child. Careful planning, close monitoring, and aggressive management should allow women with SSc to have a high likelihood of a successful pregnancy.

References

1. Levis B, Burri A, Hudson M, Baron M, Thombs BD, Canadian Scleroderma Research Group. Sexual activity and impairment in women with systemic sclerosis compared to women in the general population sample. PLoS One. 2012;7(12):e52129. doi:10.1371/journal.pone.0052129.
2. Maddali Bongi S, Del Rosso A, Mikhaylova S, Baccine M, Mattucci Cerinic M. Sexual function in Italian women with systemic sclerosis is affected by disease related and psychological concerns. J Rheumatol. 2013;40(10):1697–705.
3. Impens AJ, Rothman J, Schiopu E, Cole JC, Dang J, Gendrano N, et al. Sexual activity and functioning in female SSc patients. Clin Exp Rheumatol. 2009;27(3 Suppl 54):38–43.
4. Sampaio-Barros PD, Samara AM, Marques Neto JF. Gynaecologic history in systemic sclerosis. Clin Rheumatol. 2000;19(3):184–7.
5. Bhadauria S, Moser DK, Clements PJ, Singh RR, Lachenbruch PA, Pitkin RM, et al. Genital tract abnormalities and female sexual function impairment in systemic sclerosis. Am J Obstet Gynecol. 1995;172(2 Pt 1):580–7.
6. Englert H, Brennan P, McNeil D, Black C, Silman AJ. Reproductive function prior to disease onset in women with SSc. J Rheumatol. 1992;19(10):1575–9.
7. Ballou SP, Morley JJ, Kushner I. Pregnancy and systemic sclerosis. Arthritis Rheum. 1984;27(3):295–8.
8. Giordano M, Valentini G, Lupoli S, Giordano A. Pregnancy and systemic sclerosis. Arthritis Rheum. 1985;28(2):237–8.
9. Steen VD, Medsger Jr TA. Fertility and pregnancy outcome in women with systemic sclerosis. Arthritis Rheum. 1999;42(4):763–8.
10. Black CM, Stevens WM. SSc. Rheum Dis Clin North Am. 1989;15(2):193–212.
11. Maymon R, Fejgin M. SSc in pregnancy. Obstet Gynecol Surv. 1989;44(7):530–4.
12. Weiner SR. Organ function: sexual function and pregnancy. In: Clements PJ, Furst D, editors. Systemic sclerosis. New York: Williams and Wilkins; 1995. p. 483–99.

13. Slate WG, Graham AR. SSc and pregnancy. Trans Pac Coast Obstet Gynecol Soc. 1967;35:49–55.
14. Siamopoulou-Mavridou A, Manoussakis MN, Mavridis AK, Moutsopoulos HM. Outcome of pregnancy in patients with autoimmune rheumatic disease before the disease onset. Ann Rheum Dis. 1988;47(12):982–7.
15. Silman AJ, Black C. Increased incidence of spontaneous abortion and infertility in women with SSc before disease onset: a controlled study. Ann Rheum Dis. 1988;47(6):441–4.
16. van Wyk L, van der Marel J, Scheurwegh AJM, Schouffoer AA, Voskuyl AE, et al. Increased incidence of pregnancy complications in women who later develop scleroderma: a case control study. Arthritis Res Ther. 2011;13:R183.
17. Steen VD. Pregnancy in women with systemic sclerosis. Obstet Gynecol. 1999;94(1):15–20.
18. Chung L, Flyckt RL, Colon I, Shah AA, Druzin M, Chakravarty EF. Outcome of pregnancies complicated by systemic sclerosis and mixed connective tissue disease. Lupus. 2006;15(9):595–9.
19. Taraborelli M, Ramoni V, Brucato A, Airo P, Bajocchi G, Bellisai F, et al. Successful pregnancies but a higher risk for preterm births in patients with systemic sclerosis: an Italian multicenter study. Arthritis Rheum. 2012;64(6):1970–7.
20. Kahl LE, Blair C, Ramsey-Goldman R, Steen VD. Pregnancy outcomes in women with primary Raynaud's phenomenon. Arthritis Rheum. 1990;33(8):1249–55.
21. Chakravarty E. Pre-disease pregnancy complications and systemic sclerosis: pathogenic or pre-clinical? Arthritis Res Ther. 2012;14:102.
22. Steen VD. The many faces of SSc. Rheum Dis Clin North Am. 2008;34(1):1–15.
23. Chakravarty EF, Khanna D, Chung L. Pregnancy outcomes in systemic sclerosis, primary pulmonary hypertension, and sickle cell disease. Obstet Gynecol. 2008;111(4):927–34.
24. Chakravarty EF. Vascular complications of systemic sclerosis during pregnancy. Int J Rheumatol. 2010. pii: 287248. doi: 10.1155/2010/287248.
25. Ibba-Manneschi L, Manetti M, Milia AF, Miniati I, Benelli G, Guiducci S, et al. Severe fibrotic changes and altered expression of angiogenic factors in maternal SSc: placental findings. Ann Rheum Dis. 2010;69(2):458–61.
26. Papakonstantinou K, Hasiakos D, Kondi-Paphiti A. Clinicopathology of maternal SSc. Int J Gynaecol Obstet. 2007;99(3):248–9.
27. Doss BJ, Jacques SM, Mayes MD, Qureshi F. Maternal SSc: placental findings and perinatal outcome. Hum Pathol. 1998;29(12):1524–30.
28. Jimenez FX, Simeon CP, Fonollosa V, Espinach J, Solans R, Lima J, et al. SSc and pregnancy: obstetrical complications and the impact of pregnancy on the course of the disease (see comments). Med Clin (Barc). 1999;113(20):761–4.
29. Wanchu A, Misra R. Pregnancy outcome in systemic sclerosis. J Assoc Physicians India. 1996;44(9):637–40.
30. Lidar M, Langevitz P. Pregnancy issues in scleroderma. Autoimmun Rev. 2012;11:A515–9.
31. Steen VD. SSc renal crisis. Rheum Dis Clin North Am. 1996;22(4):861–78.
32. Altieri P, Cameron JS. SSc renal crisis in a pregnant woman with late partial recovery of renal function. Nephrol Dial Transplant. 1988;3(5):677–80.
33. Baethge BA, Wolf RE. Successful pregnancy with SSc renal disease and pulmonary hypertension in a patient using angiotensin converting enzyme inhibitors. Ann Rheum Dis. 1989;48(9):776–8.
34. Muller PR, James A. Pregnancy with prolonged fetal exposure to an angiotensin-converting enzyme inhibitor. J Perinatol. 2002;22(7):582–4.
35. Watson MA, Radford NJ, McGrath BP, Swinton GW, Agar JW. Captopril-induced agranulocytosis in systemic sclerosis. Aust N Z J Med. 1981;11(1):79–81.
36. Bullo M, Tschumi S, Bucher TS, Bianchetti MG, Simonetti GD. Pregnancy outcome following exposure to angiotensin-converting enzyme inhibitors or angiotensin receptor antagonists. Hypertension. 2012;60:444–50.
37. Steen VD, Costantino JP, Shapiro AP, Medsger Jr TA. Outcome of renal crisis in systemic sclerosis: relation to availability of angiotensin converting enzyme (ACE) inhibitors [see comments]. Ann Intern Med. 1990;113(5):352–7.
38. Steen VD. Organ involvement: renal. In: Clements PJ, Furst D, editors. Systemic sclerosis. New York: Williams and Wilkins; 1995. p. 425–40.
39. Gould JS, Wissinger HA. Carpal tunnel syndrome in pregnancy. South Med J. 1978;71(2):144–5. 154.
40. Hammar M, Larsson L, Tegler L. Calcium treatment of leg cramps in pregnancy. Effect on clinical symptoms and total serum and ionized serum calcium concentrations. Acta Obstet Gynecol Scand. 1981;60(4):345–7.
41. Fast A, Shapiro D, Ducommun EJ, Friedmann LW, Bouklas T, Floman Y. Low-back pain in pregnancy. Spine. 1987;12(4): 368–71.
42. Calhoun BC. Gastrointestinal disorders in pregnancy. Obstet Gynecol Clin North Am. 1992;19(4):733–44.
43. Ulmsten U, Sundstrom G. Esophageal manometry in pregnant and nonpregnant women. Am J Obstet Gynecol. 1978;132(3):260–4.
44. Van Thiel DH, Gavaler JS, Joshi SN, Sara RK, Stremple J. Heartburn of pregnancy. Gastroenterology. 1977;72(4 Pt 1):666–8.
45. Avrech OM, Golan A, Pansky M, Langer R, Caspi E. Raynaud's phenomenon and peripheral gangrene complicating SSc in pregnancy–diagnosis and management. Br J Obstet Gynaecol. 1992;99(10):850–1.
46. Smith CA, Pinals RS. Progressive systemic sclerosis and postpartum renal failure complicated by peripheral gangrene. J Rheumatol. 1982;9(3):455–8.
47. Fortin F, Wallaert B. Interstitial pathology and pregnancy. Rev Mal Respir. 1988;5(3):275–8.
48. Raymond R, Underwood DA, Moodie DS. Cardiovascular problems in pregnancy. Cleve Clin J Med. 1987;54(2):95–104.
49. Sullivan JM, Ramanathan KB. Management of medical problems in pregnancy–severe cardiac disease. N Engl J Med. 1985;313(5): 304–9.
50. Thompson J, Conklin KA. Anesthetic management of a pregnant patient with SSc. Anesthesiology. 1983;59(1):69–71.
51. Katz M, Gill PJ, Newman RB. Detection of preterm labor by ambulatory monitoring of uterine activity for the management of oral tocolysis. Am J Obstet Gynecol. 1986;154(6):1253–6.
52. Schachna L, Wigley FM, Chang B, White B, Wise RA, Gelber AC. Age and risk of pulmonary arterial hypertension in SSc. Chest. 2003;124(6):2098–104.
53. Madden BP. Pulmonary hypertension and pregnancy. Int J Obstet Anesth. 2009;18(2):156–64.
54. Huang S, DeSantis ER. Treatment of pulmonary arterial hypertension in pregnancy. Am J Health Syst Pharm. 2007;64(18):1922–6.
55. Bedard E, Dimopoulos K, Gatzoulis MA. Has there been any progress made on pregnancy outcomes among women with pulmonary arterial hypertension? Eur Heart J. 2009;30(3):256–65.
56. Weiner SR, Brinkman CR, Paulus HE. SSc, CREST syndrome and pregnancy. Arthritis Rheum. 1986;51:S51. Ref Type: Abstract.
57. Hadker N, Garg S, Costanzo C, Miller JD, Foster T, van der Helm W, et al. Financial impact of a novel pre-eclampsia diagnostic test versus standard practice: a decision-analytic modeling analysis from a UK healthcare payer perspective. J Med Econ. 2010;13(4):728–37.

58. Mehta N, Modi N. ACE inhibitors in pregnancy. Lancet. 1989;2(8654):96–7.
59. Pryde PG, Barr Jr M. Low-dose, short-acting, angiotensin-converting enzyme inhibitors as rescue therapy in pregnancy. Obstet Gynecol. 2001;97(5 Pt 1):799–800.
60. Easterling TR, Carr DB, Davis C, Diederichs C, Brateng DA, Schmucker B. Low-dose, short-acting, angiotensin-converting enzyme inhibitors as rescue therapy in pregnancy. Obstet Gynecol. 2000;96(6):956–61.
61. Burrows RF, Burrows EA. Assessing the teratogenic potential of angiotensin-converting enzyme inhibitors in pregnancy. Aust N Z J Obstet Gynaecol. 1998;38(3):306–11.
62. Steen VD. Pregnancy in SSc. Rheum Dis Clin North Am. 2007;33(2):345–58.
63. Steen VD. Management of pregnancy in SSc renal crisis. Arthritis Rheum. 2002;52:S45. Ref Type: Abstract.
64. Higton AM, Whale C, Musk M, Gabbay E. Pulmonary hypertension in pregnancy: two cases and review of the literature. Intern Med J. 2009;39(11):766–70.
65. Goland S, Tsai F, Habib M, Janmohamed M, Goodwin TM, Elkayam U. Favorable outcome of pregnancy with an elective use of epoprostenol and sildenafil in women with severe pulmonary hypertension. Cardiology. 2010;115(3):205–8.
66. Eisele JH, Reitan JA. SSc, Raynaud's phenomenon, and local anesthetics. Anesthesiology. 1971;34(4):386–7.
67. Younker D, Harrison B. SSc and pregnancy. Anaesthetic considerations. Br J Anaesth. 1985;57(11):1136–9.

Part VIII

Management and Outcome Assessment

Introduction to Section VIII: Management and Outcome Assessment

40

John Varga, Fredrick M. Wigley, and Christopher P. Denton

Scleroderma has complex pathogenesis, and its protean clinical and pathological manifestations reflect a disease process affecting multiple organs. In addition, scleroderma encompasses a series of related but distinct entities that are characterized by different course, severity, response to therapy, and outcomes.

Scleroderma causes pain, disfigurement, functional impairment, and a substantial decrease in life expectancy. The survival of patients with scleroderma has shown improvement during the past two decades. This improvement in survival, as well as in disease-associated morbidity and disability, is due to advances in diagnosis and early recognition of internal organ involvement, as well successful management of selected complications such as pulmonary arterial hypertension, Raynaud phenomenon, gastroesophageal reflux disease, ischemic digital ulcers, and scleroderma renal crisis. Additionally, recognition of prognostic risk factors, such as scleroderma-associated autoantibodies, has permitted better risk stratification, which is indispensible for both more effective clinical trials, as well for optimized patient management. Risk stratification in scleroderma enables the selection of more precise therapies targeted to the individual scleroderma patient while reducing potential drug toxicities.

The chapters that follow, together with preceding sections focusing on the management of specific organ-based complications, highlight our current concepts regarding the comprehensive and integrated management of the patient with scleroderma, as well as evolving considerations regarding the design of therapeutic trials. Individual chapters will describe the available immunomodulatory and biological therapies and their roles in management, as well as emerging and investigative therapies; the evaluation and management of psychosocial aspects of scleroderma, the role of occupational and physical therapy, and issues related to the design and conduct of clinical trials for scleroderma, including the selection and application of outcome measures.

The Comprehensive Approach to Patient Management

Improved outcomes for patients with scleroderma require early diagnosis and prompt initiation of appropriate treatment. Interventions are more likely to be effective if initiated before irreversible organ damage, such as digital ischemic ulcers, joint contractures, pulmonary fibrosis, or pulmonary arterial hypertension, has developed. Much recent effort has focused on accurate identification of scleroderma at a relatively early stage of the disease. The development of the revised classification criteria by the American College of Rheumatology and the European League against Rheumatism affords improved diagnostic sensitivity for scleroderma compared to previously used criteria. This in turn might facilitate accurate diagnosis, and potentially enrollment in clinical trials, at an earlier stage of disease.

Once the diagnosis of scleroderma is made, it is of importance to define the clinical phenotype, identify the disease stage, and recognize organ involvement. It is widely appreciated that scleroderma has multiple subtypes, each with distinct patterns of organ involvement, rates of disease progression, and long-term outcomes. Clinical subsetting, based largely on the pattern of skin involvement, has been moderately useful in differentiating patients into limited and

J. Varga, MD (✉)
Northwestern Scleroderma Program, John and Nancy Hughes Professor, Feinberg School of Medicine Northwestern University, Chicago, IL, USA
e-mail: J-VARGA@NORTHWESTERN.EDU

F.M. Wigley, MD
Department of Medicine/Rheumatology, The Johns Hopkins University School of Medicine, Baltimore, MD, USA

C.P. Denton, PhD, FRCP
Division of Medicine, Department of Inflammation, Centre for Rheumatology and Connective Tissue Diseases, UCL Division of Medicine, Royal Free Hospital, London, UK

J. Varga et al. (eds.), *Scleroderma*, DOI 10.1007/978-3-319-31407-5_40

diffuse cutaneous subsets. Such dichotomous classification predicts the likelihood of developing major organ manifestations and rate and extent of skin progression. Laboratory studies are increasingly useful in more nuanced phenotyping of scleroderma patients. As discussed in Chap. 15 (Kuwana and Medsger), specific autoantibodies are strongly associated with particular scleroderma subphenotypes and can identify patients with an increased risk of developing selected organ complications such as scleroderma renal crisis, pulmonary fibrosis, pulmonary hypertension, myopathy, or cancer.

It is also important to assess disease stage and activity at the earliest possible opportunity. Scleroderma patients may present with advanced skin involvement or evidence of substantial organ damage, yet have little disease activity. That is, disease severity (the cumulative burden of damage) must be distinguished from disease activity. Studies indicate that both the extent of skin involvement, as well as the rate of progression of interstitial lung disease and many other complications of scleroderma, are highest in relatively early-stage disease; therefore, therapeutic interventions for these complications are most likely to be of benefit when started promptly. Specific symptoms, and characteristic findings on physical exam, such as the presence of soft tissue edema on the extremities, are often helpful in identifying early-stage active disease. Serial evaluation by physical examination, and when indicated, pulmonary function studies, imaging, and other appropriate diagnostic tools, can also provide evidence of disease progression or stability over time. The key principle is that early recognition of organ involvement and/or disease activity affords the best opportunity to intervene and prevent further progression and minimize irreversible damage.

Gaining a clear picture of disease phenotype, stage, and activity at the earliest opportunity allows for the design of an individualized treatment protocol that is best suited for the unique needs of a particular patient. Such customized therapy carries the highest potential for effectively slowing disease progression or preventing organ damage while minimizing drug toxicity and avoiding unnecessary adverse effects. In light of the multi-organ manifestations of scleroderma, including disease affecting most vital organs, effective patient management depends on a multidisciplinary approach. Ideally this is provided at a center with adequate breadth and depth of expertise with scleroderma. The patient management team should include the rheumatologist, along with medical subspecialist depending on the pattern of organ involvement in a given patient, but com or vascular surgeons. In addition, allied health professionals can make a major contribution. Often neglected but of great importance is addressing the unique social and psychological needs of scleroderma patients. The coordination of these individual healthcare specialists permits provision of a comprehensive and harmonized management program that addresses all the patient' needs. Patient education also plays a major role in ensuring good compliance and empowering the patient to contribute to his/her care. Patient organizations, support groups, and specialist providers can furnish accurate information that empower patients to make informed decisions about their care and lifestyle. Whenever appropriate, ethically justified, and based on truly informed consent, participation in well-designed clinical trials is encouraged.

It is important to maintain continued vigilance throughout the course of the disease, which evolves over time. New organ involvement may emerge and must be continually screened for in the appropriate setting. For instance, progressive cardiac disease, pulmonary arterial hypertension, ischemic digital ulcers, calcinosis, and Barrett esophagus are often late complications, and their development mandates appropriate changes in patient management. Therefore, continued ongoing evaluation, which includes regular monitoring with appropriate laboratory, functional, and imaging tests for extended periods, is indicated in most patients with scleroderma.

Defining Outcomes

Patients with scleroderma are currently treated with a variety of therapies. These primarily target the immune, vascular, or fibrotic process. Definition of a treatment benefit in scleroderma is evolving. Obvious goals in clinical practice, as well as in clinical trials, include improved survival, improved quality of life, reducing disability, preservation or improvement of organ function, and prevention of new organ involvement. In clinical practice, continuous attention needs to be paid to the efficacy of an intervention, and decisions regarding continuation of a therapy or switching to an alternate therapy are made on the basis of regular comprehensive reevaluation. In clinical trials, a variety of outcome measures may be considered. Currently used outcome assessment tools include patient-reported outcome measures such as health assessment questionnaires, evaluation of skin involvement using the modified Rodnan skin score and other metrics, organ-specific assessment, composite measures of response, and survival and event-free (or progression-free) survival.

Immunomodulatory, Immunoablative, and Biologic Therapies

41

Jacob M. van Laar and Robert W. Simms

Introduction

Immunosuppressive drugs constitute a heterogeneous group of therapeutic compounds, each with a unique mode of action and toxicity profile (Table 41.1). Their main function is to dampen the immune system – notably T and B lymphocytes – functionally and/or numerically, hence their utility in inducing remission and control of specific rheumatic manifestations that result from inflammation. In contrast to immunoablative therapy and autologous hematopoietic stem cell transplantation (referred to as "HSCT" in the text below), immunosuppressive drugs do not permanently correct the fundamental imbalance of immune regulation in autoimmune disease and, as such, they have only limited curative potential when used in standard doses.

The use of immunosuppressive medication in systemic sclerosis (SSc) is based on the premise that the innate and/or acquired immune system plays a pivotal role in its pathogenesis. Nevertheless, their beneficial effects in SSc had been less evident than in many other rheumatological conditions such as rheumatoid arthritis (RA) and systemic lupus erythematosus (SLE) until recent evidence that HSCT for selected poor-prognosis patients with diffuse cutaneous systemic sclerosis (dcSSc) had substantial efficacy. In part this may be explained by the fact that some clinical outcome measures in SSc such as skin thickening, joint contractures, cardiac arrhythmia, and gastrointestinal (GI) dysfunction do not merely reflect acute inflammation, but are often late clinical manifestations of tissue injury and fibrogenesis triggered by inflammation. This is reminiscent of the temporal link of inflammation and fibrosis in other diseases, such as the transition from subclinical hepatitis to clinically overt liver cirrhosis. Nevertheless, methotrexate (MTX), azathioprine, glucocorticoids, cyclophosphamide (CYC), and mycophenolate mofetil (MMF) are widely used to treat specific manifestations such as skin thickening, alveolitis, and musculoskeletal signs and symptoms, even though the evidence from clinical trials or registry analyses suggests that the effectiveness of these drugs is weak [1]. The 2009 recommendations of the European League Against Rheumatism (EULAR) explicitly refer to the fact that while low-dose glucocorticoids are commonly used for the treatment of inflammatory arthritis in SSc and while uncontrolled and retrospectively controlled studies with some immunosuppressive regimens (such as azathioprine, mycophenolate mofetil, cyclosporine A) have reported efficacy in selected manifestations, their efficacy is not substantiated by RCT [2]. Clinical trials in SSc are however notoriously difficult to accomplish due to the low prevalence and the heterogeneity of the disease. This includes unique subsets of disease with different modes of onset, progression rate of disease, and varied types of organs involved. Also, determination of prognosis remains a challenge in individual cases, hampering

Table 41.1 Immunosuppressive drugs commonly used in systemic sclerosis treatment

Drug	Class	Mechanism of action
Glucocorticoids	Synthetic hormones	Pleiotropic genomic and nongenomic effects
Cyclophosphamide	Alkylating cytotoxic	Metabolites alkylate DNA
Azathioprine	Purine analogue cytotoxic	Inhibits purine synthesis
Methotrexate	Antimetabolite	Inhibits AICAR transformylase
MMF	Purine synthesis inhibitor	Inhibits inosine monophosphate dehydrogenase

MMF mycophenolate mofetil

J.M. van Laar, MD, PhD (✉)
Rheumatology and Clinical Immunology, University Medical Center Utrecht, Utrecht, The Netherlands
e-mail: j.m.vanlaar@umcutrecht.nl

R.W. Simms, MD
Department of Rheumatology, Boston Medical Center and Boston University School of Medicine, 72 East Concord Street Evans 501, Boston, MA 02118-2526, USA

J. Varga et al. (eds.), *Scleroderma*, DOI 10.1007/978-3-319-31407-5_41

efforts to identify subgroups of patients who might benefit from immunosuppressive therapy. As a result, only methotrexate and cyclophosphamide have withstood the rigor of placebo-controlled clinical trials in SSc. Despite these studies, deciding if the benefits outweigh the risks and toxicities is difficult to assess. Strategies to neutralize the pro-inflammatory cytokine tumor necrosis factor (TNF)-alpha and the pro-fibrotic cytokine transforming growth factor (TGF)-beta using monoclonal antibodies have so far not lived up to expectations. Pilot studies with rituximab have been more encouraging, and small-scale placebo-controlled clinical trials are in progress to investigate whether B-cell depletion is a more attractive target. In one of these studies, rituximab treatment resulted in a drop of serum concentrations of interleukin-6 (IL-6), a key mediator of inflammation. Several new biologicals with specific targets are currently being evaluated for their effects in SSc.

This chapter outlines the clinical pharmacology and therapeutic use of conventional immunosuppressive drugs that are most commonly used in SSc: glucocorticoids, cyclophosphamide, azathioprine, methotrexate, mycophenolate mofetil, and newer biologicals. Additionally, it will also cover the clinical pharmacology and therapeutic use of immunoablative therapy followed by autologous hematopoietic stem cell transplantation.

Glucocorticoids

Clinical Pharmacology and Mechanism of Action

Glucocorticoids have been used to treat rheumatic conditions for over 50 years, and these were the first immunosuppressive drugs used in systemic sclerosis [3]. In general, their effects and side effects are well known. Although their use as treatment for SSc is widespread, surprisingly few clinical trials have been done in this disease. Prednisone is the most commonly used oral glucocorticoid. It is a prodrug that is converted by the liver into prednisolone, which is the active drug and also a steroid.

The biological effects of glucocorticoids have been well characterized (reviewed in refs [4, 5]). Glucocorticoids cause genomic and non-genomic effects following binding to the glucocorticoid receptor (GR). The activated GR complex in turn upregulates the expression of anti-inflammatory proteins in the nucleus (a process known as transactivation), such as lipocortin 1, p11/calpactin-binding protein, and secretory leukoprotease inhibitor 1, and represses the expression of pro-inflammatory proteins in the cytosol by preventing the translocation of other transcription factors from the cytosol into the nucleus (transrepression). The interleukins IL-1, IL-2, IL-3, IL-4, IL-5, IL-6, and IL-8, interferon-gamma

Table 41.2 Unintended effects of chronic glucocorticoid use

Hyperglycemia due to increased gluconeogenesis, insulin resistance, and impaired glucose tolerance (“steroid diabetes”); caution in those with diabetes mellitus
Increased skin fragility, easy bruising
Negative calcium balance due to reduced intestinal calcium absorption
Steroid-induced osteoporosis: reduced bone density (osteoporosis, osteonecrosis, higher fracture risk, slower fracture repair)
Weight gain due to increased visceral and truncal fat deposition (central obesity) and appetite stimulation
Adrenal insufficiency (if used for long time and stopped suddenly without a taper)
Muscle breakdown (proteolysis), weakness; reduced muscle mass and repair
Expansion of malar fat pads and dilation of small blood vessels in the skin
Anovulation, irregularity of menstrual periods
Growth failure, pubertal delay
Increased plasma amino acids, increased urea formation; negative nitrogen balance
Excitatory effect on central nervous system (euphoria, psychosis)
Glaucoma due to increased cranial pressure
Cataracts

(IFN-γ), chemokines, cytokines, granulocyte-macrophage colony-stimulating factor (GM-CSF), and TNF-alpha genes and Fc receptors on macrophages are all downregulated by glucocorticoids. The aforementioned potent immunosuppressive properties of glucocorticoids translate into reduced T- and B-cell proliferation, T-cell apoptosis, antibody synthesis, and decreased phagocytosis of opsonized cells. Glucocorticoids not only suppress the immune response but also inhibit the two main products of inflammation, prostaglandins and leukotrienes.

Glucocorticoids' primary anti-inflammatory mechanism is lipocortin-1 (annexin-1) synthesis. Lipocortin-1 suppresses phospholipase A2, thereby blocking eicosanoid production, and inhibits various leukocyte inflammatory events (epithelial adhesion, emigration, chemotaxis, phagocytosis, respiratory burst, etc.). Glucocorticoids inhibit prostaglandin synthesis at the level of phospholipase A2 as well as at the level of cyclooxygenase (COX)/prostaglandin E (PGE) isomerase (COX-1 and COX-2), much like that of nonsteroidal anti-inflammatory drugs (NSAIDs). Glucocorticoids also have non-genomic effects, especially when administered in high doses, such as bolus infusions. Glucocorticoids do not selectively affect the immune system or inflammatory pathways but influence many metabolic pathways as well. This accounts for the wide variety of possible side effects that may occur in a (cumulative) dose-dependent way (Table 41.2). Adrenal suppression will begin to occur if prednisone is taken for longer than 7 days. Drug-induced, secondary adrenocortical insufficiency may be minimized by gradual reduction of dosage. This type of relative insufficiency may persist for months after discontinuation of therapy; therefore, in any situation of stress occurring during that period, hormone therapy should be reinstituted. Since mineralocorticoid secretion may be impaired, salt and/or a mineralocorticoid should be administered concurrently.

Since adequate human reproduction studies have not been done with corticosteroids, the use of these drugs in pregnancy, nursing mothers, or women of childbearing potential requires that the possible benefits of the drug be weighed against the potential hazards to the mother and embryo or fetus.

Therapeutic Use in Systemic Sclerosis

In an analysis of the German Network for Systemic Scleroderma, 577 out of 1,396 (41 %) patients were treated with glucocorticoids, especially those with diffuse skin involvement or with "overlap" clinical features (49 % and 64 %, respectively) versus 31 % of those with limited cutaneous skin involvement [1]. Glucocorticoid use was particularly prevalent in patients with kidney involvement (56.5 %) or pulmonary fibrosis (55.6 %). In addition, alone or in combination with immunosuppressive agents, glucocorticoids were used in 27 % of patients with mainly cutaneous manifestations. These registry data reflect use by usual clinical practice rather than use dictated by guidelines derived from clinical evidence. The absence of evidence should, however, not be interpreted as evidence of absence of effect. In a Japanese study [6], 23 patients with diffuse cutaneous systemic sclerosis (dcSSc) satisfying two of three criteria (early onset, edematous changes, rapid progression) were treated with prednisolone 20 mg/day as starting dose for 2–8 weeks followed by a tapering schedule to 2.5–10 mg/day as maintenance therapy and evaluated the effect using the modified Rodnan skin score (MRSS). The mean initial MRSS (20.3 ± 9.3) decreased significantly to 12.8 ± 7.0 after 1 year of treatment ($p<0.005$) and to 8.7 ± 6.1 at final evaluation ($p<0.001$). No renal crisis occurred, but one patient developed *Pneumocystis jiroveci* pneumonia requiring antibiotic therapy. Glucocorticoids have also been used to treat visceral organ involvement. In a study on cardiac function, resting radionuclide ventriculography with 99mTc was performed before and 20 days after the administration of prednisolone, 20 mg daily, in 32 patients with SSc and 32 disease controls (SLE, RA) without clinically evident myocardial dysfunction at rest [7]. An impaired left ventricular ejection fraction (LVEF) (i.e., <50 %) was found in six patients with SSc (four with diffuse and two with limited disease) and one with SLE. Prednisolone administration resulted in a significant percent improvement in the baseline LVEF (mean 18 %, $p=0.0001$) in the SSc group; this improvement was greater in the 15 patients with diffuse SSc than in the 17 with limited skin disease (27 % vs 10 %, $p=0.02$). The improvement was most prominent in the six patients with an initial impaired LVEF and significantly associated with baseline erythrocyte sedimentation rate (ESR) in the whole SSc patient group. This study suggested that prednisolone might be an effective drug in improving (subclinical) heart dysfunction, although glucocorticoid treatment-associated volume expansion may have been a confounding factor. More conclusive studies with longer follow-up are needed to determine whether and how glucocorticoids improve myocardial function. Glucocorticoids combined with i.v. pulse cyclophosphamide were also effective in a patient with rapidly progressive dcSSc with overt myocarditis, resulting in remission of the patient's symptoms [8].

The use of glucocorticoids in SSc lung disease is contentious. A small prospective study in 218 SSc patients with biopsy proven nonspecific interstitial pneumonia who were randomly allocated to either prednisolone + cyclophosphamide or cyclophosphamide treatment alone showed no difference in effects on forced vital capacity (FVC) and diffusing capacity for carbon monoxide (DLCO) at 3 years after the end of a 1-year treatment [9]. All patients received 12× i.v. cyclophosphamide 1 g/m^2; the second group also received prednisolone with a starting dose of 60 mg/day. Six bacterial infections were recorded in the whole cohort, but none was serious. No case of hemorrhagic cystitis occurred. The Rodnan skin score improved more in the second group, but the difference was not significant.

The pros and cons of the use of glucocorticoids in SSc should be carefully weighed, especially since high doses of glucocorticoids (prednisolone >30 mg/day) are implicated as a risk factor to develop a scleroderma renal crisis, although the pathophysiological mechanism in this context is unclear [10].

The benefits of medium- and low-dose glucocorticoids, for example, prednisolone ≤20 mg/day, may outweigh the risks in disabling SSc inflammatory joint disease and myositis. Glucocorticoids are also commonly prescribed for other organ manifestations, notably interstitial lung disease (ILD), pericarditis, myocarditis, and (early) diffuse cutaneous disease, but as discussed above, the scientific evidence is weak. Glucocorticoids at doses higher than 30 mg/day are best avoided.

Cyclophosphamide

Clinical Pharmacology and Mechanism of Action

Cyclophosphamide is an oxazaphosphorine-substituted nitrogen mustard and inactive prodrug requiring enzymatic bioactivation [11]. Its DNA-alkylating effects are mediated predominantly through phosphoramide mustard and, to a lesser extent, other active metabolites. These positively charged, reactive intermediates alkylate nucleophilic bases resulting in the cross-linking of DNA and of DNA proteins, breaks in DNA, and consequently decreased DNA synthesis and apoptosis. The cytotoxicity of alkylating agents correlates with the amount of DNA cross-linking, but the relationship between cytotoxicity and immunosuppressive effects is unclear. The effects of cyclophosphamide are not exclusively limited to proliferating cells or to any particular cell type. Sensitivity varies among cell populations; however, for example, hematopoietic progenitor cells are relatively resistant to even high doses of cyclophosphamide. The immunosuppressive effects of cyclophosphamide include decreased numbers of T lymphocytes and B lymphocytes, decreased lymphocyte proliferation, decreased antibody production, and suppression of delayed hypersensitivity to new antigens with relative preservation of established delayed hypersensitivity. Cyclophosphamide is rapidly metabolized, largely by the liver, to active and inactive metabolites. The formation of the active 4-hydroxycyclophosphamide is mediated by various cytochrome P-450. 4-Hydroxycyclophosphamide, which is not cytotoxic at physiologic pH, readily diffuses into cells and spontaneously decomposes into the active phosphoramide mustard. The elimination half-life of cyclophosphamide is 5–9 h. Between 30 % and 60 % of the total cyclophosphamide is eliminated in the urine, mostly as inactive metabolites, although some cyclophosphamide and active metabolites, such as phosphoramide mustard and acrolein, can also be detected in urine. Reversible myelosuppression manifesting as leukopenia and neutropenia is common and dose dependent. Platelet counts generally are not affected with intravenous pulse doses of less than 50 mg/kg, but with long-term oral use, a mild decrease in platelet count is common. After a single intravenous dose of cyclophosphamide, the approximate times to nadir and recovery of leukocyte counts are 8–14 days and 21 days. With long-term use, there is increased sensitivity to the myelosuppressive effects of cyclophosphamide, and doses usually need to be decreased over time. The bladder toxicities of cyclophosphamide, hemorrhagic cystitis, and bladder cancer are related to route of administration, duration of therapy, and cumulative cyclophosphamide dose. Of note, most of the data on cyclophosphamide-related bladder toxicity are based on studies in patients with hemato-oncological conditions treated with ifosfamide and animal studies, and very few data are available in SSc [12]. Bladder toxicity, a particular problem with long-term oral and the high intravenous doses of cyclophosphamide used in stem cell transplantation, is largely due to acrolein, a metabolite of cyclophosphamide. Bladder toxicity can be minimized in patients receiving pulse doses of intravenous cyclophosphamide by administering mesna, a sulfhydryl compound that binds acrolein in the urine and inactivates it. The short half-life of mesna renders it suboptimal for the prevention of bladder toxicity in patients receiving daily oral cyclophosphamide – but oral mesna administered three times a day with daily oral cyclophosphamide decreased the incidence of bladder toxicity to 12 % and may decrease the risk of bladder cancer. Nonglomerular hematuria, which may range from minor, microscopic blood loss to severe, macroscopic bleeding, is the most common manifestation of cyclophosphamide-induced cystitis. Cyclophosphamide increases the risk of malignancies (other than bladder cancer) twofold to fourfold. Cyclophosphamide, as used in autoimmune disease, results in significant gonadal toxicity manifesting as amenorrhea. The risk of ovarian failure depends more on age of the patient and cumulative dose of cyclophosphamide than on route of administration. The use of alkylating agents in male patients leads to azoospermia. If the clinical situation allows, referral to a fertility clinic for banking of sperm (or ova in female patients) should be considered prior to cyclophosphamide treatment. Oral cyclophosphamide is best administered as a single dose in the morning with the patient drinking plenty of fluids and emptying the bladder frequently to dilute the urinary concentration of acrolein and to minimize the time the bladder is exposed to it. Prophylaxis against *Pneumocystis jiroveci* pneumonia is often prescribed, particularly during the induction phase when doses of cyclophosphamide and corticosteroids are higher. The use of mesna to prevent bladder toxicity is described above. Urinalysis should be performed monthly, and nonglomerular hematuria should be evaluated by a urologist. All patients who receive cyclophosphamide, particularly patients who develop hemorrhagic cystitis, are at increased risk of developing bladder cancer, and lifelong surveillance is required with urinalysis, urine cytology, and, if indicated, cystoscopy. Cyclophosphamide is teratogenic, particularly in the first trimester, and should be avoided in pregnancy and during lactation.

Therapeutic Use in Systemic Sclerosis

Several nonrandomized and uncontrolled studies have shown that cyclophosphamide either as monthly i.v. bolus infusions or as daily oral treatment and with or without concomitant glucocorticoid treatment resulted in improvement of skin thickening and stabilization of pulmonary function [13–18], while one study also suggested improved survival of those patients treated with cyclophosphamide [19]. These observations formed the basis of two randomized, controlled clinical trials. In the North-American Scleroderma Lung Study I (SLS I), a randomized, controlled clinical trial in 158 patients with SSc-related interstitial lung disease of whom 145 completed at least 6 months of treatment, 1-year treatment with daily oral cyclophosphamide (2 mg/kg) resulted in statistically significant but small improvements in forced vital capacity (+2.9 % difference in the forced vital capacity at 1 year), total lung capacity (TLC), dyspnea, Rodnan skin scores, and several measures of quality of life when compared to placebo treatment [20]. However, when patients were followed for another year after completing their cyclophosphamide therapy, the beneficial effects of cyclophosphamide waned and were no longer significant by the 24-month follow-up except for a sustained improvement of dyspnea [21]. A higher number of adverse events (AE) were recorded in the cyclophosphamide group, but of all adverse events, most were not deemed treatment related, and no difference in the number of serious adverse events was found. This landmark study was the first to conclusively show a modest benefit of cyclophosphamide treatment in SSc-ILD. Of note, serum biomarkers of lung disease and fibrotic changes assessed by thoracic computed tomography (CT) scanning were also attenuated by cyclophosphamide treatment [22, 23]. On the other hand, cyclophosphamide was not more effective in ameliorating musculoskeletal symptoms [24].

Abnormal cellularity was present in 72 % of patients and defined a population with a higher percentage of men, more severe lung function, including a worse lung function (FVC, TLC, DLCO), and more extensive abnormalities on thoracic CT scan. Nevertheless, the presence or absence of an abnormal cell differential was not an independent predictor of disease progression or response to cyclophosphamide at 1 year [25].

In the other controlled trial, conducted in the UK, 45 patients were randomized to receive low-dose prednisolone (20 mg/day) and 6 monthly infusions of cyclophosphamide (600 mg) followed by oral azathioprine or placebo [26]. The primary outcome measures were change in percent-predicted forced vital capacity (FVC) and change in single-breath diffusing capacity for carbon monoxide (DLCO). Secondary outcome measures included changes in appearance on high-resolution computed tomography (HRCT) and dyspnea scores. Sixty-two percent of the patients completed the first year of treatment. Withdrawals included nine patients (six from the placebo group) with significant decline in lung function, two with treatment side effects (both from the active treatment group), and six with non-trial-related comorbidity. No hemorrhagic cystitis or bone marrow suppression was observed. Estimation of the relative treatment effect (active treatment versus placebo) adjusted for baseline FVC and treatment center revealed a favorable outcome for FVC of 4.19 % ($p=0.08$). No improvements in DLCO or secondary outcome measures were identified.

Of note, in most of the retrospective and prospective studies, patients were *not* selected on the basis of documented progression of interstitial lung disease, and it has been suggested that this should be an additional criterion in clinical trials with immunosuppressive treatment, at least in SSc lung disease [27]. In a French study in 27 SSc patients with worsening ILD (based on change in FVC and/or DLCO), 6 monthly i.v. pulse cyclophosphamide (600 mg/m^2) followed by an 18-month oral treatment with azathioprine was reportedly well tolerated and was associated with stable or improved pulmonary function test (PFT) in 70 % and 51.8 % of SSc patients at 6 months and 2 years, respectively [28]. Among the 19 (70 %) responders, 15 received azathioprine and 4 declined. Twenty-three completed 2-year follow-up, three died, and one dropped out. Further controlled studies are needed to determine whether decline in lung function is a better selection criterion in identifying those who benefit from active therapy. In a retrospective study on 28 patients with connective tissue disease-related pulmonary arterial hypertension, none of the 8 patients with systemic sclerosis had responded to treatment (according to defined response criteria) with at least three i.v. infusions of cyclophosphamide 600 mg/m^2 with or without glucocorticoids [29].

Intravenous pulse cyclophosphamide treatment was followed by remarkable clinical and endoscopic improvement of SSc-associated gastric antral vascular ectasia (GAVE) in three patients [30].

Cyclophosphamide treatment has also been shown to cause normalization of nailfold capillary abnormalities [31]. It is tempting to speculate that cyclophosphamide-induced mobilization of blood progenitor cells could explain the effects on vasculopathy [32].

Based on the above data, cyclophosphamide treatment, either oral or intravenous, should be considered in SSc patients with (progressive) interstitial lung disease. A 1-year treatment has modest symptomatic benefit and may be followed by maintenance therapy with azathioprine. Typical dosing regimens include 6–12× monthly i.v. infusions of 500–1,000 mg/m^2 or 2 mg/kg oral doses. Long-term oral treatment, arbitrarily defined as >2-year continuous treatment, should be avoided. Frequent reassessments and intensive monitoring of blood and urine are required, which should follow (inter)national guidelines. Cyclophosphamide treatment may be considered for dcSSc patients with severe and/or progressive skin disease, refractory to conventional immunosuppressive treatment. Mesna should be considered to prevent hemorrhagic cystitis especially when long oral courses are given, but evidence that this prevents bladder cancer is lacking [12].

Immunoablative Therapy with High-Dose Cyclophosphamide Followed by Autologous Hematopoietic Stem Cell Transplantation

More aggressive approaches with immunoablative therapy followed by autologous hematopoietic stem cell transplantation (HSCT) have been evaluated as a therapeutic strategy in systemic sclerosis in several pilot studies and registry analyses – the small, phase 2, randomized, controlled Autologous Stem Cell Systemic Sclerosis Immune Suppression Trial

(ASSIST) and the larger, phase 3, randomized, controlled Autologous Stem cell Transplantation International Scleroderma (ASTIS) trial [33–41]. HSCT may be seen as a means to dose-escalate cyclophosphamide to the extent that immunoablation is achieved, thus facilitating a rebooting of the immune system [42]. High-dose cyclophosphamide is not myeloablative, thus sparing hematopoietic stem cells, but is followed by reinfusion of hematopoietic stem cells nonetheless as a safety measure to shorten the duration of aplasia and reduce the risk of infection and bleeding. Several transplant regimens have been employed with most also including antithymocyte globulin and/or low-dose total body irradiation to add to the immunoablative effects of high-dose cyclophosphamide. Both unmanipulated and CD34+-selected hematopoietic stem cell transplants have been used in different trials, the latter based on the premise that enrichment for CD34-stem cells prevents reinfusion of potentially autoreactive T and B cells. The ASSIST trial was an open-label, single-center, randomized, phase 2 trial, in which 19 SSc patients with pulmonary involvement were treated with HSCT involving a regimen with high-dose cyclophosphamide, antithymocyte, and reinfusion of unmanipulated hematopoietic stem cells (treatment arm) or 6× monthly pulse intravenous cyclophosphamide (control arm). At 12-month follow-up, all ten patients treated with HSCT showed improvement in skin score (MRSS decrease by at least 25 %) and in lung function (increase of at least 10 % in FVC) compared with none of the nine patients in the control arm [72, 73]. No treatment-related mortality was observed in this small trial.

Results from the international phase 3 ASTIS trial showed that HSCT in patients with early dcSSc (disease duration 4 years or less) who had features of poor prognosis (most of whom had evidence of interstitial lung disease) experienced a survival benefit over conventional immunosuppression (40). In this study, 156 patients were randomly assigned to either 12× monthly intravenous cyclophosphamide (750 mg/m^2) ($n=77$) or to high-dose cyclophosphamide and rabbit-antithymocyte globulin ($n=79$), followed by HSCT. At a median of 5.8 years of follow-up, there was a significant event-free survival (death or irreversible organ failure) benefit in the transplantation group: of a total of 53 events, 22 had been observed in the HSCT group (19 deaths and 3 irreversible organ failures) and 31 in the control group (23 deaths and 8 irreversible organ failures) resulting in a hazard ratio of 0.34 (95 % confidence interval (CI), 0.16–0.74) at 4 years and beyond. A post hoc analysis revealed that the survival benefit after HSC transplantation was particularly noticeable in never smokers. This approach, while clearly of benefit for patients with a poor prognosis, is not for all patients, as 8 out of 78 (10.4 %) of all transplanted patients died from treatment-related mortality, most related to heart failure or respiratory insufficiency. The efficacy of HSCT was also superior on secondary end points (modified Rodnan skin score, functional ability as assessed by the health-assessment questionnaire (HAQ), vital capacity, and quality of life) over the first 2 years of follow-up. A slight, transient drop in creatinine clearance occurred in the transplant group, which was ascribed to the nephrotoxic effects of medication used during conditioning. Thus, HSCT can be viewed as a therapeutic option for patients with aggressive or poor-prognosis systemic sclerosis. Additional trials have also been initiated. For example, a large North-American multicenter trial comparing monthly intravenous cyclophosphamide compared to high-dose cyclophosphamide and total body irradiation (SCOT) has completed enrollment, but results are not yet available. Another multicenter open-label study (STAT) of HSCT and long-term immunosuppression (mycophenolate) for dcSSc is currently recruiting subjects.

Azathioprine

Clinical Pharmacology and Mechanism of Action

Azathioprine is a prodrug which is converted to 6-mercaptopurine involving the removal of an imidazole group [43]. 6-Mercaptopurine is a purine analog that acts as a cycle-specific antimetabolite chemotherapeutic agent interfering with the synthesis of nucleotides, thereby inhibiting proliferation of lymphocytes. Two enzymes, xanthine oxidase and thiopurine methyltransferase (TPMT), shunt mercaptopurine metabolites to relatively inactive compounds, whereas other enzymes, such as hypoxanthine-guanine phosphoribosyltransferase, lead to the formation of cytotoxic thiopurine nucleotides. Thiopurine metabolites, such as thioguanine nucleotides, decrease the de novo synthesis of purine nucleotides by inhibiting amidotransferase enzymes and purine ribonucleotide interconversion and are incorporated into DNA and RNA. The incorporation of thioguanine nucleotides into the nucleic acids of cells is thought to mediate the cytotoxicity of azathioprine, whereas inhibition of purine synthesis may be more important in decreasing cellular proliferation. Leukopenia is unnecessary for immunosuppression. Azathioprine decreases the circulating lymphocyte count, suppresses lymphocyte proliferation, inhibits antibody production, inhibits monocyte production, suppresses natural killer cell activity, and inhibits cell-mediated and humoral immunity.

Oral azathioprine is well absorbed and rapidly converted to 6-mercaptopurine (6-MP), which is further metabolized to several compounds including 6-thiourate, that are excreted in urine. The plasma half-life of azathioprine is less than 15 min but 1–3 h of the active derivative 6-MP. The half-life of the intracellular, active 6-thioguanine nucleotides is estimated to be 1–2 weeks, however, and concentrations do not change over the 24 h dose period in patients receiving daily azathioprine.

Azathioprine is often started at a dose of 1 mg/kg daily, and if this is tolerated, the dose is increased to 2–2.5 mg/kg after 2–4 weeks. A gradual increase in dose is often better tolerated. The onset of immunosuppressive effects is relatively slow, over several weeks, presumably because the active thioguanine metabolites slowly accumulate intracellularly. Reversible myelosuppression is dose related but varies among individuals. Low-dose azathioprine (1–2 mg/kg/day) rarely results in leukopenia or thrombocytopenia. Pure red cell aplasia is also rare. Severe myelosuppression is uncommon and caused by low or absent TPMT activity. Decreased TPMT activity leads to a decreased ability to detoxify mercaptopurine and results in increased formation of cytotoxic thioguanine metabolites and clinical toxicity. On the basis of this, some national guidelines recommend that information on TPMT genotype or activity is obtained before starting azathioprine, but this is not common practice in all countries. TPMT activity is polymorphic with a trimodal distribution. Approximately 90 % of subjects show high activity, 10 % show intermediate activity, and 0.3 % (the subjects homozygous for the poorly functional polymorphisms) show very low activity. The median TPMT activity in African-Americans is approximately 17 % lower than in white Americans. The 1 in 300 subjects with low or absent TPMT activity is at great risk of severe azathioprine-induced myelosuppression, which has a delayed but sudden onset, most commonly 4–10 weeks after azathioprine has been started. More than half of all cases of leukopenia in patients receiving azathioprine have a normal TPMT genotype and phenotype, however. Liver test abnormalities occur in 34 % but are seldom serious. Infection is less common with azathioprine than with alkylating agents; however, infections with a range of bacterial and nonbacterial pathogens, including herpes zoster and cytomegalovirus, may occur. The rate of infection when azathioprine is administered alone or with low doses of glucocorticoids is approximately 2.5 per 100 person-years of exposure. There are limited data in rheumatologic diseases, and although it is being used in pregnancy, azathioprine is better avoided in pregnancy and lactation if possible.

Therapeutic Use in Systemic Sclerosis

Azathioprine is commonly used in SSc, especially as glucocorticoid-sparing agent after induction treatment with cyclophosphamide in early diffuse SSc [44] and lung disease [26, 28]. The effects of azathioprine versus cyclophosphamide were compared head-to-head in patients with early diffuse SSc in a randomized, unblinded clinical trial where 30 patients received oral cyclophosphamide (2 mg/kg daily for 12 months and then maintained on 1 mg/kg daily) and 30 patients received oral azathioprine (2.5 mg/kg daily for 12 months and then maintained on 2 mg/kg daily) [45]. During the first 6 months of the trial, the patients also received prednisolone, which was started at a dosage of 15 mg daily and tapered to zero by the end of the sixth month. Cyclophosphamide was more effective than azathioprine in improving skin score, Raynaud's symptoms, and ESR and maintaining lung function. No life-threatening or irreversible adverse reactions were observed in either group.

With its slow mode of action, azathioprine is not the best first-line therapy to treat severe manifestations of SSc, yet it has a good track record in rheumatology as a glucocorticoid-sparing agent in inflammatory joint disease and myositis. It is also commonly used as maintenance therapy after induction with cyclophosphamide, including SSc-related interstitial lung disease. Frequent blood monitoring is recommended in accordance with (inter)national guidelines, even in those patients with normal TMPT activity.

Methotrexate

Clinical Pharmacology and Mechanism of Action

Methotrexate was originally developed as an anticancer drug and is still used in high doses to treat malignancies such as breast cancer. Methotrexate in high doses competitively inhibits dihydrofolate reductase (DHFR), an enzyme that participates in the tetrahydrofolate synthesis. The affinity of methotrexate for DHFR is about 1,000-fold that of folate for DHFR. Dihydrofolate reductase catalyzes the conversion of dihydrofolate to the active tetrahydrofolate. Folic acid is needed for the de novo synthesis of the nucleoside thymidine, required for DNA synthesis. Also, folate is needed for purine-base synthesis, so all purine synthesis will be inhibited. Methotrexate inhibits the synthesis of DNA, RNA, thymidylates, and proteins. Methotrexate acts specifically during DNA and RNA synthesis, and thus, it is cytotoxic during the S-phase of the cell cycle, thus having a more toxic effect on rapidly dividing cells. In lower doses, inhibition of dihydrofolate reductase (DHFR) is not thought to be the main mechanism. Low-dose methotrexate inhibits AICAR transformylase, which leads to increased AICA ribose (AICAR transformylase's substrate). The AICA ribose inhibits adenosine deaminase, resulting in a buildup of extracellular adenosine. Extracellular adenosine inhibits the expression of IL-2 receptors on circulating T lymphocytes, causing a suppression of the immune system and thus ameliorating the effects of the immune disorder.

Methotrexate is a highly teratogenic drug. Women must not take the drug during pregnancy, if there is a risk of becoming pregnant, or if they are breastfeeding. Men who are trying to get their partner pregnant must also not take the drug. To engage in any of these activities (after discontinuing the drug), women must wait until the end of a full ovulation cycle and men must wait 3 months.

The most common side effects are ulcerative stomatitis, leukopenia, nausea, and abdominal distress.

Therapeutic Use in Systemic Sclerosis

Methotrexate is the anchor drug in the treatment of rheumatoid arthritis, and it is also commonly used in the treatment of skin and joint manifestations of SSc patients. In a small blinded, placebo-controlled, crossover trial of intramuscular MTX (15 mg/week), the active treatment group ($n = 17$) responded better than the placebo group ($n = 12$) at 6 months, based on predefined response criteria and skin score ($p = 0.06$) [46]. The trial continued for 1 year, but most patients who initially took MTX chose not to participate in the placebo phase, so the randomized, blinded trial data that were available pertained to only 6 months. The trial included both limited and diffuse cases, whose course and responsiveness to treatment may be very different. In another placebo-controlled trial in a more homogeneous group of 71 patients with dcSSc and disease duration of 3 years or less, 12-month treatment with oral MTX (15–17.5 mg/week) was only slightly more effective than placebo [47]. When between-group differences for changes in scores from baseline to 12 months were examined using intent-to-treat methodology, MTX appeared to have a favorable effect on the MRSS (−4.3 in the MTX group versus 1.8 in the placebo group, $p < 0.009$), but differences in the degree of change in the DLCO, patient and physician global assessment, and HAQ were not significant. Dropout rates were similar in the two groups. Thirteen patients allocated to the MTX group and 11 allocated to the placebo group dropped out prior to study completion, most due to treatment inefficacy. One MTX-treated patient dropped out due to oral ulcers, and seven patients in the placebo group and three in the MTX group died during the trial and the follow-up period (median follow-up 1.5 years). MTX had no obvious effect compared with placebo in terms of proportions of responders. The significantly higher proportion of patients on glucocorticoids in the placebo group, the relative low doses of (oral) MTX in this trial, and the conventional statistical analysis may have contributed to the disappointing results. In a recent reanalysis of the data using Bayesian modeling, the authors concluded that MTX has a high probability of beneficial effects on skin score and global assessment [48].

Methotrexate should therefore be considered for patients with early dcSSc to reduce skin thickening or arrest progression of skin involvement. There is no evidence that methotrexate ameliorates signs or symptoms resulting from visceral organ involvement, myositis, or inflammatory joint disease in this subset of patients, but data are limited. In patients with RA/SSc overlap syndrome and SSc patients with demonstrable synovitis, methotrexate should be considered to treat signs and symptoms from inflammatory joint disease.

Mycophenolate Mofetil

Clinical Pharmacology and Mechanism of Action

Mycophenolate mofetil (MMF), a prodrug, is the inactive 2-morpholinoester of mycophenolic acid (MPA), which is rapidly absorbed and hydrolyzed to the active mycophenolic acid (MPA), an antibiotic with immunosuppressive effects. There are two pathways for the synthesis of guanine nucleotides: the de novo pathway and the salvage pathway. MPA reversibly inhibits inosine monophosphate dehydrogenase, a crucial enzyme for the de novo synthesis of guanosine purines [49]. T and B lymphocytes, in contrast to many other cells, are critically dependent on the de novo purine synthesis pathway and are a relatively selective target for MPA, accounting for the ability of the drug to inhibit reversibly lymphocyte proliferation and antibody formation without myelotoxicity. MPA also inhibits proliferation of fibroblasts, endothelial cells, and arterial smooth muscle cells and prevents deposition and contraction of collagen, extracellular matrix (ECM) proteins, and smooth muscle actin. MMF is rapidly and completely absorbed and de-esterified to the active MPA, which is highly (98 %) protein bound. Most MPA (>99 %) is found in plasma, with very little in cells; most is glucuronidated to the poorly active, stable phenolic glucuronide, which is eliminated in the urine. The half-life of MPA is 16 h. MPA concentrations may vary fivefold to tenfold in individuals receiving the same dose.

MMF is generally well tolerated. The most common side effects are gastrointestinal, such as diarrhea, nausea, abdominal pain, and vomiting. Occasional infections, leukopenia, lymphocytopenia, and elevated liver enzymes can occur.

Effective daily dosages of MMF range from 0.5 to 1.5 g twice a day. MMF is associated with miscarriage and congenital malformations when used during pregnancy and should therefore be avoided whenever possible by women trying to conceive. It is transferred into the mother's milk, and extreme caution should be used in women with child-bearing potential and lactating mothers.

Therapeutic Use in Systemic Sclerosis

MMF is fast becoming a popular immunosuppressive drug in rheumatology, especially in the treatment of lupus nephritis, polymyositis, dermatomyositis, and systemic sclerosis. It has also been used in the treatment of early diffuse SSc. A 1-year course of MMF after a 5-day course of i.v. rabbit antithymocyte globulin (ATG) in a small open-label study in 13 patients with early dcSSc resulted in a statistically significant drop of the mean skin score from 28 at baseline to 17 [50]. Hand contractures worsened during the study. Mean measurements of systemic disease remained stable. One patient died after a scleroderma renal crisis. Five patients developed serum sickness after ATG treatment, but this was controlled by corticosteroid therapy. MMF therapy was well tolerated. A retrospective analysis of patients with dcSSc from the same tertiary referral center showed that the 109 patients treated with MMF had a better survival than 63 matched controls treated with other immunosuppressive drugs in the same center [51]. Treatment with MMF was very well tolerated. Of all patients, 12 % experienced adverse reactions with gastrointestinal (GI) tract disturbances and infections being most frequent. MMF was discontinued due to disease stabilization in 9 %, side effects in 8 %, and no effect on the disease activity in 14 % of the patients. There was a significantly lower frequency of clinically significant pulmonary fibrosis in the MMF-treated cohort ($p=0.037$) and significantly better 5-year survival from disease onset and from commencement of treatment ($p=0.027$ and $p=0.012$, respectively). There was no significant difference between the two groups in terms of modified Rodnan skin score and forced vital capacity (FVC) change.

A regimen of glucocorticoids and MMF was evaluated in 16 SSc patients, 9 with skin disease and 7 with active ILD [52]. Patients received three consecutive daily i.v. MP pulses, followed by five additional monthly i.v. MP pulses. MMF (0.5 g bid for 1 week and then 1 g bid) and low-dose (5–10 mg/day) oral prednisolone were prescribed for 1 year. The MRSS and HAQ significantly improved over time. In ILD patients, VC, FEV1, and DLCO significantly improved. Although the difference was not statistically significant, ground-glass lesions decreased, based on semiquantitative planimetry analyses performed on chest high-resolution computed tomography. Toxicity was low and none of the patients suffered from renal crisis.

To investigate whether MMF had any effect on lung disease, five patients with dcSSc and recent-onset alveolitis were treated with MMF and small (≤10 mg/day) doses of prednisolone [53]. One patient with long-standing fibrosing alveolitis was later added to the cohort. After 4–6 months of MMF therapy, DLCO improved significantly compared with pretreatment (mean DLCO 75.4 % vs 64.2 % of predicted value, respectively, $p=0.033$). Values of FVC also improved, with the difference almost reaching levels of statistical significance (mean FVC 76.2 % vs 65.6 % of predicted value, $p=0.057$). Ground-glass opacities cleared in three of four patients with recent-onset alveolitis and were reduced in one patient after 6–8 months of treatment. Breathlessness and cough improved by 3 months. A possible treatment failure was seen in one patient. However, in five patients, functional and clinical improvement was sustained during the study period. No adverse events were recorded in this ongoing clinical trial.

In another study, 15 patients with dcSSc were treated with MMF alone over a 12-month period [54]. The MRSS significantly improved in those patients who tolerated the medication for >3 months ($p<0.0001$), and there was a statistically significant improvement in the Medsger severity scores of the general ($p=0.05$), peripheral vascular involvement ($p=0.05$), and skin ($p=0.0003$) scores. The SF-36 scores improved ($p=0.05$), and the pulmonary function studies showed a trend toward improvement, though not of statistical significance. The mean pulmonary artery pressure by 2D echocardiography did not change.

The effects of MMF on lung function were investigated in a retrospective study in 13 SSc patients with evidence of SSc-ILD on chest CT and who received >1 g/day of MMF for ≥6 months and had pulmonary function data available [55]. MMF was associated with a significant improvement in VC (mean, + 159 mL; confidence interval [CI], +30 to +289 mL and +4 % of the predicted normal value; CI, +2 to +7 %) after 12 months of treatment. In contrast, patients had a significant decrease in VC (mean, −239 mL; CI, −477 to −0.5 mL; and −5 % of the predicted normal value; CI, −11 to −0.3 %) in the 12 months prior to MMF treatment. DLCO did not change significantly during MMF treatment (mean, +1 % of the predicted normal value; CI, −2 to +5 %) but decreased significantly in the 12 months prior to treatment (mean, −5 % of the predicted normal value; CI, −10 to −1 %).

In a similar retrospective study involving 17 SSc patients with radiological evidence of ILD treated with MMF (2 g/day) for at least 12 months, demographics, bronchoalveolar lavage (BAL) findings, pulmonary physiology, and high-resolution computed tomography were recorded at baseline and after 12 and 24 months of therapy [56]. Four improved, 12 were stable, and only 1 worsened. After 12 months of therapy, radiological findings ($n=15$) were stable in 11 patients, worse in 3, and improved in 1. There were no side effects attributable to MMF therapy recorded.

In a retrospective study in ten patients with SSc-ILD treated with MMF (2 g/day) for 12 months, a significant increase in FVC and a nonsignificant increase in DLCO were found at 12 months in patients on MMF ($p=0.04$ and 0.66, respectively) but no effect on MRSS [57].

To compare the effects of different immunosuppressive strategies, a retrospective analysis of patients with dcSSc within 3 years of the onset of skin thickening was done with collection of standardized entry and follow-up data for 3 years [58]. The five different protocols were (1) intravenous cyclophosphamide followed by MMF, (2) antithymocyte globulin followed by MMF, (3) MMF alone, (4) no disease-modifying treatment, (5) and other immunosuppressant treatments. The study included 147 patients from 12 centers. Numbers of patients starting on protocols 1–5 were 29, 25, 61, 19, and 13, respectively. MRSS decreased over time from 24 (IQ 19–32) at baseline to 15.5 (IQ 9–24.5) at 3 years. Although there were differences in the magnitude of the change for different protocols, there were no significant differences between protocols in the rate of change of MRSS over time ($p=0.43$). When inverse probability weights were applied, the results remained nonsignificant ($p=0.41$).

MMF has a favorable risk-benefit ratio relative to other immunomodulatory therapies, and no specific toxicity issues have been reported in SSc patients on long-term use. MMF is used to treat SSc-related skin and lung disease, but conclusive data are lacking as to whether it is more effective in these conditions than methotrexate and cyclophosphamide, respectively.

Not all studies of MMF demonstrate benefit or improvement. Henes and colleagues assessed the impact of enteric-coated MMF on skin and pulmonary manifestations in 11 patients with dcSSc over 12 months followed by long-term follow-up [59]. Pulmonary involvement was determined by lung tissue densitometry using high-resolution computed tomography comparing baseline to 12 month. Three patients discontinued the study before month 6 (two due to side effects, one to disease progression). For the remaining eight patients, the median MRSS was nonsignificantly reduced from 13.5 to 11. Median lung density and high attenuation values were unchanged; however, intermediate attenuation values increased slightly, suggesting some degree of worsening pulmonary fibrosis. Four patients remain on MMF without clinical signs of progression after 50 months of follow-up.

Biologicals

The term "biologicals" refers to a class of medications that are produced by means of biological processes involving recombinant DNA technology. The biologicals used in rheumatology are either fusion proteins or monoclonal antibodies. In contrast to conventional immunosuppressive drugs, biologicals target a single cytokine or cell surface molecule. Biologicals are expensive due to the complex manufacturing process and quality control issues, and their use is therefore restricted in most countries due to differences in approved usage and payment systems among countries. The use of biologicals to treat SSc patients followed their successful introduction in the treatment of rheumatoid arthritis. Those now licensed for the treatment of RA neutralize pro-inflammatory cytokines such as TNF-alpha (infliximab, etanercept, adalimumab, golimumab, certolizumab) and IL-6 (tocilizumab), block co-stimulation between antigen-presenting cells and T cells (abatacept), or deplete B lymphocytes (rituximab). In SSc open-label clinical trials have been done with interferon-gamma (IFN-γ), IFN-alpha (IFN-α), human anti-transforming growth factor ß1 antibody, and more recently with infliximab, etanercept, and rituximab. These trials were preceded by preclinical work showing the potential importance of pro-inflammatory and pro-fibrotic cytokines and B lymphocytes in SSc [60–62]. Nevertheless, the clinical trials with IFN-γ, IFN-α, and anti-TGF-β yielded disappointing results [63–65], while recent studies with TNF inhibitors and B cell depletion have been more encouraging.

In a retrospective analysis of 18 patients with SSc (6 limited, 12 diffuse) with active joint disease treated with standard doses of etanercept (25 mg twice weekly or 50 mg once weekly), 15 showed marked improvement of signs and symptoms of joint disease and of HAQ, while skin scores remained stable [66]. Lung function parameters deteriorated to the same extent as untreated controls. There were no opportunistic infections, anaphylaxes, hospitalizations, or deaths attributed to etanercept therapy. Etanercept was discontinued in one patient because of a lupus-like reaction and a marked decline in lung function in another.

In another 26-week open-label pilot study, 16 dcSSc patients with substantial functional impairment and disease severity as assessed by the physician global visual analogue scale (VAS) received five infusions of infliximab (5 mg/kg) [67]. For all clinical outcome measures (including modified Rodnan skin score and HAQ-DI), there was an overall improvement between baseline and week 26, but none reached statistical significance. Serum aminoterminal propeptide of type III collagen level and secretion of type I collagen by dermal fibroblasts were significantly lower at week 26 compared with baseline. There were no deaths during the study and no suspected unexpected serious adverse reactions. Twenty-one serious adverse events (AE) occurred in seven subjects, mostly attributable to dcSSc. One hundred and twenty-seven distinct AE occurred in 16 subjects. Of these, 19 AE (15%) were probably or definitely related to infliximab treatment. Eight (50%) patients prematurely discontinued infliximab. Anti-infliximab antibodies developed during the study in five subjects and were associated with suspected infusion reactions.

B cells are increasingly thought to play a significant role in the pathogenesis of SSc. Activated B cells produce among other cytokines IL-6, IL-10, and TGF-β and may induce ECM deposition and increase inflammation as a result [62]; IL-6 secreted by B cells in particular appears to play a prominent role in promoting fibrosis and by enhancing inflammation. SSc dermal fibroblasts constitutively show a fourfold increase in IL-6 production compared to healthy control fibroblasts, and secretion of IL-6 from lung fibroblasts is induced by SSc lung-derived B cells [73]. IL-10 produced by activated B cells inhibits IL-12 production by dendritic cells, thereby promoting Th_2 differentiation. B cells thus appear to be critical for the development of Th_2 responses which characterize the cytokine milieu responsible for tissue fibrosis and antibody production.

B-cell depletion using rituximab, a chimeric monoclonal antibody directed against the B-cell marker CD20, showed potential efficacy in four open-label studies [68–71].

In one of these studies, nine patients with progressive dcSSc despite cyclophosphamide were treated with rituximab, 1 g at time 0 and after 14 days. After 6 months, patients presented a median decrease of the skin score of 43.3 % (range 21.1–64.0 %) and a decrease in disease activity index and disease severity index [60]. IL-6 levels decreased during the follow-up. After treatment, a complete depletion of peripheral blood B cells was observed in all but two patients. Only three patients presented CD20-positive cells in the biopsy of the involved skin at baseline. No major side effects were observed.

Moazedi-Fuerst et al. reported on the potential benefit of a modified rituxan (RTX) regimen in SSc-associated pulmonary disease. Five consecutive patients with dcSSc and ILD had failed conventional therapy with intravenous cyclophosphamide. All five received 500 mg RTX on day 0 and day 14 every 3 months for 12 months. All five showed decreased MRSS and improved FVC % and DLCO % from baseline to 12 months. Three of five patients showed reduced lung fibrosis by HRCT read qualitatively.

Kier et al. retrospectively reviewed the outcomes of 50 patients (excluding patients with idiopathic pulmonary fibrosis) with severe progressive ILD treated with RTX between 2010 and 2012 [74]. The connective tissue disease-ILD subgroup ($n=33$) included eight SSc patients. The other underlying CTD diagnoses included idiopathic inflammatory myopathy in ten patients, undifferentiated CTD in four patients, mixed connective tissue disease and rheumatoid arthritis in two patients, and one patient each with systemic lupus erythematosus and Sjogren's syndrome. Prior treatment included intravenous cyclophosphamide in 32 patients and mycophenolate mofetil in one patient. For this subgroup, the trajectory of FVC fell by 13 % in the 6–12 months prior to RTX treatment but then increased by 8.9 % following RTX ($p<0.01$). Similarly, the percent predicted DLCO fell 18 % pre-RTX but then stabilized post-RTX (p, 0.01) [74].

In the largest study to date of rituxan (RTX) in scleroderma, Jordan and colleagues of the European Scleroderma Trials and Research (EUSTAR) group (comprising 42 centers) evaluated 63 patients using a nested, case-control design [75]. Patients received rituxan in routine clinical practice on the decision of their physicians and were compared to matched controls within the EUSTAR dataset. Inclusion criteria included (1) fulfillment of ACR criteria for SSc, (2) treatment with rituxan, and (3) availability of follow-up data. Matching parameters for skin/lung fibrosis were the modified Rodnan skin score (MRSS), forced vital capacity (FVC), follow-up duration, scleroderma subtype, disease duration, and immunosuppressive co-treatment. The primary objective was to measure the change of MRSS from baseline to follow-up between the RTX and control group with the secondary objective being to measure the change of the FVC from baseline to follow-up between the RTX and control groups in patients with evidence for ILD and safety measures. In the dcSSc subset with mean disease duration of 5 years ($n=35$), there was a significant decrease in mean MRSS from 22.1 ± 1.6 to 17.7 ± 1.6 ($p=0.0005$) after a mean of 6 months of follow-up and a decrease of -16.7 ± 5.5 %. By confining the analysis to an enriched population of severe, dcSSc defined as MRSS ≥16 ($n=25$), the mean MRSS decreased from 26.6 ± 1.4 to 20.3 ± 1.8 ($p=0.0001$). When compared to the matched control group, the percent change in the RTX group versus baseline was above the minimal clinically important difference for the MRSS (−24.0 ± 5.2 % vs −7.7 ± 4.3 % in the control group). The effects of RTX treatment on lung function were analyzed in SSc patients with FVC<70 % predicted and with parallel evidence for ILD on HRCT ($n=9$). Compared to baseline, following RTX treatment, FVC remained stable (60.6 ± 2.4 vs 61.3 ± 4.1, $p=0.5$) and DLCO improved significantly (41.1 ± 2.8 vs 44.8 ± 2.7 %; $p=0.03$). Matched controls by contrast showed decline in FVC and when compared to RTX-treated patients, significant differences in the percent (0.4 ± 4.4 vs −7.7 ± 3.6; $p=-0.02$) and absolute change (0.8 ± 2.2 vs −4.8 ± 1.7; $p=0.01$) in FVC. There was no change in DLCO between RTX-treated and matched control-treated patients [75]. The safety data in RTX-treated patients was largely encouraging with "findings consistent with recent reports in other rheumatic autoimmune diseases." In particular, infections were noted in 21 % of the RTX-treated patients, but no serious adverse events were reported and no cases of progressive multifocal leukoencephalopathy. Furthermore, no cases of scleroderma renal crisis were reported among the RTX group despite the use of co-treatment with i.v. methylprednisolone with the RTX infusion [75].

Anti-IL-6 Tocilizumab

Tocilizumab, a humanized antibody against the IL-6 receptor, was used in two patients with progressive dcSSc. Treatment with six monthly infusions of tocilizumab 8 mg/kg resulted in a significant reduction of skin thickening paralleled by reduction of myofibroblast infiltration and thinning of collagen bundles in skin biopsies but no improvement of lung function in the one patient with ILD. No adverse events were reported [61].

In a larger observational study, Elhai et al. studied the safety and effectiveness of tocilizumab and abatacept in SSc polyarthritis or myopathy. Twenty patients with SSc with

Table 41.3 Therapeutic trials of rituximab in SSc

Reference	Design	*N*	Disease duration	Ab profile	RTX regimen	Previous therapy	Skin outcome	Lung outcome
Smith	Open label	8	<4 years	4 anti-Scl70	1 g 2 weeks apart	MTX, pen Etanercept, CYC	MRSS decrease by 40 %	Stable
Lafyatis	Open label	15	18 months	3 anti-ScL70	1 g 2 weeks apart			
Bosello	Open label	9	24 months		1 g 2 weeks apart			
Daoussis		8	6.9 years					
Daoussis								
Jordan	Open label, nested case control	63						
Moazedi-Fuerst		9						

refractory polyarthritis and seven with refractory myopathy from the EUSTAR network included 15 of who received tocilizumab and 12 abatacept [76]. After 5 months, tocilizumab induced significant improvement in the 28 joint count Disease Activity Score (DAS) with 10/15 patients achieving a EULAR good response. Treatment was stopped in two patients because of lack of efficacy. Abatacept resulted in improvement in joint scores with 6/11 patients achieving EULAR good response criteria, but had no effect on muscle outcome measures. No significant change was seen in skin or lung fibrosis in either group, and both treatments were well tolerated [76].

A phase 2/3 placebo-controlled trial in 87 dcSSc patients was recently completed, showing a trend toward improvement of the modified Rodnan skin score in the tocilizumab-treated group at 24 weeks. Exploratory analysis of change in FVC showed more placebo than tocilizumab-treated patients (81 % vs 50 %) with progression of FVC decline (≤0 %) and 27 % of placebo patients vs 3 % of tocilizumab-treated patients with ≥10 % FVC decline ($p = 0.009$) [77].

Anti-IL-1: Rilonacept

Animal models of fibrosis suggest that IL-1 plays a key role. The mechanism linking IL-1 to fibrosis involves both TGF-β and smad3-dependent stimulation. TGF-β, IL-1, and IL-6 participate in Th17 cell priming and are increased in the tissues and serum of SSc patients. Rilonacept is a dimeric fusion protein, consisting of the ligand-binding domains of the extracellular portions of the human IL-1 receptor accessory protein linked to the Fc portion of human IgG1. It is designed to attach to and neutralize IL-1 before IL-1 can bind to cell surface receptors and generate signals that trigger inflammation. Rilonacept has been shown to be effective in autoinflammatory syndromes characterized by high levels of IL-1 such as CAPS (cryopyrin-associated periodic syndromes), DIRA (deficiency of IL-1 receptor antagonist), and in systemic juvenile idiopathic arthritis (JIA) [78, 79]. Rilonacept is currently undergoing evaluation in a short-term (8 week), randomized, placebo-controlled trial with a biomarker of skin-based primary outcome (Table 41.3).

Anti-TGF-ß Fresolimumab

Fresolimumab is a first-in-class human IgG4 kappa recombinant monoclonal antibody capable of neutralizing all mammalian isoforms of TGF-β. It appears to have higher affinity for TGF-β than its predecessor CAT-192 which showed no efficacy in early dcSSc. In a phase 1 study in patients with advanced malignant melanoma or renal cell cancer, it demonstrated acceptable safety and preliminary evidence of antitumor activity [80]. It is currently undergoing evaluation in early dcSSc (MRSS >15 without significant ILD or history of scleroderma renal crisis) with a skin biomarker to detect TGF-β-responsive gene expression and MRSS as primary outcomes (Table 41.3).

Antitype 1 Interferon

Peripheral blood cells from SSc and SLE patients share a similar IFN-inducible gene expression pattern. In particular, a subset of SSc patients shows a "lupus-like" high IFN-inducible phenotype that correlates with the presence of anti-topoisomerase-1 and anti-U1RNA antibodies. Furthermore, IFN-α has been reported to induce TLR3 in dermal fibroblasts and stimulation with poly I:C resulted in increased production of the profibrotic cytokine IL-6 and increased expression of type I IFN-induced genes, and proteins are found in the blood and skin or patients with SSc. Also, IFN therapy appeared to exacerbate SSc [81]. A phase 1,

Table 41.4 Planned or ongoing studies with biologicals in systemic sclerosis, registered on ClinicalTrials.gov

Biological	Biological target	ClinicalTrials.gov ID	Phase	Patients
MEDI-546	Type I IFN receptor	NCT00930683	I	SSc
Abatacept (CTLA-4Ig)	CTLA (T cell)	NCT00442611	I/II	DcSSc
Rituximab	CD20 (B cell)	NCT01086540	II	SSc-PAH
Tocilizumab	IL-6 receptor	NCT01532869	II/III	DcSSc
Rilonacept	IL-1 receptor	NCT01538719	II	DcSSc
Fresolimumab	TGF-β	NCT01284322	I	DcSSc

open-label dose-escalation trial of MEDI-546, an antitype interferon monoclonal antibody, was evaluated in patients with predominately dcSSc (94.1 %) who had a MRSS of at least 2 on an area amenable to repeat biopsy [82]. MEDI-546 is a human IgG kappa monoclonal antibody directed against the heterodimeric type I IFN-α receptor. Following a 28-day screening period, subjects were enrolled to receive either escalating single or multiple intravenous doses of MEDI-546. Of 34 subjects, 32 completed treatment. Four treatment emergent serious adverse events occurred including a skin ulcer, osteomyelitis, vertigo, and chronic myelogenous leukemia (CML). Only CML was considered possibly treatment related. Peak inhibition of the type 1 IFN signature occurred in whole blood within 1 day and in the skin after 7 days. In patients with positive baseline skin signatures for type 1 IFN-inducible genes (15 of the total, 11 in the single-dose groups, 4 in the multiple-dose groups), there was a reduction in type 1 IFN-inducible genes in the skin seen at day 7 and day 28 [82], respectively.

Biologicals have revolutionized the field of rheumatology, and new clinical trials in systemic sclerosis are planned or in progress (Table 41.4).

Summary and Conclusions

There are now a number of immunosuppressive strategies to treat SSc or its individual manifestations but few robust clinical trial data to convincingly choose one or another or to decide on the best timing of treatment. Based on pathogenetic considerations and circumstantial evidence, it is commonly assumed that immunosuppressive therapy is more effective in early inflammatory and/or progressive disease. Immunomodulatory drugs include alkylating agents such as cyclophosphamide and purine analogue, cytotoxic drugs such as azathioprine with a long history of clinical use in rheumatology, and relatively newer noncytotoxic immunosuppressants such as MMF. Their potential efficacy and safety profiles are generally well known, and serious toxicities can usually be prevented by careful monitoring of laboratory tests – white blood counts, liver and renal function, and electrolytes. As a general rule, combination therapy of the different immunosuppressants

Table 41.5 Indications for the use of individual immunosuppressive drugs

SSc manifestation	Treatment options
Skin thickening	MTX, MMF, Pred, CTX, RTX
Myocarditis, pericarditis	Pred
Interstitial lung disease	CTX, MMF, RTX
Myositis, arthritis	Pred, MTX, RTX, TNFi

MTX methotrexate, *MMF* mycophenolate mofetil, *Pred* prednisolone, *CTX* cyclophosphamide, *RTX* rituximab, *TNFi* TNF-alpha inhibitor

discussed above should be avoided. The individual response to immunosuppressive therapy can be highly variable, and decisions to continue a chosen immunosuppressant should be revisited on a regular basis, weighing the benefits and side effects. The risks of immunosuppressive treatment should be taken into account before (usually long-term) treatment is initiated. Immunosuppressive drugs are often prescribed for long periods of time which leads to an increased risk of bacterial, viral, and fungal infection and a reduced response to vaccinations. Cytostatic agents should be avoided in pregnancy and lactation, and referral to a fertility clinic should be considered for all fertile male and female patients. Other immunosuppressive drugs should only be used in pregnancy if the potential benefits outweigh the potential risks.

Immunoablative therapy and autologous hematopoietic stem cell transplantation is the only current therapy for SSc which has been shown to improve survival over conventional immunosuppressive therapy and should be considered for poor prognosis dcSSc patients with early disease duration. This treatment approach currently has a 10 % treatment-associated mortality and therefore its use should be confined to patients with high risk of mortality from the disease itself. Biologic therapies are rapidly being deployed in clinical trials in SSc. Currently rituximab shows the greatest promise in open-label studies as a disease-modifying therapy for SSc, and TNF antagonists show preliminary benefit in joint manifestations of SSc. Additional exciting biologic agents are currently in the development pipeline.

An overview of treatment options for individual disease manifestations is shown in Table 41.5.

References

1. Hunzelmann N, Moinzadeh P, Genth E, Krieg T, Lehmacher W, Melchers I, et al. High frequency of corticosteroid and immunosuppressive therapy in patients with systemic sclerosis despite limited evidence for efficacy. Arthritis Res Ther. 2009;11:R30.
2. Kowal-Bielecka O, Landewé R, Avouac J, Chwiesko S, Miniati I, Czirjak L, et al. EULAR recommendations for the treatment of systemic sclerosis: a report from the EULAR Scleroderma Trials and Research group (EUSTAR). Ann Rheum Dis. 2009;68:620–8.
3. Rodnan GP, Black RL, Bollet AJ, Bunim JJ. Observations on the use of prednisone in patients with progressive systemic sclerosis (diffuse scleroderma). Ann Intern Med. 1956;44:16–29.
4. Stahn C, Buttgereit F. Genomic and nongenomic effects of glucocorticoids. Nat Clin Pract Rheumatol. 2008;4:525–33.
5. Rhen T, Cidlowski JA. Antiinflammatory action of glucocorticoids-new mechanisms for old drugs. N Engl J Med. 2005;353: 1711–23.
6. Takehara K. Treatment of early diffuse cutaneous systemic sclerosis patients in Japan by low-dose corticosteroids for skin involvement. Clin Exp Rheumatol. 2004;22(3 Suppl 33):S87–9.
7. Antoniades L, Sfikakis PP, Mavrikakis M. Glucocorticoid effects on myocardial performance in patients with systemic sclerosis. Clin Exp Rheumatol. 2001;19:431–7.
8. Stack J, McLaughlin P, Sinnot C, Henry M, MacEneaney P, Eltahir A, et al. Successful control of scleroderma myocarditis using a combination of cyclophosphamide and methylprednisolone. Scand J Rheumatol. 2010;39:349–50.
9. Domiciano DS, Bonfá E, Borges CT, Kairalla RA, Capelozzi VL, Parra E, et al. A long-term prospective randomized controlled study of non-specific interstitial pneumonia (NSIP) treatment in scleroderma. Clin Rheumatol. 2011;30:223–9.
10. Steen VD, Medsger Jr TA. Case-control study of corticosteroids and other drugs that either precipitate or protect from the development of scleroderma renal crisis. Arthritis Rheum. 1998;41:1613–9.
11. de Jonge ME, Huitema AD, Rodenhuis S, Beijnen JH. Clinical pharmacokinetics of cyclophosphamide. Clin Pharmacokinet. 2005;44:1135–64.
12. Monach PA, Arnold LM, Merkel PA. Incidence and prevention of bladder toxicity from cyclophosphamide in the treatment of rheumatic diseases. A data-driven review. Arthritis Rheum. 2010;62: 9–21.
13. Silver RM, Warrick JH, Kinsella MB, Staudt LS, Baumann MH, Strange C. Cyclophosphamide and low-dose prednisone therapy in patients with systemic sclerosis (scleroderma) with interstitial lung disease. J Rheumatol. 1993;20:838–44.
14. Schnabel A, Reuter M, Gross WL. Intravenous pulse cyclophosphamide in the treatment of interstitial lung disease due to collagen vascular diseases. Arthritis Rheum. 1998;41:1215–20.
15. Várai G, Earle L, Jimenez SA, Steiner RM, Varga J. A pilot study of intermittent intravenous cyclophosphamide for the treatment of systemic sclerosis-associated lung disease. J Rheumatol. 1998;25: 1325–9.
16. Davas EM, Peppas C, Maragou M, Alvanou E, Hondros D, Dantis PC. Intravenous cyclophosphamide pulse therapy for the treatment of lung disease associated with scleroderma. Clin Rheumatol. 1999;18:455–61.
17. Giacomelli R, Valentini G, Salsano F, Cipriani P, Sambo P, Conforti ML, et al. Cyclophosphamide pulse regimen in the treatment of alveolitis in systemic sclerosis. J Rheumatol. 2002;29:731–6.
18. Beretta L, Caronni M, Raimondi M, Ponti A, Viscuso T, Origgi L, et al. Oral cyclophosphamide improves pulmonary function in scleroderma patients with fibrosing alveolitis: experience in one centre. Clin Rheumatol. 2007;26:168–72.
19. White B, Moore WC, Wigley FM, Qing Xiao H, Wise RA. Cyclophosphamide is associated with pulmonary function and survival benefit in patients with scleroderma and alveolitis. Ann Intern Med. 2000;132:947–54.
20. Tashkin DP, Elashoff R, Clements PJ, Goldin J, Roth MD, Furst DE, et al. Scleroderma Lung Study Research Group. Cyclophosphamide versus placebo in scleroderma lung disease. N Engl J Med. 2006; 354:2655–66.
21. Tashkin DP, Elashoff R, Clements PJ, Roth MD, Furst DE, Silver RM, et al. Effects of 1-year treatment with cyclophosphamide on outcomes at 2 years in scleroderma lung disease. Am J Respir Crit Care Med. 2007;176:1026–34.
22. Goldin J, Elashoff R, Kim HJ, Yan X, Lynch D, Strollo D, et al. Treatment of scleroderma-interstitial lung disease with cyclophosphamide is associated with less progressive fibrosis on serial thoracic high-resolution CT scan than placebo: findings from the scleroderma lung study. Chest. 2009;136:1333–40.
23. Hant FN, Ludwicka-Bradley A, Wang HJ, Li N, Elashoff R, Tashkin DP, et al. Scleroderma Lung Study Research Group. Surfactant protein D and KL-6 as serum biomarkers of interstitial lung disease in patients with scleroderma. J Rheumatol. 2009;36:773–80.
24. Au K, Mayes MD, Maranian P, Clements PJ, Khanna D, Steen VD, et al. Course of dermal ulcers and musculoskeletal involvement in systemic sclerosis patients in the scleroderma lung study. Arthritis Care Res. 2010;62:1772–8.
25. Strange C, Bolster MB, Roth MD, Silver RM, Theodore A, Goldin J, et al. Bronchoalveolar lavage and response to cyclophosphamide in scleroderma interstitial lung disease. Am J Respir Crit Care Med. 2008;177:91–8.
26. Hoyles RK, Ellis RW, Wellsbury J, Lees B, Newlands P, Goh NS, et al. A multicenter, prospective, randomized, double-blind, placebo-controlled trial of corticosteroids and intravenous cyclophosphamide followed by oral azathioprine for the treatment of pulmonary fibrosis in scleroderma. Arthritis Rheum. 2006;54: 3962–70.
27. Bérezné A, Valeyre D, Ranque B, Guillevin L, Mouthon L. Interstitial lung disease associated with systemic sclerosis: what is the evidence for efficacy of cyclophosphamide? Ann NY Acad Sci. 2007;1110:271–84.
28. Bérezné A, Ranque B, Valeyre D, Brauner M, Allanore Y, Launay D, et al. Therapeutic strategy combining intravenous cyclophosphamide followed by oral azathioprine to treat worsening interstitial lung disease associated with systemic sclerosis: a retrospective multicenter open-label study. J Rheumatol. 2008;35:1064–72.
29. Sanchez O, Sitbon O, Jaïs X, Simonneau G, Humbert M. Immunosuppressive therapy in connective tissue diseases-associated pulmonary arterial hypertension. Chest. 2006;130:182–9.
30. Schulz SW, O'Brien M, Maqsood M, Sandorfi N, Del Galdo F, Jimenez SA. Improvement of severe systemic sclerosis-associated gastric antral vascular ectasia following immunosuppressive treatment with intravenous cyclophosphamide. J Rheumatol. 2009;36: 1653–6.
31. Caramaschi P, Volpe A, Pieropan S, Tinazzi I, Mahamid H, Bambara LM, et al. Cyclophosphamide treatment improves microvessel damage in systemic sclerosis. Clin Rheumatol. 2009;28:391–5.
32. Furuya Y, Okazaki Y, Kaji K, Sato S, Takehara K, Kuwana M. Mobilization of endothelial progenitor cells by intravenous cyclophosphamide in patients with systemic sclerosis. Rheumatology. 2010;49:2375–80.
33. Binks M, Passweg JR, Furst D, et al. Phase I/II trial of autologous stem cell transplantation in systemic sclerosis: procedure-related mortality and impact on skin disease. Ann Rheum Dis. 2001; 60:577–84.
34. Farge D, Marolleau JP, Zohar S, et al. Autologous bone marrow transplantation in the treatment of refractory systemic sclerosis: early results from a French multicentre phase I–II study. Br J Haematol. 2002;119:726–39.
35. Farge D, Passweg J, van Laar JM, et al. Autologous stem cell transplantation in the treatment of systemic sclerosis: report from the EBMT/EULAR Registry. Ann Rheum Dis. 2004;63:974–81.
36. Nash RA, McSweeney PA, Crofford LJ, Abidi M, Chen CS, Godwin JD, et al. High-dose immunosuppressive therapy and

autologous hematopoietic cell transplantation for severe systemic sclerosis: long-term follow-up of the US multicenter pilot study. Blood. 2007;110:1388–96.
37. Vonk MC, Marjanovic Z, van den Hoogen FH, et al. Long-term follow-up results after autologous haematopoietic stem cell transplantation for severe systemic sclerosis. Ann Rheum Dis. 2008;67:98–104.
38. Henes JC, Schmalzing M, Vogel W, et al. Optimization of autologous stem cell transplantation for systemic sclerosis – a single-center longterm experience in 26 patients with severe organ manifestations. J Rheumatol. 2012;39:269–75.
39. Burt RK, Shah SJ, Dill K, et al. Autologous non-myeloablative haemopoietic stem-cell transplantation compared with pulse cyclophosphamide once per month for systemic sclerosis (ASSIST): an open-label, randomised phase 2 trial. Lancet. 2011;378:498–506.
40. van Laar JM, Farge D, Sont JK, Naraghi K, Marjanovic Z, Larghero J, et al. Autologous hematopoietic stem cell transplantation vs intravenous pulse cyclophosphamide in diffuse cutaneous systemic sclerosis: a randomized clinical trial. JAMA. 2014;311(24):2490–8.
41. van Laar JM, Naraghi K, Tyndall A. Haematopoietic stem cell transplantation for poor-prognosis systemic sclerosis. Rheumatology (Oxford). 2015 Dec;54(12):2126–33.
42. Hügle T, van Laar JM. Stem cell transplantation for rheumatic autoimmune diseases. Arthritis Res Ther. 2008;10:217.
43. van Scoik KG, Johnson CA, Porter WR. The pharmacology and metabolism of the thiopurine drugs 6-mercaptopurine and azathioprine. Drug Metab Rev. 1985;16:157–74.
44. Paone C, Chiarolanza I, Cuomo G, Ruocco L, Vettori S, Menegozzo M, et al. Twelve-month azathioprine as maintenance therapy in early diffuse systemic sclerosis patients treated for 1-year with low dose cyclophosphamide pulse therapy. Clin Exp Rheumatol. 2007;25:613–6.
45. Nadashkevich O, Davis P, Fritzler M, Kovalenko W. A randomized unblinded trial of cyclophosphamide versus azathioprine in the treatment of systemic sclerosis. Clin Rheumatol. 2006;25:205–12.
46. van den Hoogen FH, Boerbooms AM, Swaak AJ, Rasker JJ, van Lier HJ, van de Putte LB. Comparison of methotrexate with placebo in the treatment of systemic sclerosis: a 24-week randomized double-blind trial, followed by a 24-week observational trial. Br J Rheumatol. 1996;35:364–72.
47. Pope JE, Bellamy N, Seibold JR, Baron M, Ellman M, Carette S, et al. A randomized, controlled trial of methotrexate versus placebo in early diffuse scleroderma. Arthritis Rheum. 2001;44:1351–8.
48. Johnson SR, Feldman BM, Pope JE, Tomlinson GA. Shifting our thinking about uncommon disease trials: the case of methotrexate in scleroderma. J Rheumatol. 2009;36:323–9.
49. Lipsky JJ. Mycophenolate mofetil. Lancet. 1996;348:1357–9.
50. Stratton RJ, Wilson H, Black CM. Pilot study of anti-thymocyte globulin plus mycophenolate mofetil in recent-onset diffuse scleroderma. Rheumatology. 2001;40:84–8.
51. Nihtyanova SI, Brough GM, Black CM, Denton CP. Mycophenolate mofetil in diffuse cutaneous systemic sclerosis–a retrospective analysis. Rheumatology. 2007;46:442–5.
52. Vanthuyne M, Blockmans D, Westhovens R, Roufosse F, Cogan E, Coche E, et al. A pilot study of mycophenolate mofetil combined to intravenous methylprednisolone pulses and oral low-dose glucocorticoids in severe early systemic sclerosis. Clin Exp Rheumatol. 2007;25:287–92.
53. Liossis SN, Bounas A, Andonopoulos AP. Mycophenolate mofetil as first-line treatment improves clinically evident early scleroderma lung disease. Rheumatology. 2006;45:1005–8.
54. Derk CT, Grace E, Shenin M, Naik M, Schulz S, Xiong W. A prospective open-label study of mycophenolate mofetil for the treatment of diffuse systemic sclerosis. Rheumatology. 2009;48:1595–9.
55. Gerbino AJ, Goss CH, Molitor JA. Effect of mycophenolate mofetil on pulmonary function in scleroderma-associated interstitial lung disease. Chest. 2008;133:455–60.
56. Zamora AC, Wolters PJ, Collard HR, Connolly MK, Elicker BM, Webb WR, et al. Use of mycophenolate mofetil to treat scleroderma-associated interstitial lung disease. Respir Med. 2008;102:150–5.
57. Koutroumpas A, Ziogas A, Alexiou I, Barouta G, Sakkas LI. Mycophenolate mofetil in systemic sclerosis-associated interstitial lung disease. Clin Rheumatol. 2010;29:1167–8.
58. Herrick AL, Lunt M, Whidby N, Ennis H, Silman A, McHugh N, et al. Observational study of treatment outcome in early diffuse cutaneous systemic sclerosis. J Rheumatol. 2010;37:116–24.
59. Henes JC, Horger M, Amberger C, Schmalzing M, Fierlbeck G, Kanz L, Koetter I. Enteric-coated mycophenolate sodium for progressive systemic sclerosis – a prospective open-label study with CT histography for monitoring of pulmonary fibrosis. Clin Rheumatol. 2013;32:673–8.
60. Varga J, Abraham D. Systemic sclerosis: a prototypic multisystem fibrotic disorder. J Clin Invest. 2007;117:557–67.
61. Koca SS, Isik A, Ozercan IH, Ustundag B, Evren B, Metin K. Effectiveness of etanercept in bleomycin-induced experimental scleroderma. Rheumatology. 2008;47:172–5.
62. Kraaij MD, van Laar JM. The role of B cells in systemic sclerosis. Biologics. 2008;2:389–95.
63. Stevens W, Vancheeswaran R, Black CM, UK Systemic Sclerosis Study Group. Alpha interferon-2a (Roferon-A) in the treatment of diffuse cutaneous systemic sclerosis: a pilot study. Br J Rheumatol. 1992;31:683–9.
64. Black CM, Silman AJ, Herrick AL, Denton CP, Wilson H, Newman J, et al. Interferon-a does not improve outcome at one year in patients with diffuse cutaneous scleroderma: results of a randomized, double-blind, placebo-controlled trial. Arthritis Rheum. 1999;42:299–305.
65. Denton CP, Merkel PA, Furst DE, Khanna D, Emery P, Hsu VM, et al. Recombinant human anti-TGF-beta 1 antibody therapy in SSc: a randomized, placebo-controlled phase I/II trial of CAT-192. Arthritis Rheum. 2007;56:323–33.
66. Lam GK, Hummers LK, Woods A, Wigley FM. Efficacy and safety of etanercept in the treatment of scleroderma-associated joint disease. J Rheumatol. 2007;34:1636–7.
67. Denton CP, Engelhart M, Tvede N, Wilson H, Khan K, Shiwen X, et al. An open-label pilot study of infliximab therapy in diffuse cutaneous systemic sclerosis. Ann Rheum Dis. 2009;68:1433–9.
68. Lafyatis R, Kissin E, York M, Farina G, Viger K, Fritzler MJ, et al. B cell depletion with rituximab in patients with diffuse cutaneous systemic sclerosis. Arthritis Rheum. 2009;60:578–83.
69. Smith V, Van Praet JT, Vandooren B, Van der Cruyssen B, Naeyaert JM, Decuman S, et al. Rituximab in diffuse cutaneous systemic sclerosis: an open-label clinical and histopathological study. Ann Rheum Dis. 2010;69:193–7.
70. Daoussis D, Liossis SC, Tsamandas AC, Kalogeropoulou C, Kazantzi A, Sirinian C, et al. Experience with rituximab in scleroderma: results from a 1-year, proof-of-principle study. Rheumatology. 2010;49:271–80.
71. Shima Y, Kuwahara Y, Murota H, Kitaba S, Kawai M, Hirano T, et al. The skin of patients with systemic sclerosis softened during the treatment with IL-6 receptor antibody tocilizumab. Rheumatology. 2010;49:2408–12.

Recommended Reading

72. Burt RK, et al. Autologous non-myeloablative haemopoietic stem-cell transplantation compared with pulse cyclophosphamide once per month for systemic sclerosis (ASSIST): an open-label, randomised phase 2 trial. Lancet. 2011;378(9790):498–506.
73. Bosello S, et al. B cells in systemic sclerosis: a possible target for therapy. Autoimmun Rev. 2011;10(10):624–30.

74. Keir GJ, et al. Severe interstitial lung disease in connective tissue disease: rituximab as rescue therapy. Eur Respir J. 2012;40(3):641–8.
75. Jordan S, Distler JH, Maurer B, Huscher D, van Laar JM, Allanore Y, Distler O; EUSTAR Rituximab study group. Effects and safety of rituximab in systemic sclerosis: an analysis from the European Scleroderma Trial and Research (EUSTAR) group. Ann Rheum Dis. 2015 Jun;74(6):1188–94.
76. Elhai M, Meunier M, Matucci-Cerinic M, Maurer B, Riemekasten G, Leturcq T, Pellerito R, Von Mühlen CA, Vacca A, Airo P, Bartoli F, Fiori G, Bokarewa M, Riccieri V, Becker M, Avouac J, Müller-Ladner U, Distler O, Allanore Y; Outcomes of patients with systemic sclerosis-associated polyarthritis and myopathy treated with tocilizumab or abatacept: a EUSTAR observational study. Ann Rheum Dis. 2013 Jul;72(7):1217–20.
77. Khanna D, Denton CP, van Laar JM, et al. Safety and efficacy of subcutaneous tocilizumab in adults with systemic sclerosis: week 24 data from a phase 2/3 trial. Arthritis Rheum. 2014;66(S3):S833.
78. Jesus AA, Goldbach-Mansky R. IL-1 blockade in autoinflammatory syndromes. Annu Rev Med. 2014;65:223–44.
79. Lovell DJ, et al. Long-term safety and efficacy of rilonacept in patients with systemic juvenile idiopathic arthritis. Arthritis Rheum. 2013;65(9):2486–96.
80. Morris JC, et al. Phase I study of GC1008 (fresolimumab): a human anti-transforming growth factor-beta (TGFbeta) monoclonal antibody in patients with advanced malignant melanoma or renal cell carcinoma. PLoS One. 2014;9(3):e90353.
81. Black CM, et al. Interferon-alpha does not improve outcome at one year in patients with diffuse cutaneous scleroderma: results of a randomized, double-blind, placebo-controlled trial. Arthritis Rheum. 1999;42:299–305.
82. Goldberg A, et al. Dose-escalation of human anti-interferon-alpha receptor monoclonal antibody MEDI-546 in subjects with systemic sclerosis: a phase 1, multicenter, open-label study. Arthritis Res Ther. 2014;16(1):R57.

42 Investigative Approaches to Drug Therapy

Voon H. Ong and Christopher P. Denton

Current approaches to disease-modifying therapy in scleroderma together with strategies that are in use to tackle individual complications of the disease are reviewed in other chapters. Here, we will consider some of the novel approaches to therapy that are under evaluation and also the extent to which some established agents may have a broader effect on the disease process than was initially expected. Immunomodulatory strategies are largely covered elsewhere and will not be a major focus of the current chapter. The majority of therapeutic interventions for scleroderma that attempt to modify the disease process are immunomodulatory, and multiple innovative compounds have now entered clinical trials. However, scleroderma is a multifaceted disease, and it is likely that other mechanisms including vascular injury and fibrosis or epithelial damage may also be logically targeted. With this in mind, it is worthwhile to explore the novel mechanisms by which a number of therapies that are already in use may be regarded as potential disease-modifying treatments. In addition, there is an emerging list of therapies that target pivotal pathways or mediators that are emerging from studies of pathogenesis including animal models, from in vitro analysis of fibroblasts and from genetic or gene expression studies. Recent trials suggest that tyrosine kinase molecules may be potential candidates for therapy especially in the fibrotic phase of the disease, but the collective experience has been mixed. Similar experience has been reported with clinical trial with a weak monospecific antibody against TGF-β despite the extensive in vitro and animal data that supports TGF-β as an important mediator of fibrosis in SSc. Based on the new insights into the key role of effecter T cells in particular Th17, T regulatory and follicular helper T subsets have T-cell-directed therapies including abatacept, halofuginone, basiliximab, alemtuzumab and rapamycin and have been proposed to be clinically beneficial. HMG-CoA reductase inhibitors, endothelin receptor antagonists and phosphodiesterase type V inhibitor have been shown to be useful to treat the vascular manifestations associated with systemic sclerosis. Table 42.1 summarises some of the targeted approaches to treating scleroderma that fall within the arena of investigative approaches to drug therapy.

As discussed elsewhere, two major clinical subsets of scleroderma are recognised: diffuse cutaneous SSc (dcSSc) and limited cutaneous SSc (lcSSc). dcSSc is typically active in the first 3 years from onset with up to 50 % of the major organ complications occurring within this period [1]. However, recent data suggests that effective assessment and screening for internal organ complications has led to the improved 5-year survival from 69 % in the early 1990 to 84 % a decade later [2]. This is supported by an increasing better understanding of SSc and wider use of disease-modifying therapies for specific organ-based manifestations [3]. However, there are no effective treatments in halting fibrosis and preventing progression of the disease. This therefore highlights the unmet clinical need for this disease. In this review, we will discuss the recent developments in the treatment for SSc.

T-Cell-Directed Strategies

There is increasing data to support the scientific rationale to target T-cell signalling pathway in scleroderma [4–7]. Recent groups have demonstrated that there is an imbalance between Th17 and T regulatory cells in patients with SSc with increased levels of circulating Th17 subpopulation and levels of Th17-inducing cytokines including IL-6 and IL-23 [8, 9]. Although there are some contradictory reports regarding which Th subset may be relevant in the aetiopathogenesis of

V.H. Ong, PhD, FRCP (✉)
Centre for Rheumatology and Connective Tissue Diseases, UCL Medical School Royal Free Hospital, London, UK
e-mail: v.ong@ucl.ac.uk

C.P. Denton, PhD, FRCP
Division of Medicine, Department of Inflammation, Centre for Rheumatology and Connective Tissue Diseases, UCL Division of Medicine, Royal Free Hospital, London, UK

J. Varga et al. (eds.), *Scleroderma*, DOI 10.1007/978-3-319-31407-5_42

Table 42.1 Table of potential targeted molecular therapies in SSc

Candidate therapy	Target pathway	
Bosentan	Et_a/Et_b receptor	Vascular
Sildenafil	PDE-5	
Treprostinil	Prostacyclin	
AMD3100	CXCL 12/	Inflammatory
Halofuginone	Th17	
MLM-1202	CCR2	
Basiliximab	IL-2Rα	
Efalizumab	LFA1/1CAM1	
Tocilizumab	IL-6R	Fibrotic
Imatinib, dasatinib, nilotinib	C-Abl, c-Kit, Src, PDGF receptor	
AM095	LPA1 receptor	
CAT-192	TGF-β1	
Fresolimumab	TGF-β1, TGF-β2, TGF-β3	
FG-3019	CTGF ligand	
P144	TGF-β ligand	
Fasudil	Rho kinase	
Terguride	5HT2A/5HT2B receptor	
Rosiglitazone, IVA337	PPAR-γ	
Rapamycin	mTOR kinase	

SSc, targeting Th17 response may be a potential immunotherapeutic avenue to intervene in the progression of SSc [10]. Interestingly, Th17 cell differentiation was recently shown to be inhibited by halofuginone via the expression of genes associated with the amino acid starvation response. Given the significance of Th17 cells in autoimmunity, there is great interest in developing drugs such as halofuginone that inhibit these cells, without interfering with the function of the other T-helper-cell lineages [11]. Halofuginone has previously been demonstrated to abrogate collagen deposition presumably by interfering with TGF-β-mediated production of collagen by fibroblasts, and its therapeutic potential has also been explored in a clinical trial in SSc [12]. However, halofuginone does not inhibit the effector function of existing Th17 cells. This may limit its clinical potential, considering that T-cell activation occurs early in disease development in SSc [13]. Nonetheless, this work may rejuvenate research interest in pursuing halofuginone as a potential treatment of SSc.

The costimulatory molecules expressed by activated T cells may represent a putative target in SSc. Abatacept is the first drug in the class of selective costimulation molecules. De Paoli et al. reported that four patients who were resistant to other treatments (including cyclophosphamide, methotrexate, prednisolone) treated with abatacept showed clinical improvement with reduction in skin score of 1.3 units per month during a period of 8–30 months [14]. All patients reported improvement in lung function and in general well-being. All patients were able to taper other immunosuppressive treatments without flare of disease.

Chakravarty et al. reported the effect of abatacept in an RCT with ten patients given either abatacept or placebo at weeks 0, 2, 4 and every 4 weeks for 24 weeks [15]. Seven patients received abatacept. At baseline, there were no significant differences in skin score, Health Assessment Questionnaire-Disability Index (HAQ-DI) and patient and physician global assessments by visual analogue scale (VAS) between the two groups. Compared to those receiving placebo, those who received abatacept reported greater improvement in patient global assessment by VAS (−8 vs. −2.7, $p = 0.023$). After adjusting for disease duration, abatacept significantly improved skin score by −9.8 points at 6 month compared to those with placebo; this improvement exceeds the minimal clinical important difference of 5.3 (threshold for significant difference in validated skin score as outcome measure in scleroderma) [16]. In this study, there was reduction in T-cell signalling gene expression that is relevant in the pathogenesis of the disease; the improvement was particularly demonstrable in the inflammatory molecular subset of the disease. No deaths or serious adverse events related to abatacept occurred and overall the study drug was well tolerated. An observational study using the European League Against Rheumatism (EULAR) Scleroderma Trials and Research (EUSTAR) database also showed that abatacept was safe and well tolerated in 12 patients with scleroderma [17]. This had led to a larger Phase 2 multicentre double-bind randomised controlled trial of abatacept in scleroderma (ClinicalTrials.gov Identifier: NCT02161406).

Blockade of Cell Trafficking: Chemokine Ligand/Receptor Axis as Potential Therapy

The initial promise of small-molecule antagonists including anti-receptor and anti-chemokine antibodies as potential candidate therapies for autoimmune diseases including SSc has yet to translate to clinical practice. Various issues have been raised to account for the apparent lack of clinical efficacy. It may be that a higher degree of receptor occupancy sufficiently abrogates chemokine activity to ensure a clinical response or that there may be redundancy in the chemokine-receptor interaction such that a blockade of multiple chemokine receptors is required.

A number of clinical trials however have reported promising outcomes in autoimmune diseases and fibrotic diseases [18, 19]. Recent studies suggest upregulation of CXCL12 and CXCR4 in the lesional skin of patients with early SSc [20]. This is also supported by the presence of CXCR4+ haematopoietic circulating progenitor cells, and it has been reported that the levels of these progenitor cells correlate with both the skin and pulmonary involvement [21, 22]. It is also now apparent that fibroblasts are derived from several cell types including circulating fibrocytes as fibrosis develops [23]. Human fibrocytes express several chemokine receptors including CXCR4, and they can migrate to area of fibrosis in response to CXCL12 gradients [24]. The administration of neutralising anti-CXCL12 antibodies to bleomycin-treated mice resulted in significantly reduced fibrocyte extravasation into the lung, reduced collagen deposition in the lungs and reduced immunohistochemical expression of a-smooth muscle actin [25]. AMD3100 that inhibits the CXCL12/CXCR4 axis was recently approved for mobilisation of haematopoietic stem cells from the bone marrow to the circulating blood for transplantation in patients with non-Hodgkin's lymphoma. Cenicriviroc is a new dual CCR2 and CCR5 antagonist that has been evaluated in NASH, and there is some evidence that CCR5 similar to CXCR4 may be important in fibrocyte biology with increased levels on lung fibrocytes compared to circulating fibrocytes [26]. It is envisaged that similar strategies may be therapeutically feasible in SSc.

Targeting Epigenetic Alterations of Immune Cell Function

In a study of heritable changes in the gene function that occurs in the absence of a change in the DNA sequence, epigenetics is increasingly recognised to play an important role in the pathogenesis of several cancers, autoimmune diseases and inflammatory bowel disease [27]. Several recent publications have reported that epigenetic modifications in gene transcription are associated with increased collagen synthesis in SSc [28, 29]. Targeting these epigenetic mechanisms with DNA methylation inhibitors (5-azacytidine), histone deacetylase inhibitors (trichostatin A) and RNA silencing strategies may reduce the excessive production of extracellular matrix proteins in SSc [30, 31]. Several histone deacetylase inhibitors are presently in clinical trials in cancer, and it is envisaged these targets may find a niche in treatment of SSc [32]. Recent preclinical experiments suggest that bromodomain proteins may be potential targets for therapeutic intervention. These proteins are important epigenetic readers of lysine acetylation, and it seems that they are well placed to regulate programmes of gene expression that may be important in a number of disease states including fibrosis [33].

Targeting Against Endothelium-Derived Mediators in Vasculopathy

Endothelin

Bosentan was shown in clinical evaluation to be ineffective in improving Raynaud's symptoms in patients without pre-existing digital ulcers, but there was improvement in the functional scores [34]. These results confirmed observations from the RAPIDS study that demonstrated the lack of efficacy of bosentan in Raynaud's attacks although it was effective in reducing the number of new digital ulcers [35, 36]. A recent observational prospective study suggests that bosentan may be a safe long-term alternative for treating the recurrence of skin ulcers in SSc patients [37]. There is some rationale that targeting ET-1 may be relevant in another important vascular complication of renal crisis. Previous studies suggest that most of the profibrotic, pro-inflammatory and proliferative effects of ET-1 are mediated via the ET-A receptor. Results from an open-label study also suggest that bosentan may be used in combination with an ACE inhibitor for renal crisis [38], and the therapeutic potential that target ET-1 pathway in renal disease is currently evaluated in a clinical study (ClinicalTrials.gov Identifier: NCT02047708). This trial evaluates a highly selective endothelin receptor antagonist specific for the ET-A receptor subtype and will explore potential benefit in mild renal impairment in SSc as well as extending experience of targeting the endothelin axis in scleroderma renal crisis with a particular focus on the recovery occurring in some cases with standard therapy.

Targeting the Nitric Oxide Pathway

NO is an important mediator of endothelium-dependent vasodilatation, and there is interest in targeting this pathway therapeutically for scleroderma vasculopathy, for Raynaud's phenomenon and also for potential broader disease-modifying effects. In line with treatments for pulmonary arterial hypertension, two approaches have been used: firstly, to reduce the breakdown of the secondary messenger compound cGMP and, secondly, through the administration of a soluble guanylate cyclase agonist riociguat. The effects of NO are mediated via cyclic guanosine monophosphate (cGMP), and sildenafil and tadalafil act as selective inhibitors of cGMP-specific phosphodiesterase V to increase NO levels. This mechanism underlies its beneficial effect in treatment of SSc-associated vasculopathy including PAH. A majority of the current studies examined sildenafil as a potential therapy in vascular complications in SSc. It was shown to be effective for treatment of Raynaud's diseases in a placebo-controlled cross-over study [39]. Similar response was noted with a modified formulation daily dose with reduction in Raynaud's attack frequency in patients with limited cutaneous SSc [40]. In addition, other studies have reported a positive effect on ulcer healing [41]. More recently, tadalafil (20 mg on alternate days over 8 weeks) as adjunctive therapy was shown to have a similar effect with improvement in Raynaud's symptoms, healing of existing digital ulcers and preventing development of new ulcers in SSc [42].

There have been suggestions that the NO pathway, or downstream mediators such as cGMP, may have broader effects on fibrosis or inflammation. This is suggested by some evidence of benefit from sildenafil in other fibrotic diseases, including improved functional outcomes in idiopathic lung fibrosis [43], and also from preclinical evidence that riociguat may benefit fibrosis, specifically in preclinical models of scleroderma [44]. This is being tested in an ongoing placebo-controlled trial that will also test potential benefit for vasculopathy in SSc [ClinicalTrials.gov Identifier:NCT02283762].

Atorvastatin

In recent years, there has been considerable interest in the hypothesis that statins via its pleiotropic effect may have a favourable benefit on the three aspects of the SSc disease process: immune dysfunction, vasculopathy and fibrosis.

Very recently, Abou-Raya et al. reported improvements in both clinical and laboratory measurements in patients with SSc treated with atorvastatin [45, 46]. Subsequent study by Kuwana suggests that these effects may be sustained with prolonged use of atorvastatin over 24 months [47]. These results were replicated in other small series of SSc patients with simvastatin and pravastatin. Treatment with pravastatin was associated with a reduction in levels of von Willebrand factor, probably the gold standard marker of endothelial cell activation [48]. However, the caveat of these studies is the small sample size and the lack of placebo-controlled studies. Louneva also found that simvastatin inhibited collagen expression in both normal and SSc fibroblasts, suggesting that statins may have a favourable effect on fibrosis [49]. This was also supported by other studies that statins may reduce the progression of hepatic fibrosis and prevent cutaneous and pulmonary fibrosis in an experimental model of SSc [50, 51].

Prostacyclin Analogues

Parenteral prostacyclin analogues are occasionally used to treat difficult SSc-associated ulcerations. An oral formulation of treprostinil compound was investigated in a randomised placebo-controlled study among patients with digital ulceration, but there was no statistically significant reduction in net ulcer burden although subgroup analysis suggested that there may be a differential effect favouring those who harbour anti-centromere antibody [52]. There is evidence that prostacyclins may have an effect on several key profibrotic pathways in systemic sclerosis through effects on expression of key mediators such as CTGF [53] or CCL2 [54]. Zhu et al. recently showed that iloprost administered as a single intraperitoneal injection inhibits lung fibrosis in the bleomycin model of lung injury and fibrosis [55].

Inhibition of Cytokine Synthesis and/or Signalling

This section reviews the recent publication on target cytokines and associated signalling pathways in SSc.

Imatinib Mesylate

Tyrosine kinases are major downstream mediators for profibrotic cytokines TGF-β and PDGF, and these may be amenable to blockade using tyrosine kinase inhibitors. Imatinib mesylate is a small-molecule tyrosine kinase inhibitor that targets c-Abl, PDGF receptor, c-kit and c-fms. c-Abl is a key downstream signalling molecule of the non-Smad TGF-β-signalling pathway. Baroni et al. demonstrated that stimulatory autoantibodies against PDGFR are present in patients with SSc and in patients with chronic graft-versus-host disease but in those with primary Raynaud's disease. These autoantibodies stimulate the production of reactive oxygen species, leading to fibroblast activation and collagen production [56]. It is however important to note that other groups have not been able to demonstrate the presence of these autoantibodies as specific to SSc cohorts. Nonetheless, there is evidence to support that PDGF is an important profibrotic cytokine in SSc, and blockade of this pathway ameliorates the fibrosis in various experimental animal models of lung, dermal, renal and hepatic fibrosis. It is likely that by targeting both TGF-β and PDGF pathways, imatinib may be a promising treatment in SSc. Several open-label and randomised controlled studies have reported its efficacy in SSc. In addition, there are initial reports that imatinib may have an antifibrotic effect in other cutaneous diseases including nephrogenic systemic fibrosis and refractory chronic graft-versus-host disease [57, 58].

In a single, large, open-label prospective study with 30 patients with dcSSc, imatinib with a median dose of 300 mg daily conferred improvement for the cutaneous and pulmonary manifestations [59]. The change in mRSS was only apparent at 6 months with a mean improvement of −4.5 points (−2.6 to −6.5, $p < 0.001$), and this was sustained at 1 year. The skin response was associated with histological improvement with loosening of connective tissue and increase in interstitial space between collagen bundles. Curiously, an improvement was also observed in the FVC particularly in those without appreciable interstitial lung disease. Khanna et al. (2011) also reported that an improvement of FVC of 1.7% and mRSS of 3.9 [60]. Over 170 adverse events possibly related to imatinib were reported in the study, including 36 episodes of infections. The common adverse events were oedema (80 %), nausea (73 %), myalgia (60 %) and fatigue (53 %). Most of these are self-limited or resolve with dose modification with a median dose of 350 mg in over 80 % of patients. These results have to be interpreted cautiously, as there was no control group and heterogeneity of the patients with variable disease duration and organ involvement.

The effect of imatinib was examined in a proof-of-concept, double-blind, randomised controlled study with early active disease SSc [61]. Similar burden of adverse events was reported with intolerance to the full dose of imatinib in more than half of the patients, and only four patients completed the trial on 400 mg daily at 6 months. In contrast to the study by Spiera et al. [60], there was no change in skin score at 6 months, and the authors concluded that it is unlikely imatinib represents a feasible treatment for early SSc. Similarly, Prey et al. did not report improvement in skin score among 28 patients with either extensive morphoea or dcSSc [62]. A particular concern with imatinib is, however, cardiotoxicity, mediated through its inhibitory effect on c-Abl particularly in patients with pre-existing heart failure. However, this has not been reported in patients with SSc [63]. Results from a complementary prospective multicentre, open-label trial of imatinib with 27 patients treated over 24 weeks reported an increase in mRSS (+9.9 %) although there was a trend towards an improvement in mRSS (9–21 %) 24 weeks after the end of treatment period [64]. Recently, the efficacy of nilotinib, a related TKI with fewer fluid-related side effects, was evaluated in a pilot study with ten patients. Accepting that the patient numbers were small, the authors reported a significant improvement in mRSS by mean of 4.2 (16 %) at 6 months and 6.3 (23 %) at 12 months with good tolerability [65]. The data so far therefore do not suggest a major superiority over existing low-intensity immunosuppressive regimens for treating scleroderma skin disease [66].

Targeting PPAR Nuclear Hormone Receptors

Initially identified in adipose tissue, the nuclear receptor peroxisome proliferator-activated receptor gamma (PPARG) was shown recently to have an antifibrotic effect. It is proposed that defects in PPARG expression and function may affect the dysregulated fibrosis in SSc. Wei et al. showed that PPARG expression was impaired in SSc [67]. In addition, it has been reported that fibroblasts exposure to pharmacological PPARG ligands resulted in suppression of collagen synthesis, myofibroblast differentiation and other TGF-β-induced fibrotic responses in vitro [68–70]. Moreover, functional studies showed that PPARG agonist attenuated dermal fibrosis in several murine models of SSc by antagonistically targeting TGF-β/Smad and Akt signalling [71]. The clinical efficacy of this approach will be investigated in a proof-of-concept study (ClinicalTrials.gov Identifier NCT02503644) that explores potential benefit of a PPAR agonist with broader activity than previous PPAR-γ-specific agonists. Recent preclinical studies have suggested that other nuclear receptors, such as the orphan nuclear receptor NR4A1, may be potential therapeutic targets in fibrosis although the toxicity or potential benefit of such approaches will need to be explored in future proof of mechanism and concept clinical trials [72].

Rapamycin

Rapamycin is a novel macrolide immunosuppressive agent, and the mechanism underlying its immunomodulatory effect is that rapamycin binds to FK-506-binding protein (FKBP12) that inhibits the function of the mammalian target of rapamycin (mTOR), which in turn reduces protein phosphorylation, cell-cycle progression and cytokine production [73]. mTOR has been shown to positively regulate collagen production in dermal fibroblasts via a P1-3-kinase-independent pathway [74], and rapamycin has been shown to inhibit collagen production by dermal and lung fibroblasts [75, 76]. More recently, rapamycin was shown to inhibit the fibrotic response and immunological abnormalities in both TSK/+ mice and bleomycin-induced SSc model mice [77].

A recent comparative pilot study between rapamycin and methotrexate in early dcSSc demonstrated improvement in skin score within individual groups [78]. However, there was no significant difference in response between the rapamycin and methotrexate groups. However, the small sample size and lack of a placebo arm limit any assessment of the efficacy of either treatment in SSc.

Anti-TGF-β1 Antibody

Although TGF-β is believed to be a key profibrotic mediator in SSc, therapeutic blockade has not yet been shown to be effective in SSc. In a randomised controlled trial with a recombinant humanised monoclonal antibody to TGF-β1 on a small cohort of patients with dcSSc, there was no change in skin score over 6 months although this was a safety study not powered for efficacy [79]. Fresolimumab on the other hand that effectively blocks all three isoforms of TGF-β when administered to 15 patients at variable doses (1–5 mg/kg) resulted in rapid reduction in mRSS with decrease in TGF-β-regulated gene expression [80]. This lends strong support to the growing evidence that TGF-β blockade may benefit in SSc and other TGF-β-mediated diseases including focal segmental glomerulosclerosis [81]. Further studies to evaluate the safety of longer-term use of fresolimumab and other TGF-β-related pathways (including topical peptide inhibitor p144) are required.

Tocilizumab as a Potential Antifibrotic Agent

IL-6 is a pleiotropic cytokine produced by multiple cell types and has multiple important roles in haematopoiesis, inflammation and immune homeostasis in addition to regulation of many biological processes including growth and differentiation of T cells and those of dermal and epidermal origin [82]. Numerous reports have documented increased production of IL-6 in fibroblasts derived from the affected skin of SSc [83]. Increased levels of IL-6 have been demonstrated in other fibrotic diseases including keloid scars and lung fibrosis with upregulation of collagen synthesis and altered response to apoptosis of fibroblasts in these diseases [84, 85]. Moreover, IL-6-deficient transgenic mice display delayed cutaneous wound healing and reduced collagen deposition [86]. Kawaguchi demonstrated that the increase procollagen type I in cultured SSc fibroblasts may be abrogated using a neutralising anti-IL-6 antibody [83]. Recently, Ong et al. observed high-level expression of sera IL-6 levels in dcSSc is associated with thrombocytosis [87]. Moreover, sera IL-6 levels correlate positively with skin score and CRP.

Taken together, these results suggest that modulation of IL-6 signalling axis may therefore be a feasible pathway for the development of a novel therapeutic intervention in fibrotic pathways. In addition, given that IL-6 regulates the balance among the Th17, Tregs and follicular T-helper cells, it is possible that targeting the IL-6 pathway may promote immune tolerance in SSc [88]. Very recently, the efficacy and safety of tocilizumab was investigated in a Phase 2 study, and a trend in improvement in mRSS was observed among treated patients compared to placebo (−39 vs. −1.2, adjusted mean difference −2.7, $p=0.09$) at week 24, and this trend remained consistent at week 48 [89]. The safety profile in this study was consistent with the natural history of SSc and the known safety profile of TCZ with no new or unexpected safety concerns. These promising results have prompted a further Phase 3 trial to evaluate the efficacy of TCZ (ClinicalTrials.gov Identifier NCT02453256).

Lipid Mediators: LPA1 Antagonist

Recently several preclinical studies have stimulated interest in the potential of an antagonist of a number of lipid-derived mediators that may have a role in fibrosis. This is analogous to the potentially beneficial effect of prostanoid mediators such as prostacyclin. The largest evidence base is that supporting antagonist of the bioactive phospholipid lysophosphatidic acid (LPA) that signals through a family of at least six G protein-coupled receptors designated LPA1. Activation of the LPA receptor axes has been demonstrated in several experimental models for fibrosis [90]. Increased LPA levels were detected in SSc serum [91]. Antagonism of LPA axes has been shown to inhibit collagen accumulation, skin thickness and myofibroblast activation in several experimental models for SSc [92, 93]. Results from a double-blind, randomised, 8-week placebo-controlled and 16-week open-label extension on a selective antagonist of LPA1 receptor demonstrated improvement in mRSS with reduction of key skin fibrotic biomarkers [94]. These data suggest that modulation of LPA pathway is feasible and these results need to be confirmed in larger controlled study.

Serotonin Receptor Blockade

Serotonin (also known as 5-hydroxytryptamine) is a vasoactive amine that is synthesised from tryptophan and stored in platelets which release the serotonin by its serotonin receptors. Serotonin has a variety of agonist effects on different cell types, including an important role as a neurotransmitter. Serotonin levels in the CNS have a profound effect on mood. However, the cardiovascular and profibrotic activity of serotonin is increasingly appreciated. Its profibrotic role has been suggested in the tissue remodelling associated with lung and liver fibrosis and cancer [95, 96]. Increased serotonin levels were also described in murine models of bleomycin-induced dermal fibrosis and tight-skin-1 mice [97]. In both models, clopidogrel inhibited platelet activation leading to reduction in dermal fibrosis and myofibroblastic differentiation. However, several trials in fibrotic diseases with targeted agents used in these models have failed in the clinical arena, and the question remains whether these models are appropriate for SSc. It is therefore absolutely necessary to confirm these results in situ in human tissues. Increased expression of serotonin receptors was recently demonstrated in human lung fibrosis and blockade of the receptors with terguride, a 5-hydroxytryptamine 2A and 2B receptor antagonist, which ameliorates experimental lung fibrosis [98]. Moreover, it is important as a candidate mediator in Raynaud's phenomenon, and drugs that lower platelet serotonin levels may be beneficial [99]. There has been a suggested potential benefit for pulmonary arterial hypertension as serotonin receptors and serotonin transporters have been implicated in remodelling of the pulmonary arteries [100]. This is an exciting area for future study especially as a number of novel serotonin receptor antagonists have been developed as potential drug therapies for a variety of indications.

Rho Kinase Inhibitors

Rho kinases are important intracellular signalling intermediates that mediate the cellular responses to the small GTPase, RhoA in reorganisation of the actin cytoskeleton that contribute to the assembly of actin filaments and contractility. These

Rho-associated coiled-coil-forming kinases (ROCKs) usually operate downstream of G protein-coupled receptors. Recent evidence suggests that blockade of ROCK inhibits activation and differentiation of a resting fibroblast into metabolically active myofibroblast in vitro, and this consequently leads to reduction of key extracellular matrix proteins including collagen and fibronectin [101]. In an animal model of unilateral urethral obstructive renal disease, tubulointerstitial fibrosis was prevented with the ROCK inhibitor Y27632 [102]. Inhibition of ROCK may therefore provide a novel therapeutic approach to target the pathological activation of fibroblasts in SSc. Moreover, ROCK signalling has been shown to be important in the induction of smooth muscle–cell contraction and therefore may provide beneficial regulatory effects on the vascular abnormalities in SSc. Fasudil, a Rho kinase inhibitor, was studied in a small clinical trial for patients with Raynaud's, and there was no discernible effect on skin temperature recovery time with no effect on digital blood flow following cold challenge [103]. Although the current data suggests a low rate of adverse effects and favourable clinical experience with fasudil in cerebral vasospasm, the balance between benefit and harmful effects in SSc will be critical in defining its potential utility.

Other Small-Molecule Inhibitors

Current studies on the physiological and pathophysiological regulatory pathways have identified other novel targeted therapies that are potentially feasible for the treatment of fibrotic diseases including SSc. Pathological activation of tyrosine kinases may drive fibrogenesis, and there are ongoing research efforts to develop monoclonal antibodies against the extracellular domains of receptor TKs and small-molecule TK inhibitors that bind the intracellular domains of both receptor and non-receptor tyrosine kinases. Src kinases might be an interesting target for antifibrotic approaches as it may be activated by known profibrotic cytokines, including TGF-β, PDGF and endothelin-1 [104]. Dasatinib that targets Abl-kinases, PDGF receptors and Src kinases was shown to abrogate the synthesis of ECM in vitro and prevent experimental fibrosis in vivo [105]. Similarly, nilotinib that targets both c-Abl and PDGF receptors may have a beneficial effect on the proliferative vasculopathy of SSc [106]. Interestingly, there is emerging evidence that Src- and Syk-related tyrosine kinases may be critical in fibrocyte differentiation [107], and this may be relevant in fibrogenesis. However, the substantial adverse effects reported in a clinical trial with Syk inhibitor in rheumatoid arthritis may limit its potential utility in SSc [108]. Similarly, the role of VEGF and EGF receptor tyrosine kinase inhibitors (semaxanib, sorafenib, erlotinib and lapatinib) in the treatment of SSc is less clear, and further careful evaluation in preclinical and clinical models is warranted. The MAPK signalling pathway is another attractive therapeutic target as a modulator of inflammatory and immune response. Although recent trials on p38 MAPK inhibitors failed to demonstrate clinical efficacy in rheumatoid arthritis, preliminary reports on selective JAK2 inhibition in rheumatoid arthritis was promising, and pharmacodynamic studies revealed inhibition of IL6-induced STAT3 phosphorylation [109].

Nintedanib is another small molecule that abrogates activation of several receptor tyrosine kinase and non-receptor tyrosine kinases including VEGFR, PDGFR, FGFR and Src family kinases; all of these have been implicated in the fibrogenesis in SSc. Nintedanib has been shown to reduced dermal microvascular endothelial cell apoptosis and modulate the pulmonary vascular remodelling by its effect on the number of vascular smooth muscle cells. Its efficacy in idiopathic lung fibrosis has been reported recently with a relative reduction of decline in FVC and reduction in the risk of acute exacerbations [110]. With the limited efficacy of cyclophosphamide in SSc-related lung fibrosis, the pharmacological potential of tyrosine kinase inhibition is promising, and this will be explored in a Phase 3 study shortly.

Galectin-3

Galectin-3, a B-galactoside-binding lectin expressed by macrophages, is an interesting molecule which has emerged as a possible target in experimental models of fibrosis [111, 112]. A Phase 2 clinical trial with galectin-3 inhibitor, GR-MD-02, has recently been announced for patients with non-alcoholic steatohepatitis (NASH) with advanced fibrosis. There is some preliminary evidence to suggest that galectin-3 may be relevant in both fibrotic and vasculopathy aspects of SSc, but it remains unclear if this molecule represents a biomarker of disease or a key pathogenic target which may lend itself as an ideal target for therapy [113–115].

Ghrelin

As an endogenous ligand for growth hormone secretagogue receptors, ghrelin has been recognised to be important for energy homeostasis. More recently, it has been shown to have anti-inflammatory effects with downregulation of pro-inflammatory cytokines including TNF-β and IL-1α. Several studies have reported its antifibrotic effects in several experimental models including bleomycin-induced dermal fibrosis [116, 117]. In addition, Ariyasu et al. reported ghrelin improved gastric emptying in a small group of patients with SSc-associated gastrointestinal involvement although clinical improvement in satiety as assessed by visual analogue score was not observed [118]. Given the limited effective treatment

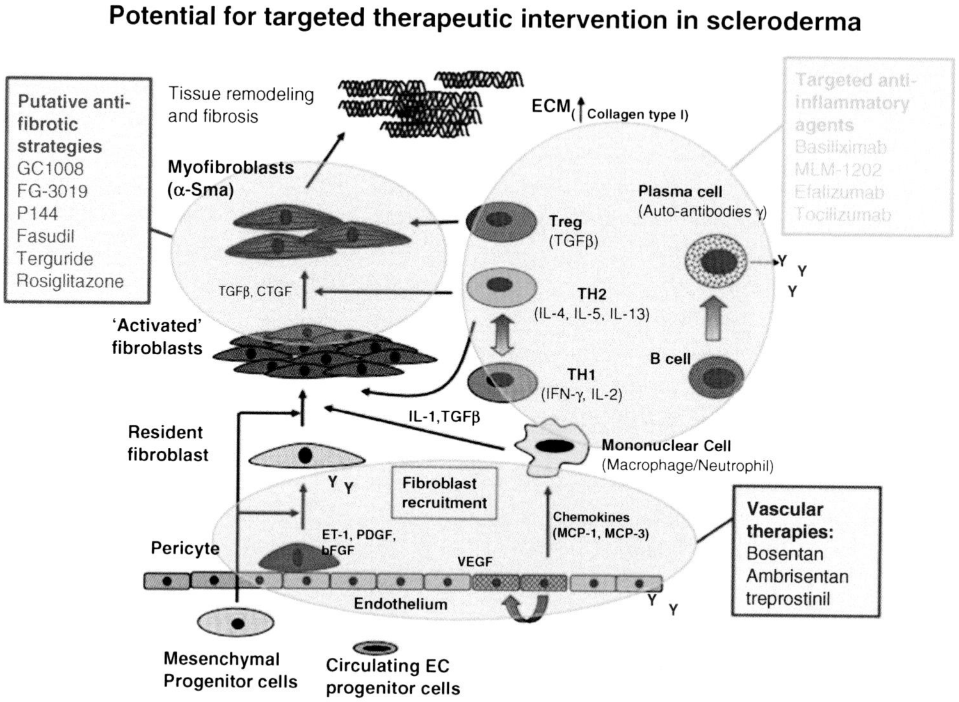

Fig. 42.1 Cellular interactions determine the pathogenic mechanisms in SSc. The multiple cell types relevant to the pathogenesis of SSc are illustrated. The different cell types and associated soluble inflammatory mediators are candidate targets for therapeutic strategies in SSc ERA endothelin receptor antagonists, PDE5 phosphodiesterase type V, *ASCT* autologous stem cell transplantation, *ET-1* endothelin-1, *TGF-β* transforming growth factor-beta, *CTGF* connective tissue growth factor, *PDGF* platelet-derived growth factor, *TNF-α* (tumour necrosis factor alpha), *IL-6* interleukin-6, *IL-4* interleukin-4 (Adapted from Denton et al. *Nature Clin Pract Rheum*, 2006)

in gastrointestinal related involvement in SSc with prokinetic agents currently available, these interesting preliminary results with ghrelin are worthy of further evaluation.

Concluding Remarks

Although many current therapeutic approaches for scleroderma are immunomodulatory, there is the potential to target broader aspects of pathogenesis. There are key mediators or pathways that are activated or dysregulated in scleroderma, and these may be amenable to therapeutic intervention using small-molecule inhibitors of biological therapeutics. Despite the complexity of the pathogenesis of SSc, there is growing understanding of the likely mechanisms that operate and link the different facets of the disease. These are highlighted in Fig. 42.1 which identifies key cell types of mediators that may be targeted. This has begun to be translated into therapeutic options such as targeted approaches in the vascular complications of SSc. Ongoing trials on broader approaches such as haematopoietic stem cell transplantation will better define the benefit of this treatment in selected patients. Research into future SSc therapies will continue to uncover a diverse multitude of prototypical targets that will include cytokines, chemokines and cellular targets. Accordingly, it is envisaged that insight into the role of Th17 and regulatory T cells and the epigenetic regulation of cytokine expression may offer novel intervention strategies to satisfy the unmet medical needs in SSc.

References

1. Shand L, Lunt M, Nihtyanova S, et al. Relationship between change in skin score and disease outcome in diffuse cutaneous systemic sclerosis: application of a latent linear trajectory model. Arthritis Rheum. 2007;56(7):2422–31.
2. Nihtyanova SI, Tang EC, Coghlan JG, et al. Improved survival in systemic sclerosis is associated with better ascertainment of internal organ disease: a retrospective cohort study. QJM. 2010;103:109–15.
3. Nihtyanova SI, Ong VH, Denton CP. Current management strategies for systemic sclerosis. Clin Exp Rheumatol. 2014;32(2 Supple 81):156–64.
4. Kalogerou A, Gelou E, Mountantonakis S. Early T cell activation in the skin from patients with systemic sclerosis. Ann Rheum Dis. 2005;64:1233–5.
5. Hasegawa M, Fujimoto M, Matsushita T, et al. Augmented ICOS expression in patients with early diffuse cutaneous systemic sclerosis. Rheumatology (Oxford). 2013;52:242–51.
6. Brembilla NC, Chizzolini C. T cell abnormalities in systemic sclerosis with a focus on Th17 cells. Eur Cytokine Netw. 2012;23:128–39.
7. Fenoglio D, Battaglia F, Parodi A, et al. Alteration of Th17 and Treg cell subpopulations co-exist in patients affected with systemic sclerosis. Clin Immunol. 2011;139:249–57.

8. Rodrigueu-Reyna TS, Furazawa-Carballeda Y, Cabiedes J, et al. Th17 polarization in systemic sclerosis is influenced by immunosuppressive treatment regardless of evolution. Arthritis Rheum 2009;60(Suppl):420.
9. Radstake TR, van Bon L, Broen J, Hussiani A, et al. The pronounced Th17 profile in systemic sclerosis together with intracellular expression of TGFbeta and IFN-gamma distinguishes SSc phenotype. PLoS One. 2009;4(6):e5903.
10. Varga J, Abraham D. Systemic sclerosis: a prototypic multisystem fibrotic disorder. J Clin Invest. 2007;117:557–67.
11. Sundrud MS, Koralov SB, Feuerer M, et al. Halofuginone inhibits TH17 cell differentiation by activating the amino acid starvation response. Science. 2009;324(5932):1334–8.
12. Pines M, Snyder D, Yarkoni S, et al. Halofuginone to treat fibrosis in chronic graft-versus-host disease and scleroderma. Biol Blood Marrow Transplant. 2003;9(7):417–25.
13. Kalogerou A, Gelou E, Mountantonakis S, et al. Early T cell activation in the skin from patients with systemic sclerosis. Ann Rheum Dis. 2005;64(8):1233–5.
14. de Paoli FV, Nielsen BD, Rasmussen F, Deleuran B, Søndergaard K. Abatacept induces clinical improvement in patients with severe systemic sclerosis. Scand J Rheumatol. 2014;43(4):342–5.
15. Chakravarty EF, Martyanov V, Fiorentino D, Wood TA, Haddon DJ, Jarrell JA, Utz PJ, Genovese MC, Whitfield ML, Chung L. Gene expression changes reflect clinical response in a placebo-controlled randomized trial of abatacept in patients with diffuse cutaneous systemic sclerosis. Arthritis Res Ther. 2015; 17:159.
16. Khanna D, Furst DE, Hays RD, Park GS, Wong WK, Seibold JR, et al. Minimally important difference in diffuse systemic sclerosis: results from the D-penicillamine study. Ann Rheum Dis. 2006;65:1325–9.
17. Elhai M, Meunier M, Matucci-Cerinic M, Maurer B, Riemekasten G, Leturcq T, Pellerito R, Von Mühlen CA, Vacca A, Airo P, Bartoli F, Fiori G, Bokarewa M, Riccieri V, Becker M, Avouac J, Müller-Ladner U, Distler O, Allanore Y, EUSTAR (EULAR Scleroderma Trials and Research group). Outcomes of patients with systemic sclerosis-associated polyarthritis and myopathy treated with tocilizumab or abatacept: a EUSTAR observational study. Ann Rheum Dis. 2013;72(7):1217–20.
18. Yellin M, Paliienko I, Balanescu A, et al. A phase II, randomized, double-blind, placebo-controlled study to evaluate the efficacy and safety of MDX-1100, a fully human anti-CXCL10 monoclonal antibody, in combination with methotrexate (MTX) in patients with rheumatoid arthritis (RA) [abstract]. Arthritis Rheum. 2012;64(6):1730–9.
19. Nishimura M, Kuboi Y, Muramoto K, et al. Chemokines as novel therapeutic targets for inflammatory bowel disease. Ann N Y Acad Sci. 2009;1173:350–6.
20. Cipriani P, Franca Milia A, Liakouli V, Pacini A, et al. Differential expression of stromal cell-derived factor 1 and its receptor CXCR4 in the skin and endothelial cells of systemic sclerosis patients: pathogenetic implications. Arthritis Rheum. 2006;54(9): 3022–33.
21. Cipriani P, Guiducci S, Miniati I, Cinelli M, et al. Impairment of endothelial cell differentiation from bone marrow-derived mesenchymal stem cells: new insight into the pathogenesis of systemic sclerosis. Arthritis Rheum. 2007;56(6):1994–2004.
22. Campioni D, Lo Monaco A, Lanza F, Moretti S, Ferrari L, et al. CXCR4 pos circulating progenitor cells coexpressing monocytic and endothelial markers correlating with fibrotic clinical features are present in the peripheral blood of patients affected by systemic sclerosis. Haematologica. 2008;93(8):1233–7.
23. Keeley EC, Mehrad B, Strieter RM. Fibrocytes: bringing new insights into mechanisms of inflammation and fibrosis. Int J Biochem Cell Biol. 2010;42:535–42.
24. Phillips RJ, Burdick MD, Hong K, et al. Circulating fibrocytes traffic to the lungs in response to CXCL12 and mediate fibrosis. J Clin Invest. 2004;114:438–46.
25. Ortiz LA, Gambelli F, McBride C, et al. Mesenchymal stem cell engraftment in lung is enhanced in response to bleomycin exposure and ameliorates its fibrotic effects. Proc Natl Acad Sci U S A. 2003;100:8407–11.
26. Reese C, Lee R, Bonner M, Perry B, Heywood J, Silver RM, Tourkina E, Visconti RP, Hoffman S. Fibrocytes in the fibrotic lung: altered phenotype detected by flow cytometry. Front Pharmacol. 2014;5:141.
27. Brooks WH, Le Dantec C, Pers JO, et al. Epigenetics and autoimmunity. J Autoimmun. 2010;34:J207–19.
28. Wang Y, Fan PS, Kahaleh B. Association between enhanced type I collagen expression and epigenetic repression of the FLI1 gene in scleroderma fibroblasts. Arthritis Rheum. 2006;54(7): 2271–9.
29. Ghosh AK, Varga J. The transcriptional coactivator and acetyltransferase p300 in fibroblast biology and fibrosis. J Cell Physiol. 2007;213:663–71.
30. Huber LC, Distler JH, Moritz F, et al. Trichostatin A prevents the accumulation of extracellular matrix in a mouse model of bleomycin-induced skin fibrosis. Arthritis Rheum. 2007;56: 2755–64.
31. Hemmatazad H, Rodrigues HM, Maurer B, et al. Histone deacetylase 7, a potential target for the antifibrotic treatment of systemic sclerosis. Arthritis Rheum. 2009;60(5):1519–29.
32. Garber K. HDAC inhibitors overcome first hurdle. Nat Biotechnol. 2007;25(1):17–9.
33. Tang X, Peng R, Phillips JE, Deguzman J, Ren Y, Apparsundaram S, Luo Q, Bauer CM, Fuentes ME, DeMartino JA, Tyagi G, Garrido R, Hogaboam CM, Denton CP, Holmes AM, Kitson C, Stevenson CS, Budd DC. Assessment of Brd4 inhibition in idiopathic pulmonary fibrosis lung fibroblasts and in vivo models of lung fibrosis. Am J Pathol. 2013;183:470–9.
34. Nguyen VA, Eisendle K, Gruber I, Hugl B, Reider D, Reider N. Effect of the dual endothelin receptor antagonist bosentan on Raynaud's phenomenon secondary to systemic sclerosis: a double-blind prospective, randomized, placebo-controlled pilot study. Rheumatology (Oxford). 2010;49:583–7.
35. Matucci-Cerinic M, Denton CP, Furst DE, Mayes MD, Hsu VM, Carpentier P, Wigley FM, Black CM, Fessler BJ, Merkel PA, Pope JE, Sweiss NJ, Doyle MK, Hellmich B, Medsger Jr TA, Morganti A, Kramer F, Korn JH, Seibold JR. Bosentan treatment of digital ulcers related to systemic sclerosis: results from the RAPIDS-2 randomised, double-blind, placebo-controlled trial. Ann Rheum Dis. 2011;70(1):32–8.
36. Korn JH, Mayes M, Matucci Cerinic M, et al. Digital ulcers in systemic sclerosis: prevention by treatment with bosentan, an oral endothelin receptor antagonist. Arthritis Rheum. 2004;50(12):3985–93.
37. García de la Peña-Lefebvre P, Rodríguez Rubio S, Valero Expósito M, Carmona L, et al. Long-term experience of bosentan for treating ulcers and healed ulcers in systemic sclerosis patients. Rheumatology (Oxford). 2008;47(4):464–6.
38. Penn H, Quillinan N, Khan K, Chakravarty K, Ong VH, Burns A, Denton CP. Targeting the endothelin axis in scleroderma renal crisis: rationale and feasibility. QJM. 2013;106(9):839–48.
39. Fries R, Shariat K, von Wilmowsky H, Böhm M. Sildenafil in the treatment of Raynaud's phenomenon resistant to vasodilatory therapy. Circulation. 2005;112(19):2980–5.
40. Herrick AL, van den Hoogen F, Gabrielli A, Tamimi N, Reid C, O'Connell D, Vazquez-Abad MD, Denton CP. Modified-release sildenafil reduces Raynaud's phenomenon attack frequency in limited cutaneous systemic sclerosis. Arthritis Rheum. 2011;63(3):775–82.

41. Brueckner CS, Becker MO, Kroencke T, et al. Effect of sildenafil on digital ulcers in systemic sclerosis – analysis from a single centre pilot study. Ann Rheum Dis. 2010;69:1475–8.
42. Shenoy PD, Kumar S, Jha LK, Choudhary SK, Singh U, Misra R, Agarwal V. Efficacy of tadalafil in secondary Raynaud's phenomenon resistant to vasodilator therapy: a double-blind randomized cross-over trial. Rheumatology (Oxford). 2010;49(12):2420–8.
43. Zisman DA, Schwarz M, Anstrom KJ, Collard HR, Flaherty KR, Hunninghake GW. A controlled trial of sildenafil in advanced idiopathic pulmonary fibrosis. Idiopathic Pulmonary Fibrosis Clinical Research Network. N Engl J Med. 2010;363(7):620–8.
44. Dees C, Beyer C, Distler A, Soare A, Zhang Y, Palumbo-Zerr K, Distler O, Schett G, Sandner P, Distler JH. Stimulators of soluble guanylate cyclase (sGC) inhibit experimental skin fibrosis of different aetiologies. Ann Rheum Dis. 2015;74(8):1621–5.
45. Abou-Raya A, Abou-Raya S, Helmii M. Statins: potentially useful in therapy of systemic sclerosis-related Raynaud's phenomenon and digital ulcers. J Rheumatol. 2008;35(9):1801–8.
46. Abou-Raya A, Abou-Raya S, Helmii M. Statins as immunomodulators in systemic sclerosis. Ann N Y Acad Sci. 2007;1110:670–80.
47. Kuwana M, Okazaki Y, Kaburaki J. Long-term beneficial effects of statins on vascular manifestations in patients with systemic sclerosis registry [abstract]. Arthritis Rheum. 2009;60 Suppl 10:448.
48. Blann AD. Plasma von Willebrand factor, thrombosis, and the endothelium: the first 30 years. Thromb Haemost. 2006;95:49–55.
49. Louneva N, Huaman G, Fertala J, Jimenez SA. Inhibition of systemic sclerosis dermal fibroblast type I collagen production and gene expression by simvastatin. Arthritis Rheum. 2006;54:1298–308.
50. Simon TG, Butt AA. Lipid dysregulation in hepatitis C virus, and impact of statin therapy upon clinical outcomes. World J Gastroenterol. 2015;21(27):8293–303.
51. Bagnato G, Bitto A, Pizzino G, Irrera N, Sangari D, Cinquegrani M, Roberts WN, Matucci Cerinic M, Squadrito F, Altavilla D, Bagnato G, Saitta A. Simvastatin attenuates the development of pulmonary and cutaneous fibrosis in a murine model of systemic sclerosis. Rheumatology (Oxford). 2013;52(8):1377–86.
52. Seibold JR, Wigley FM, Schiopu E, Denton CP, et al. Digital ischaemic ulcers in scleroderma treated with oral Treprostinil diethanolamine: a randomized, double-blind, placebo-controlled, multi-centre study [abstract]. Arthritis Rheum. 2011;63 Suppl 10:2483.
53. Stratton R, Shiwen X, Martini G, Holmes A, Leask A, Haberberger T, Martin GR, Black CM, Abraham D. Iloprost suppresses connective tissue growth factor production in fibroblasts and in the skin of scleroderma patients. J Clin Invest. 2001;108(2):241–50.
54. Carulli MT, Handler C, Coghlan JG, Black CM, Denton CP. Can CCL2 serum levels be used in risk stratification or to monitor treatment response in systemic sclerosis? Ann Rheum Dis. 2008;67(1):105–9.
55. Zhu Y, Liu Y, Zhou W, Xiang R, Jiang L, Huang K, Xiao Y, Guo Z, Gao J. A prostacyclin analogue, iloprost, protects from bleomycin-induced pulmonary fibrosis in mice. Respir Res. 2010;11:34.
56. Baroni SS, Santillo M, Bevilacqua F, Luchetti M, Spadoni T, Mancini M, Fraticelli P, Sambo P, Funaro A, Kazlauskas A, Avvedimento EV, Gabrielli A. Stimulatory autoantibodies to the PDGF receptor in systemic sclerosis. N Engl J Med. 2006;354(25):2667–76.
57. Magro L, Mohty M, Catteau B, et al. Imatinib mesylate as salvage therapy for refractory sclerotic chronic graft-versus-host disease. Blood. 2009;114:719–22.
58. Kay J, High WA. Imatinib mesylate treatment of nephrogenic systemic fibrosis. Arthritis Rheum. 2008;58(8):2543–8.
59. Spiera RF, Gordon JK, Mersten JN, Magro CM, Mehta M, Wildman HF, Kloiber S, Kirou KA, Lyman S, Crow MK. Imatinib mesylate (Gleevec) in the treatment of diffuse cutaneous systemic sclerosis: results of a 1-year, phase IIa, single-arm, open-label clinical trial. Ann Rheum Dis. 2011;70:1003–9.
60. Khanna D, Saggar R, Mayes MD, Abtin F, Clements PJ, Maranian P, Assassi S, Saggar R, Singh RR, Furst DE. A one-year, phase I/IIa, open-label pilot trial of imatinib mesylate in the treatment of systemic sclerosis-associated active interstitial lung disease. Arthritis Rheum. 2011;63(11):3540–6.
61. Pope J, McBain D, Petrlich L, Watson S, Vanderhoek L, de Leon F, Seney S, Summers K. Imatinib in active diffuse cutaneous systemic sclerosis: results of a six-month, randomized, double-blind, placebo-controlled, proof-of-concept pilot study at a single centre. Arthritis Rheum. 2011;63(11):3547–51.
62. Prey S, Ezzedine K, Doussau A, Grandoulier AS, Barcat D, Chatelus E, Diot E, Durant C, Hachulla E, de Korwin-Krokowski JD, Kostrzewa E, Quemeneur T, Paul C, Schaeverbeke T, Seneschal J, Solanilla A, Sparsa A, Bouchet S, Lepreux S, Mahon FX, Chene G, Taïeb A. Imatinib mesylate in scleroderma-associated diffuse skin fibrosis: a phase II multicentre randomized double-blinded controlled trial. Br J Dermatol. 2012;167(5):1138–44.
63. Kerkelä R, Grazette L, Yacobi R, Iliescu C, Patten R, Beahm C, Walters B, Shevtsov S, Pesant S, Clubb FJ, Rosenzweig A, Salomon RN, Van Etten RA, Alroy J, Durand JB, Force T. Cardiotoxicity of the cancer therapeutic agent imatinib mesylate. Nat Med. 2006;12(8):908–16.
64. Distler O, Distler JH, Varga J, Denton CP, Lafyatis R, Wigley F, Schett G, Matucci-Cerinic M, Wright T, Bertolino A, Gergely P. A multi-center, open-label, proof of concept study of imatinib mesylate demonstrates no benefit for the treatment of fibrosis in patients with early, diffuse systemic sclerosis. Arthritis Rheum. 2010;62 Suppl 10:560.
65. Gordon JK, Martyanov V, Magro C, Wildman HF, Wood TA, Huang WT, Crow MK, Whitfield ML, Spiera RF. Nilotinib (Tasigna™) in the treatment of early diffuse systemic sclerosis: an open-label, pilot clinical trial. Arthritis Res Ther. 2015;17(1):213.
66. Denton CP, Nihtyanova SI, Varga J, Distler O, Wigley FM, Lafyatis R, Distler JH, Schett G, Matucci-Cerinic M, Wright T, Antunes M, Racine A, Bertolino A, Gergely Jr P. Comparative analysis of change in modified Rodnan Skin score in patients with diffuse systemic sclerosis receiving imatinib mesylate suggests similar disease course to matched patients receiving standard therapy. Arthritis Rheum. 2010;62 Suppl 10:566.
67. Wei J, Ghosh AK, Sargent JL, Komura K, Wu M, Huang QQ, Jain M, Whitfield ML, Feghali-Bostwick C, Varga J. PPARgamma downregulation by TGFss in fibroblast and impaired expression and function in systemic sclerosis: a novel mechanism for progressive fibrogenesis. PLoS One. 2010;16:e13778.
68. Ghosh AK, Bhattacharyya S, Lakos G, Chen SJ, Mori Y, Varga J. Disruption of transforming growth factor beta signaling and profibrotic responses in normal skin fibroblasts by peroxisome proliferator-activated receptor gamma. Arthritis Rheum. 2004;16:1305–18.
69. Burgess HA, Daugherty LE, Thatcher TH, Lakatos HF, Ray DM, Redonnet M, Phipps RP, Sime PJ. PPARgamma agonists inhibit TGF-beta induced pulmonary myofibroblast differentiation and collagen production: implications for therapy of lung fibrosis. Am J Physiol Lung Cell Mol Physiol. 2005;16:L1146–53.
70. Kulkarni AA, Thatcher TH, Olsen KC, Maggirwar SB, Phipps RP, Sime PJ. PPAR-gamma ligands repress TGFbeta-induced myofibroblast differentiation by targeting the PI3K/Akt pathway: implications for therapy of fibrosis. PLoS One. 2011;16:e15909.
71. Wei J, Zhu H, Komura K, Lord G, Tomcik M, Wang W, Doniparthi S, Tamaki Z, Hinchcliff M, Distler JH, Varga J. A synthetic

PPAR-gamma agonist triterpenoid ameliorates experimental fibrosis: PPAR-gamma-independent suppression of fibrotic responses. Ann Rheum Dis. 2014;73(2):446–54.
72. Palumbo-Zerr K, Zerr P, Distler A, Fliehr J, Mancuso R, Huang J, Mielenz D, Tomcik M, Fürnrohr BG, Scholtysek C, Dees C, Beyer C, Krönke G, Metzger D, Distler O, Schett G, Distler JH. Orphan nuclear receptor NR4A1 regulates transforming growth factor-β signaling and fibrosis. Nat Med. 2015;21(2):150–8.
73. Harris TE, Lawrence Jr JC. TOR signaling. Sci STKE. 2003;2003(212):re15.
74. Shegogue D, Trojanowska M. Mammalian target of rapamycin positively regulates collagen type I production via a phosphatidylinositol 3-kinase-independent pathway. J Biol Chem. 2004;279:23166–75.
75. Gui YS, Wang L, Tian X, Li X, Ma A, Zhou W, Zeng N, Zhang J, Cai B, Zhang H, Chen JY, Xu KF. mTOR overactivation and compromised autophagy in the pathogenesis of pulmonary fibrosis. PLoS One. 2015;10(9):e0138625.
76. Tamaki Z, Asano Y, Kubo M, Ihn H, Tada Y, Sugaya M, Kadono T, Sato S. Effects of the immunosuppressant rapamycin on the expression of human α2(I) collagen and matrix metalloproteinase 1 genes in scleroderma dermal fibroblasts. J Dermatol Sci. 2014;74(3):251–9.
77. Yoshizaki A, Yanaba K, Yoshizaki A, Iwata Y, Komura K, Ogawa F, Takenaka M, Shimizu K, Asano Y, Hasegawa M, Fujimoto M, Sato S. Treatment with rapamycin prevents fibrosis in tight-skin and bleomycin-induced mouse models of systemic sclerosis. Arthritis Rheum. 2010;62(8):2476–87.
78. Su TI, Khanna D, Furst DE, et al. Rapamycin versus methotrexate in early diffuse systemic sclerosis: results from a randomized, single-blind pilot study. Arthritis Rheum. 2009;60(12):3821–30.
79. Denton CP, Merkel PA, Furst DE, et al. Recombinant human anti-transforming growth factor beta1 antibody therapy in systemic sclerosis: a multicenter, randomized, placebo-controlled phase I/II trial of CAT-192. Arthritis Rheum. 2007;56(1):323–33.
80. Rice LM, Padilla CM, McLaughlin SR, Mathes A, Ziemek J, Goummih S, Nakerakanti S, York M, Farina G, Whitfield ML, Spiera RF, Christmann RB, Gordon JK, Weinberg J, Simms RW, Lafyatis R. Fresolimumab treatment decreases biomarkers and improves clinical symptoms in systemic sclerosis patients. J Clin Invest. 2015;125(7):2795–807.
81. Trachtman H, Fervenza FC, Gipson DS, Heering P, Jayne DR, Peters H, Rota S, Remuzzi G, Rump LC, Sellin LK, Heaton JP, Streisand JB, Hard ML, Ledbetter SR, Vincenti F. A phase 1, single-dose study of fresolimumab, an anti-TGF-β antibody, in treatment-resistant primary focal segmental glomerulosclerosis. Kidney Int. 2011;79(11):1236–43.
82. Naka T, Nishimoto N, Kishimoto T. The paradigm of IL-6: from basic science to medicine. Arthritis Res. 2002;4 Suppl 3:S233–42.
83. Kawaguchi Y, Hara M, Wright TM. Endogenous IL-1 from systemic sclerosis fibroblasts induces IL-6 and PDGF-A. J Clin Invest. 1999;103:1253–60.
84. Moodley YP, Scaffidi AK, Misso NL, Keerthisingam C, McAnulty RJ, Laurent GJ, Mutsaers SE, Thompson PJ, Knight DA. Fibroblasts isolated from normal lungs and those with idiopathic pulmonary fibrosis differ in interleukin-6/gp130-mediated cell signaling and proliferation. Am J Pathol. 2003;163(1):345–54.
85. Ghazizadeh M, Tosa M, Shimizu H, Hyakusoku H, Kawanami O. Functional implications of the IL-6 signaling pathway in keloid pathogenesis. J Invest Dermatol. 2007;127(1):98–105.
86. Luckett LR, Gallucci RM. Interleukin-6 (IL-6) modulates migration and matrix metalloproteinase function in dermal fibroblasts from IL-6KO mice. Br J Dermatol. 2007;156(6):1163–71.
87. Khan K, Xu S, Nihtyanova S, Derrett-Smith E, Abraham D, Denton CP, Ong VH. Clinical and pathological significance of interleukin 6 overexpression in systemic sclerosis. Ann Rheum Dis. 2012;71(7):1235–42.
88. Linterman MA, Vinuesa CG. Signals that influence T follicular helper cell differentiation and function. Semin Immunopathol. 2010;32(2):183–96.
89. Khanna D, Denton CP, Jahreis A, et al. Safety and efficacy of subcutaneous tocilizumab in adults with systemic sclerosis: week 48 data from the faSScinate trial. Presented at EULAR 2015 Rome, Rome, 10–13 June 2015. Abstract # OP0054.
90. Pradère JP, Klein J, Grès S, Guigné C, Neau E, Valet P, Calise D, Chun J, Bascands JL, Saulnier-Blache JS, Schanstra JP. LPA1 receptor activation promotes renal interstitial fibrosis. J Am Soc Nephrol. 2007;18(12):3110–8.
91. Tokumura A, Carbone LD, Yoshioka Y, Morishige J, Kikuchi M, Postlethwaite A, Watsky MA. Elevated serum levels of arachidonoyl-lysophosphatidic acid and sphingosine 1-phosphate in systemic sclerosis. Int J Med Sci. 2009;6(4):168–76.
92. Ohashi T, Yamamoto T. Antifibrotic effect of lysophosphatidic acid receptors LPA1 and LPA3 antagonist on experimental murine scleroderma induced by bleomycin. Exp Dermatol. 2015;24(9):698–702.
93. Castelino FV, Seiders J, Bain G, Brooks SF, King CD, Swaney JS, Lorrain DS, Chun J, Luster AD, Tager AM. Amelioration of dermal fibrosis by genetic deletion or pharmacologic antagonism of lysophosphatidic acid receptor 1 in a mouse model of scleroderma. Arthritis Rheum. 2011;63(5):1405–15.
94. Allanore Y, Jagerschmidt A, Jasson M, Distler O, et al. Lysophosphatidic acid receptor 1 antagonist SAR100842 as a potential treatment for patients with systemic sclerosis: results from a phase 2A study. Presented at EULAR 2015 Rome, Rome, 10–13 June 2015. Abstract # OP0266.
95. Svejda B, Kidd M, Giovinazzo F, Eltawil K, Gustafsson BI, Pfragner R, Modlin IM. The 5-HT(2B) receptor plays a key regulatory role in both neuroendocrine tumor cell proliferation and the modulation of the fibroblast component of the neoplastic microenvironment. Cancer. 2010;116(12):2902–12.
96. Ruddell RG, Oakley F, Hussain Z, Yeung I, Bryan-Lluka LJ, Ramm GA, Mann DA. A role for serotonin (5-HT) in hepatic stellate cell function and liver fibrosis. Am J Pathol. 2006;169(3):861–76.
97. Dees C, Akhmetshina A, Zerr P, Reich N, Palumbo K, Horn A, Jüngel A, Beyer C, Krönke G, Zwerina J, Reiter R, Alenina N, Maroteaux L, Gay S, Schett G, Distler O, Distler JH. Platelet-derived serotonin links vascular disease and tissue fibrosis. J Exp Med. 2011;208(5):961–72.
98. Königshoff M, Dumitrascu R, Udalov S, Amarie OV, Reiter R, Grimminger F, Seeger W, Schermuly RT, Eickelberg O. Increased expression of 5-hydroxytryptamine2A/B receptors in idiopathic pulmonary fibrosis: a rationale for therapeutic intervention. Thorax. 2010;65(11):949–55.
99. Coleiro B, Marshall SE, Denton CP, Howell K, Blann A, Welsh KI, Black CM. Treatment of Raynaud's phenomenon with the selective serotonin reuptake inhibitor fluoxetine. Rheumatology (Oxford). 2001;40(9):1038–43.
100. Marcos E, Fadel E, Sanchez O, Humbert M, Dartevelle P, Simonneau G, Hamon M, Adnot S, Eddahibi S. Serotonin-induced smooth muscle hyperplasia in various forms of human pulmonary hypertension. Circ Res. 2004;94(9):1263–70.
101. Akhmetshina A, Dees C, Pileckyte M, Szucs G, Spriewald BM, Zwerina J, Distler O, Schett G, Distler JH. Rho-associated kinases are crucial for myofibroblast differentiation and production of extracellular matrix in scleroderma fibroblasts. Arthritis Rheum. 2008;58(8):2553–64.

102. Nagatoya K, Moriyama T, Kawada N, Takeji M, Oseto S, Murozono T, Ando A, Imai E, Hori M. Y-27632 prevents tubulointerstitial fibrosis in mouse kidneys with unilateral ureteral obstruction. Kidney Int. 2002;61(5):1684–95.
103. Fava A, Wung PK, Wigley FM, Hummers LK, Daya NR, Ghazarian SR, Boin F. Efficacy of Rho kinase inhibitor fasudil in secondary Raynaud's phenomenon. Arthritis Care Res (Hoboken). 2012;64(6):925–9.
104. Skhirtladze C, Distler O, Dees C, Akhmetshina A, Busch N, Venalis P, Zwerina J, Spriewald B, Pileckyte M, Schett G, Distler JH. Src kinases in systemic sclerosis: central roles in fibroblast activation and in skin fibrosis. Arthritis Rheum. 2008;58(5):1475–84.
105. Akhmetshina A, Dees C, Pileckyte M, Maurer B, Axmann R, Jüngel A, Zwerina J, Gay S, Schett G, Distler O, Distler JH. Dual inhibition of c-abl and PDGF receptor signaling by dasatinib and nilotinib for the treatment of dermal fibrosis. FASEB J. 2008;22(7):2214–22.
106. Maurer B, Reich N, Juengel A, Kriegsmann J, Gay RE, Schett G, Michel BA, Gay S, Distler JH, Distler O. Fra-2 transgenic mice as a novel model of pulmonary hypertension associated with systemic sclerosis. Ann Rheum Dis. 2012;71(8):1382–7.
107. Pilling D, Tucker NM, Gomer RH. Aggregated IgG inhibits the differentiation of human fibrocytes. J Leukoc Biol. 2006;79(6):1242–51.
108. Weinblatt ME, Kavanaugh A, Genovese MC, Musser TK, Grossbard EB, Magilavy DB. An oral spleen tyrosine kinase (Syk) inhibitor for rheumatoid arthritis. N Engl J Med. 2010;363(14):1303–12.
109. Williams W, Scherle P, Shi J, Newton R, McKeever E, Fridman J, Burn T, Vaddi K, Levy R, Moreland L. A randomized placebo-controlled study of INCB018424, a selective Janus Kinase1& 2 (JAK1&2) inhibitor in rheumatoid arthritis (RA). Arthritis Rheum. 2008;58:S431.
110. Richeldi L, du Bois RM, Raghu G, Azuma A, Brown KK, Costabel U, Cottin V, Flaherty KR, Hansell DM, Inoue Y, Kim DS, Kolb M, Nicholson AG, Noble PW, Selman M, Taniguchi H, Brun M, Le Maulf F, Girard M, Stowasser S, Schlenker-Herceg R, Disse B, Collard HR, INPULSIS Trial Investigators. Efficacy and safety of nintedanib in idiopathic pulmonary fibrosis. N Engl J Med. 2014;370(22):2071–82.
111. Traber PG, Chou H, Zomer E, Hong F, Klyosov A, Fiel MI, Friedman SL. Regression of fibrosis and reversal of cirrhosis in rats by galectin inhibitors in thioacetamide-induced liver disease. PLoS One. 2013;8(10):e75361.
112. Traber PG, Zomer E. Therapy of experimental NASH and fibrosis with galectin inhibitors. PLoS One. 2013;8(12):e83481.
113. Koca SS, Akbas F, Ozgen M, Yolbas S, Ilhan N, Gundogdu B, Isik A. Serum galectin-3 level in systemic sclerosis. Clin Rheumatol. 2014;33(2):215–20.
114. Juniantito V, Izawa T, Yuasa T, Ichikawa C, Yano R, Kuwamura M, Yamate J. Immunophenotypical characterization of macrophages in rat bleomycin-induced scleroderma. Vet Pathol. 2013;50(1):76–85.
115. Taniguchi T, Asano Y, Akamata K, Noda S, Masui Y, Yamada D, Takahashi T, Ichimura Y, Toyama T, Tamaki Z, Tada Y, Sugaya M, Kadono T, Sato S. Serum levels of galectin-3: possible association with fibrosis, aberrant angiogenesis, and immune activation in patients with systemic sclerosis. J Rheumatol. 2012;39(3): 539–44.
116. Moreno M, Chaves JF, Sancho-Bru P, Ramalho F, Ramalho LN, Mansego ML, Ivorra C, Dominguez M, Conde L, Millán C, Marí M, Colmenero J, Lozano JJ, Jares P, Vidal J, Forns X, Arroyo V, Caballería J, Ginès P, Bataller R. Ghrelin attenuates hepatocellular injury and liver fibrogenesis in rodents and influences fibrosis progression in humans. Hepatology. 2010;51(3):974–85.
117. Koca SS, Ozgen M, Sarikaya M, Dagli F, Ustundag B, Isik A. Ghrelin prevents the development of dermal fibrosis in bleomycin-induced scleroderma. Clin Exp Dermatol. 2014;39(2):176–81.
118. Ariyasu H, Iwakura H, Yukawa N, Murayama T, Yokode M, Tada H, Yoshimura K, Teramukai S, Ito T, Shimizu A, Yonezawa A, Kangawa K, Mimori T, Akamizu T. Clinical effects of ghrelin on gastrointestinal involvement in patients with systemic sclerosis. Endocr J. 2014;61(7):735–42.

43 Drug Development and Regulatory Considerations for SSc Therapies

Timothy M. Wright

Drug development is an expensive and risky endeavor with an overall failure rate of ~85 % from the time drug candidates first enter the clinic to the time they reach the market. Add to this the complexity of a systemic disease with multiple proposed pathogenic mechanisms, no proven "gold standard" therapy against which to benchmark and no validated measures of disease activity, progression, or remission, and you have described a disease that one might deliberately steer away from for the purpose of developing new therapies. These diseases are often considered "intractable," and, in the absence of a major breakthrough on disease mechanism or clinical outcome assessment, they remain the territory of post-approval exploratory and investigator-initiated trials. It is in this context that this Chapter will provide a framework for understanding the preclinical, clinical, and regulatory challenges of drug development and provide insights to guide research and development strategies to advance novel drug discovery for SSc (Table 43.1).

Drug Development Overview

From Molecule to Market: Time and Risk

The process to discover and develop a new drug (*new molecular entity* or NME) from initial concept to marketed product is lengthy and complex, typically extending over a period of 10–15 years [1, 2]. A prototypic timeline for drug discovery and development is illustrated in Fig. 43.1. Timelines will vary depending on the amount of time spent in the preclinical phase optimizing the molecule and the complexity of the development phase. Biologics and cell therapies are generally much faster than small molecules in the discovery phase. Infectious disease and orphan indications tend to have more straightforward clinical development programs and require shorter duration follow-up for initial approval.

Analyses of the success of drug development programs indicate that approximately 11 % of NMEs entering human testing will make it to the market [3–5]. The reported success rates for biologics are approximately twice the rates for small molecules, and the highest rates for success from Phase 1 (33 %) are for molecules with orphan drug designation [4, 5].

Cost of Drug Development

Considerable investments are required to develop NMEs and on average the cost to generate a single approved drug is

Table 43.1 Challenges for developing SSc therapies

Complex pathogenesis: vascular, immune, fibrotic
Disease heterogeneity – limited vs. diffuse, kinetics of disease progression, autoantibodies, organ system involvement
Lack of predictive animal models
Spontaneous improvement of the skin over time (most patients)
No validated biomarkers for disease activity, progression, and remission
Semiquantitative endpoints (e.g., MRSS)
Time for improvement of disease endpoints long (many months to a year)

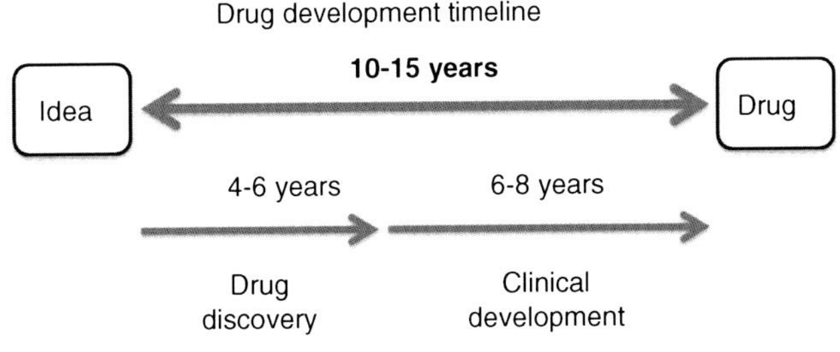

Fig. 43.1 Timeline of drug development

T.M. Wright, MD
California Institute for Biomedical Research, La Jolla, CA, USA
e-mail: twright@calibr.org

J. Varga et al. (eds.), *Scleroderma*, DOI 10.1007/978-3-319-31407-5_43

estimated to be in the range of $1.4–2.6B, depending on whether the cost of capital and failures is included [3, 6]. Also, it is more often the case than not that NMEs, once marketed, will not generate the commercial return that was needed to cover the fully loaded R&D costs.

It is worth noting that the time elapsed between when a molecule is patented to the time it is marketed may leave little patent life remaining to recoup the R&D investment. The Hatch-Waxman Act has since 1984 provided 5 years of data exclusivity to a company for approval of an NME. The Orphan Drug Act extends this to 7 years for NMEs approved for an orphan disease indication. In the EU the time frame of minimum exclusivity for orphan drugs is 10 years after approval. There are also additional financial incentives for orphan disease indications that include a 50 % US tax credit for clinical research upon approval, a waiver of the FDA PDUFA filing fee (~$2 million) and eligibility for research grants designated to support orphan product research. Similar financial incentives are in effect for EU orphan drug approvals [7, 8]. Based on the prevalence of SSc, new drugs undergoing regulatory review for this indication should be regarded as "orphan disease" therapeutics by regulators in the major markets [8]. In 2015, orphan drug status was granted to four compounds in development for the treatment of SSc [9].

Drug Discovery Phases

Initiation of New Programs

Drug discovery programs can have many roots. Initial concepts often arise from publications of research findings derived from academic laboratories. These reports cover topics ranging from basic observations in genetics, genomics, cellular, or pathway biology that point to a potentially relevant target for disease. Others may be more translational in nature and describe phenotypes in animal models or humans linked to gene or pathway perturbation. What follows these early reports can vary but is usually a replication of the findings by the investigators considering a drug discovery program (either in academia/private sector or in a pharmaceutical company laboratory). Depending on the availability of tools to accomplish this confirmation and the timing, an early drug discovery program may be initiated in parallel. The strength of the data, biologic plausibility, and ultimately independent confirmation will drive the investment for a full effort on drug discovery.

Many considerations go into the decision to embark on a new therapeutic program: (1) the degree of target validation, as mentioned above, (2) the ability to generate modulators (agonists or antagonists, as appropriate) of the target using available therapeutic modalities, (3) the likelihood that the therapeutic approach will deliver a significant benefit vs. risk for the patient, and (4) whether the profile of the drug will be acceptable for the intended use. Some companies will also initiate a commercial assessment relatively early in the drug discovery process to determine the potential future commercial value of the product (estimated net present value, eNPV, or risk-adjusted net present value, rNPV), although it is clear that such value forecasts are highly inaccurate especially for early programs [10–12]. Together these considerations shape what is often referred to as a "target product profile" or "TPP" that serves as a guide for the drug discovery team. It is important at this stage of developing novel therapeutics to remain flexible in the TPP so as not to restrict the exploration of novel therapeutics and their applications, since drug discovery involves a great deal of empiricism as well as serendipity.

New programs may originate in academic labs with the transfer of assays to central screening facilities in the private sector (e.g., NIH, NCI, some universities, and institutes), biotechs, or pharmaceutical companies. Alternatively, the screening assays may be created in the industry labs, themselves. These assays and appropriate counterscreens for selectivity, off-target effects, and cellular toxicity are used to generate the initial molecules (referred to as "compounds" until regulatory approval) for preclinical testing. The use of high-throughput (384- or 1536-well plates) robotic screening now enables the evaluation of millions of small molecules and natural products rapidly in enzyme-based or cellular assays [13]. Alternatively, monoclonal antibodies can be generated from 10^6 to 10^9 potential candidates using in vivo selection of hyperimmunized humanized mice or in vitro screening of recombinant human antibody libraries (e.g., phage or yeast display). Therapeutic peptides can be designed based on native sequences and modified to improve duration of action and potency and to alter their specificity (including dual specificity in some cases). Novel nucleic acid and cell therapeutic candidates can be generated in a matter of a few months using recombinant methods, an array of gene transduction approaches (viral and nonviral), and gene-editing techniques. For the sake of simplicity, the remainder of this Chapter will refer to new drug candidates as "compounds" and not elaborate on the differences across therapeutic modalities.

Validation and Optimization Phase

The next phase of drug discovery is a highly iterative one in which the "hits" or compounds identified from initial screens are profiled extensively in vitro using enzyme and cellular assays, as appropriate. Often significant structural modifications are made to improve compound qualities (cell permeability, plasma stability, target selectivity, etc.), and this process can continue for months to years, depending on the desired profile. Subsequently, compounds are selected for testing in animals to examine pharmacokinetics (PK), pharmacodynamics (PD), and initial toxicology assessments. These tool compounds are also used to confirm that modulating the target originally identified as linked to a human disease process or phenotype has the desired efficacy in vitro and in vivo (ideally in a relevant animal model of human disease). The other major goal of the profiling at this stage is to understand the preliminary safety and tolerability of the compound in animals (in short-term tolerability studies). Together these data are compared to the TPP described above and begin to inform the benefit-risk profile of the drug.

Years may elapse validating the new therapeutic target based on the generation of genetically modified animals, in vitro testing in cellular systems reflective of human disease processes (cellular knockdown or overexpression, in vitro) or through the evaluation of tool compounds in vitro and in vivo. Indeed, many programs never make it out of this early phase of drug discovery due to the failure of target validation or the inability to generate suitable molecules with "drug-like" properties that satisfy the TPP.

Candidate Selection and Profiling

Once advanced compounds have passed the initial battery of evaluations, a few of these are taken into the next round of more intensive preclinical profiling to determine whether they will be suitable for clinical testing. This phase includes extensive evaluation of the pharmaceutical properties of the compounds including manufacturing scalability, formulation, stability, metabolism, and more formal toxicology studies in vitro and in vivo. It is during this period using the most advanced compounds that estimates are made of human the dose, exposure and anticipated efficacy (often using PK-PD modeling). This work is greatly facilitated by having biomarkers that are associated with disease activity, response to treatment, and potential toxicity [14]. In the absence of such biomarkers and a reliable animal model reflecting the disease mechanism in humans, the program advances with great uncertainty with respect to the translatability to human efficacy and safety.

In nearly all cases, a single compound is selected as the clinical candidate for manufacturing scale up under "current good manufacturing practices" or cGMP and further preclinical testing of the compound under "good laboratory practices" or GLP. This phase of late preclinical development requires rigorous documentation and monitoring for quality, reproducibility, and reliability to meet regulatory standards to support human testing. Failure of compounds at this stage is not uncommon due to the inability to achieve consistent blood or tissue exposure (across preclinical species) at the levels projected for human efficacy or due to unacceptable toxicity in GLP preclinical safety studies. Termination of a late preclinical program due to an unexpected finding can mean going back to earlier-stage compounds with a different chemical scaffold that may have improved pharmaceutical properties or lack a specific toxicity. Alternatively, it can lead to abandonment of the entire program due to uncertainty that a backup will address the shortcomings of the initial candidate or because the timeline of the program is no longer competitive with that of other companies.

Initiating SSc Targeted Drug Discovery Programs

Considering the current state of knowledge and the apparent complexity of the pathogenesis of SSc, it would be challenging to embark on a focused de novo drug discovery program in SSc. A more likely scenario is a program that targets one of the major SSc pathogenetic mechanisms such as vascular, autoimmune, or fibrotic that would also be relevant to a wider array of related indications. Once early compounds are available from screens, it would be essential to have ready access to primary cells from SSc patients (endothelial cells, PBMCs, and fibroblasts from the skin and lung) to evaluate in secondary assays. Establishing a publicly available cell and DNA bank for SSc would greatly facilitate this process. This is particularly important since the next phase of preclinical validation, evaluation in SSc animal models, is not a straightforward (or clinically relevant) process.

Moving from in vitro cell culture assays to examining the effects of compounds in vivo in animal models is a valuable step to select compounds for advancement to the clinic. As described above, testing in animal models provides data that can enable PK-PD modeling and establish whether the degree of target modulation by the compound is likely to achieve efficacy. The big challenge with SSc in this regard is which of the many animal models reflects the human disease mechanism. Although there is no specific model that recapitulates all of the pathogenic mechanisms, existing models can be used to probe specific components of the SSc and establish a PK-PD-efficacy relationship that can serve as a guide for human testing.

In the absence of a suitable model for the mechanism of action for a compound hitting a novel disease target, it should be adequate to establish that exposures in vivo modulate the target to achieve the desired cellular or tissue effect in normal animals. The gap created by this approach can reduce confidence (and support) for pursuing the SSc indication and will no doubt cause significant uncertainty when interpreting a negative clinical trial. One way to supplement the disease-relevant preclinical information and potentially bridge to the clinic is with the use of biomarkers that are reflective of the disease activity. Further work to better define disease activity (e.g., vascular damage, immune, fibrosis) biomarkers and profiling them in preclinical models can close the gap between in vitro cellular assays and human studies.

Clinical Development Phases

Exploratory Clinical Development: Phases 1 and 2a

After compiling the package of preclinical data satisfying the requirements for safeguarding human testing and providing reasonable confidence that the compound will achieve adequate human exposure in the dosage form and route chosen, an application to perform the first in human (FIH) Phase 1 clinical trial is made to the regulatory authority and independent ethics committee (e.g., Institutional Review Board or IRB) governing the conduct of the planned human study. In the USA this is in the form of an Investigational New Drug (IND) application, and elsewhere this has other regulatory formats, such as the Clinical Trial Application (CTA) in the EU. Clinical trials worldwide are conducted according to "Good Clinical Practice" (GCP) and must adhere to the highest standards to protect human safety.

At this stage of development, it is typical to have animal toxicity studies in two species (rodent and a higher non-rodent species) that involve dosing with the compound that achieves multiples of the highest anticipated human exposure and that ideally identifies the organ system(s) sensitive to drug toxicity so as to be able to monitor for this toxicity in human testing. Exceptions can be made to two species toxicology testing depending on species cross-reactivity of the compound. The initial GLP toxicology studies are usually of 2–4 weeks duration and support human testing up to the duration of animal dosing. This is important since in most cases the duration of human dosing needed to achieve human clinical efficacy may be on the order of several months to a year. Toxicology studies are expensive to conduct and are the most demanding of the GMP compound supply in the early stage of development. Therefore, toxicology studies are usually conducted in a staggered fashion with increasing duration of dosing after Phase 1 human data have been generated.

Because of the limited ability to detect meaningful changes in disease-related parameters with single or brief (7–10 day) multiple dosing, the Phase 1 single ascending dose trial and subsequent multiple ascending dose trial are commonly performed with the dosing of healthy volunteer subjects (with appropriate safeguards and informed consent) in a domiciled setting in order to closely monitor them for safety and tolerability. The FIH trial exposes small groups of subjects to increasing single doses of compound (or placebo) with careful clinical monitoring and sampling for PK, PD, and clinical laboratory safety studies. Once a single dose has been shown to be safe and well-tolerated and has evidence of human bioavailability, a multiple ascending dose trial is conducted in healthy volunteer subjects with a similar design only dosing is repeated – typically over a period of 1–2 weeks.

In the case of compounds projected to have a narrow therapeutic index (e.g., most oncology compounds, cell and gene therapies), initial testing is performed in the intended patient population. The goal of early human testing is to establish human safety, tolerability, and pharmacokinetics of the investigational compounds. In parallel, an important secondary objective of Phase 1 studies, whenever possible, is to determine a pharmacodynamic response that corresponds to the modulation of the target intended to be achieved by the compound so that a PK-PD relationship can be established (similar to the preclinical models, above). Compounds not achieving the desired human PK exposure profile may require reformulation or may be discontinued. Safety, tolerability, PK, and PD across dose groups are carefully reviewed to assess the potential of the compound to deliver efficacy when evaluated in longer-term studies in patients.

Depending on the duration of dosing expected to be required to detect efficacy in patients, the compound may enter a Phase 2a "proof of concept" (PoC) trial immediately after Phase 1 or there may be a delay, while longer preclinical toxicology studies are performed to support chronic human dosing. The PoC study is typically a randomized, placebo-controlled, double-blind trial performed in a well-defined and often relatively homogeneous patient population (generally less than 100–200 subjects) in which the highest tolerated dose from the Phase I multiple-dose trial is tested. A lower dose may be included to get a preliminary assessment of the therapeutic range.

In designing and analyzing PoC trials, which are considered exploratory in nature, considerable flexibility is possible including planned interim analyses, exploratory analyses across dose groups, reduced statistical power, and level of statistical significance for declaring a positive study (commonly a $p<0.1$). The determination of PoC may be made on one or more endpoint (clinical, imaging, or laboratory) that gives confidence that subsequent longer duration trials will meet expectations by regulators regarding evidence of clinical efficacy. Whenever feasible, PoC trials include "registration endpoints," i.e., those established by regulatory authorities as basis for approval, although the trial design and duration may not support rigorous statistical analysis of these endpoints.

Each of the exploratory aspects of PoC trial design and data analysis comes with some risk when extrapolating results to larger studies. The tolerance for risk of replicating PoC results in subsequent Phase 2b or of accepting a false-positive POC study is established on a case-by-case basis. On average one third of compounds that reached Phase 1 (FIH) will pass PoC and enter the confirmatory phase of clinical development (Fig. 43.2).

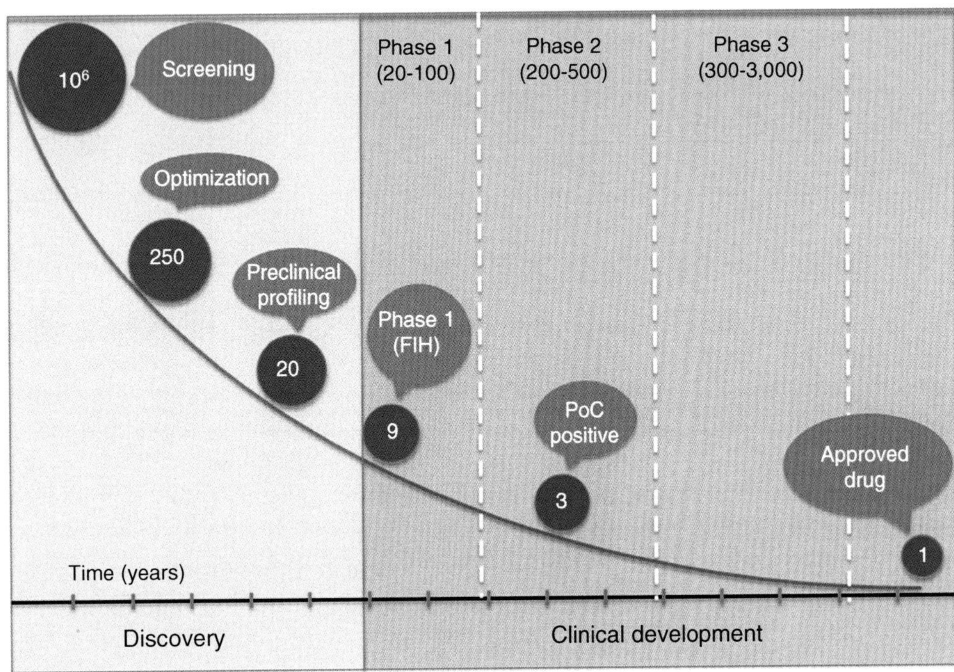

Fig. 43.2 Attrition in drug discovery and development (in part based on [15])

Confirmatory Clinical Development: Phases 2b and 3

Having achieved evidence of PoC, the next phase of clinical development is considered. This is a major inflection point in the investment for a development program and represents a period of intense analysis of available clinical and preclinical data in the context of the TPP and commercial assessment, which is more mature at this stage, factoring in the available data and the competitive landscape. In Phase 2b and 3 trials, the rigor of statistical design and analyses comes into play since these are considered trials that are core to the regulatory review and approval process. Although regulatory advice can be sought throughout the research and development process, it is a key component for the confirmatory phase of clinical development since the stakes (cost for designing an inadequate set of trials) are highest at this stage. Complicating matters is the fact that there is not global harmonization of regulatory requirements, endpoints, inclusion of comparators, and duration of follow-up for approval.

For the majority of compounds (exceptions in oncology and some orphan indications), the Phase 2b trial is a randomized placebo-controlled dose ranging study in patients designed to establish the effective dose(s) of the compound using the intended registration endpoint(s). It also serves to expand the safety database in the target population and ideally to identify a minimally effective (or ineffective) dose to guide dose selection for Phase 3. Because these studies typically extend beyond 6 months and also since continued treatment via open-label extension of dosing for patients who respond to the therapy, chronic toxicology studies need to be completed before initiating Phase 2b (6 months in rodents, 9 months in non-rodents). For most clinical indications, the sample size needed to define the dose response with a high degree of confidence ($p<0.05$) is on the order of a hundred subjects per arm, depending on many variables including the effect size, variance, the shape of the dose-response curve, and where on the curve the chosen doses fall. It is common for Phase 2b studies to require for at least 1.5–2 years for completion. At the end of Phase 2b, the data are presented to the regulatory authorities to get input and agreement on the design of the Phase 3 pivotal registration trial and whether it is required (or advisable) to conduct a single or replicate Phase 3 studies.

The final investigational leg of the clinical development journey is Phase 3 in which one or two studies (depends on the indication, design, and statistical significance for positivity) are performed in the target patient population to confirm the efficacy and safety of the compound at the proposed dose(s) for registration. The phase 3 program often involves 500–1,000+ subjects in global multicenter trials and can often last 2–3 years due to time for recruitment and duration of follow-up necessary for efficacy and safety assessments. Overall success rate for compounds entering Phase 3 is roughly 70%, and assuming no surprises, the data will support regulatory approval [4].

Regulatory Submission and Review

After the completion of a successful Phase 3 program, the sponsor completes the assembly of the dossier that documents the preclinical and clinical studies that support the regulatory review and approval process. Due to the magnitude of the databases and the complexity of collating all necessary data and supporting documents as well as cross-references and integrated assessments and interpretations, the preparation of the New Drug Application (NDA) dossier can take several months to complete. Once filed and accepted by the regulatory authorities, the review clock begins. For the USA, the review period for most applications is 10–11 months, although expedited review can occur in the case of "fast track" or breakthrough therapy designation [16]. The EMA review is usually completed over a period of 12–14 months, and faster review is possible based on the unmet medical need and data. The PMDA (Japanese regulatory authority) is similar to FDA in its review timelines and for 2014 had the fasted median approval time (10 months) of the three major health authorities [17].

Post-approval Studies: Phase 4 and Beyond

After approval, clinical research on the new drug continues and includes a variety of studies that continue to build the safety and efficacy databases for the new product. There may be a commitment on the part of the industry sponsor to perform post marketing surveillance studies to one or more health authorities. This is standard in certain countries and is more often the case when the approval has been accelerated, the primary indication is a small patient population (limited number of exposure years of safety follow-up) or if the new drug is first in a new class with a novel mechanism for which long-term safety is unknown [18–20]. Phase 4 studies build on the data generated in highly monitored and controlled trials during the earlier phases of clinical development and add to this important information generated in the "real-world" setting [20].

Once a drug has reached the market, the sponsor is more likely to entertain exploratory studies in additional patient populations. Some companies include indication expansion strategies earlier in development (e.g., Phase 2a), and this can lead to parallel Phase 2b and Phase 3 programs in more than one indication [21]. The more likely scenario is the willingness of the company to consider the evaluation of their drug following initial regulatory approval in novel indications based on preclinical (in vitro or in vivo) data, case reports, or compelling disease mechanism related rationale. These new studies may originate within the company as the result of internal scientific work or indication expansion strategy, or they may originate externally – typically from the academic community. Investigator-initiated trials (IITs, also referred to as investigator-sponsored trials) represent important mechanisms for exploratory clinical research for new drugs. These studies, if positive, can form the basis for pivotal studies that result in supplemental regulatory approvals in expanded patient populations or new indications [22].

Strategies for SSc Drug Development

As described above, the path to clinical testing of new compounds requires careful coordination of preclinical and clinical research activities and is enabled by a clear understanding of anticipated clinical and laboratory outcomes that one can define as "success" or "efficacy." It is appropriate to include patients in Phase 1 studies if there is potential to observe a measurable response to the test compound being evaluated during the period of treatment and observation (typically up to 2–4 weeks). Currently we lack evidence that SSc would exhibit a significant clinical or biomarker (laboratory or imaging) response in this time frame, making it likely that new compounds designed for SSc would be evaluated first in healthy volunteers (if safety profile was favorable) or in patients with another disease for which an earlier clinical or pharmacodynamic (e.g., biomarker) response may be observed.

In the absence of new predictive biomarkers or disease outcome measures, the earliest studies of novel compounds to measure efficacy in SSc patients will take place in Phase 2 when preliminary PK and safety for the compounds has been established and toxicology studies have been performed to support human dosing of 6 months or longer. While shorter-duration studies (e.g., 3 months) may be feasible, it may not be possible to detect clinically meaningful and statistically significant disease improvement in that time frame [23]. The identification of improved outcome measures and biomarkers for disease activity and/or response to therapy would therefore be an important enabler for SSc drug discovery and would encourage earlier exploration of novel compounds in SSc patients.

The complication of disease heterogeneity is another challenge in the design of SSc clinical trials. As noted above, most PoC trials are conducted in relatively small and homogeneous disease populations for which the mechanism of action of the compound is hypothesized to be of benefit. The desire for strict homogeneity (SSc subtype, disease duration, ANA specificity, organ system involvement) must be acknowledged and balanced with the feasibility of recruitment. It is worth noting and learning from the recent success of efforts made in trials of homogeneous patient populations with idiopathic pulmonary fibrosis leading to the approval of two NMEs [24–26].

Another approach for developing novel therapeutics for SSc is to pursue organ system specific or symptomatic therapeutics, rather than overall disease modifying drugs. There are many examples of clinical trials evaluating marketed products targeting mechanisms of relevance for the vasculopathy (Raynaud's, digital ulcer healing), gastroesophageal reflux, and pulmonary fibrosis in SSc patients. Working with companies that have novel compounds in their pipeline to conduct trials for organ-specific efficacy may lead to important therapeutic advances for SSc patients.

Conclusion

There is growing interest on the part of industry and academia to pursue the development of new drugs for orphan diseases. The recent "orphan drug" designation by the FDA for several compounds in development specifically for SSc provides optimism that new drugs may be on the horizon. Since the rate of success for compounds entering the clinic to ultimate approval is below 15 %, it likely that multiple programs will be necessary to ensure success. It is essential that basic and clinical research address gaps in our knowledge of SSc pathogenesis, markers of disease activity, and quantitative outcome measures to improve the feasibility and success of future SSc drug discovery programs.

References

1. Corr P, Williams D. The pathway from idea to regulatory approval: examples for drug development. In: Lo B, Field MJ, editors. Institute of medicine committee on conflict of interest in medical research, education, and practice. Washington, DC: National Academies Press; 2009. p. 375–83.
2. Woosley RL, Cossman J. Drug development and the FDA's critical path initiative. Clin Pharmacol Ther. 2007,81:129–33.
3. DiMasi JA, Grabowski HG, Hansen RW. Innovation in the pharmaceutical industry: new estimates of R&D costs. Tufts Center for the Study of Drug Development, 18 Nov 2014. http://csdd.tufts.edu/files/uploads/Tufts_CSDD_briefing_on_RD_cost_study_-_Nov_18,_2014..pdf. Accessed 19 Nov 2015.
4. Hay M, Thomas DW, Craighead JL, Economides C, Rosenthal J. Clinical development success rates for investigational drugs. Nat Biotechnol. 2014;32(1):40–51.
5. Kola I, Landis J. Can the pharmaceutical industry reduce attrition rates? Nat Rev Drug Discov. 2004;3:711–5.
6. Munos B. Lessons from 60 years of pharmaceutical innovation. Nat Rev Drug Discov. 2009;8:959–68.
7. EMA Website: Orphan Incentives http://www.ema.europa.eu/ema/index.jsp?curl=pages/regulation/general/general_content_000393.jsp&mid=WC0b01ac058061f017. Accessed 19 Nov 2015.
8. Field MJ, Boat TF, editors. Rare diseases and orphan products: accelerating research and development. Washington, DC: National Academies Press; 2010. p. 29–33.
9. US Food and Drug Administration. Search for orphan drug designations and approvals: http://www.accessdata.fda.gov/scripts/opdlisting/oopd/OOPD_Results_2.cfm. Accessed 22 Nov 2015.
10. Nigro GL, Morreale A, Enea G. Open innovation: a real option to restore value to the biopharmaceutical R&D. Int J Prod Econ. 2014;149:183–93.
11. Walker A, Turner S, Johnson R. Pharma and biotech valuations: divergent perspectives. Bus Dev Lic J. 2015;22:10–3.
12. Cha M, Rifai B, Sarraf P. Pharmaceutical forecasting: throwing darts? Nat Rev Drug Disc. 2013;12:737–8.
13. Hughes JP, Rees S, Kalindjian SB, Philpott KL. Principles of early drug discovery. Br J Pharm. 2011;162:1239–49.
14. Mina-Osorio P. Basics of drug development in rheumatology. Arth Rheum. 2015;67:2581–90.
15. US Food and Drug Administration. Step 3: clinical research. 2015. http://www.fda.gov/ForPatients/Approvals/Drugs/ucm405622.htm. Accessed 22 Nov 2015.
16. Kesselheim AS, Wang B, Franklin JM, Darrow JJ. Trends in utilization of FDA expedited drug development and approval programs, 1987–2014: cohort study. BMJ. 2015;351:h4633. doi:10.1136/bmj/h4633.
17. Bujar M, McAuslane N, Liberti L. New drug approvals in ICH countries 2005-2014. London: Centre for Innovation in Regulatory Science (CIRS); 2015. http://cirsci.org/sites/default/files/CIRS_R&D_57_ICH_approval_times_2005-2014_ 06072015.pdf. Accessed 19 Nov 2015.
18. Curtin F, Schultz P. Assessing the benefit:risk ratio of a drug—randomized and naturalistic evidence. Dialogues Clin Neurosci. 2011;13:183–90.
19. Glasser SP, Salas M, Delzell E. Importance and challenges of studying marketed drugs: what is a phase IV study? Common clinical research designs, registries, and self-reporting systems. J Clin Pharmacol. 2007;47:1074–86.
20. Suvarna V. Phase IV of drug development. Perspect Clin Res. 2010;1:57–60.
21. Miossec P, Kolls JK. Targeting IL-17 and T_H17 cells in chronic inflammation. Nat Rev Drug Disc. 2012;11:763–76.
22. Wang B, Kesselheim AS. Characteristics of efficacy evidence supporting approval of supplemental indications for prescription drugs in United States, 2005-14: systematic review. BMJ. 2015;351:h4679. doi:10.1136/bmj.h4679.
23. Mendoza FA, Keyes-Elstein LL, Jimenez SA. Systemic sclerosis disease modification clinical trials design: quo vadis? Arth Care Res. 2012;64:945–54.
24. Richeldi L, Costabel U, Selman M, Kim DS, Hansell DM, Nicholson AG, et al. Efficacy of a tyrosine kinase inhibitor in idiopathic pulmonary fibrosis. N Engl J Med. 2011;365:1079–87.
25. Richeldi L, du Bois RM, Raghu G, Azuma A, Brown KK, Costabel U, et al. Efficacy and safety of nintedanib in idiopathic pulmonary fibrosis. N Engl J Med. 2014;370:2071–82.
26. Aravena C, Labarca G, Venegas C, Arenas A, Rada G. Pirfenidone for idiopathic pulmonary fibrosis: a systematic review and meta-analysis. PLoS ONE. 2015;10(8):0136160.

Physical and Occupational Therapy

44

Luc Mouthon and Janet L. Poole

Systemic sclerosis (SSc) is a connective tissue disease *that causes significant* disability, handicap, and worsening of quality of life [1–3]. Management of the person with SSc requires a multidisciplinary approach including rehabilitation techniques (Table 44.1) such as occupational and physical therapy. To determine the effectiveness of rehabilitation techniques, reliability and valid outcome measures are needed. This chapter will review assessments available to measure disability (Table 44.2) and participation in persons with SSc and discuss rehabilitation techniques that have been shown to be effective in improving joint motion, hand function, strength, general conditioning, and participation in daily life.

Measuring Disability and Participation Restrictions

There are a number of assessments available to measure disability and participation in persons with SSc. These assessments offer the opportunity to study joint motion, hand function, mouth disability, strength, general conditioning, and participation in daily life in order to demonstrate the effect of drugs and/or rehabilitation techniques. These measurement tools that are helpful for determining severity and outcomes following rehabilitation therapy are reviewed in the following paragraphs.

L. Mouthon, MD, PhD (✉)
Department of Internal Medicine, Hôpital Cochin, Paris, France
e-mail: luc.mouthon@cch.aphp.fr

J.L. Poole, PhD, OTR/L
Occupational Therapy Graduate Program, School of Medicine, University of New Mexico, Albuquerque, NM, USA

Health Assessment Questionnaire

Global disability in SSc patients is usually measured by the HAQ, a self-report questionnaire consisting of 20 items divided into eight categories [35]. Items are rated from 0 (no difficulty) to 3 (unable to do). The highest scores from each category are summed and divided by 8 to yield a disability score ranging from 0 (no disability) to 3 (maximal disability). The HAQ correlates well with the extent of skin thickening, loss of ability to close the fist, proximal muscle weakness, and tendon friction rubbing but not digital ulcers [1, 28]. In SSc patients, global disability can be measured with this scale [1, 28, 35], and an acceptable sensitivity to change has been suggested [29, 36, 37]. Steen and Medsger proposed the use of the sHAQ, a more disease-specific disability scale [29] *by adding five* patient-generated visual analog scales to the original HAQ, *thus* assessing Raynaud's phenomenon, digital-tip ulcers, gastrointestinal and lung symptoms, and overall disease severity from the patient's perspective [29].

Cochin Hand Function Scale (CHFS)

Hand disability can be evaluated with the CHFS, a functional disability questionnaire about daily activities that has been validated in rheumatoid arthritis (RA) and hand osteoarthritis [38–40]. The CHFS consists of 18 items concerning daily activities; each question is scored on a scale of 0 (performed without difficulty) to 5 (impossible to do). The total score is obtained by adding the scores of all items (range 0–90). This questionnaire has been validated in SSc [2, 32].

The CHFS has good convergent validity with global disability (HAQ and sHAQ) and global hand mobility (HFI and Kapandji indexes), a weaker correlation with patient's perceived handicap (MACTAR) and disability (SF-36 for physical function and PCS), and no correlation with anxiety

J. Varga et al. (eds.), *Scleroderma*, DOI 10.1007/978-3-319-31407-5_44

Table 44.1 Summary of studies on rehabilitation techniques in for systemic sclerosis

Type of rehabilitation intervention	Authors	Description of intervention	Summary of findings
Hand exercises	Mugii et al. (2006) [4]	Stretching exercises for joints of the hand	Total passive joint motion improved at 1-month post intervention which improved or was maintained at 1 year. Total hand function did not change (HAQ), but ability to perform individual items improved
	Piga et al. (2014) [5]	Home program consisting of mobility and strengthening exercises for the hand telemonitored as to number of repetitions, force, speed, and correctness. Control group received home program booklet and instruction on 3 strengthening and 3 mobility exercises	Both groups showed improvements in hand function and pinch and MCP ROM in the dominant hand. HAQ scores and HAMIS for the dominant hand and grip and pinch for the nondominant hand improved significantly only in the telemonitoring group. There was no difference between groups
Paraffin wax treatment and hand range-of-motion exercises	Askew et al. (1983) [6]	Combination of paraffin wax, friction massage, and range-of-motion for 1 session	Joint motion, skin compliance, and hand function improved more in intervention group than control group
	Pils et al. (1991) [7]	12 treatment sessions of paraffin; paraffin wax was continued for 3 months in an intervention group but discontinued in the control group	Intervention and control group received paraffin wax; joint motion increased and skin stiffness decreased. However, improvements maintained after 3 months in intervention but not control
	Sandqvist et al. (2004) [8]	Paraffin wax and hand exercises 1 time/day to one hand; other hand served as control	In the hands receiving the intervention, finger flexion and extension, thumb abduction, wrist flexion, and perceived skin thickness and elasticity significantly improved compared to baseline. Improvements from base line were greater for the intervention hands compared to the control hands for finger extension and perceived skin stiffness and elasticity
	Mancuso et al. (2009) [9]	Paraffin wax and hand exercises 5 days/week	Series of three single-case studies. Grip and pinch strength and hand function improved in all three participants, while total active joint motion increased in 2/3 of participants
Hand massage and joint manipulation	Maddali Bongi et al. (2009) [10]	Combination of connective tissue massage and Mc Mennell joint manipulation and home range-of-motion exercise	Fist closure, joint motion (HAMIS), hand function, and quality of life improved significantly, while fist closure only improved significantly in the control group
	Vannajak et al. (2014) [11]	Combination of superficial heat, traditional Thai massage, and stretching. In addition, the experimental group wore nylon gloves 6 h/day for 2 weeks	Joint motion (HAMIS) significantly improved in both groups; however, thumb motion improved only in the group that wore the glove
Splints	Seeger et al. (1987) [12]	Dorsal splint with dynamic PIP extension outrigger worn 8 h/day for 2 months	Joint range-of-motion of the PIP joint did not improve significantly in the splinted or nonsplinted hand
Mouth and facial exercises	Naylor et al. (1984) [13]	Mouth stretching and oral augmentation exercises	At 1 month there was no significant difference in mean mouth opening between the intervention group and a control (no treatment) group
	Pizzo et al. (2003) [14]	Mouth stretching and oral augmentation exercises for 15 min twice a day	Mouth opening significantly increased; subjective improvements in eating, speaking, and ability to perform oral hygiene
	Poole et al. (2010) [15]	Mouth exercises and oral augmentation exercises in combination with education on brushing and flossing teeth and adapted dental appliances	Dental hygiene improved significantly for decreased bleeding, supragingival calculus, and increases in caries. No significant improvement in mouth opening
	Yuen et al. (2011, 2012) [16, 17]	Powered toothbrush and flosser plus mouth stretching and oral augmentation exercises if oral aperture <40 mm compared to manual toothbrush and dental floss 2 times/day for 6 months	Gingival inflammation was significantly reduced both groups. Group that used powered toothbrush showed a significantly larger reduction in inflammation than manual toothbrush group. Oral aperture significantly increased compared to controls at 3 months but not at 6 months
Massage and stretching of the face and mouth	Maddali et al. (2010) [18]	Combination of connective tissue massage, Kabat's technique, kinesitherapy, and a home exercise program	Mouth opening increased, and skin scores decreased in the intervention group compared to the home exercise only control group

(continued)

Table 44.1 (continued)

Type of rehabilitation intervention	Authors	Description of intervention	Summary of findings
Overall rehabilitation consisting of specific and global techniques	Maddali Bongi et al. (2010) [18]	Specific techniques included hand and face exercises and connective tissue massage. Those with hand edema received manual lymphatic drainage. Global techniques included respiratory exercises and land- or water-based program	Quality of life, functional ability, hand mobility and function, mouth opening, and face mobility all significantly increased at the end of the 9-week program At the 9 week follow-up, only improvements in mouth opening and hand mobility were maintained No improvements were noted in a control group who received information about scleroderma
	Schouffoer et al. (2011) [19]	Multidisciplinary intervention 1 day per week consisting of group sessions (general exercise, hand and mouth exercises, education), supervised home exercises provided by a PT 1/week, and home-based exercise program 6 days per week	Grip strength, mouth opening, distance walked in 6 min, and functional ability significantly increased at the end of the 12-week program compared to a control group who received regular outpatient care. At 24 weeks, only improvements in mouth opening was maintained
Generalized physical exercise	Oliveira et al. (2009) [20]	Progressive aerobic exercises 2 times/week consisting of 5-min warm-up, 40-min aerobics, and 5-min cooldown	Peak VO_2 increased significantly but no difference between an intervention group and control group of healthy individuals. No change in skin scores in the SSc group. No change in quality of life in both groups
	Pinto et al. (2010) [21]	Combination of 30 min of resistive training and 20 min of aerobic training. Resistive training consisted of bench press, leg press, lat pull down, leg extension, and seated row. The aerobic training was done on a treadmill	Dynamic strength (leg press, bench press) and isometric strength (hand and low back), and scores on the timed-stands test improved significantly after the 12-week training. There were no changes in peak VO_2, heart rate at rest was significantly reduced, time to exhaustion was increased, and workload and time of exercise at ventilatory thresholds and peak of exercise were increased. There were no changes in skin scores or muscle enzymes which stayed within normal limits
	Alexanderson et al. (2014) [22]	Combination of aerobic exercise on stationary bike and resistance training for the shoulder and hip flexor muscle groups 3 times/week for 14 weeks	Series of 4 single-case studies. Muscular endurance improved significantly in 3 participants, while aerobic capacity improved significantly in 2 participants
Self-management	Samuelson and Ahlmen (2000) [23]	Self-management program consisting of seven 3-h group sessions for 5 weeks. Content included medical aspects, exercise, joint protection and energy conservation, splints, activities of daily living and assistive devices, modalities and pain control, relaxation, and diet	Participants reported improvements in self-efficacy. Course evaluations showed that participants were satisfied with the content of the program and opportunities to meet others with SSc
	Brown et al. (2004) [24]	Self-management program consisting of four 3-h group sessions. Content included medical aspects, self-management, medications, relaxation, and relationships with family and health professionals	Qualitative evaluation of the program revealed that participants felt it was valuable meeting others with SSc, the involvement of a patient educator, practical tips for daily living, fatigue and time management, and the family session
	Poole et al. (2009) [25]	Self-paced self-management program consisting of a workbook and exercise DVD. Workbook content included medical aspects and management of symptoms, coping skills, exercises, activities of daily living, and advocacy	Fatigue and pain decreased while hand function increased; however, significant improvements seen for self-efficacy for pain
	Kwakkenbos et al. (2011) [26]	Multidisciplinary intervention over 6 weeks consisting of group sessions (goal setting, education, joint protection and energy conservation, psychosocial aspects, exercise, introduction to Tai Chi	Participants reported less helplessness and higher acceptance of limitations post intervention and at 6 months. No changes in mood or physical function
	Poole et al. (2014) [27]	Self-paced Internet self-management program included content on medical aspects, management of symptoms, advocacy, coping, exercise and activities of daily living, an interactive discussion board, resources, learning activities, and an exercise video	Significant improvements found for ability to manage care, health efficacy, and decreases in fatigue and depression. Evaluation of the program was positive

HAMIS hand mobility in scleroderma, *HAQ* health assessment questionnaire, *PIP* proximal interphalangeal

Table 44.2 Available/validated instruments measuring disability and participation restrictions in systemic sclerosis

	Authors	Number of patients	Reliability	Validity/construct validity	Sensitivity to change
HAQ	Poole J et al. (1991) [1]	211	Good	Good validity	NA
	Poole J et al. (1995) [28]	80	Good	Good validity	NA
	Steen et al. (1997) [29]	1,250		Good validity	Acceptable
HAMIS	Sandqvist et al. (2000) [30]	30	Good		NA
	Sandqvist et al. (2000) [31]	45	Good	Good validity	NA
CHFS	Brower et al. (2004) [32]	40	Good	Good validity	NA
	Rannou et al. (2007) [2]	50	Factor analysis extracted 2 factors that accounted for 71.63 % of the total variance: activities requiring grip and pinch strength; activities requiring pinch dexterity	Good construct validity; significant correlations between CHFS, HAQ, and HFI scores. CHFS scores contribute to 75 % of the HAQ variance	NA
MHISS	Mouthon et al. (2007) [33]	71	Excellent 3 factors explore disability due to mouth opening limitation, mouth dryness, and the aesthetic concerns	Good construct validity	NA
DASH	Varju et al. (2008) [34]	128/76[a]	Good	NA	SRM: 0.64

CHFS Cochin hand function scale, *DASH* disabilities of the arm, shoulder, and hand, *HAMIS* hand mobility in scleroderma, *HAQ* health assessment questionnaire, *MHISS* mouth handicap in systemic sclerosis, *NA* not assessed, *SRM* standardized response mean
[a]12-month follow-up

(HADa), SF-36 MCS, depression (HADd), disease duration, and age [2]. Factor analysis extracted two factors that accounted for *71.6 %* of the total variance. The first factor represented mainly activities requiring grip and pinch strength and the second represented activities requiring pinch dexterity.

The CHFS has also been used as a location-specific disability scale for hand involvement in the determination of disability in SSc [2, 32]. When assessed separately, CHFS score contributes to 75 % of the HAQ variance [2]. The mean CHSF score was 16.56 ± 16.40 and explained 75 % of the variance in HAQ global score. Significant differences were observed between patients with lcSSc and dSSc for *CHFS (11.07 ± 11.04 vs. 23.48 ± 19.45) (p = 0.01) and HAQ (0.90 ± 0.57 vs. 1.28 ± 0.75) (p = 0.05) scores* [2].

Keitel Functional Test

A German functional performance test, the Keitel Functional Test (KFT), has been developed for use in patients with RA. The KFT assesses 24 simple movement patterns for both upper and lower extremities. The 24 items are graded with a scoring system in which an index value of 100 points corresponds to normal functional ability. The test can be performed in 15–20 min and does not require any specific instrument [41]. This RA-specific measure of impairment of body functions has for several years been used by physical therapists in Denmark, for both inpatients in hospitals and outpatients in rehabilitation clinics, without prior validation. The KFT has been described as an outcome measure [42] and as a gold standard for evaluation of a new index of hand function [43]. It has been shown to have good concurrent validity [44], especially when used with the HAQ [45–47], and it has been reported to be a strong predictor of mortality [48]. *To our knowledge, this score has not been used as is in patients with SSc. However, the hand functional index (HFI), which consists of the first nine questions of the KFT, might help to evaluate hand function in these patients* [2].

Hand Function Index (HFI)

The hand functional index (HFI) consists of the first nine questions of the KFT which assesses finger and wrist flexion (four points for each hand) and extension (four points for each hand), forearm pronation and supination (three points for each forearm), and thumb abduction (three points for each thumb). The HFI score ranges from 4 (best mobility) to 42 (worst mobility). In a series of 50 patients with SSc, the HFI score was higher in patients with dSSc than in patients with lcSSc (19.35 ± 11.95 vs. 11.57 ± 8.21 ($p < 0.01$)) [2]. In this work, the correlation coefficient of the HFI with the CHFS was 0.58. This scale could be used by occupational and physical therapists for both inpatients in hospitals and outpatients in rehabilitation clinics in order to evaluate the effect of rehabilitation on hand function: finger and wrist flexion and extension, forearm pronation and supination, and thumb abduction. We have used this scale in a prospective randomized clinical trial conducted in 220 patients comparing supervised inhospital rehabilitation vs. outpatient rehabilitation. The results will be available at the end of 2011.

Kapandji Index

The Kapandji index assesses long-finger flexion (20 points for each hand) and extension (20 points for each hand) and thumb opposition (10 points for each thumb). Score ranges from 0 (worst mobility) to 100 (best mobility).

In patients with SSc, we have assessed global hand and wrist mobility by the use of the hand functional index (HFI) and the Kapandji index [2]. In SSc patients, hand global mobility was reduced, with mean HFI and Kapandji scores of *15.08±10.22* and *78.75±19.94*, respectively. Significant differences were observed between patients with lcSSc and dSSc for the Kapandji index which was higher in patients with dSSc than in patients with lcSSc (85.69±15.50 vs. 70.00±20.70 ($p<0.01$)) [2]. In this work, the correlation coefficient of the Kapandji index with the CHFS was 0.63. Whether the HFI or the Kapandji scales will be the best scale to evaluate hand and wrist mobility in patients with SSc is not known. However, these two scales have been used in a prospective randomized clinical trial conducted in 220 patients comparing supervised inhospital rehabilitation vs. outpatient rehabilitation, the results of which will be available at the end of 2011.

Hand Mobility in Scleroderma (HAMIS)

The HAMIS is a hand function test developed for adult patients with SSc. It consists of nine items designed to measure all movements assessed in an ordinary range-of-motion-measured hand test (finger and wrist flexion and extension, thumb flexion and abduction, forearm pronation and supination). HAMIS has a demonstrated concurrent validity compared with range-of-motion and skin score. Except for the pronation and supination items, the other items on the HAMIS showed significant differences between healthy individuals and persons with SSc, attesting to the discriminating ability of the HAMIS [30]. HAMIS is a reliable instrument for evaluation of hand function on SSc patients [31]. However, in order to perform the HAMIS, a number of accessories are necessary, which is not the case for HFI or Kapandji scales. Therefore, there is a need for comparison of these three approaches for the evaluation of hand function in patients with SSc.

Disabilities of the Arm, Shoulder, and Hand (DASH)

The DASH was developed for patients with upper-extremity musculoskeletal conditions. It is a self-administered measure of symptoms and functional status, with a focus on physical function, used by clinicians in daily practice and as a research tool. The DASH consists mainly of a 30-item disability/symptom scale [49]. A short version of the DASH, the QuickDASH, has also been developed. This scale has been validated in a cohort of Hungarian patients with SSc [34]. In this study, the DASH and QuickDASH correlated strongly with the HAQ-DI and with the physical dimensions of the SF-36, providing evidence that the disability of the patient with SSc is predominantly caused by the functional impairment of the upper limb. The authors recommend the shorter and simpler QuickDASH for everyday clinical use [34]. Actually, it is difficult to get a definitive idea on the interest of the QuickDASH in patients with SSc. It would probably be of interest to use this scale as a secondary outcome measure in rehabilitation trials for the evaluation of functional impairment of the upper limb in patients with SSc.

Mouth Handicap in Systemic Sclerosis Scale (MHISS)

Mouth disability can be evaluated using the MHISS scale, a self-assessment questionnaire with 12 items concerning daily activities involving the face such as eating/drinking, speaking, oral hygiene, appearance, and condition of the mouth. Each question is scored on a scale of 0 (never) to 4 (always) [33]. The total score is obtained by adding the scores of all items (range 0–48). The mean total score obtained in a cohort of 71 SSc patients was 20.3±9.7. Test-retest reliability was 0.96. Divergent validity was confirmed for global disability (Health Assessment Questionnaire [HAQ]), hand function (Cochin Hand Function Scale), interincisor distance, handicap (McMaster-Toronto Arthritis questionnaire [MACTAR]), depression (Hospital Anxiety and Depression [HAD]; HADd), and anxiety (HADa). Factor analysis extracted three factors with eigenvalues of 4.26, 1.76, and 1.47 explaining 63% of the variance. The first factor (five items) represents handicap induced by the reduction in mouth opening, the second (five items) handicap induced by sicca syndrome, and the third (three items) aesthetic concerns. In that study, the MHISS score contributed to 36% of the HAQ variance [33], highlighting the need to specifically assess mouth disability in SSc patients when evaluating treatment. To our knowledge, this scale is the only available scale that allows to measure mouth disability in patients with SSc. The interest of this scale should be evaluated in rehabilitation trials.

Evaluation of Patient Priorities

Patients' priorities in disability can be assessed by use of a French version of the McMaster-Toronto Arthritis Patient Preference Disability Questionnaire (MACTAR) as described by Tugwell et al. [50]. The MACTAR questions are open ended and cover broad areas of function such as domestic care, self-care, professional activities, leisure activities, social interaction, and roles. Patients are encouraged to add activities not already listed. Patients are asked to rank these activities in order of importance by answering "Which of these activities would you most like to be able to do?" In patients with SSc, we used a "3-item priority function" and asked patients to identify and rank three situations among activities of daily living that caused them maximal trouble. In the original MACTAR, items were not scored, but patients were asked if they had noticed changes in the problem they had identified several weeks ago. In the validation study of the MACTAR, a Likert scale was added to quantify changes [51]. In order to reflect the degree of difficulty in performing a priority activity, each item was scored on an 11-point semiquantitative scale (0–10), the global score ranging from 0 (no disability) to 30 (maximal disability).

Mouthon and colleagues provided evidence that the MACTAR adds relevant information when assessing patients with SSc and has acceptable construct validity. Its weak correlation with HAQ and the large number of activities cited and ranked by patients suggests that it adds useful information about patients' perceived disability [52]. *The evolution in MACTAR global score over time for patients with SSc reflects a general feeling of deterioration over time. However, shifts in patient priorities are common and may influence the sensitivity to change of the instrument* [53]. *Thus, additional studies are needed to better define the usefulness of the MACTAR in prospective studies.*

Rehabilitation

Rehabilitation therapies, such as occupational and physical therapy, are indicated for the person with SSc to improve joint motion, hand function, strength and general conditioning, and participation in daily activities such as self-care, home management, leisure, and work. Referral to therapy should be made early in the course of the disease especially in patients with early diffuse SSc. With disease progression, therapy referral should be made as soon as patients or physicians note decreases in joint motion and difficulty with daily tasks or work.

Hand Exercises

Because of the hand involvement and contractures observed in persons with scleroderma, range-of-motion exercises for the hand emphasize increasing flexion at the metacarpophalangeal joint, extension of the proximal interphalangeal joints, and flexion and abduction of the thumb. One study showed that total passive motion in each finger along with hand function improved after a 1-month program of stretching exercises for individual finger [4], while another study showed that hand mobility and strengthening exercises resulted in improved hand function, pinch, and metacarpophalangeal flexion [5].

Heat modalities, such as paraffin wax or hot packs, may be used before commencing range-of-motion exercises to reduce pain and increase extensibility of collagen tissue. Heat is generally applied for 20 min followed by range-of-motion and stretching exercises. Each exercise is done one to two times a day and should be held in a position for stretch for 3–5 s and repeated three to five times as directed by a therapist. Several studies have evaluated the effectiveness of hand range-of-motion exercises in conjunction with paraffin wax treatments. These studies which have varied in research design, duration, and sample size generally found increased in hand motion, dexterity, and strength after treatment [7–9, 31].

Joint motion and stretching exercises (exaggerated facial movements, manual stretching of the mouth with the thumbs, and oral augmentation exercises with tongue depressors) have also been used to improve mouth opening [5, 13, 17, 54]. Two pretest-posttest design studies and two randomized controlled trials showed increases in mouth opening after stretching, augmentation exercises [13–15, 17]. In addition, one study reported subjective improvements in eating and speaking [14], while two studies showed improvements in some aspects of dental hygiene [15, 16]. In a separate study, a combination of connective tissue massage to the face, Kabat's technique (proprioceptive neuromuscular facilitation stretch and resistive techniques for the face), and face exercises (kinesitherapy) resulted in significant improvements in mouth opening and decreases in facial skin scores in the intervention group compared to a group who received a home exercise program for the mouth and face [18].

Splints are used to maintain or increase range-of-motion, particularly in the hand. Dynamic splints, which apply a constant force over a period of time to passively stretch a joint, were not shown to be effective in maintaining or improving extension of the proximal interphalangeal joint in persons with SSc [12] *and probably not recommended.*

Massage has been investigated in two studies in combination with very different types of rehabilitation interventions. Connective tissue massage in conjunction with Mc Mennell joint manipulation and a home exercise program resulted in significant improvements in fist closure, hand function, and quality of life compared to a control group who received a home exercise program [18]. Thai massage along with stretching and heat improved joint motion; when combined with a nylon glove, the intervention also increased thumb motion [11].

While studies have shown that joint motion in the lower extremities is decreased in persons with SSc, there are no studies that have focused solely on interventions to improve joint motion for the lower extremities. The few studies listed in the next section show improvements in mobility such as walking, after conditioning exercises involving the lower extremities such as treadmill walking, riding a stationary bike, and aerobic exercises.

Strengthening and General Exercise and Conditioning

Strengthening and general conditioning exercises are indicated for the person with SSc to improve cardiovascular fitness. Resistive exercises using weights, elastic bands, exercise putty, and/or exercise machines can be used to increase muscle strength. General conditioning exercises could include water exercise, swimming, walking, cycling, or other aerobic exercises. It has only been recently that the effectiveness of multidisciplinary exercise and conditioning programs was evaluated. A 9-week program combining hand- and face-specific exercises, a global water- or land-based exercise program, showed improvements in hand and face motion, hand and overall function, and quality of life compared to a control group [10]. Antonioli et al. [55] evaluated the effectiveness of an individualized program consisting of breathing exercises, treadmill- and land-based walking, and upper-extremity exercises including stretching. At the end of 4 months, improvements were noted in quality of life and hand mobility, and decreases seen in heart rate and dyspnea after performing the 6-min walk test. A series of single-case studies using a combination of aerobic exercise and proximal muscle resistance training reported improvements in muscular endurance and aerobic capacity [22]. A slightly different multidisciplinary program involving group and individually tailored exercises in combination with group education and individualized goal setting was shown to be more effective than usual care in improving grip strength, mouth opening, distance walked, and function ability [19].

The effectiveness of an 8-week aerobic exercise program was evaluated in a group of 12 women with SSc but without lung involvement [20]. Sessions were for 40 min two times per week; each session consisted of a 5-min warm-up, aerobic exercise that was progressively increased until target heart rate was reached, followed by a 5-min cooldown. Improvements were seen in peak VO_2 and exercise intensity, but the improvements were not significantly different compared to a control group. However, a second study combining aerobic training along with a strengthening program reported improved muscle strength, function (timed-stands test), and aerobic capacity in persons with SSc without lung involvement (pulmonary artery systolic pressure>40 mmHg and forced vital capacity measured>75 % of predicted value for age and gender). There were no significant changes in peak VO2 or serum markers for muscle damage (CK, aldolase). Thus, these studies showed that aerobic exercise is safe in persons with SSc without lung involvement; those with lung involvement should probably get evaluated by their physicians and be monitored initially by a physical therapist or exercise physiologist.

Self-management Programs

Management of a complex chronic disease such as SSc requires that the person with the disease become a manager of symptoms and all aspects of treatment. Because SSc is a rare disease and the symptoms are very different from other rheumatic diseases, several disease-specific self-management programs have been developed. These programs were offered in a group format in which participants met for 3 h once a week for 4–5 weeks [23, 32]. Participants reported increases in perceived self-efficacy and confidence to manage the disease and were satisfied with content. However, the sample sizes were small in these studies so statistical analyses were not preformed (12 in Brown et al. [24]; 6 in Sandqvist [56]). Kwakkenbos and colleagues [26] reported less helplessness and higher acceptance of limitations in a group of people with SSc who participated in a psychoeducation program delivered via group format. The content included disease education, goal setting, joint protection and energy conservation, and managing psychosocial aspects of SSc. Due to the challenges of participating in group sessions, a self-management program, consisting of a workbook and exercise DVD, was developed to reach persons who did not have access to support groups or education programs. Modeled after concepts used in the Arthritis Self-Management Programs, the workbook had action plans and learning activities at the end of each chapter. While improvements in fatigue, hand function, and pain were observed, the only significant improvement was for self-efficacy for managing pain [57]. A subsequent study which converted the content to an interactive Internet format found significant improvements in the ability to manage care, health efficacy, and decreases in fatigue and depression [27]. Thus, self-management offerings exclusively for persons with SSc should be explored using methods that can be accessed remotely.

Finally, rehabilitation professionals have expertise in non-pharmaceutical modalities to manage digital ulcers. Moran et al. [58] systematically reviewed studies using modalities including intermittent compression, topical vitamin E, hyperbaric oxygen therapy, negative pressure therapy, acoustic pressure wound therapy, exercise, and iontophoresis. However, no one modality was better than others; although vitamin E gel and iontophoresis may warrant more investigation with large sample sizes and better designed and controlled studies.

Conclusions

SSc is responsible for skin, tendon, joint, and vessel damage, which leads to disability, handicap, and worsening of quality of life [1–3]. A number of assessments are available to measure disability and participation in persons with SSc. These assessments offer the opportunity to examine and monitor joint motion, hand function, mouth disability, strength, general conditioning, and participation in daily life.

The current literature on rehabilitation techniques consists of studies evaluating the effectiveness of paraffin wax treatment, hand and face stretching exercises, connective tissue massage and joint manipulation, splints, and aerobic exercise and resistance training (for a review, see [57]). Only a small number of randomized controlled trials were identified, and the majority of studies involved small sample sizes and no control groups. However, improvement in joint motion, hand function, and cardiopulmonary endurance was clear upon analysis of the results. Hand exercises seem to offer a benefit in patients with SSc.

Based on the limited number of studies available conducted in limited numbers of patients, physical and occupational therapy might increase and maintain mobility and strength and improve functional mobility and cardiopulmonary functioning. Table 44.3 provides guidelines/recommendations for rehabilitation interventions.

Table 44.3 Guidelines/recommendations for rehabilitation interventions

Limitation	Examples of interventions
Decreased ability to fully flex and extend fingers (i.e., palm of hand does not lay flat on a table)	Modalities before exercises:
	1. Paraffin
	2. Connective tissue massage
	3. Joint manipulation
	Hand exercises:
	1. Make a fist, push down on proximal phalanx
	2. Press fingers flat against table so palmer surface of hand and fingers touch table
	3. Press fingers against each other in a prayer position
	4. Touch thumb to bottom of little finger
	5. Pads of index finger and thumb of one hand against pads of index finger and thumb of other hand; attempt to stretch web space
Difficulty reaching to wash/comb hair	Shoulder exercises:
	1. Wall fingers up a wall
	2. Lie supine and flex shoulders overhead
	3. Stretching exercises to other upper-extremity joints
	4. Strengthening exercises to upper extremities with weights, elastic bands, or machines
	Assistive devices or alternate techniques:
	1. Long-handled sponge
	2. Long-handled comb or brush
Difficulty opening mouth (difficulty to brush and floss teeth or eat)	Mouth and face exercises:
	1. Exaggerated facial movements
	2. Manual stretching of mouth with the thumbs
	3. Oral augmentation exercises
	4. Massage to facial muscles
	Assistive devices or modified oral appliances:
	1. Child toothbrushes/electric
	2. Electric flossers

(continued)

Table 44.3 (continued)

Limitation	Examples of interventions
Difficulty reaching to tie shoes or cut toenails	Lower extremity stretching:
	1. Hamstring stretch
	2. Cross leg with ankle of one leg above knee of other (external rotation of hip)
	3. Yoga
	Assistive devices or alternate technique:
	1. Slip on/Velcro shoes
	2. Reachers
Difficulty walking	Strengthening and conditioning exercises:
	1. Land based – walking, treadmill walking, cycling, aerobics
	2. Water based – water exercises, swimming
	3. Yoga
	Resistive exercise – weights, elastic bands, machines:
	1. Knee extension with weights on ankles for quadriceps
	2. Sit to stand without using arms for quadriceps, hamstrings, and gluteal muscles
	3. Stand on toes for gastrocnemius muscles
	4. Exercise machines for isolated lower extremity muscles
	Assistive walking devices:
	1. Walker, cane, wheelchair
	2. Electric wheelchair, scooter
Difficulty using hands to perform daily activities	Hand exercises:
	1. See above
	2. Resistive exercises with exercise putty
	Assistive devices or alternate techniques:
	1. Built up handles on utensils
	2. Stemmed glasses
	3. Electrical appliances such as choppers
	4. Head sets for telephone, voice programs for computer
Fatigue upon doing daily activities	Education on energy conservation:
	1. Pace – alternate activity and rest
	2. Prioritize activities
	3. Plan in advance
	4. Alternate position between sit and stand
	Strengthening and conditioning exercises:
	1. See above under walking
	Assistive devices or alternate techniques:
	1. Electrical appliances
	2. Ergonomic tools
	3. Ergonomic setups at home and work
	4. Support from family, friends, or hired help

References

1. Poole JL, Steen VD. The use of the health assessment questionnaire (HAQ) to determine physical disability in systemic sclerosis. Arthritis Care Res. 1991;4(1):27–31.
2. Rannou F, Poiraudeau S, Berezné A, Baubet T, Le-Guern V, Cabane J, et al. Assessing disability and quality of life in systemic sclerosis: construct validities of the Cochin hand function scale, health assessment questionnaire (HAQ), systemic sclerosis HAQ, and MOS SF-36. Arthritis Rheum. 2007;57(1):94–102 [Epub ahead of print].
3. Hudson M, Thombs BD, Steele R, Watterson R, Taillefer S, Baron M. Clinical correlates of quality of life in systemic sclerosis measured with the world health organization disability assessment schedule II. Arthritis Rheum. 2008;59(2):279–84.
4. Mugii N, Hasegawa M, Matsushita T, Kondo M, Orito H, Yanaba K, et al. The efficacy of self-administered stretching for finger joint motion in Japanese patients with systemic sclerosis. J Rheumatol. 2006;33(8):1586–92.
5. Piga M, Tradori I, Pani D, Barabino G, Dessi A, et al. J Rheumatol. 2014;41:1324–33.
6. Askew LJ, Beckett VL, An KN, Chao EY. Objective evaluation of hand function in scleroderma patients to assess effectiveness of physical therapy. Br J Rheumatol. 1983;22(4):224–32.
7. Pils K, Graninger W, Sadil F. Paraffin hand bath for scleroderma. Phys Med Rehabil. 1991;1:19–21.
8. Sandqvist G, Akesson A, Eklund M. Evaluation of paraffin bath treatment in patients with systemic sclerosis. Disabil Rehabil. 2004;26(16):981–7.

9. Mancuso T, Poole JL. The effect of paraffin and exercise on hand function in persons with scleroderma: a series of single case studies. J Hand Ther. 2009;22(1):71–7. quiz 78.
10. Maddali Bongi S, Del Rosso A, Galluccio F, Tai G, Sigismondi F, Passalacqua M, et al. Efficacy of a tailored rehabilitation program for systemic sclerosis. Clin Exp Rheumatol. 2009;27(3 Suppl 54):44–50.
11. Vannajak K, Boonprakob Y, Eungpinichpong W, Ungpansattawong S, Nanagara T. The short term effect of gloving in combination with traditional Thai massage, heat, and stretching exercise to improve hand mobility in scleroderma patients. J Ayurveda Integr Med. 2014;5:505–55.
12. Seeger MW, Furst DE. Effects of splinting in the treatment of hand contractures in progressive systemic sclerosis. Am J Occup Ther. 1987;41(2):118–21.
13. Naylor WP, Douglass CW, Mix E. The nonsurgical treatment of microstomia in scleroderma: a pilot study. Oral Surg Oral Med Oral Pathol. 1984;57(5):508–11.
14. Pizzo G, Scardina GA, Messina P. Effects of a nonsurgical exercise program on the decreased mouth opening in patients with systemic scleroderma. Clin Oral Investig. 2003;7(3):175–8.
15. Poole J, Conte C, Brewer C, Good CC, Perella D, Rossie KM, et al. Oral hygiene in scleroderma: the effectiveness of a multi-disciplinary intervention program. Disabil Rehabil. 2010;32(5):379–84.
16. Yuen HK, Weng Y, Bandyopadhyay D, Reed SG, Leite RS, Silver RM. Effect of a multi-faceted intervention on gingival health among adults with systemic sclerosis. Clin Exp Rheumatol. 2011;29 Suppl 65:S26–32.
17. Yuen HK, Marlow NM, Reed SG, Mahoney S, Summerlin LM, et al. Effect of orofacial exercises on oral aperture in adults with systemic sclerosis. Disabil Rehabil. 2012;34:84–9.
18. Maddali-Bongi S, Landi G, Galluccio F, Del Rosso A, Miniati I, Conforti ML, et al. The rehabilitation of facial involvement in systemic sclerosis: efficacy of the combination of connective tissue massage, Kabat's technique and kinesitherapy: a randomized controlled trial. Rheumatol Int. 2010;31(7):895–901.
19. Schouffoer AA, Ninaber MK, Beaart-van de Voorde LJ, van der Giesen FJ, de Jong Z, Stolk J, et al. A randomised comparison of a multidisciplinary team care program with usual care in patients with systemic sclerosis. Arthritis Care Res (Hoboken). 2011;63(6):909–17.
20. Oliveira NC, dos Santos Sabbag LM, de Sa Pinto AL, Borges CL, Lima FR. Aerobic exercise is safe and effective in systemic sclerosis. Int J Sports Med. 2009;30(10):728–32.
21. Pinto AL, Oliveira NC, Gualano B, Christmann RB, Painelli VS, Artioli GG, et al. Efficacy and safety of concurrent training in systemic sclerosis. J Strength Cond Res. 2010;25(5):1423–8.
22. Alexanderson H, Bergegard J, Bjornadal L, Nordin A. Intensive aerobic and muscle endurance exercise in patients with systemic sclerosis; a pilot study. BMC Res Notes. 2014;7:86.
23. Samuelson UK, Ahlmen EM. Development and evaluation of a patient education program for persons with systemic sclerosis (scleroderma). Arthritis Care Res. 2000;13(3):141–8.
24. Brown SJ, Somerset ME, McCabe CS, McHugh NJ. The impact of group education on participants' management of their disease in lupus and scleroderma. Musculoskelet Care. 2004;2(4):207–17.
25. Poole J, Mendelson C, Skipper B. The effectiveness of a scleroderma self management program delivered via booklet and DVD. Arthritis Rheum. 2013;32:1393–8.
26. Kwakkenbos L, Bluyssen SJM, Vonk MC, van Helmond AF, van den Ende CHM, van den Hoogen FHJ, et al. Addressing patient health care demands in systemic sclerosis: pre-post assessment of a psycho-educational group programme. Clin Exp Rheumatol. 2011;29 Suppl 65:S60–5.
27. Poole JL, Mendelson C, Skipper B, Khanna D. Taking charge of systemic sclerosis: a pilot study to assess the effectiveness of an internet self-management program. Arthritis Care Res. 2014;66(50):778–82.
28. Poole JL, William CA, Bloch DA, Hollak B, Spitz P. Concurrent validity of the health assessment questionnaire disability index in scleroderma. Arthritis Care Res. 1995;8(3):189–93.
29. Steen VD, Medsger TA. The value of the health assessment questionnaire and special patient-generated scales to demonstrate change in systemic sclerosis patients over time. Arthritis Rheum. 1997;40(11):1984–91.
30. Sandqvist G, Eklund M. Validity of HAMIS: a test of hand mobility in scleroderma. Arthritis Care Res. 2000;13(6):382–7.
31. Sandqvist G, Eklund M. Hand Mobility in Scleroderma (HAMIS) test: the reliability of a novel hand function test. Arthritis Care Res. 2000;13(6):369–74.
32. Brower LM, Poole JL. Reliability and validity of the Duruoz Hand Index in persons with systemic sclerosis (scleroderma). Arthritis Rheum. 2004;51(5):805–9.
33. Mouthon L, Rannou F, Berezne A, Pagnoux C, Arene JP, Fois E, et al. Development and validation of a scale for mouth handicap in systemic sclerosis: the mouth handicap in systemic sclerosis scale. Ann Rheum Dis. 2007;66(12):1651–5.
34. Varju C, Balint Z, Solyom AI, Farkas H, Karpati E, Berta B, et al. Cross-cultural adaptation of the disabilities of the arm, shoulder, and hand (DASH) questionnaire into Hungarian and investigation of its validity in patients with systemic sclerosis. Clin Exp Rheumatol. 2008;26(5):776–83.
35. Merkel PA, Herlyn K, Martin RW, Anderson JJ, Mayes MD, Bell P, et al. Measuring disease activity and functional status in patients with scleroderma and Raynaud's phenomenon. Arthritis Rheum. 2002;46(9):2410–20.
36. Clements PJ, Wong WK, Hurwitz EL, Furst DE, Mayes M, White B, et al. The disability index of the health assessment questionnaire is a predictor and correlate of outcome in the high-dose versus low-dose penicillamine in systemic sclerosis trial. Arthritis Rheum. 2001;44(3):653–61.
37. Khanna D, Furst DE, Clements PJ, Park GS, Hays RD, Yoon J, et al. Responsiveness of the SF-36 and the health assessment questionnaire disability index in a systemic sclerosis clinical trial. J Rheumatol. 2005;32(5):832–40.
38. Duruoz MT, Poiraudeau S, Fermanian J, Menkes CJ, Amor B, Dougados M, et al. Development and validation of a rheumatoid hand functional disability scale that assesses functional handicap. J Rheumatol. 1996;23(7):1167–72.
39. Poiraudeau S, Lefevre-Colau MM, Fermanian J, Revel M. The ability of the Cochin rheumatoid arthritis hand functional scale to detect change during the course of disease. Arthritis Care Res. 2000;13(5):296–303.
40. Poiraudeau S, Chevalier X, Conrozier T, Flippo RM, Liote F, Noel E, et al. Reliability, validity, and sensitivity to change of the Cochin hand functional disability scale in hand osteoarthritis. Osteoarthr Cartil. 2001;9(6):570–7.
41. Keitel W, Hoffman H, Weber G, Krieger U. Development of a arm functional test for rheumatologic diseases. Dtsch Gesundheitsw. 1971;26:1901–3.
42. Keysser M, Keysser C, Keitel W, Keysser G. Loss of functional capacity caused by a delayed onset of DMARD therapy in rheumatoid arthritis. Long-term follow-up results of the Keitel function test. Brief definite report. Z Rheumatol. 2001;60(2):69–73.
43. Poole JL, Cordova KJ, Brower LM. Reliability and validity of a self-report of hand function in persons with rheumatoid arthritis. J Hand Ther. 2006;19(1):12–6. quiz 17.
44. Kalla AA, Kotze TJ, Meyers OL, Parkyn ND. Clinical assessment of disease activity in rheumatoid arthritis: evaluation of a functional test. Ann Rheum Dis. 1988;47(9):773–9.
45. Bombardier C, Raboud J. A comparison of health-related quality-of-life measures for rheumatoid arthritis research. The Auranofin

Cooperating Group. Control Clin Trials. 1991;12(4 Suppl): 243S–56.
46. Hakala M, Nieminen P, Manelius J. Joint impairment is strongly correlated with disability measured by self-report questionnaires. Functional status assessment of individuals with rheumatoid arthritis in a population based series. J Rheumatol. 1994;21(1):64–9.
47. Hakala M, Nieminen P. Functional status assessment of physical impairment in a community based population with rheumatoid arthritis: severely incapacitated patients are rare. J Rheumatol. 1996;23(4):617–23.
48. Soderlin MK, Nieminen P, Hakala M. Arthritis impact measurement scales in a community-based rheumatoid arthritis population. Clin Rheumatol. 2000;19(1):30–4.
49. Hudak PL, Cole DC, Haines AT. Understanding prognosis to improve rehabilitation: the example of lateral elbow pain. Arch Phys Med Rehabil. 1996;77(6):586–93.
50. Tugwell P, Bombardier C, Buchanan WW, Goldsmith CH, Grace E, Hanna B. The MACTAR patient preference disability questionnaire–an individualized functional priority approach for assessing improvement in physical disability in clinical trials in rheumatoid arthritis. J Rheumatol. 1987;14(3):446–51.
51. Verhoeven AC, Boers M, van der Liden S. Validity of the MACTAR questionnaire as a functional index in a rheumatoid arthritis clinical trial. McMaster Tor Arthritis J Rheumatol. 2000;27(12):2801–9.
52. Mouthon L, Rannou F, Berezne A, Pagnoux C, Guilpain P, Goldwasser F, et al. Patient preference disability questionnaire in systemic sclerosis: a cross-sectional survey. Arthritis Rheum. 2008;59(7):968–73.
53. Nguyen C, Mouthon L, Mestre-Stanislas C, Rannou F, Berezne A, Sanchez K, et al. Sensitivity to change in systemic sclerosis of the McMaster-Toronto arthritis patient preference disability questionnaire (MACTAR): shift in patient priorities over time. J Rheumatol. 2010;37(2):359–64.
54. Naylor WP. Oral management of the scleroderma patient. J Am Dent Assoc. 1982;105(5):814–7.
55. Antonioli CM, Bua G, Frige A, Prandini K, Radici S, Scarsi M, et al. An individualized rehabilitation program in patients with systemic sclerosis may improve quality of life and hand mobility. Clin Rheumatol. 2009;28(2):159–65.
56. Sandqvist G, Eklund M, Akesson A, Nordenskiold U. Daily activities and hand function in women with scleroderma. Scand J Rheumatol. 2004;33(2):102–7.
57. Poole JL. Musculoskeletal rehabilitation in the person with scleroderma. Curr Opin Rheumatol. 2010;22(2):205–12.
58. Moran ME. Scleroderma and evidence based non-pharmaceutical treatment modalities for digital ulcers: a systematic review. J Wound Care. 2014;23:510–6.

Psychosocial Issues and Care for Patients with Systemic Sclerosis

45

Lisa R. Jewett, Linda Kwakkenbos, Vanessa C. Delisle, Brooke Levis, and Brett D. Thombs

People living with chronic medical conditions face challenges not only with respect to their physical health but also to their emotional and social well-being. Chronic conditions, such as systemic sclerosis (SSc or scleroderma), often result in significant disruptions to activities of daily living, including employment and homecare, as well as social and leisure activities, and can lead to reduced health-related quality of life (HRQL). Therefore, it is important to identify factors associated with decreased HRQL and psychosocial functioning in SSc and to develop and implement strategies to help individuals with the disease manage these problems. Traditionally, there has been little research on patient-reported outcomes in SSc, and this has posed a significant clinical challenge to the field. However, recent research has highlighted important problems that have an influence on HRQL for many people living with SSc, including depression, anxiety and fear of disease progression, fatigue and sleep problems, pain, pruritus (itch), body image distress, and sexual dysfunction [1–3].

Depression

Depression is characterized by sadness, loss of interest or pleasure, feelings of guilt or low self-esteem, poor concentration, and disturbed sleep or appetite. The rate of major depressive disorder (MDD) among patients living with one or more chronic conditions is often reported to be as high as 15–20 % [4], which is substantially greater than the approximate 5 % in the general population [5] and the estimated 5–10 % in primary care settings [6]. MDD and subthreshold levels of psychological distress among patients with chronic conditions can impact physical health through biological pathways, including immune system dysfunction and inflammation, as well as through behaviors, such as poor adherence to medical treatment regimens and a reduced likelihood of adopting health-promoting lifestyles [1].

In SSc, a study from France used the Mini International Neuropsychiatric Interview (MINI) in a sample of 50 hospitalized and 50 outpatients to assess the prevalence of depression, and the authors reported rates of 19 % for current and 56 % for lifetime MDD [7]. SSc patients who were hospitalized had higher rates of a current major depressive episode (28 %) than those who were not hospitalized (10 %) [7]. In a sample of 345 SSc patients from the Canadian Scleroderma Research Group (CSRG) Registry using the Composite International Diagnostic Interview (CIDI), rates of MDD were 4 % for current (30 days), 11 % for 12 months, and 23 % for lifetime [8]. These prevalence rates were approximately twice that of the Canadian general population, as well as higher than rates reported among patients with arthritis [8]. They were lower, however, than the rates reported from France. One possible explanation for the difference in the reported rates between the French and Canadian studies is that the MINI constitutes a brief measure, rather than a comprehensive evaluation as is accomplished with the CIDI. Specifically, the MINI does not query whether symptoms of depression cause functional impairment, which could potentially result in higher rates than those reported from other diagnostic interviews, such as the CIDI.

MDD is a serious mental health condition. Many SSc patients who meet criteria for MDD, however, may have mild to moderate MDD, and their symptoms may fluctuate with time. In the Canadian study, for instance, only 3 of 12 patients with MDD at baseline still met diagnostic criteria for MDD 1 month later [9]. These results are consistent with findings from a qualitative study where 16 women with SSc were interviewed about their emotional distress [10]. Interviewed women described their distress related to SSc as distinct from the clinical diagnosis of depression and noted that their symptoms were worse in the period directly

L.R. Jewett, MSc • L. Kwakkenbos, PhD • V.C. Delisle, MSc • B. Levis, MSc • B.D. Thombs, PhD (✉)
Lady Davis Institute for Medical Research, McGill University and Jewish General Hospital, Montreal, QC, Canada
e-mail: lisa.jewett@mail.mcgill.ca

J. Varga et al. (eds.), *Scleroderma*, DOI 10.1007/978-3-319-31407-5_45

following their SSc diagnosis [10]. Given these findings, active monitoring or watchful waiting may be a good strategy for SSc patients with mild depression in order to avoid unnecessary treatment for those who experience transient symptoms that may resolve without a specific intervention.

Many studies have reported high rates of scores above cutoff thresholds on self-report measures of depressive symptoms [11], although the rates reported using these tools vary widely depending on the specific measure and cutoff that is used. For instance, one study of 566 CSRG Registry patients found that 34 % of patients scored above a standard cutoff on the 20-item Center for Epidemiologic Studies Depression Scale (CES-D), but only 21 % of the same patients exceeded the designated cutoff on the 9-item Patient Health Questionnaire (PHQ-9) [12]. Cutoffs on symptom questionnaires are designed to identify a pool of patients potentially at risk for depression but do not assess whether any particular patient meets full diagnostic criteria for a mental health condition, such as MDD. As such, when assessing MDD, standardized clinical interviews are recommended as methods of evaluation.

A number of studies have examined factors associated with depressive symptoms in SSc. Cross-sectional studies have reported that both sociodemographic factors, such as being unmarried and having less education, as well as disease variables, including more tender joints and breathing and gastrointestinal problems, are associated with higher depression symptom scores [12, 13]. Other studies have documented that factors such as overall disease severity, disability, body image, pain, sexual function, disease-related cognitions, social support, and resilience are related to mental health functioning in SSc [11].

Anxiety

Few studies have assessed anxiety and the presence of anxiety disorders among persons living with SSc, and of those conducted, samples sizes were small, and researchers often made use of self-report questionnaires [14–16]. One French study of 100 SSc patients reported that 49 % of their sample had at least one current anxiety disorder and that 64 % of patients met criteria for one lifetime anxiety disorder based on the MINI [7]. Estimates were similar among hospitalized and outpatients and were higher than those found among a general sample of the French population; however, risk for anxiety disorders was not associated with SSc disease severity [7]. Anxiety has not been reported to relate to other common correlates of SSc, including organ involvement or functional impairment [15].

Given that the course of SSc is highly unpredictable, patients may perceive the future as uncertain. As such, for patients, worry about the future, including fear of disease progression, fear of becoming physically disabled, and fear of being dependent upon others are important sources of stress [17, 18]. Because SSc is associated with serious consequences in many patients, these concerns are realistic and in themselves do not represent anxiety disorders, for which irrational fear is typically a key component. Nonetheless, fear of progression can impact HRQL substantially. In a cross-sectional study of 215 SSc patients from the Netherlands, for instance, fear of progression was highly associated with symptoms of depression [18].

Fatigue and Sleep

Fatigue is one of the most significant factors affecting HRQL across many chronic diseases, including SSc [2, 19]. In a large cohort of Canadian patients with SSc, 89 % reported fatigue at least some of the time, and 72 % described that fatigue had a moderate to severe impact on the ability to carry out daily activities [20]. Similarly, a survey across five European countries found that between 76 and 96 % of patients in each country reported fatigue at least some of the time and 63–94 % reported moderate to severe impact [21]. A systematic review concluded that fatigue ratings from SSc patients were similar to scores from patients with other rheumatic diseases and cancer patients currently undergoing treatment and higher than scores from general population samples and cancer patients in remission [22]. Factors that may be associated with greater fatigue in patients with SSc include diffuse disease subtype, breathing problems, severity of gastrointestinal problems, pain, functional disability, education level, and sleep quality [23–29].

While there is a lack of research on sleep in SSc, sleep disturbances among people with the disease appear to be higher than in the general population [30, 31]. One study reported that sleep is associated with depression, dyspnea, fatigue, and severity of acid reflux among SSc patients [30], while another found that sleep problems were only related to unmarried status and pain [31].

Pain

Between 60 and 83 % of SSc patients experience pain, which is comparable to rates found in other chronic pain conditions and rheumatic diseases [32]. Potential sources of pain vary widely in SSc and include pain associated with Raynaud's phenomenon; musculoskeletal pain; pain in distal extremities due to skin tightness, calcinosis, and ulcers; and gastrointestinal problems [1]. Pain ratings are higher among patients with diffuse SSc compared to patients with limited disease, although the difference is generally small [32]. In both cross-sectional and longitudinal studies, pain in SSc has been independently associated with physical function, activity, work disability, sleep problems, fatigue, depressive symptoms, and reduced HRQL [23, 25, 28–36].

Pruritus

Pruritus, or itch, is described as a "poorly localized, non-adapting, usually unpleasant sensation that provokes a desire to scratch" ([37], p. 5). In a recent large-scale study of 959 Canadian SSc patients, 43 % of patients reported pruritus on most days within the last month. This rate was slightly higher among patients with early SSc (<5 years since onset of non-Raynaud's phenomenon symptoms, 46 %) versus those with longer disease duration (≥5 years, 41 %), but the difference was not statistically significant [38].

Pruritus in SSc has been associated with greater skin involvement, gastrointestinal symptoms, Raynaud's phenomenon, and finger ulcers, although only gastrointestinal symptoms were found to be an independent correlate of pruritus [38]. Another study found that pruritus was associated with significantly reduced HRQL in SSc, even after controlling for disease duration, skin score, number of tender joints, gastrointestinal symptoms, breathing problems, Raynaud's phenomenon, and finger ulcers [39], although the magnitude of the relationship was small. This is consistent with a pan-Canadian patient survey, in which 69 % of 400 patients reported experiencing pruritus at least sometimes in the last month, but only 27 % reported that it had a moderate to severe impact on the ability to carry out daily activities [20].

Body Image Distress

People with an acquired disfigurement from an injury or medical illness often struggle with maintaining a healthy body image, and many experience social anxiety and avoidance due to changes in appearance [40]. The appearance changes central to SSc commonly affect visible and socially relevant body parts (e.g., the face and hands), contributing to body image distress and posing potential challenges to managing social interactions. Appearance changes to the skin have been rated by patients as one of the most significant stressors associated with the disease [17]. Furthermore, low levels of self-esteem in relation to appearance and high levels of body image dissatisfaction have been reported by SSc patients, both related to the extent of physical changes and deformities to the skin [17, 41, 42]. One study specifically examined the psychosocial impact of facial changes in 171 SSc patients from England and reported that greater mouth disability, perceived noticeability of the appearance change, and worry were all associated with body image concerns [43]. In a sample of 489 Canadian SSc patients, the extent of body and face skin involvement, the presence of telangiectasias, and hand contractures, as well as age, were associated with body image distress and social discomfort [44].

Sexual Dysfunction

Sexual dysfunction refers to problems that may include decreased desire and enjoyment, impaired arousal, and painful sex [45]. Sexual dysfunction is a common problem among women with SSc [46–49]. Compared to women in the general population, women with SSc are significantly less likely to be sexually active, and sexually active women with SSc are significantly more likely to be sexually impaired [47, 50]. Factors that are independently associated with being sexually active include younger age, fewer gastrointestinal symptoms, and less severe Raynaud's phenomenon symptoms [51]. Among women who are sexually active, sexual impairment is associated with older age, as well as more severe skin involvement and breathing problems. Vaginal pain is eight times as common among women with impairment compared to those without impairment [51].

Among men with SSc, erectile dysfunction (ED) is common, with onset typically occurring several years after the manifestation of the first non-Raynaud's phenomenon symptoms [52, 53]. While in the general population, ED is typically associated with atherosclerosis, in SSc, penile blood flow is impaired due to both myointimal proliferation of small arteries and corporal fibrosis [54]. Men with SSc who have ED are significantly more likely to be older than those without ED and tend to report non-SSc risk factors (e.g., alcohol consumption) at higher rates [53, 54]. SSc factors associated with ED include severe cutaneous, muscular, or renal involvement, diffuse disease, elevated pulmonary pressures, restrictive lung disease, endothelial dysfunction, and microvascular damage [53]. Most men with SSc who have ED do not receive treatment [54]. Among those who do, sildenafil appears to be commonly used, but its efficacy has not been established in SSc [52, 53].

Clinical Strategies for Psychosocial Care

Comprehensive, patient-centered care in chronic diseases, including SSc, involves a combination of both medical treatment of disease symptoms and services and interventions to help manage the psychological, behavioral, and social aspects of living with the disease. The European League Against Rheumatism's (EULAR) recent recommendations for the treatment of SSc [55] highlighted the need for these types of interventions, but no specific suggestions could be made, as there is currently a lack of high-quality evidence to guide recommendations. Efforts are currently underway to develop and test strategies that focus on the behavioral and psychosocial aspects of SSc [3, 56]. Meanwhile, a general stepped-care approach may be useful.

Stepped-care models of healthcare delivery involve matching interventions of differing intensities to patient needs. It entails providing services that are the least restrictive of those available but still likely to produce significant health gain, as well as care that is self-correcting [57]. Least restrictive care typically refers to the amount of treatment intensity but can also reflect the impact on patients in terms of cost and personal inconvenience. The self-correcting aspects of stepped care entail that the results and progress of treatments are systematically monitored and changes are made, or "stepped up," if these are not attaining gains in the specific area of treatment [57]. Thus, stepped-care starts off with the simplest, least intrusive intervention available and proceeds to more intense treatment approaches as necessary.

As part of a stepped-care approach, healthcare professionals should establish a relationship with a mental health practitioner, such as a psychologist, psychiatrist, or trained social worker, in order to provide more specialized treatment to patients, as needed. For instance, a skilled practitioner in cognitive behavioral therapy or a related framework would be ideal for addressing many of the psychosocial concerns common to people with SSc. This form of therapy centers on active client involvement and provides a directive and structured treatment approach to goal setting and emotional and behavioral change [58]. Cognitive behavioral therapy focuses on putting into practice strategies and techniques that will improve overall functioning and, in this way, is amenable to many conditions and settings [59]. Less intensive sources of support may include self-help resources, self-management, and local support groups.

Self-Help Resources

Self-help can be a very useful first step toward addressing relatively mild problems associated with psychosocial functioning and quality of life. Providing information to both patients and those who support them regarding issues common to people living with SSc, as well as information regarding useful resources and services to address such problems, is something that can be implemented in rheumatology clinics and doctors' offices. Nurses and rheumatologists should be aware of the important psychosocial issues that affect quality of life in order to help patients access resources and facilitate conversations that address concerns of individual patients. Additionally, links to information and educational resources can be provided in clinics regarding self-help programs that are available as a first step in providing psychosocial support.

There are a number of resources that may be particularly useful for persons living with SSc. For instance, *Positive Coping with Health Conditions, A Self-Care Workbook* [60] is a general self-care manual designed for individuals living with chronic health conditions, as well as physicians, psychologists, nurses, rehabilitation professionals, and researchers who support patients. The workbook focuses on teaching skills to manage various stressors related to living with a chronic disease. It includes sections on managing anxiety, worry, anger, depressive thinking, and low mood, problem solving, relationship building, relaxation, as well as how to apply these coping skills to various aspects of having a chronic illness, such as life changes, pain, sleep, and physical activity. The workbook is based on cognitive behavioral therapy models and framed in a manner that can be accessed by those who are not familiar with or trained in psychological interventions. Other cognitive behavioral self-help resources available for addressing negative mood, including depressive symptoms and anxiety, are the *Mind Over Mood: Change How You Feel by Changing the Way You Think* [61] and *Thoughts* and *Feelings: Taking Control of Your Moods and Your Life* [62] workbooks.

A resource that may be useful in addressing physical appearance changes and body image concerns is *Changing Faces* (www.changingfaces.org.uk). *Changing Faces* is a not-for-profit organization whose mission is to provide support for individuals touched by disfigurement and to increase public awareness regarding issues related to living with a visibly different appearance. *Changing Faces* has published a range of self-help and educational resources in the form of booklets, pamphlets, and DVDs for individuals with disfigurements, their families, as well as employers and healthcare professionals. Examples of topics covered in these resources include daily challenges when living with a different appearance, intimacy, and social life. In addition, *Changing Faces* offers workshops and training on issues surrounding disfigurement, as well as more individualized services that target social anxiety, body image distress, and, generally, adjustment to living with an altered appearance.

Self-Management Approaches

Self-management programs constitute another area that can be useful as a first step toward addressing relatively mild problems associated with the psychosocial aspects of living with a chronic condition. The Chronic Disease Self-Management Program (CDSMP) [63], which was developed by Kate Lorig and modeled on her Arthritis Self-Management Program [64], is designed to teach self-care techniques useful to persons with many chronic diseases. The CDSMP is delivered through face-to-face meetings or via the internet, in small-group settings, and led by persons who have a chronic disease. The objectives of the CDSMP are to support people living with a chronic condition in taking care of the illness, carrying out normal activities, and managing emotional changes associated with living with their condition. Topics included in the CDSMP program include managing pain, fatigue, depression, and shortness of breath; exercise; relaxation techniques; healthy eating; communication skills; medication management; advanced directives; and problem solving with specific action planning [64]. Kate Lorig also published the book *Living a Healthy Life with Chronic Conditions: Self-management of Heart Disease, Arthritis, Diabetes, Asthma, Bronchitis, Emphysema and Others* [65] that offers numerous suggestions and self-management strategies to individuals dealing with such chronic conditions, including exercise and nutrition programs, tips for symptom and medication management, help on finding community resources, and methods of working effectively with doctors.

Support Groups

A large number of patients with chronic medical illnesses, including those with SSc, join support groups in order to better cope with and manage their illness [66]. Activities of support groups include giving and receiving emotional and practical support, as well as providing education and information to patients. The specific activities and focus, as well as facilitator training and competence, may vary across support groups, which are typically organized locally. Patients may differ in the acceptability of the idea of attending a support group and the degree to which they may benefit from one. Due to their grassroots nature, support groups can be configured in a variety of ways [67]. For example, some support groups may meet face to face, whereas others may "meet" online; some groups may be facilitated by a peer, whereas others may be facilitated by a professional; and some may include structured educational activities, whereas others may not. Research on the effectiveness of support groups is scant, particularly with regard to lay-led groups. However, many people who do attend support groups describe feeling more empowered, more hopeful, and less alone following their group experience [66]. In addition, some patients who attend these groups report feeling more in control of their life, as well as more knowledgeable about their illness, coping strategies, and developments in medical and self-help treatments.

Peer-led support groups have become increasingly popular in recent years [68]. Consistent with this, most SSc support groups are peer led rather than professionally led. Given that they may be the sole source of SSc-specific support available to many patients and that they have been effective in other conditions, attending support groups may be beneficial for some patients with SSc. It is important to keep in mind, however, that support groups are meant to complement rather than supplement standard medical care. Medical professionals may want to discuss the possible benefits of attending a support group with their patients, as well as potential pitfalls. For patients who are interested in attending or joining a SSc support group, information can typically be found on local or national organization websites, such as the Scleroderma Society of Canada and the Scleroderma Foundation in the United States [69, 70].

SSc-Specific Resources

An international research consortium, the Scleroderma Patient-centered Intervention Network (SPIN), was recently established with the aim to create an infrastructure to develop, test, and disseminate a series of self-guided online psychosocial and rehabilitation interventions related to important patient-reported outcomes in SSc [3, 56]. SPIN is comprised of SSc patient organizations, clinicians, medical professionals, and researchers from Canada, the United States, Europe, Latin America, and Australia. Building on previous research [1–3] and in consultation with patient representatives, SPIN develops online programs that address previously identified problems that are important to patients, such as those reviewed in the present chapter. Once tested, SPIN's interventions will be made widely accessible to SSc partner patient organizations around the world [56].

In summary, persons living with SSc face a number of challenges that affect their psychosocial well-being and quality of life. Rather than focusing only on a single issue, such as depression, approaches to psychosocial care should take into account the different levels of issues faced by patients. Self-help resources and self-management techniques can be considered as first steps toward providing patient care for a variety of psychosocial issues. Some patients may also benefit from support from other patients via support groups. Care providers should become aware of problems faced by patients and their supporters, should facilitate discussions of these problems, and should help patients access self-help material. Beyond this, rheumatology clinics should develop a relationship with a competent mental healthcare provider to provide more focused evaluation and intervention services for patients, as needed.

Acknowledgments Ms. Jewett and Ms. Delisle were supported by Doctoral Research Awards from the Canadian Institutes of Health Research (CIHR). Dr. Kwakkenbos was supported by a Fonds de recherche du Québec – santé (FRQS) postdoctoral fellowship. Ms. Levis was supported by a FRQS Doctoral Training Award. Dr. Thombs was supported by an Investigator Salary Award from the Arthritis Society.

References

1. Thombs BD, van Lankveld W, Bassel M, Baron M, Buzza R, Haslam S, et al. Psychological health and well-being in systemic sclerosis: state of the science and consensus research agenda. Arthritis Care Res. 2010;8:1181–9.
2. Malcarne VM, Fox RS, Mills SD, Gholizadeh S. Psychosocial aspects of systemic sclerosis. Curr Opin Rheumatol. 2013;25:707–13.
3. Thombs BD, Jewett LR, Assassi S, Baron M, Bartlett SJ, Maia AC, et al. New directions for patient-centered care in scleroderma: the Scleroderma Patient-centered Intervention Network (SPIN). Clin Exp Rheumatol. 2012;30(2 Suppl 71):S23–9.
4. Evans DL, Charney DS, Lewis L, Golden RN, Gorman JM, Krishnan KR, et al. Mood disorders in the medically ill: scientific review and recommendations. Biol Psychiatry. 2005;58:175–89.
5. Blazer DG, Kessler RC, McGonagle KA, Swartz MS. The prevalence and distribution of major depression in a national community sample: the National Comorbidity Survey. Am J Psychiatry. 1994;151:979–86.
6. Pignone MP, Gaynes BN, Rushton JL, Burchell CM, Orleans CT, Mulrow CD, et al. Screening for depression in adults: a summary of the evidence for the U.S. Preventive Services Task Force. Ann Intern Med. 2002;136:765–76.
7. Baubet T, Ranque B, Taïeb O, Bérenzé A, Bricou O, Mehallel S, et al. Mood and anxiety disorders in systemic sclerosis patients. Presse Med. 2011;40(2):e111–9.
8. Jewett LR, Razykov I, Hudson M, Baron M, Thombs BD, Canadian Scleroderma Research Group. Rheumatology. 2013;52(4):669–75.
9. Thombs BD, Jewett LR, Kwakkenbos L, Hudson M, Baron M, Canadian Scleroderma Research Group. Major depression diagnoses among patients with systemic sclerosis: baseline and one-month follow-up. Arthritis Care Res. 2015;67(3):411–6.
10. Newton EG, Thombs BD, Groleau D. The experience of emotional distress among women with scleroderma. Qual Health Res. 2012;22(9):1195–206.
11. Thombs BD, Taillefer SS, Hudson M, Baron M. Depression in patients with systemic sclerosis: a systematic review of the evidence. Arthritis Rheum. 2007;57:1089–97.
12. Milette K, Hudson M, Baron M, Thombs BD, Canadian Scleroderma Research Group. Comparison of the PHQ-9 and CES-D depression scales in systemic sclerosis: internal consistency reliability, convergent validity, and clinical correlates. Rheumatology. 2010;49:789–96.
13. Thombs BD, Hudson M, Taillefer SS, Baron M, the Canadian Scleroderma Research Group. Prevalence and clinical correlates of symptoms of depression in patients with systemic sclerosis. Arthritis Rheum. 2008;59:504–9.
14. Mozzetta A, Antinone V, Alfani S, Neri P, Foglio Bonda PG, Pasquini P, et al. Mental health in patients with systemic sclerosis: a controlled investigation. J Eur Acad Dermatol Venereol. 2008;22:336–40.
15. Legendre C, Allanore Y, Ferrand I, Kahan A. Evaluation of depression and anxiety in patients with systemic sclerosis. Joint Bone Spine. 2005;72:408–11.
16. Angelopoulos NV, Drosos AA, Moutsopoulos HM. Psychiatric symptoms associated with scleroderma. Psychother Psychosom. 2001;70:145–50.
17. van Lankveld WGJM, Vonk MC, Teunissen HA, van den Hoogen FHJ. Appearance self-esteem in systemic sclerosis – subjective experience of skin deformity and its relationship with physician-assessed skin involvement, disease status and psychological variables. Rheumatology. 2007;46:972–6.
18. Kwakkenbos L, van Lankveld WGJM, Vonk MC, Becker ES, van den Hoogen FHJ, van den Ende CHM. Disease-related and psychosocial factors associated with depressive symptoms in patients with systemic sclerosis, including fear of progression and appearance self-esteem. J Psychosom Res. 2012;72:199–204.
19. Swain MG. Fatigue in chronic disease. Clin Sci. 2000;99:1–8.
20. Bassel M, Hudson M, Taillefer SS, Schieir O, Baron M, Thombs BD. Frequency and impact of symptoms experienced by patients with systemic sclerosis: results from a Canadian national survey. Rheumatology. 2011;50(4):762–7.
21. Willems LM, Kwakkenbos L, Leite CC, Thombs BD, van den Hoogen FH, Maia AC, et al. Frequency and impact of disease symptoms experienced by patients with systemic sclerosis from five European countries. Clin Exp Rheumatol. 2014;32(6 Suppl 86):S-88–93. Epub 2014 Nov 3.
22. Thombs BD, Bassel M, McGuire L, Smith MT, Hudson M, Haythornthwaite JA. A systematic comparison of fatigue levels in systemic sclerosis with general population, cancer and rheumatic disease samples. Rheumatology. 2008;47:1559–63.
23. Thombs BD, Hudson M, Bassel M, Taillefer SS, Baron M, Canadian Scleroderma Research Group. Sociodemographic, disease, and symptom correlates of fatigue in systemic sclerosis: evidence from a sample of 659 Canadian Scleroderma Research Group Registry patients. Arthritis Rheum. 2009;61:966–73.
24. Yacoub I, Amine B, Bensabbah R, Hajjaj-Hassouni N. Assessment of fatigue and its relationship with disease-related parameters in patients with systemic sclerosis. Clin Rheumatol. 2012;31:655–60.
25. Strickland G, Pauling J, Cavill C, McHugh N. Predictors of health-related quality of life and fatigue in systemic sclerosis: evaluation of the EuroQol-5D and FACIT-F assessment tools. Clin Rheumatol. 2012;31:1215–22.
26. Harel D, Thombs BD, Hudson M, Baron M, Steele R, Canadian Scleroderma Research Group. Measuring fatigue in SSc: a comparison of the short form-36 vitality subscale and functional assessment of chronic illness therapy-fatigue scale. Rheumatology. 2012;51:2177–85.
27. Sandqvist G, Archenholtz B, Scheja A, Hesselstrand R. The Swedish version of the Multidimensional Assessment of Fatigue (MAF) in systemic sclerosis: reproducibility and correlations to other fatigue instruments. Scan J Rheumatol. 2011;40:493–4.
28. Sandusky SB, McGuire L, Smith MT, Wigley FM, Haythornthwaite JA. Fatigue: an overlooked determinant of physical function in scleroderma. Rheumatology. 2009;48:165–9.
29. Assassi S, Leyva AL, Mayes MD, Sharif R, Nair DK, Fischbach M, et al. Predictors of fatigue severity in early systemic sclerosis: a prospective longitudinal study of the GENISOS cohort. PLoS ONE. 2011;6:e26061.
30. Frech T, Hays RD, Maranian P, Clements PJ, Furst DE, Khanna D. Prevalence and correlates of sleep disturbance in systemic sclerosis: results from the UCLA scleroderma quality of life study. Rheumatology. 2011;50:1280–7.
31. Milette K, Razykov I, Pope J, Hudson M, Motivala SJ, Baron M, et al. Clinical correlates of sleep problems in systemic sclerosis: the prominent role of pain. Rheumatology. 2011;50:921–5.
32. Schieir O, Thombs BD, Hudson M, Boivin JF, Steele R, Bernatsky S, et al. Prevalence, severity, and clinical correlates of pain in patients with systemic sclerosis. Arthritis Care Res. 2010;62:409–17.
33. Sandqvist G, Eklund M. Daily occupations-performance, satisfaction and time use, and relations with well-being in women with limited systemic sclerosis. Disabil Rehabil. 2008;30:27–35.
34. Hudson M, Steele R, Lu Y, Thombs BD, Canadian Scleroderma Research Group, Baron M. Work disability in systemic sclerosis. J Rheumatol. 2009;36:2481–6.
35. Müller H, Rehberger P, Günther C, Schmitt J. Determinants of disability, quality of life and depression in dermatological patients with systemic scleroderma. Br J Derm. 2012;166:343–53.
36. El-Baalbaki G, Lober J, Hudson M, Baron M, Thombs BD, Canadian Scleroderma Research Group. Measuring pain in systemic sclerosis: comparison of the short-form McGill pain questionnaire versus a single-item measure of pain. J Rheumatol. 2011;38:2581–7.

37. Weisshaar E, Kucenic MJ, Fleischer Jr AB. Pruritus: a review. Acta Derm Venereol Suppl. 2003;213:5–32.
38. Razykov I, Levis B, Hudson M, Baron M, Thombs BD, Canadian Scleroderma Research Group. Prevalence and clinical correlates of pruritus in patients with systemic sclerosis: an updated analysis of 959 patients. Rheumatology. 2011;52(11):2056–61.
39. El-Baalbaki G, Razykov I, Hudson M, Bassel M, Baron M, Thombs BD, et al. Association of pruritus with quality of life and disability in systemic sclerosis. Arthritis Care Res. 2010;62:1489–95.
40. Pruzinsky T. Social and psychological effects of major craniofacial deformity. Cleft Palate Craniofac J. 1992;29:578–84.
41. Malcarne VL, Handsdottir I, Greensbergs HL, Clements PJ, Weisman MH. Appearance self-esteem in systemic sclerosis. Cogn Ther Res. 1999;23:197–208.
42. Benrud-Larson LM, Heinberg LJ, Boiling C, Reed J, White B, Wigley FM, et al. Body image dissatisfaction among women with scleroderma: extent and relationship to psychosocial function. Health Psychol. 2003;22(2):130–9.
43. Amin K, Clarke A, Sivakumar B, Puri A, Fox Z, Brough V, et al. The psychological impact of facial changes in scleroderma. Psychol Health Med. 2011;16(3):304–12.
44. Jewett LR, Huson M, Malcarne VL, Baron M, Thombs BD, Canadian Scleroderma Research Group. Sociodemographic and disease correlates of body image distress among patients with systemic sclerosis. PLoS ONE. 2012;7(3):e:33281.
45. Bancroft J. Human sexuality and its problems. 3rd ed. Edinburgh: Churchill Livingstone; 2009.
46. Schouffoer AA, van der Marel J, Ter Kuile MM, Weijenborg PT, Voskuyl A, Vliet Vlieland CW, et al. Impaired sexual function in women with systemic sclerosis: a cross-sectional study. Arthritis Rheum. 2009;61:1601–8.
47. Knafo R, Thombs BD, Jewett L, Hudson M, Wigley F, Haythornthwaite JA. (Not) talking about sex: a systematic comparison of sexual impairment in women with systemic sclerosis and other chronic disease samples. Rheumatology. 2009;48:1300–3.
48. Schover LR, Jensen SR. Sexuality and chronic illness: a comprehensive approach. New York: Guilford; 1988. p. 74.
49. Saad SC, Behrend AE. Scleroderma and sexuality. J Sex Res. 1996;33:15–20.
50. Levis B, Burri A, Hudson M, Baron M, Thombs BD, Canadian Scleroderma Research Group. Sexual activity and impairment in women with systemic sclerosis compared to women from a general population sample. PLoS ONE. 2012;7:e52129.
51. Levis B, Hudson M, Knafo R. Rates and correlates of sexual activity and impairment among women with systemic sclerosis. Arthritis Care Res. 2012;64:640–50.
52. Walker UA, Tyndall A, Ruszat R. Erectile dysfunction in systemic sclerosis. Ann Rheum Dis. 2009;68:1083–5.
53. Foocharoen C, Tyndall A, Hachulla E, Rosato E, Allanore Y, Farge-Bancel D, et al. Erectile dysfunction is frequent in systemic sclerosis and associated with severe disease: a study of the EULAR Scleroderma Trial and Research Group. Arthritis Res Ther. 2012;14:R37.
54. Keck AD, Foocharoen C, Rosato E, et al. Nailfold capillary abnormalities in erectile dysfunction of systemic sclerosis: a EUSTAR group analysis. Rheumatology. 2014;53:639–43.
55. Kowal-Bielecka O, Landewe R, Avouac J, Chwiesko S, Miniati I, Czirjak L, et al. EULAR recommendations for the treatment of systemic sclerosis: a report from the EULAR scleroderma trials and research group (EUSTAR). Ann Rheum Dis. 2009;68:620–8.
56. Kwakkenbos L, Jewett LR, Baron M, Bartlett SJ, Furst D, Gottesman K, et al. The Scleroderma Patient-centered Intervention Network (SPIN) cohort: protocol for a cohort multiple randomised controlled trial (cmRCT) design to support trials of psychosocial and rehabilitation interventions in a rare disease context. BMJ Open. 2013;7(8):pii: e003563.
57. Bower P, Gilbody S. Stepped care in psychological therapies: access, effectiveness and efficiency: narrative literature review. B J Pysch. 2005;186:11–7.
58. Whitfield G, Davidson A. Cognitive behavioural therapy explained. Oxon: Radcliffe Publishing Ltd; 2007.
59. Lovell K, Richards D. Multiple Access Points and Levels of Entry (MAPLE): ensuring choice, accessibility and equity for CBT services. Behav Cogn Psychother. 2000;28:379–91.
60. Bilsker D, Samara J, Goldner E. Positive coping with health conditions: a self-care workbook. Vancouver: Consortium for Organizational Mental Healthcare (COMH); 2009.
61. Greenberger D, Padesky C. Mind over mood: change how you feel by changing the way you think. New York: Guilford Press; 1995.
62. McKay M, Fanning P. Thoughts and feelings: taking control of your moods and your life. Oakland: New Harbinger Publications; 1997.
63. Lorig KR, Sobel DS, Stewart AL, Brown Jr BW, Ritter PL, González VM, et al. Evidence suggesting that a chronic disease self-management program can improve health status while reducing utilization and costs: a randomized trial. Med Care. 1999;37:5–14.
64. Lorig K, Lubeck D, Kraines RG, Seleznick M, Holman HR. Outcomes of self-help education for patients with arthritis. Arthritis Rheum. 1985;28:680–5.
65. Lorig K, Holman H, Sobel D, Laurent D, González V, Minor M. Living a healthy life with chronic conditions: self-management of heart disease, arthritis, diabetes, asthma, bronchitis, emphysema, and others. Boulder: Bull Publishing Company; 2007.
66. Davison KP, Pennebaker JW, Dickerson SS. Who talks? The social psychology of illness support groups. Am Psychol. 2000;55: 205–17.
67. Uccelli MM, Mohr LM, Battaglia MA, Zagami P, Mohr DC. Peer support groups in multiple sclerosis: current effectiveness and future directions. Mult Scler. 2006;10:80–4.
68. Ussher J, Kirsten L, Butow P, Sandoval M. What do cancer support groups provide which other supportive relationships do not? The experience of peer support groups for people with cancer. Soc Sci Med. 2006;62:2565–76.
69. http://www.scleroderma.ca/Support/Find-A-Support-Group.php.
70. http://www.scleroderma.org/site/PageServer?pagename=patients_supportgroups#.VCeEoSi6pIc.

Clinical Trial Design in Systemic Sclerosis

46

Yossra A. Suliman, Harsh Agrawal, and Daniel E. Furst

Importance of Therapeutic Trials

While therapeutic trials are essential when seeking guidance in treating diseases, relying solely on open label studies or case reports may be misleading due to selection bias, reporting bias, and the lack of control group. Thus, several SSc treatments were thought to be effective until investigated in a randomized case-control manner [1, 2]. Progress in the development and validation of outcome measures, together with improved insights on SSc pathogenesis, have opened the door to establishing therapies in SSc through well-designed controlled trials.

Epidemiological Considerations

Status of Scleroderma as a Rare Disease

The Orphan Drug and Rare Disease Act of 1983 encourages pharmaceutical companies to develop drugs for "rare diseases" that otherwise have a very low prevalence and for which drug development lacks profit motive. In the US regulatory environment, "rare disease" is defined as one affecting fewer than 200,000 Americans. Given that SSc falls in the category of "rare disease", affecting about 1 in 5,000 [3], pharmaceutical companies have tax and patent incentives under the Orphan Drug and Rare Disease Act to develop drugs for this condition. In part due to the support from the abovementioned legislations, there have been 23 randomized clinical trials in SSc in the last 5 years compared to seven such trials between 1980 and 1986 [4, 8, 10].

Trial Design

Phase I–III

The principle focus of phase I trials is the safety of the tested treatment, adverse events (AE), serious adverse events (SAEs), and/or death. Even during this phase, placebo controls are necessary because only placebo controls will enable one to differentiate whether a sign or symptom is due to treatment-related adverse event or an SSc-related complication. Stopping rules during this phase are particularly important (although should be included in all trials of disease with severe consequences such as SSc). This is because it is unacceptable in some circumstances to continue the tested drug for patients who develop organ complications or nonresponders when there is available effective treatment for such organ involvement. On the other hand, it is possible to continue a drug tested in certain aspects of organ involvement when there is no known effective treatment.

Phase II trials are mainly focused on evaluating initial efficacy and establishing an appropriate dose for later trials, although safety must continue to be carefully monitored. This is also an opportunity to explore and validate clinical, laboratory and biomarker end points. End points used for clinical trials should be practical and fully validated; in SSc, the use of surrogate outcome measurements may be more feasible in selected cases. As in phase 1, there should be controls, usually placebo, to establish the true early efficacy and further safety of the drug.

Yossra A Suliman and Harsh Agrawal have no disclosures.
Daniel E. Furst. Disclosures
Grant/Research Support: AbbVie, Actelion, Amgen, BMS, Gilead, GSK, NIH, Novartis, Pfizer, Roche/Genentech, UCB
Consultant: AbbVie, Actelion, Amgen, BMS, Cytori, Janssen, Gilead, GSK, NIH, Novartis, Pfizer, Roche/Genentech, UCB
Speaker's Bureau (CME ONLY): AbbVie, Actelion, and UCB.

Y.A. Suliman, MD, MSc
Department of Rheumatology and Rehabilitation, Assiut University Hospital, Assiut, Egypt
e-mail: dr.yossra@gmail.com

H. Agrawal, MD, FACP
Department of Internal Medicine, Division of Cardiology, Paul. L. Foster School of Medicine Texas Tech University, El Paso, Texas, USA

D.E. Furst, MD (✉)
Department of Rheumatology, University of California, Los Angeles, Los Angeles, CA, USA

J. Varga et al. (eds.), *Scleroderma*, DOI 10.1007/978-3-319-31407-5_46

Phase III trials involve more patients to establish efficacy at the chosen dose(s) and establish the safety profile of the therapy for more common adverse events. This phase should be controlled, whether placebo and/or positive controls.

Phase IV: Although drugs are carefully tested in the above three phases before being marketed, postmarketing studies establish the profile of the drug in a more general population, further establish the therapy's safety profile, and attempt early discovery of less common adverse events during long-term use.

Risk evaluation and mitigation strategies (REMS) are risk management strategies initiated by the Food and Drug Administration Amendments Act of 2007 ("FDAAA"), which gave FDA the authority to request a REMS from drug companies to make sure that the benefits of a drug or biological product continue to outweigh its risks. It was specifically tailored to make sure that there is a favorable risk: benefit ratio in larger populations and in general use. The FDA website provides a list of REMS with the currently approved drugs including biologics via REMS [5].

Characteristics of Outcome Measurements in SSc

OMERACT (outcome measure in rheumatologic clinical trials) is an initiative established by a group of rheumatologists, statisticians, and epidemiologists whose main objective is to improve outcome measures in rheumatology. Clinical trials in SSc should seek to evaluate outcomes in a thorough, valid manner; the OMERACT principles of truth, discrimination, and feasibility are one approach and are frequently used [6, 7]. Those include feasibility, face, content, criterion and construct validity, reproducibility/reliability, sensitivity to change, and ability to discriminate therapy from control; it includes patient involvement and a consideration of the context (e.g., comorbidities, other medications used, cultural factors) of the measure. Certain aspects of measurement validation are particularly important, as they are critical to trial design and the ability to discern treatment effects. This applies to discrimination and responsiveness to change.

Discrimination Discriminant validity was shown in some outcome measures in SSc clinical trials. FVC percent predicted could discriminate between cyclophosphamide-treated and placebo control groups as a measure of improvement in SSc-ILD (interstitial lung disease) [8]. Johnson et al. used Bayesian model analysis of uncommon diseases to identify MRSS as an outcome measure of skin tightness in SSc. Better mean outcomes of MRSS in MTX-treated group than placebo (94 %) demonstrated the discriminant validity of MRSS in SSc [9]. Most recently, event-free survival was identified as the outcome measure in a study of long-term effects of treatment with *Hematopoietic stem cell transplantation* (HSCT) vs. cyclophosphamide in SSc. Event-free survival (time from randomization until the occurrence of death or persistent major organ failure) could discriminate the significant survival in HSCT group than in control group after 4-year follow-up [10].

Responsiveness to Change In SSc, several outcome measures may not show any change in RCTs. The reason behind the lack of change in RCTs is that most of SSc disease modification trials have been negative, although some trials showed positive change – for example, cyclophosphamide, which improved FVC and skin score [11]. Outcomes like GIT 2.0, FVC, HAQ-DI, SF-36, 6MWD, MRSS, and RCS are responsive to change and were able to show some improvement in clinical trials [12–16], while others, such as oral aperture opening, handspan, and other biomarkers, did not show any change in response to treatment [17].

Overall Measures of Scleroderma

A group of SSc experts within OMERACT started the combined response index for SSc (CRISS) as an instrument to be used for clinical trials. In an effort to develop single measure composed of a set of domains which reflect organ involvement, CRISS conducted a Delphi exercise with expert review to distinguish 11 core set items to be considered in SSc clinical trials: soluble biomarkers, cardiac, digital ulcers, gastrointestinal, global health, health-related quality of life and function, musculoskeletal, pulmonary, RP, renal, and skin. Ongoing prospective study to test the validity of CRISS against OMERACT criteria is currently being undertaken. Further revision and definition of the final set of domains will be commenced based on obtained results [18].

Another overall outcome measure in SSc is the European scleroderma study group activity index (EscSG) which evaluates both clinical domains and specific laboratory values, including the MRSS, DLCO, and presence of scleredema, digital ulcers, arthritis, ESR, hypocomplementemia, and patient-reported worsening of the skin and vascular and cardiopulmonary symptoms [19–22]. Valentini et al. evaluated the validity of EScSG activity index; face, content, and construct validity was demonstrated [20]. Further assessment of the content and construct validity was conducted by Minier et al. [22] in a larger cohort of SSc patients. Responsiveness to change, however, has not yet been evaluated for EscSG activity index, and further validation steps are still warranted.

Khanna et al. developed a consensus of 22 points to consider for evidence-based clinical trial design in SSc. They entail establishing standards for more uniform clinical trial design and improved selection of outcome measures; they also outlined areas where further research is warranted [23]. Outcome measures used in SSc clinical trials are listed in Table 46.1.

Table 46.1 Outcome measures used in SSc clinical trials

Organ system	Valid	Partially validated	Used but not completely valid	Emerging
Cardiac	Congestive heart failure clinical exam [24] Pericardial disease (EKG, clinical exam, echocardiography) [25, 26]	Tissue Doppler echocardiography [26, 27] Cardiac MRI [28, 29] Right heart catheterization [30] Left heart catheterization [31] Borg dyspnea instrument [32] Scintigraphy [33, 34] Holter [35] EKG [36] Nt-pro-BNP [37]	Cardiac conduction blocks [38] Fixed defects on perfusional scintigraphy [39] Video densitometric alterations [40]	Speckle-tracking echocardiography [41], diffuse fibrosis imaging using magnetic resonance imaging [42] Absolute perfusion magnetic resonance imaging Troponins cardiac computerized tomography [43]
Digital ulcers	Total net ulcer burden [44] HAQ pain VAS Digital Ulcer [45] HAQ disability index SF-36 [45]	Active ulcer on fingertips on the volar surface [46]	Raynaud condition score [45] Cochin hand function scale [47] Michigan hand questionnaire [48]	New ulcers Time to healing of baseline vs. largest vs. cardinal ulcer Capillaroscopy [49] Thermography Arteriography [50] MRI [51] Doppler ultrasound Laser Doppler Transcutaneous tensiometry Granulation tissue color pictures Surface area measurement
Raynaud's	Raynaud's condition score [52, 53] Frequency of RP attacks [45] Duration of RP attacks [45] Patient global assessment [45] Physician global assessment [45] Digital ulcers	VAS or Likert [45] Pain VAS or HAQ [45]		Thermography [54] Laser Doppler imaging [55] Finger systolic pressure measurements [55] Nail fold capillaroscopy [55] Plethysmography cold challenge [55]
PAH	6-min walk test [56, 57] NYHA or WHO functional class [58, 59] Right heart catheterization [60, 61] Time to clinical worsening, survival [61]	SF-36, VAS, and patient global assessments [62] SHAQ-DI NT-pro-BNP< BNP [63, 64] Pulmonary function testing [62] Anticentromere antibody [65] Dyspnea scale: Borg, Mahler [66] Telangiectasia [67] Echocardiographic parameters of RV function: TASPE, right ventricular volume, atrial volume, E/A ratio, maximum velocity of tricuspid valve regurgitation, pulmonary valve acceleration time, right ventricular systolic pressure [68, 69]	EKG [65]	High-resolution computerized tomography Exercise right heart catheterization, positron emission tomography Magnetic resonance imaging Magnetic resonance angiography Broncoalveolar lavage Encouraged 6-min walk test DETECT algorithm [69]

(continued)

Table 46.1 (continued)

Organ system	Valid	Partially validated	Used but not completely valid	Emerging
Interstitial lung disease (ILD)	Forced vital capacity [16, 70, 71] Total lung capacity [16] Diffusing capacity for carbon monoxide [16, 70, 72] HRCT [16, 70, 73, 74] Mahler dyspnea [16, 70, 75–77] VAS breathing [16, 70, 78]		Exercise oxygen desaturation [79] 6-min walking distance [70, 71, 80]	Reduced radiation HRCT [81] UCSD shortness of breath questionnaire [82]
Skin	Modified Rodnan skin score [83–85] UCLA skin score [84, 86] Kahaleh skin score [87]	Durometery [88] Skin biopsy [89] VAS [90] SHAQ [91]	Self-related VAS [92] Skin self-assessment questionnaire [93] Maximum oral aperture Hand mobility Grip strength Tendon friction rub Skin thickness progression score	Plicometery [94] Elastometry [95] Ultrasound [96, 97] Serum makers of connective tissue metabolism
Gastrointestinal tract	UCLA GIT2.0 [98, 99]. Upper gastrointestinal (UGI) endoscopy [100–102] Biopsy [103–105] Manometer [106–111] Barium [112–115] Hydrogen and methane breath tests [116, 117]	Small bowel follow-through [118]	EGG [119, 120]. SPECT [121] UGI endoscopic US [122] Anal endoscopic US [123, 124]	CT enterography MR enteroclysis (MREc) MR enterography (MREg) Video capsule (smartpill) [125] PROMIS ® GI [126]
Renal	Creatinine [127, 128] Creatinine clearance (MDRD) [129, 130]		Proteinuria [131] Renal blood flow [132, 133]	
Functional status	HAQ-DI [62, 134–137] United Kingdom functional score [138, 139] SF-36 version 2 PCS [62, 134–137] PROMIS ® physical function SF-36 version 2 MCS [62, 134–137] SF-6D [140].	SF-36 vitality scale [136, 143]	Fatigue VAS [137, 139] Pain VAS [136, 137, 139]. Sleep VAS [137, 141] Patient global assessment VAS	MOS sleep scale [142]
Joints	Cochin hand function [144, 146] HAMIS [144–146]	MSK ultrasound [147]	Tender joint count Swollen joint count Tendon friction rub Pain VAS Pt global VAS Physician global VAS ESR, CRP [146]	MRI [146]
Muscle	sysQ [148]		Manual muscle testing [149, 151] Electromyogram [149, 151] Creatine phosphokinase [127, 130] Muscle pain, tenderness [150]	

CHF congestive heart failure, *EKG* electrocardiogram, *MRI* magnetic resonance imaging, NT-pro-*BNP* N-terminal pro b-type natriuretic peptide, *HAQ* health assessment questionnaire, *VAS* visual analog scale, *SF-36* Medical Outcome Study Short-Form 36, *PCS* physical component summary, *MCS* mental component summary, *NYHA* New York Heart Association, *WHO* World Health Organization, *SHAQ* Scleroderma Health Assessment Questionnaire, *TAPSE* tricuspid annular plane systolic excursion, *E/A* ratio of the early (E) to late (A) ventricular filling velocities, *HRCT* high-resolution computed tomography, *UCSD* University of California San Diego shortness of breath questionnaire, *UCLA GIT 2.0* University of California Los Angeles gastrointestinal questionnaire, *EGG* electrogastrography, *SPECT* single-photon emission computed tomography, *PROMIS* patient-reported outcome measurement information system, *MDRD* modification of diet in renal disease, *HAMIS* hand mobility in scleroderma, *SYSQ* systemic sclerosis questionnaire, *MOS sleep scale* medical outcomes study, *CRP* C reactive protein

The Role of Surrogate Measurements

A surrogate end point is defined as a measure of a treatment effect that correlates or reflects a change in a clinical end point. Additionally, a surrogate end point is expected to predict clinical benefit based on epidemiologic, therapeutic, or pathophysiologic evidence [152]. Scleroderma is a complex disease with high rates of morbidity and case-specific mortality [153]. However, the use of mortality as a primary outcome is not feasible and requires longer study duration (years).

Surrogate end points are adopted as potential markers for clinically relevant outcomes and their response to therapy. Improved insights into the pathophysiologic pathways of SSc, in addition to identifying key cellular and molecular targets, pave the way for potential organ (pathway)-specific markers. Clinically addressed outcomes usually reflect organ function or organ-related complication. Dyspnea scales and 6-min walk distance are used as surrogate for PAH [154, 155]. FVC and HRCT are surrogates for ILD progression [8, 156]. Time to clinical worsening was considered a surrogate marker of PAH worsening in a recent study by Pulido et al. where they assessed the effect of macitentan (dual endothelin receptor antagonist) in a randomized controlled trial. They reported that macitentan significantly reduced morbidity and mortality in PAH patients [157]. Gene expression signature in the skin and peripheral blood play a major role in understanding SSc pathogenesis, identifying potential biomarkers and therapeutic targets [158]. Gene expression signatures were tested by Milano et al.; inflammatory, proliferative, limited, and normal skin patterns were identified in clustered analysis of intrinsic genes [159]. Further analyses of those intrinsic genes for changes in response to treatment were assessed by Hinchcliff et al., and differential expression was shown in MRSSs of MMF-responsive patients in comparison to nonresponders [160]. Chung et al. showed differential gene expression in the skin of two SSc patients examined before and after imatinib treatment; they also identified an imatinib-responsive signature which was differentially expressed in dcSSc (early and late) in comparison to lcSSc and normal skin [161]. Genetic studies reveal the potential value of gene signatures as surrogate markers of fibrosis and response to treatment in SSc patients, in addition to their contribution to the growing innovative field of personalized translational medicine.

Measurement Error in SSc Outcomes

Demonstration of measurable effect by a treatment in a clinical trial is of great importance. Application of treatments and diagnostic tests relies on scores obtained by the measured variable. As noted above, validated measures should adhere to the OMERACT principles or a similar approach. In a study by Pope et al. [85], of ten rheumatologist and ten Ssc patients, they found that the intraobserver reliability was better than the interobserver reliability for most variables examined. Czirjåk et al. [162] demonstrated that, with repeated teaching of rheumatologists, the coefficient of variation of the measure decreased from 54 % to 32 %, while the intraclass correlation coefficient (ICC) increased from 0.496 to the expert level of 0.722. Clinical trials in Ssc thus need a carefully validated and reliable measurement instrument to ensure accurate and clinically meaningful results. Further, training to reduce inter-investigator variability seems to improve the usefulness of some clinical surrogates.

Patient Selection

Sample Size

A limitation in clinical study design in SSc is sample size because SSc is an uncommon/rare disease, so it is hard to enroll sufficient patients to have statistical power for confidence in the results. In addition, sample size calculation is dependent on a change in validated clinically relevant measures as the primary outcome, which requires a sample size of adequate number of patients to detect the change in such an outcome. For example, an adequately powered clinical trial of cyclophosphamide versus placebo, using FVC as the primary outcome, required about 150 patients. To recruit an adequate number of SSc patients in such a clinical trial in a timely manner, multisite trial designs are often adopted. This, in turn, requires consideration of the negative aspects of multicenter design: heterogeneity among patients, increased variability in outcome measures, reduced reliability among participating sites, and high cost.

Sampling Frame

SSc is a multisystem disease with various possible phenotypes; the phenotypic variability starts with the skin which yields two distinct SSc subtypes: limited (lcSSc) and diffuse cutaneous subtypes (dcSSc). Pope et al. studied SSc patients with both SSc subtypes to calculate the baseline characteristics of commonly used outcome measures and to provide parameters for sample size calculations for SSc clinical trials. Multiple baseline characteristics were significantly different in patients with diffuse SSc in comparison to patients with limited SSc, including health assessment questionnaire (HAQ) disability score, functional Index, grip strength, skin score, and physician global assessment [163]. SSc trials to date choose to enroll patients with diffuse cutaneous disease because the primary outcomes often chosen (e.g., skin or lung changes) change more quickly in this subtype, despite the fact that the limited subtype is more common – often 60–70 % of SSc population [164]. This approach may change as serological subtyping becomes more clearly defined and differentiating [165] or as genetic signatures as a more reliable method for subtyping on a pathogenetic basis becomes validated [161]. The predominance of fibrotic and inflammatory pathways in dcSSc versus vasculopathy in lcSSc supports the dcSSc vs. lcSSc grouping. However, genotypes may differ within the same subtype, pointing to the potential for a different subgrouping [159]. The potential here, not yet proven, is that patient populations in clinical trials will have more uniform pathogenetic backgrounds and, thus, more uniform response to appropriately targeted therapies.

Thus, patient selection at baseline has a substantial effect on the outcome measured; in cases of mild to moderate ILD in SSc patients, dyspnea and decreased quality of life (QOL) may be minimal, and improvement with treatment is not practical, which is not the case in severe ILD patients. Similarly, a lower baseline renal function in a clinical trial may allow us to discern small changes to define progressive renal dysfunction progression. Subsequently, variability in baseline severity could influence the outcomes measured. Accordingly, a careful consideration of possible predictable baseline differences for defining inclusions into the study (e.g., disease duration, disease activity, medications) is appropriate, as is a plan to account for baseline differences during analysis.

Disease Duration

The preliminary ACR criteria, developed in 1980 [166] for SSc, overlook the early stages of disease, with consequent delay in treatment. Matucci-Cerinic et al. developed a consensus for very early diagnosis of systemic sclerosis (VEDOSS) in 2009 to detect early symptoms/signs of SSc before the evolution of full-blown SSc. They identified the presence of Raynaud's phenomenon (RP), abnormal capillaroscopic pattern, and abnormal laboratory values (antinuclear, anticentromere, and antitopoisomerase-I antibodies) as major criteria for VEDOSS diagnosis [167]. A recent Delphi exercise in 2011 also documented four symptoms/signs necessary for VEDOSS: Raynaud's phenomenon, puffy fingers turning to sclerodactyly, specific SSc autoantibodies, and abnormal capillaroscopy with SSc pattern [168]. The importance of early identification of such abnormalities is to detect and treat as early as possible with potential to delay progression to fully defined SSc and, perhaps, to alter the long-term course of the disease. The development of the 2013 ACR/EULAR SSc criteria [169] improved the ability to diagnose SSc patients early, yet only 44 % of the VEDOSS population fulfilled the new ACR/EULAR criteria [170]. Recently, a study by Bruni et al. [171] showed that digital lesions (ulcers and scars) are present among 26 % of 110 VEDOSS patients and demonstrated significant correlation with gastrointestinal involvement in VEDOSS patients. This actually implied that these VEDOSS patients may have had vasculopathic aspects of SSc well before being seen and diagnosed as VEDOSS patients. It is far too early to consider using VEDOSS as a criterion for trial design, but it is possible that it will be an important consideration in the future.

Trial Design

In 1995, the ACR published guidelines for designing clinical trial in patients with scleroderma [172]. Since then there have been significant advances in diagnostic testing, pathophysiological understanding, and treatment of the disease. Clinical trials should be designed using validated outcome measures, and the use of the OMERACT principles can be used to guide the use of those measures [6]. EULAR has recently put forward some point to consider when designing clinical trials in scleroderma [23] see Table 46.2.

Data Analysis

Data analysis of studies is a complex and individualized process, and a complete discussion cannot be undertaken in this section. A few points to consider are:

- Consider consulting with an expert for help with designing the trial.
- Design of the trial and outcomes will determine how the analysis is conducted and vice versa.
- The analysis should be prespecified before the trial starts, although exploratory analyses and work on validation of outcomes in early trials are encouraged.
- Critical to all trials is trying to minimize bias by using control groups and, if at all possible, blinding the trial as well as randomization of allocation.
- Sample size and power calculations for all phase III trials will depend upon the primary outcome measure(s), treatment duration, expected responses in the groups, and desired alpha and beta levels, among other factors. However, not all studies need to have a power analysis done (e.g., safety analysis, pharmacokinetics, some early phase 2 studies, and dose response trials are examples where power analysis is less important).
- Statistical analysis for in between group comparisons should consider the probability of distributions of the results (i.e., parametric vs. nonparametric variables).
- Outcome variables should be defined, using validated measures whenever possible. The characteristics of the

Table 46.2 Issues in clinical trial design

Trial design (all trials should be ethically sound)	Order of credibility:
	Fully statistically powered, randomized, controlled, double-blind trials are considered gold standard
	Possible designs:
	Active comparator
	Post trial provision of beneficial treatment
	Crossover design
	Randomized withdrawal design
	Randomized placebo phase design
	Multiple n-of-1 trials
Duration	*6 weeks to 36 months but organ specific. For example*:
	(a) 3–6 months for PAH and surrogate hemodynamic responses
	(b) 4–6 months for digital ulcer healing
	(c) 3 months for Raynaud's phenomenon
	(d) 6 weeks for GI tract-related symptoms like dyspepsia
	(e) 6 months to 2 years but usually 6–12 months for skin changes and pulmonary fibrosis
Bio sampling	Collection and storage of tissue, blood, and other material if possible should be strongly considered
Inclusion and exclusion criteria	1. Limited vs. diffuse disease and severity of disease
	2. Demographics
	3. Exclusion vs. inclusion of children
	4. Disease duration, early (<3 years) vs. late (>3 years)
	5. Excluding confounders; medications, similar disease, drug exposures, end organ damage
Data analysis	See below
Outcomes	As per OMERACT principles or similar approaches and use of validated outcome measures, as above
Surrogate outcomes	Outcomes other than mortality can be used as primary outcomes

outcomes should be considered, as they may determine the robustness of the data when not normally distributed and the power of the statistics to discriminate among therapies. In general, for example, dichotomous measures do not have as much discriminatory power as continuous measures. Continuous measures are more able to discriminate among therapies than other approaches. If the continuous measures are particularly variable, nominal, categorical, or dichotomous measures are preferable. The specific analyses available are myriad – from simple proportions tests, through ANOVA, through generalized linear regressions with many variations, through survival analyses, etc. This is a very important reason to consult early with your statistical colleagues.

- Missing data, from single variables through patient dropout, are an inevitable aspect of clinical trial design, and there are multiple methods of imputing missing data, from simple completer analysis, through nonresponder imputation, through averaging, and through general linear equation modeling. The method chosen should be chosen in advance
- Adverse event reporting is as important as reporting of benefit and should be considered before the trial begins, although the methodology of such reporting remains unsophisticated. Data safety monitoring should be considered for larger or multicenter trials.
- Criteria for early termination of the trial and interim analysis should be prespecified, if needed.

Conclusion

Clinical trials in scleroderma are inherently difficult because the disease is uncommon/rare, making recruitment problematic and requiring multisite trials; longer trials are also often needed. Partly in response to these difficulties, clinical trial methodology in SSc is evolving and has been improving. This chapter reviewed updated issues in trial design including factors such as epidemiology, phases of trial design, outcome measures, surrogate measures, patient selection, analysis, and updated guidelines for trial design.

References

1. Clements PJ, Seibold JR, Furst DE, Mayes M, White B, Wigley F, Weisman MD, Barr W, Moreland L, Medsger Jr TA, Steen V, Martin RW, Collier D, Weinstein A, Lally E, Varga J, Weiner SR, Andrews B, Abeles M, Wong WK. Semin high-dose versus low-dose D-penicillamine in early diffuse systemic sclerosis trial: lessons learned. Arthritis Rheum. 2004;33(4):249–63.
2. Furst DE, Clements PJ, Hillis S, Lachenbruch PA, Miller BL, Sterz MG, Paulus HE. Immunosuppression with chlorambucil, versus placebo, for scleroderma. Results of a three-year, parallel, randomized, double-blind study. Arthritis Rheum. 1989;32(5): 584–93.

3. Thompson AE, Pope JE. Increased prevalence of scleroderma in southwestern Ontario: a cluster analysis. J Rheumatol. 2002;29:1867–73.
4. Matucci-Cerinic M1, Denton CP, Furst DE, Mayes MD, Hsu VM, Carpentier P, Wigley FM, Black CM, Fessler BJ, Merkel PA, Pope JE, Sweiss NJ, Doyle MK, Hellmich B, Medsger Jr TA, Morganti A, Kramer F, Korn JH, Seibold JR. Bosentan treatment of digital ulcers related to systemic sclerosis: results from the RAPIDS-2 randomised, double-blind, placebo-controlled trial. Ann Rheum Dis. 2011;70(1):32–8. doi:10.1136/ard.2010.130658. Epub 2010 Aug 30.
5. http://www.fda.gov/Drugs/DrugSafety/PostmarketDrugSafetyInformationforPatientsandProviders/ucm111350.htm.
6. Boers M1, Kirwan JR2, Wells G3, Beaton D4, Gossec L5, D'Agostino MA6, Conaghan PG7, Bingham Jr CO8, Brooks P9, Landewé R10, March L11, Simon LS12, Singh JA13, Strand V14, Tugwell P15. Developing core outcome measurement sets for clinical trials: OMERACT filter 2.0. J Clin Epidemiol. 2014;67(7):745–53. doi:10.1016/j.jclinepi.2013.11.013. Epub 2014 Feb 28.
7. Williamson PR, Altman DG, Blazeby JM, Clarke M, Devane D, Gargon E, et al. Developing core outcome sets for clinical trials: issues to consider trials. J Clin Epidemiol. 2014;67(7):745–53. doi:10.1016/j.jclinepi.2013.11.013. Epub 2014 Feb 28.
8. Tashkin DP, Elashoff R, Clements PJ, Goldin J, Roth MD, Furst DE, Arriola E, Silver R, Strange C, Bolster M, Seibold JR, Riley DJ, Hsu VM, Varga J, Schraufnagel DE, Theodore A, Simms R, Wise R, Wigley F, White B, Steen V, Read C, Mayes M, Parsley E, Mubarak K, Connolly MK, Golden J, Olman M, Fessler B, Rothfield N, Metersky M, Scleroderma Lung Study Research Group. Cyclophosphamide versus placebo in scleroderma lung disease. N Engl J Med. 2006;354(25):2655–66.
9. Johnson SR, Feldman BM, Pope JE, Tomlinson GA. Shifting our thinking about uncommon disease trials: the case of methotrexate in scleroderma. J Rheumatol. 2009;36(2):323–9. doi:10.3899/jrheum.071169.
10. van Laar JM, Farge D, Sont JK, Naraghi K, Marjanovic Z, Larghero J, Schuerwegh AJ, Marijt EW, Vonk MC, Schattenberg AV, Matucci-Cerinic M, Voskuyl AE, van de Loosdrecht AA, Daikeler T, Kötter I, Schmalzing M, Martin T, Lioure B, Weiner SM, Kreuter A, Deligny C, Durand JM, Emery P, Machold KP, Sarrot-Reynauld F, Warnatz K, Adoue DF, Constans J, Tony HP, Del Papa N, Fassas A, Himsel A, Launay D, Lo Monaco A, Philippe P, Quéré I, Rich É, Westhovens R, Griffiths B, Saccardi R, van den Hoogen FH, Fibbe WE, Socié G, Gratwohl A, Tyndall A, EBMT/EULAR Scleroderma Study Group. Autologous hematopoietic stem cell transplantation vs intravenous pulse cyclophosphamide in diffuse cutaneous systemic sclerosis: a randomized clinical trial. JAMA. 2014;311(24):2490–8. doi:10.1001/jama.2014.6368.
11. Clements PJ, Roth MD, Elashoff R, Tashkin DP, Goldin J, Silver RM, Sterz M, Seibold JR, Schraufnagel D, Simms RW, Bolster M, Wise RA, Steen V, Mayes MD, Connelly K, Metersky M, Furst DE, Scleroderma Lung Study Group. Scleroderma lung study (SLS): differences in the presentation and course of patients with limited versus diffuse systemic sclerosis. Ann Rheum Dis. 2007;66(12):1641–7.
12. Frech TM, Khanna D, Maranian P, et al. Probiotics for the treatment of systemic sclerosis-associated gastrointestinal bloating/distention. Clin Exp Rheumatol. 2011;29:S22–5.
13. Khanna D, Furst DE, Clements PJ, Park GS, Hays RD, Jeonglim Y, Korn JH, Merkel PA, Naomi R, Wigley FM, Moreland LW, Richard S, Steen VD, Michael W, Mayes MD, Collier DH, Medsger Jr TA, Seibold JR, Relaxin Study Group, et al. Responsiveness of the SF-36 and the health assessment questionnaire disability index in a systemic sclerosis clinical trial. J Rheumatol. 2005;32:832–40.
14. Kaldas M1, Khanna PP, Furst DE, Clements PJ, Kee Wong W, Seibold JR, Postlethwaite AE, Khanna D, investigators of the human recombinant relaxin and oral bovine collagen clinical trials. Sensitivity to change of the modified Rodnan skin score in diffuse systemic sclerosis--assessment of individual body sites in two large randomized controlled trials. Rheumatology (Oxford). 2009;48(9):1143–6. doi:10.1093/rheumatology/kep202. Epub 2009 Jul 14.
15. Khanna PP, Maranian P, Gregory J, Khanna D. The minimally important difference and patient acceptable symptom state for the Raynaud's condition score in patients with Raynaud's phenomenon in a large randomised controlled clinical trial. Ann Rheum Dis. 2010;69:588–91.
16. Khanna D, Seibold JR, Wells A, Distler O, Allanore Y, Denton C, Furst DE. Systemic sclerosis-associated interstitial lung disease: lessons from clinical trials, outcome measures, and future study design. Curr Rheumatol Rev. 2010;6(2):138–44. PMID: 20676227. PMC2911794.
17. Merkel PA, Silliman NP, Clements PJ, Denton CP, Furst DE, Mayes MD, Pope JE, Polisson RP, Streisand JB, Seibold JR, Scleroderma Clinical Trials Consortium. Patterns and predictors of change in outcome measures in clinical trials in scleroderma: an individual patient meta-analysis of 629 subjects with diffuse cutaneous systemic sclerosis. Arthritis Rheum. 2012;64(10):3420–9. doi:10.1002/art.34427.
18. Khanna D1, Distler O, Avouac J, Behrens F, Clements PJ, Denton C, Foeldvari I, Giannini E, Huscher D, Kowal-Bielecka O, Lovell D, Matucci-Cerinic M, Mayes M, Merkel PA, Nash P, Opitz CF, Pittrow D, Rubin L, Seibold JR, Steen V, Strand CV, Tugwell PS, Varga J, Zink A, Furst DE; CRISS; EPOSS. Measures of response in clinical trials of systemic sclerosis: the Combined Response Index for Systemic Sclerosis (CRISS) and Outcome Measures in Pulmonary Arterial Hypertension related to Systemic Sclerosis (EPOSS). J. Rheumatol. 200936(10):2356-61. doi: 10.3899/jrheum.090372.
19. Valentini G, Della Rossa A, Bombardieri S, Bencivelli W, Silman AJ, D'Angelo S, et al. European multicenter study to define disease activity criteria for systemic sclerosis. II. Identification of disease activity variable and development of a preliminary activity index. Ann Rheum Dis. 2001;60:592–8.
20. Valentini G, Bencivelli W, Bombardieri S, D'Angelo S, Della Rossa A, Silman AJ, et al. European scleroderma study group to define disease activity criteria for systemic sclerosis. III. Assessment of the construct validity of the preliminary activity criteria. Ann Rheum Dis. 2003;62:ar023186.
21. Valentini G, D'Angelo S, Della Rossa A, Bencivelli W, Bombardieri S. European scleroderma study group to define disease activity criteria for systemic sclerosis IV. Assessment of skin thickening by modified rodnan skin score. Ann Rheum Dis. 2003;62:904–5.
22. Minier T, Nagy Z, Balint Z, Farkas H, Radics J, Kuma' novics G b, Czmply T, Simon D, Varju C, Nemeth P, Czirjak L. Construct validity evaluation of the European Scleroderma Study Group activity index, and investigation of possible new disease activity markers in systemic sclerosis. Rheumatology. 2010;49:1133–45.
23. Khanna D, Furst DE, Allanore Y, Bae S, Bodukam V, Clements PJ, Cutolo M, Czirjak L, Denton CP, Distler O, Walker UA, Matucci-Cerinic M, Müller-Ladner U, Seibold JR, Singh M, Tyndall A. Twenty-two points to consider for clinical trials in systemic sclerosis, based on EULAR standards. Rheumatology (Oxford). 2014. pii: keu288.
24. Owens GR, Follansbee WP. Cardiopulmonary manifestations of systemic sclerosis. Chest. 1987;91:118–27.
25. McWhorter JE, LeRoy EC. Pericardial disease in scleroderma (systemic sclerosis). Am J Med. 1974;57:566–75.

26. Smith JW, Clements PJ, Levisman J, Furst D, Ross M. Echocardiographic features of progressive systemic sclerosis (PSS). Correlation with hemodynamic and postmortem studies. Am J Med. 1979;66:28–33.
27. Antoniades L, Sfikakis PP, Mavrikakis M. Glucocorticoid effects on myocardial performance in patients with systemic sclerosis. Clin Exp Rheumatol. 2001;19:431–7.
28. Hachulla AL, Launay D, Gaxotte V, et al. Cardiac magnetic resonance imaging in systemic sclerosis: a cross-sectional observational study of 52 patients. Ann Rheum Dis. 2009;68:1878–84.
29. Di Cesare E, Battisti S, Di Sibio A, et al. Early assessment of sub-clinical cardiac involvement in systemic sclerosis (SSc) using delayed enhancement cardiac magnetic resonance (CE-MRI). Eur J Radiol. 2013;82:e268–73.
30. Hoeper MM, Bogaard HJ, Condliffe R, et al. Definitions and diagnosis of pulmonary hypertension. J Am Coll Cardiol. 2013;62:D42–50.
31. Halpern SD, Taichman DB. Misclassification of pulmonary hypertension due to reliance on pulmonary capillary wedge pressure rather than left ventricular end-diastolic pressure. Chest. 2009;136:37–43.
32. Chung L, Chen H, Khanna D, Steen VD. Dyspnea assessment and pulmonary hypertension in patients with systemic sclerosis: utility of the University of California, San Diego, Shortness of Breath Questionnaire. Arthritis Care Res. 2013;65:454–63.
33. Candell-Riera J, Armadans-Gil L, Simeon CP, et al. Comprehensive noninvasive assessment of cardiac involvement in limited systemic sclerosis. Arthritis Rheum. 1996;39:1138–45.
34. Steen VD, Follansbee WP, Conte CG, Medsger Jr TA. Thallium perfusion defects predict subsequent cardiac dysfunction in patients with systemic sclerosis. Arthritis Rheum. 1996;39:677–81.
35. Kostis JB, Seibold JR, Turkevich D, et al. Prognostic importance of cardiac arrhythmias in systemic sclerosis. Am J Med. 1988;84:1007–15.
36. Follansbee WP, Curtiss EI, Rahko PS, et al. The electrocardiogram in systemic sclerosis (scleroderma). Study of 102 consecutive cases with functional correlations and review of the literature. Am J Med. 1985;79:183–92.
37. Choi HJ, Shin YK, Lee HJ, et al. The clinical significance of serum N-terminal pro-brain natriuretic peptide in systemic sclerosis patients. Clin Rheumatol. 2008;27:437–42.
38. Assassi S, Del Junco D, Sutter K, et al. Clinical and genetic factors predictive of mortality in early systemic sclerosis. Arthritis Rheum. 2009;61:1403–11.
39. Kahan A, Devaux JY, Amor B, et al. Nifedipine and thallium-201 myocardial perfusion in progressive systemic sclerosis. N Engl J Med. 1986;314:1397–402.
40. Ferri C, Di Bello V, Martini A, et al. Heart involvement in systemic sclerosis: an ultrasonic tissue characterisation study. Ann Rheum Dis. 1998;57:296–302.
41. Geyer H, Caracciolo G, Abe H, et al. Assessment of myocardial mechanics using speckle tracking echocardiography: fundamentals and clinical applications. J Am Soc Echocardiogr: Off Publ Am Soc Echocardiogr. 2010;23:351–69; quiz 453–5.
42. Flett AS, Hayward MP, Ashworth MT, et al. Equilibrium contrast cardiovascular magnetic resonance for the measurement of diffuse myocardial fibrosis: preliminary validation in humans. Circulation. 2010;122:138–44.
43. Mok MY, Lau CS, Chiu SS, et al. Systemic sclerosis is an independent risk factor for increased coronary artery calcium deposition. Arthritis Rheum. 2011;63:1387–95.
44. Wigley FM, Wise RA, Seibold JR, et al. Intravenous iloprost infusion in patients with Raynaud phenomenon secondary to systemic sclerosis. A multicenter, placebo-controlled, double-blind study. Ann Intern Med. 1994;120:199–206.
45. Merkel PA, Herlyn K, Martin RW, et al. Measuring disease activity and functional status in patients with scleroderma and Raynaud's phenomenon. Arthritis Rheum. 2002;46:2410–20.
46. Baron M, Chung L, Gyger G, et al. Consensus opinion of a North American working group regarding the classification of digital ulcers in systemic sclerosis. Clin Rheumatol. 2014;33:207–14.
47. Rannou F, Poiraudeau S, Berezne A, et al. Assessing disability and quality of life in systemic sclerosis: construct validities of the Cochin Hand Function Scale, Health Assessment Questionnaire (HAQ), systemic sclerosis HAQ, and medical outcomes study 36-item short form health survey. Arthritis Rheum. 2007;57:94–102.
48. Impens AJ, Chung KC, Buch MH, et al. Influences of clinical features of systemic sclerosis (SSc) on the Michigan Hand Questionnaire (MHQ). Arthritis Rheum. 2006;54:S483.
49. Sebastiani M, Manfredi A, Colaci M, et al. Capillaroscopic skin ulcer risk index: a new prognostic tool for digital skin ulcer development in systemic sclerosis patients. Arthritis Rheum. 2009;61:688–94.
50. Hasegawa M, Nagai Y, Tamura A, Ishikawa O. Arteriographic evaluation of vascular changes of the extremities in patients with systemic sclerosis. Br J Dermatol. 2006;155:1159–64.
51. Allanore Y, Seror R, Chevrot A, Kahan A, Drape JL. Hand vascular involvement assessed by magnetic resonance angiography in systemic sclerosis. Arthritis Rheum. 2007;56:2747–54.
52. Black CM, Halkier-Sorensen L, Belch JJ, et al. Oral iloprost in Raynaud's phenomenon secondary to systemic sclerosis: a multicentre, placebo-controlled, dose-comparison study. Br J Rheumatol. 1998;37:952–60.
53. Wigley FM, Korn JH, Csuka ME, et al. Oral iloprost treatment in patients with Raynaud's phenomenon secondary to systemic sclerosis: a multicenter, placebo-controlled, double-blind study. Arthritis Rheum. 1998;41:670–7.
54. Chucker FD, Fowler RC, Hurley CW. Photoplethysmometry and thermography in Raynaud's disorders. A preliminary report. Angiology. 1973;24:612–8.
55. Herrick AL, Clark S. Quantifying digital vascular disease in patients with primary Raynaud's phenomenon and systemic sclerosis. Ann Rheum Dis. 1998;57:70–8.
56. Nickel N, Golpon H, Greer M, et al. The prognostic impact of follow-up assessments in patients with idiopathic pulmonary arterial hypertension. Eur Respir J. 2012;39:589–96.
57. Barst RJ, Rubin LJ, Long WA, et al. A comparison of continuous intravenous epoprostenol (prostacyclin) with conventional therapy for primary pulmonary hypertension. N Engl J Med. 1996;334:296–301.
58. Taichman DB, McGoon MD, Harhay MO, et al. Wide variation in clinicians' assessment of New York Heart Association/World Health Organization functional class in patients with pulmonary arterial hypertension. Mayo Clin Proc. 2009;84:586–92.
59. Galie N, Hoeper MM, Humbert M, et al. Guidelines for the diagnosis and treatment of pulmonary hypertension: the task force for the diagnosis and treatment of pulmonary hypertension of the European Society of Cardiology (ESC) and the European Respiratory Society (ERS), endorsed by the International Society of Heart and Lung Transplantation (ISHLT). Eur Heart J. 2009;30:2493–537.
60. Denton CP, Cailes JB, Phillips GD, Wells AU, Black CM, Bois RM. Comparison of Doppler echocardiography and right heart catheterization to assess pulmonary hypertension in systemic sclerosis. Br J Rheumatol. 1997;36:239–43.
61. McLaughlin VV, Badesch DB, Delcroix M, et al. End points and clinical trial design in pulmonary arterial hypertension. J Am Coll Cardiol. 2009;54:S97–107.
62. Khanna D, Clements PJ, Furst DE, et al. Correlation of the degree of dyspnea with health-related quality of life, functional abilities,

and diffusing capacity for carbon monoxide in patients with systemic sclerosis and active alveolitis: results from the Scleroderma Lung Study. Arthritis Rheum. 2005;52:592–600.

63. Williams MH, Handler CE, Akram R, et al. Role of N-terminal brain natriuretic peptide (N-TproBNP) in scleroderma-associated pulmonary arterial hypertension. Eur Heart J. 2006;27:1485–94.
64. Allanore Y, Borderie D, Avouac J, et al. High N-terminal pro-brain natriuretic peptide levels and low diffusing capacity for carbon monoxide as independent predictors of the occurrence of precapillary pulmonary arterial hypertension in patients with systemic sclerosis. Arthritis Rheum. 2008;58:284–91.
65. Thenappan T, Shah SJ, Rich S, Gomberg-Maitland M. A USA-based registry for pulmonary arterial hypertension: 1982–2006. Eur Respir J. 2007;30:1103–10.
66. O'Donnell DE, Chau LK, Webb KA. Qualitative aspects of exertional dyspnea in patients with interstitial lung disease. J Appl Physiol. 1998;84:2000–9.
67. Johnson SR, Fransen J, Khanna D, et al. Validation of potential classification criteria for systemic sclerosis. Arthritis Care Res. 2012;64:358–67.
68. Hachulla E, Gressin V, Guillevin L, et al. Early detection of pulmonary arterial hypertension in systemic sclerosis: a French nationwide prospective multicenter study. Arthritis Rheum. 2005;52:3792–800.
69. Coghlan JG, Denton CP, Grunig E, et al. Evidence-based detection of pulmonary arterial hypertension in systemic sclerosis: the DETECT study. Ann Rheum Dis. 2014;73:1340–9.
70. Khanna D, Brown KK, Clements PJ, Elashoff R, Furst DE, Goldin J, Seibold JR, Silver RM, Tashkin DP, Wells AU. Systemic sclerosis-associated interstitial lung disease-proposed recommendations for future randomized clinical trials. Clin Exp Rheumatol. 2010;28(2 Suppl 58):S55–62.
71. Bouros D, Wells AU, Nicholson AG, Colby TV, Polychronopoulos V, Pantelidis P, Haslam PL, Vassilakis DA, Black CM, du Bois RM. Histopathologic subsets of fibrosing alveolitis in patients with systemic sclerosis and their relationship to outcome. Am J Respir Crit Care Med. 2002;165(12):1581–6.
72. Latsi PI, du Bois RM, Nicholson AG, Colby TV, Bisirtzoglou D, Nikolakopoulou A, Veeraraghavan S, Hansell DM, Wells AU. Fibrotic idiopathic interstitial pneumonia: the prognostic value of longitudinal functional trends. Am J Respir Crit Care Med. 2003;168(5):531–7.
73. Goldin J, Elashoff R, Kim HJ, Yan X, Lynch D, Strollo D, Roth MD, Clements P, Furst DE, Khanna D, Vasunilashorn S, Li G, Tashkin DP. Treatment of scleroderma-interstitial lung disease with cyclophosphamide is associated with less progressive fibrosis on serial thoracic high-resolution CT scan than placebo: findings from the scleroderma lung study. Chest. 2009;136(5):1333–40. PMC2773360.
74. Goldin JG, Lynch DA, Strollo DC, Suh RD, Schraufnagel DE, Clements PJ, Elashoff RM, Furst DE, Vasunilashorn S, McNitt-Gray MF, Brown MS, Roth MD, Tashkin DP, Scleroderma Lung Study Research G. High-resolution CT scan findings in patients with symptomatic scleroderma-related interstitial lung disease. Chest. 2008;134(2):358–67.
75. Khanna D, Clements PJ, Furst DE, Chon Y, Elashoff R, Roth MD, Sterz MG, Chung J, FitzGerald JD, Seibold JR, Varga J, Theodore A, Wigley FM, Silver RM, Steen VD, Mayes MD, Connolly MK, Fessler BJ, Rothfield NF, Mubarak K, Molitor J, Tashkin DP, Scleroderma Lung Study G. Correlation of the degree of dyspnea with health-related quality of life, functional abilities, and diffusing capacity for carbon monoxide in patients with systemic sclerosis and active alveolitis: results from the Scleroderma Lung Study. Arthritis Rheum. 2005;52(2):592–600.
76. Khanna D, Tseng CH, Furst DE, Clements PJ, Elashoff R, Roth M, Elashoff D, Tashkin DP, for Scleroderma Lung Study I. Minimally important differences in the Mahler's Transition Dyspnoea Index in a large randomized controlled trial – results from the Scleroderma Lung Study. Rheumatology (Oxford). 2009;48(12):1537–40. PMC2777487.
77. Khanna D, Yan X, Tashkin DP, Furst DE, Elashoff R, Roth MD, Silver R, Strange C, Bolster M, Seibold JR, Riley DJ, Hsu VM, Varga J, Schraufnagel DE, Theodore A, Simms R, Wise R, Wigley F, White B, Steen V, Read C, Mayes M, Parsley E, Mubarak K, Connolly MK, Golden J, Olman M, Fessler B, Rothfield N, Metersky M, Clements PJ, Scleroderma Lung Study G. Impact of oral cyclophosphamide on health-related quality of life in patients with active scleroderma lung disease: results from the scleroderma lung study. Arthritis Rheum. 2007;56(5):1676–84.
78. Steen VD, Medsger Jr TA. The value of the health assessment questionnaire and special patient-generated scales to demonstrate change in systemic sclerosis patients over time. Arthritis Rheum. 1997;40(11):1984–91.
79. Swigris JJ, Zhou X, Wamboldt FS, du Bois R, Keith R, Fischer A, Cosgrove GP, Frankel SK, Curran-Everett D, Brown KK. Exercise peripheral oxygen saturation (SpO2) accurately reflects arterial oxygen saturation (SaO2) and predicts mortality in systemic sclerosis. Thorax. 2009;64(7):626–30. PMC3667987.
80. Buch MH, Denton CP, Furst DE, Guillevin L, Rubin LJ, Wells AU, Matucci-Cerinic M, Riemekasten G, Emery P, Chadha-Boreham H, Charef P, Roux S, Black CM, Seibold JR. Submaximal exercise testing in the assessment of interstitial lung disease secondary to systemic sclerosis: reproducibility and correlations of the 6-min walk test. Ann Rheum Dis. 2007;66(2):169–73.
81. Frauenfelder T, Winklehner A, Nguyen TD, Dobrota R, Baumueller S, Maurer B, Distler O. Screening for interstitial lung disease in systemic sclerosis: performance of high-resolution CT with limited number of slices: a prospective study. Ann Rheum Dis. 2014;73:2069–73.
82. Chung L, Chen H, Khanna D, Steen VD. Dyspnea assessment and pulmonary hypertension in patients with systemic sclerosis: utility of the University of California, San Diego, Shortness of Breath Questionnaire. Arthritis Care Res (Hoboken). 2013;65(3):454–63. doi:10.1002/acr.21827.
83. Clements PJ, Lachenbruch PA, Seibold JR, et al. Skin thickness score in systemic sclerosis: an assessment of interobserver variability in 3 independent studies. J Rheumatol. 1993;20:1892–6.
84. Clements P, Lachenbruch P, Siebold J, et al. Inter and intraobserver variability of total skin thickness score (modified Rodnan TSS) in systemic sclerosis. J Rheumatol. 1995;22:1281–5.
85. Pope JE, Baron M, Bellamy N, et al. Variability of skin scores and clinical measurements in scleroderma. J Rheumatol. 1995;22:1271–6.
86. Clements PJ, Lachenbruch PA, Ng SC, Simmons M, Sterz M, Furst DE. Skin score. A semiquantitative measure of cutaneous involvement that improves prediction of prognosis in systemic sclerosis. Arthritis Rheum. 1990;33:1256–63.
87. Kahaleh MB, Sultany GL, Smith EA, Huffstutter JE, Loadholt CB, LeRoy EC. A modified scleroderma skin scoring method. Clin Exp Rheumatol. 1986;4:367–9.
88. Merkel PA, Silliman NP, Denton CP, et al. Validity, reliability, and feasibility of durometer measurements of scleroderma skin disease in a multicenter treatment trial. Arthritis Rheum. 2008;59:699–705.
89. Furst DE, Clements PJ, Steen VD, et al. The modified Rodnan skin score is an accurate reflection of skin biopsy thickness in systemic sclerosis. J Rheumatol. 1998;25:84–8.
90. Kuhn A, Haust M, Ruland V, et al. Effect of bosentan on skin fibrosis in patients with systemic sclerosis: a prospective, open-label, non-comparative trial. Rheumatology. 2010;49:1336–45.
91. Denton CP, Engelhart M, Tvede N, et al. An open-label pilot study of infliximab therapy in diffuse cutaneous systemic sclerosis. Ann Rheum Dis. 2009;68:1433–9.

92. Sandqvist G, Akesson A, Eklund M. Evaluation of paraffin bath treatment in patients with systemic sclerosis. Disabil Rehabil. 2004;26:981–7.
93. Muellegger RR, Hofer A, Salmhofer W, Soyer HP, Kerl H, Wolf P. Extended extracorporeal photochemotherapy with extracorporeal administration of 8-methoxypsoralen in systemic sclerosis. An Austrian single-center study. Photodermatol Photoimmunol Photomed. 2000;16:216–23.
94. Basso M, Filaci G, Cutolo M, et al. Long-term treatment of patients affected by systemic sclerosis with cyclosporin A. Ann Ital Med Int: Organo Ufficiale Soc Ital Med Intern. 2001;16:233–9.
95. Balbir-Gurman A, Denton CP, Nichols B, et al. Non-invasive measurement of biomechanical skin properties in systemic sclerosis. Ann Rheum Dis. 2002;61:237–41.
96. Scheja A, Akesson A. Comparison of high frequency (20 MHz) ultrasound and palpation for the assessment of skin involvement in systemic sclerosis (scleroderma). Clin Exp Rheumatol. 1997;15:283–8.
97. Akesson A, Hesselstrand R, Scheja A, Wildt M. Longitudinal development of skin involvement and reliability of high frequency ultrasound in systemic sclerosis. Ann Rheum Dis. 2004;63:791–6.
98. Khanna D, Hays RD, Maranian P, Seibold JR, Impens A, Mayes MD, et al. Reliability and validity of the University of California, Los Angeles scleroderma clinical trial consortium gastrointestinal tract instrument. Arthritis Rheum. 2009;61:1257–63.
99. Khanna D, Hays RD, Park GS, Braun-Moscovici Y, Mayes MD, McNearney TA, et al. Development of a preliminary scleroderma gastrointestinal tract 1.0 quality of life instrument. Arthritis Rheum. 2007;57:1280–6.
100. Hung EW, Mayes MD, Sharif R, Assassi S, Machicao VI, Hosing C, St Clair EW, Furst DE, Khanna D, Forman S, Mineishi S, Phillips K, Seibold JR, Bredeson C, Csuka ME, Nash RA, Wener MH, Simms R, Ballen K, Leclercq S, Storek J, Goldmuntz E, Welch B, Keyes-Elstein L, Castina S, Crofford LJ, Mcsweeney P, Sullivan KM. Gastric antral vascular ectasia and its clinical correlates in patients with early diffuse systemic sclerosis in the SCOT trial. Rheumatology. 2013;40(4):455–60. doi:10.3899/jrheum.121087. Epub 2013 Feb 15.
101. Ghrénassia E, Avouac J, Khanna D, Derk CT, Distler O, Suliman YA, Airo P, Carreira PE, Foti R, Granel B, Berezne A, Cabane J, Ingegnoli F, Rosato E, Caramaschi P, Hesselstrand R, Walker UA, Alegre-Sancho JJ, Zarrouk V, Agard C, Riccieri V, Schiopu E, Gladue H, Steen VD, Allanore Y. Prevalence, correlates and outcomes of gastric antral vascular ectasia in systemic sclerosis: a EUSTAR case-control study. J Rheumatol. 2014;41(1):99–105. doi:10.3899/jrheum.130386. Epub 2013 Dec 1.
102. Thonhofer R, Siegel C, Trummer M, Graninger W. Early endoscopy in systemic sclerosis without gastrointestinal symptoms. Rheumatol Int. 2012;32(1):165–8. doi:10.1007/s00296-010-1595-y.
103. Hendel L1, Hage E, Hendel J, Stentoft P. Omeprazole in the long-term treatment of severe gastro-oesophageal reflux disease in patients with systemic sclerosis. Aliment Pharmacol Ther. 1992;6(5):565–77.
104. Manetti M1, Milia AF, Benelli G, Messerini L, Matucci-Cerinic M, Ibba-Manneschi L. The gastric wall in systemic sclerosis patients: a morphological study. Ital J Anat Embryol. 2010;115(1–2):115–21.
105. Hendel L. Hydroxyproline in the oesophageal mucosa of patients with progressive systemic sclerosis during an omeprazole-induced healing of reflux oesophigitis. Aliment Pharmacol Ther. 1991;5(5):471–80.
106. Horikoshi T, Matsuzaki T, Sekiguchi T. Effect of H2-receptor antagonists cimetidine and famotidine on interdigestive gastric motor activity and lower esophageal sphincter pressure in progressive systemic sclerosis. Intern Med (Tokyo, Japan). 1994;33(7):407–12.
107. Weihrauch TR, Korting GW. Manometric assessment of oesophageal involvement in progressive systemic sclerosis, morphoea and Raynaud's disease. Br J Dermatol. 1982;107(3):325–32.
108. Blom-Bülow B, Sundström G, Jonson B, Tylén U, Wollheim FA. Early changes in oesophageal function in progressive systemic sclerosis: a comparison of manometry and radiology. Clin Physiol. 1984;4(2):147–58.
109. Stentoft P, Hendel L, Aggestrup S. Esophageal manometry and pH-probe monitoring in the evaluation of gastroesophageal reflux in patients with progressive systemic sclerosis. Scand J Gastroenterol. 1987;22(4):499–504.
110. Ipsen P, Egekvist H, Aksglaede K, Zachariae H, Bjerring P, Thommesen P. Oesophageal manometry and video-radiology in patients with systemic sclerosis: a retrospective study of its clinical value. Acta Derm Venereol. 2000;80:130–3.
111. Mainie I, Tutuian R, Patel A, Castell DO. Regional esophageal dysfunction in scleroderma and achalasia using multichannel intraluminal impedance and manometry. Dig Dis Sci. 2008;53(1):210–6.
112. Owen JP, Muston HL, Goolamali SK. Absence of oesophageal mucosal folds in systemic sclerosis. Clin Radiol. 1979;30(5):489–92.
113. Dantas RO, Villanova MG, de Godoy RA. Esophageal dysfunction in patients with progressive systemic sclerosis and mixed connective tissue diseases. Arq Gastroenterol. 1985;22(3):122–6.
114. Montesi A, Pesaresi A, Cavalli ML, Ripa G, Candela M, Gabrielli A. Oropharyngeal and esophageal function in scleroderma. Dysphagia. 1991;6(4):219–23.
115. Sharma VK, Trilokraj T, Khaitan BK, Krishna SM. Profile of systemic sclerosis in a tertiary care center in North India. Indian J Dermatol Venereol Leprol. 2006;72(6):416–20.
116. Kaye SA, Lim SG, Taylor M, Patel S, Gillespie S, Black CM. Small bowel bacterial overgrowth in systemic sclerosis: detection using direct and indirect methods and treatment outcome. Br J Rheumatol. 1995;34(3):265–9.
117. Marie I, Ducrotté P, Denis P, Menard JF, Levesque H. Small intestinal bacterial overgrowth in systemic sclerosis. Rheumatology (Oxford). 2009;48(10):1314–9.
118. Weston S, Thumshirn M, Wiste J, Camilleri M. Clinical and upper gastrointestinal motility features in systemic sclerosis and related disorders. Am J Gastroenterol. 1998;93(7):1085–9.
119. Wollaston DE, Xu X, Tokumaru O, Chen JD, McNearney TA. Patients with systemic sclerosis have unique and persistent alterations in gastric myoelectrical activity with acupressure to Neiguan point PC6. J Rheumatol. 2005;32(3):494–501.
120. Franck-Larsson K1, Hedenström H, Dahl R, Rönnblom A. Delayed gastric emptying in patients with diffuse versus limited systemic sclerosis, unrelated to gastrointestinal symptoms and myoelectric gastric activity. Scand J Rheumatol. 2003;32(6):348–55.
121. Mo J, Wang C, Wang S. Gastric emptying and intragastric distribution of liquid and solid meal in patients with systemic sclerosis. Zhonghua Nei Ke Za Zhi. 1996;35(8):530–2.
122. Zuber-Jerger I, Müller A, Kullmann F, Gelbmann CM, Endlicher E, Müller-Ladner U, Fleck M. Gastrointestinal manifestation of systemic sclerosis – thickening of the upper gastrointestinal wall detected by endoscopic ultrasound is a valid sign. Rheumatology (Oxford). 2010;49(2):368–72. doi:10.1093/rheumatology/kep381. Epub 2009 Dec 14.
123. Bartosik I, Andréasson K, Starck M, Scheja A, Hesselstrand R. Vascular events are risk factors for anal incontinence in systemic sclerosis: a study of morphology and functional properties measured by anal endosonography and manometry. Scand J Rheumatol. 2014;43(5):391–7. doi:10.3109/03009742.2014.889210. Epub 2014 Apr 11.
124. Thoua NM, Schizas A, Forbes A, Denton CP, Emmanuel AV. Internal anal sphincter atrophy in patients with systemic

sclerosis. Rheumatology (Oxford). 2011;50(9):1596–602. doi:10.1093/rheumatology/ker153. Epub 2011 Apr 18.

125. Marie I, Antonietti M, Houivet E, Hachulla E, Maunoury V, Bienvenu B, Viennot S, Smail A, Duhaut P, Dupas JL, Dominique S, Hatron PY, Levesque H, Benichou J, Ducrotté P. Gastrointestinal mucosal abnormalities using videocapsule endoscopy in systemic sclerosis. Aliment Pharmacol Ther. 2014;40(2):189–99. doi:10.1111/apt.12818. Epub 2014 Jun 2.
126. Penn H, et al. Scleroderma renal crisis: patient characteristics and long-term outcomes. QJM. 2007;100(8):485–94.
127. Nagaraja V, Hays RD, Khanna PP, Spiegel BM, Chang L, Melmed GY, Bolus R, Khanna D. Construct validity of the Patient Reported Outcomes Measurement Information System (PROMIS®) gastrointestinal symptom scales in systemic sclerosis. Arthritis Care Res (Hoboken). 2014;66(11):1725–30.
128. Scheja A, et al. Renal function is mostly preserved in patients with systemic sclerosis. Scand J Rheumatol. 2009;38:1–4.
129. Mohamed RH, Zayed HS, Amin A. Renal disease in systemic sclerosis with normal serum creatinine. Clin Rheumatol. 2010;29(7):729–37. doi:10.1007/s10067-010-1389-3. Epub 2010 Feb 23.
130. Kingdon EJ, Knight CJ, Dustan K, Irwin AG, Thomas M, Powis SH, Burns A, Hilson AJ, Black CM. Calculated glomerular filtration rate is a useful screening tool to identify scleroderma patients with renal impairment. Rheumatology (Oxford). 2003;42(1):26–33.
131. Seiberlich B, Hunzelmann N, Krieg T, Weber M, Schulze-Lohoff E. Intermediate molecular weight proteinuria and albuminuria identify scleroderma patients with increased morbidity. Clin Nephrol. 2008;70(2):110–7.
132. Rivolta R1, Mascagni B, Berruti V, Quarto Di Palo F, Elli A, Scorza R, Castagnone D. Renal vascular damage in systemic sclerosis patients without clinical evidence of nephropathy. Arthritis Rheum. 1996;39(6):1030–4.
133. Scorza R, Rivolta R, Mascagni B, Berruti V, Bazzi S, Castagnone D, di Quarto PF. Effect of iloprost infusion on the resistance index of renal vessels of patients with systemic sclerosis. J Rheumatol. 1997;24(10):1944–8.
134. Khanna D, Furst DE, Clements PJ, et al. Responsiveness of the SF-36 and the health assessment questionnaire disability index in a systemic sclerosis clinical trial. J Rheumatol. 2005;32:832–40.
135. Khanna D, Yan X, Tashkin DP, et al. Impact of oral cyclophosphamide on health-related quality of life in patients with active scleroderma lung disease: results from the scleroderma lung study. Arthritis Rheum. 2007;56:1676–84.
136. Hudson M, Steele R, Lu Y, Thombs BD, Baron M. Work disability in systemic sclerosis. J Rheumatol. 2009;36:2481–6.
137. Sekhon S, Pope J, Baron M. The minimally important difference in clinical practice for patient-centered outcomes including health assessment questionnaire, fatigue, pain, sleep, global visual analog scale, and SF-36 in scleroderma. J Rheumatol. 2010;37:591–8.
138. Smyth AE, MacGregor AJ, Mukerjee D, Brough GM, Black CM, Denton CP. A cross-sectional comparison of three self-reported functional indices in scleroderma. Rheumatology (Oxford). 2003;42:732–8.
139. Sandqvist G, Scheja A, Hesselstrand R. Pain, fatigue and hand function closely correlated to work ability and employment status in systemic sclerosis. Rheumatology (Oxford). 2010;49:1739–46.
140. Khanna D, Furst DE, Wong WK, et al. Reliability, validity, and minimally important differences of the SF-6D in systemic sclerosis. Qual Life Res. 2007;16:1083–92.
141. Milette K, Razykov I, Pope J, et al. Clinical correlates of sleep problems in systemic sclerosis: the prominent role of pain. Rheumatology (Oxford). 2011;50(5):921–5.
142. Frech T, Hays RD, Maranian P, Clements PJ, Furst DE, Khanna D. Prevalence and correlates of sleep disturbance in systemic sclerosis – results from the UCLA scleroderma quality of life study. Rheumatology (Oxford). 2011;50:1280–7.
143. Thombs BD, Hudson M, Bassel M, Taillefer SS, Baron M. Sociodemographic, disease, and symptom correlates of fatigue in systemic sclerosis: evidence from a sample of 659 Canadian Scleroderma Research Group Registry patients. Arthritis Rheum. 2009;61:966–73.
144. Bongi SM, Del Rosso A, Galluccio F, Sigismondi F, Miniati I, Conforti ML, et al. Efficacy of connective tissue massage and Mc Mennell joint manipulation in the rehabilitative treatment of the hands in systemic sclerosis. Clin Rheumatol. 2009;28(10):1167–73.
145. Sandqvist G, Eklund M. Hand Mobility in Scleroderma (HAMIS) test: the reliability of a novel hand function test. Arthritis Care Res. 2000;13(6):369–74.
146. Clements PJ, Allanore Y, Khanna D, Singh M, Furst DE. Arthritis in systemic sclerosis: systematic review of the literature and suggestions for the performance of future clinical trials in systemic sclerosis. Semin Arthritis Rheum. 2012;41:801–14.
147. Scheiman-Elazary A, Ranganath VK, Ben-Artzi A, Duan L, Kafaja S, Borazan NH, Woodworth T, Elashoff D, Clements P, Furst DE. Validation of musculoskeletal us of hands and wrists in patients with systemic sclerosis abstract. Eular 2014. Annals of the Rheumatic Diseases 73(Suppl 2):651–651.
148. Ruof J, Brühlmann P, Michel BA, Stucki G. Development and validation of a self-administered systemic sclerosis questionnaire (SySQ). Rheumatology. 1999;38(6):535–42. doi:10.1093/rheumatology/38.6.535.
149. Ranque B, Bérezné A, Le-Guern V, Pagnoux C, Allanore Y, Launay D, Hachulla E, Authier FJ, Gherardi R, Kahan A, Cabane J, Guillevin L, Mouthon L. Myopathies related to systemic sclerosis: a case-control study of associated clinical and immunological features. Scand J Rheumatol. 2010;39(6):498–505. doi:10.3109/03009741003774626. Epub 2010 Aug 20.
150. Au K, Mayes MD, Maranian P, Clements PJ, Khanna D, Steen VD, et al. Course of dermal ulcers and musculoskeletal involvement in systemic sclerosis patients in the scleroderma lung study. Arthritis Care Res (Hoboken). 2010;62(12):1772–8. ms tenderness.
151. Clements PJ, Furst DE, Campion DS, Bohan A, Harris R, Levy J, Paulus HE. Muscle disease in progressive systemic sclerosis: diagnostic and therapeutic considerations. Arthritis Rheum. 1978;21(1):62–71.
152. Cohn JN. Introduction to surrogate markers. Circulation. 2004;109(25 Suppl 1):IV20–1.
153. Varga J. Systemic sclerosis. An update. Bull NYU Hosp Jt Dis. 2008;66(3):198–202.
154. Kabunga P, Coghlan G. Endothelin receptor antagonism: role in the treatment of pulmonary arterial hypertension related to scleroderma. Drugs. 2008;68(12):1635–45.
155. Launay D, Sitbon O, Le Pavec J, Savale L, Tchérakian C, Yaïci A, Achouh L, Parent F, Jais X, Simonneau G, Humbert M. Long-term outcome of systemic sclerosis-associated pulmonary arterial hypertension treated with bosentan as first-line monotherapy followed or not by the addition of prostanoids or sildenafil. Rheumatology (Oxford). 2010;49(3):490–500. doi:10.1093/rheumatology/kep398. Epub 2009 Dec 16.
156. Goh NS, Desai SR, Veeraraghavan S, Hansell DM, Copley SJ, Maher TM, Corte TJ, Sander CR, Ratoff J, Devaraj A, Bozovic G, Denton CP, Black CM, du Bois RM, Wells AU. Interstitial lung disease in systemic sclerosis: a simple staging system. Am J Respir Crit Care Med. 2008;177(11):1248–54. doi:10.1164/rccm.200706-877OC. Epub 2008 Mar 27.
157. Pulido T, Adzerikho I, Channick RN, Delcroix M, Galiè N, Ghofrani HA, Jansa P, Jing ZC, Le Brun FO, Mehta S, Mittelholzer CM, Perchenet L, Sastry BK, Sitbon O, Souza R, Torbicki A, Zeng X, Rubin LJ, Simonneau G, SERAPHIN Investigators. Macitentan and morbidity and mortality in pulmonary arterial

hypertension. N Engl J Med. 2013;369(9):809–18. doi:10.1056/NEJMoa1213917.
158. Assassi S, Mayes MD. What does global gene expression profiling tell us about the pathogenesis of systemic sclerosis? Curr Opin Rheumatol. 2013;25(6):686–91. doi:10.1097/01.bor.0000434672.77891.41.
159. Milano A, Pendergrass SA, Sargent JL, George LK, McCalmont TH, Connolly MK, Whitfield ML. Molecular subsets in the gene expression signatures of scleroderma skin. PLoS ONE. 2008;16(7):e2696. doi:10.1371/journal.pone.0002696.
160. Hinchcliff M, Huang CC, Wood TA, Matthew Mahoney J, Martyanov V, Bhattacharyya S, Tamaki Z, Lee J, Carns M, Podlusky S, Sirajuddin A, Shah SJ, Chang RW, Lafyatis R, Varga J, Whitfield ML. Molecular signatures in skin associated with clinical improvement during mycophenolate treatment in systemic sclerosis. J Invest Dermatol. 2013;133(8):1979–89. doi:10.1038/jid.2013.130. Epub 2013 Mar 14002E.
161. Chung L, Fiorentino DF, Benbarak MJ, Adler AS, Mariano MM, Paniagua RT, Milano A, Connolly MK, Ratiner BD, Wiskocil RL, Whitfield ML, Chang HY, Robinson WH. Molecular framework for response to imatinib mesylate in systemic sclerosis. Arthritis Rheum. 2009;60(2):584–91. doi:10.1002/art.24221.
162. Czirjak L, Nagy Z, Aringer M, et al. The EUSTAR model for teaching and implementing the modified Rodnan skin score in systemic sclerosis. Ann Rheum Dis. 2007;66:966–9.
163. Pope JE, Bellamy N. Sample size calculations in scleroderma: a rational approach to choosing outcome measurements in scleroderma trials. Clin Invest Med. 1995;18(1):1–10.
164. Rosa JE, Soriano ER, Narvaez-Ponce L, et al. Incidence and prevalence of systemic sclerosis in a healthcare plan in Buenos Aires. J Clin Rheumatol. 2011;17:59–63.
165. Steen VD. Autoantibodies in systemic sclerosis. Semin Arthritis Rheum. 2005;35(1):35–42.
166. Preliminary criteria for the classification of systemic sclerosis (scleroderma). Subcommittee for scleroderma criteria of the American rheumatism association diagnostic and therapeutic criteria committee. Arthritis Rheum 1980;23:581–90.
167. Matucci-Cerinic M, Allanore Y, Czirják L, et al. The challenge of early systemic sclerosis for the EULAR Scleroderma Trial and Research group (EUSTAR) community. It is time to cut the Gordian knot and develop a prevention or rescue strategy. Ann Rheum Dis. 2009;68:1377–80.
168. Avouac J, Fransen J, Walker UA, et al. Preliminary criteria for the very early diagnosis of systemic sclerosis: results of a Delphi Consensus Study from EULAR Scleroderma Trials and Research Group. Ann Rheum Dis. 2011;70:476.
169. van den Hoogen F, Khanna D, Fransen J, et al. 2013 classification criteria for systemic sclerosis: an American College of Rheumatology/European League against Rheumatism collaborative initiative. Arthritis Rheum. 2013;65:2737–47.
170. Minier T, Guiducci S, Bellando-Randone S, et al. Preliminary analysis of the Very Early Diagnosis of Systemic Sclerosis (VEDOSS) EUSTAR multicentre study: evidence for puffy fingers as pivotal sign for the suspicion of systemic sclerosis. Ann Rheum Dis. 2013. doi:10.1136/annrheumdis-2013-203716 [Epub ahead of print].
171. Bruni, Serena Guiducci, Silvia Bellando-Randone, Gemma Lepri, Francesca Braschi, Ginevra Fiori, Francesca Bartoli, Francesca Peruzzi, Jelena Blagojevic and Marco Matucci-Cerinic. Concise report Digital ulcers as a sentinel sign for early internal organ involvement in very early systemic sclerosis. Cosimo doi:10.1093/rheumatology/keu29.
172. White B, Bauer EA, Goldsmith LA, et al. Guidelines for clinical trials in systemic sclerosis (scleroderma). I. Disease-modifying interventions. The American College of Rheumatology Committee on Design and Outcomes in Clinical Trials in Systemic Sclerosis. Arthritis Rheum. 1995;38:351–60.

Measuring Disease Activity and Outcomes in Clinical Trials

47

Dinesh Khanna and Sindhu R. Johnson

Introduction

Systemic sclerosis (scleroderma, SSc) has seen a substantial progress in the development and validation of outcome measures [1]. This chapter will discuss the outcome measures ready for clinical trials in SSc.

Measurement Properties of an Instrument: Feasibility, Reliability, and Validity

An outcome measure should be feasible, reliable, and valid [2]. A feasible measure is accessible, easily interpretable, and associated with low cost. Reliability is the extent to which a measure yields the same score each time it is administered if an underlying health condition has not changed. A reliability coefficient of 0.90 or higher (means that 90 % of the score is accurate, while the remaining 10 % denotes error) is considered satisfactory for individual comparisons and 0.70 or higher is considered satisfactory for group comparisons [3]. Validity is the extent to which the score a health measure yields accurately reflects the health concept and includes face (measures what it purports to measure), content (comprehensive), construct (measures or correlates with a theorized health construct), and criterion validity (predicts or correlates with "gold standard"). Sensitivity to change (responsiveness) assesses the ability of an instrument to detect change when it has occurred. The ability of an instrument to detect clinically important change is crucial to their usefulness as an outcome measure in a clinical trial.

D. Khanna, MD, MSc (✉)
Division of Rheumatology, Department of Internal Medicine, University of Michigan, Ann Arbor, MI, USA
e-mail: khannad@umich.edu

S.R. Johnson, MD, PhD, FRCPC
Toronto Scleroderma Program, Mount Sinai Hospital, Toronto Western Hospital, Toronto, ON, Canada

Measuring Disease Activity and Severity in SSc

Investigators agree that assessment of disease activity and severity is an important goal in SSc. Based on a previous consensus reached in other rheumatic diseases [4], activity is defined as the aspect of disease that varies over time and has the potential to be reversible spontaneously or with therapy (e.g., tendon friction rubs, acute phase reactants, and inflammatory polyarthritis). Damage is a cumulative burden of a disease at a given time point and is generally irreversible (e.g., calcinosis, end-stage pulmonary fibrosis). Both activity and damage contribute to the disease severity; early in SSc, activity predominates, whereas later in the disease, damage is more likely to be the dominant part [5].

Disease Activity in SSc

The European Scleroderma Study Group has proposed a composite index to assess SSc-related disease activity in routine clinical care [6, 7]. The index is feasible as it includes measures (clinical examination, patient assessment of activity over the last month, laboratory measures, and carbon monoxide diffusing capacity or transfer factor of the lung for carbon monoxide (DLCO) percent predicted) collected in routine practice. It has face and content validity. It is scored on a 0 (no activity) to 10 (severe activity) with greatest weight assigned to deterioration of the relevant organ system as evaluated by the patient with respect to the previous month. The tests required to calculate index are inexpensive and easily carried out in routine clinical care. The index has few limitations (1): The index was developed in patients with established disease and has not yet been studied in early SSc where disease is likely to be active (2) Three patient-reported items relate to a change in their skin, vascular, and cardiopulmonary symptoms in the past month. Such change items in activity indices may be challenging because they fail to capture *persistent* activity and may be difficult to administer

J. Varga et al. (eds.), *Scleroderma*, DOI 10.1007/978-3-319-31407-5_47

every month [5]. (3) The index is not developed for clinical trials, and sensitivity to change has not been published.

Assessment of Disease Severity

A measure of disease severity encompasses both disease activity and damage and should be associated with or predict SSc-associated morbidity and mortality [5]. The revised Medsger severity index [8] was developed by international scleroderma experts using consensus methodology followed by prospective data collection. The authors identified nine organ systems and identified variables for each organ system that can be used to define severity. The nine organ systems are general, peripheral vascular, skin, joint/tendon, muscles, GI tract, lung, heart, and kidney. Each system is scored from 0 (uninvolved) to 4 (end-stage disease). The individual organ system severity scores have been shown to predict survival in large observational cohorts [9]. The severity index is not weighted and therefore should not be summed to have a "global" severity scale score.

Outcome Measures in SSc

This section outlines the outcome measures used in clinical trials (Table 47.1) that are feasible, reliable, valid, and sensitive to change [2].

Measuring Skin Disease in SSc

Modified Rodnan skin score (MRSS), a measure of skin thickness [11, 12], has been used as the primary outcome measure in clinical trials of diffuse cutaneous SSc (dcSSc). Measurement of skin thickness is used as a surrogate measure of disease severity and mortality in patients with dcSSc – an increase in skin thickening is associated with involvement of internal organs and increased mortality [12]. It is generally accepted that MRSS tends to worsen in early disease and improve in late disease, although time of peak involvement remains poorly defined. "Early" dcSSc is often defined as the rapid and severe increasing induration ("thickening") of the skin, which has been thought to peak at 1–3 years after disease onset [13]. MRSS is feasible, reliable, valid, and sensitive to change for multicenter clinical trials [11]. For example, MRSS was able to differentiate between methotrexate and placebo in early dcSSc [14] and between cyclophosphamide and placebo in dcSSc subset in the Scleroderma Lung Study [15]. However, analysis from three large RCTs in dcSSc showed that mean MRSS improved regardless of disease duration at baseline – there was a general tendency for skin to soften over time, and there was no difference in this tendency among patients with different disease durations at baseline [16]. This observation differs from the natural history of skin thickening previously reported and has important implications in the "prevention of worsening" study design, when using skin softening as an endpoint [17]. In our opinion, MRSS should be incorporated as an outcome measure in RCTs; it was recently shown to differentiate tocilizumab vs. placebo in a phase 2/3 RCT [78] and was also supported by the autologous stem cell transplant vs. cyclophosphamide and LPA-1 antagonist vs. placebo in early dcSSc, and also supports the use of MRSS as *the* primary outcome measure in early dcSSc. Approval agencies also consider MRSS as an acceptable primary outcome, but require supportive evidence for improvement in PROs and/or stabilization or prevention of internal organ involvement. If incorporated, the pivotal RCT should be at least 52 weeks.

Durometer for skin hardness: Durometers are handheld devices used to measure the hardness of materials using internationally standardized durometer units. Durometer was included in a multicenter study of early dcSSc and was found to be feasible, reliable, valid, and sensitive to change [18]. Durometer was found to have a higher intraobserver reproducibility compared to MRSS [19], suggesting a greater reliability. A moderate-to-high correlation was found (coefficient 0.44–0.81) between MRSS and durometer [18, 19]. Durometer was proposed as a core set measure in a recent Delphi exercise involving international scleroderma experts [20], although its use may be limited due to its cost.

Other methods have been proposed to measure skin disease in SSc, including skin ultrasonography, elastometry, magnetic resonance imaging, or other radiographic techniques [21], but lack data on sensitivity to change and have not been applied in a multicenter setting (lack of feasibility).

Measuring Musculoskeletal Involvement in Scleroderma

Tendon friction rubs (TFR) are a grating, "squeaking" sensation detected on passive or active motion of the affected tendon in SSc. On physical examination, TFR are most commonly present in the flexor and extensor tendons of fingers and wrists and the anterior tibial and peroneal tendons. In an RCT involving patients with early dcSSc (≤18 months from the first non-Raynaud's phenomenon symptom) [22], 14–20 % of TFR were present in these three areas. This RCT also showed the dynamic nature of TFR: only 10 % of patients having TFR at baseline continued to have TFR at subsequent visits, whereas 21 % developed new TFR over a 2-year follow-up period. The change in TFR (decrease or increase in the number of TFR compared to baseline) over 6

Table 47.1 Feasible, reliable, valid, and sensitivity to change measures that are ready for clinical trials

Instruments	Completed by patient	Completed by investigator	Laboratory
COMPOSITE INDEX			
American College of Rheumatology CRISS Index	X	X	
GLOBAL PATIENT-REPORTED OUTCOME MEASURES[A]			
SF-36	X		
Health assessment questionnaire-disability index	X		
UK functional score	X		
Pain visual analog scale (VAS) from health assessment questionnaire-disability index (HAQ-DI)	X		
SF-6D (scored using SF-36 data)	X		
GLOBAL ASSESSMENT			
Patient global assessment using VAS or Likert scale	X		
Investigator global assessment using VAS or Likert scale		X[b]	
SKIN			
Modified Rodnan skin score		X[b]	
Durometer		X[b]	
Patient assessment of skin activity	X		
Patient assessment of skin severity	X		
MUSCULOSKELETAL			
Tendon friction rubs		X[b]	
Tender joint count		X[b]	
Serum creatinine phosphokinase			X
Cochin hand function scale	X		
Hand function in scleroderma scale		X	
Mouth handicap in systemic sclerosis scale	X		
HAQ-DI	X		
CARDIAC			
Echocardiogram with Doppler			X[c]
Right heart catheterization			X
6-min walk test[d]			X
Borg dyspnea index[d] (administered immediately after the 6-min walk test)	X		
PULMONARY			
Pulmonary Function test with diffusion capacity			X
Forced vital capacity			X
			X
Total lung capacity			
High-resolution quantitative computed tomography scale			X[c]
Validated measure of dyspnea	X		
Mahler dyspnea index	X		
Saint George's X Respiratory Questionnaire	X	X	
Breathing VAS from scleroderma-health assessment questionnaire (S-HAQ)	X		
GASTROINTESTINAL			
Gastrointestinal VAS from S-HAQ	X		
UCLA scleroderma clinical trial consortium gastrointestinal instrument 2.0	X		
Body mass index		X	
Renal			
Estimated creatinine clearance			X
Systolic and diastolic blood pressure		X	

(continued)

Table 47.1 (continued)

Instruments	Completed by patient	Completed by investigator	Laboratory
Serum creatinine			X
RAYNAUD'S PHENOMENON			
Raynaud's condition score	X		
Number of Raynaud's phenomenon (RP) attacks	X		
Duration of RP attack	X		
Raynaud's VAS from S-HAQ	X		
Patient assessment of RP	X		
Physician assessment of RP		X[b]	
DIGITAL ULCER			
Active digital tip ulcer count on the volar surface		X[b]	
Digital ulcer VAS from S-HAQ	X		
BIOMARKERS			
Acute phase reactants			X
Serum B-type natriuretic peptide (BNP/NT-proBNP)			X

Modified from [2, 20]

[a]Measures such as Center for Epidemiologic Studies Depression Scale (CESD) and Functional Assessment of Chronic Illness Therapy (FACIT)-Fatigue have been found to be feasible, reliable, and valid, but their sensitivity to change has not been evaluated in SSc

[b]Assessed by the same investigator. Quality control strongly encouraged in multicenter RCT

[c]Standardized central reading mechanism strongly encouraged in multicenter RCT

[d]For patients with pulmonary arterial hypertension

and 12 months in the RCT predicted changes in skin thickening and functional disability over 12 and 24 months. In other words, an improvement/worsening of TFR at 6 and 12 months predicted an improvement/worsening in skin thickening and functional disability at 12 and 24 months. TFR should be measured by the same assessor in an RCT and incorporated as a secondary outcome measure.

Hand disability in SSc can be evaluated using the Cochin Hand Function Scale (CHFS), an 18-item instrument that relates to hand functionality or disability with various tasks in different settings (e.g., in the kitchen, dressing oneself, hygienic tasks, in the office) [23]. Each question is scored on a scale from 0 (performed without difficulty) to 5 (impossible to do), which is administered by the physician or self-administered. The total score was obtained by adding the scores from all items (range 0–90). The instrument is feasible and has shown acceptable reliability in SSc [24]. It has three scales – dexterity, rotational movement, and flexibility of the first three fingers. CHFS was sensitive to change in an intervention study that incorporated a connective tissue hand massage and home exercises [25]. CHFS is an acceptable secondary outcome measure to assess improvement in hand function and can be incorporated with MRSS in a RCT.

Hand mobility in scleroderma (HAMIS) is a nine-item performance-based test designed to examine the effects of SSc on hand mobility and hand function, and preferably administered by an occupational therapist or research physician [26, 27]. The HAMIS consists of nine items, which assess finger flexion and extension, abduction of the thumb, pincer grip, finger abduction/swelling, dorsal extension and volar flexion of the wrist, and pronation and supination. Each task is scored from 0 (no impairment) to 3 (cannot do), yielding a total possible score of 27 for each hand and a 54 total score. HAMIS has shown acceptable reliability and validity. HAMIS was sensitive to change in an intervention study with a connective tissue hand massage and home exercises [25], and complements CHFS in studies focused on the hands.

The mouth handicap in systemic sclerosis scale has been developed to assess attributes of mouth involvement in SSc [28]. It is a 12-item scale with acceptable reliability and validity. It has three scales that represent handicap associated with reduction in mouth opening, handicap associated with sicca syndrome, and esthetic concerns. The sensitivity to change was shown in an intervention program with a connective tissue massage of the face [29].

Health assessment questionnaire-disability index is a self-administered 20-question instrument that assesses a patient's level of functional ability and includes questions on fine movements of the upper extremities, locomotor activities of the lower extremities, and activities that involve both the upper and lower extremities [30]. The HAQ-DI score is determined by summing the highest item score in each of the eight domains and dividing the sum by 8, yielding a score ranging from 0 (no disability) to 3 (severe disability). Investigators should be aware that the scoring rules permit the scoring of two disability indices: the standard disability index, which takes into account the use of aids and devices; and the alternative disability index, which does not [79]. Investigators often do not specify which method is being used. Investigators should clearly delineate the method used to obtain the aggregate score [80]. The hand components of the HAQ-DI were able to differentiate bosentan from placebo in an RCT for digital ulcers in SSc [31]. HAQ-DI is also discussed in the section: Measuring Physical Function and Health-Related Quality of Life in SSc.

Measuring Lung Disease in Scleroderma

Pulmonary disease is now the leading cause of death for patients with SSc [32]. Pulmonary disease in SSc falls into two major categories: interstitial lung disease (ILD) and pulmonary hypertension (PH). There have been several recent clinical trials that specifically focus on lung disease in SSc [15, 33, 34].

Pulmonary function tests (PFTs) in patients with SSc-ILD demonstrate a restrictive lung defect with decreased forced vital capacity (FVC) and DLCO [35]. PFTs are feasible in large RCTs of SSc-ILD [15, 33, 34]. FVC has been used as the main parameter of restrictive lung disease and DLCO for pulmonary vascular disease. FVC was able to differentiate between active (cyclophosphamide [CYC]) and placebo group in the Scleroderma Lung Study I (SLS I). Low FVC predicts morbidity and mortality associated with SSc-ILD [32] and is sensitive to change in multicenter RCTs [15, 33]. Serial measurements of lung function with PFTs are also prognostic, and a 15 % decline in DLCO at 3-year follow-up corresponds to a significantly increased mortality risk in idiopathic pulmonary fibrosis [36, 37], although this has not been assessed in SSc-ILD. DLCO provides best overall estimate HRCT-ILD [81], but not specific for SSc-ILD or pulmonary hypertension and can decline in both diseases. In addition, it has high variability and did not differentiate between active vs. placebo groups in two SSc-ILD studies [38, 39]. A disproportionate decline in DLCO may indicate pulmonary hypertension [82].

Quality control programs are the key for studies in SSc-ILD and were recently discussed in detail [39]. Briefly, such programs rely on (1) the use of equipment at each participating site that meets recommended criteria for performance characteristics [40–42], as determined and affirmed by the equipment manufacturer; (2) standardized methods of calibrating the equipment with documentation that such calibrations have been carried out; (3) certification of technicians based on local or central review of the results of tests performed on an initial sample of subjects; and (4) ongoing review by a core reading center of the graphic and numeric results of tests performed on all subjects at each site with periodic feedback to the technicians concerning the quality of the tests performed, and a plan for remedial action should test quality fall below acceptable standards. Quality control programs were implemented in SLS I with satisfactory results with respect to achievement of acceptable test quality and are feasible in RCTs.

High-resolution computer tomography (HRCT) *of lungs* was incorporated successfully in recent RCTs [15, 34]. There are two key roles of HRCT imaging in clinical trials of SSc as recently discussed [39]: (1) detection and staging baseline severity that can be effectively used for cohort enrichment and adjusting for baseline severity in key treatment effect analyses (as it is likely that a treatment effect may differ in cases with mild rather than extensive lung disease) and (2) as a surrogate end point or more accurate measure of serial change. HRCT aims to diagnose and quantify the degree of fibrosis, thus supporting its face and content validity. The feasibility of HRCT for multicenter RCTs was demonstrated in two recent studies in SSc-ILD [15, 34]. The reliability of HRCT was demonstrated in the SLS trial [15] where there was good inter-reader agreement for determination of the absence or presence of pure ground-glass (kappa = 0.76) and fibrosis (kappa = 0.74), but fair agreement for honeycombing (kappa = 0.29). In the SLS, a higher degree of extent of fibrosis seen on a baseline HRCT scan was predictive of the rate of decline in FVC in subjects on placebo, as well as the response to CYC therapy; patients with the most extensive fibrosis seen on baseline HRCT scans responded the greatest to CYC treatment. A greater extent of pulmonary fibrosis on HRCT correlated well with lower FVC and DLCO values on PFTs. The extent of pulmonary fibrosis seen on HRCT scans was significantly negatively correlated with FVC ($r = -0.22$), DLCO ($r = -0.44$) and total lung capacity ($r = -0.36$) [43]. In a recent analysis of 215 patients with SSc followed for 10 years [37], an increased extent of disease (as defined by the extent and coarseness of reticulation [fibrosis] and proportion of ground-glass opacity) on HRCT >20 % correlated with an increase in mortality (hazard ratio [HR] 2.48, $P < 0.0005$).

Different scoring systems have been proposed that include two visual systems and computer-based approaches and discussed in a recent review [39]. Similar to PFTs, a rigorous standardized imaging protocol needs to be implemented across multiple sites and over several time points, and reading by central radiology core is necessary. Another important aspect is the training of technologists with respect to breathing instructions given at the time of scanning to ensure the same level of inspiration at each scan examination. This was successfully implemented in SLS I and II [81].

The 6-min Walk Test in SSc-Related ILD

The 6-min walk test (6MWT) measures the distance a person can walk in 6 min and has been extensively used as an outcome measure in various cardiac and pulmonary diseases. The 6MWT was found to be feasible and reliable in a 1-year, multicenter, double-blind, randomized control trial, comparing bosentan to placebo in 163 patients with SSc-ILD [44], but lacked construct validity and responsiveness to change in SSc-ILD. Limitations of the 6MWT were recently highlighted by various groups, showing that pain and musculoskeletal involvement can influence the walking test and that the 6MWT is not always solely reflective of changes in the lung when used in SSc [45, 46], raising doubts about its specificity in SSc-ILD and its relevance to monitoring therapy. 6MWT is not indicated for SSc-ILD trials as a primary outcome measure.

The 6MWT: An Outcome Measure for Pulmonary Arterial Hypertension

The 6MWT is presently the most widely used primary endpoint for studies investigating pulmonary arterial hypertension (PAH including SSc-related PAH). 6MWT shows good to excellent correlations with maximal cardiopulmonary exercise testing ($r \geq 0.57$) [47]. The 6MWT was able to discriminate among health controls, and patients with World Health Organization class II, III, and IV disease [47]. Criterion validity was demonstrated in patients with PAH wherein the 6MWT was the only noninvasive test that correlated with survival ($p<0.01$) [47]. The 6MWT has been successfully incorporated into trials of SSc-related PAH and was able to differentiate between active and placebo treatments in a trial of epoprostenol for SSc-related PAH [48]. Studies focusing on SSc-PAH should include hemodynamics (pulmonary vascular resistance), 6MWT, and improvement in World Health Organization functional class as outcome measures.

Dyspnea Indices

Patient-reported outcome measures are important to assess efficacy of a treatment. The *Mahler dyspnea index* [49] was used in the SLS I and assesses level of dyspnea. Baseline scores depend on ratings for three different categories: functional impairment, magnitude of task, and magnitude of effort. Baseline scores were able to discriminate between moderate and severe physiological parameters of breathing (FVC and DLCO) and correlated well with the baseline breathing visual analog scale (VAS) ($r=0.61$) [50]. Mahler's transitional dyspnea score was able to differentiate between patients on CYC and placebo in SLS at 1 year, demonstrating its sensitivity to change [51].

Saint George's respiratory questionnaire (SGRQ) was found to be reliable, valid, and responsive to change in patients with early dcSSc, both with and without ILD in a multicenter prospective study [83]. SGRQ has four scales that assess symptoms, impairment in activity, and impact and total scale. All scales showed large correlations with breathing VAS and DLCO in overall cohort and subgroup with ILD ($r>0.37$). Each scale is discriminated between presence/absence of ILD and restrictive lung disease ($p=<0.0001$–0.03). At follow-up, all scales were responsive to change using different anchors.

The breathing VAS scale in the scleroderma health assessment questionnaire (S-HAQ) allows patients to assess their degree of difficulty in performing daily activities due to shortness of breath on a continuous 100 mm scale [52]. The VAS discriminates between moderate and severe reductions in lung function and correlates well with the Mahler dyspnea index ($r=0.61$) and was shown to be sensitive to change in an SSc cohort [52]; it did not differentiate between CYC and placebo in the SLS I.

Other outcome measures for cardiopulmonary disease in SSc have been proposed – exercise echocardiography and magnetic resonance imaging – but await full validation.

Measuring Gastrointestinal Disease in SSc

Disease of gastrointestinal tract (GIT) occurs in approximately 90 % of patients with SSc. Although radiological tests are cornerstones for the diagnosis of specific GIT involvement, their feasibility is questionable in multicenter trials, and radiological tests may be positive in significant proportion of patients without symptoms [53]. Furthermore, many patients with SSc have multiple types of GIT disease with overlapping symptoms, making quantification of GIT in SSc extremely challenging. A Delphi panel [20] and separate expert consensus [54] recommended use of patient-reported outcome measures and body mass index as core set measures. Aside from a simple GIT visual analog scale (part of the S-HAQ [52]) that assesses daily interference in daily activities, a comprehensive scleroderma gastrointestinal instrument has been recently developed using Food and Drug Administration (FDA) guidelines.

University of California Scleroderma Clinical Trial Consortium Gastrointestinal Instrument (UCLA SCTC GIT 2.0) is a validated, patient-reported outcome measure to assess GIT symptoms and health-related quality of life (HRQOL) in SSc [55–57]. This 34-item instrument has seven scales: reflux, distention/bloating, diarrhea, fecal soilage, constipation, emotional well-being, and social functioning and a total GI score. The instrument is feasible and has shown acceptable reliability (test-retest and internal consistency) and validity [56]. All scales are scored from 0 (better HRQOL) to 3 (worse HRQOL) except diarrhea and constipation scales that range from 0–2 to 0–2.5, respectively. Participants who rated their GIT disease as mild had lower scores on all seven scales. Symptom scales were also able to discriminate subjects with corresponding clinical GIT diagnoses. The total GIT score is the average of six of seven scales (excludes constipation), and total GI score are scored from 0.0 (better HRQOL) to 2.8 (worse HRQOL). The instrument is sensitive to change in patient-self rated severity and is recently translated into different languages. They are available online at http://uclascleroderma.researchcore.org/.

Other outcome measures for gastrointestinal disease in SSc have been proposed or are under development, including manometry, gastric transient time, endoscopy, and measures of malabsorption [21]. There is lack of data on the sensitivity to change in SSc.

Measuring Vascular Disease in SSc: Raynaud's Phenomenon and Digital Ulcers

Raynaud's phenomenon (RP) occurs in approximately 90 % of patients with SSc. Similarly, digital ulcers (DUs) are common SSc and result in digital ischemia and gangrenous lesion as well as skin breakdown ulcers. There have been several clinical trials examining the efficacy of various interventions for RP and DUs in SSc [58–60]. The Raynaud's condition score (RCS) [58] is now the standard outcome for use in clinical trials of RP and is calculated by summing the daily score over 1 or 2 weeks to decrease day-to-day variability in RP [58]. The RCS assess the level of difficulty experienced due to RP each day (anchored from "no difficulty" to "extreme difficulty") using a 0–100 VAS or 11-point Likert scale. Other measures that are ready for RCTs include the duration of RP attacks, frequency of RP attacks, and patient and physician global assessments [58]. However, the clinical trials in RP are associated with marked variability in individual outcome measures [58]. A preliminary composite response index in RP has been recently proposed that would improve the ability to measure efficacy of an investigational drug and facilitate the ability to compare responses across trials [84]. The index includes RCS, patient global assessment, attack symptoms (pain, numbness, and tingling), physician global assessment of RP, duration of attacks, and the average number of attacks per day. The index needs to be validated in a placebo-controlled study.

S-HAQ VAS for RP (assesses interference in daily activities due to RP) is also feasible, reliable, and valid [58].

Other laboratory measures include cold stimulus fingertip lacticemy test, laser Doppler flowmetry, etc., and are discussed by A. Herrick in another chapter.

Measuring Ischemic Digital Ulcers in SSc

Methods considered for measuring DUs include standardized photographs, measuring size of ulcers, patient and physician global assessments, simple counts of ulcer frequency, and time to healing of ulcers. Definition of DU has been recently developed using a consensus methodology [31] and is defined as a loss of surface epithelialization at or distal to the proximal interphalangeal joint and did not include fissures or cracks in the skin or areas of calcium extrusion from calcinosis cutis. In a recent study aimed at assessing reliability of defining DU, a high level of intra-rater reliability (kappa = 0.81), but poor inter-rater reliability (kappa = 0.46), was noted suggesting that same observer should assess DU in an RCT [61]. The DU count was found to be feasible, reliable, valid, and sensitive to change in large RCTs of DU [31, 62]. S-HAQ VAS for DU (assesses interference in daily activities due to DUs) is feasible, reliable, valid, and sensitive to change and was shown in a large SSc cohort [52]. Current efforts are ongoing to modify CHFS (discussed in the Measuring Musculoskeletal Involvement section) for use in patients with DU [85].

Measuring Physical Function and Health-Related Quality of Life in SSc

SSc is associated with a detrimental effect on physical functioning and patients' emotional and psychological well-being, and different measures have been used.

The Short Form 36 (SF-36) and the Health Assessment Questionnaire-Disability Index (HAQ-DI)

Both the SF-36 (a measure of HRQOL) and the HAQ-DI (a measure of disability) have been extensively incorporated into multicenter clinical trials of SSc [50, 63, 64]. Both instruments have face and content validity as they measure constructs that are important to patients with SSc, and both measures are easy to administer. However, some investigators have criticized the HAQ-DI for insufficiently assessing disability caused by skin tightness and muscle weakness [87, 89]. The S-HAQ has incremental content validity to the HAQ-DI, because it contains SSc-specific domains that contribute to the multifaceted conceptual framework of disability in SSc. The addition of the S-HAQ VASs enhances the ability to capture disability secondary to internal organ involvement over the HAQ-DI alone. One threat to the content validity of the S-HAQ VASs is the phrasing of the questions. In essence, they are double-barreled questions; they require the scleroderma patient to ascertain the degree of severity of the organ in question and ascertain the degree of interference with daily activities [86]. Steen and Medsger assessed test–retest reliability of the S-HAQ in 50 scleroderma patients who completed the S-HAQ on two occasions within 1 month. The correlation coefficients for the two scores were 0.89 for the HAQ-DI and 0.78–0.87 for the Raynaud's phenomenon, finger ulceration, and breathing VASs ($P<0.001$). The pain and GI VASs were less well correlated with coefficients of 0.69 and 0.68, respectively ($P<0.001$) [88]. Poole et al. assessed concurrent validity by comparing self-reported disability on the HAQ-DI with the performance of ten of the items on the HAQ-DI scored by an occupational therapist blinded to the self-report measures. The overall ICC was 0.76, suggesting the HAQ-DI has reasonable concurrent validity [89]. Similarly, Brower and Poole evaluated the concurrent validity of the HAQ-DI and the Duruoz hand index (DHI) and reported a Spearman's rho of 0.79 ($p < 0.01$)[90]. The HAQ-DI also has good discriminant validity as SSc patients with diffuse disease have a significantly worse HAQ-DI score compared with those with limited disease (1.36 vs 0.59; $p<0.001$) [91].

Both the SF-36 and HAQ-DI have good concurrent validity as the SF-36 physical component summary and HAQ-DI score in SSc patients were adversely affected by joint involvement ($p<0.01$, $p<0.001$, respectively) ≥11 tender points ($p<0.01$, $p<0.001$), GI involvement ($p<0.01$, $p<0.01$), and high skin score ($p=0.02$, $p<0.001$) [91]. The SF-36 has good discriminant validity as SSc patients with diffuse disease had lower SF-36 scores than patients with limited disease (40.5 vs 32.4; $p=0.01$). Similarly, patients with diffuse disease have lower SF-36 physical component summary index (32.4 vs 40.5; $p=0.01$) and physical functioning domain scores (44.8 vs 64.1; $p<0.01$) than patients with limited disease [91]. Although the test-retest reliability for SF-36 has been acceptable in other rheumatologic diseases, no study has formally evaluated reliability in SSc. SF-36 and HAQ-DI were found to be responsive to change in two RCTs [63, 64]. In addition, baseline HAQ-DI scores predict mortality in early dcSSc [52, 65]. The SF-36 and HAQ-DI complement each other, and both should be incorporated as measures of HRQOL and disability in organ-specific trials in SSc [86].

UK Functional Score (UKFS) is a self-administered 11-item functional questionnaire. It includes nine items relating to upper extremity function and two items relating to muscle weakness and lower extremity function [66]. Each item is scored under four categories with both an integer and a descriptive heading, ranging from 0 (able to perform in a normal manner) to 3 (impossible to achieve) with an overall score between 0 and 33. It is a feasible and acceptable test-retest reliability (kappa ≥ 0.69). UKFS is able to differentiate between limited and dcSSc scleroderma ($p<0.05$) and is highly correlated with HAQ-DI (coefficient = 0.90). UKFS was found to change during a longitudinal study with a correlation of 0.59 with HAQ-DI [67, 68].

Patient-Reported Outcomes Measurement Information System (PROMIS)

The NIH Patient-Reported Outcomes Measurement Information System (PROMIS) Roadmap initiative is a cooperative group program of research designed to develop, evaluate, and standardize item banks to measure patient-reported outcomes relevant across common medical conditions [92]. For adults, domains have been developed in physical, mental, and social health. There is evidence to support the feasibility and construct validity of the PROMIS item banks in SSc [93], including a new GI symptoms bank [94]. PROMIS item banks are being incorporated in ongoing RCTs.

Preference-Based Measures for HRQOL in SSc: The Short Form 6D (SF-6D)

The Short Form 6D (SF-6D) is a preference-based measure that is derived from the SF-36 by using population-based utilities of health states. Preference-based measures are used in decision and cost-effectiveness analyses. SF-6D is feasible as it only requires completion of the SF-36. The test-retest reliability assessed was acceptable. The SF-36 has face and content validity as it conforms to the guidelines by the United States Public Health Service Panel on Cost-Effectiveness in Health and Medicine [69]. Construct validity was confirmed by showing good correlation with the HAQ-DI and with patient global assessment in a recent clinical trial [70]. SF-6D was able to discriminate among the baseline severity of the HAQ-DI and patient global assessment and was sensitive to change.

Other generic and disease-specific measures have been tested in SSc, including the scleroderma assessment questionnaire, and measures of anxiety, fatigue, and depression [71]. These instruments have not yet been shown to be sensitive to change in SSc.

American College of Rheumatology Provisional Composite Response Index for Clinical Trials in Early Diffuse Cutaneous Systemic Sclerosis (CRISS) index

Using a well-accepted expert consensus and data-driven approaches, the CRISS index has been developed for dcSSc trials [74, 95]. CRISS is calculated as a two-step process. The first step evaluates clinically significant decline in renal or cardiopulmonary involvement; if present, the patient is adjudicated as non-improved. The second step assesses remaining patients and calculates the predicted probability of improvement for changes in the mRSS, FVC percent predicted, patient and physician global assessments, and HAQ-DI over 1 year. The index was able to differentiate the effect of methotrexate from placebo in a 1-year RCT ($p < 0.05$).

Biomarkers for SSc

Vascular (von Willebrand factor [vWF]), T cells (soluble IL-2 receptor [Sil2R]), B cells (autoantibodies), and fibroblasts (type III procollagen N-terminal peptide propeptide [PIIINP]) candidate markers have been proposed as biomarkers in SSc. Sil2R, vWF, and PIIINP were recently assessed in an open-label trial of infliximab and SSc [72]. Serum markers were feasible, and PIIINP and vWF showed change over a 6-month period. However, marked individual variability in these markers and lack of robust data on sensitivity to change precludes their use in RCTs. A recent systematic review assessed different biomarkers in clinical trials [96]. After filtering according to the Outcome Measures in Rheumatology (OMERACT) criteria, several biomarkers sensitive to change over time and/or treatment were identified. Markers of skin fibrosis included E-selectin, thrombomodulin, interleukin-1 beta, and interleukin-6. For lung fibrosis, E-selectin, thrombomodulin, sICAM-3, sPECAM-1, KL-6, and surfactant protein D showed sensitivity to change over time or treatment. Markers of vasculopathy were as follows: pulmonary arterial hypertension (sICAM-1, sVCAM-1, sP-selectin, NT-ProBNP [75-76], MMP-9, IL-12), digital ulcers (sICAM-1, t-PA), Raynaud's (VEGF, bFGF, sVCAM-1, E-selectin, sICAM-1, t-PA, VCAM-1), and pathologic capillaroscopy (IL-6, IL-1ß).

Other readily available markers are acute phase reactants Erythrocyte sedimentation rate, C-reactive protein (ESR, CRP) that are associated with disease activity [6] and predict mortality [52, 73] and can be used for cohort enrichment [78]. Scleroderma-specific autoantibodies are valuable for predicting skin, vascular, and internal organ involvement. Autoantibodies are useful for cohort enrichment [77], but its role as an outcome measure in the context of clinical trial still needs to be demonstrated.

Conclusion

This chapter outlines the outcome measures that are feasible, reliable, and valid for RCTs in SSc.

References

1. Khanna D, Distler O, Avouac J, Behrens F, Clements PJ, Denton C, et al. Measures of response in clinical trials of systemic sclerosis: the combined response index for systemic sclerosis (CRISS) and outcome measures in pulmonary arterial hypertension related to systemic sclerosis (EPOSS). J Rheumatol. 2009;36(10):2356–61.
2. Khanna D. Assessing disease activity and outcomes in scleroderma. In: Hochberg M, Silman A, Smolen J, Weinblatt M, Weisman M, editors. Rheumatology. 5th ed. St. Louis: Mosby; 2010. p. 1367–71.
3. Khanna D, Tsevat J. Health-related quality of life – an introduction. Am J Manag Care. 2007;13 Suppl 9:S218–23.
4. Symmons DP. Disease assessment indices: activity, damage and severity. Baillieres Clin Rheumatol. 1995;9(2):267–85.
5. Medsger Jr TA. Natural history of systemic sclerosis and the assessment of disease activity, severity, functional status, and psychologic well-being. Rheum Dis Clin N Am. 2003;29(2):255–73, vi.
6. Valentini G, Della RA, Bombardieri S, Bencivelli W, Silman AJ, D'Angelo S, et al. European multicentre study to define disease activity criteria for systemic sclerosis. II. Identification of disease activity variables and development of preliminary activity indexes. Ann Rheum Dis. 2001;60(6):592–8.
7. Valentini G, D'Angelo S, Della RA, Bencivelli W, Bombardieri S. European scleroderma study group to define disease activity criteria for systemic sclerosis. IV. Assessment of skin thickening by modified rodnan skin score. Ann Rheum Dis. 2003;62(9):904–5.
8. Medsger Jr TA, Silman AJ, Steen VD, Black CM, Akesson A, Bacon PA, et al. A disease severity scale for systemic sclerosis: development and testing. J Rheumatol. 1999;26(10):2159–67.
9. Geirsson AJ, Wollheim FA, Akesson A. Disease severity of 100 patients with systemic sclerosis over a period of 14 years: using a modified Medsger scale. Ann Rheum Dis. 2001;60(12):1117–22.
10. Preliminary criteria for the classification of systemic sclerosis (scleroderma). Subcommittee for scleroderma criteria of the American Rheumatism Association Diagnostic and Therapeutic Criteria Committee. Arthritis Rheum. 1980;23(5):581–90.
11. Clements P, Lachenbruch P, Siebold J, White B, Weiner S, Martin R, et al. Inter and intraobserver variability of total skin thickness score (modified Rodnan TSS) in systemic sclerosis. J Rheumatol. 1995;22(7):1281–5.
12. Clements PJ, Hurwitz EL, Wong WK, Seibold JR, Mayes M, White B, et al. Skin thickness score as a predictor and correlate of outcome in systemic sclerosis: high-dose versus low-dose penicillamine trial. Arthritis Rheum. 2000;43(11):2445–54.
13. Clements P, Medsger TA, Feghali C. Cutaneous involvement in systemic sclerosis. In: Clements P, Furst DE, editors. Systemic sclerosis. 2nd ed. Philadelphia: Lippincott Williams and Wilkins; 2004. p. 129–50.
14. Pope JE, Bellamy N, Seibold JR, Baron M, Ellman M, Carette S, et al. A randomized, controlled trial of methotrexate versus placebo in early diffuse scleroderma. Arthritis Rheum. 2001;44(6):1351–8.
15. Tashkin DP, Elashoff R, Clements PJ, Goldin J, Roth MD, Furst DE, et al. Cyclophosphamide versus placebo in scleroderma lung disease. N Engl J Med. 2006;354(25):2655–66.
16. Amjadi S, Maranian P, Furst DE, Clements PJ, Wong WK, Postlethwaite AE, et al. Course of the modified Rodnan skin thickness score in systemic sclerosis clinical trials: analysis of three large multicenter, double-blind, randomized controlled trials. Arthritis Rheum. 2009;60(8):2490–8.
17. Clements PJ, Furst DE, Wong WK, Mayes M, White B, Wigley F, et al. High-dose versus low-dose D-penicillamine in early diffuse systemic sclerosis: analysis of a two-year, double-blind, randomized, controlled clinical trial. Arthritis Rheum. 1999;42(6):1194–203.
18. Merkel PA, Silliman NP, Denton CP, Furst DE, Khanna D, Emery P, et al. Validity, reliability, and feasibility of durometer measurements of scleroderma skin disease in a multicenter treatment trial. Arthritis Rheum. 2008;59(5):699–705.
19. Kissin EY, Schiller AM, Gelbard RB, Anderson JJ, Falanga V, Simms RW, et al. Durometry for the assessment of skin disease in systemic sclerosis. Arthritis Rheum. 2006;55(4):603–9.
20. Khanna D, Lovell DJ, Giannini E, Clements PJ, Merkel PA, Seibold JR, et al. Development of a provisional core set of response mea-

sures for clinical trials of systemic sclerosis. Ann Rheum Dis. 2008;67(5):703–9.
21. Merkel PA, Clements PJ, Reveille JD, Suarez-Almazor ME, Valentini G, Furst DE. Current status of outcome measure development for clinical trials in systemic sclerosis. Report from OMERACT 6. J Rheumatol. 2003;30(7):1630–47.
22. Khanna PP, Furst D, Clements P, Maranian P, Indulkar L, Khanna D. Tendon friction rubs in early diffuse systemic sclerosis: prevalence, characteristics and longitudinal changes in a randomized controlled trial. Rheumatology (Oxford). 2010;49(5):955–9.
23. Rannou F, Poiraudeau S, Berezne A, Baubet T, Le-Guern V, Cabane J, et al. Assessing disability and quality of life in systemic sclerosis: construct validities of the Cochin hand function scale, health assessment questionnaire (HAQ), systemic sclerosis HAQ, and medical outcomes study 36-Item short form health survey. Arthritis Rheum. 2007;57(1):94–102.
24. Brower LM, Poole JL. Reliability and validity of the Duruoz Hand Index in persons with systemic sclerosis (scleroderma). Arthritis Rheum. 2004;51(5):805–9.
25. Bongi SM, Del RA, Galluccio F, Sigismondi F, Miniati I, Conforti ML, et al. Efficacy of connective tissue massage and Mc Mennell joint manipulation in the rehabilitative treatment of the hands in systemic sclerosis. Clin Rheumatol. 2009;28(10):1167–73.
26. Sandqvist G, Eklund M. Hand Mobility in Scleroderma (HAMIS) test: the reliability of a novel hand function test. Arthritis Care Res. 2000;13(6):369–74.
27. Sandqvist G, Eklund M. Validity of HAMIS: a test of hand mobility in scleroderma. Arthritis Care Res. 2000;13(6):382–7.
28. Mouthon L, Rannou F, Berezne A, Pagnoux C, Arene JP, Fois E, et al. Development and validation of a scale for mouth handicap in systemic sclerosis: the mouth handicap in systemic sclerosis scale. Ann Rheum Dis. 2007;66(12):1651–5.
29. Maddali-Bongi S, Landi G, Galluccio F, Del RA, Miniati I, Conforti ML, et al. The rehabilitation of facial involvement in systemic sclerosis: efficacy of the combination of connective tissue massage, Kabat's technique and kinesitherapy: a randomized controlled trial. Rheumatol Int. 2010;31(7):895–901.
30. Fries JF, Spitz P, Kraines RG, Holman HR. Measurement of patient outcome in arthritis. Arthritis Rheum. 1980;23(2):137–45.
31. Korn JH, Mayes M, Matucci CM, Rainisio M, Pope J, Hachulla E, et al. Digital ulcers in systemic sclerosis: prevention by treatment with bosentan, an oral endothelin receptor antagonist. Arthritis Rheum. 2004;50(12):3985–93.
32. Steen VD, Conte C, Owens GR, Medsger Jr TA. Severe restrictive lung disease in systemic sclerosis. Arthritis Rheum. 1994;37(9): 1283–9.
33. Hoyles RK, Ellis RW, Wellsbury J, Lees B, Newlands P, Goh NS, et al. A multicenter, prospective, randomized, double-blind, placebo-controlled trial of corticosteroids and intravenous cyclophosphamide followed by oral azathioprine for the treatment of pulmonary fibrosis in scleroderma. Arthritis Rheum. 2006;54(12):3962–70.
34. Seibold JR, Denton CP, Furst DE, Guillevin L, Rubin LJ, Wells A, et al. Randomized, prospective, placebo-controlled trial of bosentan in interstitial lung disease secondary to systemic sclerosis. Arthritis Rheum. 2010;62(7):2101–8.
35. Berry CE, Wise RA. Interpretation of pulmonary function test: issues and controversies. Clin Rev Allergy Immunol. 2009;37(3):173–80.
36. Latsi PI, du Bois RM, Nicholson AG, Colby TV, Bisirtzoglou D, Nikolakopoulou A, et al. Fibrotic idiopathic interstitial pneumonia: the prognostic value of longitudinal functional trends. Am J Respir Crit Care Med. 2003;168(5):531–7.
37. Goh NS, Desai SR, Veeraraghavan S, Hansell DM, Copley SJ, Maher TM, et al. Interstitial lung disease in systemic sclerosis: a simple staging system. Am J Respir Crit Care Med. 2008;177(11):1248–54.
38. Khanna D, Seibold JR, Wells A, Distler O, Allanore Y, Denton C, et al. Systemic sclerosis-associated interstitial lung disease: lessons from clinical trials, outcome measures, and future study design. Curr Rheumatol Rev. 2010;6(2):138–44.
39. Khanna D, Brown KK, Clements PJ, Elashoff R, Furst DE, Goldin J, et al. Systemic sclerosis-associated interstitial lung disease-proposed recommendations for future randomized clinical trials. Clin Exp Rheumatol. 2010;28(2 Suppl 58):S55–62.
40. Wanger J, Clausen JL, Coates A, Pedersen OF, Brusasco V, Burgos F, et al. Standardisation of the measurement of lung volumes. Eur Respir J. 2005;26(3):511–22.
41. MacIntyre N, Crapo RO, Viegi G, Johnson DC, van der Grinten CP, Brusasco V, et al. Standardisation of the single-breath determination of carbon monoxide uptake in the lung. Eur Respir J. 2005;26(4):720–35.
42. Miller MR, Hankinson J, Brusasco V, Burgos F, Casaburi R, Coates A, et al. Standardisation of spirometry. Eur Respir J. 2005;26(2): 319–38.
43. Goldin J, Elashoff R, Kim HJ, Yan X, Lynch D, Strollo D, et al. Treatment of scleroderma-interstitial lung disease with cyclophosphamide is associated with less progressive fibrosis on serial thoracic high-resolution CT scan than placebo: findings from the scleroderma lung study. Chest. 2009;136(5):1333–40.
44. Buch MH, Denton CP, Furst DE, Guillevin L, Rubin LJ, Wells AU, et al. Submaximal exercise testing in the assessment of interstitial lung disease secondary to systemic sclerosis: reproducibility and correlations of the 6-min walk test. Ann Rheum Dis. 2007;66(2):169–73.
45. Schoindre Y, Meune C, Xuan AT, Avouac J, Kahan A, Allanore Y. Lack of specificity of the 6-minute walk test as an outcome measure for patients with systemic sclerosis. J Rheumatol. 2009;36(7):1481–5.
46. Garin MC, Highland KB, Silver RM, Strange C. Limitations to the 6-minute walk test in interstitial lung disease and pulmonary hypertension in scleroderma. J Rheumatol. 2009;36(2):330–6.
47. Miyamoto S, Nagaya N, Satoh T, Kyotani S, Sakamaki F, Fujita M, et al. Clinical correlates and prognostic significance of six-minute walk test in patients with primary pulmonary hypertension. Comparison with cardiopulmonary exercise testing. Am J Respir Crit Care Med. 2000;161(2 Pt 1):487–92.
48. Badesch DB, Tapson VF, McGoon MD, Brundage BH, Rubin LJ, Wigley FM, et al. Continuous intravenous epoprostenol for pulmonary hypertension due to the scleroderma spectrum of disease. A randomized, controlled trial. Ann Intern Med. 2000;132(6): 425–34.
49. Mahler DA, Weinberg DH, Wells CK, Feinstein AR. The measurement of dyspnea. Contents, interobserver agreement, and physiologic correlates of two new clinical indexes. Chest. 1984;85(6):751–8.
50. Khanna D, Clements PJ, Furst DE, Chon Y, Elashoff R, Roth MD, et al. Correlation of the degree of dyspnea with health-related quality of life, functional abilities, and diffusing capacity for carbon monoxide in patients with systemic sclerosis and active alveolitis: results from the scleroderma lung study. Arthritis Rheum. 2005;52(2):592–600.
51. Khanna D, Tseng CH, Furst DE, Clements PJ, Elashoff R, Roth M, et al. Minimally important differences in the Mahler's transition dyspnoea index in a large randomized controlled trial – results from the scleroderma lung study. Rheumatology (Oxford). 2009;48(12): 1537–40.
52. Steen VD, Medsger Jr TA. The value of the health assessment questionnaire and special patient-generated scales to demonstrate change in systemic sclerosis patients over time. Arthritis Rheum. 1997;40(11):1984–91.
53. Clements PJ, Becvar R, Drosos AA, Ghattas L, Gabrielli A. Assessment of gastrointestinal involvement. Clin Exp Rheumatol. 2003;21(3 Suppl 29):S15–8.

54. Baron M, Bernier P, Cote LF, Delegge MH, Falovitch G, Friedman G, et al. Screening and therapy for malnutrition and related gastro-intestinal disorders in systemic sclerosis: recommendations of a North American expert panel. Clin Exp Rheumatol. 2010;28(2 Suppl 58):S42–6.
55. Khanna D, Hays RD, Park GS, Braun-Moscovici Y, Mayes MD, McNearney TA, et al. Development of a preliminary scleroderma gastrointestinal tract 1.0 quality of life instrument. Arthritis Rheum. 2007;57(7):1280–6.
56. Khanna D, Hays RD, Maranian P, Seibold JR, Impens A, Mayes MD, et al. Reliability and validity of the University of California, Los Angeles scleroderma clinical trial consortium gastrointestinal tract instrument. Arthritis Rheum. 2009;61(9):1257–63.
57. Bodukam V, Hays RD, Maranian P, Furst DE, Seibold JR, Impens A, et al. Association of gastrointestinal involvement and depressive symptoms in patients with systemic sclerosis. Rheumatology (Oxford). 2010;50(2):330–4.
58. Merkel PA, Herlyn K, Martin RW, Anderson JJ, Mayes MD, Bell P, et al. Measuring disease activity and functional status in patients with scleroderma and Raynaud's phenomenon. Arthritis Rheum. 2002;46(9):2410–20.
59. Fries R, Shariat K, von Wilmowsky H, Bohm M. Sildenafil in the treatment of Raynaud's phenomenon resistant to vasodilatory therapy. Circulation. 2005;112(19):2980–5.
60. Wigley FM, Wise RA, Seibold JR, McCloskey DA, Kujala G, Medsger Jr TA, et al. Intravenous iloprost infusion in patients with Raynaud phenomenon secondary to systemic sclerosis. A multicenter, placebo-controlled, double-blind study. Ann Intern Med. 1994;120(3):199–206.
61. Herrick AL, Roberts C, Tracey A, Silman A, Anderson M, Goodfield M, et al. Lack of agreement between rheumatologists in defining digital ulceration in systemic sclerosis. Arthritis Rheum. 2009;60(3):878–82.
62. Matucci-Cerinic M, Denton CP, Furst DE, Mayes MD, Hsu VM, Carpentier P, et al. Bosentan treatment of digital ulcers related to systemic sclerosis: results from the RAPIDS-2 randomised, double-blind, placebo-controlled trial. Ann Rheum Dis. 2011;70:32–8.
63. Khanna D, Furst DE, Clements PJ, Park GS, Hays RD, Yoon J, et al. Responsiveness of the SF-36 and the health assessment questionnaire disability index in a systemic sclerosis clinical trial. J Rheumatol. 2005;32(5):832–40.
64. Khanna D, Yan X, Tashkin DP, Furst DE, Elashoff R, Roth MD, et al. Impact of oral cyclophosphamide on health-related quality of life in patients with active scleroderma lung disease: results from the scleroderma lung study. Arthritis Rheum. 2007;56(5):1676–84.
65. Clements PJ, Wong WK, Hurwitz EL, Furst DE, Mayes M, White B, et al. The disability index of the health assessment questionnaire is a predictor and correlate of outcome in the high-dose versus low-dose penicillamine in systemic sclerosis trial. Arthritis Rheum. 2001;44(3):653–61.
66. Silman A, Akesson A, Newman J, Henriksson H, Sandquist G, Nihill M, et al. Assessment of functional ability in patients with scleroderma: a proposed new disability assessment instrument. J Rheumatol. 1998;25(1):79–83.
67. Smyth AE, MacGregor AJ, Mukerjee D, Brough GM, Black CM, Denton CP. A cross-sectional comparison of three self-reported functional indices in scleroderma. Rheumatology (Oxford). 2003;42(6):732–8.
68. Serednicka K, Smyth AE, Black CM, Denton CP. Using a self-reported functional score to assess disease progression in systemic sclerosis. Rheumatology (Oxford). 2007;46(7):1107–10.
69. Weinstein MC, Siegel JE, Gold MR, Kamlet MS, Russell LB. Recommendations of the panel on cost-effectiveness in health and medicine. JAMA. 1996;276(15):1253–8.
70. Khanna D, Furst DE, Wong WK, Tsevat J, Clements PJ, Park GS, et al. Reliability, validity, and minimally important differences of the SF-6D in systemic sclerosis. Qual Life Res. 2007;16(6):1083–92.
71. Thombs BD, Hudson M, Taillefer SS, Baron M. Prevalence and clinical correlates of symptoms of depression in patients with systemic sclerosis. Arthritis Rheum. 2008;59(4):504–9.
72. Denton CP, Engelhart M, Tvede N, Wilson H, Khan K, Shiwen X, et al. An open-label pilot study of infliximab therapy in diffuse cutaneous systemic sclerosis. Ann Rheum Dis. 2009;68(9):1433–9.
73. Scussel-Lonzetti L, Joyal F, Raynauld JP, Roussin A, Rich E, Goulet JR, et al. Predicting mortality in systemic sclerosis: analysis of a cohort of 309 French Canadian patients with emphasis on features at diagnosis as predictive factors for survival. Medicine (Baltimore). 2002;81(2):154–67.
74. Khanna D, Lovell DJ, Giannini E, Clements PJ, Merkel PA, Seibold JR, et al. Development of a provisional core set of response measures for clinical trials of systemic sclerosis. Ann Rheum Dis. 2007;67(5):703–9.
75. Williams MH, Handler CE, Akram R, Smith CJ, Das C, Smee J, et al. Role of N-terminal brain natriuretic peptide (N-TproBNP) in scleroderma-associated pulmonary arterial hypertension. Eur Heart J. 2006;27(12):1485–94.
76. Allanore Y, Borderie D, Meune C, Cabanes L, Weber S, Ekindjian OG, et al. N-terminal pro-brain natriuretic peptide as a diagnostic marker of early pulmonary artery hypertension in patients with systemic sclerosis and effects of calcium-channel blockers. Arthritis Rheum. 2003;48(12):3503–8.
77. Steen VD. Autoantibodies in systemic sclerosis. Semin Arthritis Rheum. 2005;35(1):35–42.

Recommended Reading

78. Khanna D, Denton CP, Jahreis A, van Laar JM, Frech TM, Anderson ME, Baron M, Chung L, Fierlbeck G, Lakshminarayanan S, Allanore Y, Pope JE, Riemekasten G, Steen V, Müller-Ladner U, Lafyatis R, Stifano G, Spotswood H, Chen-Harris H, Dziadek S, Morimoto A, Sornasse T, Siegel J, Furst DE. Safety and efficacy of subcutaneous tocilizumab in adults with systemic sclerosis (faSScinate): a phase 2, randomised, controlled trial. Lancet. 2016;5. pii: S0140-6736(16)00232-4..
79. Bruce B, Fries JF. The Stanford health assessment questionnaire: a review of its history, issues, progress, and documentation. J Rheumatol. 2003;30(1):167–78.
80. Johnson SR, Lee P. The HAQ disability index in scleroderma trials. Rheumatology (Oxford). 2004;43(9):1200–1.
81. Tashkin DP, Volkmann ER, Tseng CH, Kim HJ, Goldin J, Clements P, et al. Relationship between quantitative radiographic assessments of interstitial lung disease and physiological and clinical features of systemic sclerosis. Ann Rheum Dis. 2016;75:374–81.
82. Khanna D, Gladue H, Channick R, Chung L, Distler O, Furst DE, et al. Recommendations for screening and detection of connective tissue disease-associated pulmonary arterial hypertension. Arthritis Rheum. 2013;65(12):3194–201.
83. Wallace B, Kafaja S, Furst DE, Berrocal VJ, Merkel PA, Seibold JR, et al. Reliability, validity and responsiveness to change of the Saint George's Respiratory Questionnaire in early diffuse cutaneous systemic sclerosis. Rheumatology (Oxford). 2015;54:1369–79.
84. Gladue H, Maranian P, Paulus H, Khanna D. Evaluation of test characteristics for outcome measures used in Raynaud's phenomenon clinical trials. Arthritis Care Res (Hoboken). 2013;65(4):630–6.
85. Khanna D, Denton CP, Merkel PA, Krieg T, Le Brun FO, Marr A, Papadakis K, Pope J, Matucci-Cerinic M, Furst DE; DUAL-1 Investigators; DUAL-2 Investigators. Effect of Macitentan on the

Development of New Ischemic Digital Ulcers in Patients With Systemic Sclerosis: DUAL-1 and DUAL-2 Randomized Clinical Trials. JAMA. 2016;10;315(18):1975–88.

86. Johnson SR, Hawker GA, Davis AM. The health assessment questionnaire disability index and scleroderma health assessment questionnaire in scleroderma trials: an evaluation of their measurement properties. Arthritis Rheum. 2005;53(2):256–62.
87. Silman A, Akesson A, Newman J, Henriksson H, Sandquist G, Nihill M, et al. Assessment of functional ability in patients with scleroderma: a proposed new disability assessment instrument. J Rheumatol. 1998;25(1):79–83.
88. Steen VD, Medsger Jr TA. The value of the Health Assessment Questionnaire and special patient-generated scales to demonstrate change in systemic sclerosis patients over time. Arthritis Rheum. 1997;40(11):1984–91.
89. Poole JL, Williams CA, Bloch DA, Hollak B, Spitz P. Concurrent validity of the health assessment questionnaire disability index in scleroderma. Arthritis Care Res. 1995;8(3):189–93.
90. Brower LM, Poole JL. Reliability and validity of the Duruoz Hand Index in persons with systemic sclerosis (scleroderma). Arthritis Rheum. 2004;51(5):805–9.
91. Johnson SR, Glaman DD, Schentag CT, Lee P. Quality of life and functional status in systemic sclerosis compared to other rheumatic diseases. J Rheumatol. 2006;33(6):1117–22.
92. Khanna D, Krishnan E, DeWitt EM, Khanna PP, Spiegel B, Hays RD. Patient-Reported Outcomes Measurement Information System (PROMIS(R)) – The future of measuring patient reported outcomes in rheumatology. Arthritis Care Res (Hoboken). 2011;63(S11):S486–90.
93. Khanna D, Maranian P, Rothrock N, Cella D, Gershon R, Khanna PP, et al. Feasibility and construct validity of PROMIS and "legacy" instruments in an academic scleroderma clinic. Value Health. 2012;15(1):128–34.
94. Spiegel BM, Hays RD, Bolus R, Melmed GY, Chang L, Whitman C, et al. Development of the NIH Patient-Reported Outcomes Measurement Information System (PROMIS) gastrointestinal symptom scales. Am J Gastroenterol. 2014;109(11):1804–14.
95. Khanna D, Berrocal VJ, Giannini EH, Seibold JR, Merkel PA, Mayes MD, Baron M, Clements PJ, Steen V, Assassi S, Schiopu E, Phillips K, Simms RW, Allanore Y, Denton CP, Distler O, Johnson SR, Matucci-Cerinic M, Pope JE, Proudman SM, Siegel J, Wong WK, Wells AU, Furst DE. American College of Rheumatology Provisional Composite Response Index for Clinical Trials in Early Diffuse Cutaneous Systemic Sclerosis. Arthritis Rheumatol. 2016 Feb;68(2):299-311.
96. Toniolo M DR, Moinzadeh P, Ogawa R, Furst DE, Denton CP, Khanna D, Distler O, Biomarkers sensitive to change in patients with systemic sclerosis A systematic review EULAR 2015. Paris; 2015 (abstract).

Innovative Approaches to Clinical Trials in Systemic Sclerosis

48

Rucsandra Dobrota, Ulf Müller-Ladner, and Oliver Distler

Introduction

In the last years, advances in translational and clinical research in the field of systemic sclerosis (SSc) have opened promising perspectives for new therapeutic approaches. Alongside the scientific progress and the increasing availability of specific inhibitors, interest of the pharmaceutical industry in this rare disease has also increased, leading nowadays to a dynamic and competitive field of drug development in SSc.

Nonetheless, despite several completed clinical trials to date and a clear improvement in the management of vascular complications, there is still a high unmet need for efficient anti-fibrotic and disease-modifying therapies in SSc [1]. Investigators working on clinical trial design in SSc face the challenges of dealing with a rare, multifaceted and variably progressing disease [2]. Despite that a number of trials revealed negative results in SSc, important lessons can be learned from them [2, 3]. Combining this experience with modern concepts of clinical trial design can help reshape the approach to clinical studies focusing on this disease.

Partially supported by the European Union Seventh Framework Programme [FP7/2007–2013] under Grant Agreement n° 305495 (DeSScipher) and HSM-2 grant "Gezielte und interdisziplinäre Behandlungen schwerer immunvermittelter Erkrankungen"

R. Dobrota, MD
Division of Rheumatology, University Hospital Zurich, Zurich, Switzerland

Department of Internal Medicine and Rheumatology, Cantacuzino Hospital, Carol Davila University of Medicine and Pharmacy, Bucharest, Romania

U. Müller-Ladner, MD
Internal Medicine and Rheumatology, Justus-Liebig University Giessen, Bad Nauheim, Hessia, Germany

O. Distler, MD (✉)
Division of Rheumatology, University Hospital Zurich, Zurich, Switzerland
e-mail: oliver.distler@usz.ch

J. Varga et al. (eds.), *Scleroderma*, DOI 10.1007/978-3-319-31407-5_48

Favoured strategies for an improved design of future trials in SSc are cohort enrichment strategies and a careful selection of outcome measures, with a special interest in composite outcomes reflecting the overall disease activity. In the following paragraphs, we will focus on recent data regarding study design, potential strategies for cohort enrichment and composite outcomes in SSc.

General Considerations for Clinical Study Design in Systemic Sclerosis

The lack of general agreement for outcome selection and study design has long hampered the relevance, interpretation and generalisability of clinical trials in SSc [4]. In order to foster a coherent approach to this rare disease and to allow comparison of trials, consensus-derived strategies for study design and validated outcome measures are needed.

General Guidelines for Clinical Trials in SSc

Expert-derived, consensus-based guidelines have been developed to support the development of comprehensive, consistent and reproducible protocols for SSc trials. The general guidelines for disease modification trials in SSc developed in 1995 recommended the inclusion of patients with diffuse cutaneous SSc and disease duration below 24 months, as the ones holding the worst prognosis. Other main points were long-enough study duration allowing observation of an eventual effect on disease modification and need for surrogate response measures reflecting the activity of SSc in the major target organs [5].

Recently, experts have developed a set of general points to consider for clinical trials in SSc, based on the standards of the European League Against Rheumatism (EULAR) [6]. These points consider stress key considerations for ensuring a good quality study structure and analysis. Specific recommendations focusing on the main affected organ systems in SSc will be further developed [6].

Table 48.1 Consensus-based, provisional minimal set of core domains and outcome measures/instruments for clinical trials in CTD-ILD

Core domain	Instrument/outcome measure
Dyspnoea	MRC chronic dyspnoea scale
	Dyspnoea 12 UCSD-SBQ
Cough	Leicester cough questionnaire
Health-related quality of life	Short Form 36
	St. George's Respiratory Questionnaire
	Patient global assessment (VAS)
Lung imaging	Overall extent of ILD on HRCT
Lung physiology	Forced vital capacity
	Diffusion capacity of the lung for CO
Survival	All-cause mortality

Adapted from Saketkoo et al. [4]

MRC Medical Research Council, *UCSD-SBQ* University of California San Diego Shortness of Breath Questionnaire, *VAS* visual analogue scale, *ILD* interstitial lung disease, *HRCT* high-resolution computer tomography of the chest, *CO* carbon monoxide

Additionally, important advances have been made towards standardisation of clinical trials in interstitial lung disease associated with SSc (SSc-ILD). The Connective Tissue Disease-Associated ILD (CTD-ILD) working group of the Outcome Measures in Rheumatology (OMERACT) initiative has developed a first, consensus-based set of domains to use in randomised clinical trials in CTD-ILD [4, 7]. This endeavour was achieved through a three-staged process including a Delphi exercise involving medical experts in the field, patient perspective focus groups, as well as a meeting using the nominal group technique with both medical professionals and patients. The minimal set of outcome measures for clinical trials in CTD-ILD derived from this exercise as well as the best validated and feasible instruments for their assessment are summarised in Table 48.1. In this consensus paper, the major unmet needs and points towards future research directions in the field were also highlighted [4].

Views on Clinical Trial Design in SSc

There is a general agreement that prospective, randomised, double-blind, controlled trials are needed to convincingly prove treatment efficacy [1, 5, 6, 8].

Nonetheless, in the earlier stages of drug development, such type of study design is not feasible, among others due to safety concerns, considerable costs and logistical power. As such, various study designs for proof of concept studies (POC) have been applied in SSc. The pros and cons of the various possible trial designs with respect to their application to the field of SSc are discussed in detail in several recent publications [1, 6, 8–10] and are summarised in Table 48.2.

In the context of the considerable recent developments in understanding the molecular biology of SSc, the translation of promising candidate molecular targets from basic to clinical research is nowadays a hot topic in SSc. After validating a new candidate molecule in preclinical, in vitro and in vivo studies, early clinical POC studies are needed to provide evidence for efficacy in targeting the respective pathway in patients. Such studies would need to focus on safety/tolerability and would likely include a biomarker-based main outcome measure, eventually in parallel with clinical parameters as secondary outcomes. Selected biomarkers should include those that can prove target engagement of the medication of interest. As biological responses are usually faster, early biomarker-driven POC studies have the advantage of a shorter duration and, in general, a smaller required sample size [9, 10]. Importantly, such early POC studies should be randomised, placebo controlled and double blinded [9, 10] in order to provide reliable safety and efficacy information upon which to build a potential phase II/III trial. The disadvantage of such an approach is the lack of fully validated biomarkers, making the interpretation of biomarker POC studies sometimes challenging. Alternatively, potential novel targeted therapies could be directly tested with the clinical measure of choice as the key endpoint in addition to the safety/tolerability. However, this then requires longer study duration and usually larger sample sizes because of the slower changes over time and the lower sensitivity to change of the clinical endpoints.

A recently published example is the AIMSPRO trial, a phase II, double-blind, placebo-controlled trial of hyperimmune caprine serum in patients with late-stage dcSSc [11]. The primary objective of this study was safety and feasibility of using hyperimmune caprine serum in late-stage dcSSc (>3 years disease duration), whereas the secondary objectives were (1) assessment of possible treatment effect on clinical outcomes and (2) exploration for candidate biomarkers in serum/plasma. Each arm (active therapy/placebo) included ten patients. After 26 weeks of blinded study period, tolerability of the drug was good and similar to patients on placebo. Furthermore, there was a trend towards improvement of the delta change of modified Rodnan skin score (mRSS) and of the responder rate in the treatment group compared to placebo, though none of these results achieved statistical significance. Surprisingly, despite the clinical improvement, levels of the pro-fibrotic marker PIIINP increased in the treatment group, highlighting the challenges of interpreting biomarker results in the clinical context [11].

Another recent example comes from the NCT01651143 trial of lysophosphatidic acid receptor 1 antagonist (LPA1) SAR100842 in patients with early dcSSc (<36 months disease duration) [12]. This was a shorter trial, with an 8-week, double-blind, placebo-controlled phase followed by a 16-month open-label extension period. The primary endpoint was safety, and secondary endpoints included change in biomarkers from skin biopsies and blood samples, as well

Table 48.2 Overview on various trial designs and their application in SSc research

Trial type	Main uses	Advantages	Disadvantages/challenges
Single arm, open label	Preliminary safety and possible efficacy data [1, 8, 9] Exploratory mechanistic effects and/or outcome measures [1] "Proof of concept" studies: providing rationale for later RCT [8–10] Blinding and particularly control arm strongly recommended [6, 9]	Logistically and financially less challenging [1] Biomarker-driven trials allow a shorter trial duration [9, 10]	When uncontrolled/unblinded, risk of bias (observation bias, disease course, cofounders) [1, 8]. Controlled design strongly recommended
Randomised, double blind, double arm, placebo controlled Additional designs: *Add-on* (randomised active/placebo arms, allowing background standard of care therapy) *Early escape* (randomised treatment discontinued if worsening) *Randomised withdrawal* (active, open-label phase, then randomization of responders to stay/be taken off treatment) [1, 8]	Trustworthy efficacy and safety data [1, 9] When no effective treatment is known (e.g. studies in skin fibrosis in SSc) [1] Early escape necessary when placebo controlled	Decreased bias, can prove benefit over the natural course of the disease [1, 8]	Ethical considerations Recruitment challenges (patients'/investigators' reluctance towards the placebo arm) [1]
Randomised, double blind, double arm, active controlled	To prove non-inferiority/superiority of a new agent with existing effective/standard of care therapy (e.g. studies in PAH/ renal crisis in SSc) [1, 8]	Fewer ethical concerns compared to placebo-controlled trials [1]	No unanimously accepted standard of care, overall disease-modifying drug for SSc Currently more suitable for trials in specific organ involvement; note: difficult choice of active controls (e.g. modest effect of CYC in SSc-ILD) [1]

SSc systemic sclerosis, *RCT* randomised controlled trial, *PAH* pulmonary arterial hypertension, *ILD* interstitial lung disease, *CYC* cyclophosphamide

as changes in mRSS and SHAQ score. At 8 weeks, the treated group showed a greater reduction in mRNA levels of some LPA-induced markers (e.g. Wnt2, PAI1, SFRP4) indicating successful target engagement. However, there was no significant difference in efficacy biomarkers from skin biopsies and blood samples compared to placebo. Nonetheless, the mRSS was more strongly reduced in the treatment than in the placebo arm. After 24 weeks including the open-label uncontrolled extension period, COMP and TSP1, key fibrotic biomarkers, were significantly reduced from baseline. Moreover, there was a clinically meaningful improvement in the clinical outcomes [13].

These studies reflect the fact that biomarker changes are feasible to detect in a rather short trial period. More work needs to be done to identify and fully validate biomarkers able to predict long-term clinical responses. Furthermore, these studies exemplify how including a placebo group in a small size, pilot clinical trial can offer valuable data on the safety profile of the drug.

Strategies for Cohort Enrichment

The heterogeneity of SSc, both at the clinical and pathophysiological level, makes drug development and especially proof of drug efficacy challenging. Drugs which had performed well in basic and translational science as well in early proof of concept studies have failed to show decisive effects in clinical trials in SSc [14]. Accordingly, selection of those patients who are most likely to show an effect (if any is present) is of key importance for clinical study design. This "cohort enrichment", can significantly improve the chances of success of a clinical trial [15]. Cohort enrichment can be obtained through several, partially overlapping, complementary approaches: (I) including patients with similar disease characteristics, thereby decreasing the heterogeneity of the cohort, (II) focusing on patients at risk of disease worsening (prognostic enrichment) and (III) including patients most likely to respond to the specific study drug (predictive enrichment) [15, 16].

Important recent data from the literature support these concepts and represent valuable assets for future cohort enrichment in clinical trials in SSc [14]. In the following paragraphs, we will outline the major concepts and illustrate them with suitable examples focusing on clinical studies targeting fibrosis in SSc.

Methods for Decreasing the Heterogeneity of the Study Cohort

A clinical study cohort comprised of patients with homogeneous disease characteristics can increase power of a study. This can be achieved, for example, by including subjects with similar baseline characteristics (e.g. clinical or laboratory markers within a narrow range) [15].

Given the variable clinical patterns of SSc, inclusion criteria aiming to select a clinically homogeneous cohort are recommended in clinical trials targeting fibrosis in SSc [6]. Classification criteria can also be used for this purpose. After the American College of Rheumatology (ACR) 1980 classification criteria were used for many years for SSc [17], a new set of classification criteria for SSc was recently developed through the joint effort of ACR/EULAR [18]. These were shown to perform very well in meeting their intended purpose of increasing sensibility for early and limited disease [18–20]. Nonetheless, the specificity is inherently lower than that of the old ACR1980 criteria, which makes their application as inclusion criteria in clinical trials in fibrosis possibly leading to higher cohort heterogeneity.

Approaches previously used in clinical trials in skin fibrosis which could decrease cohort heterogeneity are, for example, the inclusion of patients with dcSSc (according to the LeRoy criteria [21]) with restricted skin scores or with short disease duration [22].

Another way to decrease heterogeneity of a study cohort is to exclude spontaneous improvers and/or patients likely to drop out of the study [15].

Skin fibrosis in patients with dcSSc often regresses over time as part of the natural course of the disease. However, the factors predicting such a favourable pattern are still poorly understood. Previous analyses have not been able to identify significant predictors of skin score regression in patients with early dcSSc; however, patients with improving skin scores had a better overall outcome [23]. Recently, a longitudinal analysis including over 700 patients with dcSSc from the EUSTAR cohort showed that 22 % had a regression of the mRSS under standard of care in a 1-year observation period. This study identified a high baseline mRSS as the strongest predictor of regression of skin fibrosis suggesting that focusing on patients with higher skin scores at inclusion could actually lead to including a higher rate or improving patients into the study. Thus, if the study drug of interest is more likely to prevent worsening of skin fibrosis rather than enhancing spontaneous regression of skin fibrosis, inclusion of dcSSc patients with lower mRSS at baseline should be considered [24].

Another key strategy is to define preventive exclusion criteria in order to avoid a high drop-out rate. For example, patients with severe end-stage organ involvements which are having a high risk of adverse reactions and limited compliance to the study intervention should be excluded from clinical trials. This approach was successfully applied, for example, to the ASTIS trial, in which patients with severe organ involvement were excluded [25].

"Prognostic Enrichment": Identifying the Population at Risk

Skin Fibrosis

Clinical trials targeting skin fibrosis in dcSSc usually use the mRSS as the primary outcome measure. There is little agreement on the (upper) mRSS threshold across studies, the general approach being to include patients with higher skin scores and short disease duration as they are the ones expected to have the worst prognosis [22].

However, a retrospective analysis of the data from seven multicentre clinical trials in diffuse SSc (dcSSc) by Merkel et al. revealed a wide variability of the pattern of change in the mRSS during the studies [22]. Moreover, irrespective of the disease duration ("early"/"late"), many patients showed regression of mRSS during the study, and an overall tendency of regression to the mean was observed [22]. These data suggest that "early" disease duration on its own is not sufficient for cohort enrichment for patients with progressive skin fibrosis, as a considerable number of "early" patients showed skin improvement during the studies [22].

In a recent study, Maurer et al. identified predictors of progression of mRSS over a 1-year follow-up (the classic duration of a clinical trial) in a large EUSTAR cohort. From the almost 700 patients included in the derivation cohort, 9.7 % showed progression of skin fibrosis within 1 year. Patients with joint synovitis, disease duration ≤15 months and, interestingly, a lower skin score were more likely to progress. The cut-off mRSS value which best differentiated between progressors/non-progressors was 22/51 [26]. This offers an evidence-based mRSS threshold which can be used as an inclusion criterion for clinical trials in dcSSc. According to these data, inclusion of patients with lower mRSS values (e.g. ≤22/51 points) would result in a higher rate of progressors in clinical studies [26]. Moreover, the study analysed and validated different models for prediction of progression of skin fibrosis (mRSS), which allow an improved performance for cohort enrichment, ranging from 9.7 % progressors in the initial unselected cohort to up to 44.4 % in an optimised model [26]. These findings were confirmed in a further EUSTAR analysis from the same group. Hereby, an upper mRSS threshold ≤18 points was identified as ensuring the highest ratio of progressors over regressors [24].

Taken together, these studies highlight two important aspects: (1) in an unselected cohort of patients with dcSSc, only a small percentage of patients will progress during a standard study period, whereas a considerable proportion will improve. This is also supported by previous reports from other clinical trial cohorts [22]. (2) The initial mRSS at inclusion in the study is important for the future direction of change in skin fibrosis, either progression or regression.

From these data, it can be inferred that, in order to have a study cohort enriched for progressing patients and with fewer patients who would "naturally" regress under standard of care, the recruitment strategy for clinical trials should shift from targeting advanced cases with high mRSS values to also include dcSSc patients with milder skin involvement. This group, who is more likely to be in the progressive phase and has not yet reached the peak of their skin fibrosis, could also benefit more from therapeutic interventions.

Other reported predictors for progression of mRSS emerging from large EUSTAR studies are joint synovitis [26, 27] and tendon friction rubs [27]. These two parameters were, interestingly, also predictive of overall disease progression, dcSSc and positive anti-topoisomerase I antibodies [27].

Interstitial Lung Disease (ILD)

Decreased lung function tests are often used for risk stratification and as the primary outcome measure in clinical studies of SSc-ILD. For example, the forced vital capacity of the lung (FVC) is a validated outcome in SSc-ILD and an FVC below 50 % is a predictor of mortality [28].

Furthermore, computed tomography (CT)-based risk stratification is increasingly recognised as a key step in the assessment of SSc-ILD. This is based on several studies showing that the baseline extent of lung fibrosis on HRCT predicts further progression of ILD and also overall mortality [29, 30].

In a recent study by Nihtyanova et al. on a single-centre, unselected cohort of SSc patients, approximately half of the patients developed clinically significant ILD in the first 3 years since disease onset and up to three quarters within the first 5 years. The following predictors of development of clinically significant ILD were identified: dcSSc, greater age at disease onset, lower forced vital capacity and DLCO, and positivity for anti-topoisomerase I antibodies. In line with previous results from the literature, the presence of anti-centromere antibodies was protective [31]. A previous longitudinal analysis on the GENISOS cohort also identified anti-topoisomerase I antibodies as significantly associated with a low FVC at baseline, as well as predictive of an accelerated decline in serial FVC measurements along the first 3 years of follow-up. Interestingly, significant decrease in FVC (≥10 %) occurred mostly during the first year of follow-up [28]. This supports previous findings from Steen et al., showing that the highest rate of decline in FVC takes place in the first 4 years since disease onset [32].

However, in a post hoc analysis of the placebo group of the Scleroderma Lung Study-1 (SLS-1), there was no difference in the rate of decline in FVC between groups stratified by disease duration (0–2 years/2–4 years/>4 years). However, when stratified by the extent of fibrosis on HRCT, the rate of decline in FVC was higher in the group with extensive fibrosis [33].

Taken together, these data suggest that a low FVC at baseline, the extent of fibrosis on HRCT, positivity for anti-topoisomerase I antibodies and short disease duration could be considered as measures to enrich for progressive SSc-LD in clinical studies.

"Predictive Enrichment": Identifying a Responder Population

One of the challenges in applying targeted therapies to such heterogeneous diseases like SSc is the identification of patients in whom the specific pathway targeted by the study drug is pathologically activated. There is a strong rational to use biomarkers of pathway activation for cohort enrichment in clinical studies with targeted therapies, and similar approaches have been successfully performed in other fields like oncology and partially also in rheumatoid arthritis. For example, despite exponential use and recognised success of biological therapies in rheumatoid arthritis, these drugs are still mostly prescribed on a trial-and-error basis, and up to 40 % of patients fail to respond to these therapies [34]. In recent years, genome-wide DNA microarray analysis of peripheral mononuclear blood cells or synovial biopsies has been applied to differentiate responders from nonresponders, with promising yet still heterogeneous and not always reproducible results [34].

In terms of feasibility, biomarkers measurable in the peripheral blood would be the most suitable. In SSc, alternatives include tissue samples, in particular skin biopsies for clinical studies aiming at skin fibrosis. This could mean measurement of the activation status of targeted receptors in skin biopsies, e.g. the phosphorylation status of tyrosine kinase receptors, or more complex techniques such as gene expression analysis in tissues or circulating blood cells. However, the feasibility to identify target activation in individual patients strongly depends on the targeted pathway. It might be straighter forward in certain cases such as measurement of the activation of tyrosine kinase receptors and might be more difficult and only indirectly possible in other cases such as G protein–coupled receptors including LPA1.

In SSc, several recent studies offer interesting data for the prediction of response to therapy [16]. One example is data from recent high-throughput skin biopsy profiling studies which identify distinct inflammatory and proliferative gene expression signatures in skin biopsies; these could potentially represent different subsets of the disease, requiring distinct therapeutic approaches [35–37]. Further, an association between the inflammatory signature and therapeutic response to mycophenolate mofetil was observed in a small-scale study [37].

Before biological markers of treatment response will be validated and made available for clinical practice and clinical study design, clinical predictors remain more accessible. For example, a retrospective analysis of the Scleroderma Lung Study identified patients with more extensive reticular changes in HRCT, higher mRSS and worse dyspnoea as more likely to respond to therapy with cyclophosphamide [38].

Limitations of Cohort Enrichment

Applying cohort enrichment methods to clinical trials can successfully increase the power of a study, as well as the absolute and relative effect size [15]. Nonetheless, an excessive enrichment should be avoided, as this would make findings of the study hardly generalisable, or very difficult to apply in a real-life clinical setting [39]. Thus, different enrichment methods used for the study should be carefully balanced against generalisability of the study to the real-life clinical setting.

Another aspect to keep in mind is that, when enrichment is done through use of a special test (e.g. omics), the performance parameters of the test (sensitivity, specificity, positive and negative predictive values, analytical validity) are crucial and should be well characterised [15].

Composite Outcomes Reflecting Disease Status/Disease Activity

Single organ endpoints are accepted by agencies for registration of drugs for the treatment of the specific organ. For example, the mRSS is in general accepted as the primary endpoint for skin fibrosis and the FVC for SSc-ILD. If registration of a drug for overall SSc is sought, the mRSS is often accepted as a surrogate marker for survival and internal organ involvement, but there is an increasing request to show effects or at least trends for effects also on other key organs. This could be done by either assessing the single organ separately and adding them as co-primary or secondary endpoint or – more elegantly – by developing a composite outcome measure addressing different organs with one single measure.

For example, the autologous haematopoietic stem cell transplantation versus intravenous pulse cyclophosphamide in diffuse cutaneous systemic sclerosis (ASTIS) trial had as primary endpoint the concept of "event-free survival" [25]. This was defined as the time in days from randomization till the occurrence of death or persistent heart, lung or kidney failure. Specifically, the latter were defined as a left ventricular ejection fraction below 30% by echocardiography, hypoxemia below 60 mmHg and/or hypercapnia above 50 mmHg at rest and need for renal replacement therapy, respectively [25]. The endpoint accordingly reflects the time until a severe disease outcome, either death or a critical organ failure, occurs. Using the "event-free survival" as the primary endpoint and a long-term follow-up (median 5.8 years), the authors could demonstrate a long-term benefit in survival in the transplant group, despite an initially higher treatment-related mortality in the first year after the intervention [25].

Another approach more feasible for a 1-year clinical trial is the combined response index for systemic sclerosis (CRISS). CRISS was developed in multiple steps based on the OMERACT criteria and aims to be used as a composite outcome measure for clinical trials in SSc [40]. The final CRISS index consisting of five items with the highest face validity (MRSS, FVC predicted, Health Assessment Questionnaire-Disability Index, Patient global assessment and the Physician global assessment), was recently finalised and applied retrospectively to a clinical study cohort. It is currently in the process of publication [41].

Conclusion

Updated consensus-based guidelines, new concepts for early proof of concept studies and new prognostic as well as predictive cohort enrichment strategies have led to an improved clinical study design in SSc. Full validation of combined response indices such as CRISS will further increase the options for clinical studies in SSc. The currently ongoing advanced clinical studies with targeted therapies will show whether these strategies were successful to allow proof of efficacy of the urgently need anti-fibrotic therapies in SSc.

References

1. Mendoza FA, Keyes-Elstein LL, Jimenez SA. Systemic sclerosis disease modification clinical trials design: quo vadis? Arthritis Care Res (Hoboken). 2012;64(7):945–54.
2. Veale DJ. What can we learn from negative clinical trials in systemic sclerosis? Clin Exp Rheumatol. 2010;28(2 Suppl 58):S1–4.
3. Clements PJ, Seibold JR, Furst DE, Mayes M, White B, Wigley F, et al. High-dose versus low-dose D-penicillamine in early diffuse systemic sclerosis trial: lessons learned. Semin Arthritis Rheum. 2004;33(4):249–63.
4. Saketkoo LA, Mittoo S, Huscher D, Khanna D, Dellaripa PF, Distler O, et al. Connective tissue disease related interstitial lung

diseases and idiopathic pulmonary fibrosis: provisional core sets of domains and instruments for use in clinical trials. Thorax. 2014; 69(5):428–36.

5. White B, Bauer EA, Goldsmith LA, Hochberg MC, Katz LM, Korn JH, et al. Guidelines for clinical trials in systemic sclerosis (scleroderma). I. Disease-modifying interventions. The American College of Rheumatology Committee on Design and Outcomes in Clinical Trials in Systemic Sclerosis. Arthritis Rheum. 1995;38(3):351–60.
6. Khanna D, Furst DE, Allanore Y, Bae S, Bodukam V, Clements PJ, et al. Twenty-two points to consider for clinical trials in systemic sclerosis, based on EULAR standards. Rheumatology (Oxford). 2015;54(1):144–51.
7. Saketkoo LA, Mittoo S, Frankel S, LeSage D, Sarver C, Phillips K, et al. Reconciling healthcare professional and patient perspectives in the development of disease activity and response criteria in connective tissue disease-related interstitial lung diseases. J Rheumatol. 2014;41(4):792–8.
8. Pope JE, Khanna D, Johnson SR, Clements P. Disease modification and other trials in systemic sclerosis have come a long way, but have to go further. Arthritis Care Res (Hoboken). 2012;64(7): 955–9.
9. Chung L, Denton CP, Distler O, Furst DE, Khanna D, Merkel PA. Clinical trial design in scleroderma: where are we and where do we go next? Clin Exp Rheumatol. 2012;30(2 Suppl 71):S97–102.
10. Jordan S, Chung J, Distler O. Preclinical and translational research to discover potentially effective antifibrotic therapies in systemic sclerosis. Curr Opin Rheumatol. 2013;25(6):679–85.
11. Quillinan NP, McIntosh D, Vernes J, Haq S, Denton CP. Treatment of diffuse systemic sclerosis with hyperimmune caprine serum (AIMSPRO): a phase II double-blind placebo-controlled trial. Ann Rheum Dis. 2014;73(1):56–61.
12. Proof of Biological Activity of SAR100842 in Systemic Sclerosis. https://clinicaltrials.gov/ct2/show/NCT01651143 [24.06.2015]. Available from: https://clinicaltrials.gov/ct2/show/NCT01651143.
13. Allanore Y JA, Jasson M, Distler O, Denton C, Khanna D. Lysophosphatidic acid receptor 1 antagonist SAR100842 as a potential treatment for patients with systemic sclerosis: results from a phase 2A study. Ann Rheum Dis.2015;74(Suppl 2):172–3.
14. Allanore Y, Distler O. Systemic sclerosis in 2014: advances in cohort enrichment shape future of trial design. Nat Rev Rheumatol. 2015;11(2):72–4.
15. Enrichment strategies for clinical trials to support approval of human drugs and biological products http://www.fda.gov/downloads/Drugs/GuidanceComplianceRegulatoryInformation/Guidances/UCM332181.pdf [27.03.2015]. Available from: http://www.fda.gov/downloads/Drugs/GuidanceComplianceRegulatoryInformation/Guidances/UCM332181.pdf.
16. Dobrota R, Mihai C, Distler O. Personalized medicine in systemic sclerosis: facts and promises. Curr Rheumatol Rep. 2014;16(6):425.
17. Preliminary criteria for the classification of systemic sclerosis (scleroderma). Subcommittee for scleroderma criteria of the American Rheumatism Association Diagnostic and Therapeutic Criteria Committee. Arthritis Rheum. 1980;23(5):581–90.
18. van den Hoogen F, Khanna D, Fransen J, Johnson SR, Baron M, Tyndall A, et al. 2013 classification criteria for systemic sclerosis: an American College of Rheumatology/European League against Rheumatism collaborative initiative. Arthritis Rheum. 2013;65(11): 2737–47.
19. Jordan S, Maurer B, Toniolo M, Michel B, Distler O. Performance of the new ACR/EULAR classification criteria for systemic sclerosis in clinical practice. Rheumatology (Oxford). 2015;54(8):1454–8.
20. Andreasson K, Saxne T, Bergknut C, Hesselstrand R, Englund M. Prevalence and incidence of systemic sclerosis in southern Sweden: population-based data with case ascertainment using the 1980 ARA criteria and the proposed ACR-EULAR classification criteria. Ann Rheum Dis. 2014;73(10):1788–92.
21. LeRoy EC, Black C, Fleischmajer R, Jablonska S, Krieg T, Medsger Jr TA, et al. Scleroderma (systemic sclerosis): classification, subsets and pathogenesis. J Rheumatol. 1988;15(2):202–5.
22. Merkel PA, Silliman NP, Clements PJ, Denton CP, Furst DE, Mayes MD, et al. Patterns and predictors of change in outcome measures in clinical trials in scleroderma: an individual patient meta-analysis of 629 subjects with diffuse cutaneous systemic sclerosis. Arthritis Rheum. 2012;64(10):3420–9.
23. Steen VD, Medsger Jr TA. Improvement in skin thickening in systemic sclerosis associated with improved survival. Arthritis Rheum. 2001;44(12):2828–35.
24. Dobrota R, Maurer B, Graf N, Jordan S, Mihai C, Kowal-Bielecka O, Allanore Y, Distler O, EUSTAR coauthors. Prediction of improvement in skin fibrosis in diffuse cutaneous systemic sclerosis: a EUSTAR analysis. Ann Rheum Dis. 2016;25. [Epub ahead of print].
25. van Laar JM, Farge D, Sont JK, Naraghi K, Marjanovic Z, Larghero J, et al. Autologous hematopoietic stem cell transplantation vs intravenous pulse cyclophosphamide in diffuse cutaneous systemic sclerosis: a randomized clinical trial. JAMA. 2014;311(24):2490–8.
26. Maurer B, Graf N, Michel BA, Muller-Ladner U, Czirjak L, Denton CP, et al. Prediction of worsening of skin fibrosis in patients with diffuse cutaneous systemic sclerosis using the EUSTAR database. Ann Rheum Dis. 2015;74(6):1124–31.
27. Avouac J, Walker UA, Hachulla E, Riemekasten G, Cuomo G, Carreira PE, et al. Joint and tendon involvement predict disease progression in systemic sclerosis: a EUSTAR prospective study. Ann Rheum Dis. 2016;75(1):103–9.
28. Assassi S, Sharif R, Lasky RE, McNearney TA, Estrada YMRM, Draeger H, et al. Predictors of interstitial lung disease in early systemic sclerosis: a prospective longitudinal study of the GENISOS cohort. Arthritis Res Ther. 2010;12(5):R166.
29. Goh NS, Desai SR, Veeraraghavan S, Hansell DM, Copley SJ, Maher TM, et al. Interstitial lung disease in systemic sclerosis: a simple staging system. Am J Respir Crit Care Med. 2008; 177(11):1248–54.
30. Moore OA, Goh N, Corte T, Rouse H, Hennessy O, Thakkar V, et al. Extent of disease on high-resolution computed tomography lung is a predictor of decline and mortality in systemic sclerosis-related interstitial lung disease. Rheumatology (Oxford). 2013; 52(1):155–60.
31. Nihtyanova SI, Schreiber BE, Ong VH, Rosenberg D, Moinzadeh P, Coghlan JG, et al. Prediction of pulmonary complications and long term survival in systemic sclerosis. Arthritis Rheumatol. 2014;66(6):1625–35.
32. Steen VD. The lung in systemic sclerosis. J Clin Rheum Pract Rep Rheum Musculoskelet Dis. 2005;11(1):40–6.
33. Khanna D, Tseng CH, Farmani N, Steen V, Furst DE, Clements PJ, et al. Clinical course of lung physiology in patients with scleroderma and interstitial lung disease: analysis of the Scleroderma Lung Study Placebo Group. Arthritis Rheum. 2011;63(10):3078–85.
34. Burska AN, Roget K, Blits M, Soto Gomez L, van de Loo F, Hazelwood LD, et al. Gene expression analysis in RA: towards personalized medicine. Pharmacogenomics J. 2014;14(2):93–106.
35. Milano A, Pendergrass SA, Sargent JL, George LK, McCalmont TH, Connolly MK, et al. Molecular subsets in the gene expression signatures of scleroderma skin. PLoS ONE. 2008;3(7): e2696.
36. Pendergrass SA, Lemaire R, Francis IP, Mahoney JM, Lafyatis R, Whitfield ML. Intrinsic gene expression subsets of diffuse cutaneous systemic sclerosis are stable in serial skin biopsies. J Invest Dermatol. 2012;132(5):1363–73.
37. Hinchcliff M, Huang CC, Wood TA, Matthew Mahoney J, Martyanov V, Bhattacharyya S, et al. Molecular signatures in skin associated with clinical improvement during mycophenolate treatment in systemic sclerosis. J Invest Dermatol. 2013;133(8):1979–89.

38. Roth MD, Tseng CH, Clements PJ, Furst DE, Tashkin DP, Goldin JG, et al. Predicting treatment outcomes and responder subsets in scleroderma-related interstitial lung disease. Arthritis Rheum. 2011;63(9):2797–808.
39. Villela R, Yuen SY, Pope JE, Baron M, Canadian Scleroderma Research Group. Assessment of unmet needs and the lack of generalizability in the design of randomized controlled trials for scleroderma treatment. Arthritis Rheum. 2008;59(5):706–13.
40. Khanna D, Distler O, Avouac J, Behrens F, Clements PJ, Denton C, et al. Measures of response in clinical trials of systemic sclerosis: the Combined Response Index for Systemic Sclerosis (CRISS) and Outcome Measures in Pulmonary Arterial Hypertension related to Systemic Sclerosis (EPOSS). J Rheumatol. 2009;36(10):2356–61.
41. Khanna D, Berrocal VJ, Giannini EH, Seibold JR, Merkel PA, Mayes MD, Baron M, Clements PJ, Steen V, Assassi S, Schiopu E, Phillips K, Simms RW, Allanore Y, Denton CP, Distler O, Johnson SR, Matucci-Cerinic M, Pope JE, Proudman SM, Siegel J, Wong WK, Wells AU, Furst DE. The American College of Rheumatology Provisional Composite Response Index for Clinical Trials in Early Diffuse Cutaneous Systemic Sclerosis. Arthritis Care Res (Hoboken). 2016 Feb;68(2):167–78.

49 Molecular Stratification by Gene Expression as a Paradigm for Precision Medicine in Systemic Sclerosis

Monique Hinchcliff and Michael L. Whitfield

Introduction

Systemic sclerosis (SSc, scleroderma) is a poorly understood systemic autoimmune disease characterized by vascular injury, immunologic activation, and tissue fibrosis. A clear understanding of the fundamental biology underlying SSc pathogenesis has been impeded by these complex pathologic changes, as well as the heterogeneous clinical presentation of the disease [1]. This is further complicated by unpredictable disease progression and spontaneous remission in some individuals [2]. Thus, progressive skin fibrosis may involve mainly distal extremities and face (limited cutaneous SSc, lcSSc) or with various tempos lead to increasingly proximal, sometimes severe fibrotic skin disease (diffuse cutaneous SSc, dcSSc) [3]. Internal organ involvement accompanies each of these presentations, some with more vasculopathic features such as pulmonary arterial hypertension (PAH) [4] and others with more fibrotic features such as interstitial lung disease (ILD) [5], and adds to both the clinical and pathological disease heterogeneity. It is in this context that analysis of SSc with high-throughput, genome-wide gene expression methods has attempted to shed light on disease pathogenesis, to quantify disease heterogeneity, and to identify different molecular pathway perturbations that drive disease.

M. Hinchcliff, MD, MS
Department of Medicine, Northwestern University, Feinberg School of Medicine, Chicago, IL, USA

M.L. Whitfield, PhD (✉)
Department of Genetics, Geisel School of Medicine at Dartmouth, Hanover, NH, USA
e-mail: Michael.Whitfield@Dartmouth.edu

J. Varga et al. (eds.), *Scleroderma*, DOI 10.1007/978-3-319-31407-5_49

Clinical and Serological Markers of SSc Disease Activity

The lack of robust, objective biomarkers has made it difficult to predict clinical endpoints or to assess response to therapy. The most common outcome measure in clinical trials in SSc is the modified Rodnan skin score (mRSS) [6–8], a measure of the extent and severity of skin fibrosis [9, 10]. Some studies suggest that the mRSS correlates with disease severity [11–15], progressive skin disease, and renal involvement [16], while other studies failed to show this association [17]. Skin changes are not necessarily reflective of risk for internal organ SSc manifestations. Thus, while the mRSS is a useful marker of SSc severity, it may not be a useful marker of SSc disease activity [18, 19].

Autoantibody profiles have been associated with disease subtypes and specific clinical outcomes in SSc [16]. Up to eight autoantibodies have been identified that are associated with SSc, and in most cases, only one autoantibody is found in a given patient over the course of their disease [20, 21]. In this respect, autoantibodies are stable and consistent within a patient over time. While serum autoantibodies are useful at identifying patients at high risk for interstitial lung disease, scleroderma renal crisis, and pulmonary arterial hypertension on a population level, they are not necessarily accurate in predicting SSc disease course on a per-patient basis [22]. Additionally, no clear association between serum autoantibodies and disease pathogenesis has been established [23].

Additional efforts have been made to distinguish the heterogeneity among SSc patients using combinatorial and multivariate analysis of clinical parameters [24, 25]. Shand and colleagues used a latent trajectory model to classify patients into one of three subgroups based on skin score trajectories with different overall survival rates [26]. Another study analyzed patients with anti-topo I antibodies and divided them into five groups based on skin thickness progress rates [27]. In addition, baseline c-reactive protein, serial high-resolution computed tomography of the chest ILD combined with pulmonary function test results, and joint and tendon involvement have been suggested to be important predictors of progressive SSc [24, 28–31]. Although valuable, these studies lacked validation cohorts, and thus important work remains that will likely require large cooperative consortia in order to identify and validate a finite list of medically actionable markers of SSc disease activity and severity.

Gene Expression Profiling on the Cellular Level in SSc

Genome-wide technologies such as microarray analyses and ultra-high-throughput DNA sequencing permit broad assessments of expression levels of large numbers of mRNAs and/or other RNA species in cultured cells or a tissue simultaneously. In this way, they may provide an accurate unbiased assessment of SSc severity and activity. Gene expression differences between diseased versus healthy cells and tissues provide striking insights into the mediators, intracellular pathways, and transcriptional regulators that underlie disease. These approaches are rapidly advancing our understanding of the molecular pathogenesis in end-target cells and tissues in SSc. Gene expression in end-target tissues such as the skin has generally shown more robust and consistent differences than those found in cultured cells, a result that is true not only in SSc but also in cancer where these technologies were pioneered [32, 33]. Capturing the gene expression in affected tissues allows us to observe gene expression changes that occur in multiple cell types that may contribute to disease pathogenesis. Tissue cell type heterogeneity provides both possibilities and challenges in interpreting altered tissue gene expression. Thus, alterations in gene expression result in “signatures” comprised of the expression levels of hundreds to thousands of genes that provide information on activated, migrating, expanding, or dying cell populations. However, distinguishing these changes from altered gene expression in specific cell types within a tissue is challenging. This limitation can be overcome by complementary approaches such as immunohistochemistry and computational methods that examine tissue-specific genes [34].

A second major utility of gene expression analyses lies in its power as a clinical classification tool. This value is largely independent from its pathogenic insights and rather depends on objective analyses of the altered gene expression and combinatorial patterns that predict the underlying disease subsets. This approach has been particularly useful for defining subsets of patients with a variety of cancers (Reviewed in Chung et al. [35]) and has provided some new and very fundamental insights into patient subsets in SSc [36–41]. A variety of relevant tissues and cells from SSc patients have been analyzed including the skin [36, 38, 39, 42–44], esophagus [45], peripheral blood mononuclear cells (PBMCs) [46–50], lung [51, 52], and bronchoalveolar lavage fluid (BAL) [53, 54].

Cultured Dermal Fibroblasts

Altered behavior of SSc fibroblasts in vitro has been studied for many years and has generally been thought to provide a useful in vitro correlate for in vivo changes. Gene expression studies performed on fibroblasts isolated from SSc skin and healthy controls have provided some new insights and controversies into the utility of such studies [36, 55–57]. Zhou et al. analyzing dermal fibroblast cultures from 11 SSc (8 dcSSc and 3 lSSc) compared to 7 healthy control fibroblast cultures identified only 32 differentially expressed genes using an uncorrected *t*-test ($p<0.05$) on results from a 4,000 element microarrays [55]. Intriguingly, several of these genes included known antigens targeted by autoantibodies in SSc patients such as CENP B, RNA polymerase II, and fibrillarin. However, the absolute changes in expression levels of these genes were quite modest (1.44–1.65-fold increased in SSc compared to control fibroblasts), and the lack of correction for multiple comparisons renders these observations difficult to interpret without further validation [55].

In an alternative approach, fibroblasts from non-lesional skin of dcSSc patients were compared to matched healthy controls [56]. Using 16,659 element oligonucleotide arrays, approximately 5 % of the 8,324 genes that passed data preprocessing were found differentially expressed, but only 832 were predicted to be statistically different based on estimated false discovery rates. Of that group of 832, approximately 320 would be predicted as false positives. However, several of the genes scoring most highly (COL7A1, COL18A1, and COMP) are TGFβ targets, which is regulated and know to be increased in SSc skin. This is consistent with past observations showing persistent autocrine TGFβ activation in SSc fibroblast cultures. Other genes with significant increases in expression included lymphocyte homing antigen (CD44) and five metallothionein genes (MT1X, MT1A, MT1B, MT2A, and MT1F). Using these observations the authors were able to develop classification models composed of 26 of the differentially expressed genes, accurately predicting the class (SSc versus healthy fibroblast) to which given a fibroblast sample belonged with 99 % accuracy. These results support the notion that alterations in fibroblasts from SSc skin are preserved in vitro and that such changes can be detected in fibroblasts derived from non-lesional skin, similar to the result observed in non-lesional SSc biopsies [42]. Another study analyzing gene expression in lesional and non-lesional dcSSc fibroblasts compared to healthy controls further supports these observations [58]. Using a set of 4,193 genes, this group found that lesional and non-lesional fibroblasts from dcSSc patients were more similar to each other than to healthy controls. Collectively these data strongly support the notion that fibroblasts from lesional and non-lesional skin can replicate at least part of the altered pattern of gene expression observed in lesional and non-lesional SSc skin biopsies [36].

Table 49.1 SSc fibroblasts express increased TGFβ-regulated genes

		Gardner et al. [43]	Zhou et al. [55]	Tan et al. [56]	Zhou et al. [57]
	Culture preparation	Digested tissue	Explant tissue	Explant tissue	Explant tissue
Source cells	SSc skin source	Lesional	Lesional/non-lesional	Non-lesional	Lesional/non-lesional
Genes	COL1a2				x
	COLVIIa1	x		x	
	COLVIIIa1		—	x	x
	SPARC		x		x
	COMP			x	
	CTGF				x
	IGFBP3		x		

Further insight into the cause of SSc fibroblast gene expression was examined by studying the genetic contributions to the SSc phenotype by characterizing gene expression of fibroblasts derived from monozygotic (MZ) and dizygotic (DZ) twins discordant for SSc [57]. As in the above studies, fibroblasts from SSc patients showed altered expression of a series of genes, overlapping with those in other studies, and included genes known to be regulated by TGFβ such as connective tissue growth factor (CTGF) and secreted protein acidic and rich in cysteine/osteonectin (SPARC), COL1A2, and COL8A1. Again, fibroblasts from lesional and non-lesional skin showed similar gene expression profiles. When gene expression profiles in SSc and healthy DZ twin pairs were assessed, the differences found were similar to those found when all SSc and all healthy individuals were compared. However, remarkably, when gene expression profiles in SSc and healthy MZ twin pairs were assessed, healthy individuals with an affected monozygotic twin showed gene expression similar to SSc patients. This study suggested that ~40–50 % of unaffected MZ twins of SSc patients may have a genetic predisposition to SSc based on their genetic background that is reflected in the gene expression profiles [57]. Although the genes leading to this susceptibility have not yet been identified, important genetic susceptibilities have been identified in genome-wide surveys (see Chap. 3), implicating genes common to other autoimmune disease and/or involved in inflammation.

Despite these several studies showing consistent alterations in gene expression in SSc fibroblasts, these cells have been reported to lose their phenotype over time in culture, showing a marked reduction in collagen production in fibroblasts cultured beyond ten passages [59]. The reported differences in gene expression by SSc fibroblasts have been challenged in a study directly comparing gene expression in SSc biopsies to SSc-derived fibroblasts. Gardner et al. found that although gene expression differences were easily identified in SSc biopsies, similar changes were not found consistently in fibroblasts cultured from biopsies [43]. This is consistent with the findings of Whitfield et al., where large changes in gene expression were found in SSc skin relative to controls, but few significant differentially expressed genes were found when SSc and normal fibroblasts were analyzed by gene expression profiling [42].

Collectively, the results of these studies appear consistent on most points: (1) several groups have identified increased expression of a limited but overlapping set of genes by SSc fibroblasts many of which are known to be regulated by TGFβ (see Table 49.1); and (2) several studies indicate that changes in fibroblasts cultured from SSc-derived biopsies are less robust and identify fewer genes than studies carried out directly on SSc skin biopsies. These latter observations likely reflect both contributions of other cell types in the skin that influence gene expression, as well as the loss of phenotypic changes associated with SSc over time in culture.

Gene Expression in Skin

Because skin, lung, and esophageal diseases are cardinal SSc features and new genomic technologies can quickly and reliably measure gene expression, the body of research that examines gene expression in SSc tissues is ever expanding. Skin biopsies are simple and safe to perform during routine clinical practice and thus are amenable to study. Two early studies of dcSSc skin focusing on the gene expression differences between SSc patients and healthy controls [36, 43] showed robust and consistent changes in gene expression. In the initial DNA microarray analyses of SSc skin, lesional forearm and non-lesional back biopsies from four patients with dcSSc and four healthy controls were compared, showing more than 2700 genes differentially expressed between normal and dcSSc skin biopsies [42]. A surprising and important result from this study was that the lesional forearm samples and non-lesional back samples showed nearly identical, disease-specific patterns of gene expression, indicating that the disease was affecting skin even in areas where disease was not clinically detectable. Thus, despite the typical progression of dcSSc skin disease from distal to central skin, dcSSc is truly a systemic disease at a molecular level, likely affecting all skin from early in the disease [36]. A second important finding was that differences in gene expression could be mapped not only to fibroblasts but also to epithelial, endothelial, smooth muscle, and T and B cells [36].

In a second study, Gardner et al. analyzed lesional forearm skin biopsies from nine SSc patients (eight dcSSc and one lcSSc with forearm skin involvement) and seven healthy controls, identifying 1,800 differentially expressed probes with the SSc phenotype. Eight thousand seven hundred thirty six selected probes, with the exception of one patient, accurately grouped patients into controls and SSc (separate arms on the resulting dendrogram) using unsupervised clustering [43]. Genes representative of the TGFβ and Wnt pathways were identified among the differentially expressed genes, suggesting that these cytokines may play important roles in disease pathogenesis. In both this study and the Whitfield et al. study, genes associated with increased deposition and synthesis of the ECM were found prominently upregulated in SSc biopsies consistent with the well-described dermal fibrosis [36].

Identifying SSc Patient Subgroups by Skin Gene Expression

Although SSc patient heterogeneity is readily clinically apparent, this heterogeneity has not been well described on the molecular level. Analyzing genome-wide gene expression from dcSSc, lcSSc, localized scleroderma (morphea), and healthy control skin biopsies, Milano et al. al identified patient groups on a molecular level [36]. Assessing both lesional forearm and non-lesional back skin biopsies from the same patients, 17 of 22 subjects showed nearly identical, disease-specific gene expression. This systemic property of the biopsies was used to select 995 "intrinsic" genes showing the most consistent expression between forearm-back pairs for an individual, but the most variable across subjects, thus emphasizing consistent, patient-specific gene expression signatures rather than the differences between biopsies. The dendrogram resulting from clustering the biopsies using only these 995 "intrinsic" genes identified groups of patients (Fig. 49.1). These groups are referred to as the "intrinsic SSc subsets" (Fig. 49.1). dcSSc patients clustered mainly within two of the intrinsic subsets and lcSSc patients and control subjects each clustered primarily within two other subsets. Each of the four major subsets exhibited a unique gene expression profile, and each could be associated with specific clinical variables such as ILD, gastrointestinal involvement, and disease duration [36]. One subset of dcSSc patients showed a gene expression signature suggesting cell proliferation, which included the diffuse 1 and diffuse 2 subsets (Fig. 49.1, fibroproliferative gene cluster). A second "inflammatory" subset included dcSSc, lcSSc, and morphea patients and showed a gene expression signature suggesting inflammation (Fig. 49.1, inflammatory gene cluster). A third subset that included most of the lcSSc patients and two healthy control showed a heterogeneous gene signature (Fig. 49.1, "limited" subset). Finally, a fourth subset including most of the healthy controls and several lcSSc and dcSSc patients showed gene expression most similar to healthy controls (Fig. 49.1, the "normal-like" subset). These results have been recapitulated in two additional cohorts of dcSSc and healthy controls that show the proliferation, inflammatory, and normal-like groups are a reproducible feature of the disease [39, 60].

Both of these studies included a longitudinal analysis of skin biopsies from a subset of dcSSc patients, which suggests a patient subset is stable over periods of 6–12 months [60], although more recent studies suggest the intrinsic subsets may represent discrete stages of disease progression [40].

Meta-analysis of three independent skin cohorts was conducted and used to develop an SSc skin network (SSN) that identified the genes consistently associated with the intrinsic subsets. Mahoney et al. developed a bioinformatic method based on mutual information, an information theory concept, and performed a meta-analysis of these genome-wide gene expression datasets [40]. Using the resulting genes, an interaction network of the conserved molecular features across the intrinsic subsets, along with SSc-associated genetic polymorphisms, was created [40]. This network analysis showed that the genetic risk polymorphisms associated with SSc are connected to the aberrant gene expression we observe in SSc skin, primarily in the inflammatory subset. It further indicates that the intrinsic subsets may be long-lived, but mechanistically interconnected, and related to a patients underlying genetic risk. Specifically, these analyses suggest that one possible mechanism for SSc includes an initial environmental trigger that generates an interferon response that promotes M2 macrophage/dendritic cell/innate immune system activation, which in turn stimulates ECM production and promotes the proliferation response via TGFβ signaling.

Linking Gene Expression in SSc Skin to Biological Pathways and Pathogenesis

Gene expression data can be analyzed for data-driven groupings based solely on the expression profiles as described above for deriving intrinsic subsets, but can also be probed for pathway-specific signatures [41, 61, 62]. These analytical approaches have been described as "top-down" or "bottom-up," respectively (Fig. 49.2) [61]. In the case of the top-down approach, biological information is inferred solely from gene expression in cells or in whole tissues. On the other hand, the bottom-up approach seeks to understand gene expression signatures in samples on the basis of biological factors, commonly cytokines or other soluble mediators, known or speculatively implicated in pathogenesis.

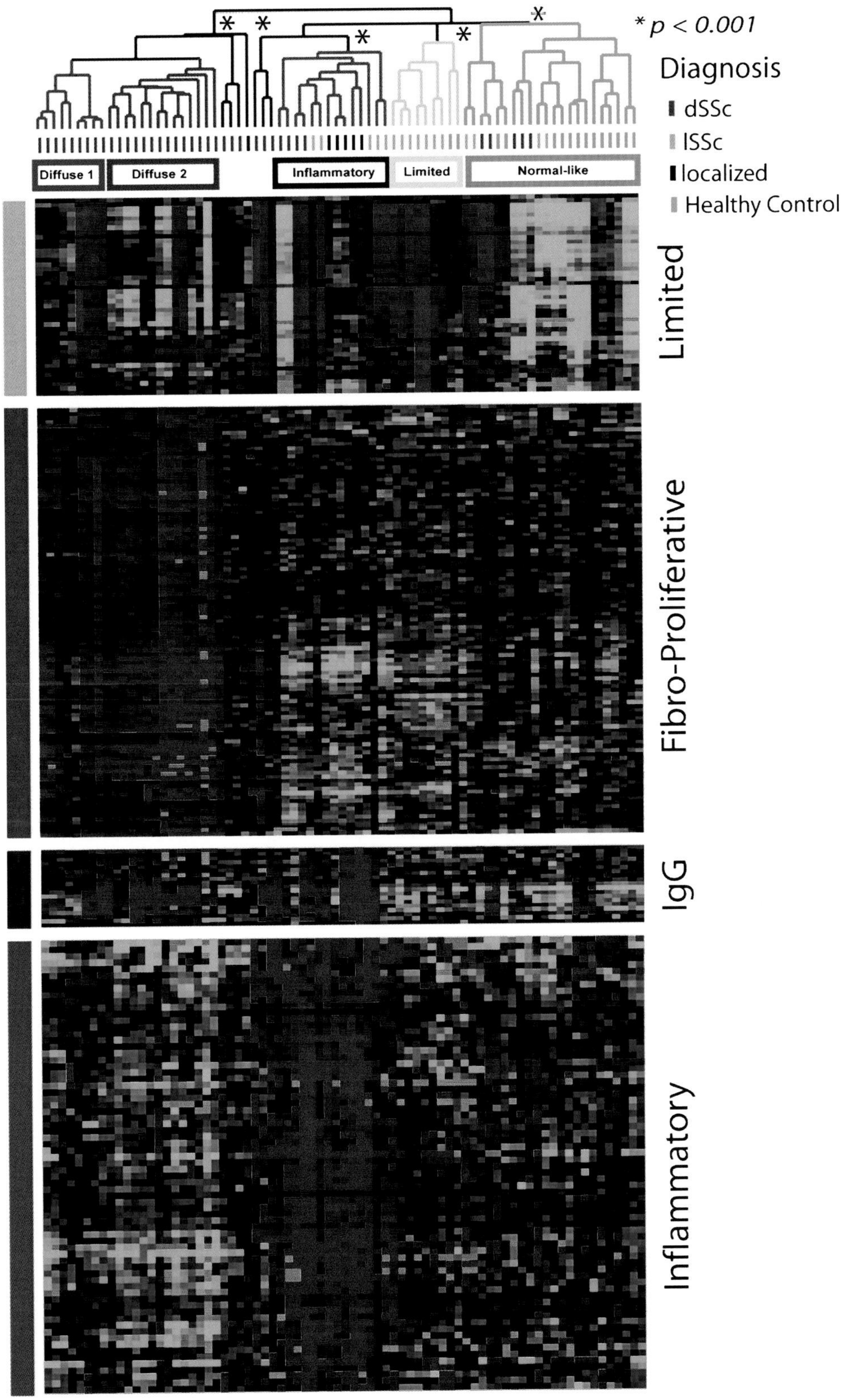

Fig. 49.1 "Intrinsic" subsets in the gene expression of SSc skin. The "intrinsic" subsets of SSc are defined by distinct gene expression signatures [36]. The dendrogram has been colored to reflect the major gene expression groups of the proliferation (*blue* and *red*), inflammatory (*purple*), limited (*gold*), and normal-like (*green*). The clinical diagnosis associated with each biopsy is indicated by the color of the hash mark below the dendrogram tree. The subset assignments of each group, diffuse proliferation (diffuse 1 and 2), inflammatory, limited, and normal-like, are indicated. A subset of the 995 intrinsic genes are shown. We refer the reader to Milano et al. [36] for a full description of the sample groupings and the underlying gene expression (Modified with permission from of Milano et al. Copyright, 2008 Milano et al.)

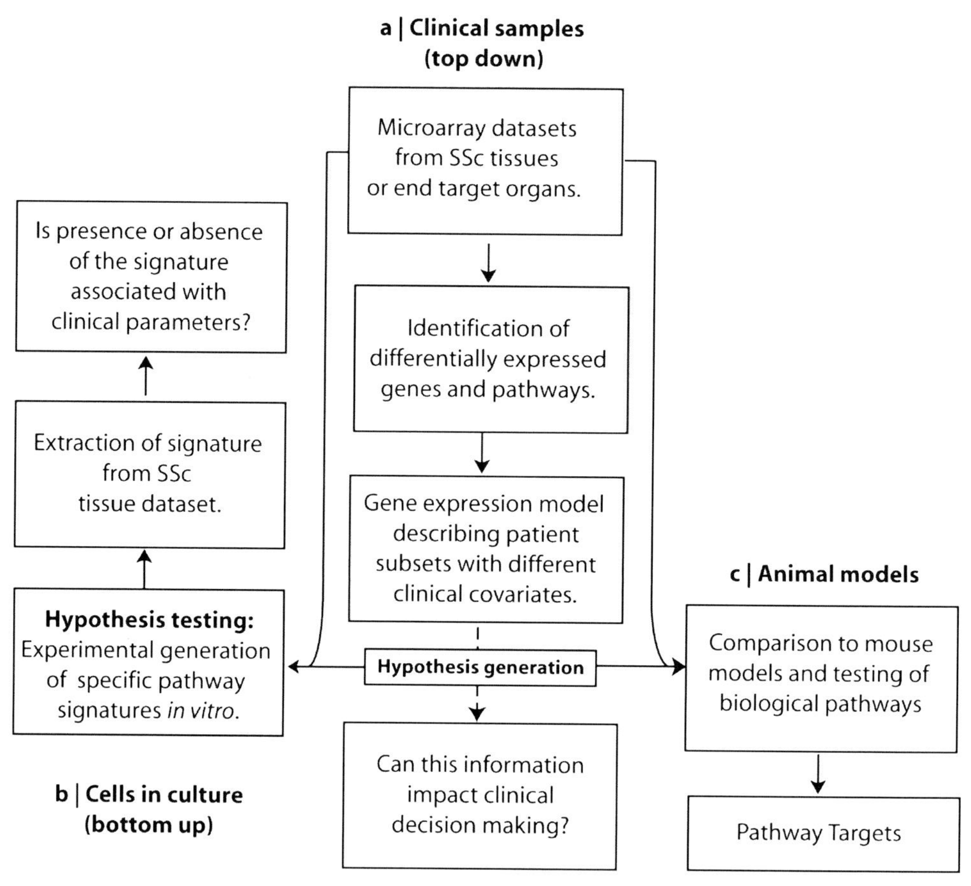

Fig. 49.2 Molecular profiling strategy for SSc. The top-down approach (**a**) begins with the profiling of SSc tissues to identify deregulated genes and pathways. Stratification of patients into molecular subsets and association with different clinical covariates may aid in treatment decisions. The bottom-up approach (**b**) provides a molecular framework to test specific hypotheses in end-target tissues using gene expression signatures derived by stimulating specific pathways such as TGFβ (see Fig. 49.3). The contribution of a specific cytokine or signaling pathway can then be assessed using the gene expression in the end-target tissues and different computational frameworks. Analysis of gene expression in end-target tissues of animal models allows for comparison of gene expression and pathways between the two, and when concordant, the pathway hypotheses can be tested more rigorously in the mouse model

The hypothesis-driven, bottom-up approach examines gene expression in clinical samples using experimentally derived gene expression signatures [63]. These signatures are identified by examining the resulting gene expression changes upon activation of a specific signaling pathway in cells in culture or in a target tissue [41, 64, 65]. The gene expression signature associated with the pathway or response of interest then provides an interpretive framework for microarray data from the target tissue, in this case SSc skin. In some cases, such as the interferon signature identified in systemic lupus erythematosus and subsequently in SSc, the gene signature can be identified relatively easily due to the pronounced alterations in gene expression, the existing databases of IFN-regulated genes, and readily recognizable gene names (e.g., interferon-induced protein 44). However, identifying a pattern of gene expression reflecting less robust or less well-characterized alterations in gene expression, particularly given the thousands of genes examined in a microarray dataset, is nontrivial, and using literature-derived gene signatures has proven error prone. This is particularly a problem in the common case in which gene signatures are derived from databases of cells or tissues that may not be entirely relevant to the tissue under examination. Therefore, the set of genes regulated after treatment of the relevant cells with a cytokine or other mediator provides a more accurate and unbiased gene signature reflective of the effect of the mediator on mRNA levels.

In order to fully understand the biology and molecular mechanisms underlying the intrinsic subsets of SSc, the analysis of skin biopsies has been coupled with a bottom-up strategy to specifically examine the role of a number of cytokines, including TGFβ previously implicated in SSc pathogenesis [41, 66]. As an example, comparing dermal fibroblast gene expression before and after treatment with TGFβ, a TGFβ-responsive gene signature was identified (Fig. 49.3). Interrogating SSc skin gene expression, this TGFβ-responsive signature identified a subset of dSSc skin biopsies (Fig. 49.3) with higher expression of TGFβ-responsive genes. This indicated that a subset of dSSc skin biopsies, but not lSSc, morphea, or healthy controls, show expression of TGFβ-responsive genes. The dSSc patients that showed high expression of the TGFβ-responsive signature were more likely to have ILD and higher skin scores than patients in whom the signature was not expressed (Fig. 49.3). A more recent meta-analysis in much larger patient cohort has confirmed the link between the expression of TGFβ-responsive genes and disease severity, at least for MRSS [41].

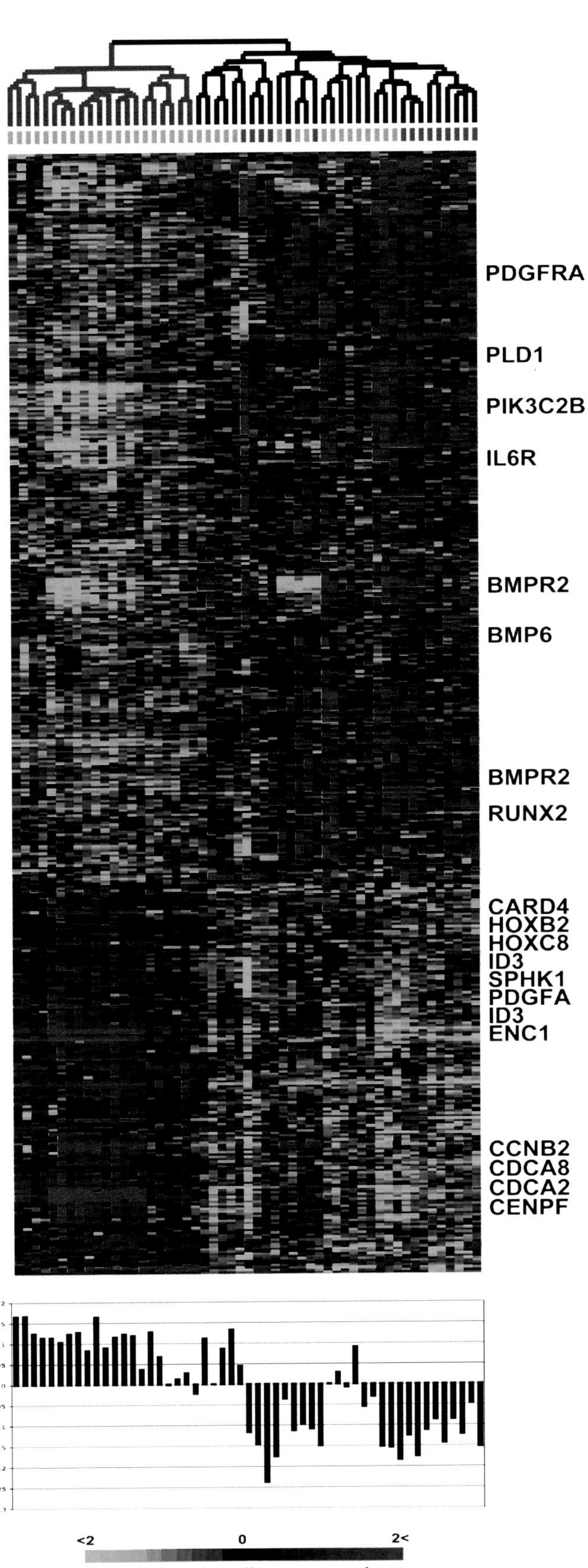

Fig. 49.3 A TGFβ-responsive gene signature is deregulated in a subset of dSSc skin biopsies. The average gene expression response derived from treating healthy and dSSc dermal fibroblasts with TGFβ is shown along the left-hand side of the figure. *Red* indicates increased gene expression and *green* shows decreased gene expression. The TGFβ-responsive gene signature was examined in gene expression measured in SSc skin [36]. The TGFβ-responsive gene signature is enriched in a subset of dSSc skin biopsies (*red* dendrogram; TGFβ-activated) as illustrated by Pearson correlations between the TGFβ-responsive centroid and each patient (*lower panel*). The TGFβ-activated group had higher mRSS (mean 26.9 ± 2.04) than the TGFβ-not-activated group (mean 17.8 ± 1.95; $p = 0.0061$) when analyzed by biopsy and was weakly significant when analyzed on a per-patient basis ($p < 0.11$). The TGFβ-activated group also had an increased prevalence of ILD with 7/16 of the TGFβ-activated group as compared to 0/10 in the not-activated group ($p = 0.014$, odds ratio of 16.58, χ-squared test). When patients rather than biopsies are considered, then five out of ten patients in the activated group had ILD, whereas 0/5 of the patients in the not-activated group had ILD ($p = 0.053$). No significant associations were found with patient age, disease duration, GI involvement, renal disease, Raynaud's severity, or digital ulcers (Reprinted with permission from Sargent et al. *J Invest Derm* 2010 [66], Copyright 2010 Sargent et al.)

An expanded analysis of pathways in SSc examined experimentally derived gene expression signatures in dermal fibroblasts for 13 different signaling pathways implicated in SSc pathogenesis [41]. These data show distinct and overlapping sets of genes induced by each pathway, allowing for a better understanding of the molecular relationship between profibrotic and immune signaling networks. Pathway-specific gene signatures were analyzed across a compendium of microarray datasets consisting of skin biopsies from three independent cohorts representing 80 SSc patients, 4 morphea, and 26 controls. IFN-α signaling showed a strong association with early disease, while TGFβ signaling spanned the fibroproliferative and inflammatory subsets, was associated with worse MRSS, and was higher in lesional than nonlesional skin. The fibroproliferative subset was most strongly associated with PDGF signaling, while the inflammatory subset demonstrated strong activation of innate immune pathways including TLR signaling upstream of NF-kB. The limited and normal-like subsets did not show associations with fibrotic and inflammatory mediators such as TGFβ and TNF-α. The normal-like subset showed high expression of genes associated with lipid signaling, which was absent in the inflammatory and limited subsets. Together, these data suggest a model by which IFN-α is involved in early disease pathology, and disease severity is associated with active TGFβ signaling [41].

Assassi et al. examined gene expression in skin biopsies from 59 SSc patients. Eighty two skin transcripts were identified that correlated with forced vital capacity % predicted (FVC) and distinguished patients with severe interstitial lung disease (ILD) defined as an FVC<70. Important genes included SELP, CCL2, and MMP3 that are known to play a role in inflammatory cell adhesion to the endothelium and extravasation. Immunofluorescence staining of SSc skin and lung revealed overexpression of these proteins compared to healthy control tissues. Plasma levels of CCL2 and sPSGL-1 correlated with FVC independent of age, sex, ethnicity, smoking status, anti-topoisomerase I antibodies status, MRSS, immune suppression treatment, disease subtype, and duration. Eight genes (CCL2, HAPLN3, GPR4, ADCYAP1, WARS, CDC25B, PLP1, and STXBP6) from the 82 skin transcripts correlated with MRSS. The authors concluded that a limited number of skin transcripts correlate with ILD in SSc patients including genes known to play a role in inflammatory cell adhesion and diapedesis [44].

Gene Expression Signatures in Esophagus

A recent study of esophageal gene expression has demonstrated that the intrinsic gene expression subsets can be found in other tissues and have a remarkable similarity to the changes we observe in the skin. In a pilot study to examine gene expression in esophageal biopsies, 16 patients with and 7 without SSc underwent an esophagogastroduodenoscopy for a clinical indication [45]. Taroni et al. identified 1,903 probes (1,350 unique genes) with significantly different expression between the two groups ($p<0.05$, *t*-test). Genes upregulated in SSc biopsies included *IL27*, *IFNAR1*, and *PDGFRA*. Genes downregulated in SSc compared to non-SSc patients included *CCL2* and several human leukocyte antigen genes. Similar to biopsies from clinically involved and uninvolved skin, paired upper and lower esophageal biopsies from 15 SSc patients showed similar expression [45]. Most importantly, intrinsic subsets (noninflammatory, inflammatory, and proliferative) were identified in esophageal biopsies that are similar to the intrinsic subsets that were previously identified in the skin (inflammatory, proliferative, normal-like, and limited) (Fig. 49.4). These data suggest that deregulated SSc molecular programs are consistent between skin and esophageal tissue [45]. This finding has important clinical implications because clinical studies to assess treatment response to immune suppression often neglect to include esophageal disease endpoints.

Gene Expression Signatures in Lung and Bronchoalveolar Lavage (BAL)

Because lung disease is prevalent and the major cause of morbidity in SSc patients, there is an important need to better understand the molecular changes associated with SSc-associated pulmonary disease. Unfortunately, the difficulty of obtaining lung tissue for these analyses is often a rate-limiting step.

One approach that has been explored is analysis of gene expression in cells from bronchoalveolar lavage (BAL). RNAs from purified T-cells of SSc or healthy control subjects were analyzed on arrays representing 4,132 cDNAs supplement with 375 gene microarrays containing primarily cytokine genes. Unsupervised clustering stratified patients into two groups: one group containing all the controls and

Fig. 49.4 Esophageal intrinsic genes. 2240 probes representing 2085 unique transcripts with the most similar expression between upper and lower biopsies for an individual but with the most dissimilar expression between individuals, termed "intrinsic," were identified (FDR<1.1 %). An asterisk indicates samples obtained at 6 months. (**a**) Sample dendrogram, leaves are colored by group membership: *red*, samples from proliferative subset; *purple*, samples from inflammatory subset; *black*, samples from noninflammatory subset. *Brackets* indicate biopsies from the upper and lower esophagus for an individual that clustered together. (**b**) Overview of hierarchically clustered probes. (**c**) Selected gene clusters: *purple*, upregulated in inflammatory patients; *red*, upregulated in a proliferative subset of patients; *black*, downregulated in inflammatory patients (Reprinted with permission from Taroni et al. *Arthritis Res Therapy* 2015 [45])

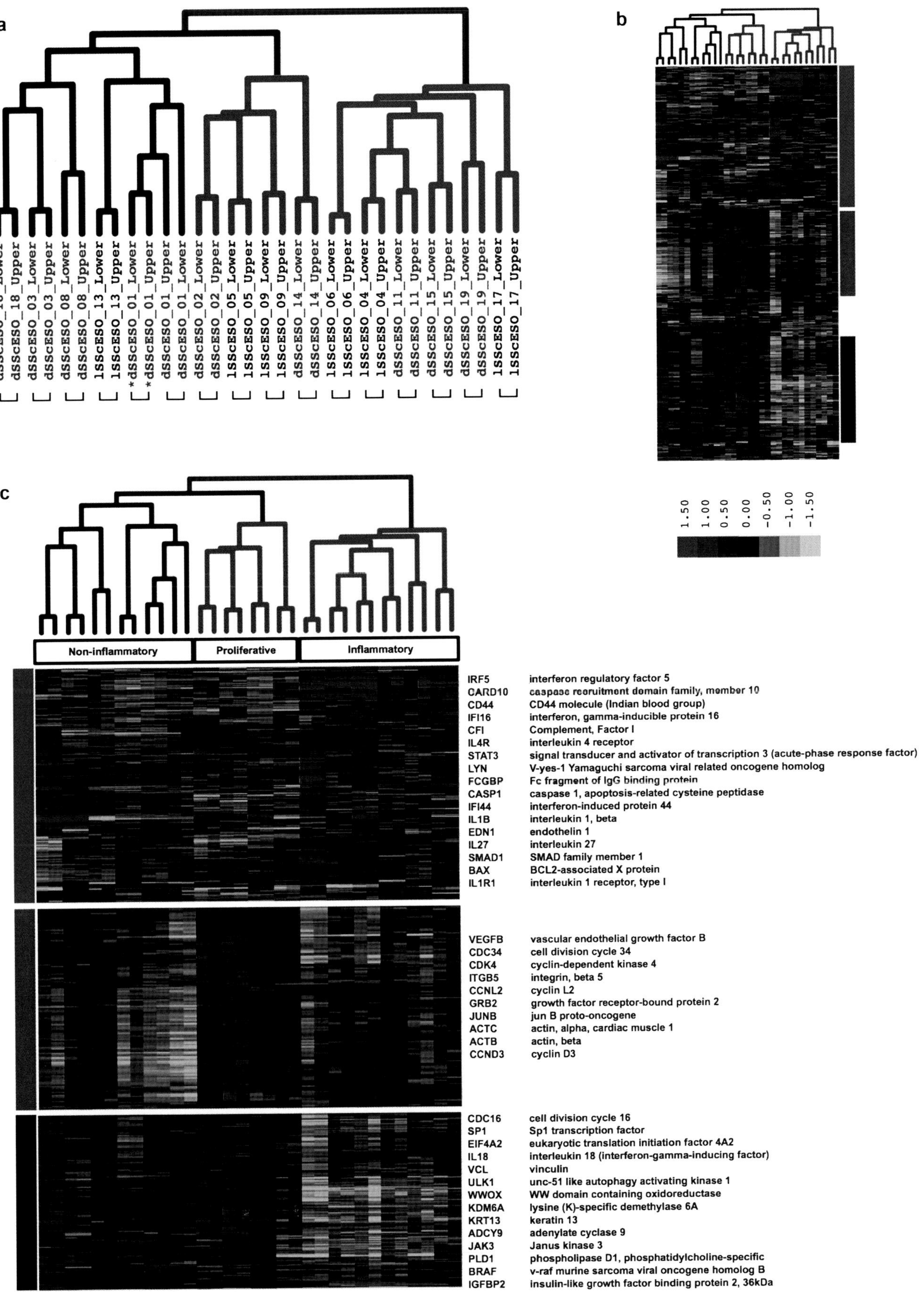
a
dSScESO_18_Lower
dSScESO_18_Upper
dSScESO_03_Lower
dSScESO_03_Upper
dSScESO_08_Lower
dSScESO_08_Upper
lSScESO_13_Lower
lSScESO_13_Upper
*dSScESO_01_Lower
*dSScESO_01_Upper
dSScESO_01_Upper
dSScESO_01_Lower
dSScESO_02_Lower
dSScESO_02_Upper
lSScESO_05_Lower
lSScESO_05_Upper
lSScESO_09_Lower
lSScESO_09_Upper
dSScESO_14_Lower
dSScESO_14_Upper
lSScESO_06_Lower
lSScESO_06_Upper
lSScESO_04_Lower
lSScESO_04_Upper
dSScESO_11_Lower
dSScESO_11_Upper
dSScESO_15_Lower
dSScESO_15_Upper
dSScESO_19_Lower
dSScESO_19_Upper
lSScESO_17_Lower
lSScESO_17_Upper
b
1.50
1.00
0.50
0.00
-0.50
-1.00
-1.50
c
Non-inflammatory
Proliferative
Inflammatory
IRF5 interferon regulatory factor 5
CARD10 caspase recruitment domain family, member 10
CD44 CD44 molecule (Indian blood group)
IFI16 interferon, gamma-inducible protein 16
CFI Complement, Factor I
IL4R interleukin 4 receptor
STAT3 signal transducer and activator of transcription 3 (acute-phase response factor)
LYN V-yes-1 Yamaguchi sarcoma viral related oncogene homolog
FCGBP Fc fragment of IgG binding protein
CASP1 caspase 1, apoptosis-related cysteine peptidase
IFI44 interferon-induced protein 44
IL1B interleukin 1, beta
EDN1 endothelin 1
IL27 interleukin 27
SMAD1 SMAD family member 1
BAX BCL2-associated X protein
IL1R1 interleukin 1 receptor, type I
VEGFB vascular endothelial growth factor B
CDC34 cell division cycle 34
CDK4 cyclin-dependent kinase 4
ITGB5 integrin, beta 5
CCNL2 cyclin L2
GRB2 growth factor receptor-bound protein 2
JUNB jun B proto-oncogene
ACTC actin, alpha, cardiac muscle 1
ACTB actin, beta
CCND3 cyclin D3
CDC16 cell division cycle 16
SP1 Sp1 transcription factor
EIF4A2 eukaryotic translation initiation factor 4A2
IL18 interleukin 18 (interferon-gamma-inducing factor)
VCL vinculin
ULK1 unc-51 like autophagy activating kinase 1
WWOX WW domain containing oxidoreductase
KDM6A lysine (K)-specific demethylase 6A
KRT13 keratin 13
ADCY9 adenylate cyclase 9
JAK3 Janus kinase 3
PLD1 phospholipase D1, phosphatidylcholine-specific
BRAF v-raf murine sarcoma viral oncogene homolog B
IGFBP2 insulin-like growth factor binding protein 2, 36kDa

some patients with noninflammatory BAL and the other group containing mainly patients with inflammatory BAL. The inflammatory group showed Th2 skewing of CD8+ T-cells, consistent with the development of fibrotic disease in these patients [54]. Such observations suggest that more complete BAL analyses using more comprehensive arrays might provide considerable additional insight into pathogenesis and possibly yield better markers for progressive lung disease.

Recent work has examined gene expression in lungs from SSc patients, exploring patterns associated with both PAH and ILD [51]. These studies revealed the expected increased expression of genes involved in fibrosis in SSc-associated ILD, including type I and type III collagen, IGFBPs, MMP7, CTGF, osteopontin, and tissue inhibitors of metalloproteases 1 (TIMP-1). SSc-PAH lungs shared functional groups with idiopathic PAH lung samples enriched in their gene expression profiles for interferon, IL-4, IL-17, and antigen presentation signaling. SSc-associated PAH also showed an increased expression of inflammatory genes including chemokines CCL2, CXCL10, and CX3CL1. Notably a significant number of genes with increased expression were shared between SSc-PF and IPF, as well as SSc-PAH and IPAH, highlighting possible overlaps in pathogenic mechanisms between these two complications that sometimes occur together in SSc.

Another prospective microarray study examined open lung biopsy specimens from 28 SSc patients with ILD and 4 healthy control subjects [52]. They found differential expression in genes involved with macrophage markers (CD68, CD163, AIF-1, and MS4A4A), chemokines (CCL13, CCL18, and CXCL5), collagen (COL1A1), TGFβ, and IFN-regulated genes (IFNAR2, OAS1, and IL-18) between SSc and healthy controls. Collagen, IFN, and macrophage gene clusters correlated with lung disease progression as assessed by changes between pre- and posttreatment pulmonary function test and maximal lung fibrosis score (FibMax = total fibrosis score in 6 lung zones). These results support the role of gene expression signatures to define unique molecular features of SSc lung disease.

Gene Expression in Cells from Patients with SSc-Peripheral Blood Mononuclear Cells (PBMCs)

PBMCs provide a source of inflammatory cells from patients with SSc that are more numerous and easier to access that inflammatory cells from tissues. Several groups have found that PBMCs from SSc patients show increased expression of genes associated with either type I and/or type II interferon (IFNs) [67, 68]. More recently, Duan and coworkers examined gene expression in purified monocytes and CD4+ T-cells from SSc patients and healthy controls, identifying 1,800 genes differentially regulated in SSc monocytes and 863 genes differentially regulated in SSc CD4+ T-cells compared to controls [47]. Of these, 361 genes were differentially expressed in both cell types suggesting that both cell types are responding similarly to the SSc microenvironment. As seen by others, the authors identified increased expression of a type I IFN-associated gene signature [47]. Liu et al. measured plasma levels of IFN-inducible chemokines (IP-10 and I-TAC) in 266 SSc patients and compared this score with a 43 gene signature composed of IFN-inducible genes identified in peripheral blood [25, 49]. They found that the plasma IFN score correlated with the peripheral blood cell IFN gene expression score and was associated with the presence of anti-U1RNP and absence of RNA polymerase III serum autoantibodies, with components of the Medsger SSc Disease Severity Scale (muscle, skin, and lung disease) but not with SSc subtype or duration. They concluded that the IFN-inducible chemokine score is a stable serologic marker of SSc disease severity and may be a useful strategy for identifying patients at high risk for severe SSc.

PBMC Gene Expression in SSc-Associated PAH

Several studies have examined genome-wide gene expression of PBMCs in SSc patients with PAH [48, 50, 69]. A study examining PBMC gene expression in patients with idiopathic PAH (IPAH) and lcSSc-PAH demonstrated a readily detectable series of genes with increased expression including inflammatory genes such as IL-1β and IL-8, vascular genes such as VEGF and ICAM1, chemokine genes such as CCL3 and CXCL2, and AP1 transcription factor genes such as JUN, JUND, and FOSB. Subgroups of lcSSc patients could be identified by gene expression correlated with PAH severity [48]. Another study focusing on lcSSc patients with or without PAH showed some of the genes noted above including ICAM1 and IL-1β [50]. Many of the genes differentially expressed showed increased expression in lcSSc patients with PAH, but then a gradient of expression associated with disease severity. For example, the highest levels of expression were found in SSc-PAH and the lowest levels of expression in healthy controls, with lcSSc without PAH showing intermediate levels of gene expression.

To understand better the role of perivascular inflammation in the pathogenesis of SSc-PAH, investigators examined gene expression in PBMCs from patients with lcSSc-PAH compared to lcSSc without PAH and healthy control subjects. Expression levels for genes involved with endoplasmic reticulum (ER) stress unfolded protein response (UPR) were evaluated. Results showed that PBMCs from patients with right-heart catheterization confirmed PAH compared to lcSSC without PAH demonstrated higher BiP (an ER chaperone protein that maintains the inactive form of three ER sensor proteins (PERK, IRE1, ATF-6), ATF-4, and ATF-6, which are proteins that play a pivotal role in the unfolded protein response signaling cascade).

Assessing the Molecular Therapeutic Response

Another and potentially even more powerful way to utilize gene expression clinically is in assessing or predicting response to therapy for an individual. Clinical trials in SSc have, for the most part, demonstrated the lack of, or minimal, therapeutic benefit. The reasons for this include clinical trial designs that include multiple molecular subsets of disease, the rarity of SSc that impedes targeted patient recruitment, a lack of sensitive outcome markers, heterogeneity in drug metabolism, and possibly not having drugs to the correct molecular targets. The molecular gene expression data suggest that SSc is an amalgamation of several different disease subtypes or pathogenic states. The finding of eight or more serum autoantibodies in SSc patients as well as ANA negative disease supports this hypothesis [22, 70].

Pilot studies that assess clinical improvement during treatment with various agents suggest that there may be gene expression signatures in patient skin that can be assessed before treatment begins and used to select targeted therapy. Two patients who demonstrated clinical improvement in skin and lung disease during 3–6 months of treatment with imatinib mesylate (Gleevec) demonstrated a specific, pretreatment, skin gene expression signature (FDR <0.001) composed of genes whose expression changed significantly during treatment [71]. Fibroblasts, endothelial cells, and B-lymphocytes were postulated to be the cells responsible for driving the specific 1,050-gene imatinib-responsive gene expression signature. This study was the first to suggest a role for analyses of gene expression in pretreatment skin biopsies from SSc patients in order to inform medical decision-making.

Specific gene expression signatures have also been associated with clinical improvement during treatment with mycophenolate mofetil (CellCept). In a study of 22 patients with SSc and 10 healthy controls, 2 specific gene expression signatures in skin were identified that were specific to patients with a clinically significant improvement in skin disease during treatment. A 321-gene signature was identified (FDR <5 %) comprised of genes whose expression differed significantly between biopsies of patients that demonstrated a clinically significant improvement in mRSS (improvers) compared to those who did not improve (non-improvers). Functional analysis of these genes revealed that they played a role in purine metabolism and response to inflammation (PRPS1, NF-KB, CXCL1, FKBP1C). Additionally, a 571-gene expression response signature was identified (FDR<10 %) only in improvers, but not in non-improvers when analyzing biopsies pre- and posttreatment. Interestingly, functional analysis of the genes whose expression increased during successful MMF treatment was involved with extracellular matrix component while the genes whose expression decreased during treatment related to cell cycle and cell division (e.g., organelle fission, mitotic cell cycle, as well as in the NOD-like receptor signaling pathway responsible for NF-KB activation, cytokine production, and apoptosis (PBEF1, CXCL1, HAT1, IL-17D, SFRP2, PDGFRL, IL-16, COL13A1, THBS2, IGFBP5, WNT3, DKK1/2, and WIF1)). There were no significant changes (FDR <50 %) in skin gene expression in non-improvers, suggesting that skin gene expression may be a sensitive and specific marker for skin disease improvement in SSc.

Hinchcliff et al. [39] was the first to demonstrate that the intrinsic gene expression subsets of SSc may predict response to therapy. The lack of a biomarker to predict MMF response results in treatment delays with other potentially effective SSc therapies. In the study of MMF, the hypothesis was that MRSS would improve during MMF therapy in patients classified in the *inflammatory intrinsic* subset because MMF impedes lymphocyte proliferation [72]. The goal was to identify biomarkers to enable targeted treatment of patients who are most likely to benefit from MMF therapy, but spare those who would not benefit the side effects of therapy. In the pilot study [39], four out of four clinical responders belonged to the *inflammatory intrinsic* subset while the three nonresponders belonged to the *fibroproliferative* or *normal-like intrinsic* subsets, supporting our preliminary hypothesis that the inflammatory patients are those most likely to improve.

Similar results have been found in two other investigator-initiated clinical trials for abatacept [73] and nilotinib [74], which appear to target one subset of patients but not another.

Chakravarty et al. [73] demonstrates that patients who improve while on abatacept therapy appear to map to the inflammatory gene expression subset. Analysis of pre- and posttreatment biopsies shows a decrease in CD28 co-stimulatory signaling which is the molecular target of abatacept. This change is only observed in patients who improve during treatment but not in those that do not or controls. The data suggest patients most likely to improve on abatacept therapy are those that are in the inflammatory subset.

A third study by Gordon et al. [74] shows that patients who improve with nilotinib therapy have high expression of genes associated with an increase in TGFβ and PDGF signaling at baseline, suggesting pathway activation in these patients. Those who do not improve do not show high-level expression of these genes. This study argues for targeting patients with TGFβ/PDGF pathway activation with TKIs.

Finally, the results of an SSc rituximab trial failed to demonstrate a significant benefit in lung and/or skin disease and lack of significant changes in skin gene expression mirrored this finding [75]. So when there is not a clinical response, a change in gene expression is also not obviously present, suggesting the changes seen above are likely to be specific to the therapy under study.

Selected Gene Biomarkers of SSc Disease Status and Progression

An alternative approach that might be viewed as either an extension of, or alternative to, high-throughput analysis of gene expression is the analysis of targeted gene expression by quantitative real-time PCR (RT-PCR) or NanoString, which can provide a potentially more economical approach for understanding underlying disease activity and/or subsets. Based on data implicating IFN and TGFβ responsive genes in SSc pathogenesis, a restricted series of genes known to be responsive to these cytokines was tested for their utility as biomarkers of the MRSS [76, 77]. Multiple linear regression permitted construction of a model using two IFN- and two TGFβ-responsive genes that correlated highly with the MRSS (see Lafyatis Chapter). Another study that used RT-PCR to measure cadherin 11 mRNA levels in SSc skin and in skin from the bleomycin scleroderma mouse model demonstrated a potential role for cadherin 11 in dermal fibrosis [78]. The expression of these genes in lesional mid-forearm skin reflects accurately the total burden of skin disease in patients and might be used as a surrogate outcome measure for clinical trials or care. Quantitative real-time PCR might also be applied to the intrinsic gene expression subsets, provided that a limited series of genes can be identified that permit accurate classification. However, until the patterns of gene expression in SSc skin and their relationship to therapies is completely defined, clinical trials will typically benefit from the more extensive gene profiling available through microarray or massively parallel deep sequencing.

Conclusions

Gene expression profiling in SSc has shown robust changes in skin, lung, and in PBMCs. The gene expression changes in fibroblasts are more variable and imperfectly reflect what is found in vivo. New advances show that gene expression profiling can capture the heterogeneity in SSc skin, showing that differing molecular patterns likely reflecting differing underlying biology can identify both patients with distinguishable clinical phenotypes (lSSc versus dSSc), but can also distinguish subsets within clinical similar phenotypes (dSSc). These analyses further show multiple gene expression subsets that point toward underlying pathogenic pathways. The TGFβ pathway has been best characterized and is deregulated in one of these groups. Further exploration of pathways promises to shed light on other pathogenic pathways. The most important future direction for clinical trials and developing treatment is that gene expression profiling can potentially measure the response to therapy and therefore could be used as a clinical outcome measure. This could be particularly important in early phase trials where the mechanism of action can be examined by examining changes in gene expression associated with treatment in the context of the known biological activity of the drug. As the gene expression subsets are refined and responses to therapy are systematically characterized, a diagnostic test could be developed to target therapies to specific patients based on their gene expression profile.

References

1. Barnett AJ, Miller MH, Littlejohn GO. A survival study of patients with scleroderma diagnosed over 30 years (1953–1983): the value of a simple cutaneous classification in the early stages of the disease. J Rheumatol. 1988;15(2):276–83.
2. Furst D, et al. Systemic sclerosis – continuing progress in developing clinical measures of response. J Rheumatol. 2007;34(5):1194–200.
3. LeRoy EC, et al. Scleroderma (systemic sclerosis): classification, subsets and pathogenesis. J Rheumatol. 1988;15(2):202–5.
4. Black CM, et al. HLA antigens, autoantibodies and clinical subsets in scleroderma. Br J Rheumatol. 1984;23(4):267–71.
5. Bolster MB, Silver RM. Lung disease in systemic sclerosis (scleroderma). Baillieres Clin Rheumatol. 1993;7(1):79–97.
6. Akesson A, Wollheim FA. Organ manifestations in 100 patients with progressive systemic sclerosis: a comparison between the CREST syndrome and diffuse scleroderma. Br J Rheumatol. 1989;28(4):281–6.
7. Merkel PA, et al. Validity, reliability, and feasibility of durometer measurements of scleroderma skin disease in a multicenter treatment trial. Arthritis Rheum. 2008;59(5):699–705.
8. Rodnan GP, Lipinski E, Luksick J. Skin thickness and collagen content in progressive systemic sclerosis and localized scleroderma. Arthritis Rheum. 1979;22(2):130–40.
9. Clements P, et al. Inter and intraobserver variability of total skin thickness score (modified Rodnan TSS) in systemic sclerosis. J Rheumatol. 1995;22(7):1281–5.
10. Furst DE, et al. The modified Rodnan skin score is an accurate reflection of skin biopsy thickness in systemic sclerosis. J Rheumatol. 1998;25(1):84–8.
11. Clements PJ, et al. Skin thickness score as a predictor and correlate of outcome in systemic sclerosis: high-dose versus low-dose penicillamine trial. Arthritis Rheum. 2000;43(11):2445–54.
12. Steen VD, Medsger Jr TA. Improvement in skin thickening in systemic sclerosis associated with improved survival. Arthritis Rheum. 2001;44(12):2828–35.
13. Verrecchia F, et al. Skin involvement in scleroderma – where histological and clinical scores meet. Rheumatology (Oxford). 2007; 46(5):833–41.
14. Sampaio-Barros PD, et al. Survival, causes of death, and prognostic factors in systemic sclerosis: analysis of 947 Brazilian patients. J Rheumatol. 2012;39(10):1971–8.

15. Hasegawa M, et al. Investigation of prognostic factors for skin sclerosis and lung function in Japanese patients with early systemic sclerosis: a multicentre prospective observational study. Rheumatology (Oxford). 2012;51(1):129–33.
16. Steen VD. Autoantibodies in systemic sclerosis. Semin Arthritis Rheum. 2005;35(1):35–42.
17. PMID 23083053.
18. Medsger TA, Steen VD. Classification, prognosis. In: Clements PJ, Furst DE, editors. Systemic sclerosis. Baltimore: Williams & Wilkins; 1996. p. 51–64.
19. Siebold JR. In: Harris ED et al., editors. Kelley's textbook of rheumatology. Philadelphia: Elsevier & Saunders; 2005.
20. Hildebrandt S, et al. A long-term longitudinal isotypic study of anti-topoisomerase I autoantibodies. Rheumatol Int. 1993;12(6): 231–4.
21. Dick T, et al. Coexistence of antitopoisomerase I and anticentromere antibodies in patients with systemic sclerosis. Ann Rheum Dis. 2002;61(2):121–7.
22. Kayser C, Fritzler MJ. Autoantibodies in systemic sclerosis: unanswered questions. Front Immunol. 2015;6:167.
23. Doering K, Rosen A. Autoantibodies in pathogenesis. In: Varga J, Denton C, Wigley F, editors. Scleroderma: from pathogenesis to comprehensive management. New York: Springer; 2012. p. 199–208.
24. Liu X, et al. Does C-reactive protein predict the long-term progression of interstitial lung disease and survival in patients with early systemic sclerosis? Arthritis Care Res (Hoboken). 2013;65(8): 1375–80.
25. Liu X, et al. Correlation of interferon-inducible chemokine plasma levels with disease severity in systemic sclerosis. Arthritis Rheum. 2013;65(1):226–35.
26. Shand L, et al. Relationship between change in skin score and disease outcome in diffuse cutaneous systemic sclerosis: application of a latent linear trajectory model. Arthritis Rheum. 2007;56(7): 2422–31.
27. Perera A, et al. Clinical subsets, skin thickness progression rate, and serum antibody levels in systemic sclerosis patients with anti-topoisomerase I antibody. Arthritis Rheum. 2007;56(8):2740–6.
28. Avouac J, et al. Joint and tendon involvement predict disease progression in systemic sclerosis: a EUSTAR prospective study. . Ann Rheum Dis. 2016;75(1):103–9. doi: 10.1136/annrheumdis-2014-205295. Epub 2014 Aug 27.
29. Domsic RT, et al. Skin thickness progression rate: a predictor of mortality and early internal organ involvement in diffuse scleroderma. Ann Rheum Dis. 2011;70(1):104–9.
30. Hoffmann-Vold AM, et al. Performance of the 2013 American College of Rheumatology/European League Against Rheumatism Classification Criteria for Systemic Sclerosis (SSc) in large, well-defined cohorts of SSc and mixed connective tissue disease. J Rheumatol. 2015;42(1):60–3.
31. Maurer B, et al. Prediction of worsening of skin fibrosis in patients with diffuse cutaneous systemic sclerosis using the EUSTAR database. Ann Rheum Dis. 2015;74(6):1124–31.
32. Perou CM, et al. Molecular portraits of human breast tumours. Nature. 2000;406(6797):747–52.
33. Ross DT, et al. Systematic variation in gene expression patterns in human cancer cell lines. Nat Genet. 2000;24(3):227–35.
34. Shen-Orr SS, et al. Cell type-specific gene expression differences in complex tissues. Nat Methods. 2010;7(4):287–9.
35. Chung CH, Bernard PS, Perou CM. Molecular portraits and the family tree of cancer. Nat Genet. 2002;32(Suppl):533–40.
36. Milano A, et al. Molecular subsets in the gene expression signatures of scleroderma skin. PLoS One. 2008;3(7):e2696.
37. Sargent JL, et al. A TGFbeta-responsive gene signature is associated with a subset of diffuse scleroderma with increased disease severity. J Invest Dermatol. 2009;130(3):694–705.
38. Pendergrass SA, et al. Intrinsic gene expression subsets of diffuse cutaneous systemic sclerosis are stable in serial skin biopsies. J Invest Dermatol. 2012;132(5):1363–73.
39. Hinchcliff M, et al. Molecular signatures in skin associated with clinical improvement during mycophenolate treatment in systemic sclerosis. J Invest Dermatol. 2013;133(8):1979–89.
40. Mahoney JM, et al. Systems level analysis of systemic sclerosis shows a network of immune and profibrotic pathways connected with genetic polymorphisms. PLoS Comput Biol. 2015;11(1):e1004005.
41. Johnson ME, et al. Experimentally-derived fibroblast gene signatures identify molecular pathways associated with distinct subsets of systemic sclerosis patients in three independent cohorts. PLoS ONE. 2015;10(1):e0114017.
42. Whitfield ML, et al. Systemic and cell type-specific gene expression patterns in scleroderma skin. Proc Natl Acad Sci U S A. 2003;100(21):12319–24.
43. Gardner H, et al. Gene profiling of scleroderma skin reveals robust signatures of disease that are imperfectly reflected in the transcript profiles of explanted fibroblasts. Arthritis Rheum. 2006;54(6):1961–73.
44. Assassi S, et al. Skin gene expression correlates of severity of interstitial lung disease in systemic sclerosis. Arthritis Rheum. 2013; 65(11):2917–27.
45. Taroni JN, Martyanov V, Huang CC, Mahoney JM, Hirano I, Shetuni B, Yang GY, Brenner D, Jung B, Wood TA, Bhattacharyya S, Almagor O, Lee J, Sirajuddin A, Varga J, Chang RW, Whitfield ML, Hinchcliff M. Molecular characterization of systemic sclerosis esophageal pathology identifies inflammatory and proliferative signatures. Arthritis Res Ther. 2015;17:194. doi: 10.1186/s13075-015-0695-1. PMID: 26220546.
46. Kimura M, et al. Cell cycle-dependent expression and spindle pole localization of a novel human protein kinase, Aik, related to Aurora of Drosophila and yeast Ipl1. J Biol Chem. 1997;272(21):13766–71.
47. Duan H, et al. Combined analysis of monocyte and lymphocyte messenger RNA expression with serum protein profiles in patients with scleroderma. Arthritis Rheum. 2008;58(5):1465–74.
48. Grigoryev DN, et al. Identification of candidate genes in scleroderma-related pulmonary arterial hypertension. Transl Res. 2008;151(4):197–207.
49. Assassi S, et al. Systemic sclerosis and lupus: points in an interferon-mediated continuum. Arthritis Rheum. 2010;62(2):589–98.
50. Pendergrass SA, et al. Limited systemic sclerosis patients with pulmonary arterial hypertension show biomarkers of inflammation and vascular injury. PLoS ONE. 2010;5(8):e12106.
51. Hsu E, et al. Lung tissues in patients with systemic sclerosis have gene expression patterns unique to pulmonary fibrosis and pulmonary hypertension. Arthritis Rheum. 2011;63(3):783–94.
52. Christmann RB, et al. Association of interferon- and transforming growth factor beta-regulated genes and macrophage activation with systemic sclerosis-related progressive lung fibrosis. Arthritis Rheumatol. 2014;66(3):714–25.
53. Luzina IG, et al. Gene expression in bronchoalveolar lavage cells from scleroderma patients. Am J Respir Cell Mol Biol. 2002; 26(5):549–57.
54. Luzina IG, et al. Occurrence of an activated, profibrotic pattern of gene expression in lung CD8+ T cells from scleroderma patients. Arthritis Rheum. 2003;48(8):2262–74.
55. Zhou X, et al. Systemic sclerosis (scleroderma): specific autoantigen genes are selectively overexpressed in scleroderma fibroblasts. J Immunol. 2001;167(12):7126–33.
56. Tan FK, et al. Classification analysis of the transcriptosome of nonlesional cultured dermal fibroblasts from systemic sclerosis patients with early disease. Arthritis Rheum. 2005;52(3):865–76.
57. Zhou X, et al. Monozygotic twins clinically discordant for scleroderma show concordance for fibroblast gene expression profiles. Arthritis Rheum. 2005;52(10):3305–14.

58. Fuzii HT, et al. Affected and non-affected skin fibroblasts from systemic sclerosis patients share a gene expression profile deviated from the one observed in healthy individuals. Clin Exp Rheumatol. 2008;26(5):866–74.
59. Vuorio T, Makela JK, Vuorio E. Activation of type I collagen genes in cultured scleroderma fibroblasts. J Cell Biochem. 1985;28(2): 105–13.
60. Pendergrass SA, Lemaire R, Francis IP, Mahoney JM, Lafyatis R, Whitfield ML. Intrinsic gene expression subsets of diffuse cutaneous systemic sclerosis are stable in serial skin biopsies. J Invest Dermatol. 2012;132(5):1363–73. doi: 10.1038/jid.2011.472. Epub 2012 Feb 9. PMID: 22318389.
61. Cabral CM, Liu Y, Sifers RN. Dissecting glycoprotein quality control in the secretory pathway. Trends Biochem Sci. 2001;26(10):619–24.
62. Wong DJ, Chang HY. Learning more from microarrays: insights from modules and networks. J Invest Dermatol. 2005;125(2):175–82.
63. Sargent JL, Whitfield ML. Capturing the heterogeneity in systemic sclerosis with genome-wide expression profiling. Expert Rev Clin Immunol. 2011;7(4):463–73.
64. Wei J, et al. PPARgamma downregulation by TGFbets in fibroblast and impaired expression and function in systemic sclerosis: a novel mechanism for progressive fibrogenesis. PLoS ONE. 2010;5(11): e13778.
65. Greenblatt MB, et al. Interspecies comparison of human and murine scleroderma reveals IL-13 and CCL2 as disease subset-specific targets. Am J Pathol. 2012;180(3):1080–94.
66. Sargent JL, et al. A TGFbeta-responsive gene signature is associated with a subset of diffuse scleroderma with increased disease severity. J Invest Dermatol. 2009;130(3):694–705.
67. York MR, et al. A macrophage marker, Siglec-1, is increased on circulating monocytes in patients with systemic sclerosis and induced by type I interferons and toll-like receptor agonists. Arthritis Rheum. 2007;56(3):1010–20.
68. Tan FK, et al. Signatures of differentially regulated interferon gene expression and vasculotrophism in the peripheral blood cells of systemic sclerosis patients. Rheumatology (Oxford). 2006;45(6): 694–702.
69. Risbano MG, et al. Altered immune phenotype in peripheral blood cells of patients with scleroderma-associated pulmonary hypertension. Clin Transl Sci. 2010;3(5):210–8.
70. Salazar GA, et al. Antinuclear antibody-negative systemic sclerosis. Semin Arthritis Rheum. 2014;44(6):680–6.
71. Chung L, et al. Molecular framework for response to imatinib mesylate in systemic sclerosis. Arthritis Rheum. 2009;60(2): 584–91.
72. Ransom JT. Mechanism of action of mycophenolate mofetil. Ther Drug Monit. 1995;17(6):681–4.
73. Chakravarty EF, Martyanov V, Fiorentino D, Wood TA, Haddon DJ, Jarrell JA, Utz PJ, Genovese MC, Whitfield ML, Chung L. Gene expression changes reflect clinical response in a placebo-controlled randomized trial of abatacept in patients with diffuse cutaneous systemic sclerosis. Arthritis Res Ther. 2015;17:159. doi: 10.1186/s13075-015-0669-3. PMID: 26071192.
74. Gordon JK, Martyanov V, Magro C, Wildman HF, Wood TA, Huang WT, Crow MK, Whitfield ML, Spiera RF. Nilotinib (Tasigna™) in the treatment of early diffuse systemic sclerosis: an open-label, pilot clinical trial. Arthritis Res Ther. 2015;17:213. doi: 10.1186/s13075-015-0721-3. PMID: 26283632.
75. Lafyatis R, et al. B cell depletion with rituximab in patients with diffuse cutaneous systemic sclerosis. Arthritis Rheum. 2009; 60(2):578–83.
76. Farina G, et al. A four-gene biomarker predicts skin disease in patients with diffuse cutaneous systemic sclerosis. Arthritis Rheum. 2010;62(2):580–8.
77. Christmann RB, et al. Interferon and alternative activation of monocyte/macrophages in systemic sclerosis-associated pulmonary arterial hypertension. Arthritis Rheum. 2011;63(6):1718–28.
78. Wu M, et al. Identification of cadherin 11 as a mediator of dermal fibrosis and possible role in systemic sclerosis. Arthritis Rheumatol. 2014;66(4):1010–21.

Part IX

Case Studies: Approach to Complex Clinical Problems

Managing the Ischemic Finger in Scleroderma

50

Fredrick M. Wigley

The case to be presented is not an actual case but was created from experience to represent an uncommon situation confounding the specialist caring for patients with scleroderma vascular disease.

Case Presentation

The patient is a 48-year-old Caucasian woman with limited scleroderma. The features of her disease include stiff puffy fingers, gastrointestinal reflux disease (GERD), severe Raynaud's phenomenon (RP), and a sicca syndrome. On her initial examination, the blood pressure was 120/69, weight 130 lb, pulse 79, temperature 98°, and normal respiratory rate. Sclerodactyly, numerous cutaneous telangiectasia on the palms and face, and definite abnormal nailfold capillaries with dilatation and areas of loss of capillaries were noted. The remainder of her examination was completely normal. The general laboratory testing was unremarkable but serology demonstrated high-titer anti-centromere antibodies. Both lung function testing and echocardiograph were normal. She was managed with a proton pump inhibitor for her GERD and artificial tears for her dry eyes.

Initial Therapy

When deciding the treatment of the RP, one must consider both improving quality of life and preventing ischemic injury to the digits and tissues. The foundation of the initial therapy for every patient with Raynaud's is nondrug management. Several daily activities, the effects of various drugs, and environmental factors greatly influence the severity of RP. Education reduces anxiety and provides the framework for the patient to avoid various aggravating factors. Patients have less Raynaud's attacks and improved quality of life after they understand why RP is happening and how to avoid the various triggers for a Raynaud's attack. A major factor in triggering events in scleroderma is the ambient temperature. In fact, managing the environmental exposures is still the most effective method to reduce the severity of RP. For example, shifting temperatures (moving into air conditioning or sitting in a cool breeze) is a major trigger for RP. Wearing layered clothing, gloves, and hat to keep the body warm is most important. Emotional stress is another factor that can trigger RP even if the patient is warm. Our patient is not a smoker, but smoking cessation is essential to reduce the risk of a severe digital ischemic event [1]. Certain drugs and agents that may cause peripheral vasoconstriction need to be avoided (see Table 50.1). Interestingly, the exact impact of managing anxiety and stress is not well studied. Interventions such as acupuncture, biofeedback, and techniques to help relaxation are not proven to be helpful, but sensible advice and good communications are clearly important.

Raynaud's phenomenon associated with scleroderma is a manifestation of peripheral vascular disease that is complicated by both abnormal vasoreactivity and structural vascular disease [2]. This vasculopathy increases the risk of ischemic-reperfu-

Table 50.1 Drugs that may aggravate Raynaud's phenomenon

Migraine headache drugs (serotonin agonist)
Cold preparations (sympathetic agonist)
Beta-blockers (controversial)
Caffeine (controversial)
ADHD: methylphenidate, dextroamphetamine-amphetamine, and atomoxetine
Weight-reducing drugs: ephedra
Estrogens (undefined)
Interferons, opiates, cocaine, polyvinyl chloride exposure, and chemotherapeutic drugs including cisplatin, bleomycin, or gemcitabine

F.M. Wigley, MD
Department of Medicine/Rheumatology,
The Johns Hopkins University School of Medicine,
5200 Eastern Avenue, Suite 4100, Mason F. Lord Building,
Center Tower, Baltimore, MD 21224, USA
e-mail: fwig@jhmi.edu

J. Varga et al. (eds.), *Scleroderma*, DOI 10.1007/978-3-319-31407-5_50

sion tissue injury due to severe repeated vasoconstriction, vascular occlusion, loss of cutaneous vessels, and defective vascular repair. While all patients with scleroderma should be considered at risk for complications from RP and peripheral vascular disease, certain subsets of patients are at greater risk for severe ischemic events which can lead to digital amputation. The patients at greatest risk of digital loss are those like our case with limited scleroderma and anti-centromere antibodies [3]. However, recurrent ischemic digital ulcers are more likely to occur in patients with diffuse skin disease [4]. Patients do appear to follow a consistent pattern of either no ischemic ulcers or one of recurring lesions.

When first seen, our patient had no signs of an ischemic event and was started on a calcium channel blocker (amlodipine 5 mg daily). Amlodipine was selected because it is a dihydropyridine-type calcium channel blocker, a class that is shown to have benefit for RP secondary to scleroderma [5]. Given the risk of occlusive vascular disease, she was also started on low-dose aspirin (81 mg daily). Studies to specifically define the role of antiplatelet therapy do not exist, but there is good rationale to use aspirin or similar agents because of the evidence of platelet activation in scleroderma [6]. She required and tolerated 15 mg of amlodipine to have a notable reduction in the severity of her RP.

The Ischemic Digital Crisis

While the patient was improved on this treatment, she suddenly developed a painful right index finger with persistent discoloration. The pain was intense and radiated from the fingertip to the palm of the hand. Despite resting and keeping very warm, the finger did not improve after several hours. On examination, the finger was ischemic with pale fingertip and hyperemia typical of ischemia from the distal interphalangeal joint extending distally (Fig. 50.1). The finger was swollen and tender to light touch. There was no capillary refilling following release of gentle pressure on the fingertip. The other fingers were cool but not ischemic. There were no lower extremity lesions and the examination of large vessels was normal. This included strong pulses in the upper and lower extremities. An Allen's test disclosed bilateral attenuation of the ulnar flow with good reflow through the radial and palmar arteries (Fig. 50.2).

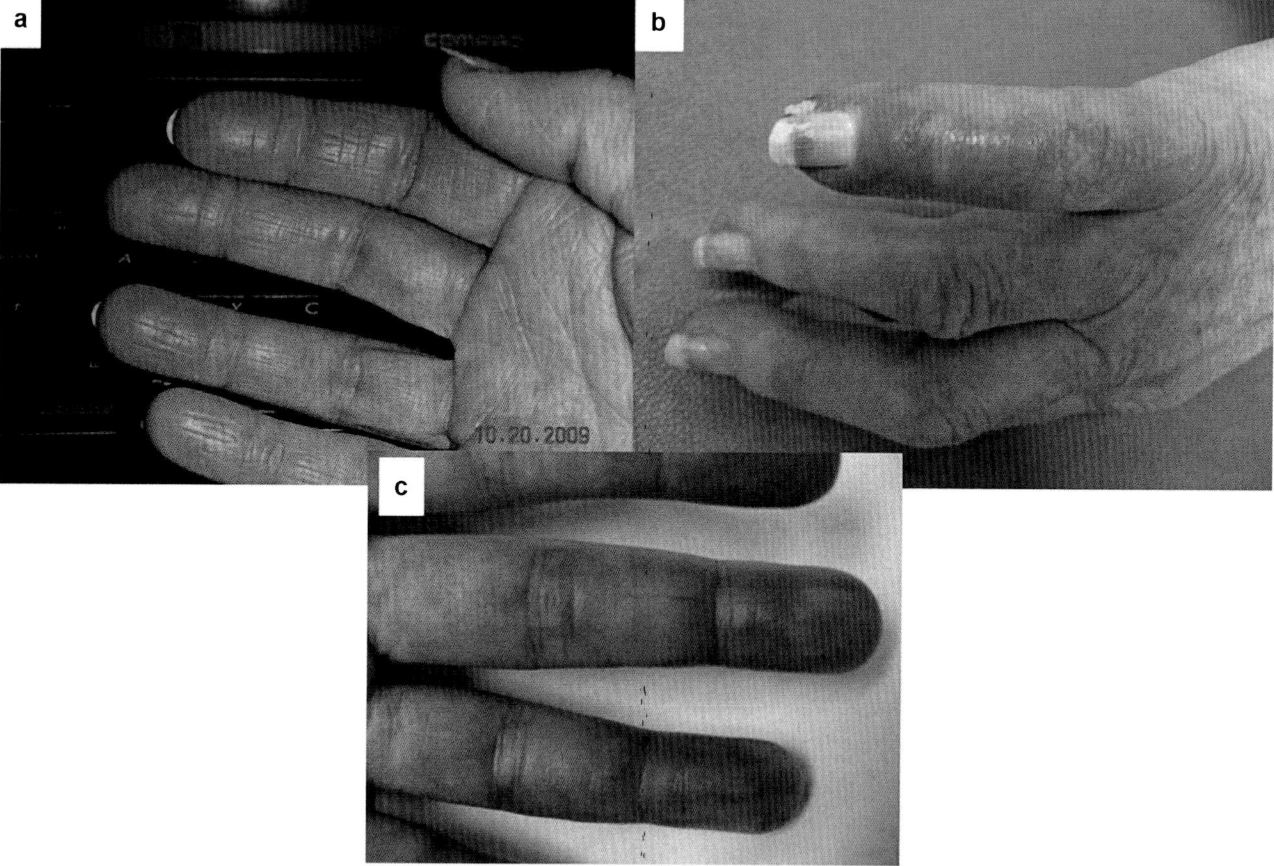

Fig. 50.1 (**a**) Cyanosis of the index finger due to digital ischemia in a patient with limited scleroderma. (**b**) Note the hyperemia of an acute ischemic finger demarcated to the distal finger. (**c**) Advancing ischemia with cyanotic fingertip

This patient presents with a medical emergency with the likelihood of acute loss of his digit due to critical ischemia secondary to underlying micro- and macrovascular disease. It is important to remember that while there is clearly significant vaso-occlusive disease in scleroderma, vasospasm plays a major role in acute ischemic events and quick action has the potential of reversing critical ischemia and tissue damage or digital loss. In this case, her amlodipine and low-dose aspirin alone failed to prevent the ischemic crisis. In order to manage the crisis, she was hospitalized. Pain control is also critical in managing this case. This was accomplished rapidly with a local digital injection of lidocaine instilled at the base of the finger. Bupivacaine is an alternative. This procedure that can be done by the rheumatologist or hand specialist may also provide a digital block to sympathetic tone and improve blood flow to the finger. Once the block dissipates, then longer-term pain control is needed with an opiate such as low-dose oxycodone (5–10 mg q6h) and/or a nonsteroidal anti-inflammatory drug.

In our case, with the local finger block, we obtained rapid but transient pain control, and we did not see immediate improvement in digital blood flow. Evaluation for a correctable lesion was done because the examination suggested ulnar artery compromise, a situation known to occur in patients with scleroderma [7]. Most of the time, both larger and diffuse small vessel disease occurs together in scleroderma, and therefore it is uncommon to find an isolated correctable lesion. The first study recommended is a Doppler ultrasound and then an angiography only if the initial evaluation suggests a high suspicion of larger vessel occlusion or thrombus. A CT angiogram is likely to not have the resolution to see smaller digital arteries and a conventional angiogram may be needed. If the imaging studies demonstrate a thrombus or correctable large vessel lesion, then immediate surgery becomes an option. Thrombolytic therapy for an acute thrombus can be done, but there is no good evidence to give specific guidance for this approach in scleroderma. In our case the Doppler confirmed that there was not a major vascular lesion that was approachable by surgical correction;

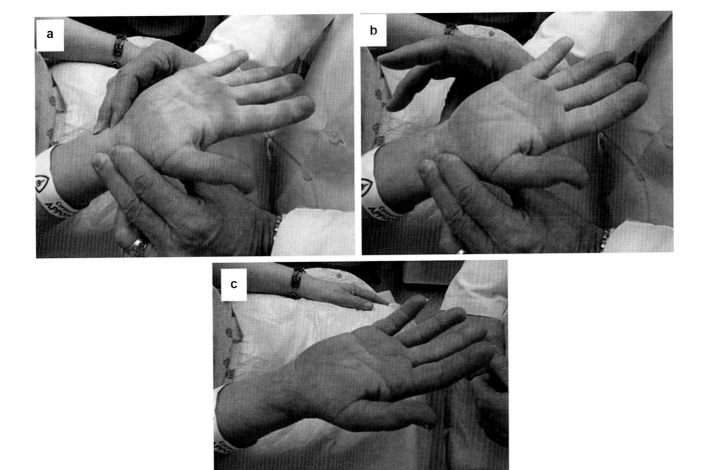

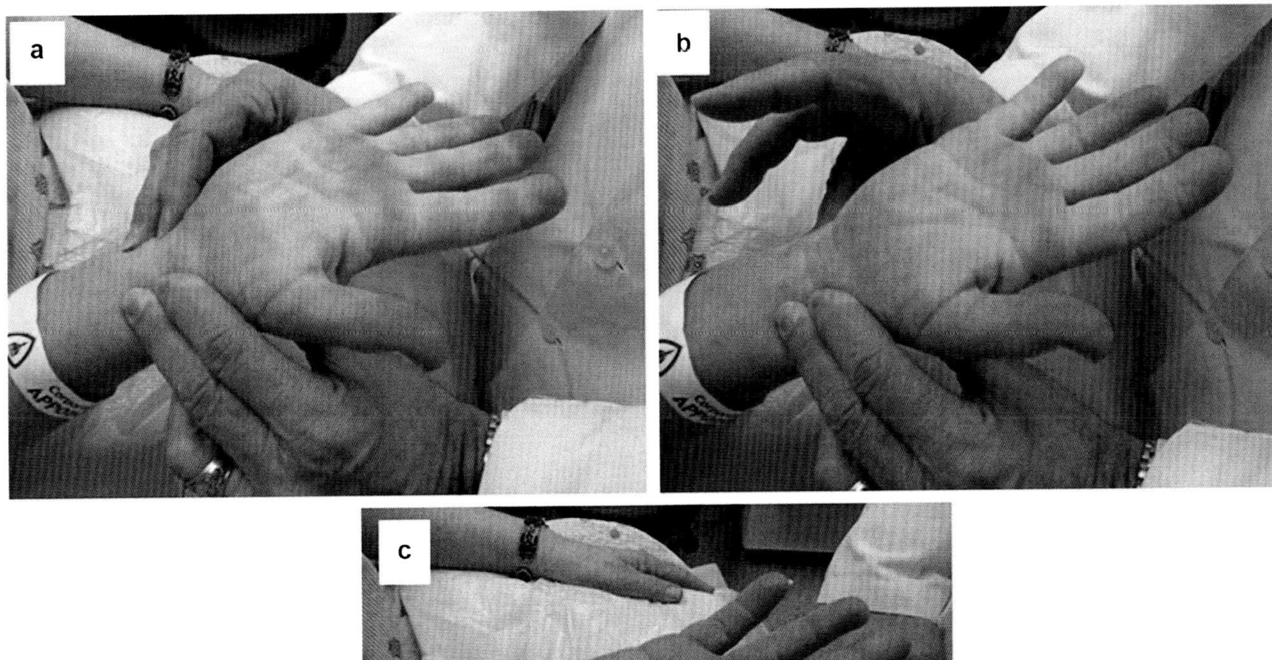

Fig. 50.2 Allen's test demonstrating compromise to ulnar flow to the hand. (**a**) Both arteries are occluded by pressure and the hand is pale. (**b**) The ulnar artery is released but the hand remains pale due to reduced blood flow. (**c**) The radial artery is released and blood flow returns and the hand flushes

nor was an isolated lesion defined that might represent a thrombus.

She had no contraindication to anticoagulation, and because the prolonged vasospasm with endothelial dysfunction is associated with thrombosis, she was acutely anticoagulated using intravenous heparin. This was continued for the next 48 h. Chronic anticoagulation in patients with scleroderma for digital ischemic events is not recommended unless a hypercoagulable state or define large thrombus is discovered.

Indication for Intravenous Therapy

Despite this therapy, the finger continued to appear ischemic and was not improving. In this situation, we begin intravenous prostacyclin (either epoprostenol or iloprost) [8]. It is best not to delay and therefore the infusion via a peripheral vein can be started while other diagnostic tests are being done. The rapid institution of the prostacyclin can stop the progression of the lesion and relieve acute vasoconstriction if occlusion or structural disease is not advanced. In non-acute situations, we administer epoprostenol (available in the USA) via a peripheral vein in an outpatient infusion center. Hospitalizing the patient provides the opportunity to deliver continuous therapy of prostacyclin (.5–2 ng/kg/min for 3–5 days). Each institution will have their own requirements and guidelines for administration of intravenous prostacyclin which is approved for the treatment of pulmonary hypertension by experts in pulmonary medicine. An observational study demonstrated that 12 % of patients in a scleroderma cohort required at least one hospitalization for administration of IV prostacyclin in an 18-month period [9]. If prostacyclin therapy is not available, then rapidly maximizing other vasodilating therapy in a controlled warm setting is an alternative. One option is to move to a rapid acting calcium channel blocker and titrating rapidly to maximum tolerated dose; for example, nifedipine 10 mg po tid increased to 20–30 mg po tid in a 24 h period. Another option is to combine the current extended release calcium channel blocker with another vasodilator. The most popular drugs to use in combination are a phosphodiesterase (PDE-5) inhibitor such as sildenafil 20–40 mg po tid or topical nitroglycerin (1/2 in. every 6 h of 2 % ointment with 12 h nitrate-free interval daily). In our case acute administration of botulinum toxin (Botox) injected locally by the skilled hand/vascular surgeon into the base of the involved finger was done, while prostaglandin infusion was underway. Our uncontrolled experience in this setting is that Botox has been helpful, usually seeing benefit in 48 h, but this recommendation is not evidence based [10]. This delayed benefit of Botox warrants the use of more acutely vasoactive agents when confronted with an acute ischemic finger. If vasoconstriction/vasospasm is not quickly reversed in patients with scleroderma, then vascular occlusion and rapid digital tissue injury will occur. The consequences can be loss of the involved digit (Fig. 50.3).

Indications for Digital Sympathectomy

If rest, pain control, and vasodilation therapy are not rapidly working, then surgical sympathectomy should be done. For example, if there is persistent digital ischemia that is not rapidly responding to a 3-day infusion of prostacyclin or if prostacyclin therapy is not available, then it is recommended to move to digital sympathectomy [11]. Delay in doing a sympathectomy may result in loss of the digit if the ischemic phase of vasospasm is not reversed quickly and irreversible thrombosis or occlusion occurs. It is no longer recommended to use a proximal sympathectomy because of the increased morbidity of the procedure and the effectiveness of an approach right at the level of the digit. If vasodilator therapy is not effective, then a digital sympathectomy can be done with or without Botox injection. In our experience, rapid intervention with digital sympathectomy can prevent digital loss and quickly reverse a critical ischemic event. In the long term, a digit or digits that have undergone a sympathectomy procedure will continue to have episodes of RP, but the severity is less and new ischemic events are much less common. A skilled vascular or hand surgeon should be able to do the procedure with low morbidity.

Prevention of Recurrent Digital Ischemic Events

In our case the prostacyclin therapy and acute anticoagulation were successful and the finger ischemia rapidly improved. The first indication of success was the resolution of pain or need for pain medications. Tissue ischemia is painful and when blood flow returns pain rapidly improves. The other signs followed with improved tissue color and decreased soft tissue swelling. The next issue then was the prevention of a relapse or new episodes. Maximizing the oral vasodilator therapy to maintain control of vasospasm is critical. In this case she was on a full dose of a calcium blocker but was tolerating it with normal blood pressure and no peripheral edema. We elected to add the PDE-5 inhibitor, sildenafil at 20 mg daily with slow titration to 20 mg tid [12]. Often sildenafil or another PDE-5 inhibitor is not available. In such cases

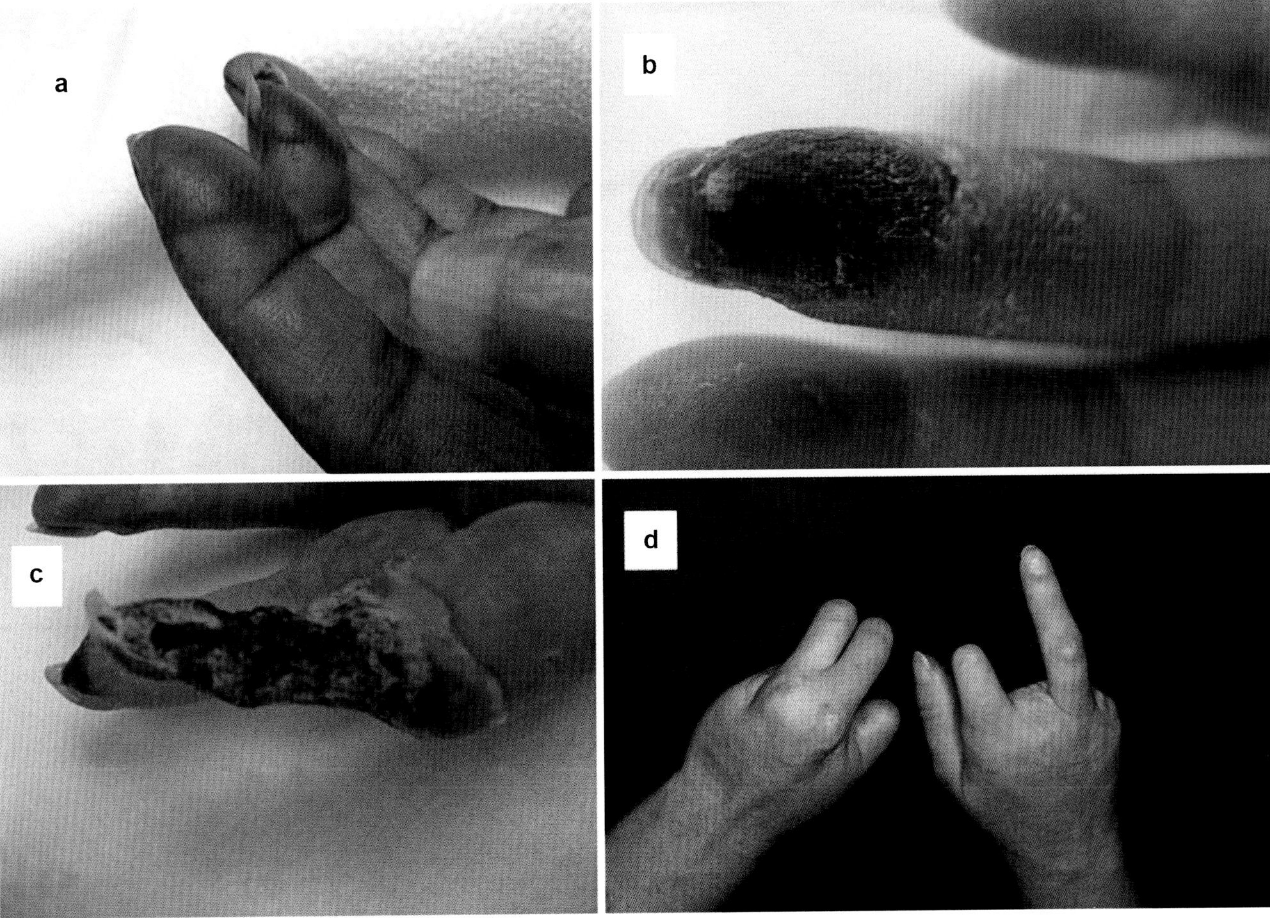

Fig. 50.3 Acute ischemic finger with advancing tissue injury and finger loss. (**a**) Early infarct of the distal finger. (**b**) Deep injury to the finger with early gangrene. (**c**) Advanced dry gangrene. (**d**) Loss of multiple fingers from scleroderma vascular disease

topical nitrates (2 % nitroglycerin cream/ointment) can be applied starting with 1/2 in. and titrating to 2 in. at 6 h intervals twice with 12 h nitrate-free interval daily [13].

In cases that cannot tolerate intense oral or topical vasodilator due to intolerance or low blood pressure, then we recommend preventive therapy with intermittent intravenous prostacyclin, for example, every 1–3 months depending on the severity of the RP. Another option is intermittent Botox injection, an attractive option especially if the Botox appeared to have an impact on first use. However, both prostacyclin and Botox may be difficult to have readily available and alternatives need to be considered. There is some evidence that a selective serotonin reuptake inhibitor (SSRI) like fluoxetine 20–40 mg daily may be helpful [14]. Another prevention strategy is the institution of a statin, a class of drugs that may protect vessels and in theory reduce the risk of ischemic digital lesions [15, 16]. Anti-platelet agents such as aspirin (81 mg po daily) or clopidogrel should be continued if there is no contraindication such as active bleeding. An endothelin receptor inhibitor (e.g., bosentan) is reported to prevent new digital ulcers from occurring in patients with scleroderma, but there is no solid evidence that this class of agents will prevent acute digital ischemia as in our case or reverse the acute vasospasm of RP [17].

In our case the finger improved after the prostacyclin infusion and continues to do well on the combination therapy of amlodipine and sildenafil with both improvement in the severity of her RP and no new severe ischemic events. In cases that do not respond to this aggressive approach and who go on to develop advanced digital injury with dry gangrene (Fig. 50.3), then surgical amputation is the only option. This procedure should be done only after the digit has completely demarcated from an occlusive event. Indications for surgery would be intractable pain or secondary infection with wet gangrene.

Key Principle Lessons of the Case

1. A subset of patients with scleroderma is at risk for major vascular events presenting with digital ischemia.
2. Rapid and aggressive intervention in cases of digital ischemia is essential to prevent tissue damage or loss of digit.
3. Rest, warm temperature, pain control, antiplatelet therapy, and vasodilation therapy are all important components of care. This may require hospitalization.
4. Intravenous prostacyclin can rapidly reverse acute vasospasm in the setting of digital ischemia.
5. Botox delivered by local injection may be helpful to prevent relapse but full evidence for this approach is still needed.
6. Acute anticoagulation may also be helpful but full evidence for this approach is still needed. Chronic anticoagulation is not recommended in the absence of a hypercoagulable state.
7. If medical therapy is not rapidly working, then digital sympathectomy should be done if vasoconstriction is still present.
8. Once the acute episode is resolved, then preventive therapy needs to be in place including either oral vasodilator therapy or intermittent intravenous prostacyclin.
9. Preventive therapy with antiplatelet therapy or statins may have a role but more evidence is needed to define their role.

References

1. Hudson M, Lo E, Lu Y, Canadian Scleroderma Research Group, et al. Cigarette smoking in patients with systemic sclerosis. Arthritis Rheum. 2011;63(1):230–8.
2. Wigley FM. Vascular disease in scleroderma. Clin Rev Allergy Immunol. 2009;36(2–3):150–75.
3. Wigley FM, Wise RA, Miller R, et al. Anticentromere antibody as a predictor of digital ischemic loss in patients with systemic sclerosis. Arthritis Rheum. 1992;35(6):688–93.
4. Denton CP, Krieg T, Guillevin L, DUO Registry investigators, et al. Demographic, clinical and antibody characteristics of patients with digital ulcers in systemic sclerosis: data from the DUO Registry. Ann Rheum Dis. 2012;71(5):718–21.
5. Thompson AE, Shea B, Welch V, et al. Calcium-channel blockers for Raynaud's phenomenon in systemic sclerosis. Arthritis Rheum. 2001;44(8):1841–7.
6. Pauling JD, O'Donnell VB, McHugh NJ. The contribution of platelets to the pathogenesis of Raynaud's phenomenon and systemic sclerosis. Platelets. 2013;24(7):503–15.
7. Park JH, Sung YK, Bae SC, et al. Ulnar artery vasculopathy in systemic sclerosis. Rheumatol Int. 2009;29(9):1081–6.
8. Wigley FM, Wise RA, Seibold JR, et al. Intravenous iloprost infusion in patients with Raynaud phenomenon secondary to systemic sclerosis. A multicenter, placebo-controlled, double-blind study. Ann Intern Med. 1994;120(3):199–206.
9. Nihtyanova SI, Brough GM, Black CM, et al. Clinical burden of digital vasculopathy in limited and diffuse cutaneous systemic sclerosis. Ann Rheum Dis. 2008;67(1):120–3.
10. Iorio ML, Masden DL, Higgins JP. Botulinum toxin A treatment of Raynaud's phenomenon: a review. Semin Arthritis Rheum. 2012; 41(4):599–603.
11. Hartzell TL, Makhni EC, Sampson C. Long-term results of periarterial sympathectomy. J Hand Surg [Am]. 2009;34(8):1454–60.
12. Brueckner CS, Becker MO, Kroencke T, et al. Effect of sildenafil on digital ulcers in systemic sclerosis: analysis from a single centre pilot study. Ann Rheum Dis. 2010;69(8):1475–8.
13. Anderson ME, Moore TL, Hollis S, et al. Digital vascular response to topical glyceryl trinitrate, as measured by laser Doppler imaging, in primary Raynaud's phenomenon and systemic sclerosis. Rheumatology (Oxford). 2002;41(3):324–8.
14. Coleiro B, Marshall SE, Denton CP, et al. Treatment of Raynaud's phenomenon with the selective serotonin reuptake inhibitor fluoxetine. Rheumatology (Oxford). 2001;40(9):1038–43.
15. Kuwana M. Potential benefit of statins for vascular disease in systemic sclerosis. Curr Opin Rheumatol. 2006;18(6):594–600.
16. Abou-Raya A, Abou-Raya S, Helmii M. Statins: potentially useful in therapy of systemic sclerosis-related Raynaud's phenomenon and digital ulcers. J Rheumatol. 2008;35(9):1801–8.
17. Matucci-Cerinic M, Denton CP, Furst DE, et al. Bosentan treatment of digital ulcers related to systemic sclerosis: results from the RAPIDS-2 randomised, double-blind, placebo-controlled trial. Ann Rheum Dis. 2011;70(1):32–8.

Scleroderma Renal Crisis

51

Edward P. Stern and Christopher P. Denton

Case

Mrs M is a 53-year-old Caucasian nurse who was previously fit and well. Her only prior medical history is of essential hypertension, for which she has taken ramipril 5 mg daily for 2 years. She was referred to a rheumatologist with a 3-month history of puffy fingers and Raynaud's phenomenon. Physical examination demonstrated skin thickening bilaterally on the upper limbs, extending proximal to the elbows—modified Rodnan skin score (MRSS) of 21/51 and palpable tendon friction rubs anteriorly at both ankles and in the right wrist. Examination of the cardiovascular, respiratory and abdominal systems was unremarkable. Her blood pressure (BP) reading was 130/70 mmHg and her urine dipstick analysis was normal.

Full blood count and routine biochemistry tests were all normal. Serum creatinine was 61 umol/L (0.69 mg/dL), giving an eGFR of >90 ml/min. Antinuclear antibodies (ANA) were strongly positive (>1:1,000) with a fine speckled/nucleolar staining pattern. Abnormal nailfold capillaroscopy with dilated capillary loops and reduced vessel density confirmed the diagnosis of diffuse cutaneous systemic sclerosis (dcSSc).

She was started on therapy with mycophenolate mofetil (MMF) primarily for active skin disease at a dose of 500 mg twice daily, which was titrated up to 1 g twice daily the following month. At this stage she was also started on prednisolone 15 mg daily for joint pain and pruritis, and omeprazole 20 mg twice daily was added for gastroesophageal reflux. Given the risk of scleroderma renal crisis (SRC) in patients with dcSSc, she was advised to buy a home BP monitor and to check her BP at least three times a week (Fig. 51.1).

Three weeks after this, she presented to the emergency department complaining of shortness of breath and headache. Her blood pressure had been at its baseline level 24 h previously, but that afternoon she had measured it at 180/110 mmHg. Oxygen saturations were 88 % on room air. On auscultation of the chest, she had coarse crepitations to the midzones bilaterally. Fundoscopy demonstrated cotton-wool spots, consistent with Grade 3 hypertensive retinopathy. Skin thickening had worsened since her last clinic visit and her fingers were poorly perfused distally.

Urinalysis was positive for both blood and protein, and serum creatinine was 195 umol/L (2.2 mg/dL). As this was >3 times her stable baseline creatinine, she was classified as having Stage 3 acute kidney injury (AKI). Haemoglobin concentration was 102 g/L, platelet count was 73 and red cell fragments were seen on her blood film.

A chest radiograph confirmed the presence of moderate pulmonary oedema and she went on to have an echocardiogram. This showed left ventricular systolic dysfunction (estimated ejection fraction 25 %) and a high estimated pulmonary artery systolic pressure of 45 mmHg.

Ramipril was titrated up over the following 48 h to 10 mg daily. She was also started on continuous low-dose iloprost infusion to treat her severe Raynaud's phenomenon. Despite this, her blood pressure remained significantly above her baseline clinic values at 160/100. In addition her renal function continued to deteriorate with a creatinine of 455 umol/L (5.2 mg/dL) on day 3 after admission and declining urine output. The angiotensin receptor blocker losartan was added in, resulting in a modest decline in systolic blood pressure and some improvement in her respiratory symptoms. On day 5 she was started on intermittent haemodialysis, initially to treat refractory hyperkalaemia.

Her BP subsequently stabilised with the addition of a third vasodilator (the alpha-blocker doxazosin); thrombocytopenia and haemolysis resolved. She continued to be oliguric and dependent on IHD. Percutaneous renal biopsy was performed

E.P. Stern, MBBS, MRCP (✉)
Centre for Rheumatology, Royal Free Hospital, London NW3 2PF, UK
e-mail: e.stern@ucl.ac.uk

C.P. Denton, PhD, FRCP
Division of Medicine, Department of Inflammation, Centre for Rheumatology and Connective Tissue Diseases, UCL Division of Medicine, Royal Free Hospital, London, UK

J. Varga et al. (eds.), *Scleroderma*, DOI 10.1007/978-3-319-31407-5_51

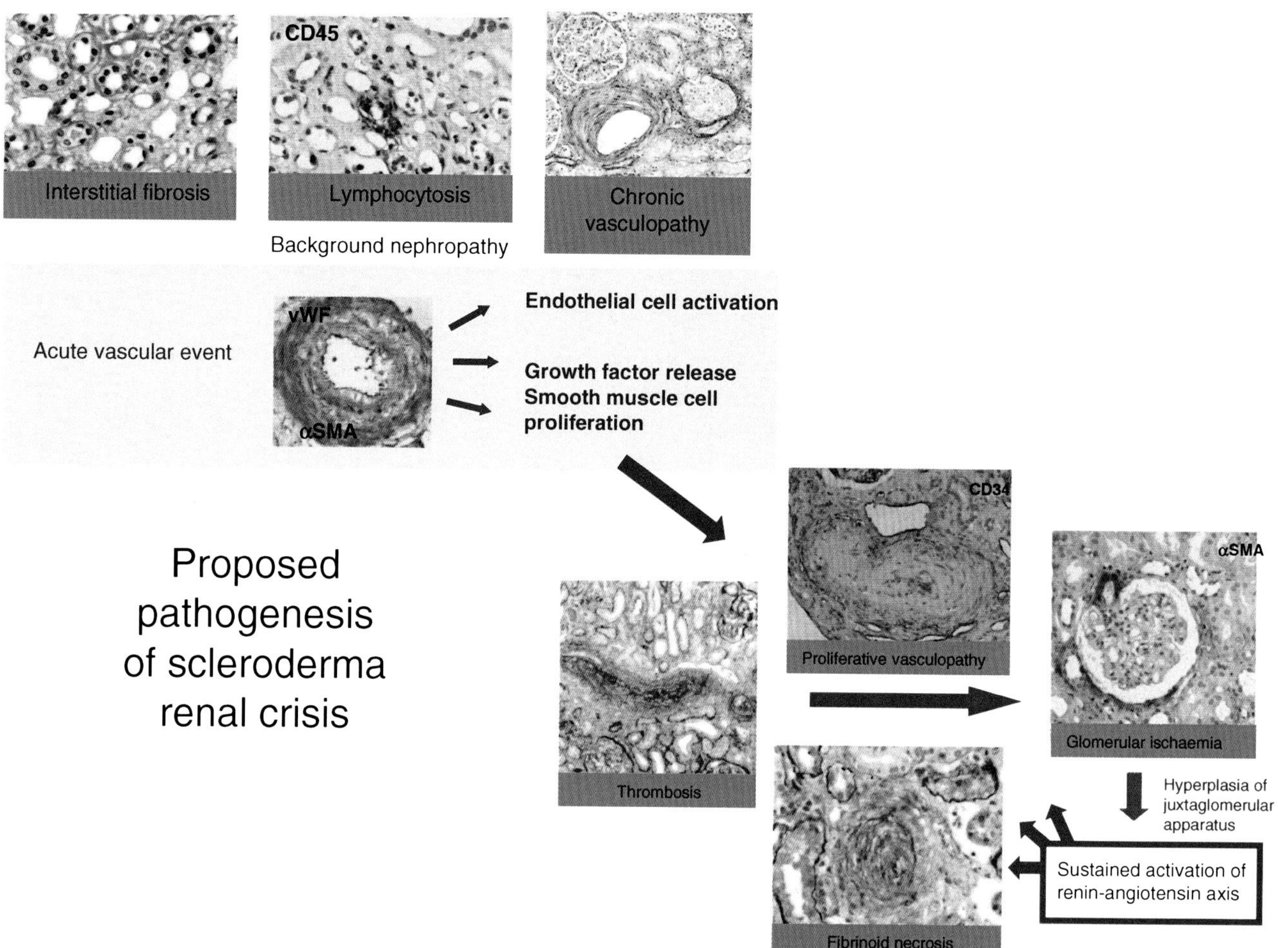

Fig. 51.1 Pathogenic processes underlying scleroderma renal crisis. Model of events that underlie development of SRC. It appears that background changes occur in many individuals but susceptibility and an acute triggering event lead to SRC. Autopsy specimens confirm that inflammation, fibrosis and chronic proliferative vasculopathy are often present in scleroderma, but it is believed that an acute vascular injury or event that triggers hypertension results in other events that lead to glomerular ischemia and increased renin-angiotensin axis activity. This results in severe proliferative vasculopathy (Courtesy of Professor Alec Howie)

on day 20: this demonstrated fibrinoid necrosis and adventitial fibrosis in the medium sized and small intrarenal arteries, occasional collapsed glomeruli and a relatively preserved tubulointerstitium (Fig. 51.2).

She was discharged home on day 30 but continued to attend for three times weekly IHD as an outpatient. Once she was established on long-term dialysis, her antihypertensive requirements reduced and losartan and doxazosin were eventually stopped. A follow-up echocardiogram demonstrated that her estimated left ventricular systolic function and pulmonary artery pressure had normalised. Pulmonary function tests were normal.

Twelve months after initial presentation with SRC, Mrs M was still on IHD. Her sister approached the nephrology team to be considered as a donor for live-related renal transplantation and was found to be a suitable donor. However, over the following months, Mrs M's urine output increased somewhat and her pre-dialysis creatinine levels were noted to be falling each week. She had a trial off IHD after 18 months, and her creatinine stabilised around 225 umol/L (2.5 mg/dL) giving her an eGFR of 21 ml/min. Renal function continued to improve over the subsequent year and was stable at 35 ml/min 3 years after diagnosis of SRC with no significant haematuria or proteinuria.

Discussion

Mrs M is an archetypal patient at high risk of SRC. At the time of presentation, she had early diffuse SSc, rapidly progressive skin score and a nucleolar staining pattern on ANA

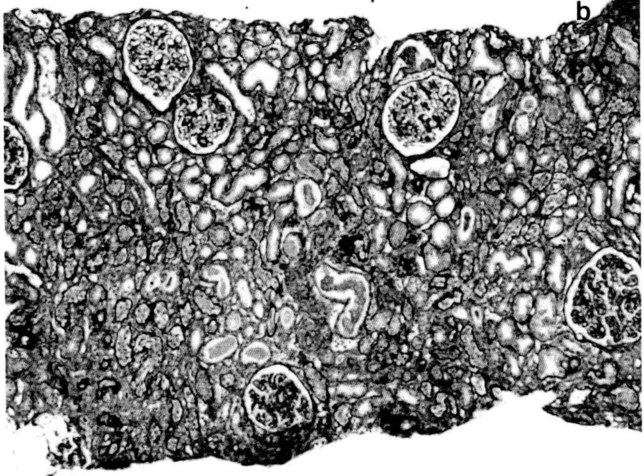

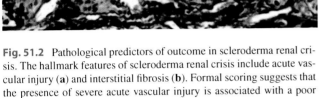

Fig. 51.2 Pathological predictors of outcome in scleroderma renal crisis. The hallmark features of scleroderma renal crisis include acute vascular injury (**a**) and interstitial fibrosis (**b**). Formal scoring suggests that the presence of severe acute vascular injury is associated with a poor prognosis and increased likelihood of permanent need for dialysis. Conversely the extent of fibrotic scar does not appear to reflect long-term renal outcome (Slides courtesy of Prof Alec Howie)

(anti-RNA polymerase III antibodies were later confirmed). Her rheumatologist appreciated this risk, choosing to minimise the dose of corticosteroid she was prescribed and arranged for her to do home BP monitoring [1, 2].

She was on angiotensin-converting enzyme (ACE) inhibitor therapy prior to the diagnosis of systemic sclerosis, for essential hypertension. There is no evidence that "prophylactic" ACE-inhibitor therapy reduces the risk of SRC, and in fact it is associated with a higher mortality (although there are many reasons that this finding may be confounded) [3].

A rise in systolic BP >20 mmHg above her baseline and an increase of >10 % from her baseline creatinine mean that she fulfilled the consensus criteria for a diagnosis of SRC when she presented to the emergency department. Pulmonary oedema, hypertensive retinopathy and microangiopathic haemolytic anaemia are all supportive of this diagnosis.

A renal biopsy was not performed at this stage because uncontrolled hypertension confers a high risk of bleeding complications. Biopsy may be considered once blood pressure and coagulation have normalised. The most important indication for this is to exclude an alternative cause for renal impairment. Differential diagnoses for AKI in this context would include allergic tubulointerstitial nephritis (TIN) caused by one of her recently introduced medications (proton pump inhibitors are among the most common causes of TIN in developed countries) or a coexisting glomerular disease, e.g. ANCA-associated vasculitis or lupus nephritis. ANCA positivity or overlap serology would be clues in such cases and they are less likely to be associated with severe hypertension [4, 5]. Biopsy may also give prognostic information regarding the chance of renal recovery [2] (Fig. 51.3).

The team caring for this patient continued to titrate up her ACE inhibitor despite worsening renal function, which is appropriate. However, her BP was not sufficiently well controlled on maximal dose of ramipril. In this setting there is no consensus regarding the best add-in agents but there are some general considerations. Beta-blockers are contraindicated in SRC as they can cause catastrophic circulatory collapse in the context of very high peripheral resistance.

Angiotensin receptor blockers (ARBs) may be beneficial given the survival benefit conferred by antagonising another part of the same renin-angiotensin system (RAS), but they have not been demonstrated to be of equivalent benefit to ACE inhibitors when used alone [6]. Furthermore, dual RAS inhibition (ARB + ACE inhibitor) is associated with a significantly increased risk of hyperkalaemia, as was seen in this case [7]. Iloprost has been demonstrated to be an effective renal vasodilator in patients with SSc, and our practice is to give 10 days of low-dose continuous iloprost in SRC; however the specific benefits in this setting are unproven [8].

Finally, this case illustrates that the uncertain long-term prognosis for patients with renal crisis has a specific impact on their renal replacement therapy planning: unlike in other causes of end-stage renal failure, early transplantation may not be appropriate. Recovery of independent renal function more than 2 years after being established on dialysis is not uncommon. In such patients, the GFR may continue to improve for several years, and they appear to be relatively protected from the gradual decline in renal function that is typical in other forms of chronic kidney disease [2, 9, 10].

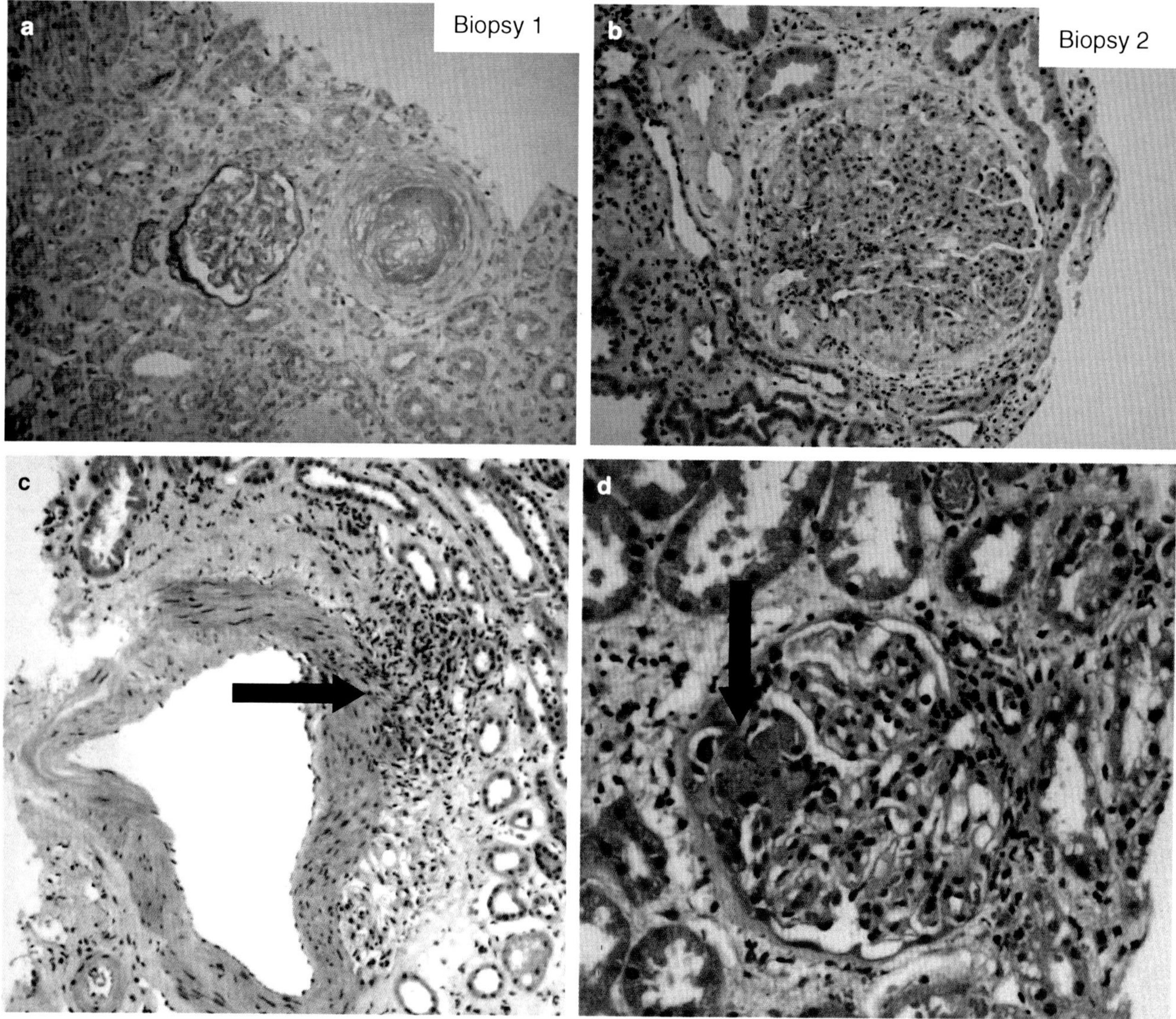

Fig. 51.3 Inflammatory renal pathology in scleroderma biopsy specimens. It is important to perform renal biopsy in cases of suspected glomerulonephritis. Clues for this included increased proteinuria and active urinary sediment or serological clues. (**a**) In the *upper case*, this was the presence of newly discovered high-titre anti-dsDNA antibodies in a case that had previously demonstrated a typical SRC on biopsy (**a**) with good outcome; there was later deterioration in renal function and increased proteinuria and the repeat renal biopsy showed membranoproliferative glomerulonephritis (**b**). The *lower case* had early dcSSc and high-titre ANCA and haematuria with normal renal function and the renal biopsy demonstrated vasculitis (**c**) and early crescentic glomerulonephritis (**d**) (Courtesy of Professor Alec Howie)

References

1. Trang G, Steele R, Baron M, Hudson M. Corticosteroids and the risk of scleroderma renal crisis: a systematic review. Rheumatol Int. 2012;32:645–53.
2. Penn H, et al. Scleroderma renal crisis: patient characteristics and long-term outcomes. QJM. 2007;100:485–94.
3. Hudson M, Baron M, Tatibouet S, Furst DE, Khanna D. Exposure to ACE inhibitors prior to the onset of scleroderma renal crisis-results from the International Scleroderma Renal Crisis Survey. Semin Arthritis Rheum. 2014;43:666–72.
4. Torpey N, Barker T, Ross C. Drug-induced tubulo-interstitial nephritis secondary to proton pump inhibitors: experience from a single UK renal unit. Nephrol Dial Transplant. 2004;19:1441–6.
5. Derrett-Smith EC, Nihtyanova SI, Harvey J, Salama AD, Denton CP. Revisiting ANCA-associated vasculitis in systemic sclerosis: clinical, serological and immunogenetic factors. Rheumatology (Oxford). 2013;52:1824–31.
6. Caskey FJ, Thacker EJ, Johnston PA, Barnes JN. Failure of losartan to control blood pressure in scleroderma renal crisis. Lancet. 1997;349:620.
7. Makani H, Bangalore S, Desouza KA, Shah A, Messerli FH. Efficacy and safety of dual blockade of the renin-angiotensin system: meta-analysis of randomised trials. BMJ. 2013;346:f360.
8. Scorza R, et al. Effect of iloprost infusion on the resistance index of renal vessels of patients with systemic sclerosis. J Rheumatol. 1997;24:1944–8.
9. Steen VD. Long-term outcomes of scleroderma renal crisis. Ann Intern Med. 2000;133:600.
10. Guillevin L, et al. Scleroderma renal crisis: a retrospective multicentre study on 91 patients and 427 controls. Rheumatology (Oxford). 2012;51:460–7.

Rapid Diffuse Skin Disease with Progressive Joint Contractures

52

Faye N. Hant and Richard M. Silver

Case Presentation

The patient is a 64-year-old female diagnosed with diffuse cutaneous systemic sclerosis (dcSSc). She developed tight swelling in her hands, feet, wrists, and arms with subsequent involvement of the face and trunk over the ensuing 2 months. The skin was intensely pruritic with superimposed burning sensation. She reported difficulty with hand grip and could not make a fist. She could not fully extend her elbows and had stiffness upon movement of her hips, knees, and ankles. She denied joint swelling or pain, but did note pain in both arms and legs along with a severe "rubbing" sensation while moving her extremities. She had Raynaud's phenomenon (RP), nonproductive cough, gastroesophageal reflux, and sicca symptoms. Physical examination was notable for sclerodactyly with loss of full range of motion of the proximal interphalangeal (PIP) and metacarpophalangeal (MCP) joints of hands (Fig. 52.1) and elbows; the involved skin was thickened and edematous with erythema over the forearms. Loss of hair was noted on the dorsum of the hands and forearms. A diffuse hyperpigmentation of the skin was noted. The modified Rodnan skin score (mRSS) was 25 (maximum 51); tendon friction rubs (TFRs) were palpable at her elbows, knees, and ankles; no joint tenderness or swelling was noted. Nailfold capillary morphology was abnormal with mildly dilated capillary loops. Laboratory evaluation revealed a positive ANA (1:160 titer, speckled pattern) and the presence of RNA polymerase III auto-antibodies. Comprehensive metabolic panel, complete blood count, CK, aldolase, thyroid testing, and urinalysis were all within normal limits. On pulmonary assessment the 6 min walk distance was limited to 316 m, forced vital capacity (FVC) was 83 % predicted, total lung capacity (TLC) was 89 % predicted, and diffusion lung capacity for carbon monoxide (DLCO) was 90 % predicted. High-resolution CT scan (HRCT) of the chest was normal, but the esophagus was dilated and gas-filled. Echocardiogram was normal except for stage 1 (mild) left ventricular diastolic dysfunction. She was started on a proton pump inhibitor for gastroesophageal reflux and a calcium channel blocker and low-dose aspirin for RP. She was placed on low-dose prednisone (10 mg daily) for her TFRs and was prescribed a blood pressure cuff and counseled on the importance of close monitoring of her blood pressure.

Introduction and Background

This case presents one of the most challenging situations in caring for a patient with scleroderma: how to manage the early rapidly progressive phase of skin disease. While there are no proven disease-modifying drugs that are approved for the management of skin disease, most believe early

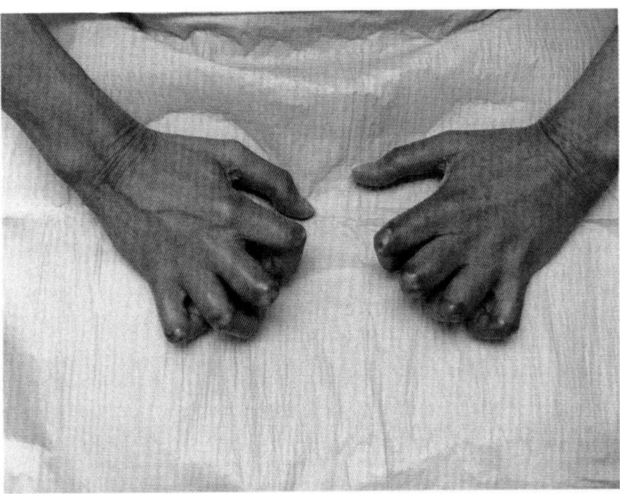

Fig. 52.1 Fixed flexion contractures of the small joints of hands in a patient who had rapidly progressive diffuse cutaneous systemic sclerosis

F.N. Hant, DO, MSCR • R.M. Silver, MD (✉)
Division of Rheumatology and Immunology, Medical University of South Carolina, Charleston, SC 29425, USA
e-mail: silverr@musc.edu

J. Varga et al. (eds.), *Scleroderma*, DOI 10.1007/978-3-319-31407-5_52

intervention with an immunosuppressive/anti-inflammatory agent can alter the course of the skin disease. Recognizing the limitations of proven options, the fact that there are no FDA-approved therapies or established standard of care, treatment is often designed by one's own experience or it is based on the current bias of the community of experts caring for patients with scleroderma. Whenever possible the authors recommend that patients in the early phase of skin disease be referred to a scleroderma specialty center to participate in organized research including clinical trials. Only by a community effort will the ideal therapy be discovered. In the absence of a research option, we recommend the following principles: (1) establish the current phase of the skin disease (i.e., is the disease active and progressive or late fibrotic inactive skin?), (2) document the extent of the disease using a modified Rodnan skin score to allow a measure of outcome, (3) consider the association with internal organ involvement and disease-related consequences, (4) take measures to prevent further morbidity and improve quality of life (e.g., control pain, physical and occupational therapy), and (5) initiate intervention.

SSc patients with diffuse cutaneous disease have a higher risk of death compared to patients with limited cutaneous involvement. Diffuse cutaneous SSc patients typically develop significant internal organ involvement, with the highest proportion of new organ systems (pulmonary, cardiac, and renal complications) affected within the first 3 years [1]. An association of scleroderma-specific auto-antibodies with certain prognostic, clinical, and laboratory characteristics is well known [2]. Joint involvement and tendon friction rubs (TFRs) are most often seen in dcSSc patients with anti-topoisomerase (Scl-70), anti-RNA polymerase III (Pol-3), or anti-U3-RNP auto-antibodies [2]. Patients with anti-Pol-3 antibodies have the highest frequency of scleroderma renal crisis and rapidly develop the most severe skin disease with the highest mRSS [2]. This particular scleroderma auto-antibody is frequently associated with the presence of a speckled ANA (can also have a nucleolar ANA), extensive skin and tendon involvement early in the disease course, negative anti-topoisomerase (Scl-70) auto-antibodies, and associated cancer and rarely is there severe interstitial lung disease [2]. There is also concern about an increased risk of gastrointestinal bleeding from GAVE. Our case presentation illustrates some of these associations.

The natural course of skin thickening in patients with dcSSc is variable. Skin thickness typically progresses over the first 2–5 years of disease and then gradually improves [3]. The prospective Pittsburgh Scleroderma Databank revealed that patients in the "improved group" (skin thickening improved by >25 % of peak skin score and a rate of change of at least 5 units/year) had an average improvement of 50 % of their peak skin score at 2 years after initial visit, and, importantly, survival was significantly better in the "improved group" at 5 and 10 years (90 % and 80 %, respectively) compared to the "unimproved group" (increased skin thickening or no improvement) (77 % and 60 %, respectively, at 5 and 10 years, ($p<0.0001$) [4]. A skin thickness progression rate (STPR), defined as the mRSS at the first patient visit divided by duration of skin thickening (in years) by patient report, may be a useful measure to perform at initial evaluation to identify patients who may be at increased risk of death and more likely to develop scleroderma renal crisis within the next 2 years [5]. A "rapid" STPR of >/= 45 has been reported to be an independent predictor of both scleroderma renal crisis within 2 years from first evaluation (OR 2.05, 95 % CI 1.10–3.85) and mortality (OR 1.72, 95 % CI 1.13–2.62) [5]. STPR is an easy measure that can be obtained at the initial visit that allows the identification of those at increased risk of scleroderma renal crisis and death [5].

Our case has findings of loss joint mobility, an early sign that joint contractures will develop if the disease is not controlled. Joint contracture is an abnormal, typically permanent shortening of scar tissue or muscle, especially within a joint, resulting in deformity [6]. Joint contractures are common in dcSSc patients, affecting large and small hand joints, and they can be a major source of morbidity and disability [7]. As the disease progresses, there may be tethering of the skin and contracture of the underlying joints, leading to a decrease in function and motor abilities [6]. The EULAR Scleroderma Trials and Research (EUSTAR) registry found in a cross-sectional examination that 31 % of patients had joint contractures, more prevalent in dcSSc patients with severe renal, muscular, vascular and interstitial lung involvement [8]. A recent study of 131 patients with 3-year follow-up found a high frequency of baseline joint contractures in the shoulders (50 %), wrists (75 %), and small joints of hands (82 %) and noted a significant decrease in ROM of the dominant hand (suggesting impaired function) compared to the nondominant hand [9].

Our case has active TFRs suggesting to us that aggressive therapy is warranted. The presence of palpable TFRs is associated with diffuse skin involvement, reduced survival, shorter disease duration, and both cardiac and renal involvement [10–12]. One study comparing early dcSSc patients having TFRs to early dcSSc patients without TFRs found that the presence of one or more TFRs was associated with an increased risk of cardiac (OR 3.26, 95 % CI 1.35–7.84), gastrointestinal (OR 5.14, 95 % CI 1.74–15.17), and renal involvement (OR 2.66, 95 % CI 1.23–5.75), as well as with increased mortality; after age and sex adjustments, TFR cases had a 5-year mortality 1.8 times greater than those without TFRs (95 % CI 1.21–2.58, $p=0.003$) [12]. SSc patients with TFRs are not more likely to have joint contractures than those SSc patients without TFRs [12].

Treatment Considerations

A number of different therapeutic agents have been assessed in the treatment of scleroderma skin disease, most with limited evidence for efficacy [13]. Limitations of the reported studies in SSc include small numbers, lack of placebo-controlled design, the heterogeneity of the stage of the skin disease under study, and the lack of appropriate timing of a therapeutic intervention [13]. We will approach our case using agents that are available as if there is no research trial option available. First, we noted that on the low-dose steroids, there was an improvement in joint pain and motion, but the nature of the skin disease was unchanged. For the pruritus, we started both an antihistamine (hydroxyzine 25 mg po q6h) and gabapentin (100 mg at bedtime). We instituted a physical therapy program to improve ADL and relieve pain. A nonsteroidal anti-inflammatory (ibuprofen 600 mg q8h) was given to use only as needed due to concerns about gastrointestinal side effects including gastrointestinal bleeding.

Methotrexate

We started our patient on methotrexate by subcutaneous injection of 1 ml at 25 mg/ml once weekly. We elected to use methotrexate because of our experience that it can help both active skin disease and the inflammatory joint/tendon process; it is our first option for early, mild skin disease. Methotrexate (MTX) has been reported to be efficacious in the treatment of skin progression in two randomized, placebo-controlled, double-blind, multicenter trials [14, 15]. In a 24-week trial followed by an observational period of 24 weeks, van den Hoogen et al. randomized 29 patients (11 dcSSc and 18 lcSSc with <3-year duration of skin thickening) to receive MTX 15 mg intramuscular weekly ($n = 17$) or placebo ($n = 12$) [15]. Patients who had a favorable response (defined as an improvement of total skin score (TSS) by >/= 30 %, of DLCO by >/= 15 %, or of the score on a visual analogue scale (VAS) of general well-being by >/= 30 %) after 24 weeks continued with the same regimen for an additional 24 weeks. Participants who showed a poor response on placebo were crossed over to MTX, and those who responded poorly to treatment with MTX 15 mg weekly had an increase in dose to 25 mg weekly [15]. After 24 weeks, a significantly greater number of patients receiving MTX ($n = 8$, 53 %) who completed the first 24 weeks of the study had responded favorably compared to patients receiving placebo ($n = 1$, 10 %, $p = 0.03$). In an intention-to-treat analysis, TSS decreased in the MTX group and increased in the placebo group ($p = 0.06$); however this difference was not stratified by subset of SSc [15]. Another study of 71 patients with dcSSc of <3 years' duration randomized 35 patients to methotrexate and 36 to placebo for 12 months, with the primary outcome being skin score and physician global assessment (PGA) [17]. At 12 months, results slightly favored the MTX group (mean ± SEM mRSS 21.4 ± 2.8 in the MTX group vs. 26.3 ± 2.1 in the placebo group, $p < 0.17$), and PGA results also favored MTX ($p < 0.035$) [14]. The authors concluded that the results of their trial demonstrated a trend in favor of MTX vs. placebo, but did not provide evidence that MTX is significantly effective in the treatment of patients with early dcSSc [14]. MTX is now considered a treatment option for skin manifestations of early dcSSc (strength of recommendation = A), based on a report from the European League Against Rheumatism (EULAR) and the EULAR Scleroderma Trials and Research group (EUSTAR) [16].

Mycophenolate Mofetil (MMF)

After 2 months of therapy, the patient clearly had progressed with advancing skin changes now on the proximal arms and legs with intense pruritus and decreased flexibility of major joints. Truncal skin on the chest and abdomen worsened with sparing of the back. At this point our options were to continue MTX and low-dose prednisone or to move to or add another agent. Given the intensity of our patient's skin disease, we elected to add mycophenolate mofetil (MMF) beginning at a dose of 500 mg twice daily and slowly titrating to full dose of 1,500 mg twice daily over several months. We check safety laboratory data (complete blood count (CBC) and liver profile) every 2 weeks during this phase of therapy. A retrospective study looked at a single-center experience using MMF comparing the change in mRSS in a MMF cohort at baseline with scores at 3, 6, 9, and 12 months to those of historical controls from a pooled analysis of three negative large, randomized controlled clinical trials of other medications (recombinant human relaxin, oral bovine type I collagen, and d-penicillamine) [21]. The mean mRSS of the patients treated with MMF decreased progressively over time from baseline, 3, 6, 9, and 12 months (mean mRSS: 24.4 ± 9.5, 23.4 ± 10.1, 21.4 ± 10.6, 17.5 ± 10.3, and 17.5 ± 10.4, respectively). Compared to baseline, there was no statistically significant change in mRSS at 3 months ($p = 0.255$); however statistical significance was reached at 6, 9, and 12 months when compared to baseline mRSS (all $p < 0.001$) [21]. The mRSS of the MMF cohort did not differ from the historical controls at 6 months but was significantly lower at 12 months (MMF −7.59 ± 10.1 vs d-penicillamine −2.47 ± 8.6, $p < 0.001$; collagen −3.4 ± 7.12, $p = 0.002$) [21]. In an open-label study to evaluate the efficacy and safety of MMF (titrated to 3,000 mg daily) to treat dcSSc patients over 12 months, 15 patients were recruited with the primary outcome being mRSS; a statistically significant improvement in mRSS was noted in those patients who tolerated the medication for >3 months ($p<0.0001$) [22]. In a pilot study of 16 patients with early SSc with either active ILD or extensive skin disease, a protocol-based treatment strategy combined the use of MMF, intravenous (IV) methylprednisolone (MP) pulses, and low-dose glucocorticoids [23]. Here, patients received three consecutive daily IV MP pulses, followed by five additional monthly IV MP pulses; MMF (titrated to 1,000 mg twice daily) and low-dose (5–10 mg daily) oral prednisolone were prescribed for 1 year; such treatment resulted in a statistically significant improvement in mRSS [23]. A 2007 retrospective analysis examined the duration, indications, and tolerability of MMF to treat dcSSc ($n=109$) compared with a control cohort ($n=63$) treated with other immunosuppressive medications [24]. MMF was well tolerated with a lower frequency of clinically significant pulmonary fibrosis in the MMF-treated cohort ($p=0.037$) and significantly better 5-year survival from disease onset and from commencement of treatment ($p=0.027$ and $p=0.012$, respectively); no significant difference between the two groups was found for mRSS [24].

Cyclophosphamide

We considered the use of cyclophosphamide (CYC) but decided to use MMF since MMF is considered to be less toxic and perhaps equally effective. A large randomized trial has recently been completed comparing CYC to MMF in the treatment of scleroderma lung disease, and preliminary analysis suggests this may be the case. The Scleroderma Lung Study (SLS-I) was a multicenter randomized, double-blind, placebo-controlled trial that looked at the safety and efficacy of daily oral CYC versus placebo for 1 year in SSc patients with ILD, followed by 1-year off therapy [18]. In the trial, 145 of 158 patients completed at least 6 months of treatment and were included in the analysis. Following a year of treatment with CYC, dyspnea, skin thickening, functional ability, and some health-related measures of the quality of life improved [18]. In an effort to assess whether these effects were sustained at 24 months, a longitudinal assessment was performed and found that the beneficial effects of CYC on pulmonary function and health status continued to increase through 18 months, after which they ceased, and skin improvements also ceased after 12 months [19]. The effect of CYC on musculoskeletal involvement was also evaluated in the SLS, and the proportion of patients with large joint contractures did not change [20]. Small hand-joint contractures did seem to improve (as measured by the ability to make a fist) over 24 months, but this was independent of treatment, either CYC or placebo [20]. Given these data and our desire to avoid side effects from CYC, we chose to use MMF instead. We expected that if MMF was to be effective, the patient would sense improvement or stabilization in 1–3 months and a decrease in the mRSS in 6–12 months. In other words, the first signs of dampening of the skin disease activity will be reduced pruritus, pain, and the lack of new areas of skin involvement. Following this the patient will note improved flexibility, new hair growth, and a sense of well-being that precedes any change in measureable skin texture or skin score.

Intravenous Immunoglobulin (IVIg)

In the next 8 weeks, the patient did not improve on this combination therapy with worsening joint flexibility and early contractures, progressive skin changes, and continued fatigue with discomfort in the muscles and soft tissues. The mRSS worsened. There was no evidence of any new internal organ disease. The options at this point were to continue on the same therapy hoping that with time there would be a response, to stop MMF and move to a new approach, or to add yet a third agent to the current regimen. Consideration of novel therapy was considered including immunoablation therapy, rituximab, other biologics, or IVIg. We elected to continue MMF and to institute IVIg. The IVIg was given monthly at 400 mg/kg daily over 5 days. IVIg is used to treat a variety of different autoimmune conditions as well as scleromyxedema, another fibrosing skin condition [25]. IVIg is also used when patients with SSc have an overlap syndrome with an inflammatory myositis. It has also been reported as adjunctive therapy for refractory skin disease. In a "tight-skin" mouse model, IVIg administration led to a significant decrease in type I collagen gene expression and collagen deposition and inhibition of TGFβ1 [26]. IVIg may also decrease fibrosis through the presence of anti-Fas and anti-fibroblast antibodies in the IVIg preparation itself [27]. In a randomized, double-blind placebo-controlled trial of a single cycle infusion dose of IVIg (400 mg/kg/day for five consecutive days: a single course) vs. placebo in 63 patients with dcSSc, there was no difference in mRSS between the groups at 12 weeks [28]. Trial participants whose mRSS did not improve by five points at 12 weeks were dosed an additional cycle of IVIg, and it was noted that those who received two IVIg treatments had a greater improvement in mRSS over time than those who received placebo followed by a later IVIg infusion. The authors concluded that although their primary outcome was not attained, repeated administration of IVIg for two courses may be effective for diffuse skin disease [28]. A retrospective study of IVIg (2 g/kg/month) to treat refractory, active dcSSc patients ($n=30$) unresponsive to current traditional therapies compared the mRSS at baseline to the mRSS at 6, 12, 18, and 24 months after starting IVIg therapy and also compared the changes in mRSS at 6 and 12 months to historical control data from three negative large, randomized controlled clinical trials of other medications (relaxin, collagen, and d-penicillamine), as well as to patients on MMF alone [29]. The authors noted significant changes in mRSS over time in patients treated with IVIg and also in comparison to historical controls in their cohort. In those treated with IVIg, the mean baseline mRSS was 29.6 ± 7.2, and this decreased to 24.1 ± 9.6 (n = 29, p = 0.0011) at 6 months, 22.5 ± 10.0 (n = 25, p = 0.0001) at 12 months, 20.6 ± 11.8 (n = 23, p = 0.0001) at 18 months, and 15.3 ± 6.4 (n = 15, $p < 0.0001$) at 24 months [29]. Compared to historical controls, the mean change in mRSS at 6 months was not significantly different in the IVIg group (-5.3 ± 7.9) compared to the relaxin trial (-4.8 ± 6.99, $p = 0.74$) or MMF group (-3.4 ± 7.4, $p = 0.26$); however, at 12 months, the mean change in mRSS was significantly better in the IVIg group (-8 ± 8.3) than in the D-pen (-2.47 ± 8.6, $p = 0.005$) and collagen (-3.4 ± 7.12, $p = 0.005$) groups, and was comparable to the group of primary MMF responders (-7.1 ± 9, p = 0.67) [29].

Tyrosine Kinase Inhibitors

We considered starting imatinib mesylate, a tyrosine kinase (TK) inhibitor with activity against c-abl, platelet-derived growth factor receptor (PDGFR), or another TK inhibitor, but we decided against using a TK inhibitor because of the lack of evidence of benefit in early skin disease and the high frequency of side effects. However, due to its ability to interfere with PDGF and TGF-β signaling, there has been interest in TK inhibitors as therapeutic agents in SSc [30–32]. In a phase IIa, single arm, open-label clinical trial, dcSSc patients were treated with imatinib mesylate 400 mg daily [32]. Of 30 participants, 24 completed 12 months of therapy. Many (171) adverse events (AE) with possible relation to imatinib mesylate were identified, 97.6 % being classified as mild to moderate. In addition, 24 serious adverse events (SAE) were identified, two of which were attributed to imatinib mesylate. The mRSS decreased by 6.6 points (22.4 %) at 12 months ($p=0.001$), and this change was noted beginning at the 6-month time point ($\Delta=-4.5$; $p<0.001$) and seen in patients with both early and late-stage disease. A 6-month, randomized, double-blind, placebo-controlled, proof-of-concept pilot study aimed to further investigate the role of imatinib mesylate in dcSSc [33]. These investigators found imatinib mesylate to be poorly tolerated due to AE which included edema, fluid retention, nausea, cramps/myalgia, and diarrhea among others, and furthermore no significant difference was observed in the mean mRSS in all patients who took imatinib mesylate (31.1 at baseline vs. 29.4 at 6 months) or in those that completed 6 months of the drug (31 at baseline vs. 30.3 at 6 months) [33]. In a recent 24-month open-label, extension phase, single-center trial to assess the long-term tolerability and safety of imatinib mesylate in dcSSc, 17 patients were enrolled. Forty of 92 AE and none of 6 serious SAEs were possibly related to medication, and overall the mRSS decreased from a median of 21–16, ($p=0.002$) [34].

Rituximab

We also considered treating our patient with rituximab (RTX) given that several small studies have investigated the efficacy of RTX for the treatment of dcSSc, including three open-label studies, one multicenter-nested case-control trial and one randomized controlled trial [35–41]. The rationale for use of this agent stems from evidence that B cells and auto-antibodies contribute to fibrosis in the lungs and skin of patients with SSc [39, 42]. Daoussis et al. performed a study to assess the efficacy of RTX in SSc and randomized eight patients with dcSSc and ILD to receive two cycles (each cycle was four weekly infusions of RTX 375 mg/m^2) at baseline and 24 weeks in addition to standard of care treatment, and six controls received standard of care treatment alone [36]. Skin scores improved significantly in the RTX group compared with the baseline score (mean ± SD = 13.5 ± 6.84 vs. 8.37 ± 6.45 at baseline vs. 1-year, respectively, $p<0.001$), contrasted to the control group, where no significant change in mRSS was noted (mean ± SD = 11.50 ± 2.16 vs. 9.66 ± 3.38 at baseline vs. 1 year, respectively, $p=0.16$) [36]. Skin tissue showed a significant reduction in dermal collagen at 24 weeks compared with baseline in the RTX-treated group (mean ± SD: 51.75 ± 19.78 vs. 31.68 ± 14.02 at baseline vs. week 24, respectively, $p=0.030$) [36]. The control group showed no change in collagen deposition at 24 weeks compared with baseline values (mean ± SD = 46.53 ± 22.43 vs. 46.27 ± 10.49 at baseline vs. week 24, respectively, $p=0.980$). In an open-label study of RTX (two doses of 1,000 mg IV, 2 weeks apart) in 15 patients with recent onset dcSSc (mean 14.5 months, range 9–18 months), there was no improvement in skin score at baseline compared to 6 months, despite noting both circulating and dermal B cell depletion [39]. In another open-label pilot study, after a two-treatment course of RTX (two doses of 1000 mg IV, 2 weeks apart, at months 0 and 6) in patients with early dcSSc, there was a clinically significant change in skin score (decrease in mRSS of 11.2 at 24 months vs. baseline, mRSS 13.6 and 24.8, respectively, $p<0.0001$), equating to a 45 % mean improvement in mRSS at month 24 vs. baseline [41]) with no significant progression in internal organ involvement [41]. In general, the studies looking at RTX are small and with inconsistent dosing regimens and trial periods. Although promising, further evaluation of RTX is necessary in the form of large randomized, placebo-controlled trials.

Immunoablation with Stem Cell Rescue

Given the aggressive nature of the skin disease in our patient and her failure to respond to MTX and MMF, we also considered immunoablation therapy, but decided not to use it due to the lack of internal organ disease and the reported treatment-related mortality risk. High-dose immunosuppressive therapy and hematopoietic autologous stem cell transplantation (HSCT) are established treatments for various hematologic and oncologic conditions, and the potential role of this as a treatment in SSc is actively being studied. The European Group for Blood and Marrow Transplantation and EULAR published results from the Autologous Stem Cell Transplantation International Scleroderma (ASTIS) trial, which was the first randomized controlled trial of autologous HSCT vs. pulse monthly cyclophosphamide in early dcSSc [43]. A total of 156 patients were randomly assigned to receive HSCT ($n = 79$) or cyclophosphamide ($n = 77$), with the primary end point being event-free survival, defined as time from randomization until the occurrence of death or persistent major organ failure [43]. During a median follow-up of 5.8 years, 53 events occurred: 22 in the HSCT group (19 deaths, 3 irreversible organ failures) and 31 in the control group (23 deaths, 8 irreversible organ failures). Time-varying hazard ratios for event-free survival were 0.35 (95 % CI, 0.16–0.74) at 2 years and 0.34 (95 % CI, 0.16–0.74) at 4 years, and the investigators concluded that among patients with early dcSSc, HSCT was associated with increased treatment-related mortality in the first year after treatment but provided a significant long-term, event-free survival benefit [43]. The results of the ongoing multicenter NIH-funded clinical trial, stem cell transplant vs. cyclophosphamide (SCOT; NCT00114530), being conducted throughout the United States are eagerly awaited to further assess efficacy and treatment-related mortality [44]. In a recent editorial, several issues are raised as to whether HSCT is ready for clinical practice [44]. The authors emphasize that the optimal conditioning regimen for autologous HSCT in SSc is unknown, and that may be a specific "window of therapeutic opportunity" in which a patient with progressive SSc and internal organ involvement might be considered for HSCT [44, 45]. Potential candidates to be considered for HSCT might include (a) patients with dcSSc within the first 4–5 years of onset with mild-moderate internal organ involvement or (b) lcSSc patients with progressive internal organ involvement, and this should be limited to patients who have failed standard immunosuppressive therapies [44].

After IVIg was started, our patient had definite improvement and the skin texture improved gradually over the next 6 months. We discontinued IVIg after 6 monthly infusions and continued the MMF. The low-dose prednisone was slowly tapered off. After 12 months the patient continued in a remission with only residual hand and finger involvement and mild skin texture changes on the forearm and dorsum of the feet (mRSS 6); more importantly, the skin did not have an inflammatory quality, new hair growth was noted on the forearms, and the patient had a marked improvement of well-being. The patient was maintained on MMF but the dose was reduced to 1000 mg twice daily for the next 6 months. The duration of MMF therapy needed is unknown, but we elect to continue therapy for 2–3 years in severe cases due to an experience of skin and disease flares following discontinuation of MMF in the early recovery phase of the disease.

Rehabilitation Therapy

Despite the lack of robust studies, we routinely engage our patients in physical and occupational therapy. Also, we try to have family members play a role in helping and understanding the needs of the patient by educating them as to what is needed. As noted above, deformities and contractures of the hand are major factors in diminished quality of life and disability in patients with SSc. Physical therapy (PT) and occupational therapy (OT) are often utilized to address impairment of hand function. A recent Canadian study sought to determine the proportion of SSc patients having hand involvement and having been referred to and used OT and PT services. Of 317 patients with hand involvement, only 90 (28 %) reported a referral to PT or OT, and only 39 (12 %)

Key Principle Lessons of the Case

1. Skin disease is best treated in the early active phase before irreversible fibrosis, skin damage, and contractures occur.
2. We strongly recommend that patients with early skin disease have a comprehensive evaluation for internal organ involvement.
3. In the absence of proven disease-modifying therapy, it is recommended that patients with early active skin disease be referred to specialty centers for the opportunity to participate in organized clinical trials.
4. Evidence suggests that immunosuppression/anti-inflammatory agents can dampen the progression of scleroderma skin disease.
5. Novel approaches to controlling the skin disease are under study and more evidence is needed to define their role.
6. Managing a patient with early skin disease requires a comprehensive approach that includes managing pain, providing physical and occupational therapy, as well as emotional support for the patient and family.

reported actually utilizing these services [46]. Much of the recent literature on rehabilitation techniques in SSc suffer from small sample sizes with no control groups and consist of studies evaluating the effectiveness of face and hand stretching exercises, paraffin wax treatment, connective tissue joint massage and manipulation, splints, and resistance training and aerobic exercise [47]. Several studies show improvement in joint motion, hand function, and cardiopulmonary endurance, except for dynamic splinting which failed to maintain PIP extension in patients with flexion contractures [47, 48]. More robust studies are required in the area of rehabilitative therapy as an adjunctive modality in the overall comprehensive care of the patient with SSc.

References

1. Steen VD, Medsger Jr TA. Severe organ involvement in systemic sclerosis with diffuse scleroderma. Arthritis Rheum. 2000;43: 2437–44.
2. Steen VD. Autoantibodies in systemic sclerosis. Semin Arthritis Rheum. 2005;35:35–42.
3. Medsger Jr TA, Steen VD, Ziegler G, Rodnan GP. The natural history of skin involvement in progressive systemic sclerosis [abstract]. Arthritis Rheum. 1980;23:720 1.
4. Steen VD, Medsger Jr TA. Improvement in skin thickening in systemic sclerosis associated with improved survival. Arthritis Rheum. 2001;44(12):2828–35.
5. Domsic RT, Rodriguez-Reyna T, Lucas M, Fertig N, Medsger Jr TA. Skin thickness progression rate: a predictor of mortality and early internal organ involvement in diffuse scleroderma. Ann Rheum Dis. 2011;70:104–10.
6. Avouac J, Clements PJ, Khanna D, Furst DE, Allanore Y. Articular involvement in systemic sclerosis. Rheumatology. 2012;51:1347–56.
7. Malcarne VL, Hansdottir I, McKinney A, Upchurch R, Greenbergs HL, Henstorf GH, et al. Medical signs and symptoms associated with disability, pain, and psychosocial adjustment in systemic sclerosis. J Rheumatol. 2007;34:359–67.
8. Avouac J, Walker U, Tyndall A, et al. Characteristics of joint involvement and relationships with systemic inflammation in systemic sclerosis: results from the EULAR Scleroderma Trial and Research Group (EUSTAR) database. J Rheumatol. 2010;37(7):1488–501.
9. Balint Z, Farkas H, Farkas N, Minier T, Kumanovics G, Horvath K, Solyom AI, Czirjak L, Varju C. A three-year follow-up study of the development of joint contractures in 131 patients with systemic sclerosis. Clin Exp Rheumatol. 2014;32(6 suppl 86):68–74.
10. Steen VD, Powell DL, Medsger Jr TA. Clinical correlations and prognosis based on serum autoantibodies in patients with systemic sclerosis. Arthritis Rheum. 1988;31:196–203.
11. Steen VD, Medsger Jr TA. The palpable tendon friction rub: an important physical examination finding in patients with systemic sclerosis. Arthritis Rheum. 1997;40:1146–51.
12. Dore A, Lucas M, Ivanco D, Medsger Jr TA, Domsic RT. Significance of palpable tendon friction rubs in early diffuse cutaneous systemic sclerosis. Arthritis Care Res. 2013;65(8):1385–9.
13. Frech TF, Shanmugam VK, Shah AA, Assassi S, Gordon JK, Hant FN, Hinchcliff ME, Steen V, Khanna D, Kayser C, Domsic RT. Treatment of early diffuse systemic sclerosis skin disease. Clin Exp Rheumatol. 2013;31:166–71.
14. Pope JE, Bellamy N, Seibold JR, Baron M, Ellman M, Carette S, Smith CD, Chalmers IM, Hong P, O'Hanlon D, Kaminska E, Markland J, Sibley J, Catoggio L, Furst DE. A randomized, controlled trial of methotrexate versus placebo in early diffuse scleroderma. Arthritis Rheum. 2001;44(6):1351–8.
15. van den Hoogen FH, Boerbooms AM, Swaak AJ, Rasker JJ, van Lier HJ, van de Putte LB. Comparison of methotrexate with placebo in the treatment of systemic sclerosis: a 24 week randomized double-blind trial, followed by a 24 week observational trial. Br J Rheumatol. 1996;35(4):364–72.
16. Kowal-Bielecka O, Landewé R, Avouac J, Chwiesko S, Miniati I, Czirjak L, Clements P, Denton C, Farge D, Fligelstone K, Földvari I, Furst DE, Müller-Ladner U, Seibold J, Silver RM, Takehara K, Toth BG, Tyndall A, Valentini G, van den Hoogen F, Wigley F, Zulian F, Matucci-Cerinic M, EUSTAR Co-Authors. EULAR recommendations for the treatment of systemic sclerosis: a report from the EULAR Scleroderma Trials and Research group (EUSTAR). Ann Rheum Dis. 2009;68(5):620–8.
17. Nadashkevich O, Davis P, Fritzler M, Kovalenko W. A randomized unblinded trial of cyclophosphamide versus azathioprine in the treatment of systemic sclerosis. Clin Rheumatol. 2006;25(2):205–12.
18. Tashkin DP, Elashoff R, Clements PJ, Goldin J, Roth MD, Furst DE, for the Scleroderma Lung Study Research Group, et al. Cyclophosphamide versus placebo in scleorderma lung disease. N Engl J Med. 2006;354:2655–66.
19. Tashkin DP, Elashoff R, Clements PJ, Goldin J, Roth MD, Furst DE, for the Scleroderma Lung Study Research Group, et al. Effects of 1-year treatment with cyclophosphamide on outcomes at 2 years in scleroderma lung disease. Am J Respir Crit Care Med. 2007;176(10):1026–34. See comment in PubMed Commons below.
20. Au K, Mayes MD, Maranian P, Clements PJ, Khanna D, Steen VD, Tashkin D, Roth MD, Elashoff R, Furst DE. Course of dermal ulcers and musculoskeletal involvement in systemic sclerosis patients in the scleroderma lung study. Arthritis Care Res. 2010;62(12):1772–8.
21. Le EN, Wigley FM, Shah AA, Boin F, Hummers LK. Long-term experience of mycophenolate mofetil for treatment of diffuse cutaneous systemic sclerosis. Ann Rheum Dis. 2011;70(6):1104–7. See comment in PubMed Commons below.
22. Derk CT, Grace E, Shenin M, Naik M, Schulz S, Xiong W. A prospective open-label study of mycophenolate mofetil for the treatment of diffuse systemic sclerosis. Rheumatology (Oxford). 2009;48(12):1595–9.
23. Vanthuyne M, Blockmans D, Westhovens R, Roufosse F, Cogan E, Coche E, Nzeusseu Toukap A, Depresseux G, Houssiau FA. A pilot study of mycophenolate mofetil combined to intravenous methylprednisolone pulses and oral low-dose glucocorticoids in severe early systemic sclerosis. Clin Exp Rheumatol. 2007;25(2):287–92.
24. Nihtyanova SI, Brough GM, Black CM, Denton CP. Mycophenolate mofetil in diffuse cutaneous systemic sclerosis – a retrospective analysis. Rheumatology (Oxford). 2007;46(3):442–5.
25. Baleva M, Nikolov K. The role of intravenous immunoglobulin preparations in the treatment of systemic sclerosis. Int J Rheumatol. 2011;2011:829751. PubMed: 22121376.
26. Blank M, Levy Y, Amital H, Shoenfeld Y, Pines M, Genina O. The role of intravenous immunoglobulin therapy in mediating skin fibrosis in tight skin mice. Arthritis Rheum. 2002;46(6):1689–90.
27. Molina V, Blank M, Shoenfeld Y. Intravenous immunoglobulin and fibrosis. Clin Rev Allergy Immunol. 2005;29(3):321–6.
28. Takehara K, Ihn H, Sato S. A randomized, double-blind, placebo-controlled trial: intravenous immunoglobulin treatment in patients with diffuse cutaneous systemic sclerosis. Clin Exp Rheumatol. 2013;31(2 Suppl 76):151–6.
29. Poelman CL, Hummers LK, Wigley FM, Anderson C, Boin F, Shah AA. Intravenous immunoglobulin may be an effective therapy for refractory, active diffuse cutaneous systemic sclerosis. J Rheumatol. 2015;42:236–42.
30. Distler JH, Distler O. Intracellular tyrosine kinases as novel targets for anti-fibrotic therapy in systemic sclerosis. Rheumatology (Oxford). 2008;47 Suppl 5:v10–1.

31. Rosenbloom J, Castro SV, Jiminez SA. Narrative review: fibrotic diseases: cellular and molecular mechanisms and novel therapies. Ann Intern Med. 2010;152:159–66.
32. Spiera RF, Gordon JK, Mersten JN, Magro CM, Mehta M, Wildman HF, Kloiber S, Kirou KA, Lyman S, Crow MK. Imatinib mesylate (Gleevec) in the treatment of diffuse cutaneous systemic sclerosis: results of a 1-year, phase IIa, single-arm, open-label clinical trial. Ann Rheum Dis. 2011;70(6):1003–9. doi:10.1136/ard.2010.143974.
33. Pope J, McBain D, Petrlich L, Watson S, Vanderhoek L, de Leon F, Seney S, Summers K. Imatinib in active diffuse cutaneous systemic sclerosis: results of a six-month, randomized, double-blind, placebo-controlled, proof-of-concept pilot study at a single center. Arthritis Rheum. 2011;63(11):3547–51.
34. Gordon J, Udeh U, Doobay K, Magro C, Wildman H, Davids M, Mersten JN, Huang WT, Lyman S, Crow MK, Spiera RF. Imatinib mesylate (Gleevec) in the treatment of diffuse cutaneous systemic sclerosis: results of a 24-month open label, extension phase, single-centre trial. Clin Exp Rheumatol. 2014;32(6 Suppl 86): S-189–93.
35. Jordan S, Distler JHW, Maurer B, et al. Effects and safety of rituximab in systemic sclerosis: an analysis from the European Scleroderma Trial and Research (EUSTAR) group. Ann Rheum Dis. 2014. doi:10.1136/annrheumdis-2013-204522.
36. Daoussis D, Liossis S-NC, Tsamandas AC, et al. Experience with rituximab in scleroderma: results from a 1-year, proof-of-principle study. Rheumatology. 2010;49:271–80.
37. Daoussis D, Liossis S-NC, Tsamandas AC, et al. Effect of long-term treatment of rituximab on pulmonary function and skin fibrosis in patients with diffuse systemic sclerosis. Clin Exp Rheumatol. 2012;30(2 Suppl 71):S17–22.
38. Bosello S, De Santis M, Lama G, et al. B cell depletion in diffuse progressive systemic sclerosis: safety, skin score modification and IL-6 modulation in an up to thirty-six months follow-up open-label trial. Arthritis Res Ther. 2010;12:R54.
39. Lafaytis R, Kissin E, York M, et al. B cell depletion with rituximab in patients with diffuse cutaneous systemic sclerosis. Arthritis Rheum. 2009;60:578–83.
40. Smith V, Van Praet JT, Vandooren B, et al. Rituximab in diffuse cutaneous systemic sclerosis: an open-label clinical and histopathological study. Ann Rheum Dis. 2010;69:193–7.
41. Smith V, Piette Y, van Praet JT, et al. Two-year results of an open label pilot study of a 2-treatment course with rituximab in patients with early systemic sclerosis with diffuse skin involvement. J Rheumatol. 2013;40:52–7.
42. McQueen FM, Solanki K. Rituximab in diffuse cutaneous systemic sclerosis: should we be using it today? Rheumatology (Oxford). 2015;54:757–67. pii: keu463.
43. van Laar JM, Farge D, Sont JK, EBMT/EULAR Scleroderma Study Group, et al. Autologous hematopoietic stem cell transplantation vs intravenous pulse cyclophosphamide in diffuse cutaneous systemic sclerosis: a randomized clinical trial. JAMA. 2014;311(24):2490–8.
44. Khanna D, Georges GE, Couriel DR. Autologous hematopoietic stem cell therapy in severe systemic sclerosis ready for clinical practice? JAMA. 2014;311(24):2485–7.
45. Khanna D, Denton CP. Evidence-based management of rapidly progressing systemic sclerosis. Best Pract Res Clin Rheumatol. 2010;24(3):387–400.
46. Bassel M, Hudson M, Baron M, Taillefer SS, Mouthon L, Poiraudeau S, Poole JL, Thombs BD. Physical and occupational therapy referral and use among systemic sclerosis patients with impaired hand function: results from a Canadian national survey. Clin Exp Rheumatol. 2012;30(4):574–7.
47. Poole JL. Musculoskeletal rehabilitation in the person with scleroderma. Curr Opin Rheumatol. 2010;22(2):205–12.
48. Seeger MW, Furst DE. Effects of splinting in the treatment of hand contractures in progressive systemic sclerosis. Am J Occup Ther. 1987;41(2):118–21.

Management of the Scleroderma Patient with Pulmonary Arterial Hypertension Failing Initial Therapy

53

Christopher J. Mullin and Stephen C. Mathai

Case

Our patient is a 53-year-old Caucasian woman with limited cutaneous systemic sclerosis (SSc) who is referred to the pulmonary hypertension clinic for evaluation of continued shortness of breath. She first developed Raynaud's phenomena around the age of 25 and was diagnosed with limited cutaneous systemic sclerosis at the age of 41 in the setting of symptoms of gastroesophageal reflux, sclerodactyly, and telangiectasias. She was found to have positive antinuclear antibody with a 1:160 titer, a positive anticentromere antibody, and negative anti Scl-70 antibody; other antibodies were all negative. She was managed with a low-dose calcium channel blocker and a proton pump inhibitor for her Raynaud's and esophageal reflux symptoms, respectively.

She initially presented to our clinic 3 months prior to this evaluation with gradually increasing dyspnea on exertion over the past 6 months. She noticed that she was becoming short of breath after walking up two flights of stairs and in retrospect noted that she had become increasingly sedentary over the past 2 years despite previously enjoying a more active lifestyle. Her physical exam was notable for an elevated jugular venous pulsation at 7 cm H_2O, a loud second heart sound, a systolic murmur at the left sternal border, fourth intercostal space, clear lungs, trace peripheral edema, sclerodactyly without digital ulcers or evidence of active synovitis, and telangiectasias on her face and chest.

Her initial evaluation included pulmonary function testing showing no evidence of obstructive or restrictive lung disease, though her diffusing capacity was moderately reduced at 60% of predicted; her forced vital capacity-to-diffusing capacity ratio was elevated at 1.7. A chest CT showed no parenchymal abnormalities or pulmonary fibrosis, and a ventilation-perfusion (VQ) scan was low probability for pulmonary embolism. A NT-proBNP was 2165 pg/ml. A transthoracic echocardiogram showed normal left ventricular size and function, normal diastolic function, a normal left atrium, but a mildly dilated right atrium (RA), a mildly dilated right ventricle (RV) with preserved RV function, and a RV systolic pressure estimated at 50 mmHg.

Given the concern for pulmonary hypertension, she underwent a right heart catheterization (RHC), which showed an RA pressure of 6, pulmonary artery (PA) pressure of 58/31 (mean PA pressure of 39), and a pulmonary arterial wedge pressure (PAWP) of 10 mmHg. Cardiac output (CO) was 3.78 ml/min, cardiac index (CI) was 2.25 ml/min/m^2, and pulmonary vascular resistance (PVR) was 7.67 Wood units. Based upon these findings, she was felt to have pulmonary arterial hypertension in the setting of SSc (SSc-PAH), World Health Organization Group I disease, with World Health Organization functional class (WHO FC) II symptoms. She was subsequently started on oral sildenafil therapy at 20 mg three times daily and furosemide 20 mg daily and was to return to pulmonary hypertension clinic in 3 months. She presents today for this 3-month follow-up.

Discussion

Our patient has a diagnosis of pulmonary arterial hypertension (PAH), with borderline cardiac function as indicated by her cardiac index of 2.25 ml/min/m^2. Based on her symptoms and current functional class, initiation of PAH-specific therapies is certainly indicated. In initiating therapy, the important aspects are first, to determine which therapy to initiate, and second, to assess the response to the initiated therapy. There are many approved PAH-specific therapies that are available by either oral, inhaled, subcutaneous, or intravenous deliveries; however for our patient, an oral therapy is the first step, based upon her functional class at diagnosis [1]. There is no consensus as to which oral agent should be used as initial therapy, and thus this decision requires an

C.J. Mullin, MD • S.C. Mathai, MD, MHS (✉)
Division of Pulmonary and Critical Care Medicine, Johns Hopkins University School of Medicine, Baltimore, MD 21205, USA
e-mail: smathai4@jhmi.edu

J. Varga et al. (eds.), *Scleroderma*, DOI 10.1007/978-3-319-31407-5_53

Table 53.1 Variables used to determine clinical response to therapy in PAH

Variable	Treatment goal
NYHA functional class	I–II
Echocardiography/cardiac MRI	Normal/near-normal RV size and function
Hemodynamics	Normalization of RV function (RAP <8 mmHg and CI >2.5–3.0 l/min/m^2)
6-Min walk distance	>380–440 m
Cardiopulmonary exercise testing	Peak oxygen consumption (VO_2) >15 ml/min/kg and ventilator equivalent for carbon dioxide ($EqCO_2$) <45 L/min/L/min
B-type natriuretic peptide level	Normal

Adapted from McLaughlin et al. [6]

understanding of the medications, data supporting their use in SSc-PAH, and treatment strategies. While initial oral therapies considered for our patient included phosphodiesterase type 5 (PDE-5) inhibitors and endothelin receptor antagonists (ERA), we selected sildenafil based upon (1) data from the SUPER-1 study demonstrating improved 6MWD and hemodynamics in patients with connective tissue-related PAH (CTD-PAH), 45 % of whom had SSc-PAH [2], and (2) our own clinical experience with this agent in SSc-PAH. Unfortunately, specific data related to SSc-PAH for other oral medications, such as the PDE-5 inhibitor tadalafil, the ERA macitentan, and the soluble guanylate cyclase stimulator riociguat, have yet to be published. Subgroup analyses of studies of both bosentan and ambrisentan have yielded mixed results in the SSc-PAH population [3–5].

As equally important as deciding on initial PAH therapy is the assessment of response to treatment. This is typically done with a combination of evaluation of a patient's symptoms and functional class, along with objective measures such as biomarkers (N-terminal pro-brain natriuretic peptide or NT-proBNP), exercise capacity as measured by distance of 6-min walk test (6MWT) or cardiopulmonary exercise testing, imaging assessment of RV structure and function, and reassessment of cardiopulmonary hemodynamics. The specifics of these assessments, as recommended in most recent guidelines [6], are included in Table 53.1.

With many of these treatment goals for PAH, there are caveats for their applications specifically in SSc-PAH. The 6MWT is a simple way to measure submaximal exercise tolerance [7] and has been used as an end point in many of the clinical trials for treatment of PAH. However, the 6MWT is influenced not only by cardiopulmonary status but also by the statuses of the peripheral vasculature, nerves, and musculature, and thus there are concerns with the use of this test in assessing response to therapies in SSc-PAH. In a study assessing limitations of 6MWT in SSc, over one third of small number of SSc-PAH patients reported limitations on 6MWT for reasons other than dyspnea, the majority of which were from lower extremity pain [8]. Therefore, interpretation of 6MWT in SSc should include considerations of pulmonary, vascular, and musculoskeletal involvement, as the distance walked may not be a direct assessment of cardiopulmonary limitations. Similarly, it is important to consider what degree of change in distance on 6MWT is clinically relevant. Using data from a large clinical trial of tadalafil in PAH, the minimal important difference for the 6MWT was determined to be around 33 m; interestingly, the estimate for CTD-PAH was smaller, around 24 m, highlighting the differences in response to therapy between these groups of PAH patients [9]. It is our practice to obtain 6MWT at 3 months after initiation of PAH-specific therapy and then subsequently at 3 or 6 month intervals thereafter. While cardiopulmonary exercise testing (CPET) can provide an integrative approach to assessing cardiac function, gas exchange, and respiratory mechanics, it has limited utility in SSc-PAH compared to IPAH and other forms of pulmonary hypertension largely due to the risk of vascular complications related to arterial line placement in SSc patients. Thus, CPET is not routinely used to assess response to treatment in SSc-PAH.

NT-proBNP is a prohormone secreted by myocardium in response to mechanical stretch, hypoxia, and stimuli by neurohormonal factors such as endothelin and catecholamines. It has a role in diagnosis, prognostication, and assessment of response to therapy in SSc-PAH. In one cohort of 109 SSc patients, an NT-proBNP level of >395 pg/ml was found to have a 95 % specificity for the diagnosis of PAH [10]. In that study, a tenfold increase in NT-proBNP while on PAH therapy was associated with a threefold increased risk of death. Another study comparing NT-proBNP levels in patients with SSc-PAH to patients with IPAH found that NT-proBNP levels 1) correlated with hemodynamics in SSc-PAH, 2) were higher in SSc-PAH despite less severe hemodynamics, and 3) were a strong predictor of mortality in SSc-PAH but not IPAH [11]. It is our practice to obtain NT-proBNP levels on SSc-PAH patients 3 months after initiating PAH-specific therapies and then at 3–6 months intervals thereafter. While no specific threshold for clinically relevant changes in NT-proBNP has been defined, in general, our goal is to attain normal or near-normal levels with therapy.

Noninvasive imaging is often used to assess response to therapy in PAH, using both echocardiography and cardiac magnetic resonance imaging (CMR). Multiple measures of RV size, structure, and function have been shown to predict outcome in PAH. Specific to SSc-PAH, the tricuspid annular plane systolic excursion (TAPSE), an echocardiographic measure of RV function, assessed prior to initiation of PAH-specific therapy, is a strong predictor of survival [12]. Similarly, the ventricular mass index (VMI), the ratio of the mass of the RV to the LV assessed by CMR, predicted survival in a small cohort of SSc patients with and without PAH [13]. However, estimates of more commonly obtained parameters, such as RV or pulmonary artery pressures, are not useful in the longitudinal evaluation of SSc-PAH, regardless of the modality with which these estimates are obtained. Importantly, to our knowledge, there are no studies describing clinically relevant responses to therapy using either echocardiography or CMR in SSc-PAH, emphasizing the need for longitudinal studies employing these modalities. While sequential RHC can be performed, the invasive nature, discomfort to the patient, and associated risks often preclude its routine use in follow-up. In our practice, we will repeat RHC if a patient is failing therapy and requires additional PAH treatment.

Case

At her visit, she reports tolerating the medications but notes worsening reflux symptoms. She has no exertional chest pain, lightheadedness, or palpitations, but has noticed new lower extremity and a 3 kg weight gain on her scale measured at home. On exam, she is normotensive with a heart rate of 96 beats per minute and a jugular venous pressure estimated at 10 cm H_2O. Her lungs are clear without any dullness to percussion at the bases, and her heart is regular with a loud s2, but without a parasternal heave or palpable P2. She has 1+ pitting edema to the midshins bilaterally, without any calf tenderness, warmth, or erythema. On a 6MWT done prior to the initiation of therapies, she walked 390 m (69 % of predicted) with a nadir oxygen saturation of 93 % with ambulation. Her distance on 6MWT today is 335 m, a decrease of 55 m since the time of her RHC, again without any ambulatory desaturations. Her NT-proBNP has increased from 2165 to 3415 pg/ml since her initial evaluation. Her echocardiogram shows a moderately dilated RV with a TAPSE of 1.8 cm; prior studies showed a TAPSE of 2.2 cm.

Discussion

At this visit, our patient has worsened, in terms of her symptoms, NYHA FC (from II to III), declining distance on 6MWT, and a rising NT-proBNP. Before labeling her as a "failure" of a single agent, it is important to think broadly about the reason for her clinical deterioration. The differential diagnosis for worsening symptoms for our patient includes issues with volume overload, hypoxemia, deconditioning, or the possibility of another disease process, such as cardiac arrhythmias, pulmonary embolism (PE), or pulmonary veno-occlusive disease (PVOD).

In addition to specific pharmacotherapies, treatment of PAH includes several general or supportive measures, such as diuretics, supplemental oxygen therapy, and rehabilitation and exercise training. Other general measures that may be appropriate for IPAH are not recommended for SSc-PAH, namely, routine anticoagulation [14]. Diuretics are not necessarily required for patients who are compensated and lack elevated filling pressures or RV failure, but they are routinely required as patients develop peripheral edema, systemic venous congestion, severe tricuspid regurgitation, and/or RV failure [15, 16]. Loop diuretics are the first line of treatment and require adequate dosing and appropriate monitoring of renal function and serum electrolytes. Spironolactone, a potassium-sparing aldosterone antagonist, is useful in patients with hypokalemia and/or ascites, and post hoc analysis of the ARIES trial showed trends toward improved exercise capacity, functional class, and clinical outcomes when spironolactone was used in conjunction with ambrisentan [17].

Supplemental oxygen therapy is used based on the assumption that hypoxia stimulates vasoconstriction in the pulmonary vasculature [18]. The role of oxygen therapy has not been specifically studied in PAH, but several published guidelines recommend supplemental oxygen be used to maintain oxygen saturations greater than 88–92 % or a partial pressure of oxygen in arterial blood of >55–60 mmHg at rest, during sleep, or with exertion [16, 19, 20]. Hypoxemia intermittently with exercise or with sleep is common in patients with PAH, and clinicians must also be aware that nocturnal hypoxemia may be seen in up to 60 % of patients with PAH who do not have exertional hypoxemia [21].

Pulmonary rehabilitation and exercise training are another form of supportive therapy in PAH. The most recent treatment guidelines for PAH [1] strongly recommend exercise training and rehabilitation based on the evidence of multiple controlled and uncontrolled trials that have shown improvements in exercise capacity, fatigue, cardiorespiratory function, and quality of life using varying models of exercise training [22–25]. One study looked at exercise training in only patients with CTD-PAH, 43 % of whom had SSc-PAH, and found improvements in distance on 6MWT, quality of life, resting heart rate, and peak oxygen consumption [24]. Thus despite the systemic and musculoskeletal manifestations of SSc, patients with SSc-PAH appear to benefit from rehabilitation and exercise training. There is no consensus as to the specific method of exercise training; however patients should be referred to rehabilitation centers that have experience with care and rehabilitation of PAH patients.

In addition to optimizing these supportive therapies, clinicians must consider other diagnostic possibilities when a patient with SSc-PAH has a clinical deterioration. The risk of pulmonary embolism (PE) is increased in systemic sclerosis; a recent population-based cohort study showed a sevenfold increased risk of PE in patients with systemic sclerosis compared to healthy controls, after adjusting for age, sex, and comorbidities [26]. Not only should the initial workup for pulmonary hypertension include an evaluation for thromboembolic disease; the possibility of PE should be considered in the setting of clinical deterioration and appropriately evaluated and treated.

Cardiac arrhythmias are an important cause of morbidity and mortality in PAH and thought to be caused by modulation in autonomic activity, delayed cardiac repolarization, and RV myocardial ischemia related to remodeling of the RV and the right atrium (RA) in response to long-standing pressure and volume overload [27]. Supraventricular arrhythmias, such as atrial fibrillation, atrial flutter, and atrioventricular reentry tachycardia (AVNRT), are typically seen in the setting of long-standing PAH, and onset of atrial tachyarrhythmias is often related to clinical deterioration [28]. Restoration of normal sinus rhythm is imperative in patients with PAH and is associated with a dramatic improvement in mortality [28]. However, in one study over 40% of patients with a first episode of supraventricular tachycardia (SVT) required an increase in their specific PAH therapy after conversion to sinus rhythm [29], suggesting that SVT is potentially a harbinger for deteriorating RV function. In addition to PAH, patients with SSc can have other mechanisms of arrhythmias such as myocardial fibrosis and autoantibody-mediated processes [30], and ventricular ectopy is associated with increased mortality [31]. The management of cardiac arrhythmias in PAH can be challenging as beta-blocker and calcium channel blocker therapies are relatively contraindicated because of their negative inotropic effects. Many antiarrhythmic agents, such as amiodarone, must be used judiciously because of their side-effect profiles and negative inotropy, but are often administered at the lowest possible effective dose given that arrhythmias are so poorly tolerated [27]. Digoxin is often used in our experience to manage atrial tachyarrhythmias. There is minimal data for its use in PAH, although one study showed an acute improvement in cardiac output and beneficial modulation of the neurohormonal axis when administered in the setting of RV failure [32]. Its use requires close monitoring of renal function and electrolytes, as it can cause hypomagnesemia and hypokalemia that can be arrhythmogenic [33].

Finally, pulmonary veno-occlusive disease (PVOD) is a rare cause of pulmonary hypertension in systemic sclerosis and is likely under-recognized because it is often difficult to distinguish from PAH. It is pathologically characterized by patchy intense capillary congestion in the alveolar parenchyma and obliterative intimal fibrosis of small veins and venules [34]. Patients typically present with severe hypoxia, pulmonary edema, and pleural effusions [35], often after initiation of PAH-specific therapies, particularly during infusions of prostacyclin [36, 37]. Diagnosis can be obtained by lung biopsy, although this is typically not done as patients are quite ill, and diagnosis can be suspected based on clinical scenario in conjunction with chest imaging that shows centrilobular ground glass nodules, septal lines, and adenopathy [38]. There is debate as to whether intravenous prostacyclin should be used as treatment [35, 37, 39], but suspected PVOD is an indication for referral for lung transplantation evaluation.

Thus, when a patient with PAH deteriorates or has worsening symptoms, the clinician must consider other diagnostic possibilities, as well as optimize volume status, correct hypoxemia, and insure adequate exercise training and rehabilitation prior to labeling that patient as a failure of PAH-specific therapy.

Case

Our patient has a chest radiograph that does not show pleural effusions, interstitial edema, or adenopathy. Her furosemide dose is increased to 40 mg daily and then to 40 mg twice daily, ultimately with improvement in her lower extremity edema, and a decrease in her weight back to her previous baseline. She is continued on sildenafil 20 mg three times daily and begins a program of pulmonary rehabilitation.

She returns to clinic after another 3 months, where she reports being improved since her previous visit, however has not noticed much, if any improvement from the time of her initial diagnosis. She can walk up about one and a half flights of stairs before stopping because of shortness of breath and on occasion will have some lightheadedness when doing so. She has no chest pain, and her peripheral edema is resolved. Her physical exam is notable for trace pedal edema, a jugular venous pulse estimated at 6 cm H_2O, and a cardiac exam with regular rate and rhythm, but now with a II/VI systolic murmur heart best at the left lower sternal border, a fixed split second heart sound, and a palpable P2. During a 6MWT she ambulates 364 m (64% predicted), with a nadir in her ambulatory saturations to 86% on room air. Her NT-proBNP is 2433 pg/ml, and a repeat echocardiogram shows moderate RA dilation, a moderately dilated RV with a TAPSE of 1.7 cm, and trace tricuspid regurgitation. She asks what the next steps are for treating her pulmonary hypertension and improving her symptoms.

Discussion

Our patient unfortunately has not had the desired response to 6 months of sildenafil. Her exercise tolerance has decreased since her diagnosis, her NT-proBNP remains elevated, and her distance on 6MWT is reduced. She now has evidence of hypoxemia with exertion, but this is a reflection of the progression of her disease. It will be important to address this with an appropriate dose of supplemental oxygen, but this may not improve her symptoms. Additionally, she has evidence of worsening RV function both on exam and on her repeat echocardiogram. When considering the treatment goals for PAH (Table 53.1), it is quite evident that she has failed single-agent therapy. It is common practice, and in accordance with treatment guidelines [1], to add additional therapies when patients fail to improve or worsen on monotherapy. Since she is already on a PDE5 inhibitor, the options for additional therapy are either an ERA or a prostanoid.

Several forms of prostaglandins are available for delivery intravenously and subcutaneously, inhaled and orally, and include epoprostenol, treprostinil, and iloprost. In SSc-PAH, continuous infusion of epoprostenol improves exercise capacity and hemodynamics [40], although in contrast to the IPAH population, a survival benefit has yet to be demonstrated [41]. Treprostinil is an epoprostenol analogue that can be delivered intravenously or subcutaneously via continuous infusion, inhaled, or orally and was shown to improve symptoms, exercise capacity, and hemodynamics in 90 patients who had CTD-PAH, 50 % of whom has SSc-PAH [42]. Less is known about the effects of either the intravenous, inhaled, or oral forms of treprostinil in CTD-PAH as disaggregated data specific to this population from the pivotal clinical trials have yet to be reported [43–46]. Intravenous and subcutaneous deliveries of prostaglandins are quite burdensome and come with the risks of catheter-associated infections for intravenous delivery and infusion site pain, bleeding, and infection for subcutaneous delivery. Manipulation of the medications and delivery devices can be challenging in SSc patients with digital ulcers and limited manual dexterity and can increase the patients' burden of their disease. Currently, intravenous prostaglandins are recommended for patients with NYHA FC IV disease, but use may be less commonly utilized in SSc-PAH compared to other forms of PAH due to these limitations [1, 47].

Using a PDE-5 inhibitor and an ERA together is an appealing combination as both agents are administered orally. Small studies of the use of bosentan with sildenafil showed improvements in exercise capacity and functional class [48, 49]; however the outcome in SSc-PAH in one small single-center study was less favorable than in IPAH [49]. The COMPASS-2 trial was a large, multicenter randomized controlled trial that evaluated the addition of bosentan therapy to PAH patients on a stable dose of sildenafil, 26 % of whom had CTD-PAH [50]. There was a minimal improvement in distance on 6MWT with bosentan compared to placebo, and NT-proBNP levels were significantly worse in the placebo group. However, there was no difference in the primary outcome of the composite end point of time to clinical worsening. In contrast, the ATHENA-1 study showed an improvement in hemodynamics and exercise capacity in 33 PAH patients treated with ambrisentan after a suboptimal clinical response to a PDE-5 inhibitor; however, no data regarding CTD-PAH was presented [51].

These results are in opposition to some of the emerging data behind using the combination of tadalafil and ambrisentan. The AMBITION trial is a recently completed, randomized controlled trial of *initial* combination therapy with ambrisentan 10 mg daily and tadalafil 40 mg daily, compared to ambrisentan 10 mg daily or tadalafil 40 mg daily [52]. The study has yet to be published; however preliminary results have been reported and show a 50 % reduction in time to clinical failure (defined as the time from randomization to the first occurrence of all-cause mortality, hospitalization for worsening PAH, disease progression, or unsatisfactory long-term clinical response) in the combination therapy compared to the monotherapy groups [52]. Additionally, a recently reported subgroup analysis of 137 patients with CTD-PAH (108 with SSc-PAH) showed that combination therapy reduced the risk of clinical failure by 57 % and resulted in greater improvements of NT-proBNP and distance on 6MWT [53]. While this appears promising, further study and careful analysis of these data must be done before an approach with dual upfront therapies can be recommended as the first line of treatment.

The difference between these seemingly discordant results may be related to trial design and primary end points or possibly from the differences in these medications themselves, including drug-drug interactions. For instance, clinicians must be aware of the interaction between bosentan and sildenafil, which results in decrease plasma levels of sildenafil and increase levels of bosentan [54]. Currently, there is insufficient evidence to recommend one combination of PDE-5 and ERA over another.

There have been several studies evaluating combining a prostaglandin with another oral PAH therapy. While the overall impact of the combination of bosentan added to intravenous epoprostenol did not show significant improvement in symptoms or functional capacity, the combination of sildenafil and epoprostenol demonstrated an improvement in exercise capacity, hemodynamics, and time to clinical worsening [45, 46]. However, no subgroup analysis for CTD-PAH patients was provided.

Similarly, combination studies with inhaled agents (iloprost and treprostinil) and various oral therapies have shown some improvement in symptoms, functional capacity, and time to clinical worsening; however, disaggregated data for CTD-PAH have not been reported [43, 44, 46]. Thus, the use of these combinations is based upon extrapolation from the PAH population in general.

A meta-analysis of the randomized controlled trials in PAH demonstrated a reduction in mortality for PAH treatments compared to control arms [55]. Combination therapy in particular was shown to improve exercise capacity and hemodynamics and decrease the risk of clinical worsening, but did not show a significant improvement in mortality. Guidelines recommend sequential therapy, with addition of a second and then third agent in the setting not only of clinical deterioration but also in the cases of inadequate responses to therapy [1]. There is no consensus as to the specifics or order of combination therapy, and in clinical practice, this is done based on provider experience and patient preference based on the mode of delivery and side-effect profiles.

Case

Our patient is started on oral ambrisentan, uptitrated to a dose of 10 mg daily, and is continued on sildenafil 20 mg three times daily. She is prescribed supplemental oxygen and with 2 L NC maintains her oxygen saturation >92 % when checked with exertion and with nocturnal oximetry. She tolerated the ambrisentan without significant adverse effects, although her furosemide needed to be increased to 80 mg twice daily because of slightly increased peripheral edema and fluid retention.

Six months after initiation of ambrisentan, she reports her exercise tolerance has slightly improved and she is able to walk up two flights of stairs again, and she has not had any chest pain, lightheadedness, or palpitations. Her exam remains generally unchanged from her previous visit, and her distance on 6MWT is 376 m. A pro-BNP is 1785 pg/ml. Her improvement with the addition of ambrisentan is marginal at best, and she certainly has not met treatment goals to suggest that she has had an adequate response. Given this, the possibility of initiation of a prostaglandin therapy is discussed with her, and the specifics of inhaled, subcutaneous, and intravenous options are reviewed. She says that she is not quite ready for another medication and asks to take some time to think about this and see if she has an additional improvement on her dual-agent therapy.

Unfortunately, at her next appointment 3 months later, she reports continued decline, with an exercise tolerance that gradual decreased to less than a full flight of stairs. She has had episodes of lightheadedness with exertion and despite feeling presyncopal has not had any episodes of syncope. She remains adherent to her medications, never missing any doses, and has not observed any changes with daily weights. Her exam is notable for a fixed split second heart sound, an increase in her systolic murmur to III/IV, and a palpable RV heave. Her lungs remain clear to auscultation and she has no peripheral edema. On a repeat 6MWT, she walks 310 m without any desaturations. A repeat transthoracic echocardiogram shows a severe RA dilation, severe RV dilation with reduced RV systolic function (TAPSE 1.4 cm), septal hypertrophy with septal bowing, and moderate tricuspid regurgitation with preserved left ventricular systolic function.

She undergoes a repeat RHC, which shows an RA pressure of 10, pulmonary artery (PA) pressure of 54/23 (mean PA pressure of 34), and a pulmonary arterial wedge pressure (PAWP) of 12 mmHg. Cardiac output (CO) was 2.64 ml/min, cardiac index (CI) was 1.57 ml/min/m^2, and pulmonary vascular resistance (PVR) was 8.33 Wood units. She is admitted to the hospital and initiated on intravenous epoprostenol. During this admission, she asks about the possibility of lung transplantation.

Discussion

Our patient has had a continuous deterioration of her cardiopulmonary status, and in the setting of relatively rapid clinical worsening and severely reduced right ventricular function, the decision was made to start her on intravenous prostanoid therapy. While this requires a gradual uptitration of dose to achieve a symptomatic benefit, at this point she will be receiving maximal medical therapy, at which point the clinician needs to consider what other therapies or interventions are available to her. Lung transplantation is considered to be the only definitive and curative treatment for PAH. PAH accounts for less than 4 % of all lung transplants, and the majority of these cases are patients with IPAH [56]. There is a reluctance to perform lung transplantation in SSc patients because of the systemic nature of the disease and the risk of peri- and postoperative complications such as renal dysfunction, impaired wound healing, and an increased risk of microaspiration due to esophageal disease that can lead to organ rejection [57, 58]. However, several cohort studies have demonstrated that for appropriately screened and approved SSc patients, outcomes for lung transplantation in patients with SSc and SSc-PAH in particular are similar to other PAH populations [57–61].

Current guidelines for referral for lung transplantation evaluation and timing of transplant listing in all pulmonary vascular diseases [62] are included in Table 53.2. There are

Table 53.2 Guidelines for referral and listing for lung transplant in pulmonary vascular diseases

Timing of referral	Timing of transplant listing
NYHA FC III or IV symptoms during escalating therapy	NYHA functional class III or IV despite a trial of at least 3 months of combination therapy including prostanoids
Rapidly progressive disease (assuming weight and rehabilitation concerns not present)	Cardiac index of <2 L/min/m^2
Use of parenteral targeted (PAH) therapy regardless of symptoms or NYHA functional class	Mean right atrial pressure of >15 mmHg
Known or suspected pulmonary veno-occlusive disease (PVOD) or pulmonary capillary hemangiomatosis	6-min walk test of <350 m
	Development of significant hemoptysis, pericardial effusion, or signs of progressive right heart failure (renal insufficiency, increasing bilirubin, brain natriuretic peptide, or recurrent ascites)

Adapted from Weill et al. [62]

no standardized guidelines for SSc-specific contraindications to lung transplantation; however several centers have proposed and implemented criteria based on skin, musculoskeletal, renal, and gastrointestinal manifestations of the disease [57, 59]. The number of lung transplant centers with significant experience in transplanting patients with SSc is small [61], and this can be a consideration when referring SSc-PAH patients for lung transplant evaluation.

Balloon atrial septostomy (BAS) is considered a last-resort therapy, and it is typically only used as a palliative procedure or as a bridging to transplantation [63]. The procedure involves creation of a right-to-left interatrial shunt which unloads the right heart, increases cardiac output, and improves systemic oxygen transport despite decreased arterial oxygen saturation [64, 65]. The procedure is contraindicated for patients with a RA pressure >20 mmHg and resting oxygen saturation <85 % on room air. Studies have shown improvement in hemodynamics and exercise capacity with BAS in IPAH patients who were NYHA FC IV with right heart failure refractory to medical therapy [64, 65]. There are case reports of the use of a BAS in SSc-PAH [66], but the impact on overall survival remains uncertain.

Finally, referral and involvement of palliative care are valuable resources that are underused in PAH. Palliative care is defined as "patient and family-centered care that optimizes quality of life by anticipating, preventing, and treating suffering" and "involves addressing physical, intellectual, emotional, social, and spiritual needs and to facilitate patient autonomy, access to information, and choice" [67]. Despite PAH and SSc-PAH portending a poor prognosis, a high degree of symptom burden, and poor or suboptimal health-related quality of life [68–71], there is very limited formal investigation of the incorporation of palliative care into a PAH treatment plan. Several surveys have shown that palliative care awareness and use by both providers and patients are low [72, 73] and that patients who die from PAH have a high degree of symptom burden, particularly dyspnea, at the time of their deaths [74]. A referral to palliative care should be considered for patients with rapidly progressing disease, NYHA FC III or IV symptoms, or who express interest, regardless of the stage of their disease. A referral to palliative care should not indicate to the clinician or the patient that either is "giving up," but instead providing an additional resource to insure that all of the patient needs and symptoms are being adequately addressed.

Case

Our patient was referred for both a lung transplant evaluation and for a palliative care consultation. She has now developed a good rapport with her palliative care physician, who has helped manage her dyspnea and provided her with many coping mechanisms for dealing with the burdens of the symptoms and treatments of her diseases. With the uptitration of epoprostenol to its effective dose, her symptoms have stabilized; however she remains NHYA FC III. She underwent a comprehensive transplant evaluation, and ultimately the decision was made to list her for double lung transplantation. She is continuing her current therapies – sildenafil, ambrisentan, and intravenous epoprostenol – and is anxiously awaiting the possibility of receiving a lung transplant.

Key Principle Lessons of the Case

1. Choice of initial therapy in SSc-PAH requires not only knowledge of the treatment guidelines in PAH, but an understanding of each individual therapy and data for its use in SSc-PAH.
2. Assessment of response to therapy in SSc-PAH is typically done with a combination of evaluation of a patient's functional class, NT-proBNP, distance on 6MWT, echocardiographic and/or CMR assessments of RV structure and function, and reassessment of cardiopulmonary hemodynamics.
3. When a SSc-PAH patient is worsening, the clinician must consider possibilities of other diagnoses such as PE, cardiac arrhythmias, and PVOD and insure that volume status, oxygenation, and exercise training and rehabilitation have been optimized prior to labeling the patient as failing PAH therapy.
4. While it is common practice and recommendation of current guidelines to sequentially add therapies to a SSc-PAH patient who is failing therapy, there is no consensus as to which combination of agents is preferred. A combination of PDE-5 inhibitor and ERA is favored in part because both drugs are administered orally.
5. Prostaglandin therapies are available by intravenous, subcutaneous, inhaled, or oral deliveries and are typically reserved for patients failing dual therapies or who are NYHA FC IV. Continuous intravenous epoprostenol has the most robust evidence in SSc-PAH, but the use of other prostaglandins in combination therapies is extrapolated from PAH population in general.
6. Referral for lung transplantation in SSc-PAH should be done in accordance with current guidelines. Despite concerns for SSc-specific-related complications, for appropriately screened SSc-PAH patients, outcomes for lung transplantation appear to be similar to other PAH populations.
7. Palliative care is an underused resource in SSc-PAH and a referral should be considered for patients with progressive or advanced disease or a high burden of symptoms and treatments from their diseases.

References

1. Galiè N, Corris PA, Frost A, Girgis RE, Granton J, Jing ZC, et al. Updated treatment algorithm of pulmonary arterial hypertension. J Am Coll Cardiol. 2013;62(25 Suppl):D60–72.
2. Galiè N, Ghofrani HA, Torbicki A, Barst RJ, Rubin LJ, Badesch D, et al. Sildenafil citrate therapy for pulmonary arterial hypertension. N Engl J Med. 2005;353(20):2148–57.
3. Denton CP, Humbert M, Rubin L, Black CM. Bosentan treatment for pulmonary arterial hypertension related to connective tissue disease: a subgroup analysis of the pivotal clinical trials and their open-label extensions. Ann Rheum Dis. 2006;65(10):1336–40.
4. Galie N, Richards D, Hutchinson T, Dufton C. Ambrisentan therapy for patients with PAH associated with connective tissue disease (PAH-CTD): one year follow-up. Eur Respir Soc Ann Congr Berl. 2008;E1418.
5. Galiè N, Olschewski H, Oudiz RJ, Torres F, Frost A, Ghofrani HA, et al. Ambrisentan for the treatment of pulmonary arterial hypertension: results of the ambrisentan in pulmonary arterial hypertension, randomized, double-blind, placebo-controlled, multicenter, efficacy (ARIES) study 1 and 2. Circulation. 2008;117(23):3010–9.
6. McLaughlin VV, Gaine SP, Howard LS, Leuchte HH, Mathier MA, Mehta S, et al. Treatment goals of pulmonary hypertension. J Am Coll Cardiol. 2013;62(25 Suppl):D73–81. Internet.
7. Guyatt GH, Sullivan MJ, Thompson PJ, Fallen EL, Pugsley SO, Taylor DW, et al. The 6-minute walk: a new measure of exercise capacity in patients with chronic heart failure. Can Med Assoc J. 1985;132(8):919–23.
8. Garin MC, Highland KB, Silver RM, Strange C. Limitations to the 6-minute walk test in interstitial lung disease and pulmonary hypertension in scleroderma. J Rheumatol. 2009;36(2):330–6.
9. Mathai SC, Puhan MA, Lam D, Wise RA. The minimal important difference in the 6-minute walk test for patients with pulmonary arterial hypertension. Am J Respir Crit Care Med. 2012;186(5):428–33.
10. Williams MH, Handler CE, Akram R, Smith CJ, Das C, Smee J, et al. Role of N-terminal brain natriuretic peptide (N-TproBNP) in scleroderma-associated pulmonary arterial hypertension. Eur Heart J. 2006;27(12):1485–94.
11. Mathai SC, Bueso M, Hummers LK, Boyce D, Lechtzin N, Le Pavec J, et al. Disproportionate elevation of N-terminal pro-brain natriuretic peptide in scleroderma-related pulmonary hypertension. Eur Respir J. 2010;35(1):95–104.
12. Mathai SC, Sibley CT, Forfia PR, Mudd JO, Fisher MR, Tedford RJ, et al. Tricuspid annular plane systolic excursion is a robust outcome measure in systemic sclerosis-associated pulmonary arterial hypertension. J Rheumatol. 2011;38(11):2410–8.
13. Hagger D, Condliffe R, Woodhouse N, Elliot CA, Armstrong IJ, Davies C, et al. Ventricular mass index correlates with pulmonary artery pressure and predicts survival in suspected systemic sclerosis-associated pulmonary arterial hypertension. Rheumatology. 2009; 48(9):1137–42.
14. Olsson KM, Delcroix M, Ghofrani HA, Tiede H, Huscher D, Speich R, et al. Anticoagulation and survival in pulmonary arterial hypertension: results from the comparative, prospective registry of newly initiated therapies for pulmonary hypertension (COMPERA). Circulation. 2014;129(1):57–65.
15. Badesch DB, Abman SH, Simonneau G, Rubin LJ, McLaughlin VV. Medical therapy for pulmonary arterial hypertension: updated ACCP evidence-based clinical practice guidelines. Chest. 2007; 131(6):1917–28.
16. McLaughlin VV, Archer SL, Badesch DB, Barst RJ, Farber HW, Lindner JR, et al. ACCF/AHA 2009 expert consensus document on pulmonary hypertension a report of the American College of Cardiology Foundation Task Force on Expert Consensus Documents and the American Heart Association developed in collaboration with the American College of. J Am Coll Cardiol. 2009;53(17):1573–619.
17. Maron BA, Waxman AB, Opotowsky AR, Gillies H, Blair C, Aghamohammadzadeh R, et al. Effectiveness of spironolactone plus ambrisentan for treatment of pulmonary arterial hypertension (from the [ARIES] study 1 and 2 trials). Am J Cardiol. 2013; 112(5):720–5.
18. Sylvester JT, Shimoda LA, Aaronson PI, Ward JPT. Hypoxic pulmonary vasoconstriction. Physiol Rev. 2012;92(1):367–520.
19. Galiè N, Hoeper MM, Humbert M, Torbicki A, Vachiery J-L, Barbera JA, et al. Guidelines for the diagnosis and treatment of pulmonary hypertension: the Task Force for the Diagnosis and Treatment of Pulmonary Hypertension of the European Society of Cardiology (ESC) and the European Respiratory Society (ERS), endorsed by the Internet. Eur Heart J. 2009;30(20):2493–537.
20. Sauler M, Fares WH, Trow TK. Standard nonspecific therapies in the management of pulmonary arterial hypertension. Clin Chest Med. 2013;34(4):799–810.
21. Minai OA, Pandya CM, Golish JA, Avecillas JF, McCarthy K, Marlow S, et al. Predictors of nocturnal oxygen desaturation in pulmonary arterial hypertension. Chest. 2007;131(1):109–17.
22. Mereles D, Ehlken N, Kreuscher S, Ghofrani S, Hoeper MM, Halank M, et al. Exercise and respiratory training improve exercise capacity and quality of life in patients with severe chronic pulmonary hypertension. Circulation. 2006;114(14):1482–9.
23. Grünig E, Ehlken N, Ghofrani A, Staehler G, Meyer FJ, Juenger J, et al. Effect of exercise and respiratory training on clinical progression and survival in patients with severe chronic pulmonary hypertension. Respiration. 2011;81(5):394–401.
24. Grünig E, Maier F, Ehlken N, Fischer C, Lichtblau M, Blank N, et al. Exercise training in pulmonary arterial hypertension associated with connective tissue diseases. Arthritis Res Ther. 2012; 14(3):R148.
25. Weinstein AA, Chin LMK, Keyser RE, Kennedy M, Nathan SD, Woolstenhulme JG, et al. Effect of aerobic exercise training on fatigue and physical activity in patients with pulmonary arterial hypertension. Respir Med. 2013;107(5):778–84.
26. Chung W-S, Lin C-L, Sung F-C, Hsu W-H, Chen Y-F, Kao C-H. Increased risks of deep vein thrombosis and pulmonary embolism in Sjogren syndrome: a nationwide cohort study. J Rheumatol. 2014;41(5):909–15.
27. Rajdev A, Garan H, Biviano A. Arrhythmias in pulmonary arterial hypertension. Prog Cardiovasc Dis. 2012;55(2):180–6.
28. Tongers J, Schwerdtfeger B, Klein G, Kempf T, Schaefer A, Knapp J-M, et al. Incidence and clinical relevance of supraventricular tachyarrhythmias in pulmonary hypertension. Am Heart J. 2007; 153(1):127–32.
29. Ruiz-Cano MJ, Gonzalez-Mansilla A, Escribano P, Delgado J, Arribas F, Torres J, et al. Clinical implications of supraventricular arrhythmias in patients with severe pulmonary arterial hypertension. Int J Cardiol. 2011;146(1):105–6.
30. Patanè S, Marte F, Sturiale M, Dattilo G, Luzza F. Atrial flutter, ventricular tachycardia and changing axis deviation associated with scleroderma. Int J Cardiol. 2011;153(2):e25–8.
31. Kostis JB, Seibold JR, Turkevich D, Masi AT, Grau RG, Medsger TA, et al. Prognostic importance of cardiac arrhythmias in systemic sclerosis. Am J Med. 1988;84(6):1007–15.
32. Rich S, Seidlitz M, Dodin E, Osimani D, Judd D, Genthner D, et al. The short-term effects of digoxin in patients with right ventricular dysfunction from pulmonary hypertension. Chest. 1998;114(3): 787–92.
33. Smith TW, Antman EM, Friedman PL, Blatt CM, Marsh JD. Digitalis glycosides: mechanisms and manifestations of toxicity. Part I. Prog Cardiovasc Dis. 1984;26(5):413–58.
34. Overbeek MJ, Vonk MC, Boonstra A, Voskuyl AE, Vonk-Noordegraaf A, Smit EF, et al. Pulmonary arterial hypertension in limited cutaneous systemic sclerosis: a distinctive vasculopathy. Eur Respir J. 2008;34(2):371–9.

35. Johnson SR, Patsios D, Hwang DM, Granton JT. Pulmonary veno-occlusive disease and scleroderma associated pulmonary hypertension. J Rheumatol. 2006;33(11):2347–50.
36. Farber HW, Graven KK, Kokolski G, Korn JH. Pulmonary edema during acute infusion of epoprostenol in a patient with pulmonary hypertension and limited scleroderma. J Rheumatol. 1999;26(5):1195–6.
37. Palmer SM, Robinson LJ, Wang A, Gossage JR, Bashore T, Tapson VF. Massive pulmonary edema and death after prostacyclin infusion in a patient with pulmonary veno-occlusive disease. Chest. 1998;113(1):237–40.
38. Resten A, Maitre S, Humbert M, Rabiller A, Sitbon O, Capron F, et al. Pulmonary hypertension: CT of the chest in pulmonary veno-occlusive disease. AJR Am J Roentgenol. 2004;183(1):65–70.
39. Okumura H, Nagaya N, Kyotani S, Sakamaki F, Nakanishi N, Fukuhara S, et al. Effects of continuous IV prostacyclin in a patient with pulmonary veno-occlusive disease. Chest. 2002;122(3):1096–8.
40. Badesch DB, Tapson VF, McGoon MD, Brundage BH, Rubin LJ, Wigley FM, et al. Continuous intravenous epoprostenol for pulmonary hypertension due to the scleroderma spectrum of disease. A randomized, controlled trial. Ann Intern Med. 2000;132(6):425–34.
41. Badesch DB, McGoon MD, Barst RJ, Tapson VF, Rubin LJ, Wigley FM, et al. Longterm survival among patients with scleroderma-associated pulmonary arterial hypertension treated with intravenous epoprostenol. J Rheumatol. 2009;36(10):2244–9.
42. Oudiz RJ, Schilz RJ, Barst RJ, Galié N, Rich S, Rubin LJ, et al. Treprostinil, a prostacyclin analogue, in pulmonary arterial hypertension associated with connective tissue disease. Chest. 2004;126(2):420–7.
43. McLaughlin VV, Oudiz RJ, Frost A, Tapson VF, Murali S, Channick RN, et al. Randomized study of adding inhaled iloprost to existing bosentan in pulmonary arterial hypertension. Am J Respir Crit Care Med. 2006;174(11):1257–63.
44. McLaughlin VV, Benza RL, Rubin LJ, Channick RN, Voswinckel R, Tapson VF, et al. Addition of inhaled treprostinil to oral therapy for pulmonary arterial hypertension: a randomized controlled clinical trial. J Am Coll Cardiol. 2010;55(18):1915–22.
45. Humbert M, Barst RJ, Robbins IM, Channick RN, Galiè N, Boonstra A, et al. Combination of bosentan with epoprostenol in pulmonary arterial hypertension: BREATHE-2. Eur Respir J. 2004;24(3):353–9.
46. Simonneau G, Rubin LJ, Galiè N, Barst RJ, Fleming TR, Frost AE, et al. Addition of sildenafil to long-term intravenous epoprostenol therapy in patients with pulmonary arterial hypertension: a randomized trial. Ann Intern Med. 2008;149(8):521–30.
47. Rubenfire M, Huffman MD, Krishnan S, Seibold JR, Schiopu E, McLaughlin VV. Survival in systemic sclerosis with pulmonary arterial hypertension has not improved in the modern era. Chest. 2013;144(4):1282–90.
48. Hoeper MM, Faulenbach C, Golpon H, Winkler J, Welte T, Niedermeyer J. Combination therapy with bosentan and sildenafil in idiopathic pulmonary arterial hypertension. Eur Respir J. 2004;24(6):1007–10.
49. Mathai SC, Girgis RE, Fisher MR, Champion HC, Housten-Harris T, Zaiman A, et al. Addition of sildenafil to bosentan monotherapy in pulmonary arterial hypertension. Eur Respir J. 2007;29(3):469–75.
50. McLaughlin V, Channick RN, Ghofrani H-A, Lemarié J-C, Naeije R, Packer M, et al. Bosentan added to sildenafil therapy in patients with pulmonary arterial hypertension. Eur Respir J. 2015;46(2):405–13.
51. Oudiz R. ATHENA-1: hemodynamic improvements following the addition of ambrisentan to background PDE5i therapy in patients with pulmonary arterial hypertension. Chest. 2011;140(4_MeetingAbstracts):905A.
52. Galiè N, Barbera J, Frost A. AMBITION: a randomised, multicentre study of the first-line ambrisentan and tadalafil combination therapy in subjects with pulmonary arterial hypertension (PAH). Eur Respir J. 2014;44 Suppl 58:A2916.
53. Coghlan JG, Galiè N, Barbera JA, Frost AE, Ghofrani HA, Hoeper MM, et al. OP0267 initial combination therapy of ambrisentan and tadalafil in Connective Tissue Disease Associated Pulmonary Arterial Hypertension (CTD-PAH): subgroup analysis from the ambition trial. Ann Rheum Dis. 2015;74 Suppl 2:173.
54. Paul GA, Gibbs JSR, Boobis AR, Abbas A, Wilkins MR. Bosentan decreases the plasma concentration of sildenafil when coprescribed in pulmonary hypertension. Br J Clin Pharmacol. 2005;60(1):107–12.
55. Galiè N, Manes A, Negro L, Palazzini M, Bacchi-Reggiani ML, Branzi A. A meta-analysis of randomized controlled trials in pulmonary arterial hypertension. Eur Heart J. 2009;30(4):394–403.
56. Yusen RD, Edwards LB, Kucheryavaya AY, Benden C, Dipchand AI, Dobbels F, et al. The registry of the International Society for Heart and Lung Transplantation: thirty-first adult lung and heart-lung transplant report – 2014; focus theme: retransplantation. J Heart Lung Transplant. 2014;33(10):1009–24.
57. Saggar R, Khanna D, Furst DE, Belperio JA, Park GS, Weigt SS, et al. Systemic sclerosis and bilateral lung transplantation: a single centre experience. Eur Respir J. 2010;36(4):893–900.
58. Schachna L, Medsger TA, Dauber JH, Wigley FM, Braunstein NA, White B, et al. Lung transplantation in scleroderma compared with idiopathic pulmonary fibrosis and idiopathic pulmonary arterial hypertension. Arthritis Rheum. 2006;54(12):3954–61.
59. Launay D, Savale L, Berezne A, Le Pavec J, Hachulla E, Mouthon L, et al. Lung and heart-lung transplantation for systemic sclerosis patients. A monocentric experience of 13 patients, review of the literature and position paper of a multidisciplinary Working Group. Presse Med. 2014;43(10 Pt 2):e345–63.
60. Bernstein EJ, Peterson ER, Sell JL, D'Ovidio F, Arcasoy SM, Bathon JM, et al. Survival of adults with systemic sclerosis following lung transplantation: a nationwide cohort study. Arthritis Rheumatol. 2015;67(5):1314–22.
61. Khan IY, Singer LG, de Perrot M, Granton JT, Keshavjee S, Chau C, et al. Survival after lung transplantation in systemic sclerosis. A systematic review. Respir Med. 2013;107(12):2081–7.
62. Weill D, Benden C, Corris PA, Dark JH, Davis RD, Keshavjee S, et al. A consensus document for the selection of lung transplant candidates: 2014 – an update from the Pulmonary Transplantation Council of the International Society for Heart and Lung Transplantation. J Heart Lung Transplant. 2015;34(1):1–15.
63. Keogh AM, Mayer E, Benza RL, Corris P, Dartevelle PG, Frost AE, et al. Interventional and surgical modalities of treatment in pulmonary hypertension. J Am Coll Cardiol. 2009;54(1 Suppl):S67–77.
64. Sandoval J, Gaspar J, Pulido T, Bautista E, Martínez-Guerra ML, Zeballos M, et al. Graded balloon dilation atrial septostomy in severe primary pulmonary hypertension. A therapeutic alternative for patients nonresponsive to vasodilator treatment. J Am Coll Cardiol. 1998;32(2):297–304.
65. Kurzyna M, Dabrowski M, Bielecki D, Fijalkowska A, Pruszczyk P, Opolski G, et al. Atrial septostomy in treatment of end-stage right heart failure in patients with pulmonary hypertension. Chest. 2007;131(4):977–83.
66. Allcock RJ, O'Sullivan JJ, Corris PA. Palliation of systemic sclerosis-associated pulmonary hypertension by atrial septostomy. Arthritis Rheum. 2001;44(7):1660–2.
67. Centers for Medicare & Medicaid Services (CMS), HHS. Medicare and medicaid programs: hospice conditions of participation. final rule. Fed Regist. 2008;73(109):32087–220.
68. Condliffe R, Kiely DG, Peacock AJ, Corris PA, Gibbs JSR, Vrapi F, et al. Connective tissue disease-associated pulmonary arterial

hypertension in the modern treatment era. Am J Respir Crit Care Med. 2009;179(2):151–7.
69. Campo A, Mathai SC, Le Pavec J, Zaiman AL, Hummers LK, Boyce D, et al. Hemodynamic predictors of survival in scleroderma-related pulmonary arterial hypertension. Am J Respir Crit Care Med. 2010;182(2):252–60.
70. Benza RL, Miller DP, Barst RJ, Badesch DB, Frost AE, McGoon MD. An evaluation of long-term survival from time of diagnosis in pulmonary arterial hypertension from the REVEAL Registry. Chest. 2012;142(2):448–56.
71. Chen H, Taichman DB, Doyle RL. Health-related quality of life and patient-reported outcomes in pulmonary arterial hypertension. Proc Am Thorac Soc. 2008;5(5):623–30.
72. Swetz KM, Shanafelt TD, Drozdowicz LB, Sloan JA, Novotny PJ, Durst LA, et al. Symptom burden, quality of life, and attitudes toward palliative care in patients with pulmonary arterial hypertension: results from a cross-sectional patient survey. J Heart Lung Transplant. 2012;31(10):1102–8.
73. Fenstad ER, Shanafelt TD, Sloan JA, Novotny PJ, Durst LA, Frantz RP, et al. Physician attitudes toward palliative care for patients with pulmonary arterial hypertension: results of a cross-sectional survey. Pulm Circ. 2014;4(3):504–10.
74. Grinnan DC, Swetz KM, Pinson J, Fairman P, Lyckholm LJ, Smith T. The end-of-life experience for a cohort of patients with pulmonary arterial hypertension. J Palliat Med. 2012;15(10):1065–70.

54 Pseudo-obstruction with Malabsorption and Malnutrition

John O. Clarke

Case Presentation

The patient is an African-American woman who initially presented to gastroenterology clinic at the age of 63 with complaints of dysphagia, reflux, diarrhea, and weight loss. She carried a diagnosis of limited scleroderma that was confirmed 1 year prior to presentation. The diagnosis was made based on Raynaud's phenomenon, esophageal dysfunction, sclerodactyly, and telangiectasia in conjunction with anticentromere antibodies. She related that the diagnosis was suspected at age 50 and that she had long-standing Raynaud's beginning in her 20s. From a gastrointestinal (GI) standpoint, she related multiple symptoms, although she overall felt her symptoms to be only mild in severity. She had solid food dysphagia which had required a prior endoscopy with dilatation of an identified peptic stricture, with only mild symptoms thereafter. Reflux symptoms were intermittently present but largely controlled with a once daily proton pump inhibitor. She would take an as needed antacid for breakthrough symptoms approximately twice per week. She related chronic loose stools, although she denied the term diarrhea at the time, with bowel movements approximately four times per day. She had lost 20 lb unintentionally within the past year.

Gastrointestinal Disease in Scleroderma

The GI tract is affected in up to 90 % of patients with systemic sclerosis (SSc) and is associated with significant morbidity. While dermatologic change is the characteristic disease hallmark, GI tract involvement is believed to be the second most common manifestation. Exact pathophysiologic mechanisms remain unclear; however, atrophy and fibrosis have both been identified on evaluation, and the leading hypothesis is that peristaltic dysfunction leads to dysmotility, gut stasis, and dilatation. Esophageal symptoms, characterized predominantly by reflux and dysphagia, are the most commonly reported GI symptoms in patients with SSc. However, involvement can occur at any level of the GI tract, and symptoms such as early satiety, postprandial fullness, nausea, distention, bloating, diarrhea, and constipation all can be present with more distal GI tract involvement. When small bowel involvement is at play, major symptoms include abdominal pain, nausea, bloating, and distention. Small bacterial intestinal overgrowth can occur with resultant malnutrition [1–4]. This is a concerning development as GI tract involvement with malnutrition carries significant risk and is the third most common cause of mortality in patients with SSc (other than cardiopulmonary and renal disease) [5]. In this case, while the patient reports heartburn and dysphagia, the worrisome aspect of her history is the report of diarrhea with weight loss – raising the question of potential malabsorption and possible malnutrition, although at the time of initial evaluation, there was no evidence to support pseudo-obstruction per se.

Chronic intestinal pseudo-obstruction (CIP) is often associated with scleroderma and is an ominous development with significant morbidity. It is recognized as a GI motility disorder with the primary defect being impaired peristalsis, such that bowel dilatation and associated symptoms occur that can mimic a bowel obstruction – although mechanical obstruction cannot be identified. It can be related to multiple etiologies, including neuropathy, myopathy, or mesenchymopathy – although it is believed to be neurogenic in the majority of patients. This is seen in conjunction with small bowel dysfunction in SSc patients and is a well-recognized manifestation of GI tract involvement. However, it is also important to note that CIP can also occur in numerous other non-rheumatic conditions, including Parkinson's disease, amyloidosis, inherited conditions, diabetes, thyroid disease, and Chagas disease and associated with adverse reactions to

J.O. Clarke, MD
Division of Gastroenterology & Hepatology, Johns Hopkins University, 4940 Eastern Avenue, A-Building, Room 344B, Baltimore, MD 21224, USA
e-mail: john.clarke@jhu.edu

J. Varga et al. (eds.), *Scleroderma*, DOI 10.1007/978-3-319-31407-5_54

numerous medications – as well as in rheumatic conditions other than SSc [6]. The most commonly reported symptoms for CIP include abdominal pain (80 %), nausea and vomiting (75 %), constipation (40 %), and diarrhea (20 %), with abdominal pain and distention often being the dominant presenting symptoms [6, 7]. One common teaching with regard to CIP is that it is intermittent, but this is in fact the exception rather than the rule. In a seminal study evaluating patients with CIP, only 11 % of patients were asymptomatic between subacute obstructive-like episodes – whereas the majority have baseline symptoms consistent with small bowel dysmotility between superimposed and relative exacerbations [7].

Diagnostic Evaluation

At a subsequent appointment the following year, the patient noted ongoing weight loss (6 lb), intermittent abdominal pain, and continued diarrhea. Reflux was well controlled at that visit after modification of her antacid regimen and dysphagia remained stable. She was also noted to have a mild normocytic anemia. She underwent an upper endoscopy and colonoscopy with random biopsies. Her endoscopy was notable for retained food in the gastric fundus, and on gastric biopsy she was noted to have inactive chronic gastritis. In addition, bacteria and cocci were identified with a morphologic appearance inconsistent with *Helicobacter pylori*. Her colonoscopy was notable for several polyps, which were tubular adenomas on pathology, with no other abnormalities noted. An abdominal CT was performed and was notable for moderate fecal burden in the colon but no other gross abnormalities. A gastric emptying study was performed and was notable for significant gastric food retention at 4 h (47 % residual, normal <10 %). Given these results and her ongoing symptoms, she was started on low-dose metoclopramide as a prokinetic and a 2-week course of rifaximin for treatment of small intestinal bacterial overgrowth.

This case highlights some of the key questions that exist with regard to the appropriate evaluation required for assessment of potential dysmotility in symptomatic SSc patients. While esophageal involvement in SSc is extremely common, involvement of the stomach, small bowel, and colon is believed to occur less frequently and is not ubiquitous. One could make an argument to pursue focused testing to evaluate mucosal integrity, motility and physiology, and absorption – with the idea that treatment would then be tailored based on the results of that evaluation. However, an equally compelling argument could be made to treat empirically based on symptoms and likely dysmotility – given the known GI manifestations associated with scleroderma and the high likelihood that symptoms stem from underlying GI impairment. If one chooses to pursue a focused diagnostic evaluation of abdominal pain, diarrhea, and weight before proceeding with treatment (or while treatment is initiated), then the workup detailed above is not unreasonable. Generally an endoscopy is reasonable to exclude other common causes of abdominal pain (such as peptic ulcer disease) and to exclude strictures or other potential causes of mechanical obstruction. A colonoscopy can be considered for colorectal cancer screening and for mucosal biopsies to exclude microscopic or gross colitis. Imaging can be justified in the context of weight loss to exclude malignancy, to exclude obstruction, and also to evaluate for fecal retention and bowel diameter. In most cases, however, the results of this limited evaluation will be relatively unremarkable, and the primary purpose of these studies is to exclude other more common conditions that may be managed in an alternative fashion.

If one wishes to evaluate physiology and motility specifically, there are three general modalities by which this can be done. The first category would be a test to evaluate transit, with the hypothesis that small bowel dysmotility will result in stasis and decreased GI transit time. A small bowel series (with either barium or water-soluble contrast) is often the first test employed in this setting, as it can be utilized to roughly evaluate transit, assess bowel diameter, exclude obstruction, and in experienced hands to also give a rough assessment of motility. A comprehensive GI transit scintigraphy study is now an option and gives a more formal objective assessment of whole gut and regional transit; however, this study encompasses multiple days and is available in only a few centers worldwide. Gastric emptying scintigraphy alone is more commonly available and does provide useful information regarding gastric transit; however, it does not assess small bowel function [8–10]. Recently, a wireless motility capsule has also become clinically available and can assess regional transit as well as regional pressure patterns; however, data with regard to this study in SSc specifically is limited and capsule retention in the context of severe dysmotility is a theoretical risk [11].

A second method to assess gastric and small bowel physiology would be via measurement of pressure patterns. Traditionally this has been done via antroduodenal manometry. During this test, a catheter is passed transnasally and positioned (using either endoscopy or fluoroscopy to ensure appropriate placement) so that pressure sensors are located in the duodenum and stomach. Prolonged pressure monitoring can be performed to allow assessment of migrating motor complex activity – in particular assessment of frequency, amplitude, and coordination of contractions. This test theoretically allows one to separate a neuropathy from a myopathy. In patients with SSc and symptoms consistent with small bowel dysfunction, the amplitude and frequency of intestinal contractions have been found to be decreased in a consistent fashion [12]. However, this test is cumbersome and only available in limited tertiary centers. Recently, the wireless motility capsule has also entered the clinical armamentarium and at least in one study has been reported to provide comparable data to antroduodenal manometry. There is no data looking at SSc specifically with this technology, however, at present [13, 14].

Finally, one could argue to evaluate small bowel physiology through assessment of intraluminal bacterial concentration and populations – in essence assessing for small intestinal bacterial overgrowth (SIBO), which is seen almost ubiquitously with small bowel dysmotility in symptomatic patients with SSc. There are several means by which this can be performed (either directly or indirectly), including breath tests (measurement of exhaled hydrogen and methane after ingestion of either glucose or lactulose), jejunal cultures for quantitative bacterial cultures, xylose absorption tests, and fecal fat collection. Unfortunately, performance characteristics for all of these tests are relatively poor. A recent systematic review of 22 articles concluded that the only fully validated test to assess for SIBO in SSc was breath tests via hydrogen and methane assessment and that there was insufficient validation for the remainder of the studies listed above [15]. A recent study from investigators in Italy using lactulose breath tests in 99 SSc patients reported abnormalities consistent with SIBO in 46 % [16]. However, both lactulose and glucose breath tests are to some extent dependent on transit and not necessarily markers of SIBO per se, with recent publications comparing both studies to scintigraphy showing high false positive rates [17–19]. In the right clinical context, one could argue to treat for bacterial dysbiosis regardless of objective breath test parameters, given the known imperfections of the diagnostic studies.

Treatment Options

The patient was started on low-dose metoclopramide and treated with a 2-week course of rifaximin. She reported prompt resolution of diarrhea and at the time of her next appointment (4 months later) had gained 7 lb. Over the next 2 years, the patient did relatively well with intermittent (2-week) courses of rifaximin as needed (three times during that period). However, by the end of that 2-year period, she noted more frequent symptoms and was initiated on an antibiotic rotation, utilizing tetracycline and ciprofloxacin (with rifaximin not being used at the time due to cost). Initially her rotation was 2 weeks on antibiotics then 2 weeks off antibiotics. However, by the following year, she was clearly feeling worse during the period that she was off antibiotics, and the rotation was changed to 3 weeks on antibiotics and then only 1 week off. The following year she developed a slight tremor and metoclopramide was discontinued. Her symptoms seemed to worsen and the time period off antibiotics was eliminated from her rotation. Metronidazole and rifaximin were also added to her rotation given fears of antibiotic resistance. Later that year, due to progressive symptoms, she was admitted to the hospital for dehydration and ongoing weight loss. She was followed closely by nutrition and started nutritional liquid supplements daily to maintain her weight. At her next appointment, she was started on domperidone and seemed to improve in the context of domperidone initiation and daily antibiotics. She was followed closely over the next 4 years but unfortunately had symptom recurrence and worsening with ongoing weight loss. She was eventually convinced to start parenteral nutrition when her body mass index reached 14 (corresponding to a weight of 70 lb). In total, she had lost 50 lb by that point since her initial presentation to the GI clinic 8 years prior to the initiation of parenteral nutrition.

This case highlights the treatment options that are available for CIP in the context of SSc with resultant malabsorption and malnutrition. While not the case for this particular patient, the first step is often to remove any medications that could potentially negatively impact bowel function. Opiates would be the classic offenders but other entities such as calcium channel blockers and anticholinergic agents could have negative potential. The next step is often lifestyle and dietary modification, with reduction in dietary fiber content and liquid nutritional supplements if appropriate. Once both of those steps have been taken, then the next steps typically involve initiation of medical therapy. There are two general options available for treatment and no consensus as to which is the best initial route to initiate.

Prokinetic agents are a mainstay of therapy in the treatment of GI dysmotility; however, data are limited with regard to long-term efficacy. Nevertheless, this approach was endorsed by a recent expert consensus panel [20]. Metoclopramide is the only agent approved by the Food and Drug Administration in the United States for treatment of gastroparesis; however, it is associated with significant side effects including potentially irreversible tardive dyskinesia. Domperidone is a peripheral dopamine receptor antagonist that is believed to cross the blood-brain barrier less effective than metoclopramide and may provide equal or superior efficacy with potentially less side effects. This medication is not approved for use in the United States; however, it can be obtained via an FDA Investigational New Drug application and is also available in at least 50 other countries. However, domperidone can be associated with QT prolongation and requires monitoring if initiated. Erythromycin is a motilin agonist and known to augment gastric emptying. Cisapride is a combined serotonin $5HT_4$ agonist/$5HT_3$ antagonist and is the most investigated prokinetic available for treatment of SSc-related dysmotility; however, it was removed from the United States market due to QT interval prolongation and numerous deaths related to arrhythmia. It is available on a limited basis for compassionate use; however, it should be used with caution and close monitoring if required [21]. Further information with regard to all of these agents can be found in the chapter "Foregut manifestations of systemic sclerosis." Other potential options include pyridostigmine, bethanechol, and prucalopride; however, data for all of these agents is limited and use is off-label.

For those patients who do not respond to conventional prokinetics, octreotide may be an option. This was evaluated in a seminal paper in *New England Journal of Medicine* in 1991, and the investigators found that low-dose octreotide stimulated intestinal motility in normal subjects and in SSc patients and that short-term use reduced bacterial overgrowth and improved symptoms. This may be an option for selected patients with CIP and malnutrition, but care needs to be taken to employ a low-dose regimen as higher doses (as often employed for treatment of diarrhea) have been shown to impair gastric emptying [22]. Octreotide administration does require subcutaneous injection and use is off-label in the United States, which can pose problems with insurance authorization – especially as the medication is expensive. This agent was not started on the patient described in this case due to logistical barriers.

Antibiotics are often a mainstay of therapy for these patients. Intestinal dysmotility, dilatation, and stasis lead to bacterial overgrowth, and decreasing enteric gut flora can often have a profound effect on absorption, distention, and other symptoms. There are no randomized controlled trials that have evaluated the efficacy of antibiotics per se for symptomatic SSc patients; however, a recent expert consensus panel felt that rotating antibiotics may be useful in SSc [20]. There are no formal recommendations as to which antibiotics are employed in practice or the duration of such therapy; however, several excellent reviews summarize treatment strategies and are available for reference [23, 24]. In practice, rifaximin is often employed as systemic absorption is minimal; however, cost is more significant. Other antibiotics commonly utilized in practice include ciprofloxacin/norfloxacin, metronidazole, tetracycline, and amoxicillin-clavulanic acid.

Ultimately, if the GI tract is unable to function appropriately despite the options detailed above, then the next most appropriate step is nutritional supplementation. Enteral supplements can be added early to a patient's regimen and are reasonable options; however, this alone (as was the case for this patient) may not be sufficient. The addition of a gastrostomy, gastrojejunostomy, or jejunostomy tube (potentially combined with a gastric decompression tube) is an option to allow directed administration of tube feeds, particularly at night when the patient is sleeping; however, if the patient has a pan-GI dysmotility, it is not surprising that this option is often not effective in clinical practice – and in my case there have only been a small handful of patients who have been successful with this route. More often, when this stage of the algorithm is achieved, the next step is parenteral nutrition. Parenteral nutrition is not without risk and can be associated with cellulitis, sepsis, thromboembolic disease, and hepatic steatosis with potential progression to fibrosis/cirrhosis and pancreatitis [6]. In addition, the cost is significant with one estimate being $120,000 USD annually plus additional expenses for any line-related complications [25]. However, generally it is only initiated when no other option exists and with careful monitoring in the context of a multidisciplinary nutritional support team. Patients on parenteral nutrition can do well with improved nutrition and quality of life; however, short-term outcomes upon initiation of parenteral nutrition are poor, with one study showing a 2-year survival rate of only 58 % [26, 27]. Ultimately, the goal of parenteral nutrition is to improve nutritional parameters while attempting to rehabilitate the gut through maximization of the therapies detailed above – in the hopes that parenteral nutrition can eventually be discontinued and the patient can resume nutrition entirely via oral means. In the case of this patient, that remains the goal and she has gained 20 lb in a slow controlled fashion since the initiation of parenteral nutrition 9 months earlier; however, it remains to be seen whether she will be able to discontinue it entirely given her ongoing symptoms and limited oral intake.

Key Points

1. While most patients with scleroderma have GI involvement, significant intestinal dysmotility leading to chronic intestinal pseudo-obstruction and malnutrition is uncommon; however, when it does occur, morbidity and mortality are high.
2. The utility of formal motility diagnostic assessment is debatable and one can argue to treat empirically based on symptoms given known pathophysiology.
3. If formal motility assessment is desired (to customize therapy), one could argue to pursue small bowel imaging, transit, and potentially pressure patterns.
4. Prokinetics are a mainstay of therapy, although these medications do not have robust long-term data and have safety concerns.
5. Antibiotics are a mainstay of therapy and long-term therapy with a rotation is often employed.
6. Octreotide can be considered for select patients with robust data to justify use.
7. Consider modifying medications if other agents have a deleterious effect on bowel function (e.g., opiates).
8. Consider dietary modification and supplements early in the disease course if applicable.
9. Parenteral nutrition may be required if all other options fail.

References

1. LeRoy EC, Black C, Fleischmajer R, et al. Scleroderma (systemic sclerosis): classification, subsets and pathogenesis. J Rheumatol. 1988;15:202–5.
2. Clements PJ, Becvar R, Drosos AA, et al. Assessment of gastrointestinal involvement. Clin Exp Rheumatol. 2003;21:S15–8.
3. Forbes A, Marie I. Gastrointestinal complications: the most frequent internal complications of systemic sclerosis. Rheumatology (Oxford). 2009;48 Suppl 3:iii36–9.
4. Butt S, Emmanuel A. Systemic sclerosis and the gut. Expert Rev Gastroenterol Hepatol. 2013;7:331–9.
5. Steen VD, Medsger Jr TA. Severe organ involvement in systemic sclerosis with diffuse scleroderma. Arthritis Rheum. 2000;43:2437–44.
6. Gabbard SL, Lacy BE. Chronic intestinal pseudo-obstruction. Nutr Clin Pract. 2013;28:307–16.
7. Mann SD, Debinski HS, Kamm MA. Clinical characteristics of chronic idiopathic intestinal pseudo-obstruction in adults. Gut. 1997;41:675–81.
8. Antoniou AJ, Raja S, El-Khouli R, et al. Comprehensive radionuclide esophagogastrointestinal transit study: methodology, reference values, and initial clinical experience. J Nucl Med. 2015;56:721–7.
9. Parkman HP. Assessment of gastric emptying and small-bowel motility: scintigraphy, breath tests, manometry, and SmartPill. Gastrointest Endosc Clin N Am. 2009;19:49–55. vi.
10. Parkman HP. Scintigraphy for evaluation of patients for GI motility disorders – the referring physician's perspective. Semin Nucl Med. 2012;42:76–8.
11. Stein E, Berger Z, Hutfless S, Shah L, Wilson LM, Haberl EB, Bass EB, Clarke JO. Wireless Motility Capsule Versus Other Diagnostic Technologies for Evaluating Gastroparesis and Constipation: A Comparative Effectiveness Review [Internet]. Rockville (MD): Agency for Healthcare Research and Quality (US); 2013 May. PMID: 23785726.
12. Weston S, Thumshirn M, Wiste J, et al. Clinical and upper gastrointestinal motility features in systemic sclerosis and related disorders. Am J Gastroenterol. 1998;93:1085–9.
13. Cassilly D, Kantor S, Knight LC, et al. Gastric emptying of a non-digestible solid: assessment with simultaneous SmartPill pH and pressure capsule, antroduodenal manometry, gastric emptying scintigraphy. Neurogastroenterol Motil. 2008;20:311–9.
14. Brun R, Michalek W, Surjanhata BC, et al. Comparative analysis of phase III migrating motor complexes in stomach and small bowel using wireless motility capsule and antroduodenal manometry. Neurogastroenterol Motil. 2012;24:332–e165.
15. Braun-Moscovici Y, Braun M, Khanna D, et al. What tests should you use to assess small intestinal bacterial overgrowth in systemic sclerosis? Clin Exp Rheumatol. 2015;33 Suppl 91:117–22.
16. Savarino E, Mei F, Parodi A, et al. Gastrointestinal motility disorder assessment in systemic sclerosis. Rheumatology (Oxford). 2013;52:1095–100.
17. Yu D, Cheeseman F, Vanner S. Combined oro-caecal scintigraphy and lactulose hydrogen breath testing demonstrate that breath testing detects oro-caecal transit, not small intestinal bacterial overgrowth in patients with IBS. Gut. 2011;60:334–40.
18. Zhao J, Zheng X, Chu H, et al. A study of the methodological and clinical validity of the combined lactulose hydrogen breath test with scintigraphic oro-cecal transit test for diagnosing small intestinal bacterial overgrowth in IBS patients. Neurogastroenterol Motil. 2014;26:794–802.
19. Lin EC, Massey BT. Scintigraphy demonstrates high rate of false-positive results from glucose breath tests for small bowel bacterial overgrowth. Clin Gastroenterol Hepatol. 2015;14:203–8.
20. Kowal-Bielecka O, Landewe R, Avouac J, et al. EULAR recommendations for the treatment of systemic sclerosis: a report from the EULAR Scleroderma Trials and Research group (EUSTAR). Ann Rheum Dis. 2009;68:620–8.
21. Acosta A, Camilleri M. Prokinetics in gastroparesis. Gastroenterol Clin N Am. 2015;44:97–111.
22. Soudah HC, Hasler WL, Owyang C. Effect of octreotide on intestinal motility and bacterial overgrowth in scleroderma. N Engl J Med. 1991;325:1461–7.
23. Gasbarrini A, Lauritano EC, Gabrielli M, et al. Small intestinal bacterial overgrowth: diagnosis and treatment. Dig Dis. 2007;25:237–40.
24. Grace E, Shaw C, Whelan K, et al. Review article: small intestinal bacterial overgrowth – prevalence, clinical features, current and developing diagnostic tests, and treatment. Aliment Pharmacol Ther. 2013;38:674–88.
25. Howard L. Home parenteral nutrition: survival, cost, and quality of life. Gastroenterology. 2006;130:S52–9.
26. Jawa H, Fernandes G, Saqui O, et al. Home parenteral nutrition in patients with systemic sclerosis: a retrospective review of 12 cases. J Rheumatol. 2012;39:1004–7.
27. Bharadwaj S, Tandon P, Gohel T, et al. Gastrointestinal manifestations, malnutrition, and role of enteral and parenteral nutrition in patients with scleroderma. J Clin Gastroenterol. 2015;49:559–64.

Progressive Interstitial Lung Disease Nonresponse to Cyclophosphamide

55

Katherine C. Silver, Kristin B. Highland, and Richard M. Silver

Case Presentation

A 27-year-old Caucasian woman presented at 23 6/7 weeks gestational age with seizure and hypoxic respiratory failure. She had no relevant past medical history, but family history was significant for a mother and sister with lupus. On initial examination, her blood pressure was 200/130 mmHg, and on chest exam, she had bibasilar crackles. Laboratory work-up revealed acute kidney injury, thrombocytopenia, and microangiopathic hemolytic anemia. She was originally thought to have eclampsia; however, she did not improve following delivery. Upon further investigation, she was found to have a positive antinuclear antibody (ANA) (1:320, homogeneous pattern), a positive anti-Scl-70 antibody, and an abnormal capillary morphology on nailfold capillaroscopy. In the absence of initial skin changes, she was diagnosed with systemic sclerosis *sine* scleroderma presenting as scleroderma renal crisis (SRC). She had complete recovery from SRC, and within several months of initial presentation, she developed diffuse scleroderma. She also had a decrease in forced vital capacity (FVC) and diffusing capacity for carbon monoxide (DLCO), so she underwent high-resolution computed tomography (HRCT) chest scan that showed mild interstitial lung disease (ILD) (Fig. 55.1a). Bronchoalveolar lavage fluid contained 12.5 % neutrophils consistent with active alveolitis.

K.C. Silver, MD
Department of Rheumatology, Medical University of South Carolina, Charleston, SC 29425, USA

K.B. Highland, MD, MSCR
Department of Pulmonary and Critical Care Medicine, Cleveland Clinic Foundation, Cleveland, OH 44195, USA

R.M. Silver, MD (✉)
Division of Rheumatology and Immunology, Medical University of South Carolina, Charleston, SC, USA
e-mail: silverr@musc.edu

Treatment Course

Eight months after her initial presentation, the patient was started on oral cyclophosphamide for systemic sclerosis-associated interstitial lung disease (SSc-ILD). She had improvement in her pulmonary function tests (PFTs) (Table 55.1), dyspnea and skin score on daily oral cyclophosphamide (2 mg/kg), but this treatment was eventually discontinued after 18 months out of concern for long-term toxicity. Within several months of discontinuing cyclophosphamide, her PFTs worsened, so she then received a course of intravenous cyclophosphamide (750 mg/m^2 body surface area monthly) for a total of 6 months. Dyspnea remained stable following treatment with intravenous cyclophosphamide; however, her PFTs continued to decline, and so she was started on mycophenolate mofetil (MMF) which was titrated up to a dose of 1.5 g twice daily. PFTs and HRCT chest scan continued to worsen (Fig. 55.1b), and she developed anemia while on mycophenolate. Therefore, MMF was stopped after just a few months, and intravenous cyclophosphamide was resumed. Despite this, PFTs continued to worsen, and repeat HRCT chest scan showed significant progression of ILD. She was then once again placed on oral cyclophosphamide. Over the next several months, the patient had decreased exercise tolerance and increasing oxygen requirement. FVC decreased to 41 % predicted, and DLCO decreased to just 23 % predicted. Thus, experimental therapy with a tyrosine kinase inhibitor (imatinib) was begun in addition to the oral cyclophosphamide which was continued. After 1 year, she developed pancytopenia, so both imatinib and oral cyclophosphamide were stopped. Her oxygen requirement had increased to 6 l/min, so she was referred for lung transplant evaluation. She was initially rejected due to severe esophageal dysmotility and gastroesophageal reflux disease (GERD). A second lung transplant center recommended surgical management of GERD prior to proceeding with lung transplant, so she underwent a Roux-en-Y gastric bypass to manage her GERD. During this time, her ILD remained stable off immunosuppressive therapy. The patient continued pulmonary rehabilitation and was able to be

J. Varga et al. (eds.), *Scleroderma*, DOI 10.1007/978-3-319-31407-5_55

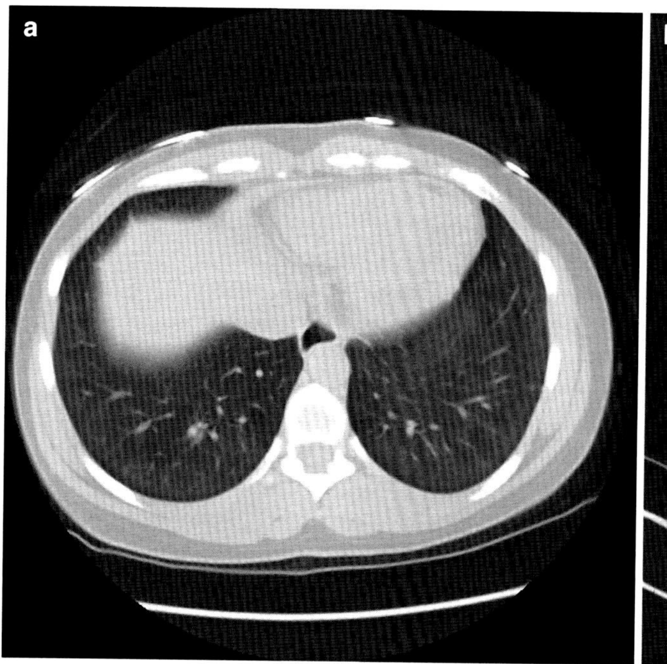

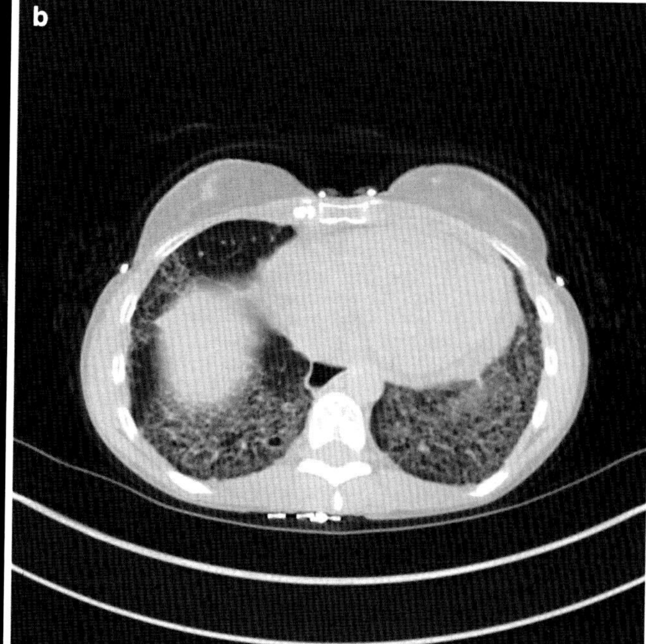

Fig. 55.1 (**a**) HRCT chest scan showing mild systemic sclerosis-associated interstitial lung disease (SSc-ILD) with ground glass opacification at both lung bases. (**b**) HRCT chest scan 8 years later and despite treatment showing honeycomb changes, traction bronchiectasis, and severe SSc-ILD

Table 55.1 Serial pulmonary function tests

Date of Study	Treatment	FVC (%)	DLCO (%)
8/2004	Oral cyclophosphamide	74	50
5/2005	Oral cyclophosphamide	67	40
6/2006	Oral cyclophosphamide	76	49
2/2007	Changed to mycophenolate	65	42
5/2008	Oral cyclophosphamide + imatinib	41	23
5/2009	Immunosuppression stopped. Evaluated for lung transplant and underwent gastric bypass	40	19
6/2010	Off immunosuppression	52	34
7/2011	Off immunosuppression	53	41
7/2012	Off immunosuppression	51	54
7/2013	Off immunosuppression	43	53
6/2014	Started back on mycophenolate	40	41

weaned off supplemental oxygen. PFTs improved as well, with FVC increasing to 51 % predicted and DLCO increasing to 52 % predicted. After doing well for several years, her FVC and DLCO began to trend downward, and she once again required supplemental oxygen. Right-heart catheterization revealed mild pulmonary hypertension with a mean PA pressure of 32 mmHg. MMF was resumed, and tadalafil was added to her medical regimen. She is once again undergoing evaluation for lung transplant.

Discussion

Since the introduction of angiotensin-converting enzyme (ACE) inhibitor therapy as the first effective treatment for scleroderma renal crisis, ILD has become a leading cause of morbidity and mortality in scleroderma (SSc) [1, 2]. Our patient had a number of risk factors for the presence and progression of SSc-ILD (Table 55.2). Interstitial lung disease occurs in all subtypes of SSc, but the prevalence of SSc-ILD is higher in patients with diffuse cutaneous systemic sclerosis (dcSSc) [3]. Although our patient originally presented as systemic sclerosis *sine* scleroderma, she quickly went on to develop a dcSSc with a high-modified Rodnan skin score. She also was found to have anti-topoisomerase I (anti-Scl-70) autoantibodies, the presence of which is strongly linked to SSc-ILD with over 85 % of Scl-70+ patients going on to develop pulmonary fibrosis [4]. Soon after her diagnosis of SSc, our patient was found to have evidence of ILD as evidenced by a decline in her FVC and abnormalities on both HRCT and bronchoalveolar lavage studies. Studies show that the greatest risk of progression of SSc is within the first

Table 55.2 Risk factors for presence and progression of interstitial lung disease

Male gender
African American
Diffuse skin involvement
Autoantibodies
Topoisomerase (Scl-70)
U1-RNP
U3-RNP
Th/To
PM/Scl
Early-onset SSc (<5 years)
Abnormal forced vital capacity
Extensive fibrosis on HRCT (>20 %)
GERD

5 years of disease with an abnormal FVC during this time frame being an important predictor for eventual end-stage lung disease [5]. Patients with more extensive fibrosis (>20 %) on HRCT are also at significantly higher risk for rapid decline in pulmonary function and death [6]. Likewise, patients with increased granulocytes on bronchoalveolar lavage have greater dyspnea and reduction in lung volumes and diffusion capacity that persists over time [7]. Although our patient did not have the classical symptoms of gastroesophageal reflux disease (GERD), she eventually was found to have severely abnormal esophageal function on testing during evaluation for lung transplantation. Aggressive treatment with proton pump inhibitors (PPIs), histamine (H2) blockers, and eventually a Roux-en-Y gastric bypass significantly improved her pulmonary function and reduced her supplemental oxygen requirement. An association between GERD and several different ILDs, including SSc-ILD, exists, and the extent of SSc-ILD as assessed by pulmonary function and HRCT is correlated with the degree of esophageal reflux [8, 9]. The sum of these risk factors may explain, in part, why our patient did not respond to conventional treatment with cyclophosphamide.

The decision to begin cyclophosphamide in our patient was based on data from the Scleroderma Lung Study I [10], which was designed as a randomized multicenter, double-blind placebo-controlled trial to evaluate the efficacy and safety of oral cyclophosphamide for 1 year in patients with symptomatic SSc-ILD and with evidence of disease activity by findings on bronchoalveolar lavage and/or HRCT chest scan. This was the first positive study in SSc-ILD and showed a modest improvement in the primary endpoint (2.53 % adjusted FVC % predicted, $p<0.03$) and improvement in a number of secondary endpoints including total lung capacity, modified Rodnan skin score, Transition Dyspnea Index, extent of fibrosis on HRCT, and several quality of life measures [10, 11]. Unfortunately, like in our patient, the treatment effect was lost by 24 months [12]. In an attempt to mitigate some of the long-term side effects of oral cyclophosphamide, we then treated our patient with intravenous cyclophosphamide, in part based on data from the Fibrosing Alveolitis in Scleroderma Trial (FAST) [13]. This small study randomized patients to receive either intravenous cyclophosphamide for 6 months followed by daily oral azathioprine or placebo infusions followed by oral placebo. At 12 months, a modest but nonstatistically significant improvement in FVC was seen in the actively treated group ($p=0.08$). At this time, the EULAR Scleroderma Trials and Research group recommends cyclophosphamide for the treatment of SSc-ILD, although there is a lack of consensus regarding strategies for induction and maintenance [14, 15].

Cyclophosphamide has been quoted as "arguably the most toxic immunosuppressive agent currently used to treat autoimmune diseases [16]," which prompted investigation into safer, less toxic alternatives. In a number of uncontrolled, prospective, or retrospective case series, mycophenolate mofetil (MMF) has been shown to stabilize or improve lung function in patients with SSc-ILD [17–28]. Scleroderma Lung Study II was designed to evaluate the efficacy and safety of MMF for 2 years in comparison with oral cyclophosphamide for 1 year followed by placebo. The results from this study are expected in 2015. Unfortunately, MMF is also not without side effects, and our patient developed anemia while on this drug.

There has been interest in the use of tyrosine kinase inhibitors, such as imatinib, in SSc-ILD because of downstream effects to inhibit transforming growth factor beta and platelet-derived growth factor, key signaling molecules in the pathogenesis of SSc-ILD. In a study of 30 consecutive SSc-ILD patients nonresponsive to cyclophosphamide, treatment with low-dose imatinib for 6 months resulted in stabilization or improvement in 73 % (22 patients) [29]. Other studies, however, have shown poor tolerability [30–35], and our patient ultimately had to discontinue imatinib because of pancytopenia.

In a post hoc analysis of Scleroderma Lung Study I (SLS I), patients like ours with severe fibrosis (>50 %) on HRCT chest scan and higher skin scores (>23 mRSS) had a greater treatment effect [36]. This supports the concept that "fibrosis begets fibrosis." Recently two antifibrotic therapies (pirfenidone [37] and nintedanib [38]) have been approved by the FDA for treatment of idiopathic pulmonary fibrosis (IPF) based on stabilization of pulmonary function. Both are currently under investigation in SSc-ILD patients. Each of these drugs is associated with significant gastrointestinal toxicity (GERD, nausea and vomiting with pirfenidone, diarrhea with nintedanib), and it remains to be seen if these drugs will be tolerable in SSc patients who already may have a myriad of gastrointestinal symptoms.

A number of other immunosuppressive agents which were not tried in our patient have recently become of interest in treating SSc-ILD. Several small studies [39, 40] suggest that rituximab may improve or stabilize PFTs and HRCT chest scan changes. An IL-6 receptor blocker (tocilizumab), a T-cell co-stimulatory blocker (abatacept), and a monoclonal antibody directed against B-cell activating factor (belimumab) are all currently being investigated. It is unclear if any of these agents will prove to be an effective therapy for SSc-ILD. Fortunately, there are many other new therapeutic agents that target growth factors, cytokines, and pathways of interest in SSc-ILD as well as existing drugs that may be repurposed for this disease.

Because both conventional and nonconventional treatments for her SSc-ILD failed, our patient chose to pursue lung transplantation. Many centers, as our patient encountered, are reluctant to perform lung transplantation in scleroderma patients because of their high prevalence of esophageal dysfunction, which is believed to contribute to allograft dysfunction. Nevertheless, transplant outcomes have been shown to be similar in carefully selected SSc patients compared to patients with IPF and with pulmonary arterial hypertension (PAH). The 2-year and 5-year survival were 72 % and 55 %, respectively [41, 42], although the severity of GERD was shown to impact the 1-year survival rate [43]. There have been no reports of recurrence of SSc-ILD in the lung allograft [44].

Autologous hematopoietic stem cell transplantation (HSCT) is another potential therapy under investigation for scleroderma. Treatment-related mortality is quite high, however, so this treatment remains experimental and is currently offered to highly selected patients considered to be at high risk for disease-related morbidity and mortality. Two phases II/III multicenter trials comparing HSCT to monthly intravenous cyclophosphamide have completed enrollment. The Autologous Stem cell Transplantation International Scleroderma (ASTIS) trial [45] included a high percentage of patients with mild to moderate restrictive lung disease (86.5 % of 156 subjects). At 5.8 years of follow-up, a statistically significant difference favoring HSCT was found in lung function (mean change in FVC 6.3 % vs −2.8 % predicted and TLC 5.1 % vs −1.3 % predicted). The Scleroderma: Cyclophosphamide or Transplantation (SCOT) study has completed enrollment, and results are expected in 2016. The Autologous Stem Cell Systemic Sclerosis Immune Suppression Trial (ASSIST) [46] was a single-center, open-label phase II trial in ten patients that demonstrated improvement in lung function as well as reduction in the extent of lung disease on HRCT. Eight of nine control patients (cyclophosphamide-treated) showed disease progression, and seven of these patients then crossed over to HSCT therapy. After 2 years, 11/18 patients showed persistent improvement in HRCT and FVC (but not TLC or DLCO). Another clinical trial, Scleroderma Treatment with Autologous Transplant (STAT) is currently enrolling patients (clinicaltrials.gov/ct2/show/NCT0141311). In this trial, selected patients with SSc-ILD who have failed conventional immunosuppressive therapy will receive autologous CD34+ stem cells followed by maintenance therapy with MMF for up to 2 years.

Table 55.3 Clinical risk factors for development of SSc-ILD-PH

Female gender
Caucasian
Diffuse skin involvement
Late age of onset of systemic sclerosis
Disease duration greater than 10 years
Presence of telangiectasias
Severe Raynaud's phenomenon
Autoantibodies
Anti-nucleolar antibody
U3RNP
Cardiolipin

Our patient recently presented with increased dyspnea and worsened exercise tolerance without substantial change in PFTs or HRCT. This prompted investigation for pulmonary hypertension, a comorbid condition that is seen in an estimated ~45 % of patients with SSc-ILD [47] and which carries a significant increase in morbidity and mortality [47–49]. Our patient had a number of clinical risk factors [48, 50, 51] (Table 55.3) for the development of SSc-ILD-PH: female, Caucasian, diffuse cutaneous systemic sclerosis, disease duration more than 10 years, presence of telangiectasias, and severe Raynaud's phenomenon. DLCO <40 % predicted or FVC % predicted/DLCO % predicted >1.6 is predictive of the presence of pulmonary hypertension in the background of interstitial lung disease [51]. The echocardiogram is notoriously inaccurate in patients with advanced lung disease [52] so the clinician should have a low threshold to obtain right-heart catheterization, the gold standard needed to establish the diagnosis of pulmonary arterial hypertension. The safety and efficacy of PAH-specific vasodilator therapy in patients with SSc-ILD-PH is not known due to the lack of high-quality clinical trials, and there is concern that these drugs could be associated with worsening hypoxemia due to V/Q mismatch. In a retrospective analysis of 70 patients with SSc-ILD-PH, there was no benefit from treatment with prostanoids, phosphodiesterase-5 inhibitors, or endothelin receptor antagonists in terms of WHO functional class, 6-min walk distance, and hemodynamics [49]. Nevertheless, in small case series, some patients have received benefit from reducing their pulmonary vascular resistance without significantly reducing oxygen tension [47, 53]. Identification of pulmonary hypertension in our patient increased her lung allocation score moving her higher up on the transplantation list.

Lastly, patients with SSc-ILD should receive supportive care including supplemental oxygen, influenza and pneumococcal vaccinations, referral for pulmonary rehabilitation, psychosocial counseling, and pregnancy prevention. Patients being treated with cyclophosphamide should also receive prophylaxis therapy to prevent *Pneumocystis jirovecii* infection.

References

1. Steen VD, Medsger Jr TA. Changes in causes of death in systemic sclerosis. Ann Rheum Dis. 2007;66:940–4.
2. Ferri C, Valentini G, Cozzi F, et al. Systemic sclerosis: demographic, clinical, and serologic features and survival in 1,012 Italian patients. Medicine (Baltimore). 2002;81:139–53.
3. Walker UA, Tyndall A, Czirják L, et al. Clinical risk assessment of organ manifestations in systemic sclerosis: a report from the EULAR scleroderma trials and research group database. Ann Rheum Dis. 2007;66:754–63.
4. Briggs DC, Vaughan RW, Welsh KI, Myers A, duBois RM, Black CM. Immunogenetic prediction of pulmonary fibrosis in systemic sclerosis. Lancet. 1991;338:661–2.
5. Morgan C, Knight C, Lunt M, Black CM, Silman AJ. Predictors of end stage lung disease in a cohort of patients with scleroderma. Ann Rheum Dis. 2003;62:146–50.
6. Goh NS, Desai SR, Veeraraghavan S, et al. Interstitial lung disease in systemic sclerosis: a simple staging system. Am J Respir Crit Care Med. 2008;177:1238–54.
7. Silver RM, Miller KS, Kinsella MB, Smith EA, Schabel SI. Evaluation and management of scleroderma lung disease using bronchoalveolar lavage. Am J Med. 1990;88:47–76.
8. Savarino E, Bazzica M, Zentilin P, et al. Gastroesophageal reflux and pulmonary fibrosis in scleroderma: a study using pH-impedance monitoring. Am J Respir Crit Care Med. 2009;179:408–13.
9. Christmann RB, Wells AU, Capelozzi VL, Silver RM. Gastroesophageal reflux incites interstitial lung disease in systemic sclerosis: clinical, radiologic, histopathologic, and treatment evidence. Semin Arthritis Rheum. 2010;40(3):241–9.
10. Tashkin D, Elashoff R, Clements P, et al. Cyclophosphamide versus placebo in scleroderma lung disease. N Engl J Med. 2006; 25(354):2655–66.
11. Goldin JG, Lynch DA, Strollo DC, et al. Follow-Up HRCT after treatment of scleroderma-interstitial lung disease with cyclophosphamide demonstrates evidence for treatment effect. Am J Respir Crit Care Med. 2008;177(A768):91.
12. Tashkin DP, Elashoff R, Clements PJ, et al. Effects of 1-year treatment with cyclophosphamide on outcomes at 2 years in scleroderma lung disease. Am J Respir Crit Care Med. 2007;176: 1026–34.
13. Hoyles RK, Ellis RW, Wellsbury J, et al. A multicenter, prospective, randomized, double-blind, placebo-controlled trial of corticosteroids and intravenous cyclophosphamide followed by oral azathioprine for the treatment of pulmonary fibrosis in scleroderma. Arthritis Rheum. 2006;54:3962–70.
14. Kowal-Bielecka O, Landewe R, Avouac J, et al. EULAR recommendations for the treatment of systemic sclerosis: a report from the EULAR Scleroderma Trials and Research group (EUSTAR). Ann Rheum Dis. 2009;60:620–8.
15. Walker KM; Pope J; participating members of the Scleroderma Clinical Trials Consortium (SCTC); Canadian Scleroderma Research Group (CSRG). Treatment of systemic sclerosis complications: what to use when first-line treatment fails--a consensus of systemic sclerosis experts. Seminars in Arthritis & Rheumatism. 2012;42(1):42–55.
16. Martinez FJ, McCune WJ. Cyclophosphamide for scleroderma lung disease. N Engl J Med. 2006;345:2707–9.
17. Swigris JJ, Olson AL, Fischer A, et al. Mycophenolate mofetil is safe, well tolerated, and preserves lung function in patients with connective tissue disease-related interstitial lung disease. Chest. 2006;130:30–6.
18. Liossis SN, Bounas A, Andonopoulos AP. Mycophenolate mofetil as first-line treatment improves clinically evident early scleroderma lung disease. Rheumatology (Oxford). 2006;45:1005–8.
19. Nihtyanova SI, Brough GM, Black CM, Denton CP. Mycophenolate mofetil in diffuse cutaneous systemic sclerosis – a retrospective analysis. Rheumatology (Oxford). 2007;46:442–5.
20. Zamora AC, Wolters PJ, Collard HR, et al. Use of mycophenolate mofetil to treat scleroderma-associated interstitial lung disease. Respir Med. 2008;102:150–5.
21. Gerbino AJ, Goss CH, Molitor JA. Effect of mycophenolate mofetil on pulmonary function in scleroderma-associated interstitial lung disease. Chest. 2008;133:455–60.
22. Derk CT, Grace E, Shenin M, Naik M, Schulz S, Xiong W. A prospective open-label study of mycophenolate mofetil for the treatment of diffuse systemic sclerosis. Rheumatology. 2009;48: 1595–9.
23. Koutroumpas A, Ziogas A, Alexiou I, Barouta G, Sakkas LI. Mycophenolate mofetil in systemic sclerosis-associated interstitial lung disease. Clin Rheumatol. 2010;29:1167–8.
24. Le EN, Wigley FM, Shah AA, Boin F, Hummers LK. Long-term experience of mycophenolate mofetil for treatment of diffuse cutaneous systemic sclerosis. Ann Rheum Dis. 2011;70:1104–7.
25. Simeon-Aznar CP, Fonollosa-Pia V, Tolosa-Vilella C, Selva-O'Callaghan A, Solans-Laque R, Vilardeli-Tarres M. Effect of mycophenolate sodium in scleroderma-related interstitial lung disease. Clin Rheumatol. 2011;30:1393–8.
26. Mendoza FA, Nagle SJ, Lee JB, Jimenez SA. A prospective observational study of mycophenolate mofetil treatment in progressive diffuse cutaneous systemic sclerosis of recent onset. J Rheumatol. 2012;39:1241–7.
27. Henes JC, Horger M, Amberger C, et al. Enteric-coated mycophenolate sodium for progressive systemic sclerosis – a prospective open-label study with CT histography for monitoring pulmonary fibrosis. Clin Rheumatol. 2013;32:673–8.
28. Panopoulos ST, Bournia VK, Trakada G, Giavri I, Kostopoulos C, Sfikakis PP. Mycophenolate versus cyclophosphamide for progressive interstitial lung disease associated with systemic sclerosis: a 2-year case control study. Lung. 2013;191:483–9.
29. Fraticelli P, Gabrielli B, Pomponio G, et al. Low-dose oral imatinib in the treatment of systemic sclerosis interstitial lung disease unresponsive to cyclophosphamide: a phase II pilot study. Arthritis Res Ther. 2014;16:R144.
30. Pope J, McBain D, Petrlich L, Watson S, Vanderhoek L, de Leon F, Seney S, Summers K. Imatinib in active diffuse cutaneous systemic sclerosis: results of a six-month, randomized, double-blind, placebo-controlled, proof-of-concept pilot study at a single center. Arthritis Rheum. 2011;63:3547–51.
31. Spiera RF, Gordon JK, Mersten JN, Magro CM, Mehta M, Wildman HF, Kloiber S, Kirou KA, Lyman S, Crow MK. Imatinib mesylate (Gleevec) in the treatment of diffuse cutaneous systemic sclerosis: results of a 1-year, phase IIa, single-arm, open-label clinical trial. Ann Rheum Dis. 2011;70:1003–9.
32. Khanna D, Saggar R, Mayes MD, Abtin F, Clements PJ, Maranian P, Assassi S, Saggar R, Singh RR, Furst DE. A one-year, phase I/IIa, open-label pilot trial of imatinib mesylate in the treatment of systemic sclerosis-associated active interstitial lung disease. Arthritis Rheum. 2011;63:3540–6.
33. Distler O, Distler JHW, Varga J, Denton CP, Lafyatis RA, Wigley FM, Schett G. A multi-center, open-label, proof of concept study of imatinib mesylate demonstrates no benefit for the treatment of fibrosis in patients with early, diffuse systemic sclerosis. [abstract]. Arthritis Rheum. 2010;62:560.
34. Guo L, Chen XX, Gu YY, Zou HJ, Ye S. Low-dose imatinib in the treatment of severe systemic sclerosis: a case series of six Chinese patients and literature review. Clin Rheumatol. 2012;31:1395–400.
35. Prey S, Ezzedine K, Doussau A, Grandoulier AS, Barcat D, Chatelus E, Diot E, Durant C, Havchulla E, de Korwin-Krokowski JD, Kostrzewa E, Quemeneur T, Paul C, Schaeverbeke T, Seneschal J, Solanilla A, Sparsa A, Bouchet S, Lepreux S, Mahon FX, Chene

G, Taïeb A. Imatinib mesylate in scleroderma-associated diffuse skin fibrosis: a phase II multicentre randomized double-blinded controlled trial. Br J Dermatol. 2012;167:1138–44.

36. Roth MD, Tseng CH, Clements PJ, et al. Predicting treatment outcomes and responder subsets in scleroderma-related interstitial lung disease. Arthritis Rheum. 2011;63(9):2797–808.
37. King TE, Bradford WZ, Castro-Bernardini S, et al. A phase 3 trial of pirfenidone in patients with idiopathic pulmonary fibrosis. N Engl J Med. 2014;370:2083–92.
38. Richeldi L, du Bois RM, Raghu G, et al. Efficacy and safety of nintedanib in idiopathic pulmonary fibrosis. N Engl J Med. 2014; 370:2071–82.
39. Daoussis D, Liossis SN, Tsamandas AC, et al. Experience with rituximab in scleroderma: results from a 1-year, proof-of-principle study. Rheumatology (Oxford). 2010;49:271–80.
40. Jordan S; Distler JH; Maurer B; Huscher D; van Laar JM; Allanore Y; Distler O; Effects and safety of rituximab in systemic sclerosis: an analysis from the European Scleroderma Trial and Research (EUSTAR) group. Rituximab study group. Annals of the Rheumatic Diseases. 2015;74(6):1188–94.
41. Shitrit D, Amitai A, Peled N, et al. Lung transplantation in patients with scleroderma: case series, review of the literature, and criteria for transplantation. Clin Transplant. 2009;23:178–83.
42. Schachna L, Medsger Jr TA, Dauber JH, et al. Lung transplantation in scleroderma compared with idiopathic pulmonary fibrosis and idiopathic pulmonary arterial hypertension. Arthritis Rheum. 2006; 54:3954–61.
43. Fisichella PM, Reder NP, Gagermeier J, Kovacs EJ. Usefulness of pH monitoring in predicting the survival status of patients with scleroderma awaiting lung transplantation. J Surg Res. 2014;189: 232–7.
44. Khan IY, Singer LG, de Perrot M, et al. Survival after lung transplantation in systemic sclerosis. A systematic review. Respir Med. 2013;107:2081–7.
45. Van Laar JM, Farge D, Sont JK, for the EBMT/EULAR Scleroderma Study Group, et al. Autologous hematopoietic stem cell transplantation vs intravenous pulse cyclophosphamide in diffuse cutaneous systemic sclerosis. A randomized clinical trial. JAMA. 2014;311: 2490–8.
46. Burt RK, Shah SJ, Dill K, et al. Autologous non-myeloablative haemopoietic stem-cell transplantation compared with pulse cyclophosphamide once per month for systemic sclerosis (ASSIST): an open-label, randomized phase 2 trial. Lancet. 2011;378:498–506.
47. Ryu JH, Krowka MJ, Pellikka PA, Swanson KL, McGoon MD. Pulmonary hypertension in patients with interstitial lung diseases. Mayo Clin Proc. 2007;82:342–50.
48. Chang B, Wigley FM, White B, Wise RA. Scleroderma patients with combined pulmonary hypertension and interstitial lung disease. J Rheumatol. 2003;30:2398–405.
49. Le Pavec J, Girgis RE, Lechtzin N, et al. Systemic sclerosis-related pulmonary hypertension associated with interstitial lung disease: impact of pulmonary arterial hypertension therapies. Arthritis Rheum. 2011;63:2456–64.
50. Shlobin OA, Nathan. Pulmonary hypertension secondary to interstitial lung disease. Expert Rev Respir Med. 2011;5:179–89.
51. Hinchcliff M, Fisher A, Schiopu E, Steen VD, PHAROS Investigators. Pulmonary hypertension assessment and recognition of outcomes in scleroderma (PHAROS): baseline characteristics and description of study population. J Rheumatol. 2011;38: 2172–9.
52. Arcasoy SM, Christie JD, Ferrari VA, Sutton MS, et al. Echocardiographic assessment of pulmonary hypertension in patients with advanced lung disease. Am J Respir Crit Care Med. 2003;167:735–40.
53. Mittoo S, Jacob T, Craig A, Bshouty Z. Treatment of pulmonary hypertension in patients with connective tissue disease and interstitial lung disease. Can Respir J. 2010;17:282–6.

56 Coping with the Disfigurement of Scleroderma: Facial, Skin, and Hand Changes

Shadi Gholizadeh, Rina S. Fox, Sarah D. Mills, Lisa R. Jewett, Brett D. Thombs, and Vanessa L. Malcarne

Case Study

A 41-year-old woman with scleroderma presented to her rheumatologist for her 12-month follow-up. At the time of her first symptoms, a little more than a year prior, she had presented to her primary care physician with fatigue, gastrointestinal complaints, and numbness in her fingertips and hands. She had also reported cold sensitivity with dramatic color changes of pallor and cyanosis of her fingers with recent onset. Due to the fact that her job as a case manager in a small law firm required many hours of typing each day, she had attributed the growing numbness and tingling in her hands to carpal tunnel syndrome. She had not been overly concerned about most of her symptoms, and had a theory that her fatigue and gastrointestinal issues resulted from an undiagnosed thyroid disorder, because her symptoms mirrored those of a friend with Hashimoto's disease. However, her cold fingers were worrisome, and she consequently had sought help from her doctor.

The patient's physician had noted puffy fingers and requested a full blood panel. General laboratory tests were normal, but serological tests were remarkable for a positive antinuclear antibody (ANA). Because the woman had been experiencing new onset of Raynaud's and had a positive ANA, the potential for an autoimmune disease, like scleroderma, was immediately recognized, and a rheumatologist was consulted. The rheumatologist had made the diagnosis of scleroderma based on abnormal skin thickening of the fingers (sclerodactyly), abnormal nailfold capillaries, and a confirmation of her positive ANA with a positive anti-Scl-70. The patient reported having been shocked, as she had no family history of autoimmune or rheumatic diseases, and she had believed that her generally healthy lifestyle would have protected her from these kinds of diseases. At the time of diagnosis, the patient had described frustration with the uncertainty around living with scleroderma, particularly in terms of its unpredictable course. Furthermore, as she was the mother of two young daughters, she had expressed anxiety about not knowing the etiology of the illness and whether it was possible that her daughters might also develop the disease. The rheumatologist had told her that scleroderma had no curative treatment and that it could shorten her life expectancy. He had ordered special testing of her lung and heart function and started her on medication to help reduce her gastrointestinal reflux and the frequency of her Raynaud's episodes.

The patient spent the next several months pursuing second opinions and consulting alternative medicine practitioners with the hope that she could discover an approach that would reverse the illness. She had returned to the rheumatologist after 3 months due to exacerbation of her symptoms, including noticeably advancing skin tightening in her fingers, hands, arms, face, and lower legs. At that appointment, she was highly distressed about the skin changes, specifically the skin thickening on her face and hands. She explained to her rheumatologist that she had searched for images associated with the disease on the Internet and had been quite shaken up by the prospect of further changes to her appearance. She also reported the onset of pruritus as well as worsening heartburn and fatigue, although she wondered if the fatigue was psychogenic and related to depression secondary to her diagnosis. The patient reported feeling "down" most days and described being unsure as to whether this was normal and expected, given her diagnosis. The rheumatologist found signs of disease progression that explained the new features and worsening of other symptoms. He ordered new testing that showed progression of lung disease with fibrosis on a high-resolution CT scan. He suggested starting

S. Gholizadeh, MS, MSc • R.S. Fox, MS, MPH • S.D. Mills, MS, MPH
V.L. Malcarne, PhD
SDSU/UC San Diego Joint Doctoral Program in Clinical Psychology, San Diego, CA, USA

L.R. Jewett, MSc • B.D. Thombs, PhD (✉)
Lady Davis Institute for Medical Research, McGill University and Jewish General Hospital, Montreal, QC, Canada
e-mail: brett.thombs@mcgill.ca

J. Varga et al. (eds.), *Scleroderma*, DOI 10.1007/978-3-319-31407-5_56

immunosuppression therapy and provided an explanation of the potential benefits, as well as the possible adverse effects, of this approach. The patient had read about various treatments on patient blogs, and she asked her rheumatologist if he would refer her to a scleroderma specialty center at a nearby large university to see if she would qualify for any experimental treatments.

Over the course of the next several months, the patient's capacity for exercise decreased due to shortness of breath. At her 12-month follow-up appointment, although her rheumatologist reported that the patient's lung function and skin thickening had stabilized, her depression and anxiety had worsened. Now, the patient described feeling "a little guilty" that she was not taking advantage of resources offered to her. She described having access to a support group, but she reported that, whereas she regularly attended her medical appointments and adhered to prescribed medication, dietary, and lifestyle regimens, she had avoided patient support groups and patient networks. She described walking into a support meeting toward the beginning of the first year after her diagnosis and feeling "absolutely terrified" after seeing several women who appeared to be close to her age who had severe manifestations of the disease in the face and hands. The patient also reported feeling guilty that she had not been able to fully perform her role as a mother and wife, as fatigue and discomfort were limiting her physical capacity.

The patient reported finding the progression of facial changes and disfigurement of her hands to be the most alarming aspects of her disease. She described avoiding mirrors and feeling a deep sense of grief around her changing appearance, as well as concerns about the potential that her appearance changes would become even more dramatic. She was interested in potentially exploring cosmetic options for her thinning lips but admitted feeling uncomfortable discussing this with her rheumatologist. She explained, "it seems petty…you know, in light of the other health problems, like my lungs."

When asked about daily activities, the patient reported avoiding social situations, especially in recent months, and spending more time alone. While she remained an active mother in the home, she had stopped going to her children's school events and was concerned about her limited involvement with her children outside of the home. Her withdrawal had impacted her level of physical activity as well, as she no longer went on the long walks that used to be her primary form of exercise. The patient described an upsetting situation in which she had been out walking and had run into someone from her neighborhood whom she had not seen for several months. When she greeted this person, the person did not initially recognize her, which the patient attributed to her changed facial features. She also was avoiding sexual encounters with her husband due to discomfort about her appearance. She reported being unable to openly discuss her distress with him for fear of rejection.

In addition, the patient reported that her appearance changes had caused her discomfort at work. She did not like discussing the disease with her coworkers but realized that it was not possible to fully conceal the visible changes in her appearance from them. She felt that people were beginning to treat her differently and also that some people seemed less comfortable interacting with her. Also, her hand contractures had become quite problematic, not only esthetically but also practically in that she can no longer be able to type. Although her supervisors had been supportive, she had had to reduce her work status to part time and relinquish many of her job duties. She described that, while her doctor had not explicitly warned her about what the progression of her contractures could mean, she had seen special devices on patient blogs for patients with hand deformities and feared the day when, "…I won't even able to open a bottle of water without help."

Discussion

Living with a serious, chronic illness can have numerous implications for a patient's self-concept and often necessitates role redefinition as the patient experiences the physical manifestations of the disease and adapts to the associated limitations (e.g., social, occupational) [1]. In the case presented above, the patient is clearly distressed by the changes in her appearance (both that have occurred and that she anticipates may occur), and this distress is contributing to lowered mood, combined with increased anxiety and social withdrawal. Despite the number and prevalence of disfiguring illnesses, the role of disease-related changes to appearance in body image and other quality of life domains in these conditions remains relatively under-investigated [2]. This is true in scleroderma, where research into body image distress remains in the early stages [3, 4]. However, greater attention to psychosocial outcomes in scleroderma, including the development of scleroderma-specific measurement tools to evaluate appearance dissatisfaction, has contributed to a growing research base in this area in recent years. Generally, research has demonstrated that body image distress, or dissatisfaction with appearance, is common in scleroderma [2, 5–9] and that changes in appearance can negatively impact psychosocial well-being and increase psychological distress [1–9], underscoring the importance of clinician awareness of the potential for significant body image concerns in scleroderma.

The word scleroderma is derived from the Greek words skleros (hard) and dermos (skin) [10]. Effects of the excessive collagen production associated with the disease and skin thickening and hardening are hallmarks of the disease. Other appearance changes in scleroderma can include [1]:

1. Loss of skinfolds
2. Shiny appearance to the skin

3. Hypo- or hyperpigmentation of the skin
4. Loss of flexibility of the lips and decreased ability to fully open the mouth
5. Pinched appearance to the nose and eyes
6. Telangiectasias
7. Subcutaneous calcinosis, often in the fingers, elbows, and knees
8. Sclerodactyly
9. Deformity of the digits
10. Limited range of motion in the hands caused by contractures and/or nonhealing ulcers, or surgical amputation to manage digital ischemia

Many scleroderma patients experience similar changes to the appearance of their face, contributing to a characteristic facial appearance. In a study of scleroderma facial involvement, standardized digital photographs of 117 patients with scleroderma were rated for degree of disfigurement by 3 independent health professionals, and these ratings were highly concordant with ratings by the patients themselves [6]. The authors suggested that this agreement may reflect the presence of a characteristic "look" in scleroderma, including common features, such as a pinched nose and shrunken mouth opening. This characteristic pattern of appearance may also contribute to the fears of future appearance changes, because patients may recognize that other patients with more advanced physical changes have the same types of involvement (e.g., thinning lips) as their own.

Although less common in scleroderma than in some other diseases (e.g., cancer), treatment may lead to changes in appearance, as well. For example, long-term steroid use can contribute to moon facies, or a rounded appearance of the face, and some of the immunosuppressant drugs (e.g., cyclophosphamide) can cause hair loss. While appearance changes are common in both limited and diffuse sclerodermas, patients with limited scleroderma tend to experience skin thickening only in the face and extremities, whereas patients with the diffuse subtype experience more widespread thickening, including trunk involvement [2, 11].

The numerous appearance changes that can occur and the variable and unpredictable nature of disfigurement in scleroderma contribute to the complexity of managing body image distress in this disease. However, advances in assessment methods and greater awareness of the role of body image distress in scleroderma have contributed to a slowly growing research base that can inform clinical practice.

Body Image Distress in Scleroderma

It is important to note that severity of visible disfigurement does not always predict distress [13, 14]. While the modified Rodnan skin score [15] is often used as a proxy for severity of disease or degree of skin involvement in research settings, in clinical settings there is no single score from which clinicians can draw inferences about body image distress. In fact, body image distress may be a concern for patients with any level of disease-related changes in appearance. For example, in a study of 93 patients with scleroderma, which investigated appearance self-esteem and treatment for disease-related changes in scleroderma, skin thickening in the right hand and fingers was the strongest predictor of appearance self-esteem [1]. In another study of 127 women with scleroderma, correlates of body image distress were identified as younger age, skin tightening above the elbows, and functional disability [2]. Another study of 171 patients with scleroderma found facial changes to be the most worrisome aspect of scleroderma [6]. In a mailed survey study of 303 patients with scleroderma who were asked more specifically about their level of concern relating to various changes in appearance, the following percentages of respondents noted concern for a specific body area: mouth furrows (80 %), thin lips (73 %), smaller mouth (77 %), telangiectasias (76 %), loss of facial lines (68 %), skin darkening (50 %), and finger ulcers (33 %) [17]. A recent study with 141 patients with scleroderma that included qualitative interviews in addition to quantitative assessment found that body image distress was higher among patients with diffuse scleroderma versus limited disease and that patients with telangiectasias reported higher levels of appearance dissatisfaction [16]. Thus, it is important to consider the role of both disease-related factors (e.g., facial involvement) and social context (e.g., younger age) in body image distress [8]. In our case study, the patient displays specific concerns about changes in her appearance, such as her telangiectasias and thinning lips, but also reports social concerns around having to explain her appearance to others, evidencing the social impacts of the disease and multidimensional nature of body image distress.

Social Impacts of Body Image Distress

Generally, problems (or perceptions of problems) with social interactions are among the most frequently endorsed challenges reported by individuals living with disfigurement [19]. Disfigurement in scleroderma often occurs in areas of the body that are both visible and socially relevant (e.g., face, hands), which can contribute to increased social anxiety and avoidance [1–3, 5, 7]. Thus, understanding and anticipating the social impacts of the disease are important, especially because dissatisfaction with appearance and social discomfort are separate, although often related, problems [8, 14]. Changes in appearance can lead to numerous challenges in social interactions to which the individual had not been exposed prior to diagnosis (e.g., staring, avoidance, negative comments, unsolicited advice or questions, unwanted attention), and these can leave patients feeling a sense of loss of control [19]. Many patients may not realize that they are engaging in social avoidance or isolation due to body image distress, and it can be difficult to disentangle these behaviors from underlying depressive symptomatology, underscoring the importance of referrals to mental health services when patients describe withdrawal or avoidance behaviors.

Examples of avoidance behaviors are present throughout our clinical case study. The patient reported limiting interactions outside of the home in an effort to avoid having to explain her condition or potentially awkward encounters with others. For individuals who are partnered or who have children, the avoidance can contribute to dyadic or family problems. The patient in the case described being a less involved parent as a result of her body image distress in that she stopped attending school events for her children. Acquired changes in appearance can also contribute to questions about one's identity and roles. There can be feelings of loss around one's previous physical appearance and ability to engage in social interactions more readily [19, 21]. That the patient in the case study avoided looking in mirrors speaks to the sense of loss that many patients have around their previous appearance and difficulty adjusting to the disease and its physical changes.

Self-Esteem and Mood Impacts of Body Image Distress

Self-esteem, or the appraisal of one's worth or significance as compared to others [22], is an important construct in that self-concept has been shown to be associated with various outcomes in chronic illness, most notably depression [1]. Appearance self-esteem is a subtype of self-esteem that is important to consider in the context of physical illnesses that cause changes in appearance [1, 24]. Appearance self-esteem has the potential to influence treatment decision-making; one study in rheumatoid arthritis demonstrated that negative self-perceptions of one's hands predicted reparative surgery desires, controlling for disease duration and objective measures of hand attractiveness [25]. There are no studies of how common cosmetic procedures are for patients with scleroderma; however, many patients do express a desire for cosmetic reconstructive options [17, 35]. The patient in the case study reported interest in cosmetic options for her thinning lips. Understanding the role of self-esteem in treatment seeking and decision-making is an important area for further exploration.

The first study exploring appearance self-esteem in scleroderma found that women with scleroderma had lower scores on self-report measures of appearance self-esteem than healthy controls, although men with scleroderma had scores similar to the healthy control group [1]. Further, appearance self-esteem was found to mediate the relationship between skin thickening and distress. Appearance self-esteem relating to acquired conditions has been most often studied in the context of acute changes (e.g., mastectomy, burns) [1], and thus there may be longitudinal processes of self-esteem changes unique to scleroderma given that the physical changes can be quite variable in severity and duration and may develop over an extended period of time. In one study, individuals with scleroderma reported lower self-esteem than hospitalized burn patients, which may be attributed to the progressive rather than stable nature of scleroderma, although another possible explanation is the relatively small scale of the burn injuries among many patients studied [6].

Body image distress has been shown to relate directly to depressive symptomatology, which has, in turn, been associated with poorer psychosocial functioning [2]; thus, depression may mediate the relationship between body image distress and psychosocial function. Further, the unpredictable and uncontrollable nature of the physical changes may cause individuals to feel helpless over their condition, which has also been associated with higher levels of depression in scleroderma [26]. In addition, there is little control over how others will react to one's changed appearance. Fear of negative evaluation by others was identified as an important contributor to the presence of anxiety symptomatology in scleroderma [28]. The patient in the case study reported depressive symptomatology associated with her body image distress in her withdrawal from social situations, feeling "down on most days," and feelings of guilt. She also described feelings of helplessness around the unclear progression of her symptoms and fears around increasing severity of her facial and hand changes.

Sexual Impacts of Body Image Distress

Sexual dysfunction is common in scleroderma, with over 50 % of women reporting impairment in sexual functioning [29] and over 80 % of men reporting erectile dysfunction [30]. Despite the prevalence of sexual dysfunction, the lack of validated measures in this area precludes a research base elucidating correlates and predictors of sexual dysfunction [3, 4]. Various physical manifestations of scleroderma, such as shrinking of the mouth, skin tightening and discomfort, and vaginal tightening and dryness, can contribute to diminished sexual function [29, 31, 32]. While one study did not find a significant association between body image distress and increased sexual impairment (dissatisfaction with appearance was associated with reduced sexual function in bivariate analysis but became nonsignificant in multivariate analysis after including pain, disease duration, and unmarried status as correlates of sexual function) [23], the strong link between body image and sexual functioning generally and in other chronic illnesses warrants further attention [33]. In the case study, the patient reports decreased sexual activity with her husband and associated feelings of guilt. Given the likely interface between physical contributors (e.g., vaginal tightening) and psychological contributors (e.g., body image distress, depressive symptomatology) to her sexual problems, it would be important to address each area of potential concern. As with body image distress in general, this may be an area that patients will not discuss unless directly assessed (i.e., "Are you experiencing sexual problems as a result of your disease?") given the sensitive nature of the topic.

Fear of Physical Progression

The unpredictable course of the disease coupled with the availability of online resources depicting severe changes in appearance in scleroderma can contribute to elevated worries and fears of progression of the physical manifestations of the disease. Indeed, many patients report avoiding potentially helpful resources, such as patient support groups, because seeing patients in more advanced stages of disease can be worry inducing. Patients may engage in comparative pursuits, assessing how their own physical changes relate to those of other patients. This type of comparison is not limited to in person support groups, and it can also occur in the context of Internet searches. Thus, asking patients about their perceptions of physical progression in scleroderma and what changes they may be expecting can be important in highlighting potential misconceptions or areas for education. This is especially important because, as described in the present case study, some patients may not feel that it is appropriate to raise concerns around body image or sexual dysfunction with their medical providers. However, given the aforementioned significant impacts of body image distress on various psychosocial domains, the importance of addressing these concerns should be evident.

Assessments of Body Image Distress

Clinicians can foster a more open environment by simply asking all patients specifically about appearance-related concerns. Clinicians should inquire about appearance-related concerns among all patients who experience changes in their appearance due to scleroderma (not just patients with the most severe disfigurement). Simply asking the patient rather than using a "screening tool" is recommended, because there are no established clinical cut offs to detect clinically significant body image distress or evidence that screening in this way would improve outcomes for patients. Being proactive in asking about body image and appearance concerns is especially important because, as described in the case study, body image may not always be an area that the patient feels comfortable broaching with the clinician. Although there is no standard protocol for how to talk to patients about appearance concerns and what to do if such concerns are voiced, it is recommended that health professionals ask patients if they have concerns about changes in appearance that have occurred or might occur, perhaps by first normalizing that such concerns are common among individuals with scleroderma. Health professionals can then engage in a dialog around this topic more openly with patients who have this concern or provide a referral to a mental health specialist as appropriate.

A consensus statement on research in scleroderma called for the development and validation of disease-specific measures that assess multiple dimensions of body image, such as social avoidance, appearance investment, and evaluation of appearance [3]. While such measures are important to researchers so that psychometrically robust instruments can be utilized to identify predictors and correlates of body image distress, there are also clinical uses for these measures. For example, in clinical care, assessments of body image can be used to track progress in treatment. However, such measures are not required, or necessarily appropriate, in all clinical settings. It is not recommended that a measure be administered unless there is a clear purpose for so doing. For many clinical encounters, simply asking the patient about concerns related to changes in their appearance or fears of changes that might occur is sufficient. However, because of the role of these measures in the growing research on body image distress in scleroderma and their potential for use by qualified professionals treating body image concerns, having an awareness of what measures exist and what constructs they assess can be important to understand.

Existing general body image distress measures may not be appropriate for use with scleroderma patients, as they include items relating to weight concerns, and often do not target disfigurement-related avoidance or social anxiety that would be important to explore in scleroderma [3]. Since the publication of the aforementioned consensus statement, the 14-item Satisfaction with Appearance Scale (SWAP) [12] and the abbreviated 6-item Brief-SWAP [7] have been validated in patients with scleroderma [7–9]. These measures require respondents to rate the extent to which they agree with items about their appearance on a seven-point scale ranging from 1 = strongly disagree to 7 = strongly agree. Higher scores indicate greater body image distress. Originally developed for body image distress relating to burn injuries, the SWAP and its abbreviated form the Brief-SWAP have been shown to yield the following two subscales: dissatisfaction with appearance and social discomfort [7, 9]. A recent study compared the two measures and concluded that both versions can be used with patients, although the Brief-SWAP is the more parsimonious option [9]. On the Brief-SWAP, the dissatisfaction with appearance subscale measures patient self-reported dissatisfaction with specific areas of the body (e.g., "I am satisfied with the appearance of my face."), while the social discomfort subscale measures the social impacts of concerns around body image (e.g., "Because of changes in my appearance caused by my scleroderma, I am uncomfortable in the presence of strangers.").

Research using these measures to explore outcomes associated with specific disease-related changes in appearance has demonstrated that there are differential impacts not only for severity of disfigurement but also for specific body areas and patient characteristics. For example, in a study examining sociodemographic correlates of body image distress in 489 patients with scleroderma using the Brief-SWAP, upper body telangiectasias and younger age were associated with greater social discomfort, finger-to-palm distance and hand contractures were associated with dissatisfaction with appearance, and extent of skin involvement and facial involvement were associated with both of these aspects of body image distress [8].

Clinical Strategies for Body Image Distress

Increasing awareness of body image distress among providers so that there can be open discourse and greater facilitation of referrals to appropriate healthcare providers and interventions is essential if patients are to receive appropriate and needed services. Psychosocial treatments for body image distress, as well as cosmetic and surgical approaches, provide important options for patients.

Psychosocial Treatments

While the need for psychosocial interventions in the treatment of scleroderma has been highlighted, there are currently no specific guidelines regarding such interventions [34]. The first strategy, as described above, is simply to evaluate the presence of body image distress. In cases where distress is present, referral to a professional may be indicated. The stepped care model has been recommended as a framework for psychosocial treatments in scleroderma [18]. Per the stepped care model, treatment may range on a spectrum ranging from self-guided intervention through online programs or books (i.e., no therapist involvement) to long-term individual face-to-face therapy with a clinical team with expertise in body image distress. Chapter 45 in this volume lists a range of self-help resources for general psychosocial distress and one resource specific to body image distress, Changing Faces (www.changingfaces.org.uk).

There are currently no evidence-based, disease-specific body image interventions available for scleroderma. A 2007 review on psychosocial interventions for individuals with visible differences [35] identified only one randomized controlled trial (RCT) [36] examining the effectiveness of a psychosocial intervention for body image distress, although this trial was too small to draw conclusions with any degree of confidence [35]. A 2015 update to the review identified only four additional studies, two of which were RCTs but similarly had methodological limitations that precluded conclusions as to the optimal type and duration of psychosocial treatment for individuals with visible differences [37]. Because the majority of the body image intervention literature is focused on appearance and weight issues in the realm of eating disorders, it is unclear how such interventions may apply to individuals with scleroderma or other disfiguring conditions. Still, there are components of therapeutic modalities that may be useful to target various components of body image distress, especially relating to social concerns. For example, cognitive behavioral therapy (CBT) for social anxiety, social skills training programs, and psychoeducational support around body image distress have been suggested as useful interventions in scleroderma, although none have been empirically tested [7, 27].

CBT focuses on the interplay among cognitions, emotions, and behaviors. In a review of studies of both acquired and congenital disfigurement, negative emotions (e.g., social anxiety), maladaptive cognitions (e.g., fear of negative judgments from others), and negative behaviors (e.g., social isolation) were frequently reported [19], underscoring the relevance of this approach. A 2013 text titled *CBT for Appearance Anxiety: Psychosocial Interventions for Anxiety due to Visible Difference* is an excellent resource for mental health professionals that can be used as a clinical manual to guide CBT-based treatment for individuals with visible differences [38]. The book is grounded in a stepped care model that is useful for health professionals hoping to deliver more intensive psychosocial interventions and those who want to deliver more basic psychological treatments. Another therapeutic approach that is increasing in popularity, particularly for chronic illnesses, is acceptance and commitment therapy (ACT). Unlike CBT, which provides tools to challenge and change unhelpful thoughts, ACT focuses on accepting these thoughts without judgment and learning how to live a valued life despite them. ACT may be useful in scleroderma, as CBT may feel invalidating for some patients because many underlying "negative" thoughts are not irrational thoughts to be challenged (e.g., "My appearance has changed quite a bit in the past five years.") but rather rational thoughts to which acceptance can be practiced.

Social skills training may also be appropriate. It is important to emphasize that this is not because individuals with scleroderma have a social deficit but rather because (1) they are now living with added social challenges that they did not have prior to their diagnosis that may necessitate new skills (e.g., how to react to rude comments or stares) and (2) these skills can be helpful in managing the negative or hurtful social reactions of others. An issue that has not received scholarly attention but may contribute to difficulties in social interactions is that of restrictions in expressing facial nonverbal emotions given limited mouth function in scleroderma. The facial changes in scleroderma can sometimes contribute to an "expressionless face," and research on facial disfigurement has suggested that this may contribute to "difficulty in 'reading' the faces of disfigured people, which in turn results in hesitancy, awkwardness, and an abbreviated interchange [19 p. 86; 20]." For patients experiencing difficulties with social interactions, it is important that interventions expand their repertoire of social skills, so that they have more available resources to respond to the myriad challenges posed by social situations rather than assuming that their social coping strategies are somehow deficient [19].

Cosmetic Camouflage and Surgical Options

As previously stated, models that assume a general, positive correlation between the severity of disfigurement and body image distress can be misleading because of individual differences that promote differential levels of distress [19]. In scleroderma, patients with the most severe changes in appearance are not necessarily the most distressed. Further, while cosmetic camouflage and surgical options, described briefly below, may sometimes be an option for some scleroderma-related appearance concerns, clinicians should offer psychosocial interventions in addition to any cosmetic camouflage or surgical options that may be available to address body image concerns.

The role of cosmetic camouflage (also referred to as makeup) has not been studied in scleroderma, although many patient support groups offer cosmetic education days with tips and guidance around downplaying or highlighting certain features (e.g., lining the lips to make them appear thicker). Experts in body image acknowledge that some conditions "…are amenable to camouflage using make-up, prosthetics, clothes or hair. However, for some, camouflage can bring its own problems in relation to issues of identity (p. 86) [19]." Clinicians hoping to educate themselves about the role of cosmetic camouflage can look to the burn literature, which includes numerous case studies and examples of how cosmetic camouflage can improve esthetic balance and help to restore symmetry to facial and bodily areas of concern [45].

Another area that has received relatively little attention in scleroderma-related body image distress is the role of surgical options to address body image concerns. There are procedures that may be of interest to patients with specific concerns. For example, lip thinning can be a very distressing change for many patients who may explore surgery as a means to recreate their previous lip thickness [43]. There has been a call for a more systematic approach to the surgical management of facial disfigurement in scleroderma. For example, some clinicians do not advise that patients with scleroderma undergo surgical procedures given concerns such as poor wound healing, while other experts argue that such concerns are unfounded [17]. Various laser and surgical options exist for patients, such as carbon dioxide laser (Coherent 5000-C Ultra Pulse laser at 300 mJ/60 W) for perioral rhytidosis [36], pulsed dye laser for treatment of telangiectasias [44, 41], and autologous fat transfer for isolated skin areas [17, 42]. There has been a call for collaboration among various clinical specialties, including plastic surgery, rheumatology, dermatology, and internal medicine, to develop guidelines for best practices for the management of patients who desire surgical treatments to address changes in appearance [17].

At present, there are no guidelines for discussing such interventions with patients who desire them. Some argue that when clinicians offer cosmetic or surgical options to patients exhibiting body image distress or assume that patients with more severe physical manifestations of the disease must be experiencing body image distress, this can be a means by which "care providers are colluding with the myth that quality of life necessarily improves when physical appearance is enhanced [p. 91; 19]." This is an area that deserves further attention so that clinicians can know how to respond to patient requests for surgical options. It is also important for health professionals to know when and how to present patients with surgical or less invasive cosmetic options when patients present with body image distress but do not know what options are available to them. Finally, clinicians who do present such options should be ready to address the clinical and psychosocial impacts of such treatments or to provide a referral to a health professional who can.

Conclusion

In summary, changes in appearance are common and distressing for many people with scleroderma. It is important for all those providing clinical care in scleroderma to be aware of body image distress and to be mindful that distress does not necessarily correlate with severity of appearance changes. As such, open communication around changes in appearance is important to ensure that patients who are not being asked about body image distress do not fall between the cracks. The recent development of scleroderma-specific body image assessments has contributed to a growing literature base that demonstrates the multidimensional nature of body image distress and the personal and social impacts that can be associated with changes in appearance. Referrals to mental health professionals may be indicated when patients have concerns related to body image distress. Further, there are resources for patients wanting to take a self-managed approach to understanding and coping with body image distress. Future efforts should focus on the identification of evidence-based scleroderma-specific interventions to aid patients with body image distress.

Acknowledgments This work was supported by a grant from the Canadian Institutes of Health Research (CIHR; #TR3-267681). Ms. Jewett was supported by a CIHR Doctoral Research Award. Dr. Thombs was supported by an Investigator Salary Award from the Arthritis Society.

References

1. Malcarne VL, Handsdottir I, Greensbergs HL, Clements PJ, Weisman MH. Appearance self-esteem in systemic sclerosis. Cogn Ther Res. 1999;23(2):197–208.
2. Benrud-Larson LM, Heinberg LJ, Boiling C, Reed J, White B, Wigley FM, et al. Body image dissatisfaction among women with scleroderma: extent and relationship to psychosocial function. Health Psychol. 2003;22(2):130–9.
3. Thombs BD, van Lankveld W, Bassel M, Baron M, Buzza R, Haslam S, et al. Psychological health and well-being in systemic sclerosis: state of the science and consensus research agenda. Arthritis Care Res. 2010;8:1181–9.
4. Malcarne VM, Fox RS, Mills SD, Gholizadeh S. Psychosocial aspects of systemic sclerosis. Curr Opin Rheumatol. 2013;25(6):707–13.
5. Heinberg LJ, Kudel I, White B, Kwan A, Medley K, Wigley F, Haythornthwaite J. Assessing body image in patients with systemic sclerosis (scleroderma): validation of the adapted satisfaction with appearance scale. Body Image. 2007;4(1):79–86.
6. Amin K, Clarke A, Sivakumar B, Puri A, Fox Z, Brough V, et al. The psychological impact of facial changes in scleroderma. Psychol Health Med. 2011;16(3):304–12.
7. Jewett LR, Hudson M, Haythornthwaite JA, Heinberg L, Wigley FM, Baron M, Thombs BD. Canadian Scleroderma Research Group. Development and validation of the Brief-Satisfaction with Appearance Scale (Brief-SWAP) for systemic sclerosis (SSc). Arthritis Care Res. 2010;62(12):1779–86.
8. Jewett LR, Huson M, Malcarne VL, Baron M, Thombs BD. Canadian Scleroderma Research Group. Sociodemographic and disease correlates of body image distress among patients with systemic sclerosis. PLoS One. 2012;7(3):e33281.
9. Mills SD, Fox RS, Merz EL, Clements PJ, Kafaja S, Malcarne VL, Furst DE, Khanna D. Evaluation of the satisfaction with appearance scale and its short form in systemic sclerosis: analysis from the UCLA scleroderma quality of life study. J Rheumatol. 2015;
10. Seibold J, Harris ED, Budd RC, Genovese MC, Sergent JS. Kelley's textbook of rheumatology. Philadelphia: Elsevier; 2007.
11. Poole JL, Steen VD. The use of the Health Assessment Questionnaire (HAQ) to determine physical disability in systemic sclerosis. Arthritis Care Res. 1991;4(1):27–31.
12. Lawrence JW, Heinberg LJ, Roca R, Munster A, Spence R, Fauerbach JA. Development and validation of the satisfaction with Appearance scale: assessing body image among burn-injured patients. Psychol Asses. 1998;10(1):64–70.
13. Robinson E. Psychological research on visible differences in adults. In: Lansdown R, Rumsey N, Bradbury E, Carr T, Partridge J, editors. Visibly different: coping with disfigurement. London: Butterworth; 1997. p. 102–11.
14. Rumsey N, Clarke A, Musa M. Altered body image: the psychosocial needs of patients. Br J Community Nurs. 2002;7(11):563–6.
15. Clements PJ, Hurwitz EL, Wong WK, Seibold JR, Mayes M, White B, Wigley F, Weisman M, Barr W, Moreland L, Medsger Jr TA, Steen VD, Martin RW, Collier D, Weinstein A, Lally E, Varga J, Weiner SR, Andrews B, Abeles M, Furst DE. Skin thickness scores as a predictor and correlate of outcome in systemic sclerosis: high-dose versus low-dose penicillamine trial. Arthritis Rheum. 2000;43(11):2445–54.
16. Ennis H, Herrick AL, Cassidy C, Griffiths CE, Richards HL. A pilot study of body image dissatisfaction and the psychological impact of systemic sclerosis-related telangiectases. Clin Exp Rheumatol. 2013;31(2 Suppl 76):12–7.
17. Paquette DL, Falanga V. Cutaneous concerns of scleroderma patients. J Dermatol. 2003;30(6):438–43.
18. Jewett LR, Haythornthwaite JA, Thombs BD. Psychosocial issues and care for patients with systemic sclerosis. In: Varga J, Denton CP, Wigley FM, editors. Scleroderma: from pathogenesis to comprehensive management. New York: Springer; 2012. p. 641–8.
19. Rumsey N, Harcourt D. Body image and disfigurement: issues and interventions. Body Image. 2004;1(1):83–97.
20. Macgregor F. After plastic surgery: adaptation and adjustment. New York: Praeger; 1979.
21. Bradbury E. Understanding the problems. In: Lansdown R, Rumsey N, Bradbury E, Carr A, Partridge J, editors. Visibly different: coping with disfigurement. Oxford: Butterworth-Heinemann; 1997. p. 180–93.
22. Coopersmith S. Studies in self-esteem. Sci Am. 1968;218(2):96–106.
23. Knafo R, Haythornthwaite JA, Heinberg L, Wigley F, Thombs BD. The association of body image dissatisfaction and pain with reduced sexual function in women with systemic sclerosis. Rheumatology. 2011;50(6):1125–30.
24. Vamos M. Body image in chronic illness: a reconceptualization. Int J Psychiat Med. 1993;23(2):163–78.
25. Vamos M. Body image in rheumatoid arthritis: the relevance of hand appearance to desire for surgery. Br J Med Psychol. 1990; 6(3):267–77.
26. Nicassio PM, Wallston KA, Callahan LF, Herbert M, Pincus T. The measurement of helplessness in rheumatoid arthritis: the development of the arthritis helplessness index. J Rheumatol. 1985;12(3):462–7.
27. Haythornthwaite JA, Heinberg LJ, McGuire L. Psychologic factors in scleroderma. Rheum Dis Clin Am. 2003;29(2):427–39.
28. Richards HL, Herrick AL, Griffin K, Gilliam PDH, Fortune DG. Psychological adjustment to systemic sclerosis—exploring the association of disease factors, functional ability, body related attitudes and fear of negative evaluation. Psychol Health Med. 2004;9(1):29–39.
29. Saad SC, Pietrzykowski JE, Lewis SS, Stepien AM, Latham VA, Messick S, et al. Vaginal lubrication in women with scleroderma and Sjögren's syndrome. Sex Disabil. 1999;17(2):103–13.
30. Walker UA, Tyndall A, Ruszat R. Erectile dysfunction in systemic sclerosis. Ann Rheum Dis. 2009;68(7):1083–5.
31. Schover LR, Jensen SR. Sexuality and chronic illness: a comprehensive approach. New York: Guilford; 1988.
32. Saad SC, Behrend AE. Scleroderma and sexuality. J Sex Res. 1996;33(3):15–20.
33. Passik SD, Newman ML, Brennan M, Tunkel R. Predictors of psychological distress, sexual dysfunction and physical functioning among women with upper extremity lymphedema related to breast cancer. Psychooncology. 1995;4(4):255–63.
34. Kowal-Bielecka O, Landewe R, Avouac J, Chwiesko S, Miniati I, Czirjak L, et al. EULAR recommendations for the treatment of systemic sclerosis: a report from the EULAR scleroderma trials and research group (EUSTAR). Ann Rheum Dis. 2009;68(5):620–8.
35. Bessell A, Moss TP. Psychosocial interventions for visible differences: a 453 systematic review. Body Image. 2007;4(3):227–38.
36. Newell R, Clarke M. Evaluation of a self-help leaflet in treatment of social difficulties following facial disfigurement. Int J Nurs Stud. 2000;37(5):381–8.

37. Norman A, Moss TP. Psychosocial interventions for adults with visible differences: a systematic review. Peer J Prepr. 2014;2:e617v1. [cited 2015 Mar 15]:available from: https://peerj.com/preprints/617v1/.
38. Clarke A, Thompson AR, Jenkinson E, Rumsey N, Newell R. CBT for appearance anxiety: psychosocial interventions for anxiety due to visible difference. Oxford: Wiley; 2013.
39. Apfelberg DB, Varga J, Greenbaum SS. Carbon dioxide laser resurfacing of peri-oral rhytids in scleroderma patients. Dermatol Surg. 1998;24:517–9.
40. Ciatti S, Varga J, Greenbaum SS. The 585 nm flashlamp-pulsed dye laser for the treatment of telangiectases in patients with scleroderma. J Am Acad Dermatol. 1996;35(3):487–8.
41. Murray AK, Moore TL, Richards H, Ennis H, Grif ths CEM, Herrick AL. Pilot study of intense pulsed light for the treatment of systemic sclerosis-related telangiectases. Br J Dermatol. 2012; 167(3):563–9.
42. Glogau RG. Microlipoinjection: autologous fat grafting. Arch Dermatol. 1988;124(9):1340–3.
43. Spackman GK. Scleroderma: what the general dentist should know. Gen Dent. 1999;47(6):576–9.
45. Sundriyal D, Kumar N, Chandrasekharan A, Gadpayle AK. Mauskopf facies. Brit Med J Case Rep [Internet]. 2013: available from: http://casereports.bmj.com/content/2013/bcr-2013-200163.full.pdf+html.
46. Rose EH. Aesthetic restoration of the severely disfigured face in burn victims: a comprehensive strategy. Plast Reconstr Surg. 1994;96(7):1573–85.

Managing Complicated Digital Ulcers

57

Robert J. Spence

Two case studies of the management of complicated scleroderma digital ulcers will be described in this chapter. These cases have been chosen to represent the two most common types of digital ulcers seen in scleroderma with the most common complications. These cases will be used to discuss the specific management of the problems associated with each case with expanded discussion of the options available, and the reasons for their use.

Case Number 1

The patient is a 36-year-old woman diagnosed with limited scleroderma at the age of 29. She was referred for management of a right index finger tip ulcer that developed after a severe episode of Raynaud's phenomenon 2.5 months prior to her referral. Immediately after the severe episode of Raynaud's phenomenon, the fingertip skin became exceedingly white, and normal color did not return for several hours. Subsequently, the patient developed hardness and discoloration of the tip skin with persistent pain. The finger became even more painful, and exudate developed around the margins of the tip eschar that had become black in color. She treated the area with triple antibiotic ointment, and the hard surface eschar softened. With time, the softened surface eschar sloughed leaving residual soft, white necrotic tissue on the fingertip covering a nonhealing ulcer.

About a week prior to her visit, she began developing more pain and her distal finger became red and swollen. Her primary care physician prescribed cephalexin by mouth and referred her for surgical management of the apparent infected fingertip ulcer. The infection improved, but she continued to have pain and redness of her distal index finger.

R.J. Spence, MD, FACS
Emeritus, MedStar Good Samaritan Hospital,
Baltimore, MD, USA
e-mail: rjs3947@gmail.com

Her current medications included nifedipine, sildenafil citrate, esomeprazole magnesium, pentoxifylline, gabapentin, low-dose acetylsalicylic acid, and cephalexin. She was not taking steroids. She had no known allergies. She did not smoke, but her husband does.

On presentation, the patient's temperature was 98.4 °F, pulse 84, blood pressure 118/70, and respirations 16. Her facial skin had multiple telangiectasias. She otherwise had no significant physical signs of her limited scleroderma physically with the exception of her hands. Sclerodactyly was present. Small pits were present on both her left ring and index fingertips with some foreshortening of her left middle finger tip suggesting previous scleroderma ulcers that had healed. A 1.4 × 1.2-cm active ulcer was present at the tip of her right index finger (Fig. 57.1). The necrotic tissue in the central wound and the base of the ulcer was a yellow-white color and fibrinous in nature. The only exception was a very small area of erythema at the volar aspect of the ulcer base. The margins were sharply demarcated with a small amount of epithelialization. There was minimal exudate, and the base was moist. The entire finger was somewhat more swollen than her other fingers. The distal phalangeal soft tissue particularly was swollen and erythematous. The rest of her

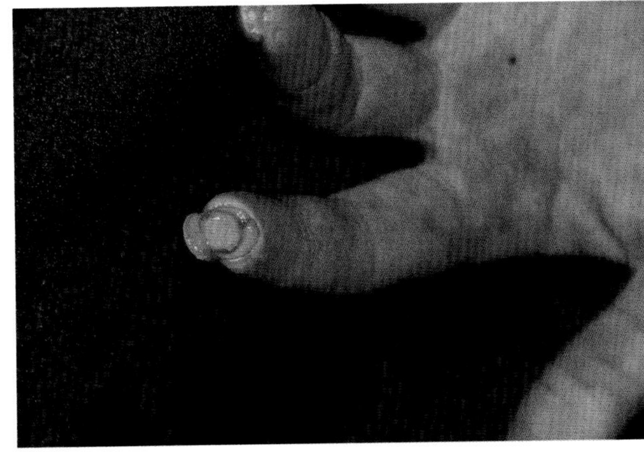

Fig. 57.1 Left index fingertip ulcer at initial presentation

J. Varga et al. (eds.), *Scleroderma*, DOI 10.1007/978-3-319-31407-5_57

hand was not swollen, and she had relatively good digital movement of her fingers with the exception of some restriction in the right index finger due to swelling. The fingers were normal in color. An Allen's test was negative, although there was mild slowing of the refill from the ulnar artery.

Management

A diagnosis of an infected scleroderma fingertip ulcer was made based on the history and physical examination. Loss of fingertip skin and subsequent development of a slowly healing or nonhealing ulcer as a result of Raynaud's phenomenon and critical digital tip ischemia with subsequent death of skin are very common in patients with limited scleroderma. A second common cause is trauma such as a sliver, a split in dry fingertip skin, or cutting or scraping the skin. The resulting small wound and possible foreign body results in inflammation in the relatively ischemic fingertip skin. The additional metabolic demand, particularly oxygen demand, caused by the inflammation cannot be satisfied by the local blood supply, and local tissue death develops. Local tissue death sets the stage for bacterial growth resulting in further inflammation and metabolic demands if the bacteria invade into the surrounding viable tissue.

Management of these ischemic fingertip ulcers is directed to optimizing the blood supply, interceding in the pathologic process described above, and reducing the factors that aggravate the situation.

On initial presentation, ulcers are routinely cultured with a surface swab done carefully due to the exquisite tenderness of these lesions. In this case, the history and physical examination has led to a clinical diagnosis of infection, so the culture is particularly important for treatment of the infection with the proper antibiotic. This diagnosis was made based on the clinical signs of increased pain, swelling, and erythema. Additionally, infection can be diagnosed on the basis of a wound exudate, particularly coming from underneath a scab or eschar.

Importantly, most scleroderma digital ulcers do not have an invasive clinical infection on presentation. However, all open wounds have bacteria living on them, and the surface swab will be positive and identify the resident bacteria. This is important information to have if clinical signs of infection develop, but the *simple presence of a positive culture from an open ulcer is not grounds for the diagnosis of infection.*

Once the wound is cultured, the question of further treating the infection and enhancing wound healing by debriding necrotic tissue is raised. In addition to debridement, removing scab or eschar in order to completely examine the ulcer is frequently necessary and desirable.

Debridement should not be attempted without providing some form of anesthesia due to the exquisite tenderness and sensitivity of these ischemic ulcers. This can be done most rapidly and effectively using a digital block with lidocaine without epinephrine [1]. If a longer-term digital block is desired, it can be mixed with the bupivacaine. One can make it a practice to inject a half-and-half mixture of 1 % lidocaine and half percent bupivacaine routinely to provide quick onset anesthesia and hours-long relief for the often very distraught patient dealing with exquisite pain on a daily basis. Furthermore, one can reduce the actual pain of injection by alkalinizing the lidocaine with sodium bicarbonate solution [2–4]. *Epinephrine should not be used in the local or regional anesthetic of vascularly compromised scleroderma digits.*

Alternatively, topical anesthetic in the form of lidocaine/prilocaine cream or 4 % lidocaine solution or gel can be applied and left in place until adequate anesthesia is established for debridement of an open wound. Given the usual exquisite pain and sensitivity of the ulcer itself, and the frequent intolerance to pain of the patient themselves, topical anesthetic is a significantly less effective alternative. Topical anesthetic rarely is effective when placed on a scab or eschar.

Once anesthesia is established, removal of scab (i.e., dried secretions) and eschar (i.e., necrotic tissue) is performed using forceps, scissors, and occasionally a #15 scalpel blade. The goal is to remove necrotic tissue with its resident microorganisms. Bleeding is rarely a problem. Even debridement to apparently viable tissue is problematic because the bases of these ischemic ulcers tend to be avascular on initial presentation. One must remember that if clearly viable and bleeding tissue is reached, the poor vascularity of the tissues will commonly cause this newly exposed viable tissue to die as a result of exposure to the cooling and drying effect of the air. The debrided ulcer should be immediately covered with a dressing that will protect and maintain a physiologic environment on the surface of the wounds, but even this is often unsuccessful in keeping newly exposed viable tissue alive.

The wound is covered with the best dressing available once it has been debrided and the surface and surrounding skin washed with soap and water. Although sterile wound cleansing solutions are promoted, there is no evidence that any is better than gentle soap and water, and most do not have the detergent action that soap provides.

Dressings and Medications

Scleroderma ulcers heal over several months rather than the weeks that we expect in normal tissue wounds. One must have patience, read the appearance of the wound, and listen to the patient to determine what particular dressing is indicated. Scleroderma patients frequently have a long history of multiple ulcers treated over many months and years. These patients frequently know what works in their wounds and for them, so they should not be ignored. However, there are some principles that should be used in deciding which dressings and topical medication to use. They are as follows:

1. Wounds heal best in a physiological, occluded, sterile, moist environment. Such an environment is present under a stable, dry eschar or scab (i.e., "Nature's bandage") [5]. Providing such an environment for an open wound requires a dressing that can be a topical medication and/or a device.
2. Decide whether the patient prefers a *moist or dry wound* with regard to comfort and their belief on how well the wound will heal with each. As indicated above, a dry eschar or scab is frequently a very comfortable, beneficial, and convenient cover to allow healing to proceed under it.
3. For those patients who are most comfortable with moist ulcers either from a pain standpoint, protection of the wound, or simply to have a dressing on the ulcer, the following dressings and topical medications should be considered.

Dressings

The patient's own skin graft (i.e., autograft) is the gold standard to which all dressings should be compared. A skin graft occludes the wound providing a moist, physiological environment. It prevents desiccation and allows wound-healing processes to proceed. In addition, the cut surface of the graft gives off growth factors that stimulate the wound to heal [6]. If the resident bacterial flora is less than 10^5 per gram of tissue, a fibrin bond is established between the graft and the wound bed that helps leukocytes phagocytize bacteria without opsonization, reducing the bacterial count.

It is impractical to place patient's skin grafts on wounds, but all substitutes for it should be assessed with it in mind. Skin allograft (i.e., "skin bank skin" or cadaver skin) is an excellent substitute but also generally impractical for general clinical use. After these, the dressings that provide the most physiological environment and any stimulus to wound healing should be the next considered. Regrettably, placing anything on a wound that does not provide normal pH, moisture, and salt balance has some negative effect on wound healing than those more ideal dressing above. Table 57.1 lists various classes of occlusive wound dressings.

Modern dressings, including the occlusive dressings listed in Table 57.1, frequently have silver impregnated into them as an option. Silver has been found to have antimicrobial effect against a very broad spectrum of microorganisms and is thought to minimize bacteria in the wound. Further, the antimicrobial action frequently continues for several days allowing for many fewer dressing changes [8]. This, of course, is of great benefit to scleroderma digital ulcer patients trying to maintain a physiological environment to avoid desiccation and avoid pain.

The inclusion of cellophane as a dressing may be somewhat surprising. It is included because of its excellent occlusion properties of those commercially available products that adhere to the skin. The patient has easy access to these products, and they can be used as an outer dressing to prevent desiccation and protest the inner dressing from water, dirt, and other contaminants when appropriate. Self-adhering cellophane dressings can also be used in place of tape or Band-Aid-type dressings to hold other dressings or devices in place.

When infection is present in the wound, occlusive dressings may aggravate the infection by keeping the wound moist and warm. It is best to use occlusion in wounds that are not exudative and have no other signs of invasive infection. These nonocclusive dressings include Band-Aid-type dressings and dressings made of nonadherent dressing pads and tape.

Topical Medications

For various reasons, topical medications may be beneficial when applied to the scleroderma digital ulcer, frequently under one of the dressings or devices listed. The common medications to consider include:

(a) *Bacitracin or "triple antibiotic" ointment* is frequently used by scleroderma patients to provide a good wound-healing environment and a small amount of antibacterial action that provides some prophylaxis from more serious infection. The petroleum vehicle is relatively benign in its effect on wound healing. It is also inexpensive and easily available over the counter.

(b) *Silver hydrogel* is used to provide a good wound-healing environment in a wound that tends to be dry or is more painful to the patient when it is dry. It provides prophylaxis from infection by keeping resident bacterial flora in check because of the presence of the heavy metal, silver. It is more expensive and frequently requires a prescription.

Silver alginate and hydrofiber dry foam dressings are one of the most commonly used dressings for chronic ulcers in the non-scleroderma setting. However, they are rarely used, as most scleroderma ulcers are arterial/ischemic ulcers, and are usually dry and not exudative unless they are infected.

(c) *Mupirocin ointment* is an ointment similar to bacitracin ointment, but with a more powerful antibiotic component that is particularly effective against staphylococcus and methicillin-resistant staphylococcus, which are the most common pathogens in scleroderma digital ulcers [9]. It is best saved for use when there is definite evidence of an infection in the ulcer. Routine use will lead to the development of resistant bacteria in the wound that will be more difficult to treat if invasive infection develops.

Table 57.1 Dressings [5, 7]

Type	Composition	Examples
Films	Polyurethane or co-polyester with adhesive backing	Op-site™ (Smith & Nephew) Tegaderm™ (3M)
Hydrogels	80–99 % water in cross-linked polymer with polyethylene oxide, polyvinyl	Elastogel™ (SW Technologies) FlexiGel™ (Smith & Nephew) Hypergel® (Molnylcke Health Care)
Calcium alginate	Nonwoven composite of fibers from calcium alginate, a cellulose-like polysaccharide	Melgisorb® (Molnylcke Health Care) Kaltostat® (ConvaTec)
Hydrocolloids	Cross-linked polymer matrices with integrated starches and adhesives	Duoderm® (ConvaTec) Comfeel® (Coloplast) Tegasorb™ (3M)
Hydrofibers	Highly absorbent ribbons of carboxymethyl cellulose	Aquacel® (ConvaTec)
Cellophane	Cellulose with glycerine or glycerol plasticizer added	Saran wrap® (Johnson) Press'n Seal® (Glad)

(d) *Silver sulfadiazine cream* is an excellent broad-spectrum antibiotic cream used in the treatment of acute burns. It can be used to advantage when there is definite evidence of infection in the wound, and broad-spectrum coverage is desired before the sensitivity of the organism causing the infection is known. Its disadvantage is that it is known to inhibit wound healing by inhibition of fibroblast activity apparently related to its cold cream base. It is therefore used for as little time as possible, usually a week, to get control of a wound infection before the results of the culture are back.

(e) *Mafenide acetate (Sulfamylon) cream* is similar to silver sulfadiazine cream, but it penetrates eschar better to attack underlying bacterial infection. However, it is more painful on the wound and more difficult to obtain than silver sulfadiazine cream.

(f) *A&D ointment* contains vitamin A and vitamin D. Vitamin A is known to inhibit the negative wound-healing effect of steroids [10]. It is advantageous in those patients who have uninfected wounds and are taking prednisone or some other systemic steroid.

(g) *Collagenase* is an enzymatic debriding ointment in white petrolatum. It digests collagen in necrotic tissue. A several-day course of application may be effective in removing thin layers of residual necrotic tissue that may be left after surgical debridement.

Systemic Medications

The following systemic medications are of particular importance in the surgical treatment of scleroderma-related wounds:

1. *Antibiotics*: The use of systemic antibiotics to treat wounds should generally be reserved for those wounds with evidence of invasive infections. As indicated above, the signs of infection looked for in managing scleroderma digital ulcers include purulent exudate and/or marginal erythema around the base of an eschar or scab and tenderness, swelling, and erythema in the local tissues around an eschar, scab, or open ulcer. With clear evidence of infection, a broad-spectrum antibiotic such as a fluoroquinolone can be given until the results of the wound culture are known. Alternatively, a sulfamethoxazole and trimethoprim combination is given if suspicion of methicillin-resistant staphylococcus exists.

   Occasionally systemic use of antibiotics empirically is warranted to treat an ulcer that does not seem to be responding to usual ulcer management to rule out subclinical infection as the cause of its failure to heal. Invasive infections can be masked in patients taking steroids, so the threshold for giving systemic antibiotics is lower in such patients with nonhealing ulcers generally and particularly when they fail to heal after usual wound healing management for such ulcers, as described above.

   A systemic antibiotic such as cephalosporin is generally recommended for perioperative prophylaxis unless the patient has a history of allergy, or there is suspicion of methicillin-resistant organisms. Another appropriate antibiotic is then used instead.
2. *Steroids*: Steroids are important in surgical treatment for their negative wound-healing effect. It is therefore important to be aware of the patient taking steroids, so that one may use topical vitamin A, usually in the form of A&D ointment, and systemic vitamin A to counteract the negative wound-healing effect of steroids [10].
3. *Vitamin A*: As indicated above, vitamin A counteracts the negative wound-healing effect of steroids [10]. High doses are required. Typically, scleroderma patients taking steroids with one or more ulcers or new surgical wounds are given doses of 20,000–25,000 international units of vitamin A daily. This high dosage should not be continued any more than 6 weeks. After 6 weeks, the patient discontinues the vitamin A for 4 weeks before resuming it for another 6 weeks if the ulcer or wound has not healed. Incidentally, when vitamin A in these dosages is not available in pharmacies, it may be obtained through health food stores.
4. *Other medications to optimize blood flow*: The patient with ischemic scleroderma ulcers must have optimal medical management to optimize blood flow to the

patient's ulcer. These include calcium channel blockers and medications to increase the flow characteristics of the patient's blood. Occasionally, the use of nitroglycerin paste or botulinum toxin injection might be added to the patient's optimized systemic medication regimen. These medications should be carefully reviewed at the beginning of scleroderma ulcer management, and close coordination with the patient's rheumatologist is important to maintain this optimal blood flow management.

Continued Management

After debridement and washing of her ulcer, our Case Number 1 patient was dressed with mupirocin ointment and a gentle, nonocclusive Band-Aid-type dressing over the tip of her finger, reinforced with gentle but securing tape circumferentially. *It is particularly important in scleroderma patients that any circumferential tape or dressing must be place carefully to avoid compromise of the blood flow.*

She was given instructions to remove the dressing and soak her finger in warm–tepid water and reapply a similar dressing with mupirocin ointment twice daily. Further, she was instructed to avoid environmental factors that would aggravate her ulcer and relative digital ischemia. Particularly, she was told to keep herself and her finger warm, to avoid stress, and to avoid cigarette smoke [11, 12]. She should avoid secondary smoke and ask her husband to smoke outside the home. She was given a list of signs that would suggest worsening of her infection including increased pain, increased swelling, extension of the swelling or erythema into her hand, or significant increase in the size of the ulcer. She was further instructed to call if any of the signs develop or if she had any questions regarding her care. Lastly, she was instructed to return in 1 week for continued, careful follow-up.

When she returned, the patient stated that her hand felt much better. Examination showed that the ulcer was the same size and continued to have a white-yellow base. The finger swelling was less, although not normal, and the distal finger erythema had resolved. No debridement was performed, as viable tissue exposed by the debridement would most likely become necrotic due to the innate ischemia of the fingertip. *In ischemic ulcers, repeated debridements tend to make the wound larger and cause unnecessary pain offsetting any wound-healing benefit from the debridement.*

She felt most comfortable keeping the ulcer moist, so she was changed to a silver hydrogel dressing covered with the Band-Aid-type dressing that she was now used to. She was instructed to cover her dressing further with adherent cellophane if her wound tended to dry out with the new silver hydrogel dressing or she wished to protect it from dirt or water.

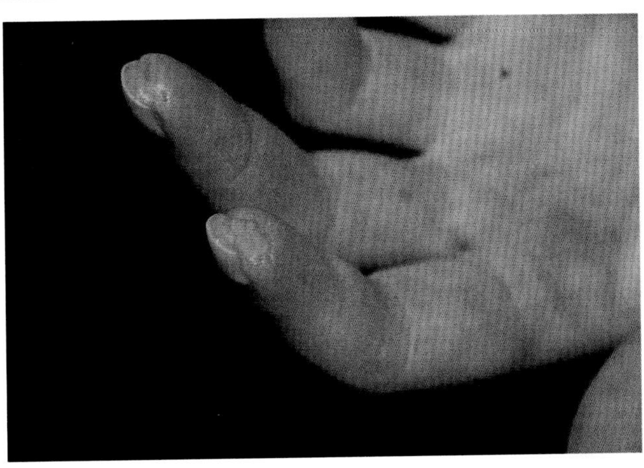

Fig. 57.2 Case number 1: left index fingertip ulcer 5 weeks after initial presentation

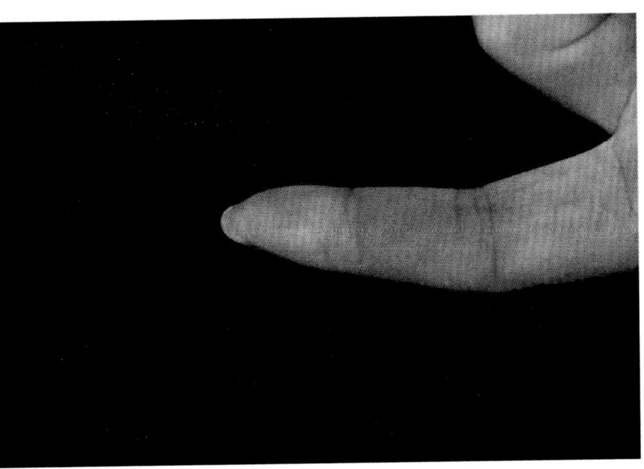

Fig. 57.3 Case number 1: left index fingertip ulcer healed with some soft tissue loss on long-term follow-up

With the resolution of the infection, the patient's office visits were reduced to every 2 weeks. Over the subsequent 6 weeks, no evidence of infection returned. There was an increase in epithelialization of the ulcer margins (Fig. 57.2). Over subsequent weeks, there was a very slow increase in the amount of red granulation tissue in the base of the ulcer. These signs are an indication of healing, and her office visits were reduced to once monthly.

At her office visit approximately 3 months after her original visit, examination showed that the ulcer was 0.2 × 0.2 cm in size and covered with a dry, very adherent tan-colored scab with no evidence of surrounding drainage, erythema, or swelling. With obvious substantial healing, the patient was given an appointment for the following month, but she subsequently called to report that her finger was completely healed and did not return for a final visit. She was subsequently seen in the office for a small subungual ulcer, and complete healing of some fingertip atrophy of the right index fingertip was confirmed (Fig. 57.3).

If after 2–3 months of optimal wound management there had been minimal evidence of healing or no healing, an MRI would have been obtained to check for osteomyelitis of the distal phalanx. If osteomyelitis were found, a debridement of the distal phalanx would have been performed under digital block anesthesia in the office. All of the bone that is typically soft from osteomyelitis is excised with a rongeur or similar bone-excising instrument. Further hard bone is removed if necessary to make sure that the surrounding viable soft tissue is in relative excess to allow healing over the shortened distal phalanx. Optimal wound care would then be continued. Nonhealing ulcers will frequently heal once the nidus of osteomyelitis is removed. If the osteomyelitis persists, amputation of the distal phalanx is frequently necessary for final healing.

In the absence of osteomyelitis, treatment with botulinum toxin injection around the digital neurovascular bundles at the base of the finger to augment her vasodilatation therapy would have been considered [13, 14]. With continued failure to heal in the absence of osteomyelitis, digital sympathectomy to further treat her distal ischemia would have been considered [15]. Amputation is, obviously, the last resort.

Case Number 2

The patient is a 64-year-old woman with systemic sclerosis initially diagnosed 27 years prior to her referral. She was referred by her rheumatologist for evaluation of a nonhealing ulcer of the left index finger proximal interphalangeal (PIP) joint. She had a history of development of interphalangeal (IP) joint contractures of her right-hand fingers, particularly, with previous occasional ulceration of the skin over the contracted joints that had healed. The ulcer for which she was referred developed 5 months prior to her referral. This coincided with worsening of her left index finger PIP joint contracture to the point where it became a fixed right angle. Within the last month, the patient developed redness and swelling of her finger, and the ulcer became significantly larger. The finger improved on antibiotics, but the ulcer continued to remain open. On a recent consultation, a hand surgeon recommended amputation of her left index finger. The development of the infection, the nonhealing of the ulcer, and the recommendation for the amputation led to her referral for a second opinion for this complicated digital scleroderma ulcer.

Her medications included esomeprazole magnesium, triamterene–hydrochlorothiazide, celecoxib, sildenafil citrate, nifedipine, pentoxifylline, gabapentin, and sulfamethoxazole–trimethoprim. She had no known allergies. She did not smoke.

On examination, the patient's temperature was 97.1° F, pulse 90, blood pressure 118/66, and respirations 18.

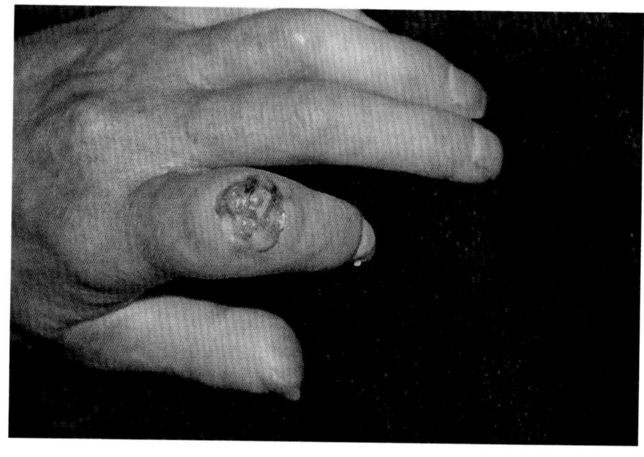

Fig. 57.4 Case number 2: left index finger dorsal PIP joint ulcer on initial presentation

Pertinent examination showed a 1.5 × 1.5-cm ulcer of the dorsal skin of the left index finger PIP joint (Fig. 57.4). The joint was exposed. The extensor tendon was absent, and the head of the proximal phalanx is seen in the base of the wound. The wound was generally clean, and there was no pus in the joint or drainage from the wound itself. The surrounding skin was normal without significant erythema. The finger was only mildly swollen. The PIP joint was flexed to more than 90°. Finger contractures of the PIP joints close to 90° were present in all the fingers of her right hand. The PIP joints of the left hand were more flexible and not contracted as much as the right with the exception of the left index finger. Skin tightness was present over both hands. The finger skin was normal in color with the exception of whiteness of the skin over the contracted PIP joints. Allen's test was normal bilaterally.

Management

Unlike patients with limited scleroderma who may develop severe Raynaud's phenomenon causing distal finger ischemia (as in Case Number 1), patients with the generalized systemic sclerosis form of scleroderma tend to have a lower incidence of ulcers from distal finger ischemia. The most common digital ulcer in systemic sclerosis patients is the dorsal interphalangeal joint ulcer. These ulcers develop from the underlying bony pressure from the sharply contracted joint into the tight skin over the dorsal aspect of interphalangeal joint contractures. Not only is the dorsal skin ischemic due to the constant stretching of the tight skin in this area, but also the area is very frequently traumatized during normal hand use in daily activities because of the contractures. This patient presented with such a digital ulcer.

Generally, the wound management of the dorsal digital ulcer itself is similar to that of the digital ulcers in general, as

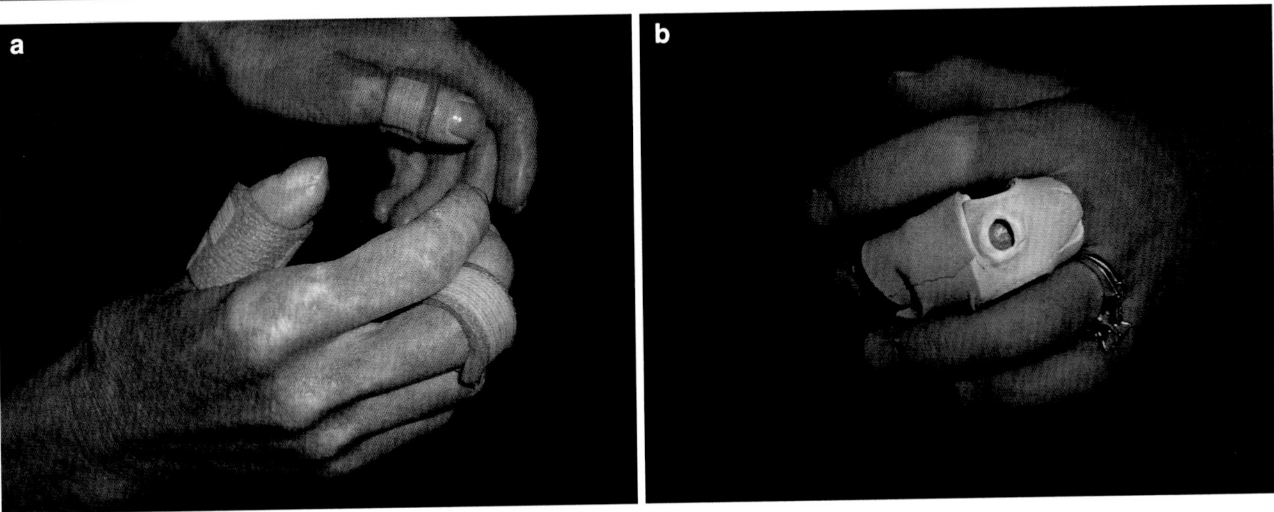

Fig. 57.5 Examples of protective devices. (**a**) Mepilex AG silver foam wraps. (**b**) Thermoplast protector

discussed above with Case Number 1. What distinguishes the management of the two types of ulcers otherwise is addressing the primary etiology of each type of ulcer. After the direct wound care itself, the primary focus of the systemic sclerosis PIP joint ulcer is to protect the ulcer from further trauma and, when severe or nonhealing, address the severe contracture of the PIP joint surgically. This contrasts with the distal digital ischemic ulcers most commonly seen in limited scleroderma patients where optimizing blood flow through medications, elimination of aggravating factors, and sometimes the use of botulinum toxin and sympathectomy is paramount.

Protection from trauma can be achieved using several dressings/devices. Several such devices that can be considered are:

Protective Dressings and Devices

1. *Silver-containing, adherent foam dressings*: Silver-containing, adherent foam dressings (e.g., Mepilex AG ™) are protective dressings that provide silver for broad-spectrum antimicrobial action (Fig. 57.5a). Its silicone interface on one side allows adherence to the surrounding skin of an ulcer but does not adhere to the wound, so that it can be removed gently without trauma to healing tissue or pain. The silver minimizes wound bacteria, and the foam acts as a mechanical protection from further wound trauma. It is particularly good for patient with dorsal IP joint ulcers. Some patients without ulcers use it simply as a convenient protection of the easily traumatized dorsal PIP joint skin.
2. *Silver alginate and hydrofiber wound dressings*: Silver alginate and hydrofiber wound dressings in either the hydrogel or solid foam form provide excellent wound-healing environments for uninfected ulcers and broad-spectrum antimicrobial action (see Silver hydrogel in Topical Medications). However, the solid foam provides the additional benefit of trauma protection.
3. *Hydrocolloid dressings* (see Table 57.1): Hydrocolloid dressings also provide a good wound-healing environment with trauma protection.
4. *Hard cover-type devices*: Hard cover-type devices can be made by occupational therapists from Thermoplast™-type moldable plastic that protects easily traumatized areas, such as dorsal PIP joint skin, from trauma. Holes can be made over ulcers to avoid pressure. Velcro straps make them secure and easily removable while making excess circumferential pressure less likely than tape (Fig. 57.5b).
5. *Negative-pressure wound therapy (NPWT)*: Judicious use of negative-pressure wound dressings has succeeded in assisting wound healing on selected scleroderma patients [unpublished data]. Typically one can prepare a chronic ulcer with an avascular base and increase neovascularity with NPWT by placing it directly on the wound and changing every other day. Additionally, NPWT can be used as the overlying dressing after applying either skin allograft to prepare the wound or skin autograft to get final healing. When placed over grafts the NPWT is applied with a lower negative pressure (e.g., −75 mmHg.) than when used for direct wound application.

A word of caution: NPWT dressing is not for all scleroderma ulcers. It should not be used for ischemic ulcers that are still progressing due to ischemia and those in which ongoing significant ischemia is a concern.

Further, many studies of various other modes of wound therapy are present in the literature, but no one therapeutic intervention has been found to be clinically superior to any other [16]. The therapies listed as options above have been successful for the author.

In this patient, a diagnosis of a nonhealing ischemic scleroderma ulcer of the left index finger PIP joint associated with severe finger contracture was made. Additionally, the PIP joint was found to be open in the wound, and the extensor tendon central slip was absent. In this case, there was no evidence of infection, and there was no significant necrotic tissue to debride.

Given the several complications associated with this ulcer, it was unlikely that the ulcer would heal. Various options were presented to the patient with amputation being a last resort. One option discussed was arthrodesis of her PIP joint with excision of the ulcer and closure of the wound if the size of the ulcer could be reduced somewhat more than on initial presentation. In the absence of infection, there was time for an attempt at reducing the size of the ulcer by adjusting her ulcer management. Her finger was dressed with an occlusive dressing of silver hydrogel, and she was given instructions to change the dressing daily after washing her wound. She was also given instructions to avoid aggravating the ulcer by carefully protecting the ulcer from trauma and cold exposure.

When she returned 6 weeks after her initial visit, the ulcer was found to be 0.8×0.7-cm in size. The PIP joint was still open, and the proximal phalangeal head and middle phalangeal base were exposed and desiccated. There was no evidence of red granulation tissue. However, there was also no evidence of infection within the joint or in the surrounding skin. The impression was that the ulcer had healed to the point where it could no longer contract over the dry, bony ulcer base. At this point, it was decided to proceed with arthrodesis of her PIP joint with excision of the residual ulcer and wound closure as the digit became shorter with excision of the joint.

The operation was performed under sedation and digital block as an outpatient 3 months after the patient's first office visit. Cephalexin was given as a preoperative prophylactic antibiotic. A "cup and cone" arthrodesis was performed to obtain fixation with no exposed metal in the area of the wound closure itself [17]. The patient's Kirschner wire fixation device was removed 7 weeks after the arthrodesis with good union of the arthrodesis and the PIP joint fused in a much more functional position. The skin had healed without complications (Fig. 57.6).

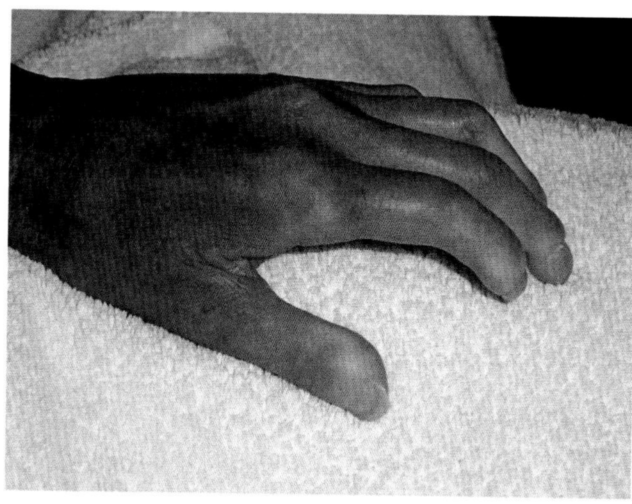

Fig. 57.6 Case number 2: healed left index finger after excision of ulcer and arthrodesis

References

1. Latham JL, Martin SN. Infiltrative anesthesia in office practice. Am Fam Physician. 2014;89(12):956–62.
2. Cepeda MS, Tzortzopoulou A, Thackrey M, Hudcove J, Arora Gandhi P, Schumann R. Adjusting the pH of lidocaine for reducing pain in injection. Cochrane Database Syst Rev. 2010;12:CD006581.
3. Malamed SF, Tavana S, Falkel M. Faster onset and more comfortable injection with alkalinized 2% lidocaine with epinephrine 1:100,000. Compend Contiun Educ Dent. 2013;34(Spec no 1):10–20.
4. Welch MN, Czyz CN, Kalwerisky K, Holck DE, Mihora LD. Double-blind, bilateral pain comparison with simultaneous injection of 2% lidocaine versus buffered 2% lidocaine for periocular anesthesia. Ophthalmology. 2012;119(10):2048–52.
5. Broussard KC, Powers JG. Wound dressings: selecting the most appropriate type. Am J Clin Dermatol. 2013;14:449–59.
6. Rennekampff HO, Kiessig V, Loomis W, Hansbrough JF. Growth peptide release from biologic dressings: a comparison. J Burn Car Rehabil. 1996;17(6 Pt 1):522–7.
7. Kannon GA, Garrett AB. Moist wound healing with occlusive dressings: a clinical review. Dermatol Surg. 1995;21:583–90.
8. Percival SL, Cooper R, Lipsky B. Antimicrobial interventions for wounds. In: Percival SL, Cutting K, editors. Microbiology of wounds. Boca Raton: CRC Press; 2010. p. 293–310.
9. Giuggioli D, Manfredi A, Colaci M, et al. Scleroderma digital ulcers complicated by infection with fecal pathogens. Arthritis Care Res (Hoboken). 2012;64:295–7.
10. Ehrlich HP, Hunt TK. Effects of cortisone and vitamin A on wound healing. Ann Surg. 1968;167:324–8.
11. Cappelli L, Wigley FM. Management of Raynaud's phenomenon and digital ulcers in scleroderma. Rheum Dis Clin N Am. 2015;41:410–38.
12. Hudson M, Lo E, Lu Y, Canadian Scleroderma Research Group, et al. Cigarette smoking in patients with systemic sclerosis. Arthritis Rheum. 2011;63:230–8.
13. Van Beek AL, Lim PK, Gear AJ, et al. Management of vasospastic disorders with botulinum toxin A. Plast Reconstr Surg. 2007; 119:217–26.
14. Neumeister MW. Botulinum toxin type A in the treatment of Raynaud's phenomenon. J Hand Surg Am. 2010;35:2085–92.
15. Kotsis SV, Chung KC. A systematic review of the outcomes of digital sympathectomy for treatment of chronic digital ischemia. J Rheumatol. 2003;30:1788–92.
16. Moran ME. Scleroderma and evidence-based non-pharmaceutical treatment modalities for digital ulcer: a systematic review. J Wound Care. 2014;23(10):510–6.
17. Carroll RE, Hill NA. Small joint arthrodesis in hand reconstruction. J Bone Joint Surg. 1969;51A:1219–21.

Index

J. Varga et al. (eds.), *Scleroderma*, DOI 10.1007/978-3-319-31407-5

B

D

J

K

L